The International Consensus Classification of Myeloid and Lymphoid Neoplasms

Daniel A. Arber, MD
Donald West and Mary Elizabeth King Professor and Chair
Department of Pathology
University of Chicago
Chicago, Illinois

Michael J. Borowitz, MD, PhD
Professor of Pathology and Oncology
Johns Hopkins Medical Institutions
Baltimore, Maryland

James R. Cook, MD, PhD
Hematopathology Section Head
Department of Pathology and Laboratory Medicine
Cleveland Clinic
Cleveland, Ohio

Laurence de Leval, MD, PhD
Professor and Chair
Institute of Pathology
Department of Laboratory Medicine and Pathology
Lausanne University Hospital and Lausanne University
Lausanne, Switzerland

John R. Goodlad, MBChB, MD, FRCPath
Department of Pathology
NHS Greater Glasgow and Clyde
Glasgow, Scotland

Robert P. Hasserjian, MD
Professor of Pathology
Department of Pathology
Massachusetts General Hospital
Boston, Massachusetts

Rebecca L. King, MD
Professor
Division of Hematopathology
Mayo Clinic
Rochester, Minnesota

Hans Michael Kvasnicka, MD, PhD
Chair, Professor of Pathology
Institute of Pathology and Molecular Pathology
University Clinic Wuppertal, University of Witten/Herdecke
Wuppertal, Germany

Attilio Orazi, MD, FRCPath
Professor and Chair
Department of Pathology
Texas Tech University Health Sciences Center, El Paso
El Paso, Texas

Wolters Kluwer

Philadelphia • Baltimore • New York • London
Buenos Aires • Hong Kong • Sydney • Tokyo

Acquisitions Editor: Nicole Dernoski
Senior Development Editor: Ariel Winter
Editorial Coordinator: Vinodhini Varadharajalu
Marketing Manager: Kirsten Watrud
Production Project Manager: Bridgett Dougherty
Manager, Graphic Arts & Design: Stephen Druding
Manufacturing Coordinator: Lisa Bowling
Prepress Vendor: TNQ Tech

10 9 8 7 6 5 4 3 2

Printed in Mexico

Library of Congress Cataloging-in-Publication Data

ISBN-13: 978-1-975222-59-8

Cataloging in Publication data available on request from publisher.

shop.lww.com

QUADM0425

Contributors

Ranjana Hira Advani, MD
Professor
Department of Medicine
Stanford University
Stanford, California

Carl E. Allen, MD, PhD
Professor
Department of Pediatrics
Baylor College of Medicine
Houston, Texas

Steve M. Ansell, MD, PhD
Division Chair
Division of Hematology
Mayo Clinic
Rochester, Minnesota

Emmanuel Bachy, MD, PhD
Professor of Hematology
Department of Clinical Hematology
Lyon Sud Hospital Center
Oullins-Pierre-Bénite, France

Chris M. Bacon, BMedSci, MBChB, PhD, FRCPath
Senior Lecturer in Haematopathology
Translational and Clinical Research Institute
Newcastle University
Newcastle upon Tyne, United Kingdom

Adam Bagg, MD
Professor
Department of Pathology and Laboratory Medicine
University of Pennsylvania
Philadelphia, Pennsylvania

Carmen Barcena, MD
Associate Pathologist
Institute of Pathology
Department of Laboratory Medicine and Pathology
Lausanne University Hospital and Lausanne University
Lausanne, Switzerland

Carlos Barrionuevo, MD, PhD
Pathologist
Department of Pathology
Instituto Nacional De Enfermedades Neoplasicas School of Medicine
Universidad Nacional Mayor de San Marcos
Lima, Peru

Silvia Bea, PhD
Senior Specialist
Department of Pathology
Hospital Clinic
Barcelona, Spain

Marie C. Béné, PharmSciD, PhD
Immunology and Hematology Professor Emeritus
Faculty of Medicine
Nantes University
Nantes, France

John M. Bennett, MD
Physician
Division of Hematopathology
Department of Pathology
Laboratory Medicine and Medicine
University of Rochester Medical Center
Rochester, New York

P. Leif Bergsagel, MD
Professor of Medicine
Department of Medicine
Mayo Clinic
Phoeniz, Arizona

Bettina Bisig, MD, PhD
Senior Staff Pathologist
Institute of Pathology
Department of Laboratory Medicine and Pathology
Lausanne University Hospital and Lausanne University
Lausanne, Switzerland

Pierre Brousset, MD, PhD
Head, Professor of Pathology
Pathology Department
University Hospital of Toulouse
Toulouse, France

Julie Bruneau, MD, PhD
Associate Professor
Department of Pathology
University Hospital Necker
Paris Cite University
Paris, France

Rena Buckstein, MD, FRCPC
Head, Hematology Clinical Trials, Chair MDS-CAN
Department of Hematologist/Oncology
Odette Cancer Center, Sunnybrook Health Sciences Center
Toronto, Ontario, Canada

Carlos E. Bueso-Ramos, MD, PhD
Professor of Pathology
Department of Hematopathology
The University of Texas MD Anderson Cancer Center
Houston, Texas

Eduardo Calonje, MD
Consultant
Department of Dermatopathology
St John's Institute of Dermatology
London, United Kingdom

Katherine R. Calvo, MD, PhD
Acting Chief, Hematology Section
Department of Laboratory Medicine
National Institute of Health, Clinical Center
Bethesda, Maryland

Elias Campo, MD
Professor of Pathology
Senior Consultant
Pathology Department Hospital Clinic of Barcelona
Institute of Biomedical Research August Pi i Sunyer (IDIBAPS)
University of Barcelona
Barcelona, Spain

Antonino Carbone, MD
Former Chair
Department of Pathology
Centro di Riferimento Oncologico di Aviano
National Cancer Institute
Aviano, Italy

Mario Cazzola, MD
Professor of Hematology
Fondazione IRCCS Policlinico San Matteo
University of Pavia
Pavia, Italy

Lorenzo Cerroni, MD
Director
Dermatopathalogy Unit
Department of Dermatology
Medical University of Graz
Graz, Austria

Devon Chabot-Richards, MD
Associate Professor
Vice Chair for Education
Department of Pathology and Laboratory Medicine
University of New Mexico
Albuquerque, New Mexico

Wing C. Chan, MD
Director
Anatomic Pathology MC
City of Hope National Medical Center
Duarte, California

Sindhu Cherian, MD
Professor
Laboratory Medicine and Pathology
University of Washington
Seattle, Washington

Junhun Cho, MD, PhD
Assistant Professor
Department of Pathology
Samsung Medical Centre
Seoul, South Korea

Fina Climent, MD, PhD
Haematopathologist
Department of Pathology
Hospital Universitari de Bellvitge-IDIbell
L'Hospitalet de Llobregat
Barcelona, Spain

Jeffrey I. Cohen, MD
Chief, Laboratory of Infectious Diseases
Chief, Medical Virology Section
National Institutes of Health
Bethesda, Maryland

Nneka I. Comfere, MD
Professor
Department of Dermatology and Laboratory Medicine and Pathology
Mayo Clinic
Rochester, Minnesota

Genevieve M. Crane, MD, PhD
Staff Pathologist
Pathology and Laboratory Medicine Institute
Cleveland Clinic
Cleveland, Ohio

Christine Cserti-Gazdewich, MD, FRCPC
Assistant Professor
Transfusion Medicine and Clinical Hematology
University Health Network and University of Toronto
Toronto, Ontario, Canada

Paola Dal Cin, PhD
Professor of Pathology
Department of Pathology
Brigham and Women's Hospital
Boston, Massachusetts

Francesco d'Amore, MD, OMSC
Clinical Professor and Chair, Head Physician
Department of Hematology
Aarhus University
Aarhus, Denmark

Andrew Davies, Bsc (Hons), BM (Hons), PhD, FRCP
Professor of Haematological Oncology
Cancer Sciences Unit
Faculty of Medicine
University of Southampton
Southampton, United Kingdom

Claire Dearden, MD, FRCP, FRCPath
Consultant Haematologist
The Royal Marsden and Institute of Cancer Research
London, United Kingdom

Jan Delabie, MD, PhD
Division Head,
Department of Hematopathology, Transfusion Medicine and Histocompatibility
Laboratory Medicine and Pathology
University Health Network and University of Toronto
Toronto, Ontario, Canada

Amy E. DeZern, MD, MHS
Professor of Oncology
Division of Hematologic Malignancies
Sidney Kimmel Comprehensive Cancer Centre
The John Hopkins University School of Medicine
Baltimore, Maryland

Courtney D. DiNardo, MD
Associate Professor
Department of Leukemia
The University of Texas MD Anderson Cancer Center
Houston, Texas

David Dingli, MD, PhD
Professor
Division of Hematology
Mayo Clinic
Rochester, Minnesota

Stefan Dirnhofer, MD
Deputy Chief Physician
Institute of Medical Genetics and Pathology
University of Basel Hospital
Basel, Switzerland

Angela Dispenzieri, MD
Professor
Division of Hematology
Mayo Clinic
Rochester, MN

Ahmet Dogan, MD, PhD
Professor of Pathology and Laboratory Medicine
Pathology and Laboratory Medicine
Memorial Sloan Kettering Cancer Center
New York, New York

Hartmut Döhner, MD
Medical Director
Internal Medicine III
Ulm University Hospital
Ulm, Baden-Württemberg, Germany

Stefan Dojcinov, MD, FRCPath
Professor/Consultant Pathologist
Department of Pathology
Swansea Bay University Health Board/Swansea University
Swansea, Wales

Martin Dreyling, MD, PhD
Professor of Medicine
Department of Medicine III
LMU University Hospital
Munich, Germany

Amy Duffield, MD, PhD
Professor
Department of Pathology, Molecular and Cell-Based Medicine
Icahn School of Medicine at Mount Sinai Hospital
Mount Sinai, New York

Eric Duncavage, MD
Professor
Department of Pathology and Immunology
Washington University
St. Louis, Missouri

Kieron Dunleavy, MD
Director of Hematology
Department of Hematology and Oncology
Georgetown University
Washington DC

Benjamin H. Durham, MD
Assistant Attending Pathologist/Assistant Member, Level 1
Department of Pathology and Laboratory Medicine
Memorial Sloan Kettering Cancer Center
New York, New York

Benjamin L. Ebert, MD, PhD
Professor of Medicine, Chair of Medical Oncology
Department of Medical Oncology
Dana-Farber Cancer Institute
Boston, Massachusetts

Caoimhe Egan, MB, BCh, BAO, FRCPath
Consultant Haematopathologist
Haematopathology and Oncology Diagnostic Service
Cambridge University Hospital NHS Foundation Trust
Cambridge, Cambridgeshire, United Kingdom

Harry Paul Erba, MD, PhD
Professor
Department of Medicine
Hematologic Malignancies and Cellular Therapy
Duke University
Durham, North Carolina

Mark D. Ewalt, MD
Associate Attending
Department of Pathology and Laboratory Medicine
Memorial Sloan Kettering Cancer Center
New York, New York

Fabio Facchetti, MD, PhD
Former Full Professor of Pathology
Department of Molecular and Translational Medicine, Pathology Unit
University of Brescia School of Medicine-Spedali Civili of Brescia
Brescia, Italy

Brunangelo Falini, MD
Institute of Hematology and CREO
University of Perugia
Perugia, Italy

Andrew L. Feldman, MD
Professor
Division of Hematopathology
Rochester, Minnesota

Falko Fend, MD
Professor and Chairman
Institute of Pathology and Neuropathology
University Hospital Tübingen
Tübingen, Germany

Kathryn Foucar, MD
Distinguished Professor
Department of Pathology
University of New Mexico School of Medicine
Albuquerque, New Mexico

Sylvie Fraitag, MD
Head Consultant Dermatopathology
Department of Pathology
Necker-Enfants Malades Hospital
Paris, France

Jonathan W. Friedberg, MD, MMSc
Director, Wilmot Cancer Institute
Samuel Durand Professor of Medicine
University of Rochester
Rochester, New York

Philippe Gaulard, MD
Professor
Department of Pathology
Henri Mondor University Hospital
Creteil, France

Tracy I. George, MD
Professor
Department of Pathology
University of Utah School of Medicine
Salt lake City, Utah

Umberto Gianelli, MD
Professor of Pathology
University of Milan
Milan, Italy

Sarah E. Gibson, MD
Associate Professor
Department of Laboratory Medicine and Pathology
Mayo Clinic Arizona
Phoenix, Arizona

Jason Gotlib, MD, MS
Professor of Medicine
Stanford Cancer Institute
Stanford University School of Medicine
Stanford, California

John G. Gribben, MD, DSc
Professor
Department of Medical Oncology
Centre for Haemato-Oncology
Barts Cancer Institute
Queen Mary University of London
London, United Kingdom

Sandeep Gurbuxani, MBBS, PhD
Professor of Pathology
Section of Hematopathology
Department of Pathology
University of Chicago
Chicago, Illinois

Thomas M. Habermann, MD
Professor of Medicine
Division of Hematology
Department of Medicine
Mayo Clinic College of Medicine and Science
Mayo Clinic
Rochester, Minnesota

Eva Hellström-Lindberg, MD, PhD
Professor, Senior Consultant, Research Group Leader
Department of Medicine
Karolinska Institute
Huddinge, Sweden

Jason L. Hornick, MD, PhD
Director of Surgical Pathology and Immunohistochemistry
Professor of Pathology
Department of Pathology
Brigham and Women's Hospital
Harvard Medical School
Boston, Massachusetts

Steven M. Horwitz, MD
Attending Physician and Member
Professor of Medicine
Department of Medicine
Memorial Sloan Kettering Cancer Center
New York, New York

Eric D. Hsi, MD
Professor and Chair
Department of Pathology
Department of Laboratory Medicine and Pathology
Mayo Clinic
Rochester, Minnesota

Stephen Hunger, MD
Chief, Division of Oncology
Department of Pediatrics
Children's Hospital of Philadelphia
Philadelphia, Pennsylvania

Elias Jabbour, MD
Professor of Medicine
Leukemia Department
The University of Texas MD Anderson Cancer Center
Houston, Texas

Elaine S. Jaffe, MD
NIH Distinguished Investigator
Head, Hematopathology
Laboratory of Pathology
Center for Cancer Research
National Cancer Institute
National Institutes of Health
Bethesda, Maryland

Siddhartha Jaiswal, MD, PhD
Assistant Professor
Department of Pathology
Stanford University
Palo Alto, California

Dragan Jevremovic, MD, PhD
Professor
Division of Hematopathology
Mayo Clinic
Rochester, Minnesota

Benjamin A. Kaumeyer, MD
Clinical Assistant Professor of Pathology
Department of Pathology and Laboratory Medicine
Nationwide Children's Hospital
Columbus, Ohio

Rashmi Kanagal-Shamanna, MD
Associate Professor, Hematopathology
Director, Molecular Diagnostic Laboratory
Department of Hematopathology
The University of Texas MD Anderson Cancer Center
Houston, Texas

Won Seog Kim, MD, PhD
Professor
Division of Hematology-Oncology
Sungkyunkwan University School of Medicine, Samsung Medical Center
Seoul, South Korea

Jeffery M. Klco, MD, PhD
Associate Member, Department of Pathology
Director, Division of Hematopathology and Molecular Pathology
St. Jude Children's Research Hospital
Memphis, Tennessee

Rami Komrokji, MD
Professor and Vice Chair
Department of Malignant Hematology
H Lee Moffitt Cancer Center and Research Institute
Tampa, Florida

Young-Hyeh Ko, MD, PhD
Emeritus Professor
Sungkyunkwan University
Seoul, South Korea

Nicole E. Kucine, MD, MS
Associate Professor
Department of Pediatrics
Weill Cornell Medicine
New York, New York

Ann LaCasce, MD, MMSc
Associate Professor of Medicine
Department of Medical Oncology
Dana Farber Cancer Institute
Needham, Massachusetts

Angela M. Lager, PhD, FACMG
Assistant Professor
Department of Pathology
University of Chicago
Chicago, Illinois

Andrew A. Lane, MD, PhD
Associate Professor
Department of Medical Oncology
Dana-Farber Cancer Institute
Boston, Massachusetts

Richard A. Larson, MD
Professor of Medicine
Section of Hematology/Oncology
The University of Chicago
Chicago, Illinois

Camille Laurent, MD, PhD
Professor
Department of Pathology
University Hospital of Toulouse
Toulouse, France

Roos Leguit, MD
Haematopathologist
Department of Pathology
University Medical Center Utrecht
Utrecht, Netherlands

François Lemonnier, MD, PhD
Professor
Lymphoid Hematology
Henri Mondor Hospital
Créteil, France

George Lenz, MD
Professor, Director
Medical Department A for Hematology, Oncology and Pneumology
University Hospital Münster
Münster, Germany

John P. Leonard, MD
Senior Associate Dean for Innovation and Initiatives
Richard T. Silver Distinguished Professor of Hematology and Medical Oncology
Weill Cornell Medicine
New York, New York

Pei Lin, MD
Professor
Department of Hematopathology
The University of Texas MD Anderson Cancer Center
Houston, Texas

Michael Link, MD
Professor of Pediatrics
Department of Pediatrics
Stanford University School of Medicine
Stanford, California

Yen-Chun Liu, MD, PhD
Associate Professor
Department of Pathology
St. Jude Childern's Research Hospital
Memphis, Tennessee

Cristina López, MD, PhD
Postdoc
Molecular Pathology Laboratory
IDIBAPS, Hospital Clínic
Barcelona, Spain

Luisa Lorenzi, MD, PhD
Pathologist, Researcher
Pathology Unit
Department of Molecular and Translational Medicine
University of Brescia School Medicine
Brescia, Italy

Robert B. Lorsbach, MD, PhD
Clinical Professor of Pathology
Department of Pathology and Laboratory Medicine
University of Cincinnati College of Medicine
Cincinnati Children's Hospital Medical Center
Cincinnati, Ohio

Selina Luger, MD, FRCPC
Professor of Medicine
Department of Hematology Oncology
Abramson Cancer Center
University of Pennsylvania
Philadelphia, Pennsylvania

Jarek P. Maciejewski, MD, PhD, FACP
Chair
Translational Hematology and Oncology Research Department
Cleveland Clinic
Cleveland, Ohio

Luca Malcovati, MD
Assistant Professor of Pathology
Professor of Hematology
Section of Molecular Medicine
University of Pavia & IRCCS San Matteo Foundation
Pavia, Italy

Estella Matutes, MD, PhD
Haematopathology
Hospital Clinic de Barcelona
Barcelona, Spain

Ellen D. McPhail, MD, CM
Professor
Division of Hematopathology
Mayo Clinic
Rochester, Minnesota

Christopher Melani, MD
Assistant Research Physician
Lymphoid Malignancies Branch
Center for Cancer Research
National Cancer Institute
National Institute of Health
Bethesda, Maryland

Ari Melnick, MD
Laurel Gebroe Family Professor of Hematology and Oncology
Sanford and Joan Weill Department of Medicine
Professor of Immunology and Pharmacology
Weill Cornell Medicine
New York, New York

Charles G. Mullighan, MBBS(Hons), MSc, MD, FRACP, FRCPA
Member
Department of Pathology
St. Jude Children's Research Hospital
Memphis, Tennessee

Shigeo Nakamura, MD
Professor Emeritus
Department of Pathology and Laboratory Medicine
Nagoya University Hospital
Nagoya, Japan

Megan O. Nakashima, MD
Associate Professor
Department of Laboratory Medicine
Cleveland Clinic
Cleveland, Ohio

Arianna di Napoli, MD
Associate Professor of Pathology
Clinical and Molecular Medicine
Sapienza University of Rome
Roma, Italy

Marina Narbaitz, MD
Chief of Service
Hematopathologist
Diagnosis Department
FIHEMA Academia De Medicina
Buenos Aires, Argentina

Charlotte M. Niemeyer, MD
Professor
Division of Pediatric Hematology and Oncology
Department of Pediatrics
University Medical Center Freiburg
Freiburg im Breisgau, Germany

Olatoyosi M. Odenike, MD, FASCO
Professor of Medicine
Section of Hematology/Oncology
Department of Medicine
The University of Chicago
Chicago, Illinois

Robert S. Ohgami, MD, PhD
Professor and Vice President of the ARUP Institute for Research and Innovation
Department of Pathology
University of Utah and ARUP Laboratories
Salt Lake City, Utah

Koichi Ohshima, MD, PhD
Professor
Department of Pathology
School of Medicine
Kurume University
Kurume, Fukuoka

Sarah L. Ondrejka, DO
Associate Professor of Pathology
Department of Laboratory Medicine
Cleveland Clinic
Cleveland, Ohio

Francesco Onida, MD
Associate Professor of Hematology
Department of Oncology and Hemato-Oncology
University of Milan
Milan, Italy

Etan Orgel, MD, MS
Professor of Clinical Pediatrics
Cancer and Blood Disease Institute
Children's Hospital Los Angeles/University of Southern California
Los Angeles, California

Neval Ozkaya, MD
Assistant Professor of Pathology
Department of Pathology
Section of Hematopathology
The University of Chicago Medicine
Chicago, Illinois

Michele E. Paessler, DO
Division Chief of Hematopathology, Immunology
Medical Director of Clinical Immunology Laboratory and Attending Hematopathologist
Department of Pathology and Laboratory Medicine
Children's Hospital of Philadelphia
Philadelphia, Pennsylvania

Elli Papaemmanuil, PhD
Associate Attending
Department of Epidemiology-Biostatistics
Computational Oncology Service
Memorial Sloan Kettering Cancer Center
New York, New York

Sanjay S. Patel, MD, MSc, MPH
Assistant Professor of Pathology and Laboratory Medicine
Division of Hematopathology
Department of Pathology and Laboratory Medicine
Weill Cornell Medical College
New York, New York

Jay L. Patel, MD, MBA
Professor
Department of Pathology
University of Utah and ARUP Laboratories
Salt Lake City, Utah

Astrid Pavlovsky, MD
Medical Director- Staff Hematology Department
Department of Hematology
Centro de Hematología Pavlovsky, Hematóloga en FUNDALEU
Buenos Aires, Argentina

Anamarija M. Perry, MD
Professor of Pathology
Department of Pathology
University of Michigan
Ann Arbor, Michigan

Tony Petrella, MD
Associate Professor
Department of Pathology
Hôpital Maisonneuve-Rosemont
Montreal, Quebec, Canada

Stefano A. Pileri, MD
Professor of Pathology, H. C. Medical Degree
Scientific Board of the University Hospital St. Orsola Polyclinic IRCCS
Department of Haematology
Bologna University/European Institute of Oncology IRCCS
Bologna/Milano, Italy

Miguel A. Piris, MD, PhD
Emeritus Researcher
Department of Pathology
Fundacion Jimenez Diaz
Madrid, Spain

Stefania Pittaluga, MD, PhD
Senior Research Physician
Laboratory of Pathology
National Cancer Institute
Bethesda, Maryland

Marco Pizzi, MD, PhD
Pathology Unit, Department of Medicine - DIMED
University of Padova School of Medicine
Padova, Italy

Nikolai A. Podoltsev, MD, PhD
Associate Professor of Medicine (Hematology)
Department of Medicine
Yale University School of Medicine
New Haven, Connecticut

Anna Porwit, MD, PhD
Professor Emerita
Department of Clinical Sciences, Oncology and Pathology
Lund University, Faculty of Medicine
Lund, Sweden

Olga Pozdnyakova, MD, PhD
Professor of Pathology
Division of Hematopathology
Department of Pathology and Laboratory Medicine
Hospital of the University of Pennsylvania
Philadelphia, Pennsylvania

Sonam Prakash, MBBS
Clinical Professor
Department of Laboratory Medicine
University of California, San Francisco
San Francisco, California

Barbara Pro, MD
Professor of Medicine
Director of Lymphoma Program
Department of Medicine
Columbia University
New York, New York

Leticia Quintanilla-Martinez, MD
Professor
Institute of Pathology and Neuropathology
University Hospital Tübingen
Tübingen, Germany

Kaaren Reichard, MD
Professor
Division of Hematopathology
Mayo Clinic
Rochester, Minnesota

Andreas Reiter, MD
Professor of Medicine
Department of Hematology and Oncology
University Hospital Mannheim
Heidelberg University
Mannheim, Germany

Socorro Maria Rodriguez-Pinilla, MD, PhD
Associate Chief Physician
Haematopathology Section Chief
Department of Pathology
Fundación Jiménez Díaz
Madrid, Spain

Heesun J. Rogers, MD, PhD
Associate Professor of Pathology
Laboratory Medicine Institute
Cleveland Clinic
Cleveland, Ohio

Steven T. Rosen, MD
Ex VP, Emeritus
Beckman Research Institute of City of Hope Cancer Center
Professor Hematology
Department of Hematopoietic Transplantation
Duarte, California

Maria Rozman, MD, PhD
Senior Consultant
Department of Hematopathology
Hospital Clinic Barcelona
Barcelona, Spain

Martina Rudelius, MD
Assistant Professor
Department of Pathology
Ludwig-Maximilians University
Munich, Germany

Leonie Saft, MD, PhD
Senior Consultant Hematopathologist
Department of Clinical Pathology and Cancer Diagnostics
Karolinska University Laboratory
Stockholm, Sweden

Itziar Salaverria, PhD
Junior Group Leader
Instituto de Investigaciones Biomédicas August Pi i Sunyer
Barcelona, Spain

Gilles Salles, MD, PhD
Service Chief
Department of Medicine
Memorial Sloan Kettering Cancer Center
New York, New York

David A. Sallman, MD
Associate Member, Myeloid Section Head
Department of Malignant Hematology
Moffitt Cancer Center
Tampa, Florida

Birgitta Sander, MD, PhD
Professor
Department of Laboratory Medicine, Pathology
Karolinska Institute and Karolinska University Hospital
Stockholm, Sweden

Jesus F. San-Miguel, MD, PhD
Professor
Director of Clinical and Translational Medicine
University of Navarra
Pamplona, Spain

Kerry J. Savage, BSc, MD, MSc
Medical Oncologist
Department of Medical Oncology
BC Cancer Center
Vancouver, British Columbia, Canada

Annette Schmitt-Graeff, MD
Professor of Pathology
University of Freiburg
Freiburg, Germany

Anne-Roos Schrader, MD, PhD
Pathologist
Department of Pathology
Leiden University Medical Center
Leiden, Netherlands

David W. Scott, MBchB, PhD
Associate Professor
Department of Medicine
University of British Columbia/BC Cancer
Vancouver, British Columbia, Canada

Laurie H. Sehn, MD, MPH
Medical Oncologist
BC Cancer
Vancouver, British Columbia, Canada

John F. Seymour, MBBS, PhD, FRACP
Director
Department of Haematology
Peter MacCallum Cancer Centre & Royal Melbourne Hospital
Melbourne, Victoria

Min Shi, MD, PhD
Consultant and Professor
Department of Laboratory Medicine and Pathology
Mayo Clinic
Rochester, Minnesota

Akiko Shimamura, MD, PhD
Professor of Pediatrics
Harvard Medical School
Pediatric Hematology/Oncology
Boston Children's Hospital and Dana Farber Cancer Institute
Boston, Massachusetts

Margaret A. Shipp, MD
Professor of Medicine, Harvard Medical School
Medical Oncology
Dana-Farber Cancer Institute
Boston, MA

Alexa J. Siddon, MD
Hematopathologist
Department of Laboratory Medicine and Pathology
Yale University
New Haven, Connecticut

Jorge Sierra, MD, PhD
Director
Department of Hematology
Hospital de la Santa Creu i Sant Pau
Barcelona, Spain

Lauren B. Smith, MD
Professor
Department of Pathology
University of Michigan
Ann Arbor, Michigan

Lorinda A. Soma, MD
Professor, Division of Hematopathology
Department of Pathology
City of Hope Medical Center
Duarte, California

Louis Staudt, MD, PhD
Chief, Lymphoid Malignancies Branch
Director, Center for Cancer Genomics
National Cancer Institute
Bethesda, Maryland

Elliot Stieglitz, MD
Associate Professor
Department of Pediatric Oncology
UCSF Benioff Children's Hospitals
San Francisco, California

Richard M. Stone, MD
Professor of Medicine
Harvard Medical School
Department of Medical Oncology
Dana-Farber Cancer Institute
Boston, Massachusetts

Charlotte Syrykh, MD
Pathology
Toulouse University Hospital Center
Cancer Institute University of Toulouse-Oncopole
Toulouse, France

Natasha Szuber, MSc, MD
Associate Professor of Medicine
University of Montreal
Division of Hematology
Department of Medicine
Maisonneuve-Rosemont Hospital
Montreal, Quebec, Canada

Martin S. Tallman, MD
Professor of Medicine
Northwestern University Feinberg School of Medicine
Robert H. Lurie Comprehensive Cancer Center
Chicago, Illinois

Wayne Tam, MD, PhD
Senior Director
Division of Hematopathology
Professor of Pathology and Laboratory Medicine
Department of Pathology and Laboratory Medicine
Donald and Barbara Zucker School of Medicine at Hofstra/Northwell
Hempstead, New York

Sarah K. Tasian, MD
Associate Professor of Pediatrics
Pediatrics, Division of Oncology and Center for Childhood Cancer Research
Children's Hospital of Philadelphia
University of Pennsylvania School of Medicine
Philadelphia, Pennsylvania

David T. Teachey, MD
Professor
Department of Pediatric Oncology
The Childern's Hospital of Philadelphia
University of Pennsylvania Perelman School of Medicine
Philadelphia, Pennsylvania

Ayalew Tefferi, MD
Barbara Woodward Lips Professor of Medicine
Division of Hematology
Department of Medicine
Mayo Clinic
Rochester, New York

Catherine Thieblemont, MD, PhD
Professor
Department of Hémato-oncologie
Assistance Publique - Hôpitaux de Paris and Université de Paris
Paris, France

Juergen Thiele, MD, PhD
Professor of Pathology
Institute of Pathology
University of Cologne
Cologne, Germany

Anne Tierens, MD, PhD
Hematopathologist
Laboratory Medicine Program
University Health Network
Toronto, Ontario, Canada

Thomas A. Tousseyn, MD, PhD
Hematopathologist
Department of Pathology
Translational Cell and Tissue Research Lab
University Hospitals Leuven; KU Leuven
Leuven, Belgium

Steven Treon, MD, MA, MS, PhD, FACP, FRCP
Professor of Medicine
Department of Medicine
Harvard Medical School
Boston, Massachusetts

Alexandar Tzankov, MD
Professor of Pathology
Department of Histopathology and Autopsy
Institute of Medical Genetics and Pathology
University Hospital Basel
Basel, Switzerland

Alessandro Maria Vannucchi, MD
Professor of Hematology
Department of Experimental and Clinical Medicine
University of Florence, Aou Careggi
Florence, Italy

Luis Veloza, MD, PhD
Assistant Pathologist
Institute of Pathology
Department of Laboratory Medicine and Pathology
Lausanne University Hospital and Lausanne University
Lausanne, Switzerland

Girish Venkataraman, MD, MBBS
Professor of Pathology
Department of Pathology
The University of Chicago Medicine
Chicago, Illinois

Julie M. Vose, MD, MBA
Chief, Hematology/Oncology
Department of Internal Medicine
University of Nebraska Medical Center
Omaha, Nebraska

Roland B. Walter, MD, PhD, MD
Professor
Division of Translational Science and Therapeutics
Fred Hutchinson Cancer Center
Seattle, Washington

Sa A. Wang, MD
Professor of Pathology
Department of Hematopathology
The University of Texas MD Anderson Cancer Center
Houston, Texas

Andrew H. Wei, MBBS, PhD
Department of Haematology
Peter MacCallum Cancer Centre
Royal Melbourne Hospital
Walter and Eliza Hall Institute of Medical Research
Melbourne, Victoria

Oliver Weigert, MD
Professor for Translational Lymphoma Research
Medical Department 3
Ludwig-Maximilians-University (LMU) Hospital
Munich, Germany

Olga K. Weinberg, MD
Professor of Pathology
UT Southwestern Medical Center
Dallas, Texas

Wyndham H. Wilson, MD, PhD
Chief, Lymphoid Malignancies Therapeutic Section
Lymphoid Malignancies Branch
National Cancer Institute
Bethesda, Maryland

Jane N. Winter, MD
Professor
Department of Medicine
Feinberg School of Medicine, Northwestern University
Chicago, Illinois

Mina L. Xu, MD
Associate Professor
Director of Hematopathology
Pathology & Laboratory Medicine
Yale University
New Haven, Connecticut

Mariko Yabe, MD, PhD
Attending Hematopathologist
Department of Pathology and Laboratory Medicine
Memorial Sloan Kettering Cancer Center
New York, New York

Tadashi Yoshino, MD, PhD
Honorary Professor and Specially Appointed Professor
Department of Pathology
Okayama University Medical School
Okayama, Japan

Alberto Zamò, MD, PhD
Consultant Pathologist, Honorary Professor
Institute of Pathology
University of Würzburg
Würzburg, Bavaria, Germany

Andrew D. Zelenetz, MD, PhD
Attending Physician, Lymphoma Service
Professor, Weill Cornell Med College
Department of Medicine
Memorial Sloan Kettering Cancer Center
New York, New York

Gina Zini, MD, PhD
Professor of Hematology
Università Cattolica Sacro Cuore
Rome, Italy

Pier Luigi Zinzani, MD, PhD
Professor
Institute of Hematology
University of Bologna
Bologna, Italy

Emanuele Zucca, MD, PhD
Professor
Oncology Institute of Southern Switzerland
Ente Ospedaliero Cantonale
Bellinzona, Switzerland

Preface

Pathology classifications inexorably must evolve over time as we learn more about specific disease entities. New discoveries provide us information about disorders we thought we knew well but turn out to be more complicated than we had imagined. These discoveries and their influence on disease classification have helped lead to novel therapies and improved outcomes for patients afflicted with hematologic neoplasms. The International Consensus Classification (ICC) presented in this book was developed by over 200 experts in the continued pursuit of defining relevant disease entities. The ICC is the latest phase of a process that started following the publication of the Revised European-American Classification of Lymphoid Neoplasms (REAL classification) created by the International Lymphoma Study Group in 1994. The REAL classification differed from prior lymphoma classifications—which were generally put forth by individuals or small regional groups—and represented a consensus among a large cohort of pathologists from around the world. The classification incorporated all available data and techniques at that time, including morphology, immunophenotype, genetics, and clinical features, to define disease entities. Following the publication of the REAL classification, the World Health Organization (WHO) began planning for a 3rd edition series on *Pathology and Genetics of Tumours*, to be published by its affiliate International Agency for the Research on Cancer (IARC). This series of books ultimately became known as the *WHO Blue Books*. Prior to the 3rd edition, the WHO classification series were not widely used. The first edition contained only a list of disease names and images, while the 2nd edition did not include a book on hematopoietic neoplasms.

Les Sobin, a co-editor with Paul Kleihues of the 3rd edition Blue Book series, approached Elaine Jaffe, a co-author of the REAL Classification, to develop a similar classification for the WHO 3rd edition series. Dr Jaffe at that time was also President of the Society for Hematopathology. Dr Jaffe and the Society for Hematopathology Executive Committee recommended that the 3rd edition WHO effort also include myeloid neoplasms and acute leukemia; be overseen by the two major hematopathology societies, the Society for Hematopathology (SH) and the European Association for Haematopathology (EA4HP); and incorporate input from a Clinical Advisory Committee (CAC) of leading international pathologists, oncologists, hematologists, and geneticists. Although a significant departure from prior hematopathology classifications, and unique among the 3rd edition series Blue Books, this approach was embraced by the WHO/IARC.

The first CAC meeting was held at Arlie House, Virginia in 1997. The organizers outlined key issues in advance for discussion among pathologists, scientists, and treating physicians to arrive at a broad consensus for diagnostic criteria and definitions of entities. The concept of provisional entities was introduced, in which there was compelling evidence to include in the classification but for which more data were needed before including as a full entity. After the CAC, the lead pathologists were tasked with resolving remaining areas of controversy and finalizing criteria. Once complete, the proceedings of the CAC meetings were published in leading journals, and the results published as the 3rd edition *WHO Classification of Tumors of Hematopoietic and Lymphoid Tissues* in 2001, with 75 contributing authors from across the globe. The 1997 CAC format set the standard for future classifications: similar CACs were held in 2007 and 2014 in Chicago and resulted in WHO Classification publications in 2008 (4th edition) and 2017 (revised 4th edition), respectively. The revised 4th edition, which had more than 200 contributors from 24 countries, was necessary due to delays in finalizing the remaining disease group volumes of the 4th edition Blue Book series, and reflected the significant scientific advances in hematologic neoplasms that had occurred in the interim.

The partnership between the hematopathology societies (including the CAC process that was devised and organized by the societies) and the WHO was an overwhelming success. The 3rd, 4th, and revised 4th editions of *Tumours of Haematopoietic and Lymphoid Tissues* Blue Books were best sellers and moved the field away from the historic classifications to a more widely accepted consensus approach.

As preparations began for the 5th edition WHO Blue Book, it became clear IARC intended to follow a different process for this series, one that would not involve an initial CAC meeting; would not maintain continuity with the leadership of prior editions; and would not involve a collaboration with the SH and EA4HP. Accordingly, the leaders of the revised 4th edition WHO Blue Book decided to move ahead with a CAC at the University of Chicago in 2021 and to publish the ICC first in the journal *Blood* in 2022 and then in this book as a complete classification.

Thus, development of the ICC classification of hematologic neoplasms followed the same process used for the prior successful REAL classification and 3rd, 4th, and revised 4th edition WHO publications and is intended as an update in continuity with those classifications. The book follows a format similar to the prior Blue Books and is authored by hundreds of experts in the field, most of whom were involved with the revised 4th edition Blue Book. In recognition of their prior work, we thank the editors of those editions, Elias Campo, Nancy Lee Harris, Elaine S. Jaffe, Stefano A. Pileri, Harald Stein, Steven Swerdlow, Jürgen Thiele, and James W. Vardiman, some of whom participated as co-authors of chapters in this book. The editors hope that this publication will assist pathologists in diagnosing and understanding cases in daily practice, as well as physicians who treat patients with hematologic malignancies. As the readers use the book, they will begin to identify new questions that future classifications will need to address, emphasizing the continued evolution and refinement of the way we categorize myeloid and lymphoid neoplasms.

Daniel A. Arber
Michael J. Borowitz
James R. Cook
Laurence de Leval
John R. Goodlad
Robert P. Hasserjian
Rebecca L. King
Hans Michael Kvasnicka
Attilio Orazi

Contents

Contributors iii
Preface xv
The International Consensus Classification of Myeloid and Lymphoid Neoplasms xxix

INTERNATIONAL CONSENSUS CLASSIFICATION OF MYELOID DISORDERS AND ACUTE LEUKEMIAS

Introduction to the International Consensus Classification of Myeloid Disorders and Acute Leukemias **1**
Robert P. Hasserjian, Daniel A. Arber, Mario Cazzola, Hartmut Döhner, Hans Michael Kvasnicka, Richard A. Larson, Attilio Orazi, and Ayalew Tefferi

SECTION 1 Myeloproliferative Neoplasms

1 **Chronic Myeloid Leukemia** **22**
Hans Michael Kvasnicka, Carlos E. Bueso-Ramos, Attilio Orazi, Annette Schmitt-Graeff, and Ayalew Tefferi

2 ***BCR::ABL1*-Negative Myeloproliferative Neoplasms** **31**
Hans Michael Kvasnicka, Attilio Orazi, Ayalew Tefferi, Juergen Thiele, and Alessandro Maria Vannucchi

Polycythemia Vera 33
Essential Thrombocythemia 38
Primary Myelofibrosis 42

3 **Chronic Neutrophilic Leukemia** **52**
Attilio Orazi, Carlos E. Bueso-Ramos, Hans Michael Kvasnicka, Marco Pizzi, Natasha Szuber, and Ayalew Tefferi

4 **Chronic Eosinophilic Leukemia, Not Otherwise Specified** **56**
Sa A. Wang, Attilio Orazi, Kaaren Reichard, and Ayalew Tefferi

5 **Myeloproliferative Neoplasms, Unclassifiable** **61**
Umberto Gianelli, Hans Michael Kvasnicka, Attilio Orazi, Ayalew Tefferi, and Juergen Thiele

SECTION 2 Myeloid/Lymphoid Neoplasms With Eosinophilia and Tyrosine Kinase Gene Fusions

6 Myeloid/Lymphoid Neoplasms With Eosinophilia and Tyrosine Kinase Gene Fusions **68**
Sa A. Wang, Jason Gotlib, Kaaren Reichard, Andreas Reiter, and Alexandar Tzankov

Myeloid/Lymphoid Neoplasms With Eosinophilia and Rearrangement of *PDGFRA* 70
Myeloid/Lymphoid Neoplasms With Eosinophilia and Rearrangement of *PDGFRB* 73
Myeloid/Lymphoid Neoplasms With Eosinophilia and Rearrangement of *FGFR1* 74
Myeloid/Lymphoid Neoplasms With Eosinophilia and *PCM1::JAK2* and Genetic Variants *ETV6::JAK2* and *BCR::JAK2* 76
Myeloid/Lymphoid Neoplasms With Eosinophilia and *FLT3* Rearrangement 77
Myeloid Lymphoid Neoplasms With Eosinophilia and *ETV6::ABL1* 78

SECTION 3 Mastocytosis

7 Mastocytosis **84**
Kaaren Reichard, Tracy I. George, Roos Leguit, Attilio Orazi, Andreas Reiter, Ayalew Tefferi, Alexandar Tzankov, and Sa A. Wang

SECTION 4 Myelodysplastic/Myeloproliferative Neoplasms

8 Chronic Myelomonocytic Leukemia **102**
Sonam Prakash, Daniel A. Arber, Kathryn Foucar, Robert P. Hasserjian, Luca Malcovati, Attilio Orazi, and Alexa J. Siddon

9 Atypical Chronic Myeloid Leukemia **110**
Marco Pizzi, Francesco Onida, Attilio Orazi, Sonam Prakash, and Sa A. Wang

10 Myelodysplastic/Myeloproliferative Neoplasm With *SF3B1* Mutation and Thrombocytosis **114**
Sonam Prakash, Robert P. Hasserjian, Luca Malcovati, Attilio Orazi, and Annette Schmitt-Graeff

11 Myelodysplastic/Myeloproliferative Neoplasm, Not Otherwise Specified **118**
Carlos E. Bueso-Ramos, Rashmi Kanagal-Shamanna, and Attilio Orazi

SECTION 5 Premalignant Clonal Cytopenias and Myelodysplastic Syndromes

Introduction to Premalignant Clonal Cytopenias and Myelodysplastic Syndromes **124**
Robert P. Hasserjian

12 Clonal Cytopenia of Undetermined Significance and Other Clonal Cytopenias **127**
Jay L. Patel, Benjamin L. Ebert, Siddhartha Jaiswal, and Luca Malcovati

13 Myelodysplastic Syndrome With Mutated *SF3B1* **132**
Alexa J. Siddon, Eva Hellström-Lindberg, and Luca Malcovati

14 Myelodysplastic Syndrome With del(5q) **136**
Leonie Saft and Rami Komrokji

15 **Myelodysplastic Syndrome With Mutated *TP53*** 140
Mariko Yabe, Robert P. Hasserjian, David A. Sallman, and Olga K. Weinberg

16 **Myelodysplastic Syndrome, Not Otherwise Specified** 145
Olga Pozdnyakova, John M. Bennett, Amy E. DeZern, and Sa A. Wang

17 **Myelodysplastic Syndrome With Excess Blasts** 150
Mina L. Xu, Rena Buckstein, and Robert P. Hasserjian

18 **Myelodysplastic Syndrome/Acute Myeloid Leukemia** 153
Robert P. Hasserjian and Hartmut Döhner

SECTION 6 Pediatric and/or Germline Disorders

19 **Juvenile Myelomonocytic Leukemia** 160
Martina Rudelius, Katherine R. Calvo, Charlotte M. Niemeyer, Elliot Stieglitz, and Olga K. Weinberg

20 **Refractory Cytopenia of Childhood and Pediatric Myelodysplastic Syndromes** 166
Olga K. Weinberg, Katherine R. Calvo, Robert P. Hasserjian, Nicole E. Kucine, Charlotte M. Niemeyer, Attilio Orazi, and Martina Rudelius

21 **Hematologic Malignancies With Germline Predisposition** 171
Katherine R. Calvo, Courtney D. DiNardo, Jeffery M. Klco, Charlotte M. Niemeyer, Martina Rudelius, and Akiko Shimamura

SECTION 7 Acute Myeloid Leukemias

22 **Acute Promyelocytic Leukemia With t(15;17)(q24.1;q21.2)/*PML::RARA* and Acute Promyelocytic Leukemia With Other *RARA* Rearrangements** 190
Kathryn Foucar, Devon Chabot-Richards, Jeffery M. Klco, and Martin S. Tallman

23 **Acute Myeloid Leukemia With t(8;21)(q22;q22.1/*RUNX1::RUNX1T1*** 194
Sandeep Gurbuxani, Tracy I. George, Angela M. Lager, and Olatoyosi M. Odenike

24 **Acute Myeloid Leukemia With inv(16)(p13.1q22) or t(16;16)(p13.1;q22)/ *CBFB::MYH11*** 198
Sandeep Gurbuxani, Tracy I. George, Angela M. Lager, and Olatoyosi M. Odenike

25 **Acute Myeloid Leukemia With t(9;11)(p21.3;q23.3)/*KMT2A::MLLT3* and Other *KMT2A* Rearrangements** 202
Wayne Tam, Harry Paul Erba, and Yen-Chun Liu

26 **Acute Myeloid Leukemia With t(6;9)(p22.3;q34.1)/*DEK::NUP214*** 208
Genevieve M. Crane, Heesun J. Rogers, and Martin S. Tallman

27 **Acute Myeloid Leukemia With inv(3)(q21.3q26.2) or t(3;3)(q21.3;q26.2)/ *GATA2*; *MECOM*(*EVI1*) and Acute Myeloid Leukemia With Other *MECOM* Rearrangements** 211
Genevieve M. Crane, Hartmut Döhner, and Heesun J. Rogers

28 Acute Myeloid Leukemia With Other Rare Recurring Translocations **215**
Jeffery M. Klco and Daniel A. Arber

29 Acute Myeloid Leukemia With t(9;22)(q34.1;q11.2)/*BCR::ABL1* **218**
Adam Bagg, Sandeep Gurbuxani, and Selina Luger

30 Acute Myeloid Leukemia With Mutated *NPM1* **221**
Sanjay S. Patel, Andrew H. Wei, and Olga K. Weinberg

31 Acute Myeloid Leukemia With In-Frame bZIP *CEBPA* Mutations **224**
Alexa J. Siddon, Nikolai A. Podoltsev, Jorge Sierra, and Olga K. Weinberg

32 Acute Myeloid Leukemia and Myelodysplastic Syndrome/Acute Myeloid Leukemia With Mutated *TP53* **228**
Olga K. Weinberg, Maria Rozman, and Richard M. Stone

33 Acute Myeloid Leukemia and Myelodysplastic Syndrome/Acute Myeloid Leukemia With Myelodysplasia-Related Gene Mutations **231**
Olga K. Weinberg, Courtney D. DiNardo, Hartmut Döhner, Eric Duncavage, and Elli Papaemmanuil

34 Acute Myeloid Leukemia and Myelodysplastic Syndrome/Acute Myeloid Leukemia With Myelodysplasia-Related Cytogenetic Abnormalities **234**
Olga K. Weinberg, Daniel A. Arber, Paola Dal Cin, and Olatoyosi M. Odenike

35 Acute Myeloid Leukemia and Myelodysplastic Syndrome/Acute Myeloid Leukemia, Not Otherwise Specified **237**
Daniel A. Arber, John M. Bennett, Kathryn Foucar, Attilio Orazi, Roland B. Walter, and Gina Zini

Pure Erythroid Leukemia 239
Acute Basophilic Leukemia 241
Acute Panmyelosis With Myelofibrosis 242

36 Myeloid Sarcoma **245**
Marco Pizzi, Richard A. Larson, Attilio Orazi, and Stefano A. Pileri

SECTION 8 Myeloid Proliferations Associated With Down Syndrome

37 Myeloid Proliferations Associated With Down Syndrome **250**
Michele E. Paessler, Benjamin A. Kaumeyer, and Sarah K. Tasian

Transient Abnormal Myelopoiesis of Down Syndrome 250
Myeloid Leukemia Associated With Down Syndrome 252

SECTION 9 Blastic Plasmacytoid Dendritic Cell Neoplasm

38 Blastic Plasmacytoid Dendritic Cell Neoplasm **256**
Fabio Facchetti, Andrew A. Lane, Luisa Lorenzi, and Stefano A. Pileri

SECTION 10 Lymphoblastic Neoplasms

Introduction to Lymphoblastic Neoplasms **262**
Amy Duffield, Michael J. Borowitz, Sindhu Cherian, Mark D. Ewalt, Elias Jabbour, Charles G. Mullighan, Leonie Saft, and David T. Teachey

39 Acute Leukemias of Ambiguous Lineage **275**
Anna Porwit, Marie C. Béné, Michael J. Borowitz, Etan Orgel, and Olga K. Weinberg

Acute Undifferentiated Leukemia 282
Mixed-Phenotype Acute Leukemia With Recurrent Genetic Abnormalities 283
Mixed-Phenotype Acute Leukemia With Defining Immunophenotypic Changes 285

40 B-Lymphoblastic Leukemias/Lymphomas **289**
Amy Duffield, Michael J. Borowitz, Sindhu Cherian, Mark D. Ewalt, Stephen Hunger, Elias Jabbour, Charles G. Mullighan, and Leonie Saft

B-ALL/LBL With Recurrent Genetic Abnormalities 289
B-ALL/LBL With t(9;22)(q34.1;q11.2)/*BCR::ABL1* With Lymphoid Only Involvement 289
B-ALL/LBL With t(9;22)(q34.1;q11.2)/*BCR::ABL1* With Multilineage Involvement 290
B-ALL/LBL With t(v;11q23.3)/*KMT2A*-Rearranged 293
B-ALL/LBL With t(12;21)(p13.2;q22.1)/*ETV6::RUNX1* 294
B-ALL/LBL, Hyperdiploid 296
B-ALL/LBL, Low Hypodiploid 297
B-ALL/LBL, Near Haploid 297
B-ALL/LBL With t(5;14)(q31.1;q32.1)/*IGH::IL3* 299
B-ALL/LBL With t(1;19)(q23;p13.3)/*TCF3::PBX1* 299
B-ALL/LBL, *BCR::ABL1*-Like, *ABL1*-Class Rearranged 301
B-ALL/LBL, *BCR::ABL1*-Like, JAK-STAT Activated 301
B-ALL/LBL, *BCR:ABL1*-Like, Not Otherwise Specified 302
B-ALL/LBL With Intrachromosomal Amplification of Chromosome 21 (iAMP21) 303
B-ALL/LBL with *DUX4*-Rearrangement 304
B-ALL/LBL With *ZNF384*-Rearrangement 304
B-ALL/LBL With *MEF2D*-Rearrangement 305
B-ALL/LBL With *MYC*-Rearrangement 305
B-ALL/LBL With *NUTM1*-Rearrangement 306
B-ALL/LBL with *UBTF::ATXN7L3/PAN3,CDX2* (*CDX2/UBTF*) 307
B-ALL/LBL With *HLF*-Rearrangement 307
B-ALL/LBL With PAX5 P80R 308
B-ALL/LBL With IKZF1 N159Y 308
B-ALL/LBL, NOS 309
B-ALL/LBL: Provisional Entities 309

41 T-Lymphoblastic Leukemias/Lymphomas **315**
Amy Duffield, Michael J. Borowitz, Sindhu Cherian, Mark D. Ewalt, Elias Jabbour, Charles G. Mullighan, Leonie Saft, and David T. Teachey

Early T-Cell Precursor Lymphoblastic Leukemia/Lymphoma, *BCL11B*-Activated 315
Early T-Cell Precursor Lymphoblastic Leukemia/Lymphoma, NOS 317
T-Lymphoblastic Leukemia/Lymphoma, NOS 318
T-Acute Lymphoblastic Leukemia/Lymphoblastic Lymphoma: Provisional Entities 318

42 **NK-Cell Acute Lymphoblastic Leukemia** 323
Olga K. Weinberg, and Michael J. Borowitz

INTERNATIONAL CONSENSUS CLASSIFICATION OF MATURE LYMPHOID AND HISTIOCYTIC/DENDRITIC CELL NEOPLASMS

Introduction to the International Consensus Classification of Mature Lymphoid Neoplasms 327
James R. Cook, Laurence de Leval, John R. Goodlad, and Rebecca L. King

SECTION 11 Mature B-Cell Neoplasms

43 **Chronic Lymphocytic Leukemia/Small Lymphocytic Lymphoma and Monoclonal B-Cell Lymphocytosis** 340
Birgitta Sander, Silvia Bea, John G. Gribben, Eric D. Hsi, Estella Matutes, and Andrew D. Zelenetz

44 **B-Cell Prolymphocytic Leukemia** 348
Birgitta Sander, Elias Campo, Martin Dreyling, and Estella Matutes

45 **Splenic Marginal Zone Lymphoma** 351
Alexandar Tzankov, Stefan Dirnhofer, and Emanuele Zucca

46 **Hairy Cell Leukemia** 356
Miguel A. Piris, Brunangelo Falini, and Catherine Thieblemont

47 **Splenic B-Cell Lymphoma/Leukemia, Unclassifiable** 360
Miguel A. Piris, Brunangelo Falini, and Catherine Thieblemont

Splenic Diffuse Red Pulp Small B-Cell Lymphoma 360
Hairy Cell Leukemia Variant 361

48 **Lymphoplasmacytic Lymphoma** 367
James R. Cook, Pei Lin, and Steven Treon

49 **IgM Monoclonal Gammopathy of Undetermined Significance** 373
James R. Cook, Megan O. Nakashima, and Steven Treon

50 **Primary Cold Agglutinin Disease** 375
Jan Delabie, Christine Cserti-Gazdewich, Ahmet Dogan, and Anne Tierens

51 **Heavy Chain Diseases** 377
James R. Cook, David Dingli, and Elaine S. Jaffe

Gamma Heavy Chain Disease 377
Mu Heavy Chain Disease 379
Alpha Heavy Chain Disease 380

52 Plasma Cell Neoplasms **384**
Falko Fend, P. Leif Bergsagel, Dragan Jevremovic, Robert B. Lorsbach, Megan O. Nakashima, and Jesus F. San-Miguel

Non-IgM Monoclonal Gammopathy of Undetermined Significance 384
Multiple Myeloma 385
Plasmacytoma 396

53 Monoclonal Immunoglobulin Deposition Diseases **403**
Ellen D. McPhail, Angela Dispenzieri, and Falko Fend

Systemic Immunoglobulin Light Chain Amyloidosis 403
Localized Immunoglobulin Light Chain Amyloidosis 405
Light Chain and Heavy Chain Deposition Disease 406

54 Extranodal Marginal Zone Lymphoma of Mucosa-Associated Lymphoid Tissue (MALT Lymphoma) **409**
Sarah E. Gibson, Ahmet Dogan, and Gilles Salles

55 Primary Cutaneous Marginal Zone Lymphoproliferative Disorder **417**
John R. Goodlad, Sarah E. Gibson, Steven T. Rosen, and Alberto Zamò

56 Nodal Marginal Zone Lymphoma **421**
Ahmet Dogan, Adam Bagg, and Emanuele Zucca

57 Follicular Lymphoma **427**
Camille Laurent, Steve M. Ansell, Leticia Quintanilla-Martinez, and Gilles Salles

Early Lesions of Follicular Lymphoma 435

58 *BCL2*-Rearrangement Negative, CD23-Positive Follicle Center Lymphoma **441**
Leticia Quintanilla-Martinez, Itziar Salaverria, and Oliver Weigert

59 Primary Cutaneous Follicle Center Lymphoma **446**
John R. Goodlad, and Steven T. Rosen

60 Pediatric-Type Follicular Lymphoma **450**
Elaine S. Jaffe, Junhun Cho, Robert S. Ohgami, and Leticia Quintanilla-Martinez

61 Testicular Follicular Lymphoma **454**
Chris M. Bacon, and Ahmet Dogan

62 Large B-Cell Lymphoma With *IRF4* Rearrangement **458**
Stefania Pittaluga, Jan Delabie, and Itziar Salaverria

63 Mantle Cell Lymphoma: Conventional and Leukemic Nonnodal Subtypes **462**
Elias Campo, Martin Dreyling, Birgitta Sander, and Andrew D. Zelenetz

64 Diffuse Large B-Cell Lymphoma, Not Otherwise Specified **472**
Elias Campo, Andrew Davies, Stefan Dirnhofer, George Lenz, John P. Leonard, Ari Melnick, Astrid Pavlovsky, Stefano A. Pileri, Gilles Salles, David W. Scott, Laurie H. Sehn, Margaret A. Shipp, Louis Staudt, Wyndham H. Wilson, and Jane N. Winter

65 Large B-Cell Lymphoma With 11q Aberration **481**
Eric D. Hsi, Leticia Quintanilla-Martinez, and Jane N. Winter

66 Nodular Lymphocyte Predominant B-Cell Lymphoma **484**
Stefano A. Pileri, Ranjana Hira Advani, Astrid Pavlovsky, and Lauren B. Smith

67 T-Cell/Histiocyte-Rich Large B-Cell Lymphoma **490**
Stefano A. Pileri, Ranjana Hira Advani, Margaret A. Shipp, and Lauren B. Smith

68 Primary Diffuse Large B-Cell Lymphoma of the Central Nervous System **494**
Lorinda A. Soma, Andrew Davies, Stefan Dirnhofer, and Gilles Salles

69 Primary Diffuse Large B-Cell Lymphoma of the Testis **499**
Lorinda A. Soma, Andrew Davies, Stefan Dirnhofer, and Gilles Salles

70 Primary Cutaneous Diffuse Large B-Cell Lymphoma, Leg Type **502**
John R. Goodlad, Steven T. Rosen, and Anne-Roos Schrader

71 Intravascular Large B-Cell Lymphoma **505**
Shigeo Nakamura and Girish Venkataraman

72 HHV8- and EBV-Negative Primary Effusion-Based Lymphoma **508**
Lorinda A. Soma, George Lenz, and Leticia Quintanilla-Martinez

73 Epstein-Barr Virus–Positive Mucocutaneous Ulcer **510**
Stefan Dojcinov, Jeffrey I. Cohen, and Elaine S. Jaffe

74 Epstein-Barr Virus–Positive Diffuse Large B-Cell Lymphoma, Not Otherwise Specified **514**
Elaine S. Jaffe, Stefania Pittaluga, and Wyndham H. Wilson

75 Diffuse Large B-Cell Lymphoma Associated With Chronic Inflammation **518**
Philippe Gaulard, Ellen D. McPhail, and Ari Melnick

Fibrin-Associated Diffuse Large B-Cell Lymphoma 520

76 Lymphomatoid Granulomatosis **523**
Elaine S. Jaffe, Christopher Melani, and Stefania Pittaluga

77 Epstein-Barr Virus–Positive Polymorphic B-Cell Lymphoproliferative Disorder, Not Otherwise Specified **527**
Stefan Dojcinov, Genevieve M. Crane, Elaine S. Jaffe, Leticia Quintanilla-Martinez, and Wyndham H. Wilson

78 ALK-Positive Large B-Cell Lymphoma **532**
Eric D. Hsi, Philippe Gaulard, and Astrid Pavlovsky

79 Plasmablastic Lymphoma **535**
Camille Laurent, Stefan Dirnhofer, and George Lenz

80 Human Herpesvirus 8–Associated Lymphoproliferative Disorders **538**
Miguel A. Piris, Elias Campo, and Antonino Carbone

HHV8-Positive Multicentric Castleman Disease 539
HHV8-Positive Germinotropic Lymphoproliferative Disorder 541
HHV8-Positive Diffuse Large B-Cell Lymphoma, NOS 542
Primary Effusion Lymphoma 543

81 Burkitt Lymphoma **546**
Eric D. Hsi, Jonathan W. Friedberg, Michael Link, and Anamarija M. Perry

82 High-Grade B-Cell Lymphoma With *MYC* and *BCL2* Rearrangements **552**
Rebecca L. King, Ellen D. McPhail, David W. Scott, and John F. Seymour

83 High-Grade B-Cell Lymphoma With *MYC* and *BCL6* Rearrangements **558**
Rebecca L. King, Ellen D. McPhail, David W. Scott, and John F. Seymour

84 High-Grade B-Cell Lymphoma, Not Otherwise Specified **561**
Anamarija M. Perry, Rebecca L. King, and David W. Scott

85 Primary Mediastinal Large B-Cell Lymphoma **564**
Sarah L. Ondrejka, Adam Bagg, and Kerry J. Savage

86 Mediastinal Gray Zone Lymphoma **569**
Elaine S. Jaffe, Kieron Dunleavy, and Stefania Pittaluga

87 Classic Hodgkin Lymphoma **573**
Pierre Brousset, Steve M. Ansell, Ann LaCasce, Lauren B. Smith, Charlotte Syrykh, Thomas A. Tousseyn, and Girish Venkataraman

SECTION 12 Mature T- and NK-Cell Neoplasms

88 T-Cell Prolymphocytic Leukemia **588**
Claire Dearden, Emmanuel Bachy, Cristina López, and Sa A. Wang

89 T-Cell Large Granular Lymphocytic Leukemia **594**
Eric D. Hsi, Jarek P. Maciejewski, Min Shi, and Sa A. Wang

90 Chronic Lymphoproliferative Disorder of Natural Killer Cells **600**
Eric D. Hsi, Jarek P. Maciejewski, Min Shi, and Sa A. Wang

91 Adult T-Cell Leukemia/Lymphoma **604**
Koichi Ohshima, Philippe Gaulard, Steven M. Horwitz, and Shigeo Nakamura

92 Epstein-Barr Virus-Positive T- and Natural Killer-Cell Lymphoproliferative Disorders of Childhood **613**
Leticia Quintanilla-Martinez, Carlos Barrionuevo, Jeffrey I. Cohen, Young-Hyeh Ko, and Stefania Pittaluga

Hydroa Vacciniforme Lymphoproliferative Disorder 613
Severe Mosquito Bite Allergy 616
Chronic Active Epstein-Barr Virus Disease, Systemic 617
Systemic Epstein-Barr Virus-Positive T-Cell Lymphoma of Childhood 621

93 Extranodal Natural Killer/T-Cell Lymphoma, Nasal Type **627**
Wing C. Chan, Won Seog Kim, Young-Hyeh Ko, and Stefania Pittaluga

94 Aggressive Natural Killer-Cell Leukemia **635**
Wing C. Chan, Won Seog Kim, Young-Hyeh Ko, and Stefania Pittaluga

95 Primary Nodal Epstein-Barr Virus-positive T-Cell/NK-Cell Lymphoma **640**
Shigeo Nakamura, Carlos Barrionuevo, Fina Climent, and Won Seog Kim

96 Type II Refractory Celiac Disease and Enteropathy-Associated T-Cell Lymphoma **644**
Laurence de Leval, Julie Bruneau, Francesco d'Amore, and Ahmet Dogan

Type II Refractory Celiac Disease 644
Enteropathy-Associated T-Cell Lymphoma 646

97 Monomorphic Epitheliotropic Intestinal T-Cell Lymphoma **655**
Luis Veloza, Laurence de Leval, Won Seog Kim, and Tadashi Yoshino

98 Intestinal T-Cell Lymphoma, Not Otherwise Specified and Indolent Lymphoproliferative Disorders of the Gastrointestinal Tract **660**
Laurence de Leval, Anamarija M. Perry, Luis Veloza, Andrew L. Feldman, Steven M. Horwitz, Won Seog Kim, and Tadashi Yoshino

Intestinal T-Cell Lymphoma, Not Otherwise Specified 660
Indolent Clonal T-Cell Lymphoproliferative Disorder of the Gastrointestinal Tract 661
Indolent Natural Killer-Cell Lymphoproliferative Disorder of the Gastrointestinal Tract 664

99 Hepatosplenic T-Cell Lymphoma **667**
Philippe Gaulard, Carmen Barcena, Andrew L. Feldman, and Barbara Pro

100 Mycosis Fungoides **672**
Nneka I. Comfere, Eduardo Calonje, and Lorenzo Cerroni

101 Sézary Syndrome **680**
Nneka I. Comfere, Eduardo Calonje, and Lorenzo Cerroni

102 Primary Cutaneous CD30-Positive T-Cell Lymphoproliferative Disorders **684**
Andrew L. Feldman and Lorenzo Cerroni

Lymphomatoid Papulosis 684
Primary Cutaneous Anaplastic Large Cell Lymphoma 688

103 Primary Cutaneous CD4-Positive Small/Medium T-Cell Lymphoproliferative Disorder **695**
Socorro Maria Rodriguez-Pinilla and Lorenzo Cerroni

104 Subcutaneous Panniculitis-Like T-Cell Lymphoma **697**
Philippe Gaulard, John R. Goodlad, and Barbara Pro

105 Primary Cutaneous Gamma-Delta T-Cell Lymphoma **702**
Socorro Maria Rodriguez-Pinilla and Barbara Pro

106 Primary Cutaneous Acral CD8-Positive T-Cell Lymphoproliferative Disorder **706**
Tony Petrella, John R. Goodlad, and Barbara Pro

107 Primary Cutaneous CD8-Positive Aggressive Epidermotropic Cytotoxic T-Cell Lymphoma **709**
John R. Goodlad, Lorenzo Cerroni, and Barbara Pro

108 Peripheral T-Cell Lymphoma, Not Otherwise Specified **712**
Philippe Gaulard, Wing C. Chan, Fina Climent, Laurence de Leval, Andrew L. Feldman, Miguel A. Piris, and Julie M. Vose

109 Follicular Helper T-Cell Lymphoma **720**
Ahmet Dogan, Philippe Gaulard, François Lemonnier, Sarah L. Ondrejka, and Pier Luigi Zinzani

110 Anaplastic Large Cell Lymphoma, ALK Positive **733**
Andrew L. Feldman, Bettina Bisig, Steven M. Horwitz, Marina Narbaitz, and Kerry J. Savage

111 Anaplastic Large Cell Lymphoma, ALK Negative **741**
Andrew L. Feldman, Bettina Bisig, Steven M. Horwitz, Marina Narbaitz, and Kerry J. Savage

112 Breast Implant–Associated Anaplastic Large Cell Lymphoma **749**
Camille Laurent, Arianna Di Napoli, Andrew L. Feldman, and Steven M. Horwitz

SECTION 13 Immunodeficiency-Associated Lymphoproliferative Disorders

113 Posttransplant Lymphoproliferative Disorders **754**
Thomas A. Tousseyn, Genevieve M. Crane, Thomas M. Habermann, Elaine S. Jaffe, and Rebecca L. King

114 Other Iatrogenic Immunodeficiency-Associated Lymphoproliferative Disorders **769**
Thomas A. Tousseyn, Genevieve M. Crane, Thomas M. Habermann, Elaine S. Jaffe, and Rebecca L. King

SECTION 14 Histiocytic and Dendritic Cell Neoplasms

Introduction to Histiocytic and Dendritic Cell Neoplasms **778**
Laurence de Leval, Elaine S. Jaffe, and Stefano A. Pileri

115 Histiocytic Sarcoma **783**
Stefano A. Pileri, Caoimhe Egan, and Jason L. Hornick

116 Langerhans Cell Histiocytosis **787**
Stefano A. Pileri, Carl E. Allen, and Alberto Zamò

117 Indeterminate Dendritic Cell Histiocytosis **791**
Neval Ozkaya and Elaine S. Jaffe

118 Interdigitating Dendritic Cell Sarcoma **794**
Andrew L. Feldman and Wayne Tam

119 ALK-Positive Histiocytosis **798**
Elaine S. Jaffe and Benjamin H. Durham

120 Juvenile Xanthogranuloma **803**
John R. Goodlad and Sylvie Fraitag

121 Erdheim-Chester Disease **806**
Neval Ozkaya and Ahmet Dogan

122 Rosai-Dorfman-Destombes Disease **811**
Neval Ozkaya and Ahmet Dogan

123 Follicular Dendritic Cell Sarcoma **816**
Laurence de Leval, Caoimhe Egan, Elaine S. Jaffe, and Alberto Zamò

124 Fibroblastic Reticular Cell Sarcoma **820**
Laurence de Leval, Caoimhe Egan, Elaine S. Jaffe, and Alberto Zamò

125 Epstein-Barr Virus–Positive Inflammatory Follicular Dendritic Cell/Fibroblastic Reticular Cell Tumor **822**
Daniel A. Arber, Laurence de Leval, Elaine S. Jaffe, and Alberto Zamò

Index 825

The International Consensus Classification of Myeloid and Lymphoid Neoplasms

Myeloproliferative Neoplasms
Chronic myeloid leukemia
Polycythemia vera
Essential thrombocythemia
Primary myelofibrosis
  Early/prefibrotic primary myelofibrosis
  Overt primary myelofibrosis
Chronic neutrophilic leukemia
Chronic eosinophilic leukemia, not otherwise specified (NOS)
Myeloproliferative neoplasm, unclassifiable

Myeloid/Lymphoid Neoplasms With Eosinophilia and Tyrosine Kinase Gene Fusions
Myeloid/lymphoid neoplasm with *PDGFRA* rearrangement
Myeloid/lymphoid neoplasm with *PDGFRB* rearrangement
Myeloid/lymphoid neoplasm with *FGFR1* rearrangement
Myeloid/lymphoid neoplasm with *JAK2* rearrangement
Myeloid/lymphoid neoplasm with *FLT3* rearrangement
Myeloid/lymphoid neoplasm with *ETV6::ABL1*

Mastocytosis

Myelodysplastic/Myeloproliferative Neoplasms
Chronic myelomonocytic leukemia
  Clonal monocytosis of undetermined significance
Atypical chronic myeloid leukemia
Myelodysplastic/myeloproliferative neoplasm with thrombocytosis and *SF3B1* mutation
Myelodysplastic/myeloproliferative neoplasm with ring sideroblasts and thrombocytosis, NOS
Myelodysplastic/myeloproliferative neoplasm, NOS
  Myelodysplastic/myeloproliferative neoplasm with isolated isochromosome (17q)

Myelodysplastic Syndromes and Premalignant Clonal Cytopenias
Clonal cytopenia of undetermined significance and other clonal cytopenias
Myelodysplastic syndrome with mutated *SF3B1*
Myelodysplastic syndrome with del(5q)
Myelodysplastic syndrome with mutated *TP53*
Myelodysplastic syndrome, NOS (MDS, NOS)
  MDS, NOS without dysplasia
  MDS, NOS with single lineage dysplasia
  MDS, NOS with multilineage dysplasia
Myelodysplastic syndrome with excess blasts
Myelodysplastic syndrome/acute myeloid leukemia (MDS/AML)
  MDS/AML with mutated *TP53*
  MDS/AML with myelodysplasia-related gene mutations
  MDS/AML with myelodysplasia-related cytogenetic abnormalities
  MDS/AML, NOS

Pediatric or Germline Mutation–Associated Disorders
Juvenile myelomonocytic leukemia
Juvenile myelomonocytic leukemia-like neoplasms
Noonan syndrome–associated myeloproliferative disorder
Refractory cytopenia of childhood
Hematologic neoplasms with germline predisposition

Acute Myeloid Leukemias
Acute promyelocytic leukemia (APL) with t(15;17)(q24.1;q21.2)/*PML::RARA*
APL with other *RARA* rearrangements
AML with t(8;21)(q22;q22.1)/*RUNX1::RUNX1T1*
AML with inv(16)(p13.1q22) or t(16;16)(p13.1;q22)/*CBFB::MYH11*
AML with t(9;11)(p21.3;q23.3)/*MLLT3::KMT2A*
AML with other *KMT2A* rearrangements
AML with t(6;9)(p22.3;q34.1)/*DEK::NUP214*
AML with inv(3)(q21.3q26.2) or t(3;3)(q21.3;q26.2)/*GATA2*; *MECOM(EVI1)*
AML with other *MECOM* rearrangements
AML with other rare recurring translocations
AML with t(9;22)(q34.1;q11.2)/*BCR::ABL1*
AML with mutated *NPM1*
AML with in-frame bZIP *CEBPA* mutations
AML and MDS/AML with mutated *TP53*
AML and MDS/AML with myelodysplasia-related gene mutations
AML with myelodysplasia-related cytogenetic abnormalities
AML NOS
Myeloid Sarcoma

Myeloid Proliferations Associated With Down Syndrome

Blastic Plasmacytoid Dendritic Cell Neoplasm

Acute Leukemia of Ambiguous Lineage
Mixed phenotype acute leukemia (MPAL) with t(9;22)(q34.1;q11.2); *BCR::ABL1*
MPAL, with t(v;11q23.3); *KMT2A* rearranged
MPAL with *ZNF384* rearrangement
MPAL with *BCL11B* activation
MPAL with defining immunophenotypic changes
Acute undifferentiated leukemia
Acute leukemia of ambiguous lineage, NOS

B-Lymphoblastic Leukemias/Lymphomas (B-ALL)
B-ALL with recurrent genetic abnormalities
  B-ALL with t(9;22)(q34.1;q11.2)/*BCR::ABL1*
    with lymphoid only involvement
    with multilineage involvement
  B-ALL with t(v;11q23.3)/*KMT2A* rearranged
  B-ALL with t(12;21) (p13.2;q22.1)/*ETV6::RUNX1*
  B-ALL, hyperdiploid
  B-ALL, low hypodiploid

B-ALL, near haploid
B-ALL with t(5;14)(q31.1;q32.3)/*IL3::IGH*
B-ALL with t(1;19)(q23.3;p13.3)/*TCF3::PBX1*
B-ALL, *BCR::ABL1*–like, ABL-1 class rearranged
B-ALL, *BCR::ABL1*–like, JAK-STAT activated
B-ALL, *BCR::ABL1*–like, NOS
B-ALL with iAMP21
B-ALL with *MYC* rearrangement
B-ALL with *DUX4* rearrangement
B-ALL with *MEF2D* rearrangement
B-ALL with *ZNF384* rearrangement
B-ALL with *NUTM1* rearrangement
B-ALL with *HLF* rearrangement
B-ALL with *UBTF::ATXN7L3/PAN3,CDX2* ("CDX2/UBTF")
B-ALL with PAX5 P80R
B-ALL with IKZF1 N159Y
B-ALL, NOS
B-ALL, provisional entities*

T-Lymphoblastic Leukemias/Lymphomas

Early T-cell precursor ALL with *BCL11B*-activated
Early T-cell precursor ALL, NOS
T-ALL, NOS
T-ALL, provisional entities*

NK-Lymphoblastic Leukemia/Lymphoma*

Mature B-Cell Neoplasms

Chronic lymphocytic leukemia/small lymphocytic lymphoma
Monoclonal B-cell lymphocytosis
  CLL type
  Non-CLL type
B-cell prolymphocytic leukemia
Splenic marginal zone lymphoma
Hairy cell leukemia
Splenic B-cell lymphoma/leukemia, unclassifiable*
  Splenic diffuse red pulp small B-cell lymphoma*
  Hairy cell leukemia-variant*
Lymphoplasmacytic lymphoma
  Waldenström macroglobulinemia
IgM monoclonal gammopathy of undetermined significance (MGUS)
  IgM MGUS, plasma cell type
  IgM MGUS, NOS
Primary cold agglutinin disease
Heavy chain diseases
  Mu heavy chain disease
  Gamma heavy chain disease
  Alpha heavy chain disease
Plasma cell neoplasms
  Non-IgM monoclonal gammopathy of undetermined significance
  Multiple myeloma (Plasma cell myeloma)
    Multiple myeloma, NOS
    Multiple myeloma with recurrent genetic abnormalities
      Multiple myeloma with *CCND* family translocation
      Multiple myeloma with *MAF* family translocation
      Multiple myeloma with *NSD2* translocation
      Multiple myeloma with hyperdiploidy
  Solitary plasmacytoma of bone
  Extraosseous plasmacytoma
Monoclonal immunoglobulin deposition diseases
  Immunoglobulin light chain amyloidosis (AL)
  Localized AL amyloidosis
  Light chain and heavy chain deposition disease
Extranodal marginal zone lymphoma of mucosa-associated lymphoid tissue (MALT lymphoma)
Primary cutaneous marginal zone lymphoproliferative disorder
Nodal marginal zone lymphoma
Follicular lymphoma
  In situ follicular neoplasia
  Duodenal-type follicular lymphoma
BCL2-R-negative, CD23-positive follicle center lymphoma*
Primary cutaneous follicle center lymphoma
Pediatric-type follicular lymphoma
Testicular follicular lymphoma
Large B-cell lymphoma with *IRF4* rearrangement
Mantle cell lymphoma
  In situ mantle cell neoplasia
  Leukemic nonnodal mantle cell lymphoma
Diffuse large B-cell lymphoma (DLBCL), NOS
  Germinal center B-cell subtype
  Activated B-cell subtype
Large B-cell lymphoma with 11q aberration*
Nodular lymphocyte predominant B-cell lymphoma
T cell/histiocyte rich large B-cell lymphoma
Primary DLBCL of the central nervous system
Primary DLBCL of the testis
Primary cutaneous DLBCL, leg type
Intravascular large B-cell lymphoma
Human herpesvirus 8 (HHV-8) and Epstein-Barr virus (EBV)–negative primary effusion-based lymphoma*
EBV-positive mucocutaneous ulcer
EBV-positive DLBCL, NOS
DLBCL associated with chronic inflammation
  Fibrin-associated DLBCL
Lymphomatoid granulomatosis
EBV-positive polymorphic B-cell lymphoproliferative disorder, NOS
ALK-positive large B-cell lymphoma
Plasmablastic lymphoma
HHV-8–associated lymphoproliferative disorders
  Multicentric Castleman disease
  HHV-8–positive germinotropic lymphoproliferative disorder
  HHV-8–positive DLBCL, NOS
  Primary effusion lymphoma
Burkitt lymphoma
High-grade B-cell lymphoma with *MYC* and *BCL2* rearrangements
High-grade B-cell lymphoma with *MYC* and *BCL6* rearrangements*
High-grade B-cell lymphoma, NOS
Primary mediastinal large B-cell lymphoma
Mediastinal gray zone lymphoma

Classic Hodgkin Lymphoma

Nodular sclerosis classic Hodgkin lymphoma
Lymphocyte-rich classic Hodgkin lymphoma
Mixed cellularity classic Hodgkin lymphoma
Lymphocyte-depleted classic Hodgkin lymphoma

Mature T-Cell and NK-Cell Neoplasms

T-cell prolymphocytic leukemia
T-cell large granular lymphocytic leukemia
Chronic lymphoproliferative disorder of NK cells*
Adult T-cell leukemia/lymphoma
EBV-positive T/NK lymphoproliferative disorders of childhood
  Hydroa vacciniforme LPD
    Classic
    Systemic
  Severe mosquito bite allergy
  Chronic active EBV disease (T-cell and NK-cell phenotype)
  Systemic EBV-positive T-cell lymphoma of childhood
Extranodal NK/T-cell lymphoma, nasal type
Aggressive NK-cell leukemia
Primary nodal EBV-positive T/NK-cell lymphoma*
Enteropathy-associated T-cell lymphoma
  Type II refractory celiac disease
Monomorphic epitheliotropic intestinal T-cell lymphoma
Intestinal T-cell lymphoma, NOS
Indolent clonal T-cell lymphoproliferative disorder of the gastrointestinal tract
Indolent NK-cell lymphoproliferative disorder of the gastrointestinal tract
Hepatosplenic T-cell lymphoma
Mycosis fungoides
Sézary syndrome
Primary cutaneous CD30-positive T-cell lymphoproliferative disorders
  Lymphomatoid papulosis
  Primary cutaneous anaplastic large cell lymphoma
Primary cutaneous CD4-positive small/medium T-cell lymphoproliferative disorder
Subcutaneous panniculitis-like T-cell lymphoma
Primary cutaneous gamma-delta T-cell lymphoma
Primary cutaneous acral CD8-positive T-cell lymphoproliferative disorder
Primary cutaneous CD8-positive aggressive epidermotropic cytotoxic T-cell lymphoma
Peripheral T-cell lymphoma, NOS
Follicular helper T-cell lymphoma
  Follicular helper T-cell lymphoma, angioimmunoblastic type (Angioimmunoblastic T-cell lymphoma)
  Follicular helper T-cell lymphoma, follicular type
  Follicular helper T-cell lymphoma, NOS
Anaplastic large cell lymphoma, ALK positive
Anaplastic large cell lymphoma, ALK negative
Breast implant-associated anaplastic large cell lymphoma

Immunodeficiency-Associated Lymphoproliferative Disorders

Posttransplant lymphoproliferative disorders (PTLD)
  Nondestructive PTLD
    Plasmacytic hyperplasia PTLD
    Infectious mononucleosis PTLD
    Florid follicular hyperplasia PTLD
  Polymorphic PTLD
  Monomorphic PTLD (B-cell and T/NK-cell types)
  Classic Hodgkin lymphoma PTLD
Other iatrogenic immunodeficiency–associated lymphoproliferative disorders

Histiocytic and Dendritic Cell Neoplasms

Histiocytic sarcoma
Langerhans cell histiocytosis
Langerhans cell sarcoma
Indeterminate dendritic cell histiocytosis
Interdigitating dendritic cell sarcoma
ALK-positive histiocytosis
Disseminated juvenile xanthogranuloma
Erdheim-Chester disease
Rosai-Dorfman-Destombes disease
Follicular dendritic cell sarcoma
Fibroblastic reticular cell sarcoma
EBV-positive inflammatory follicular dendritic cell/fibroblastic reticular cell tumor

* Provisional entity

INTERNATIONAL CONSENSUS CLASSIFICATION OF MYELOID DISORDERS AND ACUTE LEUKEMIAS

Introduction to the International Consensus Classification of Myeloid Disorders and Acute Leukemias

Robert P. Hasserjian, Daniel A. Arber, Mario Cazzola, Hartmut Döhner, Hans Michael Kvasnicka, Richard A. Larson, Attilio Orazi, and Ayalew Tefferi

The 2001 *WHO Classification of Tumours: Pathology and Genetics of Tumours of Haematopoietic and Lymphoid Tissues* (3rd edition) reflected a paradigm shift in the approach to the classification of myeloid neoplasms: this classification was the first to incorporate genetic information into the diagnostic algorithms for various entities and was also the first to engage a large group of pathologists, geneticists, hematologists, and oncologists through the Clinical Advisory Committee (CAC) process, supported by the Society for Hematopathology and the European Association for Haematopathology, in developing the classification. The publication predicted that future revisions would be necessitated by rapidly emerging genetic information relevant to the diagnosis and classification of myeloid malignancies. The 4th edition (published in 2008)[1] and the 4th edition revision (published in 2017)[2] reflected the significant new molecular insights that became available since the publication of the 3rd edition, proving that prediction to be correct. The CAC process and continued engagement of the hematopathology societies helped to foster the huge successes and global acceptance of the 3rd, 4th, and revised 4th edition classifications.[3,4]

The International Consensus Classification (ICC) adopted the same approach to classification as the prior World Health Organization (WHO) classifications, including further integration of new genetic discoveries. The CAC convened as a hybrid meeting at the University of Chicago in September 2021, with initial publication of the classification in the fall of 2022 in the journal *Blood*.[5] With the approval of numerous new therapies for acute myeloid leukemia (AML),[6] myelodysplastic syndromes (MDSs),[7] and other myeloid neoplasms in recent years, clinical input is even more essential to making informed decisions around many of the changes in the classification. Indeed, clinicopathologic discussions in the CAC that preceded the ICC fostered the development of a more genetically-defined approach to MDS, incorporation of entities with mutated *TP53* in both MDS and AML, and creation of a new category of MDS/AML in adults.[5] The multidisciplinary consensus approach used by the ICC promotes its applicability and clinical utility to the current classification of myeloid neoplasms.

General Principles for the International Consensus Classification of Myeloid Neoplasms

As with the prior revised 4th edition WHO classification, the ICC recognizes several broad groups of myeloid neoplasms: the *acute leukemias*, characterized by a proliferation of blasts, and several groups of *chronic myeloid neoplasms* (which can themselves progress to acute leukemias/blast transformation, with varying propensities). The ICC also recognizes clonal myeloid proliferations (clonal hematopoiesis) that are precursor states for myeloid neoplasms. The organization of these groups is shown in Figure 1.

The ICC continues to integrate clinical features (blood counts, splenomegaly), morphology, and genetic features into the diagnostic criteria of nearly all entities; immunophenotype impacts the classification of acute leukemias. An important principle retained in the ICC is that a myeloid neoplasm diagnosis in a given patient is always rendered with the knowledge of that patient's prior history. Generally, the first diagnosis of a myeloid neoplasm will dictate how any subsequent diagnostic samples are classified, as discussed in each chapter. The initial diagnosis should be made prior to any therapy that may alter the patient's blood counts or disease morphology. In some cases, the effects of comorbid conditions such as an infection or concurrent nonmyeloid neoplasm involving the bone marrow must be taken into account.

The final diagnostic pathology report for all myeloid neoplasms should provide the precise ICC diagnosis wherever possible, integrating all necessary diagnostic modalities including any required genetic studies. Any progression (change in diagnosis) from a known prior myeloid neoplasm should be stated in the report (see Figure 1). Ideally, all supportive clinical, morphologic, genetic, and immunophenotypic information should be included in the report to allow comparison with any subsequent samples. If a definitive classification cannot be determined, whether because of unknown clinical history, inadequate or suboptimal material for diagnosis, or

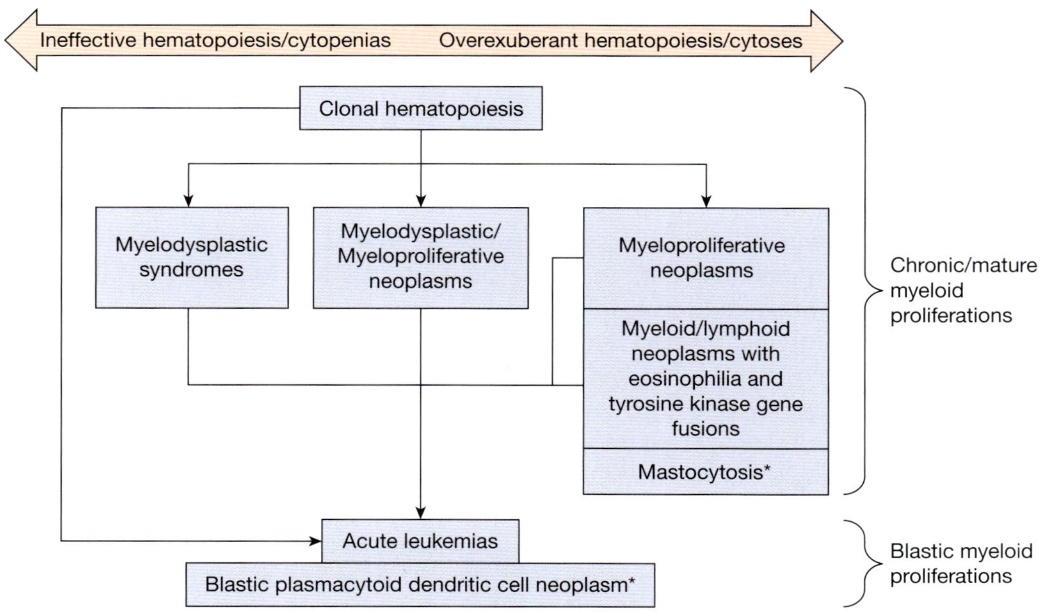

FIGURE 1 Organization of myeloid neoplasms groups in the International Consensus Classification, including preneoplastic clonal hematopoiesis, and their patterns of progression. Once diagnosed with a chronic/mature myeloid proliferation, a case should remain in its initial diagnostic group unless it progresses from clonal hematopoiesis to any myeloid neoplasm or from any chronic/mature myeloid neoplasm to an acute leukemia, as indicated by the arrows. *Mastocytosis and blastic plasmacytoid dendritic cell neoplasm can co-occur with other myeloid neoplasms.

ambiguity in applying the diagnostic criteria, the report should provide guidance of what information or additional studies may be needed to clarify the diagnosis.

Guidelines for the Use of Testing That Impacts the Classification of Myeloid Neoplasms

Clinical features

Peripheral blood counts

Specific abnormalities of the blood counts (cytopenias and/or cytoses) are critical defining features in many myeloid neoplasms, and thus knowledge of the peripheral blood counts is critical in their diagnosis. Minimal information should include hemoglobin, hematocrit, white blood cell count (including white blood cell count differential, discussed under Peripheral Blood Morphology), and platelet count. While peripheral blood count parameters used in the ICC are in large part based on historic precedent,[8] they are necessary to define (1) the ineffective hematopoiesis that is inherent to MDS and MDS/myeloproliferative neoplasm (MPN); (2) the overexuberant mature hematopoiesis that characterize MPN, MDS/MPN, and myeloid/lymphoid neoplasms with eosinophilia and tyrosine kinase gene fusions; and (3) the maturation arrest and blast expansion inherent to acute leukemias. Cytopenias are used as major diagnostic features of MDS and MDS/MPN and in the ICC are defined as the presence of anemia (hemoglobin <13 g/dL in males/<12 g/dL in females), neutropenia (absolute neutrophil count $<1.8 \times 10^9$/L), or thrombocytopenia (platelets $<150 \times 10^9$/L). Cytoses are used as diagnostic features for MPN, MDS/MPN, and myeloid/lymphoid neoplasms with eosinophilia and tyrosine kinase gene fusions and are defined as erythrocytosis (hemoglobin ≥16.5 g/dL or hematocrit ≥49% g/dL in males/ hemoglobin ≥16.0 g/dL or hematocrit ≥48% in females, or red blood cell mass >25% above mean predicted value), leukocytosis (white blood count $\geq 13 \times 10^9$/L, not due to a lymphocytosis), thrombocytosis (platelets $\geq 450 \times 10^9$/L), monocytosis (monocytes $\geq 0.5 \times 10^9$/L and ≥10% of all leukocytes), or hypereosinophilia (eosinophil count $\geq 1.5 \times 10^9$/L and ≥10% of all leukocytes). Leukocytosis, thrombocytosis, and monocytosis are also used as exclusionary features in MDS. Importantly, blood counts should always be interpreted in the context of any growth factors, drugs, or infections that may cause alterations. Although diagnostic criteria are by convention based on blood counts obtained at the time of the diagnostic bone marrow sample, in some cases, access to multiple antecedent time points can help clarify a true cytopenia or cytosis in the presence of conditions that temporarily alter the blood counts.

Splenomegaly

The presence or absence of splenomegaly, detected by either physical exam or imaging studies, is included in the diagnostic criteria for chronic neutrophilic leukemia and juvenile myelomonocytic leukemia. It also represents a minor criterion for the diagnosis of primary myelofibrosis and an additional cocriterion used in establishing a diagnosis of post-essential thrombocythemia/post-polycythemia myelofibrosis. Additionally, knowledge of splenomegaly is also helpful in differential diagnosis of other entities, for example, MDS (in which splenomegaly is relatively uncommon) versus MPN.

Prior cytotoxic therapy

Certain myeloid neoplasms (MDS, MDS/MPN, and AML) that develop in patients previously treated with cytotoxic chemotherapy or radiotherapy are designated as "therapy-related" (t-MN). In the revised 4th edition WHO classification, t-MN represented a distinct category within myeloid neoplasms. The underlying mechanism by which cytotoxic therapies precipitate the development of t-MN is still uncertain: recent data suggest that these therapies alter the bone marrow microenvironment, facilitating the selection and expansion of preexisting myeloid clonal hematopoiesis.[9] In particular, these therapies select for clones bearing mutations in DNA-damage response genes, such as *TP53* and *PPM1D*.[10,11] The specific agents that are implicated in t-MN are shown in Table 1. Based on recent evidence, Poly (ADP-ribose) polymerase inhibitors and radioimmunoconjugates have been added to the list of agents associated with the development of myeloid neoplasms.[12,13] Some individuals may have genetic susceptibility to develop t-MN due

TABLE 1 Cytotoxic agents implicated in therapy-related myeloid neoplasms

Alkylating agents	Melphalan, cyclophosphamide, nitrogen mustard, chlorambucil, busulfan, carboplatin, cisplatin, dacarbazine, procarbazine, carmustine, mitomycin C, thiotepa, lomustine
Topoisomerase II inhibitors	Etoposide, teniposide, doxorubicin, daunorubicin, mitoxantrone, amsacrine, actinomycin
Antimetabolites	Thiopurines, mycophenolate mofetil, fludarabine, PARP inhibitors
Antitubulin agents	Vincristine, vinblastine, vindesine, paclitaxel, docetaxel
Radiation therapy	Large fields exposing hematopoietic bone marrow, radioimmunoconjugates

PARP, Poly (ADP-ribose) polymerase.

to certain underlying germline predisposition syndromes (such as germline *TP53* mutation) that affect DNA repair or polymorphisms in genes that affect metabolism of cytotoxic agents.[14]

t-MN have more aggressive biologic behavior compared with their de novo counterparts, which largely appears to reflect a higher incidence of adverse genetic aberrations such as complex karyotype and/or *TP53* mutation. Recent studies have shown that, in MDS and AML, the underlying genetic characteristics influence outcome more than therapy-relatedness.[15-17] In effect, whether a given myeloid neoplasm develops as a consequence of iatrogenic cytotoxic therapy or arises stochastically, its clinical features and behavior depend more on its specific portfolio of mutations and cytogenetic aberrations than on its actual etiology. Moreover, there is no specific morphologic or genetic signature of therapy-relatedness, and it is likely that many myeloid neoplasms designated as therapy-related may arise as coincidence rather than being incited by the prior therapy, particularly when they occur after a very long latency (>10 years).[18] For these reasons, the ICC has removed therapy-relatedness as an overarching disease category and instead classifies t-MN according to their morphologic and genetic features as for de novo disease. Nevertheless, t-MN are more likely to fall into higher-risk disease categories and may have reduced tolerance to intensive therapies used to treat some myeloid neoplasms. The ICC thus recommends to apply a therapy-related qualifier to the diagnosis of any MDS, MDS/MPN, or AML that develops in a patient previously exposed to any of the agents shown in Table 1. Since causation by the prior cytotoxic therapy cannot always be proven, this term does not imply that a myeloid neoplasm was induced by the therapy, but rather merely that it occurred in a patient exposed to a cytotoxic therapy with the potential to cause myeloid neoplasia.

Germline conditions predisposing to myeloid neoplasms

Any known germline mutation or syndrome that predisposes to myeloid malignancy (specific entities discussed in Chapter 21) is also noted as a qualifier to the diagnosis in the ICC. In some instances, a germline condition may be suspected based on the patient's family or personal history, morphology, or results of genetic testing. In such cases, this possibility may be noted in a comment with a suggestion for genetic counseling and/or additional genetic testing to investigate for a germline predisposition.

Other clinical features

As discussed earlier, the diagnostician should be aware of any antecedent myeloid neoplasm as well as any clinical conditions or treatments that could affect the blood counts or morphologic appearance, potentially leading to misclassification.

Morphology

Peripheral blood specimen

A well-prepared and well-stained peripheral blood smear should be examined and correlated with the patient's blood counts. Cytology of leukocytes, red blood cells, and platelets should be evaluated. A manual 200-cell leukocyte differential count (or counting of all available cells in markedly leukopenic cases) should be performed as part of the evaluation of all myeloid neoplasms. The following cells should be enumerated as a proportion of peripheral blood leukocytes (excluding nucleated red blood cells [nRBCs]): *segmented neutrophils, bands, myelocytes, metamyelocytes, promyelocytes, blasts, monocytes, promonocytes, basophils, eosinophils*, and *lymphocytes*. The nRBC count should be expressed as the number of nRBCs counted per 100 leukocytes. If circulating neoplastic cells from a concomitant nonmyeloid neoplasm (such as a lymphoma or plasma cell leukemia) are present, they should be excluded from the white blood count and leukocyte differential count when applying thresholds for the diagnosis of myeloid neoplasms.

Bone marrow aspirate specimen

Well-prepared direct smears or buffy coat smears from aspirated bone marrow should be prepared and examined. If spiculated aspirate material cannot be obtained due to "dry tap," touch preparations of the biopsy should be prepared (taking care to avoid damage to the core biopsy). Aspirate and touch preparations should be stained with Wright-Giemsa or May-Grünwald-Giemsa, and extra unstained smears should be prepared for possible iron or cytochemical stains.

At least 500 nucleated bone marrow cells should be counted from areas close to spicules to avoid hemodilution or from more cellular areas of buffy coat smears, ideally obtaining counts from several different areas of the smear(s). The following cells should be individually enumerated as a proportion of all nucleated cells: *segmented neutrophils, bands, myelocytes, metamyelocytes, promyelocytes, blasts, monocytes, promonocytes, basophils, eosinophils, lymphocytes, plasma cells,* and *erythroid precursors*; it is acceptable to count segmented neutrophils, bands, myelocytes, and metamyelocytes together in one group of *granulocytes and myeloid precursors*, since the relative proportion of these cells does not impact classification of any myeloid neoplasm. Mast cells should only be included in the differential if mastocytosis is under diagnostic consideration. In cases where pure erythroid leukemia is a diagnostic consideration (see Chapters 32 and 35), *pronormoblasts* should be enumerated separately from maturing erythroid precursors. Although megakaryocytes are not included in the formal cell count, their presence and estimated frequency should be mentioned in the report. If a concomitant nonmyeloid neoplasm is present, these neoplastic cells should be excluded when applying thresholds for the purpose of classifying a myeloid neoplasm.

Cytology of megakaryocytes, nucleated erythroids, and myeloid elements should be evaluated, as well as the cytology of blasts if increased and any other cell types that appear morphologically abnormal. The differential counts obtained from marrow aspirates should be compared with an estimate of the cells observed in corresponding biopsy sections in order to determine possible sampling artifacts, including hemodilution of the aspirate specimen.

Bone marrow trephine biopsy specimen

The bone marrow biopsy provides information that is critical to the classification of myeloid neoplasms: hematopoietic cellularity, hematopoietic architecture, the relative proportions, maturation, and cytology of hematopoietic cells, and abnormalities of bone marrow stroma, particularly increased marrow fibrosis. The biopsy also provides material for immunohistochemical studies that may aid in diagnosis and classification. The biopsy specimen should optimally be taken at a right angle to the cortical bone, and be at least 1.5 cm in length, to enable evaluation of multiple intertrabecular areas of hematopoietic marrow.[19] The bone marrow specimen should be well fixed, decalcified by a method that preserves cytomorphology and antigen immunogenicity, and thinly sectioned (at 2-4 μm). The biopsy should be stained with hematoxylin and eosin; Giemsa stain (which facilitates visualization of mast cells) and/or periodic acid-Schiff stain (which facilitates the visualization of megakaryocytes) also may be performed. A cell block prepared from clotted aspirate material may be fixed and evaluated similarly to the bone marrow biopsy specimen.

The bone marrow biopsy cellularity should be provided as part of the pathology report for all myeloid neoplasms. The cellularity should be expressed as a percentage, calculated as the proportion of the intertrabecular marrow area (excluding vascular spaces) occupied by hematopoietic cells (both neoplastic and nonneoplastic). Cellularity estimation should optimally be performed in areas devoid of artifacts such as intertrabecular hemorrhage and crushed tissue and should exclude subcortical areas of nonhematopoietic fatty marrow. When variable, the overall cellularity across the entire evaluable marrow should be reported. Marrow may be normocellular, hypocellular, or hypercellular based on the percentage cellularity relative to the patient's age (age-adjusted cellularity); the recommended ranges are shown in Table 2. Although there is good interobserver reproducibility in estimating bone marrow cellularity, in the future artificial intelligence technologies may provide more accurate assessments.[20] Machine learning–based analysis of bone marrow biopsy images may also inform the future diagnosis and classification of MDS and other myeloid neoplasms, by revealing novel morphologic features and mitigating subjectivity in interpreting well-established cytologic abnormalities.[21,22]

TABLE 2 Age-adjusted bone marrow cellularity (adults)

Age	Hypocellular	Hypercellular
20-<40 years	<30% cellularity	>70%
40-<60 years	<30% cellularity	>65%
60-70 years	<30% cellularity	>60%
≥70 years	<20% cellularity	>60%

Data from Wong J, Jackson R, Chen L, et al. Determination of age-dependent bone marrow normocellularity. *Am J Clin Pathol.* 2024;161(2):170-176; and Bono E, McLornan D, Travaglino E, et al. Clinical, histopathological and molecular characterization of hypoplastic myelodysplastic syndrome. *Leukemia.* 2019;33(10):2495-2505.

Megakaryocytes typically occur as single cells distributed evenly in the marrow space; approximately 3 to 4 megakaryocytes are seen per 40× field on average. Megakaryocytes can be regarded as increased or decreased if they are appreciably higher or lower in number. Megakaryocyte topography and cytology should be carefully evaluated and are key features in the classification of myeloid neoplasms, particularly MPN. Definitions of abnormalities in megakaryocyte number, topography, and cytology are shown in Table 3. The relative proportion (myeloid:erythroid ratio) and maturation of erythroid and myeloid elements in the biopsy should also be evaluated.

Identification and morphologic evaluation of blasts in the biopsy and aspirate smear

Morphologic identification and enumeration of blasts in the bone marrow and peripheral blood is critical for the classification of all myeloid neoplasms.[23] Marrow blast enumeration should be performed on the aspirate

TABLE 3 Megakaryocyte morphology

Abnormality	Definition	Association
Increased number	>4 per 40 × field	Many myeloid neoplasms
Small nuclear size	Nucleus smaller than normal, usually with rounded nuclear contour	Many myeloid neoplasms
Micromegakaryocyte	15 µm or less diameter or similar in size to promyelocyte	MDS
Small cluster	4-6 cells in contact	Ph- MPN
Large cluster	7-9 cells in contact	PMF
Giant cluster	≥10 cells in contact	PMF
Endosteal translocation	Megakaryocytes closely apposed to bone trabecular surface	PMF
Bulbous nucleus	Large nucleus with scalloped border, often hyperchromatic	PMF
Staghorn-type nucleus	Large, multilobulated nucleus	ET and PV
Naked nucleus	Hyperchromatic nucleus without cytoplasm	Ph- MPN
Hypolobated nucleus	Nucleus with one lobe or round or oval nonlobated nucleus	MDS and CML
Separated nuclei	Two or more round or oval nuclei detached from one another	MDS

CML, chronic myeloid leukemia; ET, essential thrombocythemia; MDS, myelodysplastic syndrome; Ph- MPN, Philadelphia-chromosome negative myeloproliferative neoplasms; PMF, primary myelofibrosis; PV, polycythemia vera.

smear or touch preparation if an aspirate is unobtainable or markedly hemodilute. Immunohistochemical staining for CD34 on the biopsy specimen highlights $CD34^+$ blasts that can be enumerated, although in some myeloid neoplasms the blasts do not express CD34. It may be appropriate to use the $CD34^+$ blast estimate on the biopsy specimen in lieu of the aspirate blast count in the following instances: (1) The aspirate smear is unobtainable due to dry tap and a touch preparation is not available or not evaluable; (2) the aspirate smear/touch prep are compromised due to hemodilution or other artifacts; (3) sampling artifact is suggested by a larger number of blasts seen in the biopsy compared with the aspirate smear, including cases with focal aggregates or sheets of blasts in the biopsy. In cases where blasts are known to be CD34 negative and are $CD117^+$, CD117 immunostaining can be used to estimate blasts; however, CD117 also stains early erythroid elements, promyelocytes, and mast cells and thus blasts may be overestimated based on CD117 immunostaining. Flow cytometry determination of blast percentage should not be used as a substitute for visual counting of blasts: flow cytometry samples of bone marrow aspirate can be hemodilute and can also be affected by a number of preanalytic variables, such as loss or exclusion of nucleated erythroid cells.

For the purposes of myeloid neoplasm classification, the following cells are counted as blasts: *myeloblasts, monoblasts,* and *megakaryoblasts.*[24] Additionally, *promonocytes* are considered as blast equivalents and included in the overall blast count for all myeloid neoplasms, although caution must be exercised to correctly identify promonocytes and distinguish them from immature or reactive monocytes[25]; monocytes, whether cytologically normal or abnormal, are never considered as blast equivalents.[26] *Promyelocytes* are only regarded as blast equivalents in the setting of *PML::RARA* rearrangement (acute promyelocytic leukemia). *Pronormoblasts* are only regarded as blast equivalents in the setting of pure erythroid leukemia (see Chapters 32 and 35). Descriptions and immunophenotypes of the various blast and blast equivalent cell types are shown in Table 4.

Cytochemical stains

Cytochemical studies performed on bone marrow or blood smears can be useful in determining the lineage of blasts and maturing hematopoietic elements; however, in most laboratories they have been supplanted by immunological studies using flow cytometry and are not required for the diagnosis of any ICC entities. The morphologic and cytochemical features of blasts and blast equivalents are summarized in Table 4. In cases of MDS/MPN, nonspecific esterase (NSE) and myeloperoxidase (MPO) staining may be helpful in distinguishing monocytes from dysplastic granulocytic precursors. The presence of MPO or NSE staining by cytochemistry, in addition to immunophenotypic features, can also be used to establish a myeloid lineage component in the diagnosis of a mixed-phenotype acute leukemia (see Chapter 39).[27]

Reticulin and trichrome stains

A silver impregnation method to evaluate reticulin fibrosis should be performed on all myeloid

TABLE 4 Blasts and blast equivalents

Type	Morphology	Cytochemistry
Myeloblast	Size from slightly larger than mature lymphocytes to the size of monocytes or larger, with scant to abundant dark-blue to bluish-gray cytoplasm. Nuclei round to oval, with finely granular chromatin and usually several nucleoli; in some, nuclear irregularities are prominent. The cytoplasm may contain a few azurophilic granules.	MPO often positive, usually granular or Golgi pattern staining.
Monoblast	Large with abundant cytoplasm, light gray to deep blue and may show pseudopod formation. Nuclei are usually round, with delicate, lacy chromatin and one or more prominent nucleoli.	NSE strongly positive (diffuse cytoplasmic), MPO weak or negative.
Promonocyte	Large with delicately convoluted, folded, or grooved nucleus and finely dispersed chromatin, a small, indistinct, or absent nucleolus, and finely granulated cytoplasm.	NSE positive (diffuse cytoplasmic), often some MPO activity in the form of fine granules.
Abnormal monocyte	Medium to large size with clumped chromatin, variably indented and folded nuclei, and gray cytoplasm with abundant lilac-colored granules. Nucleoli are usually absent or indistinct.	NSE positive (diffuse cytoplasmic), often some MPO activity.
Megakaryoblast	Small with dispersed chromatin, may have pseudopods.	MPO negative.
Pronormoblast	Large with deeply basophilic cytoplasm, often with large vacuoles (when neoplastic)	MPO negative. PAS-positive large cytoplasmic globules.

MPO, myeloperoxidase; NSE, nonspecific esterase; PAS, periodic acid-Schiff.

neoplasms to quantify the presence and degree of any bone marrow fibrosis. Trichrome stain assists in fibrosis assessment and should be performed in any cases with significantly increased reticulin fibrosis (grade 2 or 3). Bone marrow fibrosis (reticulin and trichrome) should be graded according to the European consensus scoring system[28,29] (see Tables 2.2 and 2.3 in Chapter 2).

Iron stain

Although iron stains can be performed on both aspirate and biopsy tissue specimens, evaluation for ring sideroblasts and storage iron should always be performed on the bone marrow aspirate (or touch prep), since iron is leached out in the decalcification and processing of the biopsy specimen. Iron staining should be performed in all possible MDS and MDS/MPN cases to evaluate for ring sideroblasts, defined as erythroid precursors with at least five granules of iron, encircling one-third or more of the nucleus.[24] When present, ring sideroblasts should be enumerated as a percentage of all nucleated erythroid elements. Although ring sideroblasts are most sensitively detected in the aspirate smears, they may be identified in some cases in nondecalcified bone marrow clot sections. Iron staining also evaluates for the presence of storage iron, which may be helpful in separating polycythemia vera (which typically lacks stainable iron in the bone marrow) from other types of MPN.

Immunophenotype

Immunophenotypic analysis by multiparameter flow cytometry is a useful tool in the characterization of many myeloid neoplasms and is of crucial importance in assessing acute leukemias. Immunophenotyping has a central role in distinguishing the subtypes of acute leukemias, including acute leukemias of ambiguous lineage (see Chapter 39) and blast phases of MPN. Aberrant blast immunophenotypes occur in over 90% of cases of AML and in most B-cell acute lymphoblastic leukemia (B-ALL) and T-cell acute lymphoblastic leukemia (T-ALL) cases. Although not impacting classification at diagnosis, these abnormal immunophenotypes are used in follow-up specimens from patients with B-ALL, T-ALL, and AML to assess for measurable residual disease.[30] Aberrant immunophenotypes of blasts and abnormal antigen expression patterns on maturing cell populations also occur in MDS and MDS/MPN.[31] These abnormal immunophenotypes can facilitate the diagnosis of MDS and chronic myelomonocytic leukemia,[32] although they are not formally part of the diagnostic criteria for MDS.

In cases where aspirate material is not available and lesional cells are absent from the peripheral blood, immunohistochemistry (IHC) can be used in lieu of flow cytometry, although IHC may not be as sensitive as flow cytometry to detect some antigens and is not available for all antigens relevant to the classification of myeloid neoplasms and acute leukemias. Immunohistochemical staining can also be a valuable adjunct to identifying cell types that are not readily identified by flow cytometry in the aspirate smear, particularly in the following instances: (1) CD61, CD42, or factor VIII to identify abnormal small megakaryocytes, which may not be readily visible on routine stains; (2)

CD123 to highlight mature plasmacytoid dendritic cell nodules as well as blastic plasmacytoid dendritic cell neoplasm; (3) CD117 and tryptase to highlight the number, distribution, and cytology of mast cells. In instances when evaluation of maturing hematopoietic elements is compromised due to fibrosis or crush artifact, lineage-specific markers for erythroid elements (Glycophorin A, Glycophorin C, CD71, hemoglobin, spectrin, E-cadherin), megakaryocytes (CD61, CD42b, factor VIII), myeloid/monocytic elements (CD33, CD68, lysozyme), granulocytic elements (MPO), and monocytes (CD14) may be helpful.

Genetics

The ICC incorporates specific genetic abnormalities in the diagnostic criteria of many entities, both as defining and exclusionary features. Specific genetic abnormalities incorporated into the classification include gene fusions and chromosomal rearrangements; unbalanced chromosomal alterations such as trisomies, monosomes, or deletions; and gene mutations.

A complete cytogenetic analysis of bone marrow by conventional karyotyping should be performed at the time of initial evaluation of all myeloid neoplasms.[33] Additional diagnostic genetic studies to detect gene fusions or numerical chromosomal abnormalities should be guided by the diagnosis suspected based on the clinical and morphologic features, as discussed in each section below. Targeted reverse transcription polymerase chain reaction (RT-PCR), fluorescence in situ hybridization (FISH), and RNA-based fusion assays can detect gene rearrangements that are cytogenetically cryptic and can also be useful if conventional karyotyping fails or is inadequate. Quantitative RT-PCR performed at the time of diagnosis can also provide a baseline to monitor a specific disease-defining genetic fusion. Recently, more comprehensive genetic analyses such as optical genomic mapping (OGM) or whole genome sequencing are providing more detailed karyotypic assessment that may in the future supplant conventional karyotyping for the detection of gene fusions and numerical cytogenetic aberrations.[34,35]

Almost all myeloid neoplasms are characterized by somatic gene mutations, which include both aberrations that are relatively specific for certain entities and those that are seen across many myeloid neoplasm subtypes. These mutations are usually assessed by next-generation sequencing (NGS), which allows simultaneous assessment of mutations across a large number of genes that are commonly mutated in myeloid neoplasms. Current approaches to genomic profiling include (1) the interrogation of a single genetic lesion (such as *JAK2* V617F) by PCR or a small NGS panel (such as *JAK2*, *MPL*, and *CALR*) for a specific suspected myeloid neoplasm; or (2) a panel-based NGS assay that queries many genes (from 30 to over 400) implicated across all myeloid malignancies, or even including other hematopoietic malignancies such as lymphomas.[33] Although the latter approach is usually costlier, its advantage is to provide a more comprehensive analysis when the diagnosis is unclear and also to provide genetic information that is helpful in prognosis and may guide the use of targeted therapies. Importantly, somatic mutations can occur in hematopoietic cells in individuals without a myeloid neoplasm. Thus, the identification of a mutation, even in a gene commonly mutated in myeloid neoplasia, does not necessarily indicate a hematopoietic neoplasm; the ICC recognizes such nonneoplastic clonal states in a section on clonal hematopoiesis (see Chapter 12).

The ICC includes some criteria that rely on technologies that are not yet widely available. Single nucleotide polymorphism array assessment for loss of heterozygosity at the *TP53* locus is important in classifying MDS in which a *TP53* mutation is identified, since presence or absence of loss of the wild-type *TP53* allele impacts the classification.[36] RNA microarray assessment defines several new provisional entities in B-ALL, which have distinct biologic behaviors and risk profiles.[37] Since these assessments identify biologically and prognostically relevant disease biomarkers, it will be important for laboratories to adopt these new technologies in order to accurately diagnose these new and emerging entities.[33]

A listing of recommended genetic testing for each group of myeloid neoplasms, for both diagnosis and risk stratification, is shown in Table 5. Of note, the ICC applies variant allele fraction (VAF) cutoffs for several myeloid neoplasm categories and also notes certain mutations where highly sensitive VAF testing is recommended, as discussed in each relevant disease section. The purpose of including minimal VAF thresholds in diagnostic criteria is to avoid misdiagnosis due to the presence of a small, incidental mutation that either may be present in a separate, nonneoplastic clone or may be a small secondary subclone rather than a true disease driver. For example, *TP53* mutations can occur as small, stable mutations in clonal hematopoiesis and are unlikely to be driver mutations if they occur at low VAF levels.[38,39] Future classifications may have different VAF thresholds based on individual genes, as more studies are performed to interrogate the applicability of specific VAF thresholds to diagnosis. The

TABLE 5 Recommended genetic testing for myeloid neoplasm categories

Category	Gene mutation testing	Karyotype/structural variants
Clonal cytopenias, MDS, MDS/MPN	*ASXL1, BCOR, BCORL1, CBL, CEBPA, CSF3R, DDX41, DMNT3A, ETV6, ETNK1, EZH2, FLT3*-ITD, *FLT3*-TKD, *GATA2, GNB1, IDH1, IDH2, JAK2, KIT, KRAS, KMT2A*-PTD, *NF1, NPM1, NRAS, PHF6, PPM1D, PRPF8, PTPN11, RAD21, RUNX1, SAMD9,*[a] *SAMD9L,*[a] *SETBP1, SF3B1, SRSF2, STAG2, TET2, TP53,*[b] *U2AF1, UBA1, WT1, ZRSR2*	Conventional karyotype
MPN (except CEL)	*ASXL1, CALR, CBL, CSF3R, DNMT3A, EZH2, IDH1, IDH2, JAK2, KIT, KRAS, MPL, NRAS, PTPN11, RUNX1, SETBP1, SF3B1, SH2B3, SRSF2, TET2, U2AF1, ZRSR2*	Conventional karyotype, *BCR::ABL1* FISH and/or RT-PCR
Mastocytosis	*KIT*[c]	Conventional karyotype
JMML	*PTPN11, NRAS, KRAS, NF1, CBL*	Conventional karyotype
MLNEo-TK and CEL	*ASXL1, CBL, DNMT3A, EZH2, KRAS, NRAS, RUNX1, SF3B1, SRSF2, STAT5B, TET2, U2AF1*	Conventional karyotype; FISH or fusion panel testing for *BCR::ABL1, FGFR1::R, FLT3::R, JAK2::R, PDGFRA::R, PDGFRB::R, ABL1::R*
AML and ALAL	*ASXL1, BCOR, CEBPA, DDX41, EZH2, FLT3*-ITD, *FLT3*-TKD, *IDH1, IDH2, NPM1, RUNX1, SF3B1, SRSF2, STAG2, TP53, U2AF1, ZRSR2*	Conventional karyotype; consider FISH or fusion panel testing for cryptic *BCR::ABL1, CBFB::MYH11, DEK::NUP214, MECOM::R, KMT2A::R, NUP98::R, RUNX1::RUNX1T1, PML::RARA*
BPDCN	Not required	Conventional karyotype

ALAL, acute leukemia of ambiguous lineage; AML, acute myeloid leukemia; BPDCN, blastic plasmacytoid dendritic cell neoplasm; CEL, chronic eosinophilic leukemia; FISH, fluorescence in situ hybridization; JMML, juvenile myelomonocytic leukemia; MDS, myelodysplastic syndrome; MLNEo-TK, myeloid/lymphoid neoplasm with eosinophilia and tyrosine kinase gene fusion; MPN, myeloproliferative neoplasm; RT-PCR, reverse transcription polymerase chain reaction.

Adapted from Duncavage EJ, Bagg A, Hasserjian RP et al Genomic profiling for clinical decision making in myeloid neoplasms and acute leukemia. *Blood.* 2022;140(21):2228-2247.

[a]For pediatric patients.

[b]Recommend assessment for copy-neutral loss of heterozygosity at *TP53* locus.

[c]If associated with a myeloid neoplasm, consider additional genetic testing appropriate for the type of the other neoplasm.

purpose of specifying highly sensitive testing for *KIT* and *JAK2* in mastocytosis and classic MPN, respectively, is to ensure detection of small neoplastic clones in the bone marrow that might not be well represented in the bone marrow aspirate, despite causing a clinically significant myeloid proliferation.[40]

Updates to the Classification of Myeloid Neoplasm Disease Groups

Myeloproliferative neoplasms

MPNs encompass clonal hematopoietic stem cell disorders characterized by overproduction of one or more mature myeloid blood cell types (neutrophils, platelets, red cells, or eosinophils). The vast majority of MPNs show bone marrow hypercellularity, with varied morphology that depends on the specific disease type. Splenomegaly and hepatomegaly, typically due to extramedullary proliferation of the clonal myeloid cells, are commonly seen in MPN.

Most MPNs are associated with genetic aberrations resulting in activated tyrosine kinase signaling, which drives the myeloproliferation. These abnormalities include translocations (such as *BCR::ABL1*), mutations of genes encoding tyrosine kinase receptors (such as *MPL* and *CSF3R*), and mutations in genes that promote abnormal, constitutively activate protein tyrosine signaling (such as *JAK2* and *CALR*). The specific types of genetic events variably impact disease categorization: for example, *BCR::ABL1* rearrangement in a chronic myeloid neoplasm essentially defines chronic myeloid leukemia (CML), while *JAK2* mutation is seen in several different MPN subtypes and can also be found in other types of myeloid neoplasms, such as MDS and MDS/MPN. Importantly, aside from CML, other MPN subtypes are not fully defined by the presence of a specific genetic abnormality and the molecular pathogenesis of subsets of MPN lacking a known tyrosine kinase gene is unknown. Such cases may still be classified as a specific MPN subtype based on their clinical, laboratory, and morphologic features, even in the absence of the typically associated genetic aberration. For example, the MPN entity chronic eosinophilic leukemia, not otherwise specified (CEL, NOS) is not associated with any specific genetic abnormality and is diagnosed based on the absence of other disease-defining genetic abnormalities, the presence of unexplained eosinophilia, and an abnormal bone marrow myeloproliferation, often with one or more gene mutations to support the clonal nature of the myeloproliferation.[41]

Although biologically related to CML by virtue of a gene fusion that activates a tyrosine kinase, hematopoietic neoplasms with other (non-*BCR::ABL1*) tyrosine kinase gene fusions are classified apart from the MPN in a separate group of "myeloid/lymphoid neoplasms with eosinophilia and tyrosine kinase gene fusions" (discussed later). These neoplasms are typically, but not invariably, associated with eosinophilia and, like CML, display myeloid:lymphoid lineage plasticity due to origin in a multipotent stem cell.[42]

Patterns of progression in MPN

Although many MPNs exhibit an indolent disease course, all have the potential to undergo progression that culminates in an aggressive acute leukemia. By convention, any acute leukemia originating in a patient with a prior confirmed diagnosis of an MPN is diagnosed as *blast phase* of the MPN. Although the vast majority of these transformations exhibit a myeloid phenotype, in CML up to one-third of blast phase disease displays a precursor B-lymphoid phenotype. MPN cases of any type with 10% to 19% blasts in the peripheral blood or bone marrow are considered to represent accelerated phase; CML has additional criteria defining accelerated phase (see Chapter 1). Increased bone marrow fibrosis may be seen at initial diagnosis or as a manifestation of disease progression, and thus, assessment of bone marrow fibrosis is a critical aspect in the analysis of all MPNs. Finally, although not usually present at diagnosis, dysplastic morphology in one or more lineages may develop secondarily in "pure MPN."[43] While such dysplastic changes should be noted in the pathology report and could represent a type of progression (often due to acquisition of additional mutations),[44,45] these cases should not be reclassified as MDS/MPN. The types of progression in the each of the MPN are shown in Table 6.

TABLE 6 Nomenclature for patterns of progression (disease phases) in MPN subtypes

Disease	Grade 2-3 fibrosis	10%-19% blasts	≥20% blasts
CML	NA	Accelerated phase[b]	Blast phase
ET	Post-ET MF[a]	Accelerated phase	Blast phase
PV	Post-PV MF[a]	Accelerated phase	Blast phase
Primary myelofibrosis	Overt PMF[a]	Accelerated phase	Blast phase
CEL	NA	Accelerated phase	Blast phase
CNL	NA	Accelerated phase	Blast phase
MPN, unclassifiable	NA	Accelerated phase	Blast phase

CEL, chronic eosinophilic leukemia; CML, chronic myeloid leukemia; CNL, chronic neutrophilic leukemia; ET, essential thrombocythemia; MF, myelofibrosis; MPN, myeloproliferative neoplasm; NA, not applicable; PMF, primary myelofibrosis; PV, polycythemia vera.

[a]Other cocriteria are required for diagnosing post-ET or post-PV MF.

[b]Accelerated phase of CML can also be established by additional cytogenetic abnormalities or increased basophils.

Main updates from the revised 4th edition WHO classification

Overall, the classification of MPN in the ICC is largely unchanged from the prior revised 4th edition WHO classification. Listed are several minor changes:

1. Owing to well-established recognition of the defining *BCR::ABL1* gene rearrangement, this translocation has been removed from the name of CML.
2. The criteria for accelerated phase of CML (CML-AP) have been simplified and are now limited to blood or bone marrow blasts of 10% to 19%, peripheral blood basophils ≥20%, or the presence of several specific additional cytogenetic abnormalities in addition to the *BCR::ABL1*. Regarding blast phase of CML, it has been noted that >5% morphologically apparent lymphoblasts warrants close follow-up and consideration of impending lymphoid blast phase; the threshold for myeloid blast phase of CML remains at ≥20% myeloblasts in blood or bone marrow.
3. Owing to the strong association of *CSF3R* mutation with chronic neutrophilic leukemia, the minimal white blood cell count requirement for this diagnosis has been reduced from 25×10^9/L to 13×10^9/L if an activating *CSF3R* mutation is documented; all other diagnostic requirements are the same.
4. Morphologic criteria (increased cellularity and dysplastic megakaryocytes, often associated with other dysplastic features, increased fibrosis, bone marrow eosinophilic infiltrate, and/or increased blasts) have been added to the diagnostic criteria for CEL, NOS.
5. So-called lymphocyte variant hypereosinophilic syndrome, in which the eosinophilia is driven by an immunophenotypically abnormal T-cell population, has been excluded from idiopathic hypereosinophilic syndrome.
6. The morphologic criteria for essential thrombocythemia, polycythemia vera, and primary myelofibrosis have been refined with additional distinguishing features based on recent evidence.[46,47]

7. Since relatively small *JAK2, CALR*, or *MPL*-mutated clones may be associated with significant blood count elevations and clinical sequelae, warranting diagnoses of overt MPN, the use of highly sensitive assays to evaluate for mutations in these genes is recommended.

Myeloid/lymphoid neoplasms with eosinophilia and tyrosine kinase gene fusions

Myeloid/lymphoid neoplasms with eosinophilia and tyrosine kinase gene fusions (MLNEo-TK) represent a group of clonal hematopoietic stem cell disorders characterized by fusions of specific tyrosine kinase genes, usually associated with overproduction of eosinophils. The neoplastic stem cell is primitive and exhibits lineage plasticity, with the capacity to differentiate along B-lymphoid, T-lymphoid, and/or myeloid lines. Accordingly, these cases may progress to or present initially as acute lymphoid or myeloid leukemias, which must be distinguished from de novo ALL and AML. The specific tyrosine kinase genes defining the entities within this group are *PDGFRA, PDGFRB, FGFR1, JAK2*, and *FLT3*, which are fused with various partners that create a constitutively activate chimeric tyrosine kinase protein. The specific *ETV6::ABL1* fusion is also included within this category; however, other alternative *ABL1* translocations typically present as *BCR::ABL1*-like B-ALL or de novo T-ALL and would thus be classified in those categories rather than among the MLNEo-TK.[48,49]

These rare MLNEo-TK entities are critical to accurately diagnose, as they often respond to specific targeted therapies. However, they may be challenging to diagnose because many of the lesions are cytogenetically cryptic and alternate partners may not be cytogenetically well-characterized or may overlap with similar lesions on conventional G-banded karyotype. Some subtypes, but not all, can be recognized by interphase cytogenetics (FISH). Thus, if MLNEo-TK is suspected and cytogenetic analysis is negative or unclear, more comprehensive genetic analysis to detect specific gene fusions is recommended, such as RNA sequencing, RNA-based fusion assays, or OGM.[50]

Patterns of progression

MLNEo-TK may present as chronic myeloid neoplasms, usually with eosinophilia, or as an acute blastic disease, which may display a B-lymphoid, T-lymphoid, or myeloid phenotype. Chronic phase MLNEo-TK may also subsequently progress to acute leukemias. Conventionally, chronic phase diseases have 0–19% bone marrow and blood blasts, while acute leukemic manifestations of MLNEo-TK are defined as either ≥20% bone marrow or blood myeloid or lymphoid blasts, or the presence of an extramedullary blastic infiltrate (myeloid sarcoma or lymphoblastic lymphoma).

Main updates from the revised 4th edition WHO classification

1. Recognition of any *JAK2* gene fusions, in addition to the most common *PCM1::JAK2* gene fusion recognized in the 4th edition WHO classification.[51]
2. Addition of *FLT3* and *ETV6::ABL1* fusions to this group of diseases.

Mastocytosis

Mastocytosis is a neoplasm of mast cells, characterized by infiltration of various tissue types by the clonal mast cell proliferation. In cutaneous mastocytosis (usually affecting children) the disease is limited to the skin, while in systemic mastocytosis (SM) there is by definition extracutaneous involvement, with the diagnosis most commonly made by identifying mast cell infiltrates in the bone marrow. Several subtypes of SM are recognized based on their clinical and morphologic features. An activating *KIT* mutation is typically seen in SM; however, it is not present in all cases. Additional mutations (other than *KIT*) characterize cases of advanced SM, particularly cases of SM with an associated myeloid neoplasm.

Main updates from the revised 4th edition WHO classification

1. The name of the SM subtype "SM with an associated hematological neoplasm" has been changed to "SM with an associated myeloid neoplasm" (SM-AMN), excluding from this category cases of nonmyeloid neoplasms that may occur together with SM but are not generally genetically related to the underlying SM.[52]
2. Updates have been made to the diagnostic criteria for mast cell leukemia, to allow for the presence of a suboptimal bone marrow aspirate that hampered the application of the prior diagnostic criteria; the subcategories of aleukemia versus leukemic mast cell leukemia have been eliminated.
3. A chronic form of mast cell leukemia is no longer recognized, since mast cell leukemia is now defined specifically as a proliferation of atypical immature mast cells.
4. The presence of any gene fusions defining MLNEo-TK entities found in the absence of a concomitant *KIT* mutation now excludes a diagnosis of SM, since many of the MLNEo-TK have an abnormal mast cell proliferation that might otherwise meet morphologic criteria for SM.

Myelodysplastic/myeloproliferative neoplasms

The MDS/MPN encompass clonal myeloid disorders characterized by overproduction of neutrophils, monocytes, or platelets together with ineffective hematopoiesis in one or more lineages, resulting in cytopenia(s).[53] These neoplasms are usually characterized by bone marrow hypercellularity, in most cases with a predominance of granulocytes; variable degrees of morphologic dysplasia are characteristic, but significant dysplasia may be absent in some cases. Mutations in epigenetic regulators such as *TET2* and *ASXL1* are common in MDS/MPN, and the spliceosome gene *SRSF2* is commonly mutated in chronic myelomonocytic leukemia (CMML). However, although the presence of mutation(s) (if at a VAF of at least 10%) can be used to establish clonality and have been incorporated into the diagnostic criteria for CMML, they are neither diagnostic nor specific for CMML or for MDS/MPN in general.[54] Combined mutations of *SF3B1* and *JAK2* (or much less commonly, *MPL* or *CALR*) are characteristic of the entity MDS/MPN with *SF3B1* mutation and thrombocytosis (MDS/MPN-SF3B1-T), while the mutation profiles of other MDS/MPN entities overlap significantly. Thus, the MDS/MPN entities are distinguished mainly by morphologic and clinical features, particularly blood counts at presentation.

Patterns of progression

Any of the MDS/MPN may progress to AML, defined as the presence of ≥20% bone marrow or blood blasts (including promonocytes as blast equivalents); in such cases, the AML is classified as for de novo AML with the diagnosis qualified as having progressed from prior MDS/MPN. Cases of CMML with 10% to 19% blasts in bone marrow (or the presence of Auer rods) are diagnosed as CMML-2. CMML may also undergo progression from myelodysplastic to the myeloproliferative subtype, often due to the acquisition of RAS-pathway mutations.[55] Progression of MDS-SF3B1 to MDS/MPN-SF3B1-T due to the acquisition of a *JAK2* V617V mutation has also been reported.[56] Unlike the MPN, a formal accelerated phase is not recognized in any of the MDS/MPN entities.

Main updates from the revised 4th edition WHO classification

1. The requirement for at least one cytopenia (in addition to a defining cytosis) has been added to the diagnostic criteria of all MDS/MPN, with the exception of rare cases of early CMML that may show borderline or no cytopenia.[57]
2. The threshold of monocytosis defining CMML has been lowered from 1.0×10^9/L to 0.5×10^9/L, with monocytes still required to comprise at least 10% of circulating white blood cells.[58,59] Although these new "oligomonocytic" CMML cases with ≥0.5-<1.0 $\times 10^9$/L monocytes generally have genetic profiles similar to those of "conventional" CMML with ≥1.0 x 10^9/L monocytes and likely represent an earlier phase of the disease,[60] the ICC applies more rigid criteria for their diagnosis: the presence of clonality documented by a cytogenetic abnormality and/or one or more somatic mutations in genes associated with myeloid neoplasia at VAF of ≥10% is required.
3. The prior category of CMML-0 (defined by <5% bone marrow and <2% blood blasts) has been eliminated and combined with CMML-1, given that recent large-scale studies have shown that such cases are biologically and prognostically similar to CMML-1 cases with ≥5%-<10% bone marrow or ≥2-<5% blood blasts.[61,62] Thus, there are now only two blast count tiers for CMML: CMML-1 and CMML-2.
4. The presence of an abnormal monocyte immunophenotype has been added as one of the diagnostic cocriteria to diagnose CMML for cases that lack documented evidence of clonality.[32]
5. Bone marrow morphologic findings have been incorporated into the diagnostic criteria for CMML as an absolute requirement, to exclude clonal monocytosis of undetermined significance (see later discussion), cases of AML that may present with a mature monocytosis, or other myeloid neoplasms that may show monocytosis.
6. The precursor lesion "clonal monocytosis of undetermined significance" (CMUS) has been added as a nonneoplastic counterpart to clonal monocytic proliferations that do not meet criteria for CMML or other myeloid neoplasms.[63,64]
7. The "*BCR-ABL1* negative" suffix has been removed from the name of atypical CML (aCML) given the well-established recognition that this entity, by definition, lacks *BCR::ABL1*.
8. Eosinophilia has been added as an exclusionary criterion for atypical CML (aCML). In the absence of defining genetic lesions of CML or MLNEo-TK, such cases would be classified as chronic eosinophilic leukemia, NOS (which may show significant dysplasia despite classification as a "pure MPN").[41]
9. MDS/MPN-SF3B1-T has been added as a new entity, encompassing most cases previously classified as "MDS/MPN with ring sideroblasts and thrombocytosis" (MDS/MPN-RS-T), since the vast majority of MDS/MPN-RS-T are associated with

SF3B1 mutation. "MDS/MPN with ring sideroblasts and thrombocytosis" is retained as a repository for the uncommon cases that have ≥15% ring sideroblasts but lack *SF3B1* mutation at a VAF of ≥10%.

10. The name of "MPN, unclassifiable" has been changed to "MDS/MPN, not otherwise specified" (MDS/MPN, NOS).
11. Cases of MDS/MPN, NOS (not fulfilling features of other MDS/MPN subtypes, MDS, or MPN) that exhibit an isolated isochromosome 17q abnormality are placed in a new provisional entity "MDS/MPN with isolated iso(17q)," since they appear to have distinct molecular features and worse prognosis compared with MDS/MPN, NOS.[65]
12. Because of its unique association with childhood and strong association with RAS pathway mutations, juvenile myelomonocytic leukemia has been moved out of the MDS/MPN category into a new category of pediatric myeloid neoplasms (discussed later).

Myelodysplastic syndromes and clonal cytopenias

MDSs are characterized by a proliferation of a neoplastic myeloid clone displaying morphologic dysplasia and ineffective hematopoiesis, resulting in peripheral blood cytopenias. In recent years, large-scale population studies and studies of patients coming to clinical attention due to cytopenia have revealed that clonal myeloid proliferations can occur in the absence of defining dysplasia, with an incidence that increases with age.[66,67] This general phenomenon has been termed clonal hematopoiesis, which encompasses several variants based on the presence or absence of cytopenias and other clinical associations. Although not strictly considered as myeloid neoplasms, these clonal hematopoiesis entities have been included in this classification, as they have variable propensity to progress to MDS and other myeloid neoplasms.[38,39,68] Moreover, some types of clonal hematopoiesis are associated with nonhematologic morbidities, such as cardiovascular disease and autoimmunity.[69]

Distinction between clonal hematopoiesis and MDS is diagnostically challenging, as it relies largely on the presence or absence of morphologic dysplasia in 10% of cells in at least one hematopoietic lineage, an arbitrary threshold that can be subjective and difficult to apply reproducibly in practice. Moreover, some recent studies have shown that clonal hematopoiesis displaying cytopenia and certain mutation profiles is similar to lower-risk MDS subtypes in terms of its clinical behavior and patient outcome.[70] At the other end of the MDS spectrum, the 20% blast threshold used to define AML in the 3rd, 4th, and revised 4th WHO classifications is also arbitrary, and many MDS cases with high blast counts show significant overlap in molecular features, responses to therapies, and patient outcomes when compared with patients presenting with overt AML.[71] For these reasons, the ICC has (1) maintained from the revised 4th edition classification many genetic features that define MDS in a cytopenic patient irrespective of dysplasia; (2) expanded the list of AML-defining genetic aberrations that allow a diagnosis of AML with a blast count of <20%; (3) introduced a new category of adult "MDS/AML," representing a transitional group between MDS and AML encompassing cases with 10% to 19% blasts that lack AML-defining genetics.

Based on a large amount of accumulating genetic evidence since the revised 4th edition WHO classification, the ICC has also introduced two new entities within MDS defined by two genetic features: mutations in *SF3B1* and *TP53*. These two gene mutations engender MDS subtypes with distinct prognoses and clinical features; although often associated with particular morphologies (ring sideroblasts with *SF3B1* and increase in blasts with *TP53*), these new genetic definitions create better-defined and more clinically relevant entities.[36,72]

Patterns of progression

MDS progression is determined by an increase in bone marrow and/or peripheral blood blasts beyond defined thresholds or presence of Auer rods, which remain the same as for the revised 4th edition WHO classification. Cases of lower-grade MDS that subsequently are found to have ≥5% bone marrow or ≥2% blood blasts (either with or without treatment) are diagnosed as having progressed to MDS with excess blasts (MDS-EB), and cases with lower-grade MDS or MDS-EB that develop 10% to 19% blasts in blood or bone marrow have progressed to MDS/AML. Rare cases of MDS may subsequently develop secondary, persistent proliferations of neutrophils, monocytes, or platelets that cross levels defining MDS/MPN. The ICC recommends that these cases not be reclassified as MDS/MPN, but rather retain designation as MDS, with the new proliferative features (sometimes accompanied by the acquisition of RAS-pathway or signaling mutations)[43] noted in the diagnostic report.

Main updates from the revised 4th edition WHO classification

1. "MDS with mutated *SF3B1*" has been added as a new entity, encompassing most cases previously

classified as "MDS with ring sideroblasts" (with or without multilineage dysplasia). Ring sideroblasts, although strongly associated with *SF3B1* mutation, are no longer used to define any specific MDS subtype. However, ring sideroblasts do represent a type of erythroid dysplasia and thus can be used to establish a primary diagnosis of MDS.

2. "MDS with mutated *TP53*" has been added as a new entity, encompassing cases between 0% and 9% blasts that have multihit mutations or mutation plus deletion of the *TP53* gene.
3. Cases lacking excess blasts that do not meet defining features for MDS with mutated *SF3B1*, MDS with mutated *TP53*, or MDS with del(5q) are now termed "MDS, NOS" and are further separated by the presence of single lineage or multilineage dysplasia, as in the revised 4th edition classification.
4. The prior category of "MDS, unclassifiable" (MDS-U) has been eliminated. Cases previously classified as MDS-U due to defining cytogenetic abnormalities are now classified as "MDS, NOS-without dysplasia," those with exactly 1% peripheral blasts remain within MDS, NOS (unless measured on two separate occasions, which now qualify for MDS-EB), and those with single lineage dysplasia and pancytopenia now remain within MDS, NOS with single lineage dysplasia. Severe cytopenias are already captured in risk stratification schemes such as the Revised International Scoring System (IPSS-R) and Molecular International Scoring System (IPSS-M) and thus do not need to impact the classification.[15,73]
5. A new entity "MDS/AML" has been created to encompass prior MDS with excess blast cases with 10% to 19% blasts in bone marrow or peripheral blood. Accordingly, there is now only a single category of MDS with excess blasts: cases with 5% to 9% bone marrow blasts, 2% to 9% blood blasts, or Auer rods. MDS/AML is considered an intermediate category between MDS and AML, including both patients who may be best treated as MDS and others who may be treated more effectively with intensive AML-type therapy. Further study is needed to determine which factors should determine treatment decisions for this group of patients on the MDS-AML spectrum, but these decisions are more likely to be impacted by genetic features of individual cases rather than an arbitrary numeric blast threshold.[71,74]

Pediatric myeloid neoplasms

MDS in children has features that differ from those of MDS in adults, including more frequent presentation with hypoplastic marrow, different mutation profiles, and more frequent association with underlying congenital bone marrow failure conditions. Thus, pediatric MDS is now formally separated from adult MDS in a new section of pediatric myeloid neoplasms. Most cases fall into the category of "refractory cytopenia of childhood" (RCC). RCC is now a full pediatric disease entity versus the provisional entity in the revised 4th edition WHO classification, given the accumulation of evidence supporting clearer diagnostic features. The adult MDS entities MDS with mutated *SF3B1* and MDS with del(5q) are exceedingly rare in children. Unlike in adult MDS, there is no MDS/AML entity in children (<18 years old): pediatric MDS with excess blasts is a single category encompassing cases with 5% to 19% bone marrow blasts, 2% to 19% blood blasts, or Auer rods.

As mentioned previously, juvenile myelomonocytic leukemia (JMML) has now been included within this category of pediatric myeloid neoplasms and has been removed from the MDS/MPN category. A diagnosis of JMML now requires the presence of a somatic RAS pathway mutation, with pediatric myeloid neoplasms resembling JMML but lacking such a mutation being classified as "JMML-like" neoplasms.

Acute myeloid leukemia

AML is an aggressive myeloid neoplasm characterized by impaired maturation of the neoplastic clone, resulting in an expansion of myeloid blasts in the bone marrow, peripheral blood, and/or extramedullary tissue. Importantly, any of the chronic myeloid neoplasm groups discussed earlier may manifest variable numbers of increased blasts, but the number is always <20%: by convention, any patient diagnosed with a chronic myeloid neoplasm is considered to have progressed to AML (or blastic phase, in the case of MPN) if blasts reach 20% or more in bone marrow or blood or if there is an extramedullary mass-forming proliferation of myeloid blasts (myeloid sarcoma). Several genetic lesions are strongly associated with impaired maturation and rapid accumulation of myeloblasts, and such genetic abnormalities are considered to be AML defining, even if myeloblasts are <20%. Historically, three cytogenetic findings—a t(8;21)(q22;q22.1) (*RUNX1::RUNXT1*), inv(16)(p13.1q22) or t(16;16)(p13.1;q22)(*CBFB::MYH11*), or *PML::RARA*—were considered to be sufficient to diagnose AML irrespective of the blast count. The ICC has expanded the list of such AML-defining genetic aberrations, as delineated later. The significance of recognizing certain genetic findings as AML defining is that these patients could be considered eligible for intensive AML-type therapy and may benefit from this approach earlier in the course of disease rather than waiting until the blast count reaches 20%.[71] This expansion in AML-defining genetic abnormalities enforces the concept that an arbitrary blast percentage may not capture cases that have an underlying AML-like genetic signature; recent evidence indicates that such cases behave similarly to bona fide AML cases and should be grouped together with them for the purposes of prognosis and therapeutic approach.[75-77] The ICC imposes a minimum 10% blast threshold for these AML-defining genetic aberrations in order to document some degree of maturation impairment; rare cases that present with an AML-defining genetic lesion and <10% blasts should be followed closely, and repeat biopsy and genetic testing may be warranted to clarify the diagnosis and dictate the optimal therapeutic approach in these instances. Within the group of AML with genetic aberrations, AML with *BCR::ABL1* represents a single exception by requiring ≥20% blasts. Myeloid neoplasms with *BCR::ABL1* that present de novo with 10% to 19% blasts are diagnosed as CML in accelerated phase.

The ICC has refined the prior WHO revised 4th edition group of AML with recurrent genetic abnormalities by adding several more recently recognized entities and has also divided the prior "AML with myelodysplasia-related changes" into several genetic categories, most notably with the addition of a new entity of AML with mutated *TP53*. While AML, NOS remains as a category, it is expected that this group will be smaller than the revised 4th edition AML, NOS group due to the recognition of these new genetic entities.[78] The ICC does not formally require that AML, NOS be subcategorized based on the blast immunophenotype or morphology. However, it is recommended to determine blast immunophenotypes for all AML cases and include this information in the diagnostic reports in order to better identify the neoplastic blasts after treatment and potential different sensitivities to therapies in cases with monocytic differentiation[79] (see Chapter 35). Specifically, megakaryoblastic and minimal differentiation AML subtypes may pose diagnostic challenges, and, in adults, pure erythroid leukemia almost always occurs as a morphologic/immunophenotypic subtype of AML with mutated *TP53*.

Main updates from the revised 4th edition WHO classification

1. Several new recurrent genetic abnormalities have been added, including alternate *KMT2A*, *RARA*, and *MECOM* rearrangements and rare abnormalities such as *NUP98* rearrangements; all of the recurrent genetic abnormalities (except for *BCR::ABL1*) are considered to be AML defining for any blood or bone marrow blast count of ≥10%.
2. The name of AML with biallelic *CEBPA* mutations has been changed to AML with in-frame bZIP *CEBPA* mutation, and this new entity requires at least one *CEBPA* mutation that involves the N-terminal bZIP domain and is not a frameshift mutation.[80,81]
3. The prior group of AML with myelodysplasia-related changes (AML-MRC) has been dissolved: most cases now fall into several new entities based on their genetic signatures, and there is no longer a specific AML subtype defined by dysplastic morphology affecting nonblast cells or history of MDS or MDS/MPN. These new entities are AML with myelodysplasia-related gene mutations, AML with myelodysplasia-related cytogenetic abnormalities, and AML with mutated *TP53*.
4. The AML, NOS category, which fails to exhibit any recurrent genetic abnormalities, MDS-related genetic abnormalities, or mutated *TP53*, no longer is formally subdivided into morphologic/immunophenotypic subtypes.
5. As discussed in the MDS section, a new category of MDS/AML has been created for cytopenic myeloid neoplasms with 10% to 19% blood or bone marrow blasts that lack AML-defining genetic aberrations.
6. Although many of the new genetic categories in the ICC tend to be mutually exclusive, there may occasionally be overlap; thus, the ICC has established a hierarchy of the categories to determine which category supersedes for classification purposes when multiple genetic lesions are present (Figure 2).

Blastic plasmacytoid dendritic cell neoplasm

Blastic plasmacytoid dendritic cell neoplasm (BPDCN) is a very rare hematologic malignancy characterized by a proliferation of immature blastic plasmacytoid dendritic cells. It represents a distinct myeloid neoplasm and is not part of any other myeloid neoplasm group, although it shares its blastic nature and aggressive natural history with the acute leukemias. There are no significant changes to the diagnostic criteria for BPDCN in the ICC compared with the prior revised 4th edition definition.

Acute leukemias of ambiguous lineage

This category of acute leukemias encompasses genetically diverse cases that either show commitment to

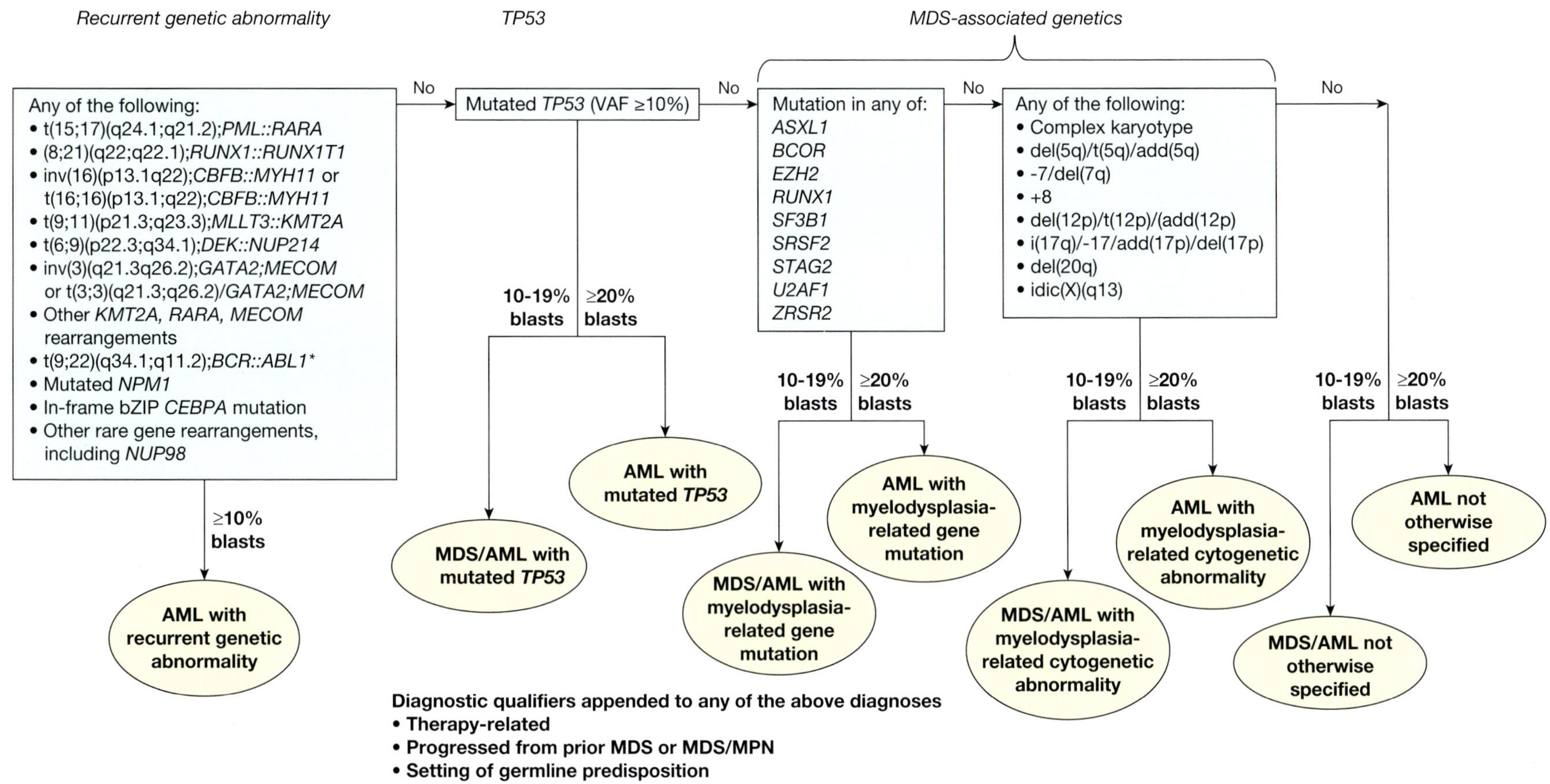

FIGURE 2 Hierarchy of AML and MDS/AML subtypes (≥10% blasts in blood or bone marrow) based on genetic features. *Requires at least 20% blasts in blood or bone marrow. AML, acute myeloid leukemia; MDS, myelodysplastic syndrome. (Adapted from Figure 1 Döhner H, Wei AH, Appelbaum FR, et al. Diagnosis and management of AML in adults: 2022 recommendations from an international expert panel on behalf of the ELN. *Blood*. 2022;140(12):1345-1377.

multiple lineages (myeloid and lymphoid, or T-cell and B-cell), termed mixed phenotype acute leukemias (MPAL), or fail to demonstrate commitment to any hematopoietic lineage, termed acute undifferentiated leukemia (AUL). The immunophenotypic markers defining each lineage remain unchanged from the revised 4th edition WHO; however, now it is noted that at least 5% of the blasts must show commitment to a lineage to diagnose MPAL.[27] MPAL continues to be divided into categories based on recurrent genetic features, including the prior MPAL with *BCR::ABL1* and MPAL with *KMT2A* rearrangement as well as new entities MPAL with *ZNF384* rearrangement and MPAL with *BCL11B* alteration. The ICC has also updated exclusionary features of MPAL or AUL that mandate classification as AML: acute leukemias with a mixed myeloid/lymphoid lineage and presence of myelodysplasia-related gene mutations or cytogenetic abnormalities, or *TP53* mutations are classified as AML, not MPAL.

Diagnostic qualifiers to myeloid neoplasm diagnoses

A general concept of the ICC is that myeloid neoplasms are classified based on their genetic features and morphology; accordingly, factors that reflect the disease history or genetic background are superimposed on this genetic-morphologic classification as disease *qualifiers*. Qualifiers that can be applied to myeloid neoplasms include therapy-relatedness, a background inherited germline predisposition, or (in the case of AML only) progression from an antecedent chronic myeloid neoplasm. This use of qualifiers differs from the prior 4th edition WHO classification, in which therapy-relatedness and progression from an antecedent myeloid neoplasm often superseded genetic features in assigning a disease group. A given myeloid neoplasm diagnosis in the ICC thus now includes the diagnosis according to the diagnostic criteria for de novo disease, followed by the relevant qualifier(s), if any.

As mentioned earlier, a *therapy-related* qualifier can be applied to any clonal cytopenia, AML, MDS, or MDS/MPN entity diagnosed in a patient exposed to prior cytotoxic chemotherapy and/or radiation therapy that exposed hematopoietic marrow. A *germline predisposition* qualifier can be applied to any clonal cytopenia or myeloid neoplasm occurring in a background of a germline mutation or syndrome that predisposes to the development of myeloid neoplasia or acute lymphoblastic leukemia. Additionally, any diagnosis of AML following a known diagnosis of MDS or MDS/MPN is classified as for de novo AML, but with the diagnosis qualified by having *progressed from the antecedent myeloid neoplasm*. An exception is made for acute leukemias progressing from any MPN, which are termed *blast phase* disease rather than AML. AML progressed from MDS or MDS/MPN usually shows MDS-related gene mutations and/or cytogenetic abnormalities, or *TP53* mutation, and typically maintains the same mutations as the prior MDS while often acquiring new RAS-pathway or signaling mutations.[82,83]

It should be noted that multiple qualifiers could be applied to a given case: for example, if a patient with germline *TP53* mutation (Li-Fraumeni syndrome) and a prior history of chemotherapy for lung cancer develops MDS and then progresses to AML with mutated *TP53*, the diagnosis in the ICC would be "AML with mutated *TP53*, therapy-related, progressed from MDS, in the setting of germline *TP53* mutation." Such a structured diagnosis fully expresses the disease ontogeny and provides the best guidance to optimize the clinical approach in this complex situation.

Key References

1. Swerdlow SH, Campo E, Harris NL, eds. WHO Classification of Tumours of Haematopoietic and Lymphoid Tissues (4th ed). IARC Press; 2008.
2. Swerdlow SH CE, Harris NL, Jaffe ES, eds. WHO Classification of Tumours of Haematopoietic and Lymphoid Tissues. (ed Revised 4th edition). International Agency for Research on Cancer; 2017.
3. Swerdlow SH, Campo E, Arber DA, et al. Response to "The WHO classification of haematolymphoid tumours" (Editorial). *Leukemia.* 2022;36(11):2748-2749.
4. Arber DA, Hasserjian RP, Orazi A, et al. Classification of myeloid neoplasms/acute leukemia: Global perspectives and the international consensus classification approach. *Am J Hematol.* 2022;97(5):514-518.
5. Arber DA, Orazi A, Hasserjian RP, et al. International consensus classification of myeloid neoplasms and acute leukemias: integrating morphologic, clinical, and genomic data. *Blood.* 2022;140(11):1200-1228.
6. Roman Diaz JL, Vazquez Martinez M, Khimani F. New approaches for the treatment of AML beyond the 7+3 regimen: current concepts and new approaches. *Cancers (Basel).* 2024;16(3):677.
7. Karel D, Valburg C, Woddor N, Nava VE, Aggarwal A. Myelodysplastic Neoplasms (MDS): the current and future treatment landscape. *Curr Oncol.* 2024;31(4):1971-1993.
8. Greenberg PL, Tuechler H, Schanz J, et al. Cytopenia levels for aiding establishment of the diagnosis of myelodysplastic syndromes. *Blood.* 2016;128(16):2096-2097.

9. Wong TN, Ramsingh G, Young AL, et al. Role of TP53 mutations in the origin and evolution of therapy-related acute myeloid leukaemia. *Nature.* 2015;518(7540):552-555.
10. Hsu JI, Dayaram T, Tovy A, et al. PPM1D mutations drive clonal hematopoiesis in response to cytotoxic chemotherapy. *Cell Stem Cell.* 2018;23(5):700-713.e6.
11. Bolton KL, Ptashkin RN, Gao T, et al. Cancer therapy shapes the fitness landscape of clonal hematopoiesis. *Nat Genet.* 2020;52(11):1219-1226.
12. Marmouset V, Decroocq J, Garciaz S, et al. Therapy-related myeloid neoplasms following PARP inhibitors: real-life experience. *Clin Cancer Res.* 2022;28(23):5211-5220.
13. Molenaar RJ, Sidana S, Radivoyevitch T, et al. Risk of hematologic malignancies after radioiodine treatment of well-differentiated thyroid cancer. *J Clin Oncol.* 2018;36(18):1831-1839.
14. Shih AJ, Jun T, Skol AD, et al. Inherited cancer predisposing mutations in patients with therapy-related myeloid neoplasms. *Br J Haematol.* 2023;200(4):489-493.
15. Bernard E, Tuechler H, Greenberg PL, Hasserjian RP, Arango JE, et al. Molecular international prognostic scoring system for myelodysplastic syndromes. *N Engl J Med Evid.* 2022;1(7):EVIDoa2200008.
16. Bernard E, Hasserjian RP, Greenberg PL, et al. Molecular taxonomy of myelodysplastic syndromes and its clinical implications. *Blood.* 2024;2024:blood.2023023727.
17. Kuendgen A, Nomdedeu M, Tuechler H, et al. Therapy-related myelodysplastic syndromes deserve specific diagnostic sub-classification and risk-stratification-an approach to classification of patients with t-MDS. *Leukemia.* 2021;35(3):835-849.
18. Granfeldt Østgård L S, Medeiros BC, Sengelov H, et al. Epidemiology and clinical significance of secondary and therapy-related acute myeloid leukemia: a National Population-Based Cohort Study. *J Clin Oncol.* 2015;33(31):3641-3649.
19. Lee SH, Erber WN, Porwit A, Tomonaga M, Peterson LC; International Council for Standardization In Hematology. ICSH guidelines for the standardization of bone marrow specimens and reports. *Int J Lab Hematol.* 2008;30(5):349-364.
20. D'Abbronzo G, D'Antonio A, De Chiara A, et al. Development of an artificial-intelligence-based tool for automated assessment of cellularity in bone marrow biopsies in Ph-negative myeloproliferative neoplasms. *Cancers (Basel).* 2024;16(9):1687.
21. Bruck OE, Lallukka-Bruck SE, Hohtari HR, et al. Machine learning of bone marrow histopathology identifies genetic and clinical determinants in patients with MDS. *Blood Cancer Discov.* 2021;2(3):238-249.
22. Sirinukunwattana K, Aberdeen A, Theissen H, et al. Artificial intelligence-based morphological fingerprinting of megakaryocytes: a new tool for assessing disease in MPN patients. *Blood Adv.* 2020;4(14):3284-3294.
23. Chen X, Fromm JR, Naresh KN. "Blasts" in myeloid neoplasms - how do we define blasts and how do we incorporate them into diagnostic schema moving forward? *Leukemia.* 2022;36(2):327-332.
24. Mufti GJ, Bennett JM, Goasguen J, et al. Diagnosis and classification of myelodysplastic syndrome: International Working Group on Morphology of myelodysplastic syndrome (IWGM-MDS) consensus proposals for the definition and enumeration of myeloblasts and ring sideroblasts. *Haematologica.* 2008;93(11):1712-1717.
25. Goasguen JE, Bennett JM, Bain BJ, et al. Morphological evaluation of monocytes and their precursors. *Haematologica.* 2009;94(7):994-997.
26. Foucar K, Hsi ED, Wang SA, et al. Concordance among hematopathologists in classifying blasts plus promonocytes: a bone marrow pathology group study. *Int J Lab Hematol.* 2020;42(4):418-422.
27. Weinberg OK, Arber DA, Dohner H, et al. The International Consensus Classification of acute leukemias of ambiguous lineage. *Blood.* 2023;141(18):2275-2277.
28. Kvasnicka HM, Beham-Schmid C, Bob R, et al. Problems and pitfalls in grading of bone marrow fibrosis, collagen deposition and osteosclerosis - a consensus-based study. *Histopathology.* 2016;68(6):905-915.
29. Thiele J, Kvasnicka HM, Facchetti F, Franco V, van der Walt J, Orazi A. European consensus on grading bone marrow fibrosis and assessment of cellularity. *Haematologica.* 2005;90(8):1128-1132.
30. Heuser M, Freeman SD, Ossenkoppele GJ, et al. 2021 Update on MRD in acute myeloid leukemia: a consensus document from the European LeukemiaNet MRD Working Party. *Blood.* 2021;138(26):2753-2767.
31. van de Loosdrecht AA, Kern W, Porwit A, et al. Clinical application of flow cytometry in patients with unexplained cytopenia and suspected myelodysplastic syndrome: A report of the European LeukemiaNet International MDS-Flow Cytometry Working Group. *Cytometry B Clin Cytom.* 2023;104(1):77-86.
32. Selimoglu-Buet D, Wagner-Ballon O, Saada V, et al. Characteristic repartition of monocyte subsets as a diagnostic signature of chronic myelomonocytic leukemia. *Blood.* 2015;125(23):3618-3626.
33. Duncavage EJ, Bagg A, Hasserjian RP, et al. Genomic profiling for clinical decision making in myeloid neoplasms and acute leukemia. *Blood.* 2022;140(21):2228-2247.
34. Duncavage EJ, Schroeder MC, O'Laughlin M, et al. Genome sequencing as an alternative to cytogenetic analysis in myeloid cancers. *N Engl J Med.* 2021;384(10):924-935.
35. Akkari YMN, Baughn LB, Dubuc AM, et al. Guiding the global evolution of cytogenetic testing for hematologic malignancies. *Blood.* 2022;139(15):2273-2284.
36. Bernard E, Nannya Y, Hasserjian RP, et al. Implications of TP53 allelic state for genome stability,

clinical presentation and outcomes in myelodysplastic syndromes. *Nat Med*. 2020;26(10):1549-1556.

37. Paietta E, Roberts KG, Wang V, et al. Molecular classification improves risk assessment in adult BCR-ABL1-negative B-ALL. *Blood*. 2021;138(11):948-958.
38. Weeks LD, Niroula A, Neuberg D, et al. Prediction of risk for myeloid malignancy in clonal hematopoiesis. *NEJM Evidence*. 2023;2(5):EVIDoa2200310.
39. Cargo C, Bernard E, Beinortas T, et al. Predicting cytopenias, progression, and survival in patients with clonal cytopenia of undetermined significance: a prospective cohort study. *Lancet Haematol*. 2024;11(1):e51-e61.
40. Jovanovic JV, Ivey A, Vannucchi AM, et al. Establishing optimal quantitative-polymerase chain reaction assays for routine diagnosis and tracking of minimal residual disease in JAK2-V617F-associated myeloproliferative neoplasms: a joint European LeukemiaNet/MPN&MPN-EuroNet (COST action BM0902) study. *Leukemia*. 2013;27(10):2032-2039.
41. Wang SA, Hasserjian RP, Tam W, et al. Bone marrow morphology is a strong discriminator between chronic eosinophilic leukemia, not otherwise specified and reactive idiopathic hypereosinophilic syndrome. *Haematologica*. 2017;102(8):1352-1360.
42. Reiter A, Gotlib J. Myeloid neoplasms with eosinophilia. *Blood*. 2017;129(6):704-714.
43. Faria C, Tzankov A. Progression in Myeloid Neoplasms: Beyond the Myeloblast. *Pathobiology*. 2024;91(1):55-75.
44. Barraco D, Elala YC, Lasho TL, et al. Molecular correlates of anemia in primary myelofibrosis: a significant and independent association with U2AF1 mutations. *Blood Cancer J*. 2016;6(5):e416.
45. Boiocchi L, Hasserjian RP, Pozdnyakova O, et al. Clinicopathological and molecular features of SF3B1-mutated myeloproliferative neoplasms. *Hum Pathol*. 2019;86:1-11.
46. Jeryczynski G, Thiele J, Gisslinger B, et al. Pre-fibrotic/early primary myelofibrosis vs. WHO-defined essential thrombocythemia: the impact of minor clinical diagnostic criteria on the outcome of the disease. *Am J Hematol*. 2017;92(9):885-891.
47. Gisslinger H, Jeryczynski G, Gisslinger B, et al. Clinical impact of bone marrow morphology for the diagnosis of essential thrombocythemia: comparison between the BCSH and the WHO criteria. *Leukemia*. 2017;31(3):774-775.
48. Yao J, Xu L, Aypar U, et al. Myeloid/lymphoid neoplasms with eosinophilia/basophilia and ETV6-ABL1 fusion: cell-of-origin and response to tyrosine kinase inhibition. *Haematologica*. 2021;106(2):614-618.
49. Tasian SK, Loh ML, Hunger SP. Philadelphia chromosome-like acute lymphoblastic leukemia. *Blood*. 2017;130(19):2064-2072.
50. Saft L, Kvasnicka HM, Boudova L, Gianelli U, Lazzi S, Rozman M. Myeloid/lymphoid neoplasms with eosinophilia and tyrosine kinase fusion genes: a workshop report with focus on novel entities and a literature review including paediatric cases. *Histopathology*. 2023;83(6):829-849.
51. Bain BJ, Ahmad S. Should myeloid and lymphoid neoplasms with PCM1-JAK2 and other rearrangements of JAK2 be recognized as specific entities? *Br J Haematol*. 2014;166(6):809-817.
52. Wang SA, Hutchinson L, Tang G, et al. Systemic mastocytosis with associated clonal hematological non-mast cell lineage disease: clinical significance and comparison of chomosomal abnormalities in SM and AHNMD components. *Am J Hematol*. 2013;88(3):219-224.
53. Orazi A, Germing U. The myelodysplastic/myeloproliferative neoplasms: myeloproliferative diseases with dysplastic features. *Leukemia*. 2008;22(7):1308-1319.
54. Mughal TI, Cross NC, Padron E, et al. An International MDS/MPN Working Group's perspective and recommendations on molecular pathogenesis, diagnosis and clinical characterization of myelodysplastic/myeloproliferative neoplasms. *Haematologica*. 2015;100(9):1117-1130.
55. Ricci C, Fermo E, Corti S, et al. RAS mutations contribute to evolution of chronic myelomonocytic leukemia to the proliferative variant. *Clin Cancer Res*. 2010;16(8):2246-2256.
56. Malcovati L, Cazzola M. Refractory anemia with ring sideroblasts. *Best Pract Res Clin Haematol*. 2013;26(4):377-385.
57. Cargo C, Cullen M, Taylor J, et al. The use of targeted sequencing and flow cytometry to identify patients with a clinically significant monocytosis. *Blood*. 2019;133(12):1325-1334.
58. Geyer JT, Tam W, Liu YC, et al. Oligomonocytic chronic myelomonocytic leukemia (chronic myelomonocytic leukemia without absolute monocytosis) displays a similar clinicopathologic and mutational profile to classical chronic myelomonocytic leukemia. *Mod Pathol*. 2017;30(9):1213-1222.
59. Calvo X, Garcia-Gisbert N, Parraga I, et al. Oligomonocytic and overt chronic myelomonocytic leukemia show similar clinical, genomic, and immunophenotypic features. *Blood Adv*. 2020;4(20):5285-5296.
60. Calvo X, Roman-Bravo D, Garcia-Gisbert N, et al. Outcomes and molecular profile of oligomonocytic CMML support its consideration as the first stage in the CMML continuum. *Blood Adv*. 2022;6(13):3921-3931.
61. Xicoy B, Triguero A, Such E, et al. The division of chronic myelomonocytic leukemia (CMML)-1 into CMML-0 and CMML-1 according to 2016 World Health Organization (WHO) classification has no impact in outcome in a large series of patients from the Spanish group of MDS. *Leuk Res*. 2018;70:34-36.

62. Loghavi S, Sui D, Wei P, et al. Validation of the 2017 revision of the WHO chronic myelomonocytic leukemia categories. *Blood Adv.* 2018;2(15):1807-1816.

63. Valent P. Oligo-monocytic CMML and other pre-CMML states: clinical impact, prognostication and management. *Best Pract Res Clin Haematol.* 2020;33(2):101137.

64. Valent P, Orazi A, Savona MR, et al. Proposed diagnostic criteria for classical chronic myelomonocytic leukemia (CMML), CMML variants and pre-CMML conditions. *Haematologica.* 2019;104(10):1935-1949.

65. Kanagal-Shamanna R, Orazi A, Hasserjian RP, et al. Myelodysplastic/myeloproliferative neoplasms-unclassifiable with isolated isochromosome 17q represents a distinct clinico-biologic subset: a multi-institutional collaborative study from the Bone Marrow Pathology Group. *Mod Pathol.* 2022;35(4):470-479.

66. Valent P, Orazi A, Steensma DP, et al. Proposed minimal diagnostic criteria for myelodysplastic syndromes (MDS) and potential pre-MDS conditions. *Oncotarget.* 2017;8(43):73483-73500.

67. Steensma DP, Bejar R, Jaiswal S, et al. Clonal hematopoiesis of indeterminate potential and its distinction from myelodysplastic syndromes. *Blood.* 2015;126(1):9-16.

68. Cargo CA, Rowbotham N, Evans PA, et al. Targeted sequencing identifies patients with preclinical MDS at high risk of disease progression. *Blood.* 2015;126(21):2362-2365.

69. Jaiswal S, Natarajan P, Silver AJ, et al. Clonal hematopoiesis and risk of atherosclerotic cardiovascular disease. *N Engl J Med.* 2017;377(2):111-121.

70. Malcovati L, Galli A, Travaglino E, et al. Clinical significance of somatic mutation in unexplained blood cytopenia. *Blood.* 2017;129(25):3371-3378.

71. Estey E, Hasserjian RP, Dohner H. Distinguishing AML from MDS: a fixed blast percentage may no longer be optimal. *Blood.* 2022;139(3):323-332.

72. Malcovati L, Stevenson K, Papaemmanuil E, et al. SF3B1-mutant MDS as a distinct disease subtype: a proposal from the International Working Group for the Prognosis of MDS. *Blood.* 2020;136(2):157-170.

73. Greenberg PL, Tuechler H, Schanz J, et al. Revised international prognostic scoring system for myelodysplastic syndromes. *Blood.* 2012;120(12):2454-2465.

74. DiNardo CD, Garcia-Manero G, Kantarjian HM. Time to blur the blast boundaries. *Cancer.* 2022;128(8):1568-1570.

75. Montalban-Bravo G, Kanagal-Shamanna R, Sasaki K, et al. NPM1 mutations define a specific subgroup of MDS and MDS/MPN patients with favorable outcomes with intensive chemotherapy. *Blood Adv.* 2019;3(6):922-933.

76. Falini B, Martelli MP, Brunetti L, Gjertsen BT, Andresen V. The NPM1 mutant defines AML irrespective of blast count. *Am J Hematol.* 2023;98(7):E187-E189.

77. Siddiqui M, Konoplev S, Issa G, et al. Biologic features and clinical outcomes in newly diagnosed myelodysplastic syndrome with KMT2A rearrangements. *Am J Hematol.* 2023;98(4):E91-E94.

78. Huber S, Baer C, Hutter S, et al. AML classification in the year 2023: How to avoid a Babylonian confusion of languages. *Leukemia.* 2023;37(7):1413-1420.

79. Garciaz S, Hospital MA, Collette Y, Vey N. Venetoclax resistance in acute myeloid leukemia. *Cancers (Basel).* 2024;16(6):1091.

80. Zhao D, Zhou Q, Zarif M, et al. AML with CEBPA mutations: a comparison of ICC and WHO-HAEM5 criteria in patients with 20% or more blasts. *Leuk Res.* 2023;134:107376.

81. Taube F, Georgi JA, Kramer M, et al. CEBPA mutations in 4708 patients with acute myeloid leukemia: differential impact of bZIP and TAD mutations on outcome. *Blood.* 2022;139(1):87-103.

82. Guess T, Potts CR, Bhat P, et al. Distinct patterns of clonal evolution drive myelodysplastic syndrome progression to secondary acute myeloid leukemia. *Blood Cancer Discov.* 2022;3(4):316-329.

83. Menssen AJ, Khanna A, Miller CA, et al. Convergent clonal evolution of signaling gene mutations is a hallmark of myelodysplastic syndrome progression. *Blood Cancer Discov.* 2022;3(4):330-345.

SECTION 1

Myeloproliferative Neoplasms

Chapter 1
Chronic Myeloid Leukemia

Hans Michael Kvasnicka, Carlos E. Bueso-Ramos, Attilio Orazi, Annette Schmitt-Graeff, and Ayalew Tefferi

Definition

Chronic myeloid leukemia (CML) is caused by the chromosomal translocation (9;22)(q34.1;q11.2) resulting in the formation of the Philadelphia (Ph) chromosome containing the *BCR::ABL1* fusion gene.[1] The resulting *BCR::ABL1* oncoprotein is a constitutively active tyrosine kinase that activates multiple signaling pathways that collectively lead to malignant transformation.[1] Granulocytes are the major proliferative component, but all myeloid lineages and some lymphoid and endothelial cells carry the abnormal gene.[2] The natural history of untreated CML is biphasic or triphasic: an initial chronic phase (CML-CP) is followed by an accelerated phase (CML-AP) and a blast phase (CML-BP).[3,4] Importantly, progression to blast phase can occur directly from CML-CP without a prior CML-AP.

Diagnosis of CML requires detection of the Ph chromosome or the *BCR::ABL1* fusion gene in an appropriate clinical and laboratory setting.[5] A complete blood count with leukocyte differential and bone marrow examination are required to obtain material for a complete karyotype and morphologic evaluation to assess disease phase.[6] Bone marrow biopsy is particularly valuable in patients suspected of disease progression and is always necessary to evaluate for the presence and extent of bone marrow fibrosis.[7] Karyotype analysis of bone marrow cells is indicated to confirm the diagnosis of CML.[5] At least 20 metaphase spreads should be analyzed. More than 95% of patients with CML carry the Ph chromosome, but in about 3% to 5% of patients the Ph chromosome is part of complex translocations involving additional chromosomes. Rarely, a silent Ph occurs that cannot be identified by classical karyotyping and requires molecular testing to establish the diagnosis. In addition, quantitative reverse transcriptase polymerase chain reaction for baseline measurement of *BCR::ABL1* transcripts is necessary for disease monitoring.[5,6]

Epidemiology

The annual incidence of CML is 1.0 to 1.5/10^5 with no significant racial or geographic differences[8] and accounts for approximately 15% of newly diagnosed adult leukemia cases.[9] Patients treated with modern therapies that block the tyrosine kinase activity of *BCR::ABL1* have a life expectancy close to that of age-matched controls.[10] As a result, the prevalence of CML is increasing and it is predicted to become the most common myeloid neoplasm.[11,12] The only well-documented risk factor for the development of CML is ionizing radiation.[13]

General Clinical Features

Patients with CML may present with constitutional symptoms including fatigue, weight loss, and night sweats. Splenomegaly is common, while hepatomegaly may be present and, like splenomegaly, reflects extramedullary hematopoiesis.[6] Significant lymphadenopathy is uncommon, and if present, a lymph node biopsy should be considered to exclude blast transformation.[14] The median age at diagnosis is 65 years, but CML can occur at any age, including childhood.[8,15-17] There is a slight male predominance. More than 50% of newly diagnosed patients are asymptomatic and diagnosed in the setting of a persistent unexplained leukocytosis.[17] The diagnosis is established by the characteristic Ph chromosome t(9;22)(q34;q11), assessed either by routine cytogenetics or the detection of a *BCR::ABL1* abnormality by fluorescence in situ hybridization or molecular studies.[6,17] Most patients are diagnosed in CMP-CP, but about 5% of patients initially present with CML-AP or CML-BP without previously recognized chronic phase.[8] Bone marrow examination is required to obtain material for karyotype and morphologic evaluation to assess disease phase.[5,6]

Without effective therapy patients progress with gradual but persistent deterioration in hematologic parameters. Disease progression is invariably associated with additional genetic abnormalities.[6] Recognition of progressive disease is important, but the clinical and morphologic boundaries between CML-CP, CML-AP, and CML-BP are not sharp, and the parameters to define these phases vary among different guidelines.[18-21] However, recent data suggest that among patients with CML-CP who have evolved into CML-AP, the definition of the latter retains critical importance in evaluating the response to tyrosine kinase inhibitor (TKI)-based treatments or novel therapies, as well as for monitoring patients, including consideration of allogeneic stem cell transplantation.[22]

Morphology

Chronic phase, CML-CP

Peripheral blood in CML-CP typically shows neutrophilic leukocytosis (Figure 1.1), with the majority of cells in the mature neutrophil and myelocyte stages (the latter has been referred to as "myelocyte bulge"). Cellular function is mostly normal, and patients with CML-CP are not at increased risk of infection or bleeding (Table 1.1). Significant dysplasia is absent, and blasts usually account for less than 2% of white blood cells.[8] Absolute basophilia is a typical finding and mildly elevated eosinophils may be present, but significant eosinophilia raises the question of an alternative diagnosis. The absolute monocyte count may

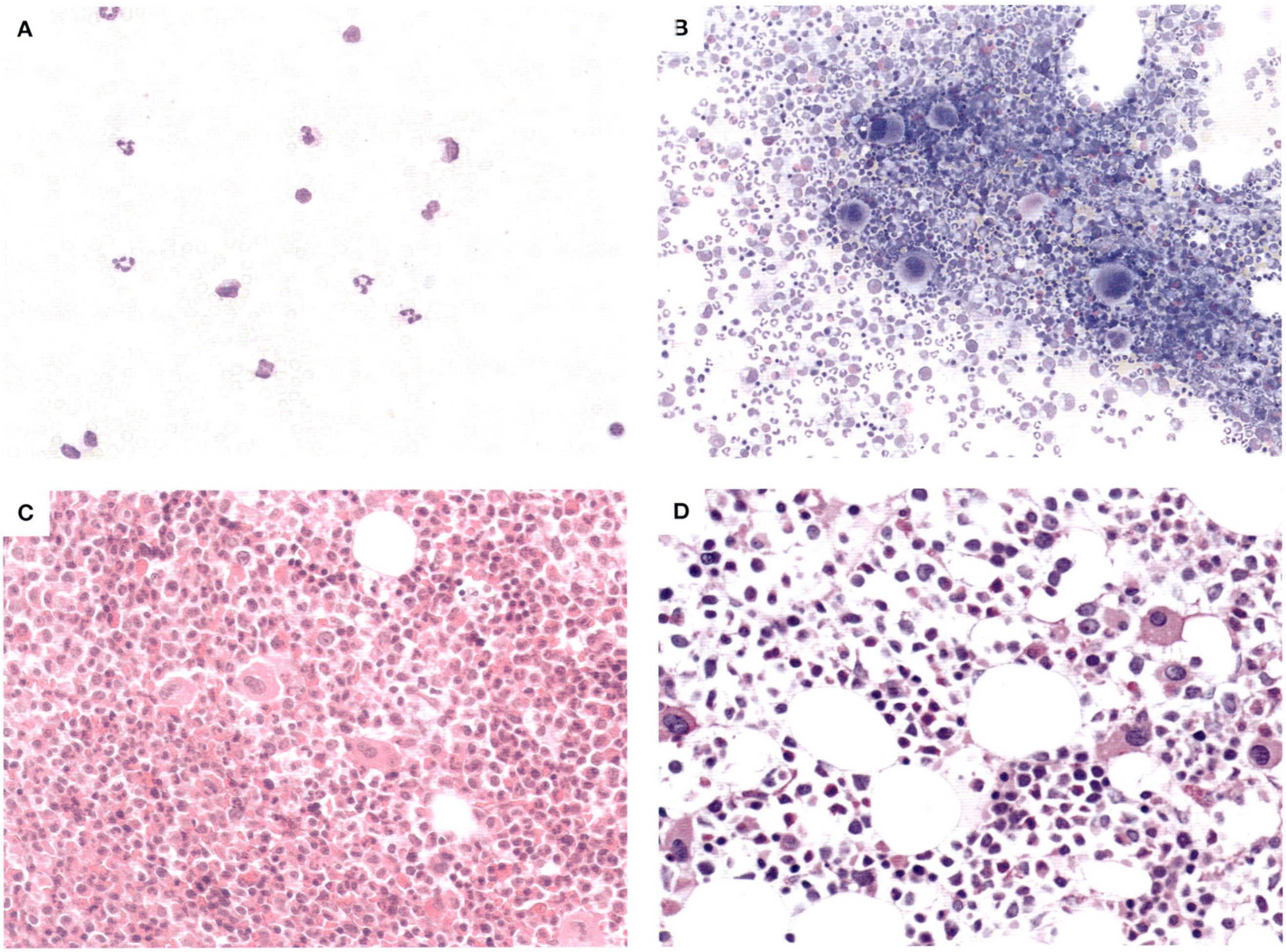

FIGURE 1.1 Chronic myeloid leukemia, chronic phase (CML-CP). **A:** Peripheral blood smear with marked leukocytosis showing a spectrum of neutrophil maturation, including a prominence of myelocytes and segmented neutrophils. **B:** Hypercellular bone marrow aspirate with granulocytic proliferation and increased numbers of megakaryocytes, many of which are "dwarf" megakaryocytes. **C:** The trephine core biopsy illustrates the significant shift of myeloid/erythroid ratio; increased numbers of eosinophils; small, dwarf megakaryocytes with hypolobated nuclei. **D:** CML-CP with the p190-*BCR::ABL1* isoform reveals small megakaryocytes with dysplastic, small rounded nuclei. In the background Gaucher-like cells with foamy and striated cytoplasm can be seen. (**A** and **B:** Wright-Giemsa; **C** and **D:** hematoxylin and eosin; **A** and **B:** 60×; **C** and **D:** 40×).

TABLE 1.1 Diagnostic features of chronic phase chronic myeloid leukemia

Peripheral blood
• Leukocytosis • Platelets normal or increased • Anemia often present • Spectrum of maturing granulocytes with a "myelocyte bulge" • Blasts usually <2% of white blood cells • Absolute basophilia • No significant dysplasia
Bone marrow morphology
• Hypercellularity with increased myeloid/erythroid ratio • Pronounced layer of immature granulocytes around bone trabeculae • Blasts usually <5%, always <10% • Megakaryocytes normal or increased in number, but with hypolobated nuclei ("dwarf" morphology) • Reticulin fibers normal (MF-0) or minimally increased (MF-1)
Genetics
• *BCR::ABL1* fusion gene (or Philadelphia chromosome)

be elevated (>1 × 10^9/L), but the percentage of monocytes is usually less than 3%.[6,8,17] Anemia is common, but hemoglobin levels below 10 g/dL at initial presentation are rare. The platelet count is mildly or moderately elevated, but in about 10% of cases marked thrombocytosis (>1000 × 10^9/L) is seen, suggesting another diagnosis. These cases have a normal or only slightly elevated white blood count and may mimic other subtypes of myeloproliferative neoplasms such as essential thrombocythemia.[23] In addition, leukocytosis composed almost exclusively of segmented neutrophils may resemble chronic neutrophilic leukemia (CNL)[24] and cases with absolute monocytosis may resemble chronic myelomonocytic leukemia (CMML).[25] These unusual presentations of CML often correlate with variations in the size of the *BCR::ABL1* fusion protein due to different breakpoints within the BCR gene.[26]

In CML-CP, the bone marrow is almost always hypercellular (Figure 1.1) with marked granulocytic proliferation and expansion of the myelocytic and segmented neutrophilic stages.[27-31] There is no significant dysplasia.[32] Blasts typically account for less than 5% of the bone marrow cells,[27-30] while 10% or more immature cells indicate progression to CML-AP (Table 1.2).[19] An expansion of myelocytes is typically seen. Eosinophils and basophils are usually increased while erythroid precursors are reduced. Histiocytes resembling Gaucher cells or "sea-blue" histiocytes (Figure 1.1) are often observed and are

TABLE 1.2 Diagnostic criteria for accelerated phase and blast phase chronic myeloid leukemia

Accelerated phase
• Bone marrow or peripheral blood blasts 10%-19% • Peripheral blood basophils ≥20% • Presence of additional clonal cytogenetic abnormality in Philadelphia chromosome+ cells[a]
Blast phase
• Bone marrow or peripheral blood myeloid blasts ≥20% • Myeloid sarcoma[b] • Bone marrow or peripheral blood lymphoid blasts ≥5% is consistent with lymphoblastic crisis[c]

[a]Second Philadelphia chromosome, trisomy 8, isochromosome 17q, trisomy 19, complex karyotype ≥3 cytogenetic abnormalities, or abnormalities of 3q26.2.
[b]Extramedullary blast proliferation, for lesions showing a diffuse (non–mass forming) blast proliferation.
[c]Immunophenotypic analysis is required to confirm lymphoid lineage.

attributed to an increased cellular burden and turnover.[29] The frequency of megakaryocytes may be normal or decreased, but nearly 50% of cases show moderate to marked megakaryocytic proliferation.[30] In most cases, the megakaryocytes are rather small and have hypolobated nuclei (ie, "dwarf megakaryocytes"), but they differ from the "micromegakaryocytes" seen in myelodysplastic syndromes.[29,30] The finding of significant numbers of myelodysplasia-like micromegakaryocytes should raise concern for disease progression.[29,30]

Bone marrow biopsy sections (Figure 1.1) show in chronic phase an increased number of immature granulocytes often layered along the bony trabeculae (usually 5-10 cells in thickness) with progressive granulocytic maturation toward the center of the intertrabecular spaces.[30] A minimal number of blasts may be seen immediately adjacent to the bone and/or scattered among the maturing cells, but clusters of immature cells are not present in CML-CP, although aggregates of myelocytes may be observed. Minimal (MF-1) to marked reticulin fibrosis (MF-2) is seen in 30% to 40% of cases at diagnosis[29] and may be accompanied by increased numbers of megakaryocytes and splenomegaly (Figure 1.2).[27]

Accelerated phase, CML-AP

While the diagnosis of CML is mainly based on the detection of the *BCR::ABL1* rearrangement, the clinical and morphologic boundaries between CML-CP and CML-AP are not sharp, and the parameters used to define this transition phase vary between different guidelines.[18,19,21,33] Furthermore, the gene expression profiles of CML-AP and CML-BP are similar, with

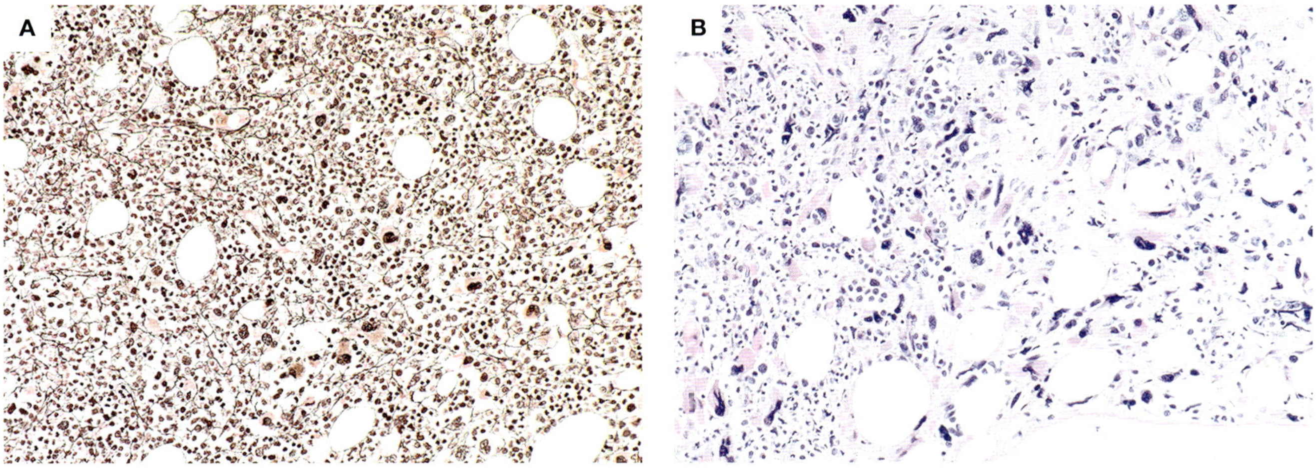

FIGURE 1.2 Chronic myeloid leukemia, chronic phase (CML-CP). **A:** Hypercellular bone marrow trephine with minimal reticulin fibrosis (grade MF-1) and increased numbers of small, atypical megakaryocytes. **B:** Overt bone marrow fibrosis (grade MF-3) at CML diagnosis mimicking other myeloproliferative neoplasm subtypes, small grossly atypical megakaryocytes. (**A** and **B:** hematoxylin and eosin; **A** and **B:** 40×).

changes in the expression profile occurring late in CML-CP or early in CML-AP before clinical or morphologic evidence of overt progression.[14] However, as recent data highlight, accurate detection of disease progression remains important because patients with CML-AP who progress from CML-CP have a worse overall prognosis, even in the era of modern TKI therapy.[22] These patients need to be identified by easy-to-use criteria in order to be referred to investigational trials offering alternative therapies, including consideration of allogeneic stem cell transplantation.[21] In addition, 20% to 30% of patients receiving TKI therapy have apparent disease progression due to acquired mutations in *BCR::ABL1* that affect the tyrosine kinase–binding domain and render the TKI ineffective.[5,34] Less commonly, subclones of leukemic cells with amplification of *BCR::ABL1* or mutations in the SH3-SH2 domain lead to disease progression, or there may be genetic alterations that occur in *BCR::ABL1*-independent signaling pathways.[34,35]

CML-AP (Table 1.2) is defined by 10% to 19% bone marrow or peripheral blood blasts, peripheral blood basophilia ≥20%, or the identification of additional clonal cytogenetic abnormalities in Ph+ cells, ie, second Ph, trisomy 8, isochromosome 17q, trisomy 19, complex karyotype, or abnormalities of 3q26.2.[19] Previous criteria for AP such as therapy-unrelated thrombocytopenia (≤100 × 10^9/L) or therapy-unresponsive thrombocytosis (>1000 × 10^9/L) and/or splenomegaly have been discarded,[33] and failure to achieve a complete hematologic response or resistance to sequential TKIs or the occurrence of >2 mutations on *BCR::ABL1* during treatment have also been eliminated in the definition of CML-AP.

Bone marrow specimens of patients with CML-AP show variable cellularity, and there may be dysplastic features in the granulocytic and other myeloid lineages.[30,32] An increase in myeloid lineage blasts (10% to 19%) may be appreciated on aspirate smears or in biopsy sections, in which they can be highlighted with immunohistochemical stains for CD34 (Figure 1.3). Large clusters of megakaryocytes are sometimes seen, including true myelodysplasia-like micromegakaryocytes, often associated with significant reticulin or collagen fibrosis.[30] The presence of lymphoblast in the blood or bone marrow (confirmed by flow cytometry) should raise concern for an impending lymphoblastic crisis (Figure 1.3), as lymphoblastic CML-BP is reported to sometimes have an abrupt onset and usually lacks a preceding CML-AP.[20,36,37]

Blast phase, CML-BP

CML-BP is characterized by 20% or more myeloid blasts or extramedullary proliferation of blasts that disrupts the architecture of the infiltrated tissue, ie, extramedullary myeloid sarcoma (Table 1.2). Importantly, the presence of ≥5% lymphoid blasts in peripheral blood or bone marrow defines lymphoblastic crisis and should prompt further laboratory and genetic studies.[38,39] Of note, other classification and risk stratification systems, including the International Blood and Marrow Transplant Registry, MD Anderson Cancer Center, and the European LeukemiaNet, have defined a higher blast threshold of more than 30% for CML-BP and are often used as eligibility criteria in clinical trials.[5,6,40] In addition, if blasts occupy focal but significant areas of the marrow, such as an entire intertrabecular bone marrow biopsy space, a presumptive diagnosis

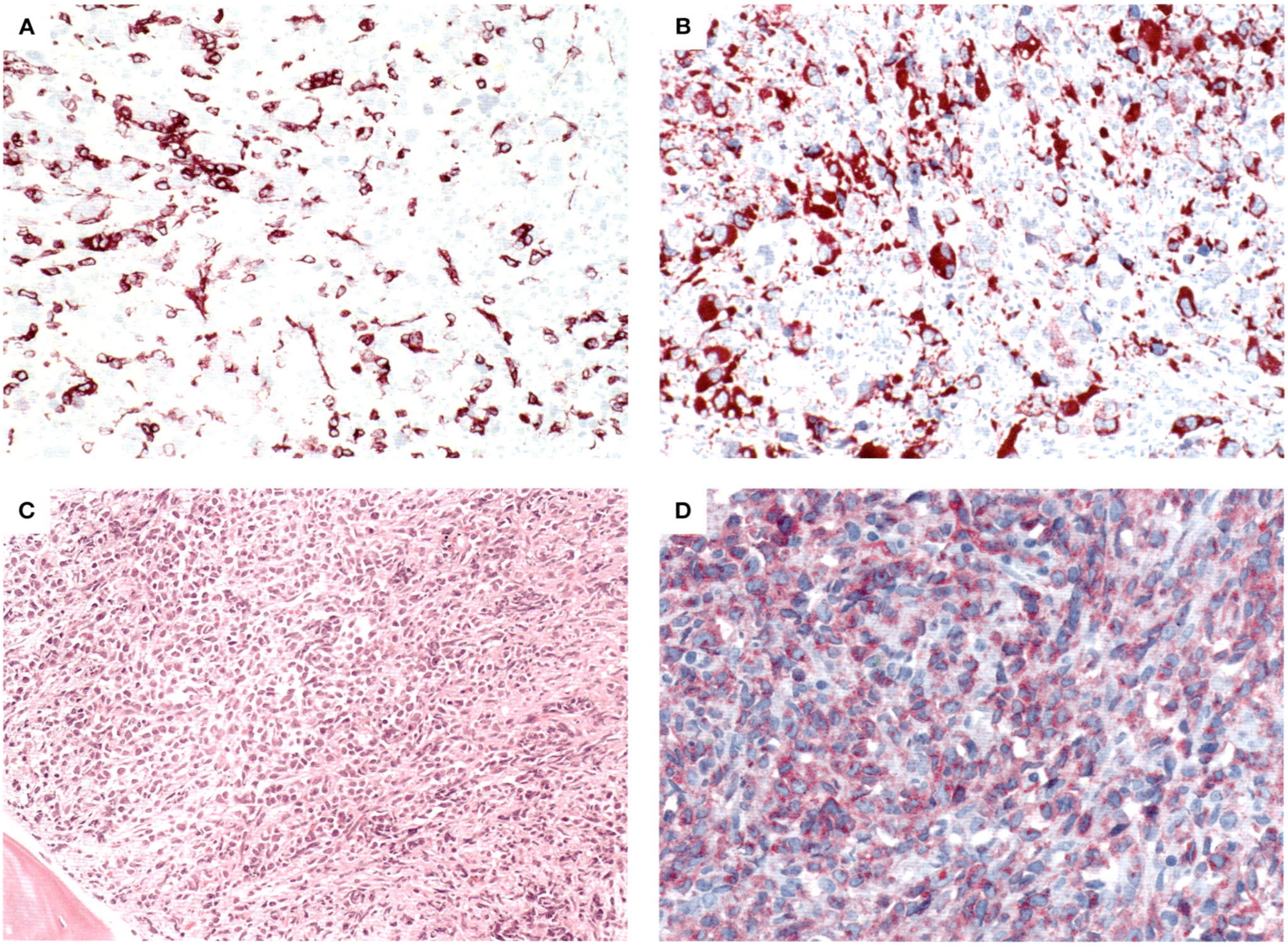

FIGURE 1.3 Chronic myeloid leukemia, accelerated and blast phase (CML-AP, CML-BP). **A:** CML-AP with increased numbers of CD34$^+$ blasts in the bone marrow biopsy. **B:** Accelerated phase of CML is in many cases associated with an increased number of highly atypical megakaryocytes with myelodysplasia-like morphology. **C:** Lymphoid blast phase shows increased blast proliferation with lymphoid/lymphoblastic morphology. **D:** The blasts express CD19. (**A:** CD34; **B:** CD61; **C:** hematoxylin and eosin; **D:** CD19; **A-D:** 40×).

of CML-BP is warranted even if the remainder of the marrow shows CML-CP.[19]

In the majority of CML-BP cases, the blasts are of myeloid lineage (neutrophilic, monocytic, megakaryocytic, basophilic, eosinophilic, erythroid blasts, or any combination thereof)[14,30,41,42]; however, 20% to 30% of cases are composed of lymphoblasts, usually of B-cell origin (Figure 1.3), although cases of T-lymphoblastic and NK-cell transformation have been reported.[37] Sequential lymphoblastic and myeloblastic crises may also occur. The origin of the blasts is often morphologically obvious, but sometimes the blasts are primitive or heterogeneous and mixed phenotypes are common; therefore, immunophenotypic analysis, preferably by multiparameter flow cytometry, is recommended. Rare cases of myeloid CML-BP have cytogenetic abnormalities in which a specific recurrent chromosomal rearrangement associated with acute myeloid leukemia, such as inv(16)(p13.1q22) or t(16;16)(p13.2;q22), is found in the same cells as the Ph chromosome. In such cases, however, these chromosomal abnormalities, which are often associated with favorable outcomes in acute leukemia, are reported to have no favorable effect when found with the Ph chromosome.[43]

Extramedullary tissues

In CML-CP the spleen is variably enlarged because of infiltration of the red pulp cords by granulocytes.[30] A similar infiltrate is seen in the hepatic sinuses and occasionally in lymph nodes.[31] These extramedullary infiltrates are composed of a mixture of immature and mature granulocytes; any significant shift toward immaturity with an increased percentage of blasts (≥10%) indicates progressing or transformed disease. In CML-BP any extramedullary tissue can be infiltrated, but spleen, liver, lymph node, skin, and soft tissues are most commonly involved.[31] Regardless of blood and marrow findings, clinical evidence of an infiltrative process in any extramedullary site should be investigated to exclude CML-BP.

Immunophenotype

Immunophenotypic analysis in CML-CP has only limited diagnostic value, although some data suggest that abnormal expression of CD7, CD56, or CD11b on CD34+ stem cells may impact response to TKI therapy.[44,45] The main role of flow cytometry, however, is phenotypic analysis of CML-BP including the detection of mixed phenotypes.[46] Immunohistochemical stains can also be helpful if there are insufficient numbers of blasts in the blood and a marrow aspirate cannot be obtained.[36]

In the myeloid blast phase, the blasts have strong, weak, or no myeloperoxidase activity but express one or more antigens associated with granulocytic, monocytic, megakaryocytic, or erythroid differentiation (eg, CD33, CD13, CD14, CD11c, CD11b, CD117, CD15, CD41, CD61, CD71, glycophorin A or C). However, in many cases of myeloid origin, the blasts also express one or more lymphoid-related antigens. Most lymphoblastic cases are of B precursor origin and express terminal deoxynucleotidyl transferase in addition to B-related antigens (CD19, CD10, CD79a, PAX5, CD20), but a minority of cases express T-cell-related antigens (CD3, CD2, CD5, CD4, CD8, CD7).[41,46] Expression of one or more myeloid-related antigens is common in B- and T-cell-derived blast phases. An increased incidence of unusual immunophenotypes and types of blasts (eg, basophil blasts, megakaryoblasts) has been described in the era of TKIs.[19]

Genetics

CML is characterized by the chromosomal translocation (9;22)(q34;q11), yielding the Philadelphia chromosome (Ph) and generating the *BCR::ABL1* fusion gene that encodes a constitutively active protein tyrosine kinase.[1] The Philadelphia chromosome is not specific for CML but is also present in 15% to 30% of adults and 5% of children with B-lymphoblastic leukemia, in some cases of mixed phenotype acute leukemia, and in rare cases of acute myeloid leukemia. The fusion protein encoded by the *BCR::ABL1* fusion gene has abnormal tyrosine kinase activity, leading to increased cell proliferation through its activation of downstream signaling pathways such as *JAK/STAT*, *PI3K/AKT*, *RAS/MEK*, *mTOR*, and *Src* kinases.[47] Different breakpoints and rearrangements determine the phenotype of the disease: in 95% of patients with CML and 25% to 30% of cases of Ph+ acute lymphoblastic leukemia the breakpoint occurs in the major breakpoint cluster region, spanning exons 12 to 16, and an abnormal fusion protein, p210, is formed; rarely the breakpoint in BCR is in the mu breakpoint region, spanning exons 17 to 20, resulting in a larger fusion p230 protein.[48,49] These patients usually demonstrate marked peripheral blood neutrophilia or thrombocytosis[24]; in about 1% to 2% of patients a break in the minor breakpoint region results in a short fusion protein (p190) that is usually also found in Ph+ acute lymphoblastic leukemia, although small amounts of the p190 transcript can be detected in most patients with CML because of alternative splicing of the BCR gene.[26,50] Patients carrying the short p190 transcript may present with increased numbers of monocytes resembling CMML.[25]

About 30% of patients with CML in CML-CP with resistance to first or second generation of TKIs harbor mutations in the *BCR::ABL1* kinase domain.[51] Currently more than 100 mutations have been found, in which the T315I mutation is the most common mutation (about 13%-16%); E255K and M351T mutations account for 9% to 14% of mutations; Y253F, Q252H, F317L, and other mutations account for 3% to 6% of mutations, while V299L mutations are rare.[47,51] Compound mutations (variants containing ≥2 mutations within the same *BCR::ABL1* allele that presumably arise sequentially or simultaneously) exhibit different spectra of resistance from single mutations. In *BCR::ABL1*-independent mechanisms of TKI resistance stem cells can survive through activation of alternative signaling pathways, such as *Src*, *JAK/STAT*, *RAS/MAPK*, and *PI3K/AKT*; genomic instability; epigenetic dysfunction; and dysfunction of the immune system.[47] Activation of alternative pathways may reveal why the disease still recurs in patients who achieved an excellent response to treatment.[52,53]

During progression to CML-AP and CML-BP secondary chromosomal abnormalities can be detected, most commonly +8 (34% of cases with additional changes), +Ph (30%), i(17q) (20%), +19 (13%), -Y (8% of males), +21 (7%), +17 (5%), and monosomy 7 (5%), which are often associated with an unfavorable prognosis.[54] The acquisition of major-route additional chromosomal abnormalities on treatment is considered as hallmark of disease progression[14] with higher rate of relapse on second or subsequent line of therapy.

Gene mutations additional to *BCR::ABL1* can be identified in 30% to 40% of Ph+ clones at diagnosis.[53,55,56] Most commonly epigenetic regulator genes such as *ASXL1*, *DNMT3A*, *EZH2*, *IDH1*, *IDH2*, and *TET2* are affected.[56,57] While *ASXL1* mutations may be present in CML-CP, patients with *ASXL1* mutations acquire other additional variants during progression to CML-BP, including *RUNX1*, *TP53*, *BCOR*, and *SETD1B*.[58] In rare cases mutations have been identified in Ph+ and Ph− clones simultaneously, raising the possibility that the mutation preceded the acquisition of *BCR::ABL1*.[39,57] In this context, next-generation sequencing is highly sensitive to identify emerging resistant mutations and should be incorporated in clinical decision making in high-risk patients with CML.[52,59]

Prognosis and Clinical Comment

The development of TKIs that target the constitutively activated tyrosine kinase domain of the *BCR::ABL1* fusion protein is a remarkable advance that led to dramatic improvements in survival and quality of life in patients afflicted with CML.[17] Now, most patients with newly diagnosed CML can be expected to live a nearly normal life span if treated with TKI therapy. In the current age of TKI therapy, the most important prognostic indicator is the response to therapy at the hematologic, cytogenetic, and molecular levels. Overall, the complete cytogenetic response rate to first-line TKI is 70% to 90% with a 5-year progression-free and overall survival between 80% and 95%. At 10 years, the survival rate is still 82% to 85%.[60] A major molecular response (MMR: *BCR::ABL1* < 0.1% on the international scale) and a deeper molecular response (*BCR::ABL1* < 0.01% or less) are achieved faster and more frequently with second-generation TKIs and the resistance rate to second-generation TKI is <10%.[5,6,20] The key to the success of TKI therapy is regular and continual assessment of the hematologic, cytogenetic, and molecular status of the patient to detect changes indicative of drug failure or resistance. The morphologic features in blood and bone marrow specimens of patients receiving TKI therapy reflect the changes in the cytogenetic and molecular events as the patient responds, with normalization of the white blood cell count and return to a normal cellular bone marrow with relatively normal morphology, usually during a period of 3 to 6 months.[61,62] Although morphologic features are not sensitive enough to reflect early increases in the burden of the *BCR::ABL1* transcript that usually indicate drug resistance, the persistence or reappearance of any morphologic features indicative of CML in follow-up specimens of patients receiving TKI therapy should raise concern for drug resistance and prompt further evaluation of the cytogenetic or molecular status.[17] In patients with CML-CP with tyrosine kinase domain mutations or *BCR::ABL1* amplification, disease progression may be circumvented or reversed by increasing the dosage or switching to a newer-generation TKI. Recently, a new class of small molecules targeting the myristoyl pocket of ABL1 has been introduced into the treatment of CML.[63,64]

References

1. Chereda B, Melo JV. Natural course and biology of CML. *Ann Hematol.* 2015;94:S107-S121.
2. Gunsilius E, Duba HC, Petzer AL, et al. Evidence from a leukaemia model for maintenance of vascular endothelium by bone-marrow-derived endothelial cells. *Lancet.* 2000;355(9216):1688-1691.
3. Osman AEG, Deininger MW. Chronic Myeloid Leukemia: modern therapies, current challenges and future directions. *Blood Rev.* 2021;49:100825.
4. Cortes J. Natural history and staging of chronic myelogenous leukemia. *Hematol Oncol Clin North Am.* 2004;18(3):569-584, viii.
5. Deininger MW, Shah NP, Altman JK, et al. Chronic myeloid leukemia, version 2.2021, NCCN clinical practice guidelines in oncology. *J Natl Compr Canc Netw.* 2020;18(10):1385-1415.
6. Cross NCP, Ernst T, Branford S, et al. European LeukemiaNet laboratory recommendations for the diagnosis and management of chronic myeloid leukemia. *Leukemia.* 2023;37(11):2150-2167.
7. Hidalgo-Lomicronpez JE, Kanagal-Shamanna R, Quesada AE, et al. Bone marrow core biopsy in 508 consecutive patients with chronic myeloid leukemia: assessment of potential value. *Cancer.* 2018;124(19):3849-3855.
8. Hoffmann VS, Baccarani M, Hasford J, et al. The EUTOS population-based registry: incidence and clinical characteristics of 2904 CML patients in 20 European Countries. *Leukemia.* 2015;29(6):1336-1343.
9. American Cancer Society. Cancer Facts & Figures 2019. American Cancer Society; 2019.
10. Hochhaus A, Larson RA, Guilhot F, et al. Long-Term outcomes of imatinib treatment for chronic myeloid leukemia. *N Engl J Med.* 2017;376(10):917-927.
11. Delord M, Foulon S, Cayuela JM, Rousselot P, Bonastre J. The rising prevalence of chronic myeloid leukemia in France. *Leuk Res.* 2018;69:94-99.
12. Huang X, Cortes J, Kantarjian H. Estimations of the increasing prevalence and plateau prevalence of chronic myeloid leukemia in the era of tyrosine kinase inhibitor therapy. *Cancer.* 2012;118(12):3123-3127.

13. Ali Hailan YM, Al-Dubai HN, Yassin MA. Chronic myeloid leukemia following exposure to radioactive iodine (I131): a systematic review. *Oncology.* 2023;101(6):362-368.
14. Senapati J, Jabbour E, Kantarjian H, Short NJ. Pathogenesis and management of accelerated and blast phases of chronic myeloid leukemia. *Leukemia.* 2023;37(1):5-17.
15. Millot F, Traore P, Guilhot J, et al. Clinical and biological features at diagnosis in 40 children with chronic myeloid leukemia. *Pediatrics.* 2005;116(1):140-143.
16. Suttorp M, Eckardt L, Tauer JT, Millot F. Management of chronic myeloid leukemia in childhood. *Curr Hematol Malig Rep.* 2012;7(2):116-124.
17. Jabbour E, Kantarjian H. Chronic myeloid leukemia: 2022 update on diagnosis, therapy, and monitoring. *Am J Hematol.* 2022;97(9):1236-1256.
18. Khoury JD, Solary E, Abla O, et al. The 5th edition of the World Health Organization classification of haematolymphoid tumours: myeloid and histiocytic/dendritic neoplasms. *Leukemia.* 2022;36(7):1703-1719.
19. Arber DA, Orazi A, Hasserjian RP, et al. International consensus classification of myeloid neoplasms and acute leukemias: integrating morphologic, clinical, and genomic data. *Blood.* 2022;140(11):1200-1228.
20. Hochhaus A, Baccarani M, Silver RT, et al. European LeukemiaNet 2020 recommendations for treating chronic myeloid leukemia. *Leukemia.* 2020;34(4):966-984.
21. Lauseker M, Bachl K, Turkina A, et al. Prognosis of patients with chronic myeloid leukemia presenting in advanced phase is defined mainly by blast count, but also by age, chromosomal aberrations and hemoglobin. *Am J Hematol.* 2019;94(11):1236-1243.
22. Kantarjian HM, Tefferi A. Classification of accelerated phase chronic myeloid leukemia in the era of the BCR::ABL1 tyrosine kinase inhibitors: a work in progress. *Am J Hematol.* 2023;98(9):1350-1353.
23. Sora F, Autore F, Chiusolo P, et al. Extreme thrombocytosis in chronic myeloid leukemia in the era of tyrosine kinase inhibitors. *Leuk Lymphoma.* 2014;55(12):2958-2960.
24. Pane F, Frigeri F, Sindona M, et al. Neutrophilic-chronic myeloid leukemia: a distinct disease with a specific molecular marker (BCR/ABL with C3/A2 junction). *Blood.* 1996;88(7):2410-2414.
25. Melo JV, Myint H, Galton DA, Goldman JM. P190BCR-ABL chronic myeloid leukaemia: the missing link with chronic myelomonocytic leukaemia? *Leukemia.* 1994;8(1):208-211.
26. Melo JV. The diversity of BCR-ABL fusion proteins and their relationship to leukemia phenotype. *Blood.* 1996;88(7):2375-2384.
27. Thiele J, Kvasnicka HM, Fischer R. Bone marrow histopathology in chronic myelogenous leukemia (CML)—evaluation of distinctive features with clinical impact. *Histol Histopathol.* 1999;14(4):1241-1256.
28. Thiele J, Kvasnicka HM, Fischer R. Histochemistry and morphometry on bone marrow biopsies in chronic myeloproliferative disorders—aids to diagnosis and classification. *Ann Hematol.* 1999;78(11):495-506.
29. Thiele J, Kvasnicka HM, Schmitt-Graeff A, et al. Bone marrow features and clinical findings in chronic myeloid leukemia—a comparative, multicenter, immunohistological and morphometric study on 614 patients. *Leuk Lymphoma.* 2000;36(3-4):295-308.
30. Thiele J, Kvasnicka HM, Vardiman J. Bone marrow histopathology in the diagnosis of chronic myeloproliferative disorders: a forgotten pearl. *Best Pract Res Clin Haematol.* 2006;19(3):413-437.
31. Cotta CV, Bueso-Ramos CE. New insights into the pathobiology and treatment of chronic myelogenous leukemia. *Ann Diagn Pathol.* 2007;11(1):68-78.
32. Xu Y, Dolan MM, Nguyen PL. Diagnostic significance of detecting dysgranulopoiesis in chronic myeloid leukemia. *Am J Clin Pathol.* 2003;120(5):778-784.
33. Arber DA, Orazi A, Hasserjian R, et al. The 2016 revision to the World Health Organization classification of myeloid neoplasms and acute leukemia. *Blood.* 2016;127(20):2391-2405.
34. Hochhaus A, Ernst T, Eigendorff E, La Rosee P. Causes of resistance and treatment choices of second- and third-line treatment in chronic myelogenous leukemia patients. *Ann Hematol.* 2015;94:S133-S140.
35. Vaidya S, Vundinti BR, Shanmukhaiah C, Chakrabarti P, Ghosh K. Evolution of BCR/ABL gene mutation in CML is time dependent and dependent on the pressure exerted by tyrosine kinase inhibitor. *PLoS One.* 2015;10(1):e0114828.
36. El Rassi F, Bergsagel JD, Arellano M, et al. Predicting early blast transformation in chronic-phase chronic myeloid leukemia: is immunophenotyping the missing link? *Cancer.* 2015;121(6):872-875.
37. Efstathopoulou M, Zoi K, Siakantaris MP, et al. A case report of chronic myelogenous leukemia presenting as blastic crisis with a T-cell acute lymphoblastic leukemia phenotype: awareness of a rare entity. *Acta Haematol.* 2023;146(6):530-537.
38. How J, Venkataraman V, Hobbs GS. Blast and accelerated phase CML: room for improvement. *Hematology Am Soc Hematol Educ Program.* 2021;2021(1):122-128.
39. Schmidt M, Rinke J, Schafer V, et al. Molecular-defined clonal evolution in patients with chronic myeloid leukemia independent of the BCR-ABL status. *Leukemia.* 2014;28(12):2292-2299.
40. Cortes JE, Talpaz M, O'Brien S, et al. Staging of chronic myeloid leukemia in the imatinib era: an evaluation of the World Health Organization proposal. *Cancer.* 2006;106(6):1306-1315.
41. Reid AG, De Melo VA, Elderfield K, et al. Phenotype of blasts in chronic myeloid leukemia in blastic phase—analysis of bone marrow trephine biopsies and correlation with cytogenetics. *Leuk Res.* 2009;33(3):418-425.

42. Shi Y, Rand AJ, Crow JH, Moore JO, Lagoo AS. Blast phase in chronic myelogenous leukemia is skewed toward unusual blast types in patients treated with tyrosine kinase inhibitors: a comparative study of 67 cases. *Am J Clin Pathol.* 2015;143(1):105-119.

43. Wu Y, Slovak ML, Snyder DS, Arber DA. Coexistence of inversion 16 and the Philadelphia chromosome in acute and chronic myeloid leukemias: report of six cases and review of literature. *Am J Clin Pathol.* 2006;125(2):260-266.

44. Kosugi N, Ebihara Y, Nakahata T, Saisho H, Asano S, Tojo A. CD34+CD7+ leukemic progenitor cells may be involved in maintenance and clonal evolution of chronic myeloid leukemia. *Clin Cancer Res.* 2005;11(2 pt 1):505-511.

45. Yong AS, Szydlo RM, Goldman JM, Apperley JF, Melo JV. Molecular profiling of CD34+ cells identifies low expression of CD7, along with high expression of proteinase 3 or elastase, as predictors of longer survival in patients with CML. *Blood.* 2006;107(1):205-212.

46. Khalidi HS, Brynes RK, Medeiros LJ, et al. The immunophenotype of blast transformation of chronic myelogenous leukemia: a high frequency of mixed lineage phenotype in "lymphoid" blasts and a comparison of morphologic, immunophenotypic, and molecular findings. *Mod Pathol.* 1998;11(12):1211-1221.

47. Sun J, Hu R, Han M, et al. Mechanisms underlying therapeutic resistance of tyrosine kinase inhibitors in chronic myeloid leukemia. *Int J Biol Sci.* 2024;20(1):175-181.

48. Zenebe B, Nigussie H, Belay G, Seboka N. A review on characterization of BCR—ABL transcript variants for molecular monitoring of chronic myeloid leukemia phenotypes. *Hematology.* 2023;28(1):2284038.

49. Abdelmagid MG, Litzow MR, McCullough KB, et al. Chronic phase CML with sole P190 (e1a2) BCR::ABL1: long-term outcome among ten consecutive cases. *Blood Cancer J.* 2022;12(7):103.

50. van Rhee F, Hochhaus A, Lin F, Melo JV, Goldman JM, Cross NC. p190 BCR-ABL mRNA is expressed at low levels in p210-positive chronic myeloid and acute lymphoblastic leukemias. *Blood.* 1996;87(12):5213-5217.

51. Soverini S. Resistance mutations in CML and how we approach them. *Hematology Am Soc Hematol Educ Program.* 2023;2023(1):469-475.

52. Krishnan V, Kim DDH, Hughes TP, Branford S, Ong ST. Integrating genetic and epigenetic factors in chronic myeloid leukemia risk assessment: toward gene expression-based biomarkers. *Haematologica.* 2022;107(2):358-370.

53. Shahrin NH, Wadham C, Branford S. Defining higher-risk chronic myeloid leukemia: risk scores, genomic landscape, and prognostication. *Curr Hematol Malig Rep.* 2022;17(6):171-180.

54. Wang W, Cortes JE, Tang G, et al. Risk stratification of chromosomal abnormalities in chronic myelogenous leukemia in the era of tyrosine kinase inhibitor therapy. *Blood.* 2016;127(22):2742-2750.

55. Branford S, Wang P, Yeung DT, et al. Integrative genomic analysis reveals cancer-associated mutations at diagnosis of CML in patients with high-risk disease. *Blood.* 2018;132(9):948-961.

56. Duncavage EJ, Bagg A, Hasserjian RP, et al. Genomic profiling for clinical decision making in myeloid neoplasms and acute leukemia. *Blood.* 2022;140(21):2228-2247.

57. Makishima H, Jankowska AM, McDevitt MA, et al. CBL, CBLB, TET2, ASXL1, and IDH1/2 mutations and additional chromosomal aberrations constitute molecular events in chronic myelogenous leukemia. *Blood.* 2011;117(21):e198-e206.

58. Ochi Y. Genetic landscape of chronic myeloid leukemia. *Int J Hematol.* 2023;117(1):30-36.

59. Soverini S, Abruzzese E, Bocchia M, et al. Next-generation sequencing for BCR-ABL1 kinase domain mutation testing in patients with chronic myeloid leukemia: a position paper. *J Hematol Oncol.* 2019;12(1):131.

60. Iezza M, Cortesi S, Ottaviani E, et al. Prognosis in chronic myeloid leukemia: baseline factors, dynamic risk assessment and novel insights. *Cells.* 2023;12(13):1703.

61. Kvasnicka HM, Thiele J, Staib P, et al. Reversal of bone marrow angiogenesis in chronic myeloid leukemia following imatinib mesylate (STI571) therapy. *Blood.* 2004;103(9):3549-3551.

62. Thiele J, Kvasnicka HM, Schmitt-Graeff A, et al. Effects of the tyrosine kinase inhibitor imatinib mesylate (STI571) on bone marrow features in patients with chronic myelogenous leukemia. *Histol Histopathol.* 2004;19(4):1277-1288.

63. Hughes TP, Mauro MJ, Cortes JE, et al. Asciminib in chronic myeloid leukemia after ABL kinase inhibitor failure. *N Engl J Med.* 2019;381(24):2315-2326.

64. Rea D, Mauro MJ, Boquimpani C, et al. A phase 3, open-label, randomized study of asciminib, a STAMP inhibitor, vs bosutinib in CML after 2 or more prior TKIs. *Blood.* 2021;138(21):2031-2041.

Chapter 2

BCR::ABL1-Negative Myeloproliferative Neoplasms

Hans Michael Kvasnicka, Attilio Orazi, Ayalew Tefferi, Juergen Thiele, and Alessandro Maria Vannucchi

Introduction

The classical *BCR::ABL1*-negative myeloproliferative neoplasms (MPN), essential thrombocythemia (ET), primary myelofibrosis (PMF), and polycythemia vera (PV) are characterized by clonal myeloproliferation with effective maturation in the bone marrow, which leads to accumulation of terminally differentiated cells in the peripheral blood and in various organs.[1] Splenomegaly and hepatomegaly are common and in advanced stages of PMF are mainly caused by extramedullary hematopoiesis (EMH).[2] Despite an insidious onset, each MPN subtype has the potential to progress to bone marrow failure due to myelofibrosis, ineffective hematopoiesis, transform to a blast phase, or any combination of these events.[3]

Disease progression is usually accompanied by genetic evolution. Clonal hematopoiesis is driven in most cases by upregulation of the Janus kinase (JAK) and signal transducer and activator of transcription (STAT) pathway.[4] The cause of MPN is unknown and most cases of MPN are sporadic, but an inherited susceptibility has been described.[5] Relatives of patients with MPN have an increased risk of developing polycythemia vera, essential thrombocythemia, or PMF, and many families with multiple affected members have been reported.[5,6] A germline *JAK2* 46/1 haplotype may be a predisposing factor, but this haplotype is relatively common, and most affected individuals do not develop MPN.[7] Polycythemia vera and essential thrombocythemia are relatively indolent, and most patients have a near normal life expectancy, in contrast to patients with PMF.[8] Therefore, an accurate diagnosis of the MPN subtype is clinically relevant.[9] Furthermore, identification of early-stage disease is of importance allowing early therapeutic intervention to prevent disease-related complications.[10] It is important to recognize that major thrombotic and other complications may sometimes precede a definitive clinical diagnosis of MPN, particularly in patients with positive driver mutation status, usually with low variant allele frequency (VAF) presenting with cerebral or splanchnic vein thrombosis, including Budd-Chiari syndrome.[11]

The diagnosis of MPN in its initial stage may be clinically challenging, particularly because typical hematological features and symptoms generally found in cases of overt MPN may not be present in the early stages (Table 2.1).[9,10] Careful evaluation of clinical features, peripheral blood counts and smear review, bone marrow morphology, karyotype, and molecular genetic testing allow diagnosis of MPN and guide further subtyping. The detection of one of the characteristic driver mutations such as *JAK2* V617F, Calreticulin (*CALR*), and *MPL* is an important diagnostic feature, but is not specific to the MPN subtypes.[4] Therefore, bone marrow morphology remains the core diagnostic platform, but it is important to emphasize that bone marrow morphologic features should only be interpreted in the context of appropriate clinical, laboratory, and molecular findings (see Table 2.1).[1,12,13]

Assessment of Driver Mutations

Accurate assessment of MPN-associated driver mutations, *JAK2* V617F, *JAK2* exon 12, *CALR* type1/2, and *MPL* W515L/K by highly sensitive single-target (RT-qPCR, ddPCR) or multitarget panel (NGS) assays is important to support the diagnosis of MPN and to separate clonally undefined (wild-type or triple-negative) cases.[14,15] The optimal source for DNA preparation are purified peripheral blood granulocytes, particularly if using assays with a sensitivity >3% as in these instances the use of whole blood may lead to underestimation of VAF or even false negative results. Therefore, it is recommended to use *JAK2* V617F assays with a sensitivity of <1%, whereas a sensitivity of 1% to 3% may be satisfactory for *CALR* and *MPL* mutation testing.[1,15] In negative cases, the search for noncanonical *JAK2* (including *MPL* in essential thrombocythemia and PMF) mutations is encouraged, whereas a *JAK2* V617F VAF of <1% should prompt the search for coexisting canonical *CALR* (and *MPL*) mutations.[5]

TABLE 2.1 Clinical and morphological features of *BCR::ABL1*-negative MPN subtypes

	PV	ET	Pre-PMF	Overt-PMF	Post-PV MF Post-ET MF
Clinical features					
Hb/Hct	increased	normal	in most cases normal	Anemia	Anemia
Platelets	often increased	increased	increased	variable, often decreased	variable, often decreased
WBC	increased	normal	increased	variable, mostly increased	variable, mostly increased
LDH	increased	normal	increased	Increased	Increased
Splenomegaly	±	–	±	++	++
Morphology					
Peripheral blood	normochromic, normocytic red blood cells	platelet anisocytosis	platelets may be abnormally large with altered granulation	often teardrop cells	often teardrop cells
Leukoerythroblastosis	–	–	–	+	+
Bone marrow					
Cellularity	increased	normal	hypercellular	variable, can be hypocellular in patients in advanced stage	variable, often hypocellular can be hypocellular in patients in advanced stage
Myeloid/erythroid ratio	shift toward erythropoiesis	normal	shift toward granulopoiesis	variable, often dyserythropoiesis	variable, often dyserythropoiesis and dysgranulopoiesis
Megakaryocytes	variable in size	predominance of large cells	variable, small to giant	variable, small to medium sized, often micromegakaryocytes	variable, dysmegakaryopoiesis is common
Clustering	loose grouping	infrequent small clusters	large clusters	large clusters	large clusters
Nuclear features	hyperlobation, staghorn	hyperlobation, staghorn	hypolobation, bulbous	hypolobation, bulbous, bizarre shaped	hypolobation, bulbous, bizarre shaped

ET, essential thrombocythemia; Overt-PMF, overt primary myelofibrosis; Post-ET MF, post-essential thrombocythemia myelofibrosis; Post-PV MF, post-polycythemia vera myelofibrosis; Pre-PMF, prefibrotic primary myelofibrosis; PV, polycythemia vera.

Grading of Bone Marrow Fibrosis

Accurate assessment of the bone marrow stromal matrix is clinically relevant in the diagnostic workup of MPN and other myeloid neoplasms.[16,17] There is compelling evidence that the amount of bone marrow fibrosis is associated with overall survival in patients with MPN, particularly in overt PMF, where the clinical phenotype is closely correlated with the development of bone marrow fibrosis.[18,19] In addition, a more complete analysis of the bone marrow stroma, including assessment of collagen deposition and osteosclerosis, has become important in evaluating the therapeutic effects of potentially disease-modifying agents.[17] Therefore, separate grading systems for reticulin, collagen deposition, and osteosclerosis are recommended to better assess bone marrow stromal changes present at the time of diagnosis or after therapy (Tables 2.2 and 2.3, Figure 2.1).[20-22]

The quality of staining techniques and their adherence to appropriate laboratory standards are key to achieving high reproducibility of grading.[17] A core biopsy taken at right angle (90°) from cortical bone of sufficient length (≥1 cm) without fragmentation is generally considered mandatory for all proposed grading schemes. Scoring of bone marrow samples with a heterogeneous pattern, which is more common after therapy, is defined by the highest grade of fibrosis seen in at least 30% of the total bone marrow evaluable area. Grading of collagen fibrosis distinguishes a focal deposition seen in earlier disease stage from a more extensive collagenization with a coarse meshwork of collagen fibers seen in the later stages (see Table 2.3), whereas grading of osteosclerosis reflects a progressively more

TABLE 2.2 Grading of bone marrow fibrosis.[16,21]

Grade[a]	Description
MF-0	Scattered linear reticulin fibers with no intersections (crossovers), corresponding to normal bone marrow
MF-1	Loose network of reticulin with many intersections, especially in perivascular areas
MF-2[b]	Diffuse and dense increase in reticulin fibers with extensive intersections, occasionally with focal bundles of thick fibers mostly consistent with collagen or focal osteosclerosis
MF-3[b]	Diffuse and dense increase in reticulin with extensive intersections and coarse bundles of thick fibers consistent with collagen, usually associated with osteosclerosis

[a]Should be assessed only in hematopoietic areas. If the fibrosis pattern is heterogeneous, the final score is determined by the highest grade present in at least 30% of the marrow area.
[b]In grades MF-2 and MF-3, trichrome staining is recommended to confirm the presence of collagen.
Adapted from Thiele J, Kvasnicka HM, Facchetti F, Franco V, van der Walt J, Orazi A. European consensus on grading bone marrow fibrosis and assessment of cellularity. *Haematologica.* 2005;90(8):1128-1132. and Swerdlow SH, Campo E, Harris NL, et al. *WHO Classification of Tumours of Haematopoietic and Lymphoid Tissues.* 4th ed. International Agency for Research on Cancer; 2017.

severe degree of new bone formation, which results in thickening of the bony trabeculae (see Table 2.3). Initial grades of osteosclerosis include irregularity of the trabecular bone surface with focal osteosclerotic buds, hooks, or spikes that eventually coalesce into an extensive interconnected network.

POLYCYTHEMIA VERA

Definition

Polycythemia vera is a MPN defined by increased red blood cell (RBC) production independent of normal regulatory mechanisms.[23] Virtually all polycythemia vera patients have an acquired somatic gain-of-function mutation of the Janus 2 kinase gene, *JAK2* V617F, or, less commonly, a functionally similar *JAK2* exon 12 mutation, leading to autonomous proliferation resulting in panmyelosis in the bone marrow.[23]

Synonyms

None.

Epidemiology

Polycythemia vera usually occurs in elderly patients with an annual incidence of 1 to 3 per 100,000 in the Western world and less frequently in Asia.[24] Median age at diagnosis is 62 years,[25] and patients younger than 20 years are rarely described.[23]

General Clinical Features

Polycythemia vera is characterized by an increase in hemoglobin, hematocrit, and RBC. Diagnostic thresholds include an acquired increase in hemoglobin and/or hematocrit greater than 16.5 g/dL and/or 49% in men and 16 g/dL and/or 48% in women, in the context of a *JAK2* mutation and characteristic bone marrow morphology (Table 2.4).[1,9,20,23] Although not commonly measured in clinical practice, the red cell mass is increased >25% above the mean predicted normal value.[23] Most of the symptoms associated with polycythemia vera are because of an increased blood viscosity and reduced blood flow. Thirty to fifty percent of patients present with constitutional symptoms such as headache, weakness, pruritus, fatigue, dizziness, and sweating.[23] These symptoms are often associated

TABLE 2.3 Grading of bone marrow collagen deposition and osteosclerosis[17,21]

Grade[a]	Bone marrow collagen deposition[b]	Bone marrow osteosclerosis[c]
0	Perivascular collagen only (normal)	Regular bone trabeculae (distinct paratrabecular borders)
1	Focal paratrabecular or/and central collagen deposition without connecting meshwork	Focal budding, hooks, spikes or paratrabecular apposition of new bone
2	Paratrabecular or/and central deposition of collagen with focally connecting meshwork or generalized paratrabecular apposition of collagen	Diffuse paratrabecular new bone formation with thickening of trabeculae, occasionally with focal interconnections
3	Diffuse (complete) connecting meshwork of collagen	Extensive interconnecting meshwork of new bone with overall effacement of marrow spaces

[a]if the pattern is heterogeneous, the final score is determined by the highest grade present in at least 30% of the marrow area.
[b]trichrome staining (Masson trichrome or Martius scarlet blue [MSB]) with positive internal control by perivascular staining of collagen required.
[c]bone marrow core biopsy taken at right angle (90°) from the cortical bone of sufficient length without fragmentation is mandatory for grading of osteosclerosis, H&E or silver impregnation.
Kvasnicka HM, Beham-Schmid C, Bob R, et al. Problems and pitfalls in grading of bone marrow fibrosis, collagen deposition and osteosclerosis—a consensus-based study. Histopathology. 2016;68(6):905-915. and Swerdlow SH, Campo E, Harris NL, et al. *WHO Classification of Tumours of Haematopoietic and Lymphoid Tissues.* 4th ed. International Agency for Research on Cancer; 2017.

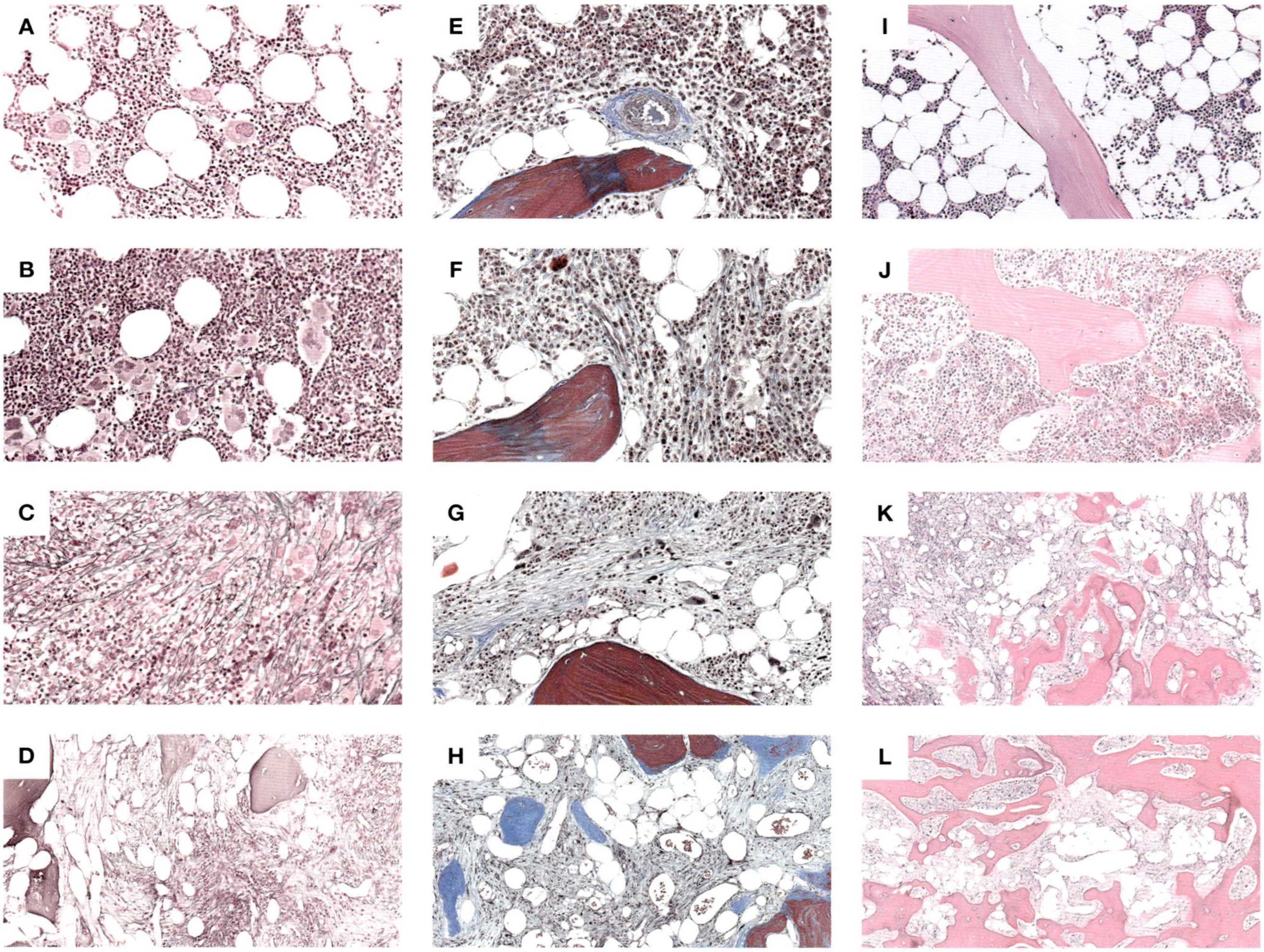

FIGURE 2.1 Grading of bone marrow fibrosis, collagen deposition, and osteosclerosis. **A-D: Bone marrow fibrosis: A:** MF-0 with scattered linear reticulin showing no intersections (cross-overs) corresponding to a normal bone marrow pattern. **B:** MF-1 with slight increase in reticulin with a loose network revealing many intersections, especially in perivascular areas. **C:** MF-2 with a diffuse and dense increase in reticulin with extensive intersections, occasionally with focal bundles of thick fibers. **D:** MF-3 showing a diffuse and dense increase in reticulin with extensive intersections and coarse bundles of thick fibers and initial osteosclerosis. **E-H: Collagen deposition: E:** Grade 0 corresponds to a normal bone marrow pattern with positive internal control by perivascular staining. **F:** Grade 1 with a focal paratrabecular and only minimal central collagen deposition without connecting meshwork. **G:** Grade 2 reveals a paratrabecular and prominent central deposition of collagen with focally connecting meshwork. **H:** Grade 3 represents a diffuse and complete connecting meshwork of collagen. **I-L: Osteosclerosis: I:** Grade 0 corresponds to a regular architecture of bone trabeculae with distinct paratrabecular borders. **J:** Grade 1 shows initial paratrabecular apposition of new bone with focal buddings (hooks, spikes). **K:** Grade 2 represents a diffuse paratrabecular new bone formation with thickening of trabeculae and focal interconnections. **L:** Grade 3 is characterized by an extensive interconnecting meshwork of new bone with overall effacement of marrow space (**A-D:** Gomori stain; **E-H:** Masson trichrome staining; **I-L:** hematoxylin & eosin; **A-L:** 40×.)

with increased blood viscosity and/or microvascular thrombotic events, but thrombosis involving major arteries or veins may also occur and can pose life-threatening events.[25] In the case of splanchnic vein thrombosis and Budd-Chiari syndrome, a differential diagnosis of polycythemia vera should always be considered.[11,26] However, a significant proportion of patients are asymptomatic and are diagnosed following a routine blood count examination showing erythrocytosis often associated with elevated white blood cell (WBC) and platelet counts.[10,27] Mild splenomegaly is often present. In the polycythemic phase of polycythemia vera, splenomegaly, which is usually of a moderate degree is primarily due to splenic red pulp congestion. Progression to secondary myelofibrosis, known as post-polycythemia vera myelofibrosis (post-PV MF) or post-polycythemic myeloid metaplasia (clinically also termed spent phase), heralds an aggressive disease course with median survival not different from overt PMF.[28]

TABLE 2.4 Diagnostic criteria for Polycythemia Vera

Major criteria
1. Elevated hemoglobin concentration or elevated hematocrit or increased red blood cell mass[a]
2. Bone marrow biopsy showing age-adjusted hypercellularity with trilineage proliferation (panmyelosis), including prominent erythroid, granulocytic, and megakaryocytic proliferation with pleomorphic, mature megakaryocytes lacking atypia[b]
3. Presence of *JAK2* V617F or *JAK2* exon 12 mutation[c]
Minor criterion
Subnormal serum erythropoietin level
The diagnosis of polycythemia vera requires either all three major criteria or the first two major criteria plus the minor criterion.

[a] Diagnostic thresholds: hemoglobin: >16.5 g/dL in men and >16.0 g/dL in women; hematocrit: >49% in men and >48% in women; red blood cell mass: >25% above mean normal predicted value.

[b] A bone marrow biopsy may not be required in patients with sustained absolute erythrocytosis (hemoglobin concentrations of >18.5 g/dL in men or >16.5 g/dL in women and hematocrit values of >55.5% in men or >49.5% in women) and the presence of a *JAK2* V617F or *JAK2* exon 12 mutation.

[c] It is recommended to use highly sensitive assays for *JAK2* V617F (sensitivity level <1%); in negative cases, consider searching for noncanonical or atypical *JAK2* mutations in exons 12 to 15.

Morphology

The diagnosis of polycythemia vera requires the integration of clinical, laboratory, and molecular data with morphologic findings in adequate, well-prepared peripheral blood smear and bone marrow biopsy specimens.[1]

Peripheral blood

Peripheral blood smears usually show a mild to overall excess of normochromic, normocytic erythrocytes. Because of iron deficiency due to erythroid overactivity in the bone marrow, occult mucosal bleeding, decreased iron absorption or other mechanisms, plus iron loss with phlebotomies, the red cells are often hypochromic and microcytic.[23] Circulating blasts are usually absent. Frankly polycythemic patients characteristically show increased hemoglobin and hematocrit; however, these levels may be decreased if iron deficiency occurs. If the hematocrit exceeds 60%, an elevated RBC volume is almost always documented.[23] The WBCs are in most patients only moderately increased; left-shifted granulocytosis may be seen in some cases. The platelet count is often markedly elevated, a finding that may suggest a possible diagnosis of essential thrombocythemia. This is especially true in the early stages of polycythemia vera, as both hematocrit and RBC volume may not be markedly elevated in these patients.[10,20]

Bone marrow

Bone marrow aspirate smears are generally characterized by the presence of age-adjusted hypercellularity due to trilineage proliferation (ie, panmyelosis) of erythroid and granulocytic precursors associated with increased megakaryopoiesis (Figure 2.2).[29] The diagnostic morphologic features may not be as readily appreciated on smears as on biopsy sections, and therefore bone marrow histology is key to establishing a valid diagnosis (see Table 2.4).[1] The histopathology of the bone marrow is defined by increased hematopoiesis extending into the normally hypocellular subcortical marrow spaces.[22] Although a panmyelotic proliferation is seen in most instances, an increased number of nucleated erythroid progenitors and megakaryocytes can also occur in a proportion of the cases. Erythropoiesis is usually normoblastic with erythroid precursors forming large aggregates or confluent sheets.[22] Granulopoiesis is usually morphologically normal. Megakaryopoiesis is characterized by a higher than normal degree of pleomorphism, ie, a mixture of small, medium size, and large to giant megakaryocytes. Megakaryocytes appear dispersed or in loose clusters around bone marrow sinusoids or close to bony trabeculae and do not show significant degrees of atypia or maturation defects as seen in PMF.[22] They are often surrounded by maturing erythroid cells.

Iron staining, preferably performed on smears of bone marrow aspirates, is an important diagnostic tool in the workup of polycythemia vera, as iron-containing macrophages are rarely observed (<6%). Cases with a high platelet count may be clinically suggestive of essential thrombocythemia, but in essential thrombocythemia there is only a prominent proliferation of medium to giant megakaryocytes with hyperlobulated nuclei and loose clustering and no increase in overall bone marrow cellularity.[20] A minimal increase in bone marrow reticulin (MF-1) is found in 10% to 20% of patients at the time of diagnosis and is significantly associated with a higher prevalence of splenomegaly and faster progression to post-polycythemia vera myelofibrosis.[30]

Post-polycythemia vera myelofibrosis

Post-polycythemia vera myelofibrosis (post-PV MF), the advanced and often terminal phase of polycythemia vera (Table 2.5), develops in approximately 15% of patients usually 10 to 15 years after initial diagnosis.[25,31,32] Post-PV MF is characterized by anemia, leukoerythroblastic blood smear, grade 2 or 3 bone marrow fibrosis, and splenomegaly due to EMH.[1,33] Bone marrow

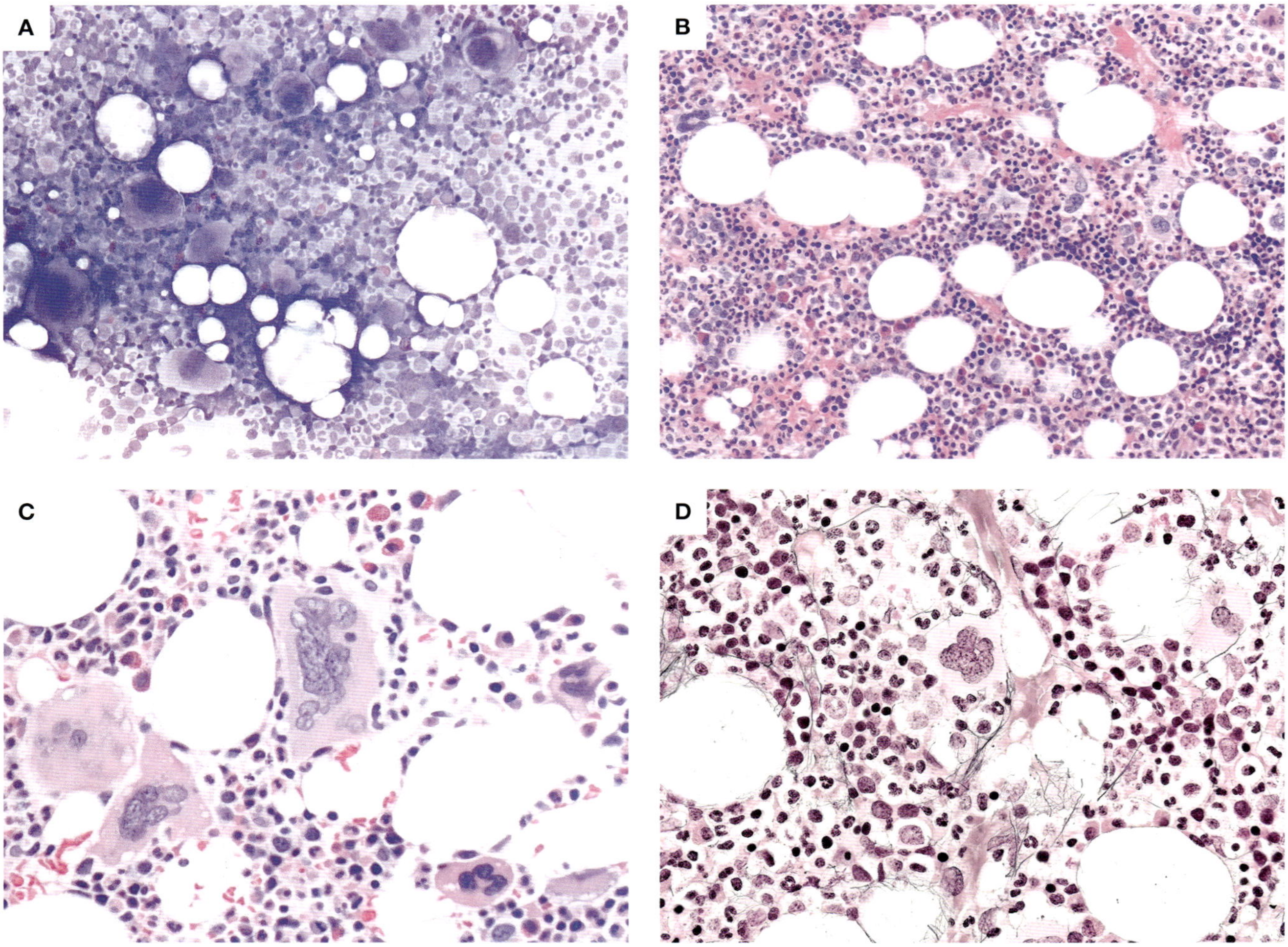

FIGURE 2.2 Polycythemia vera. **A:** Bone marrow aspirate with increased cellularity and prominent megakaryocytes. **B:** Hypercellular bone marrow biopsy with panmyelosis, randomly arranged megakaryocytes. **C:** Megakaryocytes show increased pleomorphism with significant size variation (small to giant cells), but no relevant maturation defects or clustering. **D:** Initial increase in bone marrow reticulin (MF-1). (**A:** Wright-Giemsa, **B**-**D:** hematoxylin & eosin; **A** and **C:** 60×, **B** and **D:** 40×).

TABLE 2.5 Diagnostic criteria for post-polycythemia vera myelofibrosis (post-PV MF)

Required criteria
1. Previous established diagnosis of polycythemia vera
2. Bone marrow fibrosis of grade 2 or 3[16,21]
Additional criteria
1. Anemia (ie, below the reference range given age, sex, and altitude considerations) or sustained loss of requirement of either phlebotomy (in the absence of cytoreductive therapy) or cytoreductive treatment for erythrocytosis
2. Leukoerythroblastosis
3. Increase in palpable splenomegaly of >5 cm from baseline or the development of a newly palpable splenomegaly
4. Development of any 2 (or all 3) of the following constitutional symptoms: >10% weight loss in 6 mo, night sweats, unexplained fever (>37.5 °C)

The diagnosis of post-polycythemia vera myelofibrosis is established by all required criteria and at least two additional criteria.

specimens are variably cellular (Figure 2.3), but often show decreased erythropoiesis and, in the terminal stage, decreased overall marrow cellularity.[34] Peripheral blood changes are similar or identical to those observed in overt PMF including teardrop-shaped RBCs.[23] Bone marrow histologic findings are generally indistinguishable from those seen in advanced stages of PMF, and differentiation of these two conditions in *JAK2* V617F mutant cases may be impossible without a documented history of polycythemia vera.[34] Granulopoiesis may be reduced, and large clusters of abnormal megakaryocytes of variable size with hyperchromatic, bizarre nuclei are often the predominant bone marrow component. Bone marrow sinuses are dilated and filled with hematopoietic progenitors and megakaryocytes.[22] Bone marrow fibrosis is at least MF-2 but often is MF-3 with diffuse stromal collagenization and pronounced osteosclerosis.

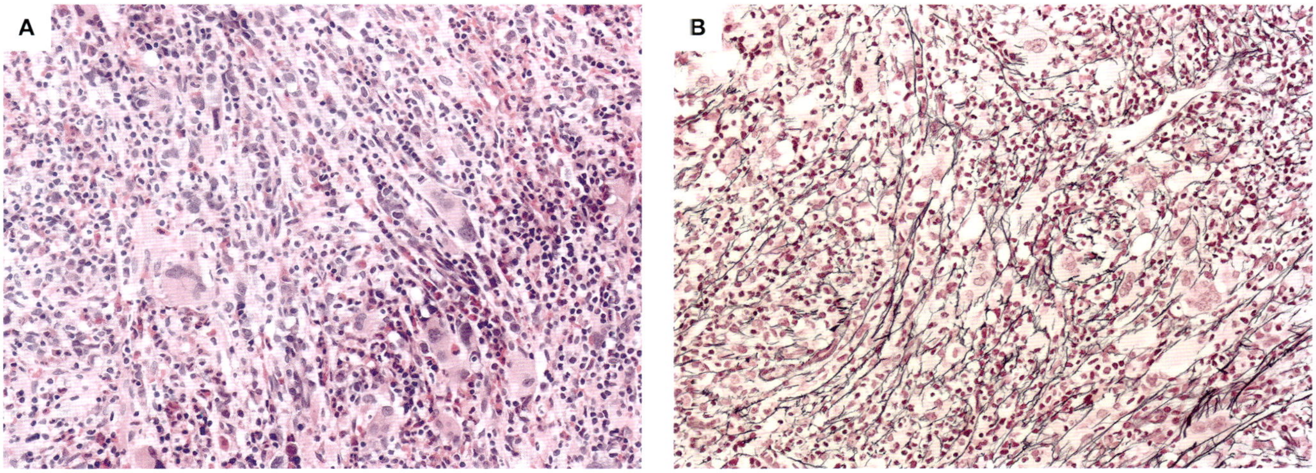

FIGURE 2.3 Post-polycythemia vera myelofibrosis. **A:** Hypercellular bone marrow with streaming of atypical megakaryocytes and increased erythropoiesis. **B:** Manifest bone marrow fibrosis (MF-2). (**A:** hematoxylin & eosin, **B:** Gomori stain; **A and B:** 40×.)

Accelerated and blast phase

The finding of more than 10% blasts in the blood or bone marrow or severe myelodysplastic features, especially in the granulocytic and erythroid lineages, generally supports accelerated phase, whereas 20% or more blasts indicate blast phase.[35] Almost all patients with myelodysplastic features or leukemic transformation show karyotypic evolution, often with the acquisition of complex chromosomal abnormalities. Development of blast phase is rare, with an incidence of 1% to 2% in patients treated with phlebotomy alone and may occur in the setting of post-polycythemia vera myelofibrosis.[32] The risk of progression appears to be higher in older patients. In virtually all cases, the blast phase is myeloid.[35] In grossly fibrotic bone marrow specimens that prevent aspiration, detection of blasts in the biopsy may be facilitated by immunostaining for CD34 and CD117. Splenic myeloid sarcoma or other type of extramedullary blast transformation can also be observed.

Although myelofibrotic progression and accelerated/blast phase are the most commonly recognized types of progression in polycythemia vera, in some cases of post-polycythemia vera myelofibrosis, the concurrence of elevated peripheral neutrophil counts and marked mature myeloid proliferation in the bone marrow may pose diagnostic difficulties.[36] Some of these cases may morphologically resemble chronic neutrophilic leukemia (CNL), a rare subtype of *BCR::ABL1* negative MPN characterized by the prevalence of normally segmented, nondysplastic neutrophils. Bone marrow biopsy in these neutrophilic polycythemia vera cases shows a striking proliferation of mature neutrophils, but there is no mutation in the cytoplasmic domain of the *CSF3R* receptor, a highly sensitive molecular marker for chronic neutrophilic leukemia. In addition, there are cases of progressive post-polycythemia vera myelofibrosis presenting with neutrophilic leukocytosis (WBC $\geq 13 \times 10^9$/l) with ≥10% immature myeloid cells in the peripheral blood, morphologically overlapping with atypical chronic myeloid leukemia (aCML).[36] In these cases, the history of polycythemia vera, the absence of severe dysplastic features and wild-type *SETBP1* may help exclude such an alternative diagnostic possibility.

Extramedullary tissues

Splenomegaly becomes prominent in post-polycythemia vera myelofibrosis in contrast to the polycythemic phase, where minimal to moderate splenomegaly is due to the increased number of RBCs in the sinuses with minimal or no EMH. A similar pattern of EMH is seen in the liver. EMH needs to be distinguished from extramedullary blast transformation (ie, myeloid sarcoma). Immunohistochemistry with CD34 and other myeloid markers can be useful in confirming a blast preponderant proliferation.

Immunophenotype

In general, immunophenotyping does not facilitate the diagnosis of polycythemic polycythemia vera. However, advanced-stage disease eg, post-polycythemia vera myelofibrosis, can be associated with increased blasts and immunohistochemistry can be useful in documenting progression to accelerate/blast phase. The main role of flow cytometry in polycythemia vera is in the blast phase. In almost all cases flow cytometry reveals a population of early committed CD34+ myeloid blasts.[35]

Genetics

Virtually all cases of polycythemia vera are driven by a mutation in the Janus kinase 2 (*JAK2*) gene.[4] Approximately 95% of patients have the activating *JAK2V* 617F mutation in exon 14, and most of the remaining cases reveal a *JAK2* mutation in exon 12.[37] Considering the central role of *JAK2* mutations in polycythemia vera, it is important to recognize the need for diagnostic assays with <1% sensitivity.[15] Also, the possibility of other noncanonical *JAK2* mutations should be considered in *JAK2* V617F-negative cases. The *JAK2* V617F is not unique to polycythemia vera but is present in 50% to 60% of cases of essential thrombocythemia and PMF, occasionally in MDS/MPN, and in rare cases of acute myeloid leukemia.[4] Homozygosity for *JAK2* V617F is more common in polycythemia vera than in other MPN subtypes carrying the mutation.[5] Additional somatic mutations such as *TET2*, *ASXL1*, *SRSF2*, *IDH2*, and *EZH2* can be found in patients with polycythemia vera and are generally associated with poorer survival.[38] Karyotype abnormalities that are not specific for polycythemia vera, may be detected in 10% to 20% of patients at diagnosis, the most common of which are +9 (5%), loss of Y (4%), +8 (3%), and del(20q) (3%).[38] An abnormal karyotype has been associated with inferior overall survival.[38]

Prognosis and Clinical Comment

Thrombotic events are the major clinical complications in polycythemia vera, affecting overall survival and contributing to disease-related comorbidity.[25] The rate of thrombosis in polycythemia vera is estimated to be between 2.6% and 4.4% of patients per year.[31,39] Age over 65 years and a history of thrombosis are both associated with an increased risk (so-called high-risk patients) and shorter survival. In addition, WBC $\geq 15 \times 10^9$/L is also an independent risk factor for thrombosis and reduced survival,[40] whereas the *JAK2* V617F allele burden has been variably associated with thrombotic risk.[31,41] Median overall survival in treated polycythemia vera exceeds 13 years but is generally much higher in patients diagnosed younger than 40 years.[25,42] The reported overall mortality rate is 3.7 deaths per 100 persons/year.[43] Cardiovascular mortality, solid tumors, and hematologic transformation account for 45%, 20%, and 13% of the deaths, respectively.[43] The cumulative risk of the blast phase is 2.3%, 5.5%, and 7.9% at 10, 15, and 20 years, respectively.[25] Prognostic stratification is enhanced by the inclusion of molecular data, especially *SRSF2* mutations and abnormal karyotype, and allows separation of distinct risk groups with an estimated median survival range of 5.4 to 25.3 years for high- and low-risk patients.[38]

ESSENTIAL THROMBOCYTHEMIA

Definition

Essential thrombocythemia (ET) is characterized by a sustained thrombocytosis ($\geq 450 \times 10^9$/L) that is not associated with any of the known reactive causes and a characteristic proliferation of megakaryocytes in the bone marrow.[1] Nearly 90% of patients with essential thrombocythemia have a mutation in one of the three driver genes and additional mutations and cytogenetic abnormalities are rare (<10% of patients).[4]

Synonyms

None.

Epidemiology

The incidence of essential thrombocythemia is estimated to be 1.2 to 3.0 per 100,000 population per year with a slight predominance among women.[9] The age distribution is broad, ranging from adolescents to elderly patients; most cases are seen in patients older than 50 years, but well-documented cases in young adults and children with a relatively benign course have been reported.[44] Rare familial forms of essential thrombocythemia may also occur, and when it is diagnosed in a child, it is reasonable to determine whether the disorder is acquired or familial by examining and testing the parents and other family members.[45] Although patients with essential thrombocythemia have a near-normal life expectancy, they have an increased risk of thrombosis and/or hemorrhage.[46,47]

General Clinical Features

Up to 50% of patients with essential thrombocythemia are diagnosed incidentally when thrombocytosis is noted on a complete blood count obtained for another reason or a routine check-up.[47] Others may present with disease-related symptoms such as headache, dizziness, visual changes, or complications related to thrombosis, bleeding, or first-trimester fetal loss.[23] The risk of cerebrovascular events, myocardial infarction, superficial thrombophlebitis, deep vein thrombosis, pulmonary embolism, and hemorrhage at diagnosis is modulated by qualitative and quantitative platelet alterations and patient comorbidities.[47] Importantly, patients with platelet counts >1000 × 10^9/L are at high risk of bleeding due to an acquired von Willebrand disease, which most likely results from adsorption of von Willebrand factor to abnormal blood cells, in particular platelets. Reported incidence rates of thrombosis and hemorrhage at diagnosis range from 9% to 22% and 3% to 37%, respectively.[39,48] During follow-up, the reported rates of subsequent thrombosis and hemorrhage range from 7% to 31% and 8% to 14%, respectively, with a median follow-up of 3 to 11 years.[49] Splenomegaly is typically absent but mild splenomegaly may be seen in approximately 15% to 20% of the cases, whereas hepatomegaly is rare.[26]

Morphology

The diagnosis of essential thrombocythemia requires integration of clinical, morphologic, laboratory, and molecular data and adequate, well-prepared peripheral blood smear and bone marrow biopsy specimens (Table 2.6).[1]

Peripheral blood

In essential thrombocythemia, peripheral blood smears show an overall excess of platelets that can range from 450 to more than 2000 × 10^9/L.[50] Platelets often show anisocytosis, ranging from tiny forms to abnormally large or giant platelets that may display bizarre shapes, pseudopods, and rarely agranularity. The mean platelet volume is significantly increased due to the large platelet size, whereas the observed high platelet distribution width reflects the broad spectrum of platelet sizes.[47] Circulating megakaryocyte nuclei and cytoplasmic fragments may be observed. WBC and leukocyte differential counts are usually normal. RBCs may be hypochromic and microcytic as a consequence of iron deficiency secondary to hemorrhages. A leukoerythroblastic picture with teardrop-shaped RBCs (dacryocytes), poikilocytosis, and circulating nucleated red cells and maturing myeloid precursors suggests transformation to post-essential thrombocythemia myelofibrosis (post-ET MF).[51] Patients with mutated *CALR* have been reported to have lower Hb levels but higher platelet counts than those with mutated *JAK2*.[50]

Bone marrow

Bone marrow aspirate smears may not be as informative as the mandatory bone marrow biopsy. The smears usually show large megakaryocytes, often associated with large pools of platelets. Emperipolesis of

TABLE 2.6 Diagnostic criteria for Essential Thrombocythemia (ET)

Major Criteria

1. Platelet count ≥ 450 × 10^9/L
2. Bone marrow biopsy showing proliferation mainly of the megakaryocytic lineage, with increased numbers of enlarged, mature megakaryocytes with hyperlobulated staghorn-like nuclei, infrequently dense clusters;[a] no significant increase or left shift in neutrophil granulopoiesis or erythropoiesis; no relevant BM fibrosis[b]
3. Diagnostic criteria for *BCR::ABL1*-positive chronic myeloid leukemia, polycythemia vera, primary myelofibrosis or other myeloid neoplasms are not met
4. *JAK2*, *CALR*, or *MPL* mutation[c]

Minor Criteria

Presence of a clonal marker[d] or absence of evidence of reactive thrombocytosis[e]

The diagnosis of essential thrombocythemia requires either all major criteria or the first three major criteria plus the minor criteria.

[a]Three or more megakaryocytes lying adjacent without other BM cells in between; in most of these rare clusters < 6 megakaryocytes may be observed, increase in large clusters (≥6 cells) accompanied by granulocytic proliferation is a morphological hallmark of pre-PMF.

[b]Very rarely a minor increase in reticulin fibers may occur at initial diagnosis (MF-1).[16,21]

[c]Highly sensitive assays for *JAK2* V617F (sensitivity level < 1%) and *CALR* and *MPL* (sensitivity level 1% to 3%) are recommended; in negative cases, search for noncanonical *JAK2* and *MPL* mutations should be considered.

[d]Assessed by cytogenetics or sensitive NGS techniques.

[e]Reactive causes of thrombocytosis include a variety of underlying conditions such as iron deficiency, chronic infection, chronic inflammatory disease, medication, neoplasia, or history of splenectomy.

neutrophils is sometimes seen; however, this is not specific and may be seen in megakaryocytes from normal or reactive bone marrow samples. Bone marrow biopsy is key for diagnosing essential thrombocythemia and to distinguish it from prefibrotic primary myelofibrosis (pre-PMF), polycythemia vera, and other MPNs, as well as other myeloid neoplasms associated with thrombocytosis, and last, from reactive thrombocytosis.[52] Characteristically, the bone marrow is normocellular for the patient's age with moderate hypercellularity only being seen in rare patients (Figures 2.4 and 2.5). The myeloid to erythroid ratio is usually normal, but in a few cases a preponderance of erythroid precursors may be found, especially if the patient has had recurrent major bleeding or is pretreated with hydroxyurea, but granulocytic proliferation is highly unusual.[10,22] Megakaryopoiesis is always increased with random distribution of megakaryocytes or very loose groupings within the bone marrow space. Megakaryocytic cytology includes mostly large to giant forms with abundant mature cytoplasm and deeply lobulated and hyperlobulated (staghorn) nuclei.[13] Dense megakaryocytic

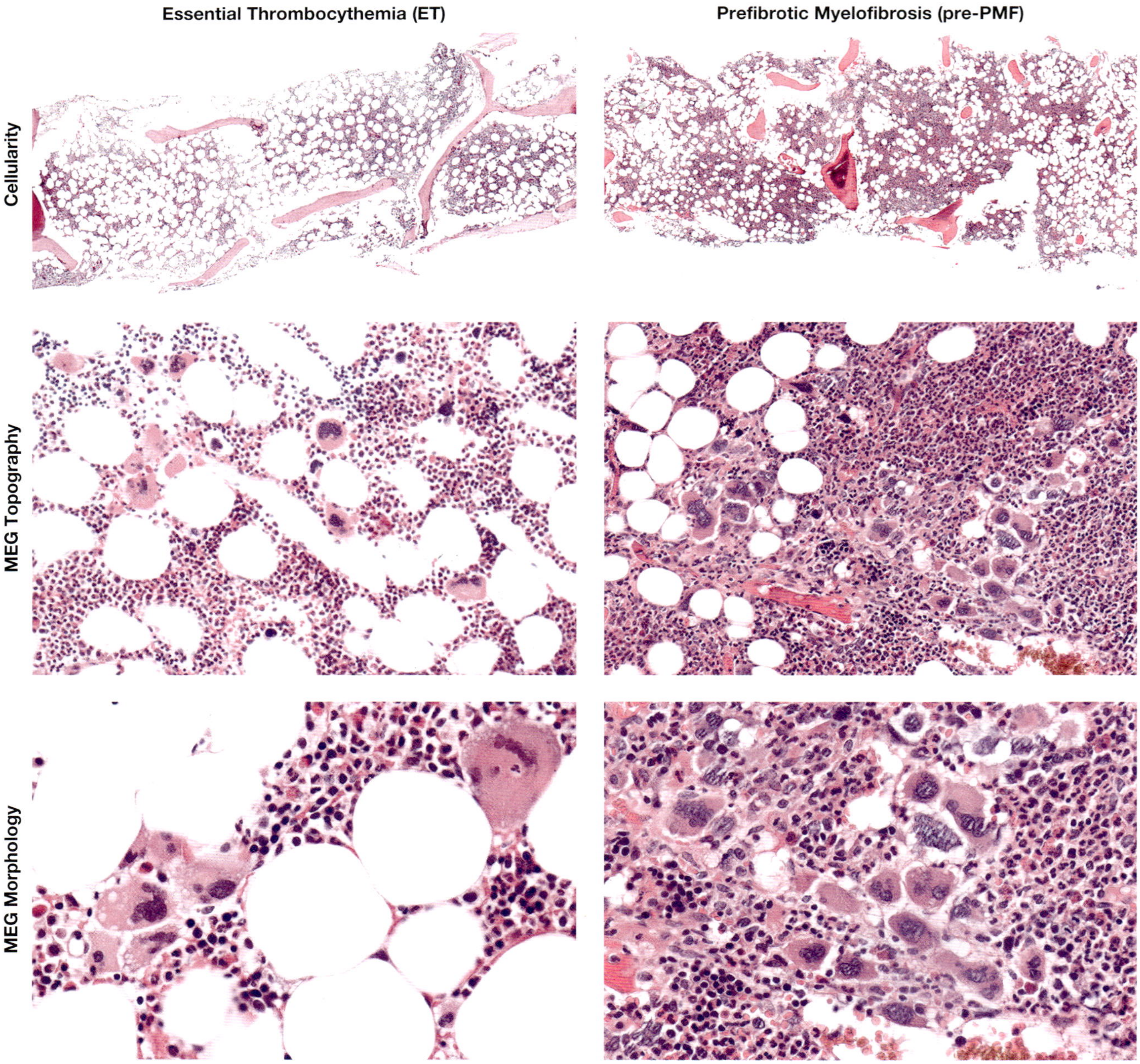

FIGURE 2.4 Morphological features of essential thrombocythemia and prefibrotic myelofibrosis. Key morphologic differences between essential thrombocythemia and pre-PMF include cellularity, megakaryocyte topography, and especially megakaryocyte morphology with characteristic clustering in pre-PMF. In essential thrombocythemia, small clusters (<6 megakaryocytes) may be seen, but no morphologic atypia. In contrast, megakaryocytes in pre-PMF show an altered nuclear/cytoplasmic ratio with hypolobated (bulky, cloud-like) nuclei and an overall bizarre appearance. (hematoxylin & eosin, top 10×, middle 20×, bottom 40×.)

clusters, defined as three or more megakaryocytes with no other marrow cells in between, are rare. The finding of bizarre, highly atypical megakaryocytes or frequent large dense clusters (≥6 megakaryocytes) is not seen in essential thrombocythemia. When present, differential diagnosis with pre-PMF can be challenging, but the lack of megakaryocyte atypia (increased nuclear/cytoplasmic ratio, irregular chromatin clumping, and bulbous appearance), lack of granulocytic proliferation, and lack of clinical features such anemia, leukocytosis, elevated LDH, or splenomegaly are key to distinguishing these cases from pre-PMF.[2] In addition, the finding of even a mild degree of combined granulocytic and erythroid proliferation should raise the possibility of an early stage of polycythemia vera. The network of reticulin fibers is usually normal or very rarely (less than 5%) minimally increased (MF-1), and the finding of significant reticulin fibrosis (ie, ≥MF-2) or any

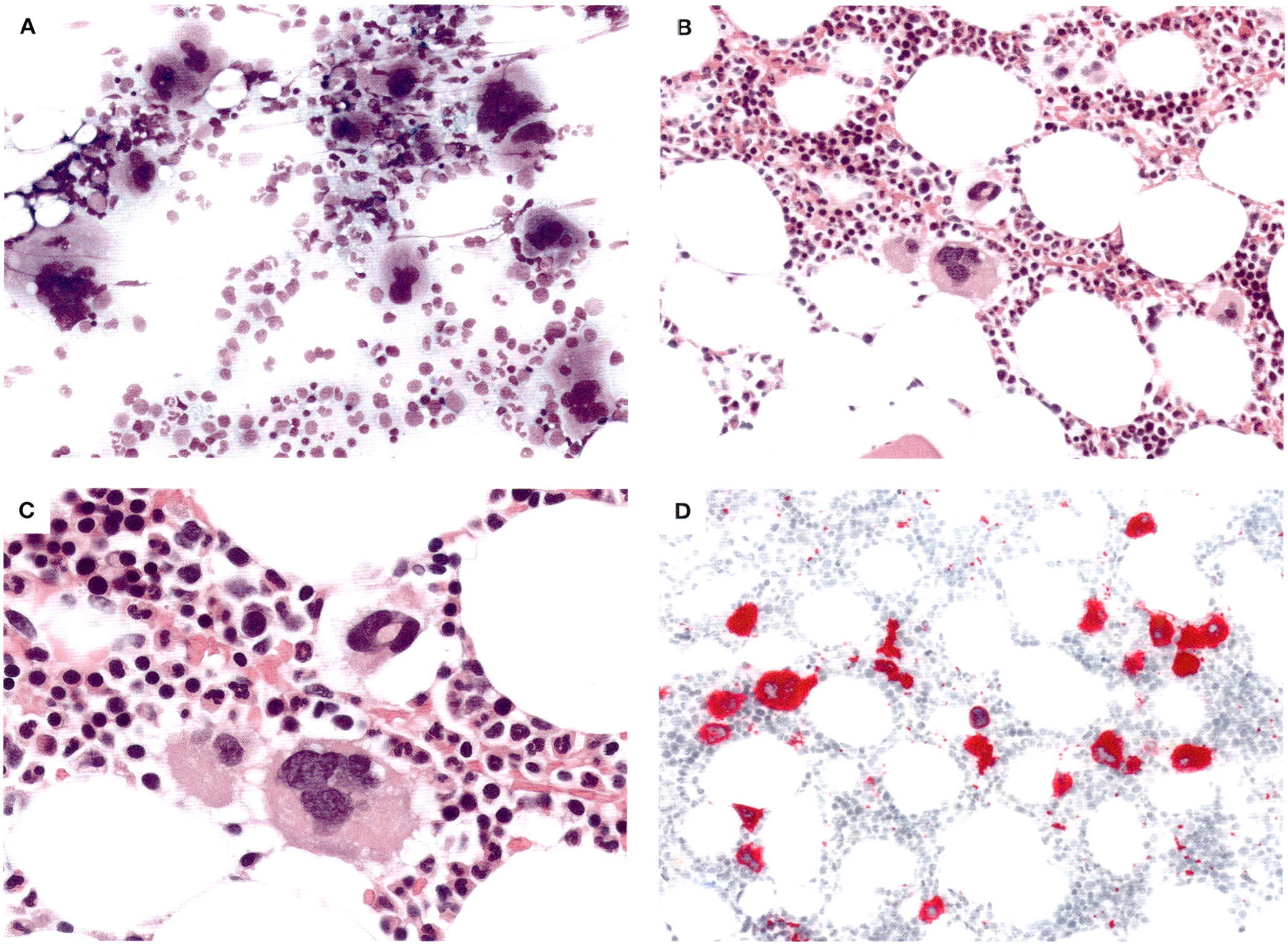

FIGURE 2.5 Essential thrombocythemia (ET). **A:** Bone marrow aspirate smear generally shows an increase in the number and size of the megakaryocytes with deeply lobulated megakaryocytic nuclei. **B:** Bone marrow biopsy shows normal cellularity but increased numbers of medium to large megakaryocytes with hyperlobulated nuclei, no significant increase in erythropoiesis or granulopoiesis is seen. **C:** Loose clusters of megakaryocytes may be observed; enlarged megakaryocytes show abundant amounts of mature cytoplasm, and nuclei are deeply lobulated (staghorn-like) nuclei. **D:** Dense clustering of megakaryocytes is not seen in essential thrombocythemia. (**A:** Wright-Giemsa, **B** and **C:** hematoxylin & eosin; **D:** CD61; **A** and **C:** 60×, **B:** 40×, **D:** 20×.)

collagen fibrosis excludes the diagnosis of essential thrombocythemia.[52]

Post-essential thrombocythemia myelofibrosis

The exact incidence of secondary myelofibrotic transformation into post-essential thrombocythemia myelofibrosis remains controversial and is certainly influenced by clinical risk status and diagnostic criteria used but is generally very low. The 15-year cumulative risk has been reported to be 4%, but the risk of myelofibrotic transformation in essential thrombocythemia is much lower than the risk of thrombosis (17% at 15 years).[9] Disease transformation should be suspected in patients with unexpected cytopenias, circulating blasts, and other immature forms, and worsening of essential thrombocythemia-associated symptoms.[53] In these patients, careful bone marrow evaluation is critical, as the presence of MF-2 or MF-3 bone marrow fibrosis is a prerequisite for diagnosis (Table 2.7).[33]

Accelerated and blast phase

Very rarely, essential thrombocythemia may progress to blast phase, which is defined by 20% or more blasts in the blood or bone marrow, whereas the finding of 10% to 19% blasts indicates an accelerated phase. The risk of blast transformation has been documented with a range of 2% to 3.3% at 15-year follow-up.[54] Low hemoglobin levels (<12 g/dL in women, <13.5 in men) and platelet counts $\geq 1000 \times 10^9$/L were identified as major risk factors in multivariate analysis, whereas *JAK2* V617F mutation levels or treatment with cytoreductive

TABLE 2.7 Diagnostic criteria for post-essential thrombocythemia myelofibrosis (post-ET MF)

Required criteria
1. Previous established diagnosis of essential thrombocythemia
2. Bone marrow fibrosis of grade 2 or 3[16,21]
Additional criteria
1. Anemia (ie, below the reference range given age, sex, and altitude considerations) and a >2 g/dL decrease from baseline hemoglobin concentration
2. Leukoerythroblastosis
3. Increase in palpable splenomegaly of >5 cm from baseline or the development of a newly palpable splenomegaly
4. Elevated lactate dehydrogenase (LDH) level above the reference range
5. Development of any two (or all three) of the following constitutional symptoms: >10% weight loss in 6 mo, night sweats, unexplained fever (>37.5 °C)
The diagnosis of post-essential thrombocythemia myelofibrosis is established by all required criteria and at least two additional criteria.

agents were not associated with progression. Similarly to polycythemia vera, immunohistochemistry and flow cytometry may be helpful in confirming the presence of an increased number of myeloid blasts.

Extramedullary tissues

Splenic enlargement is uncommon at the time of diagnosis; if present, it may be largely due to pooling and sequestration of platelets. EMH is absent or minimal.[26]

Immunophenotype

No aberrant phenotype has been described.

Genetics

Acquired gain-of-function mutations in *JAK2* V617F (50%-70%), *CALR* (20%-25%), and *MPL* (3%-8%) are found in most patients, but up to 10% of cases may be clonally undefined, ie, wild-type or triple-negative.[4,5,15] The type of driver mutation is not helpful in differentiating essential thrombocythemia from other MPN subtypes presenting with thrombocytosis, especially pre-PMF, although it may be associated with clinically relevant consequences: *JAK2* V617F is associated with older age, higher hemoglobin level, leukocytosis, lower platelet count and increased risk of thrombosis.[50] In contrast, *CALR* mutation is associated with higher platelet count, younger age, but lower incidence of thrombotic events. Platelet count is significantly higher in type 2 versus type 1 *CALR*-mutated patients and male sex is more often associated with only type 1. Patients with *CALR*-mutated essential thrombocythemia belong more frequently to the low-risk group. Additional somatic mutations are seen in a small number of patients, the most common being *TET2* and *ASXL1*. The presence of high-molecular-risk mutations (eg, *TP53*, *SF3B1*, *SRSF2*, *U2AF1*) has been shown to affect overall survival, myelofibrosis-free survival, and leukemia-free survival.[38] Less than 7% of patients with essential thrombocythemia show an abnormal karyotype at diagnosis, including loss of chromosome Y only (-Y) in 2%, and abnormalities other than -Y in 4.8%, the most frequent being del(20q).[55] Abnormal karyotype, other than -Y, is associated with older age, higher leukocyte count, history of arterial thrombosis, and overall reduced survival.[55]

Prognosis and Clinical Comment

Life expectancy is normal for most patients with essential thrombocythemia, but thrombotic and hemorrhagic complications can be the major cause of morbidity and mortality.[9,39,46,47,49] Median survival shows a range of approximately 11 to 35 years, with a median of 35 years for patients 40 years of age or younger, and 11 years for patients >60 years of age.[56] Thrombotic risk is increased in older patients with a history of thrombosis, *JAK2* V617F mutation, and cardiovascular risk factors.[57] Transformation to blast phase is considerably low (2%-3% at 15 years) and is often associated with advanced age, extreme thrombocytosis, anemia, leukocytosis, and mutations involving *TP53* and *EZH2*.[32,54] Accordingly, the cumulative probability of myelofibrotic progression to post-essential thrombocythemia myelofibrosis is approximately 4% at 15 years but is increased in patients with *JAK2* V617F allele burden >35% and *CALR* type 1/1-like or *MPL* mutations.[53]

PRIMARY MYELOFIBROSIS

Definition

Primary myelofibrosis (PMF) is a clonal hematopoietic stem cell disorder characterized by proliferation of abnormal megakaryocytes and granulocytes in the bone marrow and associated in its full-blown stage with variable degrees of bone marrow fibrosis, cytopenias, constitutional symptoms, hepatosplenomegaly, and/or EMH.[58] Its initial prefibrotic stage (pre-PMF) is defined by absent or minimal bone marrow fibrosis. Pre-PMF may clinically mimic ET by presenting with isolated thrombocytosis and thrombohemorrhagic complications[52]; however, the distinction from essential thrombocythemia is clinically relevant because pre-PMF has a higher risk of major bleeding, arterial and venous thrombotic events, and an increased risk of leukemic progression.[9,49,59-63] Many, but not all, patients with pre-PMF develop a stepwise progression to overt myelofibrosis (overt PMF) in which a marked reticulin or collagen fibrosis often associated with osteosclerosis is seen in the bone marrow.[52] It is important to note that bone marrow fibrosis alone is not diagnostic of PMF, as other myeloid malignancies may present with varying degrees of bone marrow fibrosis.[16] Among the classical MPN subtypes, PMF has the overall worst prognosis due to a higher frequency of disease progression including leukemic transformation, thrombohemorrhagic complications, and infections.[8,58] The diagnosis of PMF, both prefibrotic and overt stage, requires the integration of clinical, morphologic, and genetic findings.[1]

Synonyms

None.

Epidemiology

PMF most commonly affects middle-aged to elderly individuals and is rarely seen in younger age. The median age at diagnosis is in the sixth to seventh decade, and less than 10% of patients are younger than 40 years.[42] The overt fibrotic phase is estimated to occur in 0.5 to 1.5 per 100,000 persons per year, with approximately equal incidence in men and women.[8] Valid data on the incidence of pre-PMF are not available, as many of these cases were previously diagnosed as essential thrombocythemia.[9] In larger reclassification studies, the incidence of pre-PMF is estimated to range between 14% and 18% in patients clinically presenting as essential thrombocythemia.[9] PMF is extremely rare in children and some cases have been described suggesting a familial predisposition.[45] Pediatric patients show lower rates of the driver mutations typically found in adults and less frequently experience thrombotic events, disease progression to overt myelofibrosis, and acute leukemia.[44,45] The exact cause of PMF is unknown, but exposure to benzene or ionizing radiation has been documented in some cases.

Prefibrotic Primary Myelofibrosis

Pre-PMF is defined as a distinct entity within the group of classical *BCR::ABL1*-negative MPNs that must be distinguished from other subtypes (Table 2.8),[1] particularly essential thrombocythemia, by its clinical complications, progression profile, and characteristic morphologic features.[9] Bone marrow biopsy is an integral part of the diagnostic process, and laboratory parameters are used to complement and not replace the morphologic diagnosis.[10]

TABLE 2.8 Diagnostic criteria for Prefibrotic Primary Myelofibrosis (pre-PMF)

Major criteria
1. Bone marrow biopsy showing megakaryocytic proliferation and atypia,[a] bone marrow fibrosis grade <2,[16,21] increased age-adjusted bone marrow cellularity, granulocytic proliferation, and (often) decreased erythropoiesis
2. *JAK2*, *CALR*, or *MPL* mutation[b]
or
presence of another clonal marker[c]
or
absence of reactive bone marrow reticulin fibrosis[d]
3. Diagnostic criteria for *BCR::ABL1*-positive chronic myeloid leukemia, polycythemia vera, essential thrombocythemia, myelodysplastic syndromes, or other myeloid neoplasms are not met
Minor criteria
1. Anemia not attributed to a comorbid condition
2. Leukocytosis ≥11 × 10^9/L
3. Palpable splenomegaly
4. Lactate dehydrogenase level above the reference range

The diagnosis of pre-PMF requires all three major criteria and at least one minor criterion confirmed in two consecutive determinations.

[a]Morphology of megakaryocytes in pre-PMF demonstrates a high degree of megakaryocytic atypia including small to giant megakaryocytes with a prevalence of severe maturation defects (cloud-like, bulbous-like hypolobulated, and hyperchromatic nuclei) and presence of abnormal large dense clusters (>6 megakaryocytes lying strictly adjacent).

[b]Highly sensitive assays for *JAK2* V617F (sensitivity level <1%) and *CALR* and *MPL* (sensitivity level 1%-3%) are recommended; in negative cases, search for noncanonical *JAK2* and *MPL* mutations should be considered.

[c]Assessed by cytogenetics or sensitive NGS techniques; detection of mutations associated with myeloid neoplasms (eg, *ASXL1*, *EZH2*, *IDH1*, *IDH2*, *SF3B1*, *SRSF2*, and *TET2* mutations) supports the clonal nature of the disease.

[d]Minimal reticulin fibrosis (MF-1) can be seen secondary to infection, autoimmune disorder or other chronic inflammatory conditions, hairy cell leukemia or another lymphoid neoplasm, metastatic malignancy, or toxic (chronic) myelopathies.

General clinical features

At diagnosis, approximately 30% to 40% of patients with pre-PMF are asymptomatic and present with significant thrombocytosis as a prominent feature.[61,63,64] The clinical presentation may also include mild anemia, leukocytosis, and especially elevated LDH levels, whereas significant anemia or leukoerythroblastosis with circulating immature WBCs are very rare.[52] Compared with overt PMF, patients with pre-PMF are younger and have higher hemoglobin, leukocyte, and platelet counts.[62] Symptomatic cases are characterized by constitutional symptoms (fatigue, weight loss, night sweats, and dyspnea). The degree of splenomegaly varies with the duration of the disease and is present in approximately 45% of patients.[2] A higher rate of hemorrhagic complications has been reported in pre-PMF than in essential thrombocythemia, particularly in patients on aspirin medication.[49] In addition, elevated WBC counts have a significant impact on the incidence of arterial and venous thrombotic events.

Morphology

Morphologic examination is an integral part of the diagnostic process in pre-PMF.[10,52] The presence of laboratory features of pre-PMF in an otherwise suspected case of essential thrombocythemia should raise the possibility and suggest further evaluation, including bone marrow biopsy (see Table 2.8).[61]

Peripheral blood

The most common finding is a marked increase in platelets; mild neutrophilia with a left shift and anemia may also occur. A leukoerythroblastic blood picture with nucleated erythrocytes and circulating myeloid precursors as well as teardrop-shaped RBCs, however, is not seen in pre-PMF.[62] Most patients present with moderate to marked thrombocytosis (mean platelet count, 962×10^9/L; range, 104-3215 $\times 10^9$/L), borderline anemia, mild leukocytosis, and elevated LDH levels.[63]

Bone marrow

The bone marrow usually reveals age-adjusted hypercellularity characterized by a variably prominent megakaryocytic and granulocytic proliferation with increased myeloid/erythroid ratio usually associated with a slight reduction of erythropoiesis (Figures 2.5 and 2.6).[10,52] By definition, reticulin fibrosis is absent (MF-0) or mild (MF-1).[1] Therefore, the demonstration of reticulin fibrosis is not a required criterion for the diagnosis of pre-PMF. The identification of abnormal megakaryocytic histotopography (distribution within the bone marrow space) and megakaryocytic atypia are key features to recognize pre-PMF.[52] The megakaryocytes often form dense and large clusters (the latter defined as ≥6 megakaryocytes) frequently adjacent to bone marrow vascular sinuses or bony trabeculae. Most megakaryocytes show a large size, but small megakaryocytes may also be seen. Deviations from the normal nuclear/cytoplasmic ratio, abnormal patterns of chromatin clumping with cloud-like, hypolobulated and hyperchromatic nuclei, and the frequent occurrence of bare (naked) megakaryocytic nuclei are all typical features. In terms of distinguishing pre-PMF from essential thrombocythemia (as mentioned before the latter may occasionally display rare clusters of megakaryocytes), a diagnosis of pre-PMF should not be focused just on the megakaryocytic morphology but rather following a holistic approach based on a multiparametric assessment by evaluating the complete histologic pattern, including bone marrow cellularity, myeloid/erythroid ratio, the morphology of megakaryocytes, and size of their clusters, in conjunction with clinical and laboratory data.[2,10,52]

Immunophenotype

No abnormal phenotypic features have been reported.

Genetics

The incidence of MPN driver mutations in pre-PMF has been estimated to be 52% to 67% for *JAK2* V617F; 12.2% and 5.8% for *CALR* type 1 and type 2 mutations, respectively, and 4% to 6% for *MPL* W515L/K mutation.[9,63] Approximately 10% of patients are triple negative, which is generally associated with poorer survival.[65] In contrast, the presence of a *CALR* type 1 mutation is associated with a better prognosis.[62] Nondriver mutations are seen in pre-PMF in a subset of patients. These include high-risk mutations whose presence would place a patient in the so-called high mutation risk category (any mutation in *ASXL1*, *SRSF2*, *IDH1*, *IDH2*, *EZH2*), which occur in approximately 27% of cases. Their frequency is, however, higher in overt PMF.[62] Degree of fibrosis has been associated with higher frequencies of *ASXL1* and *EZH2* mutations, whereas the allelic burden of driver mutations is not associated with disease stage.[62] Overall, the observed combined pattern of driver and nondriver myeloid gene mutations may contribute to prognosis in pre-PMF. Abnormal cytogenetics can be found in approximately 18% of pre-PMF cases and unfavorable karyotypes in 4% to 8% (complex karyotype or single or two abnormalities including +8, −7/7q-, i(17q), −5/5q-, 12p-, inv(3), or 11q23 rearrangement).[62]

Prognosis and clinical comment

Median survival in pre-PMF is 11 to 17 years, compared to only 6 to 7 years in overt PMF.[63,64] The calculated overall incidences of overt myelofibrotic progression in pre-PMF after 5 and 10 years of follow-up are 2.3% and 12.3%, respectively. In contrast, the calculated risk in essential thrombocythemia cases is only 0.2% at 5 years and 0.8% at 10 years of follow-up.[9] Grade 1 reticulin fibrosis and anemia at initial diagnosis were identified as risk factors. Transformation to blast phase at 10 and 15 years is seen in 5.8% and 11.7%,

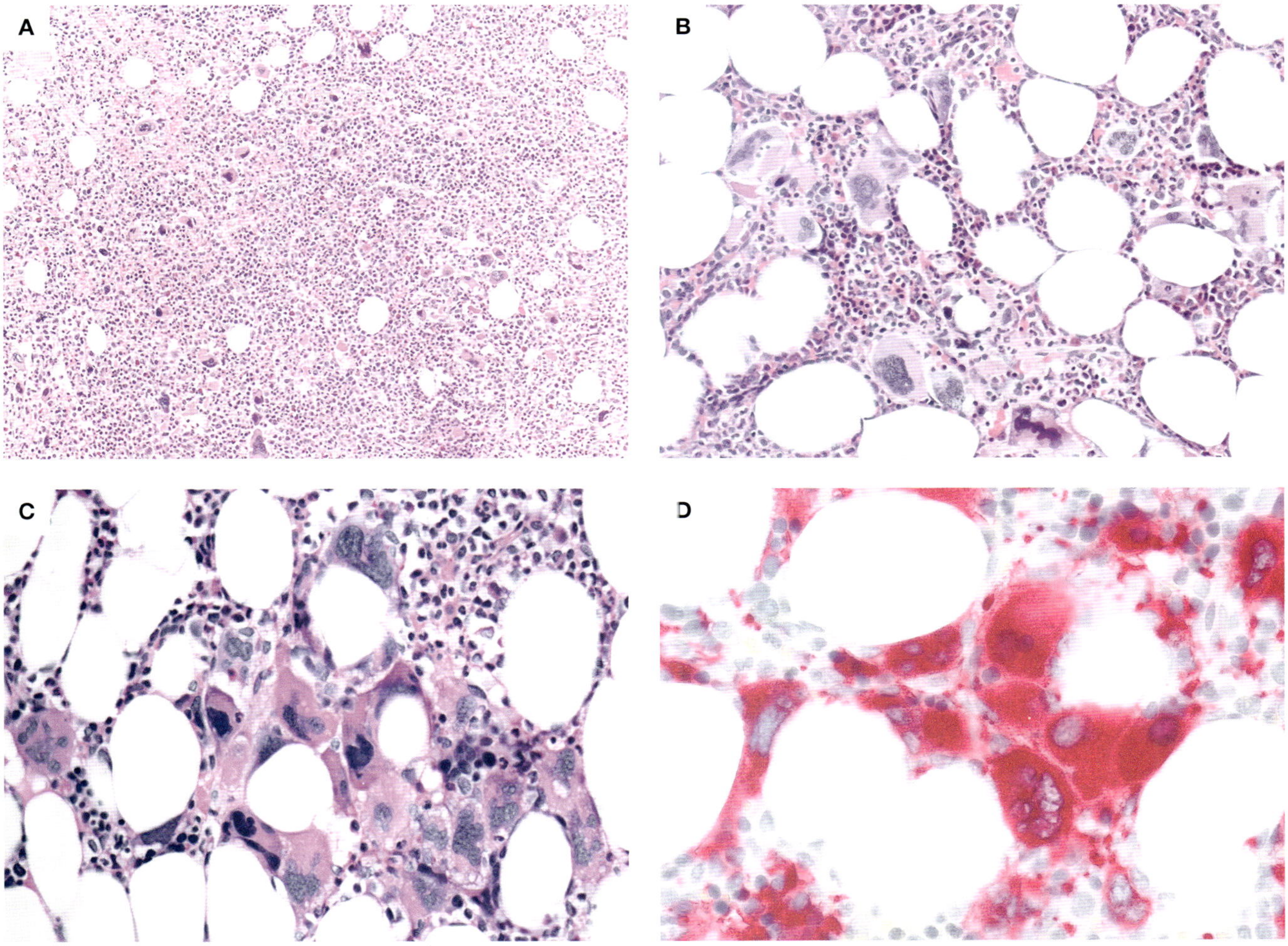

FIGURE 2.6 Prefibrotic myelofibrosis (pre-PMF). **A.** The bone marrow is hypercellular and shows a megakaryocytic and granulocytic proliferation. **B.** Increased numbers of atypical megakaryocytes with condensed nuclei revealing conspicuously clumped chromatin and abnormal nuclear-cytoplasmic ratio. **C.** Megakaryocytic abnormalities and extensive clustering (large clusters of ≥6 atypical cells) are key to the diagnosis. **D.** Abnormalities of megakaryopoiesis include anisocytosis, size variation, abnormal nuclear/cytoplasmic ratio, hyperchromatic, and hypolobated nuclei. (**A** and **B:** hematoxylin & eosin; **C:** PAS; **D:** CD61; **A:** 20×, **C** and **D:** 40×, **D:** 60×.)

respectively.[9] Variables associated with blast phase progression include age >65 years, leukocytosis (WBC > 15 × 10^9/L), LDH ratio >1.5 times the institutional norm, and cytogenetic abnormalities. The risk of major hemorrhagic complications is increased in pre-PMF, whereas the risk of arterial and venous thrombosis is similar to essential thrombocythemia.[49]

Overt PMF

PMF in its overt fibrotic stage (overt PMF) is an MPN subtype associated with bone marrow fibrosis, cytopenias, constitutional symptoms, hepatosplenomegaly, and/or EMH (Table 2.9).[26] Approximately 10% to 15% of cases of overt PMF represent progression from pre-PMF.[18] Overt-PMF has the worst prognosis among the MPNs, and patients are at higher risk for disease progression, leukemic transformation, thrombohemorrhagic complications, and infections.[8] Bone marrow fibrosis is the hallmark of PMF and contributes to the impaired hematopoiesis. It is a secondary phenomenon induced by growth factors abnormally released from clonally expanded, atypical megakaryocytes and an inflammatory signature of the bone marrow microenvironment, which collectively result in abnormal deposition of excess collagen derived from nonclonal fibroblasts.[26,58] Microenvironmental changes are also at least partially responsible for altering the hematopoietic stem cell niche resulting in increased mobilization into the peripheral blood of marrow-derived progenitors and myeloid precursors, which in turn are responsible for the production of clonally related EMH.

TABLE 2.9 Diagnostic criteria for Overt Primary Myelofibrosis (Overt-PMF)

Major criteria

1. Bone marrow biopsy showing megakaryocytic proliferation and atypia,[a] accompanied by reticulin and/or collagen fibrosis grades 2 or 3[16,21]
2. *JAK2*, *CALR*, or *MPL* mutation[b]

   or

   presence of another clonal marker[c]

   or

   absence of reactive bone marrow reticulin fibrosis[d]
3. Diagnostic criteria for *BCR::ABL1*-positive chronic myeloid leukemia, polycythemia vera, essential thrombocythemia, myelodysplastic syndromes, or other myeloid neoplasms[e] are not met

Minor criteria

1. Anemia not attributed to a comorbid condition
2. Leukocytosis ≥11 × 10^9/L
3. Palpable splenomegaly
4. Lactate dehydrogenase level above the reference range
5. Leukoerythroblastosis

The diagnosis of PMF requires all three major criteria and at least one minor criterion confirmed in two consecutive determinations.

[a]Morphology of megakaryocytes in PMF demonstrates a high degree of megakaryocytic atypia including small to giant megakaryocytes with a prevalence of severe maturation defects (cloud-like, hypolobulated, and hyperchromatic nuclei) and presence of abnormal large dense clusters (mostly >6 megakaryocytes lying strictly adjacent).
[b]Highly sensitive assays for *JAK2* V617F (sensitivity level <1%) and *CALR* and *MPL* (sensitivity level 1%-3%) are recommended; in negative cases, search for noncanonical *JAK2* and *MPL* mutations should be considered.
[c]Assessed by cytogenetics or sensitive NGS techniques; detection of mutations associated with myeloid neoplasms (eg, *ASXL1*, *EZH2*, *IDH1*, *IDH2*, *SF3B1*, *SRSF2*, and *TET2* mutations) supports the clonal nature of the disease.
[d]Reticulin fibrosis secondary to infection, autoimmune disorder or other chronic inflammatory conditions, hairy cell leukemia or another lymphoid neoplasm, metastatic malignancy, or toxic (chronic) myelopathies.
[e]Monocytosis can be present at diagnosis or develop during the course of PMF; in these cases, a history of MPN excludes chronic myelomonocytic leukemia (CMML). Furthermore, a higher variant allelic frequency for MPN-associated driver mutations supports the diagnosis of PMF with monocytosis rather than CMML. In contrast, multi-hit *TET2* mutations, often in combination with mutated *ASXL1* and *SRSF2*, are very common in CMML.

General clinical features

The most common clinical manifestations of PMF include severe anemia, hepatosplenomegaly, constitutional symptoms (eg, fatigue, night sweats, fever), cachexia, bone pain, splenic infarction, pruritus, thrombosis, and bleeding.[62] Approximately 15% to 30% of patients with overt PMF are asymptomatic at the time of initial presentation, and the diagnosis is made during evaluation for splenomegaly, hepatomegaly, or abnormal blood findings.[26] Splenomegaly and hepatomegaly are due to the presence of EMH associated with PMF. Elevated serum concentrations of alkaline phosphatase, lactate dehydrogenase, uric acid, leukocyte alkaline phosphatase, and vitamin B12 are common findings.[64] Anemia with hemoglobin less than 10 g/dL is seen in about 50% of cases.[62] Platelet and leukocyte counts are variable. Marked leukocytosis (>30 × 10^9/L) and thrombocytosis (>500 × 10^9/L) occur in approximately 11% to 13% of patients at diagnosis, whereas leukopenia and thrombocytopenia become more common in disease progression.[54] The incidence of arterial and venous thrombotic events is approximately 2 per 100 patient-years.[66] Ineffective erythropoiesis and hepatosplenic EMH are the major causes of anemia and organomegaly, respectively. Causes of death in overt PMF include leukemic progression, which occurs in approximately 20% of patients, and comorbid conditions, including cardiovascular events and consequences of cytopenias, including infection or bleeding.[58,67]

Morphology

Myelofibrosis is characterized by an increase in the amount of reticulin and collagen fibers, which is associated with the clonal proliferation of hematopoietic stem cells.[2] Although bone marrow fibrosis is a hallmark of overt PMF, any subtype of MPN can progress to myelofibrosis, and accumulation of fibers can be observed in a wide variety of other diseases, both benign and malignant. Therefore, integrating clinical features, laboratory data, molecular profile, and bone marrow morphology is the cornerstone of diagnosing PMF (see Table 2.9).[1]

Peripheral blood

The peripheral smear in overt PMF is characterized by anisocytosis, poikilocytosis, and variable numbers of teardrop-shaped RBCs (dacrocytes). Hypersegmented neutrophils and fragmented megakaryocytes are common. Platelets may be abnormally large with altered granulation. The presence of normoblasts and circulating immature myeloid cells is common as part of the leukoerythroblastic blood picture (Figure 2.7). Blasts generally account for less than 5% of the WBC.[1,12,13] In addition, the absolute number of circulating $CD34^+$ hematopoietic progenitor cells is increased.[58] Any increase in the blast count should prompt careful monitoring for further evidence of progression to an accelerated or blast phase.[54] A small subset of patients can present at onset or develop during the course of their disease sustained absolute monocyte counts greater than 1 × 10^9/L, which is generally considered indicative of progression and poor prognosis.[68]

Bone marrow

Bone marrow aspiration in overt PMF usually results in a dry tap due to the fibrotic marrow. In addition, the result of aspiration alone, if successful, is not diagnostic.

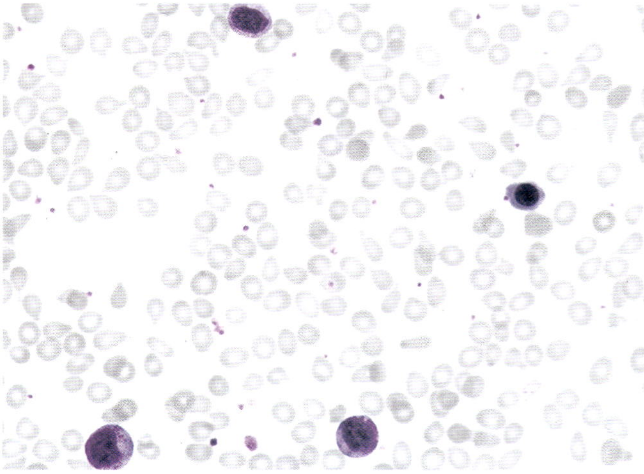

FIGURE 2.7 Leukoerythroblastic blood picture. Peripheral blood smear demonstrates leukoerythroblastosis with numerous tear-drop-shaped red blood cells (dacryocytes), immature neutrophils and a normoblast. (Wright-Giemsa, 60×.)

The most common findings include the presence of a neutrophilic proliferation in association with a proliferation of morphologically atypical megakaryocytes often forming dense clusters (Figure 2.8). Therefore, a bone marrow biopsy is essential for the diagnosis of overt PMF. In most cases, the bone marrow is hypercellular for the age, with increased granulopoiesis and decreased erythropoiesis.[22] The megakaryocytes form clusters of different sizes. However, a few large clusters (defined as ≥6 atypical megakaryocytes) are almost always observed. In some cases, a sheet-like proliferation of megakaryocytes can also occur. In a subset of cases showing prominent vascular ectasia megakaryocytes together with immature hematopoietic cells can be found predominantly localized within dilated vascular sinuses. Megakaryocytes, which vary from small- to large-sized cells, mostly display a hyperlobulated nucleus with a higher than normal nuclear/cytoplasmic

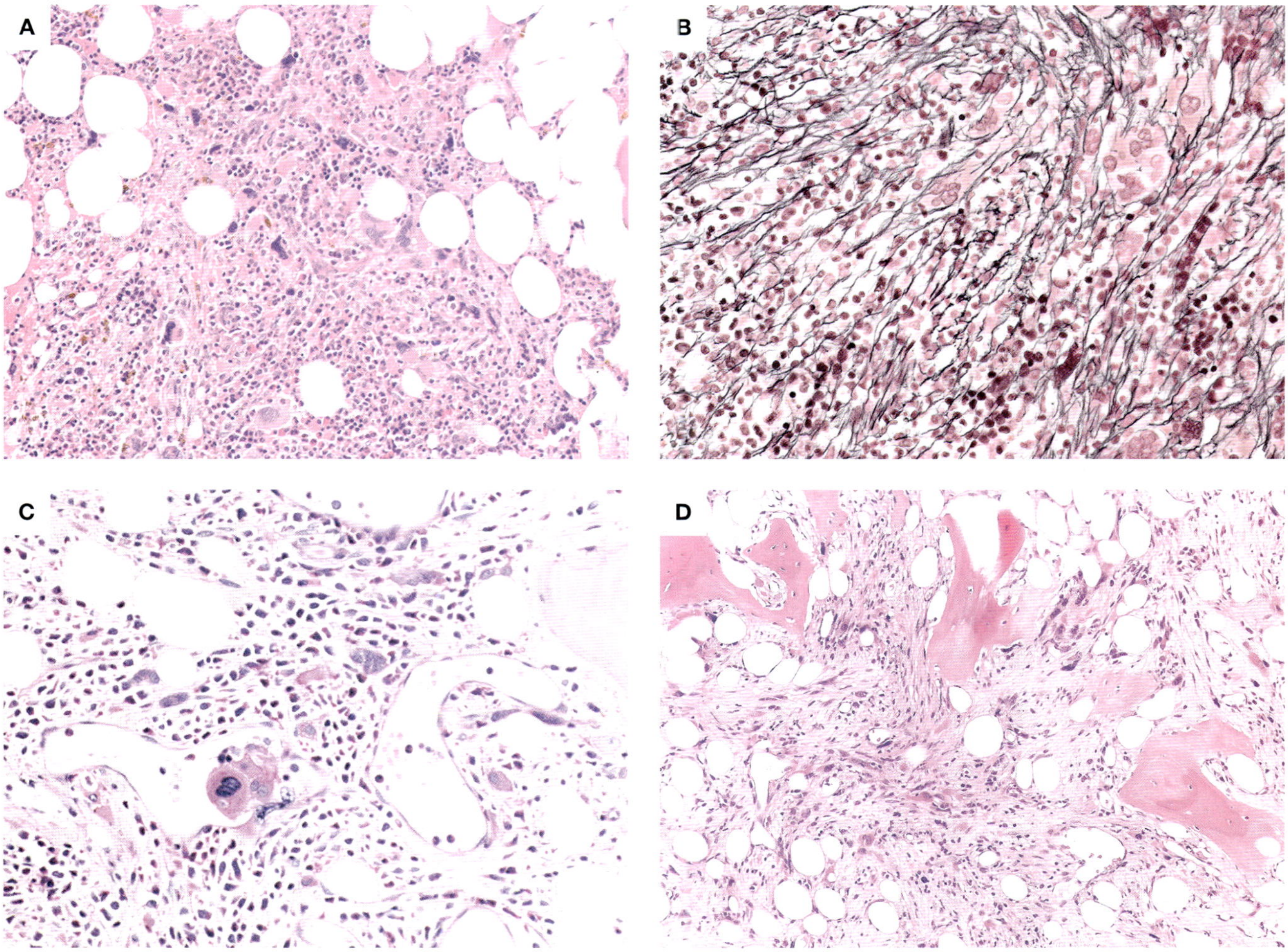

FIGURE 2.8 Overt myelofibrosis (PMF). **A:** Bone marrow biopsy specimen showing hypocellularity and grossly atypical megakaryocytes, often arranged in clusters. **B:** Overt reticulin and collagen fibrosis (MF-2). **C:** In more advanced, terminal stages dilated sinus containing megakaryocytes or immature hematopoietic elements are a common finding. **D:** Osteosclerotic stage of disease (MF-3, osteosclerosis grade 2) characterized by broad, irregular bone trabeculae and cellular depletion. (**A, C, D:** hematoxylin & eosin, **B:** Gomori's stain; **A** and **B:** 20×; **C** and **D:** 40×).

ratio. The nuclei may show plump cloud-like, or balloon-like features or may appear hyperchromatic. Numerous naked megakaryocytic nuclei may also be seen.[22]

Overt reticulin or collagen fibrosis (MF-2 or MF-3) is a hallmark of PMF and is often associated with varying degrees of osteosclerosis.[17] Trichrome staining is useful in identifying collagen deposition. With disease progression, the marrow cellularity decreases, and occasionally the bone marrow is almost devoid of hematopoietic cells, showing mainly dense reticulin or collagen fibrosis, with small islands of nucleated hematopoietic progenitors located mostly in vascular sinuses.[22] Osteoid seams or appositional new bone formation in bud-like endophytic plaques may be observed. In this osteosclerotic phase, the bone may form broad, irregular trabeculae that may occupy >50% of the bone marrow space. Lymphoid aggregates composed predominantly of reactive T lymphocytes may also be seen in many patients.

Accelerated and blast phase

The presence of 10% to 19% blasts in the blood or bone marrow indicates an accelerated stage of the disease, whereas 20% or more blasts define transformation to blast phase. Adverse cytogenetics and variants/mutations as well as the presence of *JAK2* variants are associated with a significant leukemogenic potential and reflect genomic instability.[69]

Extramedullary tissues

In advanced PMF, the development of EMH is common and foci of EMH may occur in almost any organ. Common sites of involvement include the spleen, liver, lymph nodes, lungs, kidneys, and gastrointestinal tract. EMH may also be found in soft tissues, body cavities, serosal surfaces, central nervous system, skin, and other sites. Many of the morphologic abnormalities seen in the peripheral blood of overt PMF, such as teardrop cells and leukoerythroblastosis, are caused by the abnormal release of cells into the blood from the sites of EMH, particularly the spleen and liver.[70] In the spleen, EMH causes expansion of the red pulp by a proliferation of erythroid, granulocytic, and megakaryocytic cells in association with increased neoangiogenesis. Occasionally, large aggregates of atypical megakaryocytes, growing cohesively, can produce macroscopically evident tumor lesions. Consistent with peripheral blood findings, a slight increase in $CD34^+$ cells can also be demonstrated in the spleen.[22,70] Because EMH is rarely as effective as medullary hematopoiesis, cytopenias are often seen in overt PMF. Diffuse granulocytic predominance appears to be associated with a worse prognosis. The spleen may be the site of extramedullary blast transformation. In the presence of nodular lesions and large amounts of EMH, the possibility of progression to myeloid sarcoma should be considered and carefully excluded by performing immunohistological studies with CD34 and CD117 and myeloid markers.[71]

Immunophenotype

No abnormal phenotypic features have been reported. Immunohistochemistry and flow cytometry play an important role in detecting and confirming leukemic transformation (ie, blast phase disease).

Genetics

Approximately 90% of PMF patients carry one of the MPN driver mutations (*JAK2* V617F: 57%-65%, *CALR*: 20%-25%, *MPL*: 5%-10%). *CALR* mutations are more common in younger patients with higher platelet counts, and patients with type 1 *CALR* mutations generally have the best clinical outcomes. Mutations other than *JAK2*, *CALR*, or *MPL*, including *ASXL1*, *SRSF2*, *IDH1*, *IDH2*, *EZH2*, *SF3B1*, and *TET2*, have been reported in up to 80% of patients.[5] Therefore, advanced molecular testing, including assessment for the presence of these mutations, may help confirm the clonal nature of triple-negative PMF cases.[4] However, in triple-negative cases showing pronounced dysplastic changes of erythro- and/or granulocytic cells and/or a preponderance of micromegakaryocytes and no prior history of MPN, a diagnosis of MDS/MPN may be more appropriate.[65] In addition, somatic noncanonical variants or germline *MPL* or *JAK2* variants have been identified in some patients with triple-negative PMF.[5]

In overt PMF, an abnormal karyotype is seen in 35% to 40% of patients, which is higher than reported for pre-PMF.[72] The most common abnormalities include del(20q), del(13q), +8, +9, and abnormalities of 1q. Complex karyotypes are found in about 15% of cases.[64] More than 90% of patients with transformation to blast phase have cytogenetic abnormalities, which are often complex and include abnormalities of chromosomes 5 and 7.[72] Knowledge of cytogenetics and somatic mutations not only facilitates the diagnosis of MPN, but is also used as a prognostic factor.

Prognosis and clinical comment

The natural evolution of PMF is a gradual progression toward a markedly fibrotic, often osteosclerotic, and cellular depleted bone marrow clinically associated with the presence of worsening anemia, marked degrees of hepatosplenomegaly, profound constitutional symptoms, and cachexia. Median survival for patients with overt PMF is 6 to 7 years[8]; however, patients with low-risk features may have a median survival of 11 to 15 years, whereas those with high-risk features may have a median survival of 1 to 2 years.[73] Progression to blast phase is the most common cause of death, accounting for up to 20%.[57] Other causes include thromboembolic and cardiovascular complications, infection, hemorrhage, portal hypertension, and second cancers. The overall cumulative incidence of blast phase transformation is 11% at 5 years and 23% at 10 years.[54] Older age, *IDH1/ASXL1/SRSF2* mutations, very high-risk karyotype, circulating blasts >3%, presence of moderate or severe anemia, and constitutional symptoms contribute to a higher risk.[74] Median overall survival rates for patients with a mutation in *JAK2*, *CALR*, and *MPL* are 5.9, 15.9, and 9.9, respectively, in contrast to triple-negative disease with a median survival of only 2.3 years.[65] The number of additional mutations defining the high mutation risk category (*ASXL1*, *SRSF2*, *U2AF1Q157*, *EZH2*, *IDH1*, *IDH2*) adversely affects prognosis.[72] Therefore, expanded mutation testing by next-generation sequencing and cytogenetic assessment is important for risk stratification and facilitates the treatment decision process, especially with regard to the timing of allogeneic hematopoietic stem cell transplant.[72,73]

References

1. Arber DA, Orazi A, Hasserjian RP, et al. International consensus classification of myeloid neoplasms and acute leukemias: integrating morphologic, clinical, and genomic data. *Blood*. 2022;140(11):1200-1228.
2. Kvasnicka HM, Thiele J. The impact of clinicopathological studies on staging and survival in essential thrombocythemia, chronic idiopathic myelofibrosis, and polycythemia rubra vera. *Semin Thromb Hemost*. 2006;32(4 pt 2):362-371.
3. Patel AA, Odenike O. Genomics of MPN progression. *Hematology Am Soc Hematol Educ Program*. 2020;2020(1):440-449.
4. Moliterno AR, Kaizer H. Applied genomics in MPN presentation. *Hematology Am Soc Hematol Educ Program*. 2020;2020(1):434-439.
5. Luque Paz D, Kralovics R, Skoda RC. Genetic basis and molecular profiling in myeloproliferative neoplasms. *Blood*. 2023;141(16):1909-1921.
6. Landgren O, Goldin LR, Kristinsson SY, Helgadottir EA, Samuelsson J, Björkholm M. Increased risks of polycythemia vera, essential thrombocythemia, and myelofibrosis among 24,577 first-degree relatives of 11,039 patients with myeloproliferative neoplasms in Sweden. *Blood*. 2008;112(6):2199-2204.
7. Masselli E, Pozzi G, Carubbi C, Vitale M. The genetic makeup of myeloproliferative neoplasms: role of germline variants in defining disease risk, phenotypic diversity and outcome. *Cells*. 2021;10(10):2597.
8. Szuber N, Mudireddy M, Nicolosi M, et al. 3023 mayo clinic patients with myeloproliferative neoplasms: risk-stratified comparison of survival and outcomes data among disease subgroups. *Mayo Clin Proc*. 2019;94(4):599-610.
9. Barbui T, Thiele J, Passamonti F, et al. Survival and disease progression in essential thrombocythemia are significantly influenced by accurate morphologic diagnosis: an international study. *J Clin Oncol*. 2011;29(23):3179-3184.
10. Kvasnicka HM, Thiele J. Prodromal myeloproliferative neoplasms: the 2008 WHO classification. *Am J Hematol*. 2010;85(1):62-69.
11. Sant'Antonio E, Guglielmelli P, Pieri L, et al. Splanchnic vein thromboses associated with myeloproliferative neoplasms: an international, retrospective study on 518 cases. *Am J Hematol*. 2020;95(2):156-166.
12. Thiele J, Kvasnicka HM, Orazi A, et al. The international consensus classification of myeloid neoplasms and acute Leukemias: myeloproliferative neoplasms. *Am J Hematol*. 2023;98(1):166-179.
13. Gianelli U, Thiele J, Orazi A, et al. International Consensus Classification of myeloid and lymphoid neoplasms: myeloproliferative neoplasms. *Virchows Arch*. 2023;482(1):53-68.
14. Jovanovic JV, Ivey A, Vannucchi AM, et al. Establishing optimal quantitative-polymerase chain reaction assays for routine diagnosis and tracking of minimal residual disease in JAK2-V617F-associated myeloproliferative neoplasms: a joint European LeukemiaNet/MPN&Nr-EuroNet (COST action BM0902) study. *Leukemia*. 2013;27(10):2032-2039.
15. Loscocco GG, Coltro G, Guglielmelli P, Vannucchi AM. Integration of molecular information in risk assessment of patients with myeloproliferative neoplasms. *Cells*. 2021;10(8):1962.
16. Thiele J, Kvasnicka HM, Facchetti F, Franco V, van der Walt J, Orazi A. European consensus on grading bone marrow fibrosis and assessment of cellularity. *Haematologica*. 2005;90(8):1128-1132.
17. Kvasnicka HM, Beham-Schmid C, Bob R, et al. Problems and pitfalls in grading of bone marrow fibrosis, collagen deposition and osteosclerosis—a consensus-based study. *Histopathology*. 2016;68(6):905-915.
18. Thiele J, Kvasnicka HM. Grade of bone marrow fibrosis is associated with relevant hematological findings—a clinicopathological study on 865 patients with chronic idiopathic myelofibrosis. *Ann Hematol*. 2006;85(4):226-232.
19. Guglielmelli P, Vannucchi AM; AGIMM Investigators. The prognostic impact of bone marrow fibrosis in primary myelofibrosis. *Am J Hematol*. 2016;91(10):E454-E455.

20. Kvasnicka HM, Orazi A, Thiele J, et al. European LeukemiaNet study on the reproducibility of bone marrow features in masked polycythemia vera and differentiation from essential thrombocythemia. *Am J Hematol.* 2017;92(10):1062-1067.
21. Swerdlow SH, Campo E, Harris NL, et al. WHO Classification of Tumours of Haematopoietic and Lymphoid Tissues. 4th ed. International Agency for Research on Cancer; 2017.
22. Thiele J, Kvasnicka HM, Orazi A. Bone marrow histopathology in myeloproliferative disorders—current diagnostic approach. *Semin Hematol.* 2005;42(4):184-195.
23. Tefferi A, Barbui T. Polycythemia vera: 2024 update on diagnosis, risk-stratification, and management. *Am J Hematol.* 2023;98(9):1465-1487.
24. Titmarsh GJ, Duncombe AS, McMullin MF, et al. How common are myeloproliferative neoplasms? A systematic review and meta-analysis. *Am J Hematol.* 2014;89(6):581-587.
25. Tefferi A, Rumi E, Finazzi G, et al. Survival and prognosis among 1545 patients with contemporary polycythemia vera: an international study. *Leukemia.* 2013;27(9):1874-1881.
26. Tremblay D, Yacoub A, Hoffman R. Overview of myeloproliferative neoplasms: history, pathogenesis, diagnostic criteria, and complications. *Hematol Oncol Clin North Am.* 2021;35(2):159-176.
27. Kiladjian JJ, Cassinat B. Myeloproliferative neoplasms and splanchnic vein thrombosis: contemporary diagnostic and therapeutic strategies. *Am J Hematol.* 2023;98(5):794-800.
28. Passamonti F, Giorgino T, Mora B, et al. A clinical-molecular prognostic model to predict survival in patients with post polycythemia vera and post essential thrombocythemia myelofibrosis. *Leukemia.* 2017;31(12):2726-2731.
29. Combaluzier S, Quessada J, Abbou N, et al. Cytological diagnosis of classic myeloproliferative neoplasms at the age of molecular biology. *Cells.* 2023;12(6):946.
30. Barbui T, Thiele J, Passamonti F, et al. Initial bone marrow reticulin fibrosis in polycythemia vera exerts an impact on clinical outcome. *Blood.* 2012;119(10):2239-2241.
31. Passamonti F, Rumi E, Pietra D, et al. A prospective study of 338 patients with polycythemia vera: the impact of JAK2 (V617F) allele burden and leukocytosis on fibrotic or leukemic disease transformation and vascular complications. *Leukemia.* 2010;24(9):1574-1579.
32. Cerquozzi S, Tefferi A. Blast transformation and fibrotic progression in polycythemia vera and essential thrombocythemia: a literature review of incidence and risk factors. *Blood Cancer J.* 2015;5(11):e366.
33. Barosi G, Mesa RA, Thiele J, et al. Proposed criteria for the diagnosis of post-polycythemia vera and post-essential thrombocythemia myelofibrosis: a consensus statement from the International Working Group for Myelofibrosis Research and Treatment. *Leukemia.* 2008;22(2):437-438.
34. Boiocchi L, Mathew S, Gianelli U, et al. Morphologic and cytogenetic differences between post-polycythemic myelofibrosis and primary myelofibrosis in fibrotic stage. *Mod Pathol.* 2013;26(12):1577-1585.
35. Dunbar AJ, Rampal RK, Levine R. Leukemia secondary to myeloproliferative neoplasms. *Blood.* 2020;136(1):61-70.
36. Boiocchi L, Gianelli U, Iurlo A, et al. Neutrophilic leukocytosis in advanced stage polycythemia vera: hematopathologic features and prognostic implications. *Mod Pathol.* 2015;28(11):1448-1457.
37. Tefferi A, Lavu S, Mudireddy M, et al. JAK2 exon 12 mutated polycythemia vera: Mayo-Careggi MPN Alliance study of 33 consecutive cases and comparison with JAK2V617F mutated disease. *Am J Hematol.* 2018;93(4):E93-E96.
38. Tefferi A, Guglielmelli P, Lasho TL, et al. Mutation-enhanced international prognostic systems for essential thrombocythaemia and polycythaemia vera. *Br J Haematol.* 2020;189(2):291-302.
39. Hultcrantz M, Bjorkholm M, Dickman PW, et al. Risk for arterial and venous thrombosis in patients with myeloproliferative neoplasms: a population-based Cohort study. *Ann Intern Med.* 2018;168(5):317-325.
40. Carobbio A, Vannucchi AM, De Stefano V, et al. Neutrophil-to-lymphocyte ratio is a novel predictor of venous thrombosis in polycythemia vera. *Blood Cancer J.* 2022;12(2):28.
41. Guglielmelli P, Loscocco GG, Mannarelli C, et al. JAK2V617F variant allele frequency >50% identifies patients with polycythemia vera at high risk for venous thrombosis. *Blood Cancer J.* 2021;11(12):199.
42. Szuber N, Vallapureddy RR, Penna D, et al. Myeloproliferative neoplasms in the young: mayo Clinic experience with 361 patients age 40 years or younger. *Am J Hematol.* 2018;93(12):1474-1484.
43. Marchioli R, Finazzi G, Specchia G, et al. Cardiovascular events and intensity of treatment in polycythemia vera. *N Engl J Med.* 2013;368(1):22-33.
44. Sobas M, Kiladjian JJ, Beauverd Y, et al. Real-world study of children and young adults with myeloproliferative neoplasms: identifying risks and unmet needs. *Blood Adv.* 2022;6(17):5171-5183.
45. Kucine N. Myeloproliferative neoplasms in children, adolescents, and young adults. *Curr Hematol Malig Rep.* 2020;15(2):141-148.
46. Tefferi A, Guglielmelli P, Larson DR, et al. Long-term survival and blast transformation in molecularly annotated essential thrombocythemia, polycythemia vera, and myelofibrosis. *Blood.* 2014;124(16):2507-2615. quiz 2615.
47. Tefferi A, Pardanani A. Essential thrombocythemia. *N Engl J Med.* 2019;381(22):2135-2144.
48. Gangat N, Singh A, Szuber N, et al. Site-specific venous thrombosis in essential thrombocythemia: impact on subsequent vascular events and survival. *J Thromb Haemost.* 2022;20(10):2439-2443.

49. Finazzi G, Carobbio A, Thiele J, et al. Incidence and risk factors for bleeding in 1104 patients with essential thrombocythemia or prefibrotic myelofibrosis diagnosed according to the 2008 WHO criteria. *Leukemia.* 2012;26(4):716-719.
50. Rumi E, Pietra D, Ferretti V, et al. JAK2 or CALR mutation status defines subtypes of essential thrombocythemia with substantially different clinical course and outcomes. *Blood.* 2014;123(10):1544-1551.
51. Puglianini OC, Peker D, Zhang L, Papadantonakis N. Essential thrombocythemia and post-essential thrombocythemia myelofibrosis: updates on diagnosis, clinical aspects, and management. *Lab Med.* 2023;54(1):13-22.
52. Thiele J, Kvasnicka HM, Mullauer L, Buxhofer-Ausch V, Gisslinger B, Gisslinger H. Essential thrombocythemia versus early primary myelofibrosis: a multicenter study to validate the WHO classification. *Blood.* 2011;117(21):5710-5718.
53. Loscocco GG, Guglielmelli P, Gangat N, et al. Clinical and molecular predictors of fibrotic progression in essential thrombocythemia: a multicenter study involving 1607 patients. *Am J Hematol.* 2021;96(11):1472-1480.
54. Tefferi A, Alkhateeb H, Gangat N. Blast phase myeloproliferative neoplasm: contemporary review and 2024 treatment algorithm. *Blood Cancer J.* 2023;13(1):108.
55. Gangat N, Jadoon Y, Szuber N, et al. Cytogenetic abnormalities in essential thrombocythemia: clinical and molecular correlates and prognostic relevance in 809 informative cases. *Blood Cancer J.* 2022;12(3):44.
56. Gangat N, Guglielmelli P, Betti S, et al. Cerebral venous thrombosis and myeloproliferative neoplasms: a three-center study of 74 consecutive cases. *Am J Hematol.* 2021;96(12):1580-1586.
57. Carobbio A, Thiele J, Passamonti F, et al. Risk factors for arterial and venous thrombosis in WHO-defined essential thrombocythemia: an international study of 891 patients. *Blood.* 2011;117(22):5857-5859.
58. Tefferi A. Primary myelofibrosis: 2023 update on diagnosis, risk-stratification, and management. *Am J Hematol.* 2023;98(5):801-821.
59. Buxhofer-Ausch V, Gisslinger H, Thiele J, et al. Leukocytosis as an important risk factor for arterial thrombosis in WHO-defined early/prefibrotic myelofibrosis: an international study of 264 patients. *Am J Hematol.* 2012;87(7):669-672.
60. Carobbio A, Vannucchi AM, Rumi E, et al. Survival expectation after thrombosis and overt-myelofibrosis in essential thrombocythemia and prefibrotic myelofibrosis: a multistate model approach. *Blood Cancer J.* 2023;13(1):115.
61. Gisslinger H. Pre-PMF emerging as important subgroup of MPN. *Blood.* 2017;129(24):3142-3144.
62. Guglielmelli P, Pacilli A, Rotunno G, et al. Presentation and outcome of patients with 2016 WHO diagnosis of prefibrotic and overt primary myelofibrosis. *Blood.* 2017;129(24):3227-3236.
63. Jeryczynski G, Thiele J, Gisslinger B, et al. Pre-fibrotic/early primary myelofibrosis vs. WHO-defined essential thrombocythemia: the impact of minor clinical diagnostic criteria on the outcome of the disease. *Am J Hematol.* 2017;92(9):885-891.
64. Mudireddy M, Shah S, Lasho T, et al. Prefibrotic versus overtly fibrotic primary myelofibrosis: clinical, cytogenetic, molecular and prognostic comparisons. *Br J Haematol.* 2018;182(4):594-597.
65. Al-Ghamdi YA, Lake J, Bagg A, et al. Triple-negative primary myelofibrosis: a bone marrow pathology group study. *Mod Pathol.* 2023;36(3):100016.
66. Barbui T, Carobbio A, Cervantes F, et al. Thrombosis in primary myelofibrosis: incidence and risk factors. *Blood.* 2010;115(4):778-782.
67. Dores GM, Curtis RE, Linet MS, Morton LM. Cause-specific mortality following polycythemia vera, essential thrombocythemia, and primary myelofibrosis in the US population, 2001-2017. *Am J Hematol.* 2021;96(12):E451-E454.
68. Boiocchi L, Espinal-Witter R, Geyer JT, et al. Development of monocytosis in patients with primary myelofibrosis indicates an accelerated phase of the disease. *Mod Pathol.* 2013;26(2):204-212.
69. Benton CB, Boddu PC, DiNardo CD, et al. Janus kinase 2 variants associated with the transformation of myeloproliferative neoplasms into acute myeloid leukemia. *Cancer.* 2019;125(11):1855-1866.
70. Thiele J, Kvasnicka HM, Czieslick C. CD34+ progenitor cells in idiopathic (primary) myelofibrosis: a comparative quantification between spleen and bone marrow tissue. *Ann Hematol.* 2002;81(2):86-89.
71. Coltro G, Mannelli F, Vergoni F, et al. Extramedullary blastic transformation of primary myelofibrosis in the form of disseminated myeloid sarcoma: a case report and review of the literature. *Clin Exp Med.* 2020;20(2):313-320.
72. Tefferi A, Guglielmelli P, Nicolosi M, et al. GIPSS: genetically inspired prognostic scoring system for primary myelofibrosis. *Leukemia.* 2018;32(7):1631-1642.
73. Tefferi A, Guglielmelli P, Lasho TL, et al. MIPSS70+ version 2.0: mutation and karyotype-enhanced international prognostic scoring system for primary myelofibrosis. *J Clin Oncol.* 2018;36(17):1769-1770.
74. Vallapureddy RR, Mudireddy M, Penna D, et al. Leukemic transformation among 1306 patients with primary myelofibrosis: risk factors and development of a predictive model. *Blood Cancer J.* 2019;9(2):12.

Chapter 3
Chronic Neutrophilic Leukemia

Attilio Orazi, Carlos E. Bueso-Ramos, Hans Michael Kvasnicka, Marco Pizzi, Natasha Szuber, and Ayalew Tefferi

Definition

Chronic neutrophilic leukemia (CNL) is a rare, often aggressive, myeloproliferative neoplasm (MPN) defined by persistent mature neutrophilic leukocytosis, marked granulocyte proliferation in the bone marrow (BM), and frequent hepatosplenomegaly.[1] Driver mutations in colony-stimulating factor 3 receptor (*CSF3R*), which are present in the vast majority of cases, represent a key diagnostic feature. The presence of *BCR::ABL1* fusion including the variant fusion gene and p230 BCR::ABL1 protein, which is associated with prominent neutrophilic maturation (ie, neutrophil-rich chronic myeloid leukemia [CML]), excludes the diagnosis. Also excluded are cases with genetic abnormalities associated with myeloid/lymphoid neoplasms with eosinophilia and tyrosine kinase gene fusions (M/LN-Eo-TK) (Table 3.1).

Synonyms

None.

Epidemiology

CNL is a rare disease, and its true incidence remains largely unknown. A recent population-based study addressing CNL epidemiology found an overall incidence of 0.1 cases/million individuals, using combined Surveillance, Epidemiology, and End Results and National Cancer Database data.[2] CNL typically presents in elderly patients with a median age at diagnosis of 66.5 years (range: 15-86) and slight male preponderance (56%-58% of cases).[3] The etiology of CNL is unknown.

General Clinical Features

CNL most commonly presents as incidental neutrophilic leukocytosis in an asymptomatic subject. In the large majority of the patients, leukocytosis precedes the diagnosis by several months. More rarely, patients present with symptoms such as fatigue, bone pain, pruritus, easy bruising, or gout. Splenomegaly is detected in about 36% of cases and can be symptomatic. Hepatomegaly may occur, while lymph node involvement is relatively uncommon. Bleeding manifestations, including an appreciable incidence of cerebral hemorrhage, have also been related to CNL.[3] Lactate dehydrogenase levels are typically elevated. The leukocyte alkaline phosphatase score is high, unlike what is observed in CML. Vitamin B_{12} levels are often elevated due to transcobalamin release from granulocytes and their precursors.

Pronounced neutrophilia can be caused by both benign and malignant disorders, and a diagnosis of CNL requires exclusion of reactive neutrophilia/leukemoid reaction. About a quarter of CNL cases reported prior to the 2016 World Health Organization (WHO) classification were associated with an underlying neoplasm, most often multiple myeloma (MM) or monoclonal gammopathy of undetermined significance (MGUS). The majority of such cases most likely constituted a neutrophilic leukemoid reaction mediated by granulocyte colony stimulating factor or other cytokines secreted by the neoplastic plasma cells. However, rare patients may develop true CNL with concurrent MM/MGUS, suggesting that both clonal and nonclonal neutrophilia may exist in such cases.[3] As for other myeloid neoplasms, CNL needs to be separated from CML, MPN with marked neutrophilia (more often observed during disease progression of primary myelofibrosis or polycythemia vera), and myelodysplastic/myeloproliferative neoplasms, such as atypical chronic myeloid leukemia (aCML) and chronic myelomonocytic leukemia (CMML). In this context, integration of clinical, morphological, and above all molecular findings is mandatory to support an evidence-based diagnosis of CNL.

Morphology

The peripheral blood shows leukocytosis with neutrophilia (Figure 3.1). In a 2015 series of WHO-defined CNL cases, the median white blood cell (WBC) count was 54×10^9/L (range: 21.7-176.2).[4] A diagnosis of CNL

TABLE 3.1 Diagnostic criteria for chronic neutrophilic leukemia (CNL)

1.	Peripheral blood white blood cell count ≥13 × 10^9/L[a] • Segmented neutrophils plus banded neutrophils constitute ≥80% of the white blood cells • No significant dysgranulopoiesis • Neutrophil precursors (promyelocytes, myelocytes, and metamyelocytes) constitute <10% of the white blood cells • Circulating blasts only rarely observed[b] • Monocyte count <10% of all leukocytes
2.	Hypercellular bone marrow with neutrophil granulocytes increased in percentage and absolute number, showing normal maturation
3.	*CSF3R* T618I or another activating *CSF3R* mutation ---or--- Persistent neutrophilia (≥3 months), splenomegaly, and no identifiable cause of reactive neutrophilia including absence of a plasma cell neoplasm or, if a plasma cell neoplasm is present, demonstration of clonality of myeloid cells by cytogenetic or molecular studies
4.	Not meeting diagnostic criteria for *BCR::ABL1*-positive chronic myeloid leukemia, polycythemia vera, essential thrombocythemia, or primary myelofibrosis, or of a myeloid/lymphoid neoplasm with eosinophilia and tyrosine kinase gene fusions

The diagnosis of CNL requires all four criteria

[a]≥25 × 10^9/L in cases lacking *CSF3R* T618I or another activating *CSF3R* mutation.

[b]10% to 19% blasts in peripheral blood or bone marrow represent CNL in accelerated phase; ≥20% blasts represent blast phase.

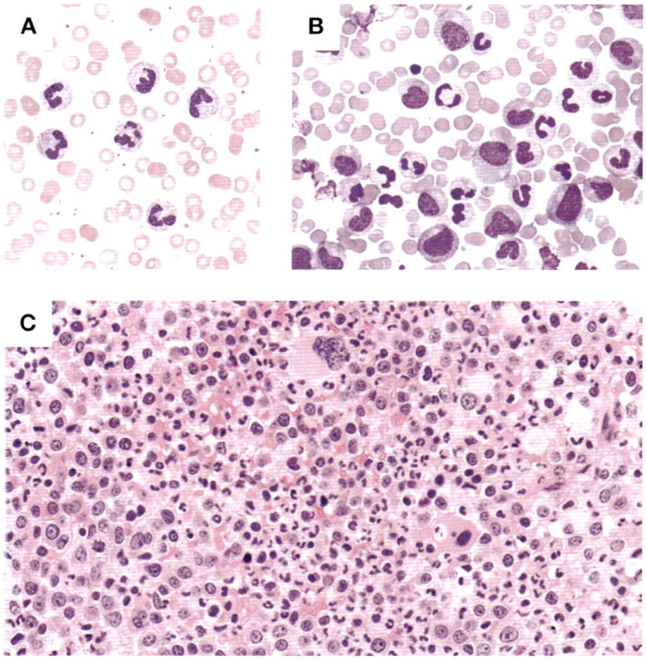

FIGURE 3.1 Chronic neutrophilic leukemia. **A:** Peripheral blood smear showing the characteristic neutrophilia. No neutrophilic precursors are present. The neutrophils lack dysplasia. **B:** Bone marrow (BM) aspirate smear demonstrates a preponderant, slightly left-shifted neutrophil proliferation with no significant cytologic abnormalities. **C:** The BM is hypercellular with a markedly elevated myeloid to erythroid ratio due to the proliferation of granulocytic forms, in particular mature segmented neutrophils (Wright-Giemsa and hematoxylin & eosin stains; original magnification, smears: 60× and 100×; biopsy: 40×).

requires WBC ≥13 × 10^9/L in cases with T618I or other activating mutations of *CSF3R*.[1,3] In their absence, WBC must be ≥25 × 10^9/L (Table 3.1). The neutrophilic granulocytes constitute ≥80% of the differential count.[1,3] Most of the neutrophils are normally segmented, but an increased number of band forms is frequently seen. Granulocytic dysplasia is not detected. Unless disease progression is present, the neutrophil precursors (promyelocytes, myelocytes, and metamyelocytes) are <10% and myeloblasts are only rarely encountered. While most cases have <1% blasts and <10% myeloid precursors in the peripheral blood, values in excess of these should not disqualify a working diagnosis of CNL, if T618I or other activating *CSF3R* mutations are present. Instead, any case with 1% to 9% blasts and/or increased myeloid precursors in the peripheral blood should raise concerns regarding disease progression toward accelerated or blast phase.

In CNL, the neutrophils either are normal or show toxic granulations and/or Döhle bodies. The latter, however, have been reported mostly in the past, when cases of leukemoid reaction associated with MM or other causes were included in the CNL spectrum.

The majority of patients present with mild anemia. In one series,[4] the median hemoglobin value was 10.8 g/dL (range: 8.5-16.0). Although thrombocytopenia may occur, platelet counts may be normal or increased, with a reported platelet range of 25 to 476 × 10^9/L.[4] Monocytosis, basophilia, or eosinophilia is typically absent. Their occurrence should prompt a critical review of the original diagnosis.

The BM is markedly hypercellular (>90% cellularity) due to increased granulopoiesis with prevalence of myelocytes, metamyelocytes, and segmented granulocytes. The myeloid to erythroid ratio is high and may exceed 20:1. Monocytes, basophils, and eosinophils are not increased. Erythropoiesis is usually decreased with normal maturation, while megakaryocytes, which are often morphologically normal, may be normal or slightly increased in number. Myeloblasts are typically <5% with absence of Auer rods. Significant dysplasia is absent. Mild increase of reticulin fibrosis can be seen in a minority of the cases.

Increased numbers of circulating or BM blasts (10%-19%) indicate transformation to an accelerated phase, while ≥20% blasts define blast phase. Progressive splenomegaly and worsening of thrombocytopenia are typical features of disease progression or blast transformation.

The International Consensus Classification diagnostic criteria of CNL are reported in Table 3.1.

Immunophenotype

Despite being nonspecific to CNL, immunophenotypic and cytochemical studies may be useful by complementing the morphological evaluation. Particularly in *CSF3R*-unmuted cases, strong myeloperoxidase (MPO) positivity and the lack of CD14 or other monocytic antigens may facilitate separation from CMML. Similarly, cytochemistry for MPO and nonspecific esterase can be of help in distinguishing neutrophilic cells from monocytes. CD61, CD41, and/or CD42b facilitate the recognition of micromegakaryocytes, which are usually absent in CNL but may occur in aCML.

Genetics

The incidence of cytogenetic abnormalities is variable in different studies.[3,5] In one of those,[5] 37% of CNL cases presented cytogenetic abnormalities, which included trisomy 8, trisomy 21, deletion of 11q, and deletion of 20q. There is no *BCR::ABL1* fusion and no genetic abnormalities associated with M/LN-Eo-TK.[1]

Mutations of *CSF3R* are found in 80% to 90% of the cases and are the characteristic genetic signature of CNL.[1,3,6,7] Their absence, however, does not exclude the possibility of CNL.[1,3] *CSF3R* mutations lead to the receptor constitutive activation, promoting neutrophil proliferation and differentiation. Two main mutational variants of *CSF3R* have been reported: the more common membrane proximal mutations, consisting primarily of T618I and T615A point mutations, and frameshift or nonsense mutations leading to premature truncation of the cytoplasmic tail of *CSF3R* (eg, D771fs, S783fs, Y752X, and W791X).[6,8] Compared with other *CSF3R* mutations, T618I-mutated cases show adverse clinical and laboratory features, including more advanced age at diagnosis, higher WBC counts, lower hemoglobin values and platelet counts at diagnosis, more frequent cytogenetic abnormalities, and shorter overall survival (OS).[9]

In *CSF3R*-mutated CNL concurrent mutations are observed in many cases.[3] *ASXL1, SETBP1,* and *SRSF2* are among the most commonly affected genes. The presence of *ASXL1* comutation has been shown to be independently associated with reduced survival.[4] The prognostic relevance of concurrent *SETBP1* and *CSF3R* mutations remains to be determined, although some evidence suggests a detrimental impact on prognosis. Mutations in spliceosome complex components such as *SRSF2* and *U2AF1* are less commonly reported in CNL. Their cooperative role in the pathogenesis of CNL or in its prognostic assessment still remains obscure.[3] Comutations in *JAK2* and *CALR* have been rarely reported, and whether those cases represent true CNL rather than "classical" MPN with neutrophilia remains controversial.[10,11]

Prognosis and Clinical Comment

Overall prognosis of CNL is variable, with a median reported OS of between 21 and 30 months[4,5] with that of T618I-mutated cases specifically documented as 24 months.[12] Natural history may recapitulate accelerated and blast phases analogous to those observed in untreated CML. Potentially fatal complications include intracranial hemorrhage, progressive disease, transformation to acute myeloid or rarely lymphoblastic leukemia, and treatment-related toxicities.[3] Disease progression is often heralded by resistance to therapy, uncontrolled refractory neutrophilia, worsening anemia, and organomegaly, with eventual blast crisis concomitant with acquisition of new molecular or cytogenetic abnormalities. Leukemic transformation rates vary between 10% and 21% with median time to acute myeloid leukemia transformation of 21 months (range: 3-94 months).[9] A risk stratification model for survival established prognostically relevant variables with commensurate adverse risk points as follows: platelet count $<160 \times 10^9$/L (2 points), WBC $>60 \times 10^9$/L (1 point), and presence of *ASXL1* mutation (1 point), with high-risk cases (2-4 points) displaying significantly reduced OS compared with low-risk ones (0-1 point) (22.4 months vs "not yet reached").[9]

There is currently no standard of care for the management of CNL. While JAK inhibitor therapy has emerged as a novel potential adjunct to the therapeutic arsenal,[13] with conventional oral chemotherapy (eg, hydroxyurea) remaining the standard frontline, allogeneic hematopoietic stem cell transplant (HSCT) remains the only curative option, although typically with limited applicability to a minority of eligible patients. It is thus recommended that patients with CNL first and foremost be evaluated for eligibility and disposition for HSCT, with the remaining therapeutic agents being aimed at controlling myeloproliferation (targeting leukocytes <25-30 × 10^9/L) and alleviating symptoms.[9] Development of disease-modifying therapies for CNL and inclusion of these rare disease cohorts in randomized clinical trials constitute major unmet needs.

References

1. Arber DA, Orazi A, Hasserjian RP, et al. International consensus classification of myeloid neoplasms and acute leukemias: integrating morphologic, clinical, and genomic data. *Blood.* 2022;140(11):1200-1228.
2. Ruan GJ, Smith CJ, Day C, et al. A population-based study of chronic neutrophilic leukemia in the United States. *Blood Cancer J.* 2020;10(6):68.
3. Szuber N, Orazi A, Tefferi A. Chronic neutrophilic leukemia and atypical chronic myeloid leukemia: 2024 update on diagnosis, genetics, risk stratification, and management. *Am J Hematol.* 2024;99(7):1360-1387.
4. Elliott MA, Pardanani A, Hanson CA, et al. ASXL1 mutations are frequent and prognostically detrimental in CSF3R-mutated chronic neutrophilic leukemia. *Am J Hematol.* 2015;90(7):653-656.
5. Reilly JT. Chronic neutrophilic leukaemia: a distinct clinical entity? *Br J Haematol.* 2002;116(1):10-18.
6. Maxson JE, Gotlib J, Pollyea DA, et al. Oncogenic CSF3R mutations in chronic neutrophilic leukemia and atypical CML. *N Engl J Med.* 2013;368(19):1781-1790.
7. Pardanani A, Lasho TL, Laborde RR, et al. CSF3R T618I is a highly prevalent and specific mutation in chronic neutrophilic leukemia. *Leukemia.* 2013;27(9):1870-1873.
8. Fleischman AG, Maxson JE, Luty SB, et al. The CSF3R T618I mutation causes a lethal neutrophilic neoplasia in mice that is responsive to therapeutic JAK inhibition. *Blood.* 2013;122(22):3628-3631.
9. Szuber N, Finke CM, Lasho TL, et al. CSF3R-mutated chronic neutrophilic leukemia: long term outcome in 19 consecutive patients and risk model for survival. *Blood Cancer J.* 2018;8(2):21.
10. Boiocchi L, Gianelli U, Iurlo A, et al. Neutrophilic leukocytosis in advanced stage polycythemia vera: hematopathologic features and prognostic implications. *Mod Pathol.* 2015;28(11):1448-1457.
11. Gao J, Han S, Deng B, Deng Y, Gao X. Research progress of additional pathogenic mutations in chronic neutrophilic leukemia. *Ann Hematol.* 2023;103(8):2591-2600.
12. Cui YJ, Jiang Q, Liu JQ, et al. The clinical characteristics, gene mutations and prognosis of chronic neutrophilic leukemia. *Zhonghua Xue Ye Xue Za Zhi.* 2017;38(1):28-32.
13. Dao KT, Gotlib J, Deininger MMN, et al. Efficacy of Ruxolitinib in patients with chronic neutrophilic leukemia and atypical chronic myeloid leukemia. *J Clin Oncol.* 2020;38(10):1006-1018.

Chapter 4

Chronic Eosinophilic Leukemia, Not Otherwise Specified

Sa A. Wang, Attilio Orazi, Kaaren Reichard, and Ayalew Tefferi

Definition

Chronic eosinophilic leukemia, not otherwise specified (CEL, NOS) is a myeloproliferative neoplasm, characterized by a clonal proliferation of eosinophils and persistent eosinophilia in peripheral blood and bone marrow. Eosinophilia in CEL, NOS requires an absolute eosinophil count (AEC) $\geq 1.5 \times 10^9/L$ (hypereosinophilia) and eosinophils ≥10% of white blood cells (WBCs) in blood to ensure that eosinophilia is a dominant hematological abnormality. Acute myeloid leukemia (AML) must be excluded, including cases with peripheral blood and bone marrow ≥20% blasts and cases meeting the criteria of AML with recurrent genetic abnormalities. Organ damage may occur as a result of leukemic infiltration or the release of cytokines, enzymes, or other proteins by the eosinophils. A closely related entity is idiopathic hypereosinophilic syndrome (iHES), defined as persistent (≥6 months) peripheral blood eosinophilia in which eosinophilic infiltration and mediator release cause damage to multiple organs, and an underlying cause, either reactive or a clonal myeloid process, cannot be identified.[1] If unexplained hypereosinophilia is not associated with tissue damage/dysfunction, the designation "idiopathic hypereosinophilia" (iHE) is appropriate.[1] Given the difficulty to prove clonality in some cases of true CEL, NOS with current diagnostic modalities, and the prevalence of clonal hematopoiesis of unknown significance, bone marrow morphology[2,3] is now incorporated in the diagnostic criteria for both CEL, NOS and iHES/iHE. The diagnostic criteria for CEL, NOS and iHES/iHE are summarized in Table 4.1 and Table 4.2, respectively. A diagnosis of CEL, NOS and iHES/iHE must exclude cases with a *BCR::ABL1* rearrangement or other tyrosine kinase gene fusions such as *PDGFRA, PDGFRB, FGFR1, JAK2, FLT3,* and *ETV6::ABL1* in myeloid/lymphoid neoplasms with eosinophilia (M/LN-eo-TK). CEL, NOS requires abnormal bone marrow morphology with features supporting the presence of a myeloid neoplasm or an increase in myeloblasts in the peripheral blood or bone marrow. On the contrary, iHES/iHE exhibits unremarkable bone marrow morphology except for increased eosinophils. In the classification hierarchy, CEL, NOS will trump a diagnosis of atypical chronic myeloid leukemia (aCML), myeloproliferative neoplasm (MPN)-unclassifiable, and myelodysplastic syndrome/myeloproliferative neoplasm (MDS/MPN), NOS.

Synonyms

None.

Epidemiology

CEL, NOS is rare, with an incidence of 1.2% among patients with hypereosinophilia.[4] According to the Surveillance, Epidemiology, and End Results (SEER) data between 2004 and 2015, the incidence of CEL, NOS (which did not differentiate M/LN-eo-TK and some iHES) is less than 0.4

TABLE 4.1 Diagnostic criteria for chronic eosinophilic leukemia, not otherwise specified (CEL, NOS)

Peripheral blood hypereosinophilia (eosinophil count $\geq 1.5 \times 10^9/L$ and eosinophils ≥10% of white blood cells)
Blasts constitute <20% cells in peripheral blood and bone marrow, not meeting any other diagnostic criteria for AML[a]
No tyrosine kinase gene fusion including *BCR::ABL1*, other *ABL1*, *PDGFRA, PDGFRB, FGFR1, JAK2, FLT3* fusions
Not meeting criteria for other well-defined MPN; chronic myelomonocytic leukemia, or systemic mastocytosis[b]
Bone marrow shows increased cellularity with dysplastic megakaryocytes with or without dysplastic features in other lineages and often significant fibrosis, associated with an eosinophilic infiltrate, or there are increased blasts ≥5% in the bone marrow and/or ≥2% in the peripheral blood
Demonstration of a clonal cytogenetic abnormality and/or somatic mutation(s)[c]

AML, acute myeloid leukemia; MPN, myeloproliferative neoplasm.
[a]AML with recurrent genetic abnormalities with <20% blasts is excluded.
[b]CEL, NOS may occur as SM-AMN (systemic mastocytosis associated with myeloid malignancies).
[c]In the absence of a clonal cytogenetic abnormality and/or somatic mutation(s) or increased blasts, bone marrow findings supportive of the diagnosis will suffice in the presence of persistent eosinophilia, provided other causes of eosinophilia having been excluded.

TABLE 4.2 Diagnostic criteria for idiopathic hypereosinophilic syndrome

Persistent peripheral blood hypereosinophilia (eosinophil count ≥1.5 × 10^9/L and ≥10% eosinophils)[a]
Organ damage and/or dysfunction attributable to tissue eosinophilic infiltrate[b]
No evidence of a reactive, well-defined autoimmune disease or neoplastic condition/disorder underlying the hypereosinophilia
Exclusion of lymphocyte variant hypereosinophilic syndrome[c]
Bone marrow morphologically within normal limits except for increased eosinophils
No molecular genetic clonal abnormality, with the caveat of clonal hematopoiesis of indeterminate potential

[a]Preferably a minimal duration of 6 months if documentation is available.
[b]Idiopathic hypereosinophilia has no tissue damage; otherwise, should follow the same diagnostic criteria.
[c]The abnormal T-cell population needs to be detected immunophenotypically with or without TCR clonality by PCR.

cases per 1,000,000 population.[5] CEL, NOS is more common in men, with a reported median age of 60 to 70 years; while the median age of iHES is in the 40 to 50 years and shows no significant gender preference.[3,6,7]

General Clinical Features

For CEL, NOS, a few patients may be asymptomatic, and eosinophilia and leukocytosis are detected incidentally. However, over half of the patients present with constitutional symptoms such as weight loss, night sweats, fever, fatigue, dyspnea; 20% to 30% with organomegaly, and approximately 60% with elevated lactate dehydrogenase. Unlike iHES, eosinophilia-related organ damage/dysfunction is not required for diagnosis but may be seen in 50% to 60% of patients with symptoms such as pruritus/skin rash, muscle and/or joint pain, diarrhea, and cough. Endomyocardial fibrosis, scarring of cardiac valves with subsequent thrombosis and cardiac failure, and central nervous system (CNS) dysfunction are serious complications. In contrast, patients with iHES[3,7] often present with symptoms of allergy/hypersensitivity, skin rashes, upper respiratory symptoms such as asthma/cough, rheumatoid symptoms, symptoms related with gastrointestinal, and/or endocrine involvement. Cardiac and CNS involvement may occur in a small subset of patients.

Morphology

The peripheral blood smear of CEL, NOS shows hypereosinophilia and leukocytosis. The median WBC is 20 to 30 × 10^9/L and median absolute eosinophil count is 6 to 12 × 10^9/L. In addition to eosinophilia, anemia, thrombocytopenia, or thrombocytosis may be seen in over two-thirds of patients. Eosinophils are mostly mature and may show a range of abnormal morphologic features including hypogranulation, uneven granulation, cytoplasmic vacuoles, abnormal nuclear lobation (hypolobated or hypersegmented) (Figure 4.1C), and large forms. Of note, eosinophil abnormalities are not specific to CEL, NOS and can be seen in other clonal eosinophilic conditions and, occasionally, in reactive conditions, although to a milder degree. Some cases may have basophilia. Blasts if present, are usually low (<1%). Monocytes are <10%. Compared with CEL, NOS, patients with iHES/iHE generally have a significantly lower WBC (median 10-11 × 10^9/L) and AEC (3.0-4.0 × 10^9/L) with mature normal bilobed eosinophils (Figure 4.1A).[3,7] While some patients with iHES may present with mild anemia and/or mild thrombocytopenia, the majority have a normal platelet count and hemoglobin level.

Bone marrow aspirate smears and core biopsies in CEL, NOS are mostly hypercellular, predominantly due to an increase in eosinophils and granulocytic cells, resulting in a significantly increased myeloid:erythroid ratio (Figure 4.1E and F). Megakaryocytes are usually abnormal, frequently myelodysplasia (MDS)-like (small, hypolobated or megakaryocytes with widely separated nuclear lobes) (Figure 4.1E). In some cases, there may be a spectrum of megakaryocytic morphology including larger, hyperlobulated MPN-like megakaryocytes (Figure 4.1F). Bone marrow eosinophils are often left-shifted with increased eosinophilic precursors (Figure 4.1D) and may have cytologic abnormalities similar to those described in peripheral blood, but often less prominent. Dysgranulopoiesis and dyserythropoiesis may be present but are not invariable findings. Bone marrow blasts are often less than 5% of total nucleated cells. Increased reticulin fibrosis (≥MF-2) may be observed in approximately 20% to 30% of cases. Overall, CEL, NOS bone marrows show features consistent with a chronic myeloid neoplasm. In contrast, the bone marrow of iHES is typically unremarkable[3,8-10] except for increased eosinophils. Cellularity is normal or only slightly increased. Granulopoiesis, erythropoiesis, and megakaryopoiesis should be adequate without significant dysplastic features (Figure 4.1B). Blasts are not increased, and eosinophils are morphologically unremarkable.

Immunophenotype

Immunohistochemical studies for CD117, tryptase, and CD25 will help to exclude the presence of systemic mastocytosis, which may be associated with CEL, NOS.

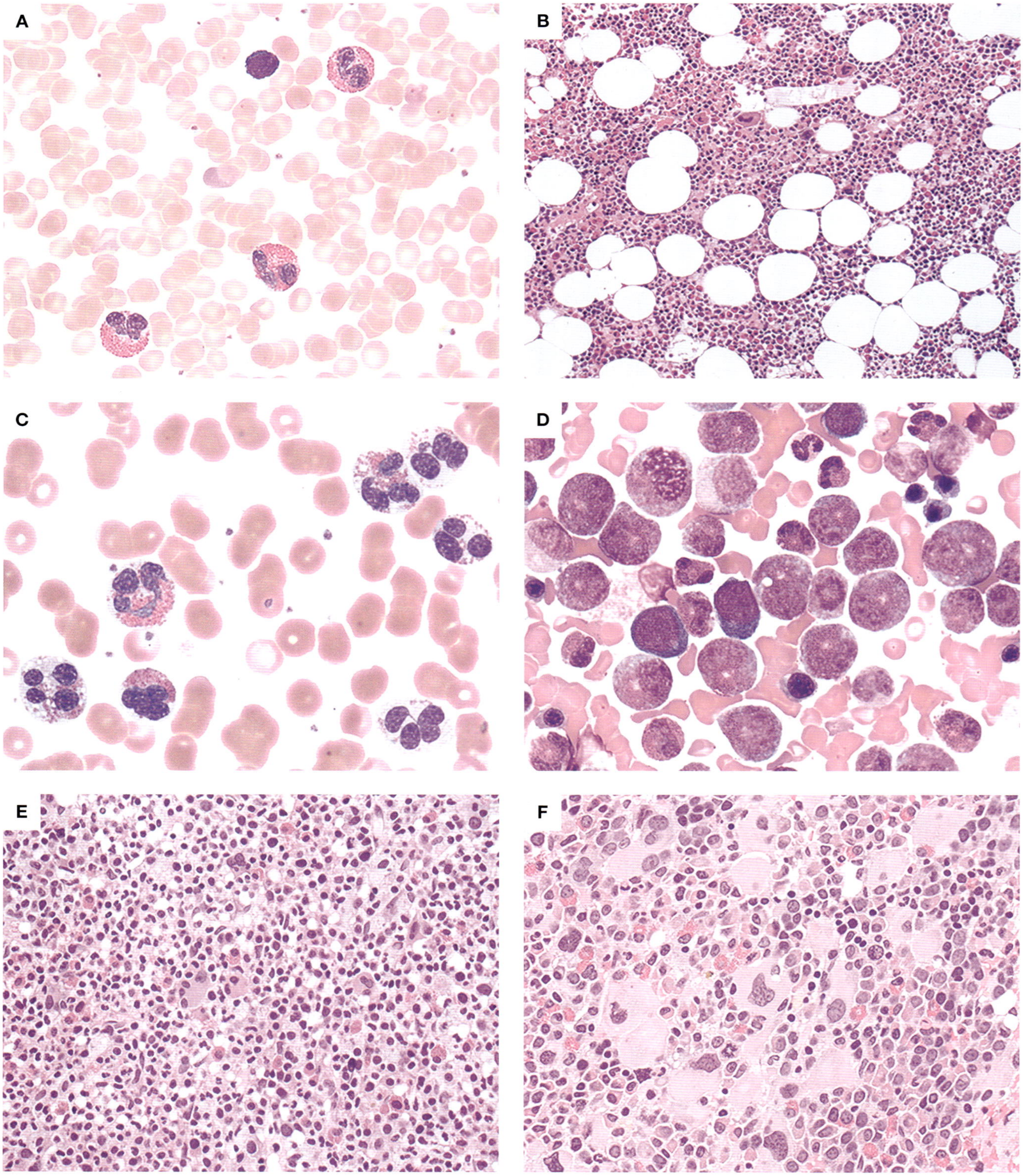

FIGURE 4.1 Morphological features of idiopathic hypereosinophilic syndrome (iHES) (**A** and **B**) and chronic eosinophilic leukemia, not otherwise specified (CEL, NOS) (**C-F**). The peripheral blood (PB) of iHES typically shows mild eosinophilia with normal bilobed eosinophils (**A**). Bone marrow (BM) of iHES (35-year-old) is normal or slightly hypercellular with normal trilineage hematopoiesis except for increased eosinophils (**B**). PB smear of CEL, NOS often shows numerous abnormal eosinophils, in this case with nuclear hypersegmentation and marked hypogranulation. BM aspirate may show increased eosinophil precursors (**D**). BM is almost always hypercellular (**E** and **F**), mostly with small dysplastic megakaryocytes (**E**); occasional cases may show large megakaryocytes (**F**). (**A, C, D:** Wright-Giemsa; **B, E, F:** hematoxylin and eosin; **A, C, D:** 100×; **B:** 10×; **E:** 20×; **F:** 40×.)

Flow cytometry to analyze T and NK cells and evaluation of their immunophenotypic abnormalities should be performed, especially before making a diagnosis of iHES, to rule out eosinophilia due to a T/NK cell lymphoproliferation, including lymphocytic variant (LV-HES). LV-HES is an uncommon eosinophilic disorder due to clonal or aberrant phenotypic T cells that secrete T helper type 2 cytokines.

Genetics

Cytogenetic abnormality is reported in 40% to 90% of CEL, NOS[3,4,11] depending on the study inclusion criteria. Abnormalities include trisomy 8, a complex karyotype, and other numerical and structural abnormalities, none of which is unique to this entity. iHES, theoretically, should not show clonal cytogenetic abnormalities, but rare cases may carry clonal cytogenetic abnormality of unknown significance.[8]

By next-generation sequencing, mutations have been identified in cases previously diagnosed as iHES/iHE.[6,7,12,13] Commonly mutated genes include *ASXL1, TET2, EZH2, SETBP1, STAT5B N642H, CBL, NOTCH, IDH2, JAK2 (exon 13), KIT, STAG2, JAK1,* and *CCT6B.* In the setting of abnormal bone marrow morphology, these mutations will help solidify a diagnosis of CEL, NOS rather than iHES/iHE. Two or more mutations and mutations involving *SETBP1, STAT5B, EZH2, NRAS, CSF3R, JAK2, and TP53* are reported to correlate with abnormal bone marrow morphology.[3] It is also acknowledged that like other myeloid neoplasms, some CEL, NOS cases may not demonstrate a molecular genetic alteration with current available testing methods. In such situations, the presence of persistent unexplained hypereosinophilia, abnormal bone marrow morphology, and clinical features of a chronic myeloid neoplasm (eg, splenomegaly) should suffice to support a diagnosis of CEL, NOS. On the other hand, some mutations may be observed in iHES/iHE.[3,13] These mutations tend to be single mutations involving DTA (*DNMT3A, TET2,* and *ASXL1*) or genes not commonly reported in myeloid neoplasms[13,14] with a variant allele frequency frequently <10%. A multidisciplinary approach is required to discriminate such cases from true clonal eosinophilia.

Prognosis and Clinical Comment

The prognosis in patients with CEL, NOS with karyotypic abnormality and/or increased blasts is unfavorable with a short median overall survival of less than 2 years.[4,6,11] The median overall survival is better (4 years) when CEL, NOS also includes cases with a normal karyotype but clonality demonstrated by mutations.[3] AML progression occurs in <20% of patients. Death is often due to infection, bleeding, disease-related organ failure, or AML transformation. In iHES, after clonal eosinophilia is excluded, the disease is often chronic in nature, and the prognosis is favorable through long-term disease control with chronic corticosteroid therapy, anti-IL5, and better management of disease/treatment complications and supportive care.[15] Long-term disease-related mortality of iHES is 10% to 15%, attributable to serious eosinophilia-related tissue damage, such as myocardial infarction or heart failure, chronic obstructive lung disease, or complications due to long-term steroid use.

References

1. Valent P, Degenfeld-Schonburg L, Sadovnik I, et al. Eosinophils and eosinophil-associated disorders: immunological, clinical, and molecular complexity. *Semin Immunopathol.* 2021;43(3):423-438. doi:10.1007/s00281-021-00863-y
2. Arber DA, Orazi A, Hasserjian RP, et al. International consensus classification of myeloid neoplasms and acute leukemias: integrating morphologic, clinical, and genomic data. *Blood.* 2022;140(11):1200-1228. doi:10.1182/blood.2022015850
3. Wang SA, Hasserjian RP, Tam W, et al. Bone marrow morphology is a strong discriminator between chronic eosinophilic leukemia, not otherwise specified and reactive idiopathic hypereosinophilic syndrome. *Haematologica.* 2017;102(8):1352-1360. doi:10.3324/haematol.2017.165340
4. Morsia E, Reichard K, Pardanani A, Tefferi A, Gangat N. WHO defined chronic eosinophilic leukemia, not otherwise specified (CEL, NOS): a contemporary series from the Mayo Clinic. *Am J Hematol.* 2020;95(7):E172-E174. doi:10.1002/ajh.25811
5. Ruan GJ, Smith CJ, Day C, et al. A population-based study of chronic eosinophilic leukemia-not otherwise specified in the United States. *Am J Hematol.* 2020;95(10):E257-E260. doi:10.1002/ajh.25906
6. Wang SA, Tam W, Tsai AG, et al. Targeted next-generation sequencing identifies a subset of idiopathic hypereosinophilic syndrome with features similar to chronic eosinophilic leukemia, not otherwise specified. *Mod Pathol.* 2016;29(8):854-864. doi:10.1038/modpathol.2016.75
7. Pardanani A, Lasho T, Wassie E, et al. Predictors of survival in WHO-defined hypereosinophilic syndrome and idiopathic hypereosinophilia and the role of next-generation sequencing. *Leukemia.* 2016;30(9):1924-1926. doi:10.1038/leu.2016.73

8. Fang H, Ketterling RP, Hanson CA, et al. A test utilization approach to the diagnostic workup of isolated eosinophilia in otherwise morphologically unremarkable bone marrow: a single institutional experience. *Am J Clin Pathol*2018;150(5):421-431. doi:10.1093/ajcp/aqy064
9. Kim H, Cho YU. Diagnostic spectrum of hypereosinophilia based on bone marrow pathology: 10 years' experience at a tertiary care hospital. *Int J Lab Hematol.* 2023;45(3):328-336. doi:10.1111/ijlh.14025
10. Kelemen K, Saft L, Craig FE, et al. Eosinophilia/hypereosinophilia in the setting of reactive and idiopathic causes, well-defined myeloid or lymphoid leukemias, or germline disorders. *Am J Clin Pathol.* 2021;155(2):179-210. doi:10.1093/ajcp/aqaa244
11. Helbig G, Soja A, Bartkowska-Chrobok A, Kyrcz-Krzemien S. Chronic eosinophilic leukemia-not otherwise specified has a poor prognosis with unresponsiveness to conventional treatment and high risk of acute transformation. *Am J Hematol.* 2012;87(6):643-645. doi:10.1002/ajh.23193
12. Cross NCP, Hoade Y, Tapper WJ, et al. Recurrent activating STAT5B N642H mutation in myeloid neoplasms with eosinophilia. *Leukemia.* 2019;33(2):415-425. doi:10.1038/s41375-018-0342-3
13. Lee JS, Seo H, Im K, et al. Idiopathic hypereosinophilia is clonal disorder? Clonality identified by targeted sequencing. *PLoS One.* 2017;12(10):e0185602. doi:10.1371/journal.pone.0185602
14. Choudhuri J, Eskandari M, Shi Y, Wang Y. Intermediate between idiopathic hypereosinophilia and chronic eosinophilic leukemia: a report of two hypereosinophilic cases with possible novel molecular mutations. *Case Rep Hematol.* 2021;2021:1142124. doi:10.1155/2021/1142124
15. Shomali W, Gotlib J. World Health Organization-defined eosinophilic disorders: 2022 update on diagnosis, risk stratification, and management. *Am J Hematol.* 2022;97(1):129-148. doi:10.1002/ajh.26352

Chapter 5

Myeloproliferative Neoplasms, Unclassifiable

Umberto Gianelli, Hans Michael Kvasnicka, Attilio Orazi, Ayalew Tefferi, and Juergen Thiele

Definition

Myeloproliferative neoplasms unclassifiable (MPN-U) represent a heterogeneous group with clinical, morphologic, or molecular features consistent with a diagnosis of myeloproliferative neoplasm (MPN) but lacking or overlapping the diagnostic criteria for one of the specific MPN subtypes.[1]

In practice, cases of MPN-U can be divided into several phenotypic categories: (1) MPN at a very early (prodromal) stage of the disease, when the morphologic and/or clinical features of a specific entity are not fully developed[2]; (2) MPN at an advanced stage, in which the presence of severe myelofibrosis (MF), osteosclerosis, and/or cell depletion does not allow accurate subclassification[3,4]; (3) MPN cases with thrombosis at unusual sites, such as splanchnic or cerebral vein thrombosis, associated with one of the driver mutations in which the bone marrow does not have fully developed or overlapping morphologic characteristics,[5] or in cases where discrepancies between the clinical and morphologic presentation occur due to hemodilution, thrombosis, and hypersplenism[6]; (4) MPN cases in which the presence of a coexisting inflammatory or neoplastic condition obscures the clinical and/or morphologic features of a specific subtype. A dynamic review over time is recommended, and cases should be reclassified to one of the defined MPN subtypes if diagnostic criteria are met after initial evaluation.[7,8]

Importantly, the diagnosis of MPN-U should not be made when laboratory data necessary for classification are incomplete or never obtained, bone marrow sample size or quality is inadequate for complete evaluation, or the patient has received prior cytotoxic or growth factor therapy.[9] In these cases, suggestions for additional clinical and laboratory information needed to accurately diagnose and subclassify the case should be provided along with a description of the morphologic features.[10]

Synonyms

None.

Epidemiology

While the incidence of MPN-U was initially reported to be 10% to 15% in earlier studies,[3] the correct application of clinical, morphologic, and molecular criteria has reduced the percentage to approximately 5%.[4,11-13]

General Clinical Features

Patients with MPN-U tend to be in the fifth or sixth decade of life.[11] Clinical features are variable and depend on the stage of disease and the underlying phenotypic category. Constitutional symptoms such as pruritus, night sweats, and weight loss are present in about one-third of cases,[10] while the presence of hepatosplenomegaly with extramedullary hematopoiesis is usually associated with advanced fibrotic cases.[14] In most patients, laboratory features are characterized by persistent thrombocytosis with or without leukocytosis.[2] Hemoglobin levels tend to remain within normal limits in early-stage cases, while anemia is a common finding in the fibrotic phase of MPN-U. Thrombotic complications, including unusual sites such as splanchnic vein thrombosis (Budd-Chiari syndrome; portal, splenic, or mesenteric vein thrombosis) or cerebral vein thrombosis (cortical or deep cerebral veins, dural venous sinuses), are common in MPN-U.[5,12] Approximately 40% of patients with MPN presenting with splanchnic vein thrombosis have discrepancies between clinical and morphologic features because the resulting portal hypertension and hypersplenism may mask the increase in blood cell counts.[6,15] In these cases, the presence of a *JAK2*, *CALR*, or *MPL* mutation helps to establish the diagnosis of an MPN. Cerebral venous thrombosis occurs in less than one percent of patients but is closely associated with *JAK2* mutation, younger age, and female gender.[5] Notably, these patients have a high risk of recurrent thrombosis, including a propensity for splanchnic venous events despite antithrombotic therapy.[5] Significant cytopenia is uncommon and suggests an alternative diagnosis such as myelodysplastic syndrome (MDS) with fibrosis or an MDS/MPN overlap.[1,9]

Morphology

Basic diagnostic evaluation requires the integration of complete blood counts, peripheral blood smear, bone marrow aspirate and trephine biopsy for morphological assessment, cytogenetic evaluation, and MPN driver mutation screening (Table 5.1).[1]

Morphologic features are variable and related to the heterogeneity of MPN-U cases. Early-phase (prodromal) MPN is more often characterized by increased, sometimes left-shifted, granulopoiesis in the bone marrow,[2] whereas a predominant erythropoiesis is seen in less than 30% of cases.[12] Megakaryocytes are usually increased in number and tend to form clusters, more often loose, although dense and large clusters may be seen in some cases. Giant forms with hyperlobulated or bulbous nuclei and maturation defects are common. A mild increase in bone marrow fibrosis is seen in most cases. In this early stage category, three possible differential diagnoses should be considered[2]: (1) essential thrombocythemia (ET), (2) prefibrotic primary myelofibrosis (pre-PMF), and (3) early (prepolycythemic) phase of polycythemia vera (PV). A normocellular or mildly hypercellular bone marrow with an increased number of megakaryocytes, predominantly characterized by large to giant elements with hyperlobulated nuclei and mature cytoplasm that tend to form loose clusters, is morphologically compatible with ET.[16] In contrast, a hypercellular bone marrow with expanded left-shifted granulopoiesis, increased myeloid/erythroid ratio, and increased number of morphologically atypical megakaryocytes (increased nuclear/cytoplasmic ratio, irregular chromatin clumping, bulbous appearance, hyperchromatic nuclei) that predominantly form dense and large clusters is morphologically indicative of pre-PMF.[2,16] However, sometimes there is a true morphologic overlap between the two patterns (Figure 5.1). In these cases, the bone marrow is only mildly hypercellular due to expanded granulopoiesis and the proliferating megakaryopoiesis does not reveal the full spectrum of morphologic abnormalities, especially dense clustering. In addition, there may be an overlap of clinical features, such as splenomegaly and/or borderline anemia. Therefore, it is important to emphasize that the diagnosis of ET and especially pre-PMF must be supported by additional clinical criteria.[1,9,16] Otherwise, a diagnosis of MPN-U with a comment on the morphologic pattern found is more appropriate. In *JAK2*-mutated cases with borderline elevated hemoglobin and hematocrit values below the defined diagnostic thresholds for PV, but hypercellular bone marrow with increased erythrocytosis and granulopoiesis and pleomorphic megakaryopoiesis, a very early (prepolycythemic) phase of PV could be suspected and a final diagnosis of MPN-U with a morphologic pattern of PV should be made (Figure 5.2).[17] Of note, patients presenting with thrombotic complications in unusual

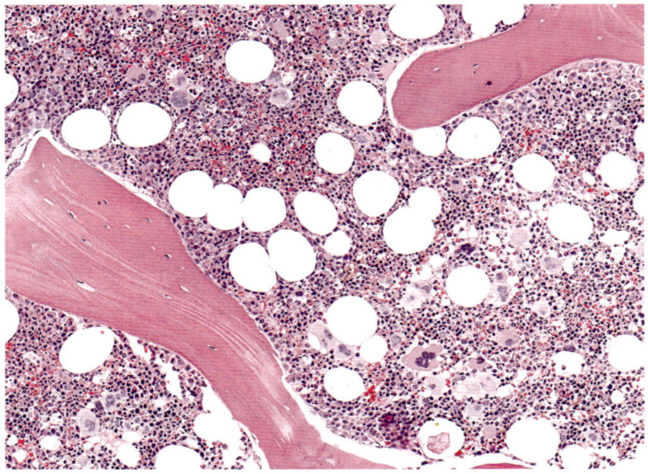

FIGURE 5.1 Male, 16 years old, presenting with thrombocytosis *JAK2* V617F positive; WBC 13.5 × 10^9/L, Hb 15.1 g/dL, PLT 823 × 10^9/L, LDH 342, spleen: 13.3 cm. The bone marrow is slightly hypercellular for the patient's age with hyperplastic granulopoiesis (especially in paratrabecular location) and increased number of polymorphic megakaryocytes with large to giant forms with hyperlobulated nuclei and few elements with bulbous atypical nuclei, increased nuclear/cytoplasmic ratio, and initial reticulin fibrosis (MF-1). The differential diagnosis is between essential thrombocythemia and prefibrotic primary myelofibrosis, but there is an overlap in morphologic features. The diagnosis of myeloproliferative neoplasms unclassifiable is appropriate (Hematoxylin and eosin, 20×).

TABLE 5.1 Diagnostic criteria of myeloproliferative neoplasms, unclassifiable (MPN-U)

1. Clinical and hematological features of an MPN are present[a]
2. *JAK2*, *CALR*, or *MPL* mutation[b] or presence of another clonal marker[c]
3. Diagnostic criteria for any other MPN, MDS, MDS/MPN[d] or *BCR::ABL1*-positive CML are not met

The Diagnosis of MPN-U Requires all three Criteria

[a]In cases presenting with bone marrow fibrosis reactive causes must be excluded (eg, bone marrow fibrosis secondary to infection, autoimmune disorder or another chronic inflammatory condition, hairy cell leukemia or another lymphoid neoplasm, metastatic malignancy, or toxic myelopathy).
[b]It is recommended to use highly sensitive assays for *JAK2* V617F (sensitivity level, 1%) and *CALR* and *MPL* (sensitivity level 1%-3%); in negative cases, consider searching for noncanonical *JAK2* and *MPL* mutations.
[c]Assessed by cytogenetics or sensitive next-generation sequencing techniques; detection of variants associated with myeloid neoplasms (*ASXL1*, *EZH2*, *IDH1*, *IDH2*, *SF3B1*, *SRSF2*, and *TET2* mutations) supports the clonal nature of the disease.
[d]In cases presenting with myelodysplastic features effects of any previous treatment, severe comorbidity, and changes during the natural progression of the disease process must be carefully excluded.

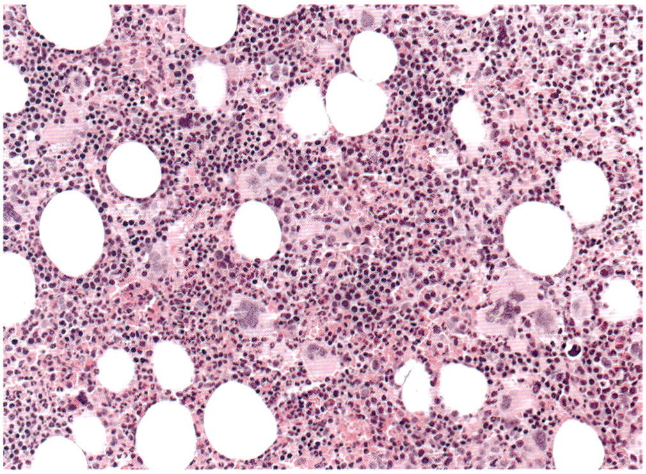

FIGURE 5.2 Male, 38 years old, presenting with splanchnic vein thrombosis *JAK2* V617F positive, hemoglobin 13.2 g/dL, hematocrit 42%, WBC 6.7 × 10^9/L, PLT 270 × 10^9/L. The bone marrow is hypercellular with prominent erythropoiesis and increased number of megakaryocytes with a marked polymorphism suggestive of polycythemia vera, but clinical thresholds for hemoglobin and hematocrit are not met. The diagnosis of myeloproliferative neoplasms unclassifiable is appropriate. (Hematoxylin and eosin, 40x).

sites, such as splanchnic or cerebral vein thrombosis, may have a very low variant allele frequency for *JAK2* and no significant increase in bone marrow cellularity and/or other morphologic features suggestive of PV.[6,18] However, it is important to recognize these patients as they have the same clinical risk of thromboembolic complications as fully established (polycythemic) PV.[7,19]

Diagnostic difficulties may also occur in advanced stages of MPN with overt MF and osteosclerosis.[3] In these cases, bone marrow cellularity ranges from hypercellular to very hypocellular (cell-depleted) patterns, often accompanied by grossly atypical megakaryopoiesis, myelodysplastic changes in erythropoiesis and granulopoiesis, and/or increased blasts. At this stage of the disease, it may be difficult or impossible to distinguish between overt PMF and secondary MF due to progression of PV or ET (post-PV MF or post-ET MF), without knowledge of the clinical history.[10,12] A detailed description of all morphologic and stromal changes including immunohistochemistry with CD34 and CD117 to highlight blasts would be appropriate, and a diagnosis of MPN-U should be made.

The differential diagnosis of MDS with bone marrow fibrosis can be challenging and requires careful integration of clinical, morphologic, and molecular data.[1,7,20] The presence of dyserythropoiesis and/or dysgranulopoiesis mandates classification as MDS, whereas persistent monocytosis should prompt a differential diagnosis of myelodysplastic/myeloproliferative neoplasm (MDS/MPN). Anemia and ineffective erythroid proliferation with dyserythropoiesis and the presence of ring sideroblasts and/or the detection of an *SF3B1* mutation are key diagnostic features of MDS/MPN-RS-T, NOS and MDS/MPN-T-SF3B1 and thus exclude the diagnosis of MPN-U.[1] In contrast, the presence of at least some degree of cytosis (more commonly thrombocytosis) and organomegaly associated with the morphology of megakaryocytes presenting as large to giant cells with hyperlobulated nuclei and the detection of driver mutations (*JAK2*, *CALR*, or *MPL*) strongly support the diagnosis of MPN-U.[13]

A chronic inflammatory or neoplastic condition (lymphoid or myeloid neoplasm, solid tumor) that extensively involves the bone marrow may obscure the diagnostic features of an underlying MPN.[3] The presence of megakaryocytes with MPN-like features (especially large to giant megakaryocytes with hyperlobulated nuclei or atypically clustered megakaryocytes with bulbous nuclei) along with the detection of an MPN driver mutation may help support the diagnosis of coexisting MPN-U.

In line with the other MPN subtypes, an increase in peripheral blood or bone marrow blasts between 10% and 19% is classified as MPN-U in accelerated phase, and any blast count of 20% or more is defined as blast phase.[1] Immunohistochemical evaluation of the bone marrow biopsy by CD34 or CD117 is recommended in grossly fibrotic bone marrow specimens that prevent aspiration.

Immunophenotype

In most cases, immunophenotyping does not facilitate the diagnosis of MPN-U, but in the blast phase, a population of early committed CD34+ myeloid blasts can almost always be detected by flow cytometry. Immunohistochemistry of the bone marrow biopsy with lineage-specific markers such as glycophorin C, CD71, E-cadherin, myeloperoxidase, and CD61 or CD42b may be helpful to evaluate the morphological pattern. In the accelerated or blast phase, immunohistochemistry for CD34 and CD117 facilitates the assessment of immature elements. Pan-B- and pan-T-cell markers can be useful in characterizing lymphoid aggregates, and tryptase helps in the differential diagnosis of mast cell infiltrates.[20]

Genetics

Genetic and molecular abnormalities are not specific for the diagnosis of MPN-U, but MPN-associated driver mutations involving *JAK2*, *CALR*, or *MPL* genes are found in approximately 70% to 80% of patients.[11,12] In so-called triple-negative cases, the detection of additional variants such as *ASXL1*, *EZH2*, *TET2*, *IDH1*, *IDH2*, *IDH2*, and *SF3B1* supports the diagnosis of a clonal disease.[9] Approximately 20% to 30% of patients have cytogenetic abnormalities.[10,12] The finding of a *BCR::ABL1* fusion gene or rearrangements of *PDGFRA*, *PDGFRB*, or *FGFR1* or *PCM1::JAK2* precludes the diagnosis of MPN-U.[1] It is important to emphasize that the identification of a driver mutation or the detection of another clonal driver is a necessary diagnostic criterion for the diagnosis of MPN-U. Documentation of the clonal nature is particularly important to separate some MPN-mimicking reactive conditions such as infections, morphologic changes due to toxins and chemotherapy, and administration of growth factors, cytokines, and immunosuppressive agents.[7]

Prognosis and Clinical Comment

The prognosis of patients diagnosed with MPN-U is highly variable and depends on the stage of the disease as well as the clinical setting.[10] In general, early-stage disease with overlapping morphologic and/or clinical features has a favorable prognosis with an estimated 10-year overall survival of 88%.[12] Consistent with other MPN subtypes, high-risk molecular status and triple-negative disease have been identified as negative prognostic parameters in these patients.[21] Major arterial and venous thrombotic events including splanchnic vein thrombosis (Budd-Chiari syndrome, portal, splenic, or mesenteric vein thrombosis) are common and affect the overall morbidity and mortality in MPN-U.[6] Patients with advanced, overtly fibrotic MPN-U are likely to have significant disease-related symptoms and a poor prognosis, with estimated overall survival ranging from 1.5 to 4 years. Clinical features such as platelet count $<500 \times 10^9$/L and leukocytosis $>12 \times 10^9$/L may also influence event-free survival.[12] Prognostic stratification in these patients should always include clinical, cytogenetic, and molecular features by calculating an individual risk score.[21] Patients with MPN-U with concurrent malignancy are expected to have a worse prognosis.[12]

References

1. Arber DA, Orazi A, Hasserjian RP, et al. International consensus classification of myeloid neoplasms and acute leukemias: integrating morphologic, clinical, and genomic data. *Blood*. 2022;140(11):1200-1228.
2. Kvasnicka HM, Thiele J. Prodromal myeloproliferative neoplasms: the 2008 WHO classification. *Am J Hematol.* 2010;85(1):62-69.
3. Gianelli U, Cattaneo D, Bossi A, et al. The myeloproliferative neoplasms, unclassifiable: clinical and pathological considerations. *Mod Pathol.* 2017;30(7):1043-1179.
4. Yun J, Kim JA, Park J, et al. Reclassification of subtypes in Philadelphia chromosome-negative myeloproliferative neoplasm by 2016 WHO diagnostic criteria: focus on the cases classified as myeloproliferative neoplasm, unclassifiable by the 2008 version. *Leuk Lymphoma.* 2020;61(14):3498-3502.
5. Gangat N, Guglielmelli P, Betti S, et al. Cerebral venous thrombosis and myeloproliferative neoplasms: a three-center study of 74 consecutive cases. *Am J Hematol.* 2021;96(12):1580-1586.
6. Gianelli U, Iurlo A, Cattaneo D, et al. Discrepancies between bone marrow histopathology and clinical phenotype in BCR-ABL1-negative myeloproliferative neoplasms associated with splanchnic vein thrombosis. *Leuk Res.* 2015;39(5):525-529.
7. Barbui T, Thiele J, Gisslinger H, et al. The 2016 WHO classification and diagnostic criteria for myeloproliferative neoplasms: document summary and in-depth discussion. *Blood Cancer J.* 2018;8(2):15.
8. Kvasnicka HM. WHO classification of myeloproliferative neoplasms (MPN): a critical update. *Curr Hematol Malig Rep.* 2013;8(4):333-341.
9. Thiele J, Kvasnicka HM, Orazi A, et al. The international consensus classification of myeloid neoplasms and acute Leukemias: myeloproliferative neoplasms. *Am J Hematol.* 2023;98(3):544-545.
10. McLornan DP, Hargreaves R, Hernández-Boluda JC, Harrison CN. How I manage myeloproliferative neoplasm-unclassifiable: practical approaches for 2022 and beyond. *Br J Haematol.* 2022;197(4):407-416.
11. Iurlo A, Gianelli U, Cattaneo D, Thiele J, Orazi A. Impact of the 2016 revised WHO criteria for myeloproliferative neoplasms, unclassifiable: comparison with the 2008 version. *Am J Hematol.* 2017;92(4):E48-E51.
12. Deschamps P, Moonim M, Radia D, et al. Clinicopathological characterisation of myeloproliferative neoplasm-unclassifiable (MPN-U): a retrospective analysis from a large UK tertiary referral centre. *Br J Haematol.* 2021;193(4):792-797.
13. Pizzi M, Croci GA, Ruggeri M, et al. The classification of myeloproliferative neoplasms: Rationale, Historical background and Future Perspectives with focus on unclassifiable cases. *Cancers.* 2021;13(22):5666.
14. Kvasnicka HM, Thiele J. The impact of clinicopathological studies on staging and survival in essential thrombocythemia, chronic idiopathic myelofibrosis, and polycythemia rubra vera. *Semin Thromb Hemost.* 2006;32(4 pt 2):362-371.
15. Cattaneo D, Bucelli C, Marchetti A, et al. Pathological and genomic features of myeloproliferative neoplasms

associated with splanchnic vein thrombosis in a single-center cohort. *Ann Hematol.* 2023;102(6):1409-1420.

16. Thiele J, Kvasnicka HM, Mullauer L, Buxhofer-Ausch V, Gisslinger B, Gisslinger H. Essential thrombocythemia versus early primary myelofibrosis: a multicenter study to validate the WHO classification. *Blood.* 2011;117(21):5710-5718.
17. Kvasnicka HM, Orazi A, Thiele J, et al. European LeukemiaNet study on the reproducibility of bone marrow features in masked polycythemia vera and differentiation from essential thrombocythemia. *Am J Hematol.* 2017;92(10):1062-1067.
18. Greenfield G, McMullin MF. Splanchnic venous thrombosis in JAK2 V617F mutation positive myeloproliferative neoplasms—long term follow-up of a regional case series. *Thromb J.* 2018;16:33.
19. Barbui T, Thiele J, Gisslinger H, Carobbio A, Vannucchi AM, Tefferi A. Diagnostic impact of the 2016 revised who criteria for polycythemia vera. *Am J Hematol.* 2017;92(5):417-419.
20. Gianelli U, Thiele J, Orazi A, et al. International Consensus Classification of myeloid and lymphoid neoplasms: myeloproliferative neoplasms. *Virchows Arch.* 2023;482(1):53-68.
21. Tefferi A, Guglielmelli P, Lasho TL, et al. MIPSS70+ version 2.0: mutation and karyotype-enhanced international prognostic scoring system for primary myelofibrosis. *J Clin Oncol.* 2018;36(17):1769-1770.

SECTION 2

Myeloid/Lymphoid Neoplasms With Eosinophilia and Tyrosine Kinase Gene Fusions

Chapter 6

Myeloid/Lymphoid Neoplasms With Eosinophilia and Tyrosine Kinase Gene Fusions

Sa A. Wang, Jason Gotlib, Kaaren Reichard, Andreas Reiter, and Alexandar Tzankov

The disease category made its debut in the 2008 (4th edition) World Health Organization (WHO) classification with the original name of "myeloid/lymphoid neoplasm with eosinophilia and abnormalities of *PDGFRA, PDGFRB or FGFR1.*" *PCM1::JAK2* and its genetic variants were introduced as provisional entities to the category in the revised 4th edition WHO classification. In the current classification, this category is further expanded to include rearrangements of *FLT3* and t(9;12)(q34;p13)/*ETV6::ABL1* as new members and to promote *PCM1::JAK2* and its genetic variants (*ETV6::JAK2* and *BCR::JAK2*) to formal entities. In addition, the category name is changed to myeloid/lymphoid neoplasms with eosinophilia and tyrosine kinase gene fusions (M/LN-eo-TK)[1] to emphasize that the molecular genetic changes underlying these hematopoietic neoplasms lead to constitutive tyrosine kinase (TK) signaling, amenable to targeted therapy.[2,3] These neoplasms originate from mutated pluripotent bone marrow stem cells and may differentiate along myeloid and/or lymphoid lineages, often leading to complex and heterogeneous clinical manifestations. Eosinophilia is frequently, although not invariably present; retaining "eosinophilia" in the category name helps to raise suspicion of these genetically defined lesions, particularly in cases with cryptic rearrangements. Other potential candidates for M/LN-eo-TK include, but are not limited to, rearrangements involving *LYN, FGFR2, NTRK3, RET, SKY, ALK*, and *KIT*. Such cases so far are limited to individual case studies, and more data will be needed to understand their clinicopathological features, overlap with other genetically defined entities, and response to tyrosine kinase inhibitor (TKI) therapy. However, for cases presenting as a myeloid neoplasm in chronic or blast phase, or a hematopoietic neoplasm involving both myeloid and lymphoid lineages, often accompanied by eosinophilia and responsive to TKI, a diagnosis of M/LN-eo-TK would be appropriate. With the increased use of RNA sequencing in clinical practice, more tyrosine kinase gene fusions may be discovered and added to this evolving disease category. One important note is that the diagnosis of M/LN-eo-TK applies to hematopoietic neoplasms bearing the specific genetic aberration at initial presentation, not cases (rare) that have acquired such abnormalities during disease progression/evolution.

M/LN-eo-TK share many common clinical and pathological features, although the frequencies of certain features may differ by the underlying TK fusions. The disease presentations are often heterogeneous, most commonly as a chronic myeloid neoplasm (CMN) with varying degrees of eosinophilia. It must be noted that, overall, eosinophilia ($\geq 0.5 \times 10^9$/L) is present in 70% to 80% of M/LN-eo-TK and hypereosinophilia only in 30% to 50% of cases ($\geq 1.5 \times 10^9$/L).[4-6] Abnormal eosinophils can be seen in about 30% to 50% of cases, including abnormal nuclei, granulations, and cell size, which are not unique and can be observed in other clonal eosinophilia and some reactive eosinophilia, although the latter often at a milder degree. Eosinophilia-associated tissue damage/organ dysfunction may be seen in some patients but is not universally present. Variable proportions of patients present with blast phase of CMN, or extramedullary diseases (EMDs), and the blasts can be myeloid, lymphoid, or mixed phenotype (MPAL). The EMD lesions often have an accompanied eosinophilic infiltrate. The peripheral blood and bone marrow features vary from case to case. Before a TK gene is identified, based on peripheral blood and bone marrow findings, these cases may be diagnosed as chronic eosinophilic leukemia, not otherwise specified (CEL, NOS), myeloproliferative neoplasm, unclassifiable (MPN-U), chronic myelomonocytic leukemia (CMML), atypical chronic myeloid leukemia (aCML), myelodysplastic/myeloproliferative neoplasm, not otherwise specified (MDS/MPN, NOS), myelodysplastic syndrome (MDS), acute myeloid leukemia (AML)/myeloid sarcoma, acute B- or T-lymphoblastic leukemia/lymphoma (B- or T-ALL/LBL), rarely juvenile chronic myelomonocytic leukemia (JMML), or systemic mastocytosis (SM) with or without an associated myeloid neoplasm (SM-AMN). Increased spindle mast cells have been described in almost all types of TK fusions except for *PCM1::JAK2*, and immunohistochemistry for mast cells (CD117, tryptase) with aberrant expression of CD25 may provide diagnostic hints for clonal eosinophilia.

M/LN-eo-TK may present as B- or T-lymphoblastic leukemia/lymphoma (ALL), whereas *BCR::ABL1*-like B-ALL, de novo T-ALL, and even mature T-cell lymphoma may involve one of the TK genes. The differences may be at least in part attributable to the partner genes fused with the TK genes. For example, t(5;12)(q32;p13.2)/*ETV6::PDGFRB* often manifests with multilineage involvement, characteristic of M/LN-eo-TK, whereas *PDGFRB* with partners such as *EBF1*, *SSBP2*, *TNIP1*, *ZEB2*, and *ATF7IP* often presents as de novo B-ALL without involvement of the myeloid lineage and should be diagnosed as *BCR::ABL1*-like B-ALL.[7] Similarly, *JAK2* fusions with certain partner genes, such as t(5;9)(q14.1;p24.1)/*STRN3::JAK2*, and *PAX5::JAK2* are usually seen in *BCR::ABL1*-like B-ALL, which are, by definition, not M/LN-eo-TK. To complicate the issue, some fusion partners, such as *ETV6::JAK2* and *ETV6::ABL1*, are observed in both entities.[8-10] This overlap occurs in all TK genes, and the diagnosis should be driven by the general rule that, for cases of M/LN-eo-TK that initially present as B- or T-ALL, the TK gene fusion should involve the myeloid lineage in addition to lymphoblasts. In such instances, the CMN of M/LN-eo-TK may manifest prior to or concomitantly with or emerge after therapy for the ALL (Figure 6.1). This concept is similar to the distinction between CML presenting in lymphoid blast crisis and de novo adult *BCR::ABL1*+ ALL. For practical purposes, fluorescence in situ hybridization (FISH) studies detecting respective gene fusions in a clearly myeloid population is helpful in distinguishing M/LN-eo-TK from ALL.

As mentioned earlier, abnormal mast cells are commonly observed in M/LN-eo-TK. In rare cases, especially in cases with a high serum tryptase, the mast cell proliferation can be florid and mimic SM. However, these cases consistently lack the *KIT* D816V mutation and show similar responses to TKI as other M/LN-eo-TK.[6,11] In the current classification, such cases are classified under M/LN-eo-TK if one of the TK gene fusions is detected.[1,10,12] It is highly recommended to test cases of putative SM for TK gene fusions in cases associated with eosinophilia and lacking a *KIT* mutation (using high-sensitivity molecular methods). In rare cases, a TK gene fusion and a *KIT* D816V mutation may coexist, and these may represent co-occurrence of two diseases with separate clones or a subclone with an acquired activating *KIT* mutation, which fall within the spectrum of SM-AMN with M/LN-eo-TK being the associated myeloid neoplasm (AMN).

Key points in differentiating these overlapping entities are illustrated in Figure 6.1.

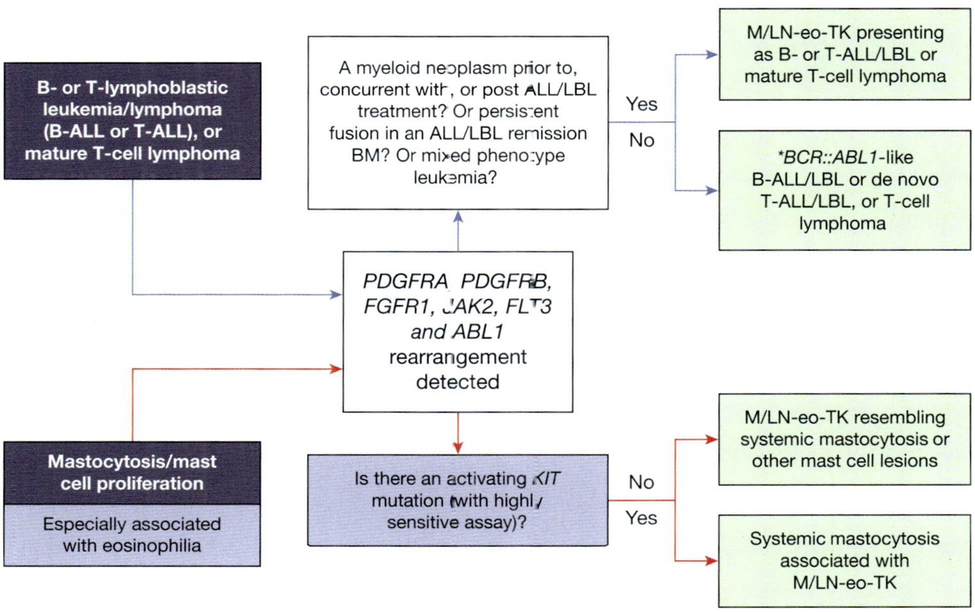

FIGURE 6.1 Addressing the overlapping entities. (1) Myeloid/lymphoid neoplasm with eosinophilia and tyrosine kinase fusion(M/LN-eo-TK) versus *BCR::ABL1*-like B-ALL/LBL, de novo T-ALL/LBL, or mature T-cell lymphoma; (2) M/LN-eo-TK versus systemic mastocytosis with associated M/LN-eo-TK. *Certain partner genes, such as *EBF1, SSBP2, TNIP1, ZEB2, and ATF7IP with PDGFRB; ATF7IP, EBF1, GOLGA5, HMBOX1, OFD1, PAX5, PPFIBP1, RFX3, SMU1, SNX29, SSBP2, STRN3, TERF2, TPR, USP25, ZBTB46, ZNF274, ZNF340* with *JAK2*, are almost exclusively reported in *BCR::ABL1*-like B-ALL, not M/LN-eo-TK.

MYELOID/LYMPHOID NEOPLASMS WITH EOSINOPHILIA AND REARRANGEMENT OF *PDGFRA*

Definition

A myeloid and/or lymphoid neoplasm derived from a pluripotent (lymphoid/myeloid) stem cell bearing a rearrangement of *PDGFRA* or rarely an activating mutation leading to constitutive activation of the TK. Most cases (approximately 90%) harboring the *FIP1L1::PDGFRA* fusion present as a chronic myeloid neoplasm (CMN) with eosinophilia. A minority of cases show alternative gene partners.

Synonyms

None.

Epidemiology

There is a marked male predominance with a male:female ratio of approximately 17:1. The median age of presentation is in the late 40s, peak 25 to 55 years. It is the most common rearrangement among M/LN-eo-TK.

General Clinical Features

Patients may present with fatigue, shortness of breath, and constitutional symptoms, some with pruritus, respiratory, and, rarely, cardiac or gastrointestinal symptoms.[6,13] The latter symptoms are likely related to end-organ damage due to an eosinophilic infiltrate or the release of enzymes and other proteins by the eosinophils. Splenomegaly is common, seen in 40% to 50% of patients, and hepatomegaly may be seen in some patients. Some patients may present with extramedullary diseases (EMDs). Eosinophilia is present in 90% of patients, essentially in all patients with *FIP1L1::PDGFRA*,[4] although some may not reach hypereosinophilia (1.5×10^9/L). Some patients have anemia, thrombocytopenia, and monocytosis.[4] Other laboratory features include a marked increase in serum vitamin B_{12} and elevated serum tryptase.

Morphology and Immunophenotype

Eosinophils in peripheral blood are increased with mostly mature morphology. Marked eosinophil abnormalities are seen in >50% of cases,[6] including hypo- and/or uneven granulation, abnormal large or small granules, cytoplasmic vacuolation, nuclear hyper- or hyposegmentation, and increased eosinophil size (Figure 6.2).[6,13,14] Blasts, basophils, and monocyte counts are usually not increased but may be seen in some cases with partner genes other than *FIP1L1*.

The bone marrow is hypercellular with markedly increased numbers of eosinophils. Eosinophils are mainly of mature forms, but in some cases, they may be left-shifted with increased eosinophil precursors. Eosinophil abnormalities, if present, are usually less pronounced than those observed in peripheral blood. Megakaryocytes are frequently decreased but can be adequate or increased and morphologically may be unremarkable, large with separate nuclear lobes, small dysplastic forms, or exhibiting a spectrum of morphology (Figure 6.2).[6] Focal necrosis, and Charcot-Leyden crystals may be seen. Mast cells are often increased and spindled, mostly scattered, or in loose noncohesive clusters, but in some cases, the mast cell proliferation may form aggregates resembling SM.[6,11] Mild myelofibrosis is common, but MF-2 or MF-3 fibrosis is only seen in 20% cases.

A minor proportion of patients present with acute leukemia, such as AML or T-ALL/LBL, which may be preceded by eosinophilia. Extramedullary infiltrates or tumoral lesions are not infrequent, commonly involving lymph nodes, epidural and/or paraspinal spaces, bones, and cutaneous tissue. These lesions are often myeloid, ranging from immature to mature; in some cases, they can be T-ALL/LBL, and rarely B-ALL/LBL. Eosinophils are variably present. These EMD lesions may present at initial diagnosis or later in the course of the disease. If blasts are increased, or EMD lesions are biopsied, flow cytometric immunophenotyping and/or immunohistochemistry should be utilized to characterize their phenotype. The presence of abnormal mast cells often helps to confirm clonal eosinophilia.

Genetics

The *PDGFRA* rearrangement is usually due to an interstitial deletion of approximately 800 kb (including *CHIC2*) on chromosome 4q12 that leads to the *FIP1L1::PDGFRA* fusion. This rearrangement is cryptic on conventional karyotyping and requires FISH, reverse transcription polymerase chain reaction (RT-PCR) or RNA sequencing (RNAseq) for identification. Seven other partner genes have been reported, including *CDK5RAP2*/ins(9;4)(q33;q12q25), *ETV6*/t(4;12)(q12;p13), *FOXP1*/t(3;4)(p13;q12), *KIF5B*/t(4;10)(q12;p11), *STRN*/t(2;4)(p22;q12), *TNKS2*/t(4;10)(q12;q23), *BCR*/t(4;22)(q12;q11) (Table 6.1). These

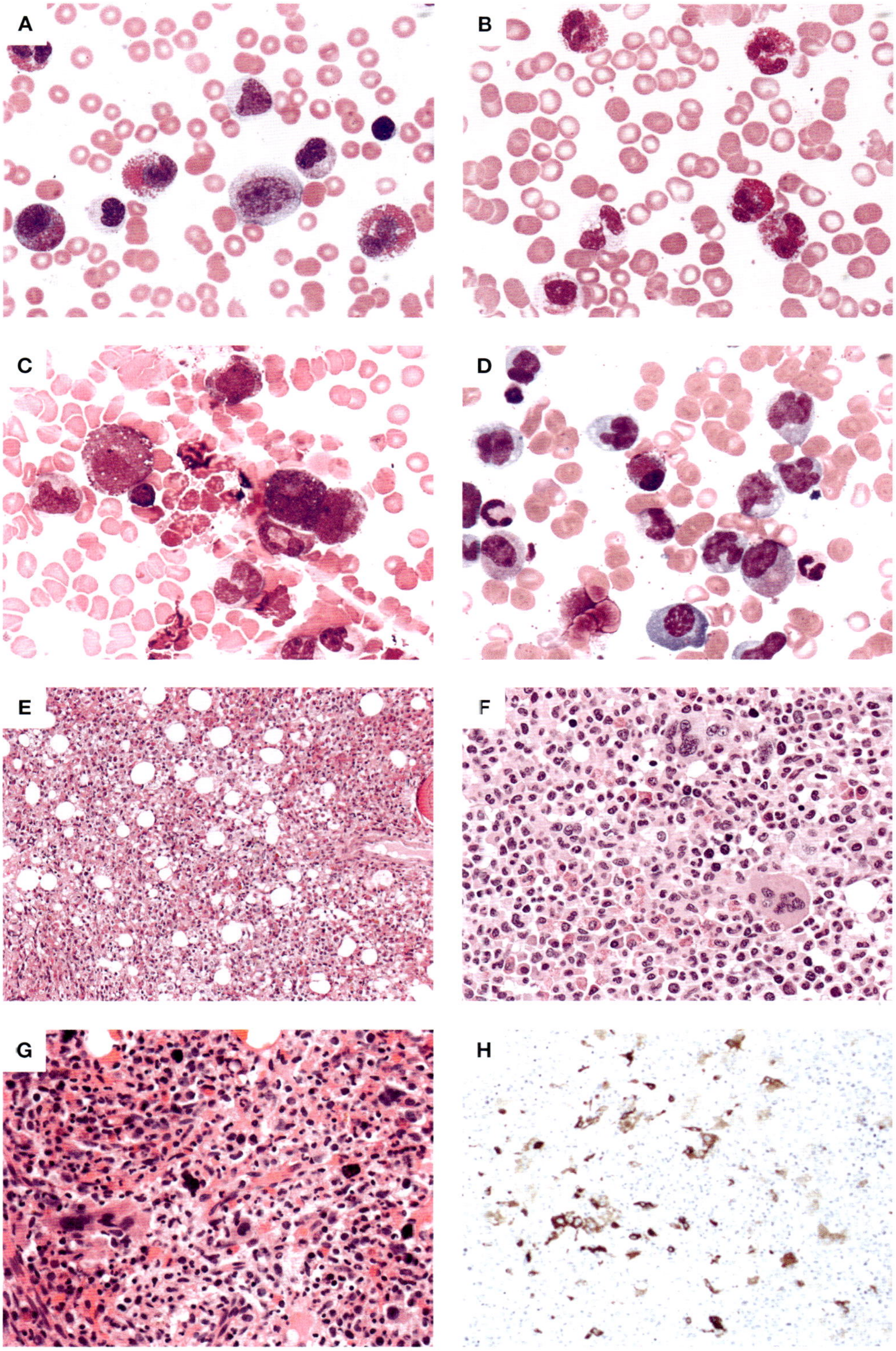

FIGURE 6.2 Common peripheral blood (PB) and bone marrow (BM) findings of M/LN-eo-TK, illustration using cases of *PDGFRA* (A, C, E, F) and *PDGFRB* (B, D, F, H). PB frequently shows eosinophilia (**A** and **B**); eosinophil abnormalities can be frequently observed, such as nuclear hypo- (**A**) or hyper- (**B**) segmentation, abnormal granulation (**A** and **B**), large forms (**A**). Some cases may also show granulocytic abnormalities, such as dysgranulopoiesis and the presence of granulocytic precursors (**A**). BM eosinophilic abnormalities are usually less striking than that of PB but frequently show increased eosinophilic precursors. Monocytosis can be seen in 15% to 20% *PDGFRB* rearranged cases; in this case, also shown in BM (D). BM trephine biopsy is usually hypercellular (**E-G**); megakaryocytes may be significantly decreased (**E**) or large with widely separated nuclei (**F**) or small dysplastic forms (**G**). Increased scatter spindle mast cells are common and may be seen in any M/LN-eo-TK (**H**). (**A-D:** Wright-Giemsa; **E-G:** hematoxylin and eosin; **H:** tryptase; **A-D:** 100×, **E:** 20×, **F-H:** 40×).

TABLE 6.1 Genetic abnormalities, clinical presentations, and targeted therapy of myeloid/lymphoid neoplasms with eosinophilia and tyrosine kinase gene fusions (M/LN-eo-TK)

TK gene	Most common fusion	Other partner genes/variants	Typical clinical and bone marrow (BM) manifestations	Accompanying mutations	Targeted therapy
PDGFRA	Cryptic deletion 4q12/ *FIP1L1::PDGFRA*[a]	*BCR; CDK5RAP2; ETV6; FOXP1; KIF5B; STRN; TNKS2*	Most common M/LN-eo-TK with a male-to-female ratio: 17:1; median age in the late 40s; eosinophilia in >90%.Most commonly presenting as CEL-like CMN with extramedullary involvement.	20%-50%, including *ASXL1, BCOR, DNMT3A, RUNX1, SRSF2, TET2, PTPN11*	Durable and complete hematologic, cytogenetic, and molecular remissions to the first-generation TKI (imatinib).
PDGFRB	t(5;12)(q32;p13.2)/ *ETV6::PDGFRB*	>30 partners, may be cryptic	Male-to-female ratio: 2:1; median age in the late 40s, PB eosinophilia in around 80%. Common presentations are CEL- or CMML-, aCML-like CMN, less commonly MDS, SM.	30%-50%, including *ASXL1, BCOR, DNMT3A, NRAS, STAG2, STAT5B, TET2, ZSRS2*	Durable and complete hematologic, cytogenetic, and molecular remissions to the first-generation TKI (imatinib).
FGFR1	t(8;13)(p11.1;q12.1)/ *ZMYM2::FGFR1*	15 other partners, including *BCR*	Male-to-female ratio: 1.5:1; median age in the late 40s to 50s; PB eosinophilia in around 70%.Commonly presenting with nodal T-ALL/LBL with BM MPN-like features or blast phase (myeloid, B-ALL/LBL or mixed phenotype) of MPN in the BM.	70%, including *RUNX1, ASXL1, CSFR3, STAG2, FBXW7*	Complete clinical and cytogenetic responses to pemigatinib (anti-FGFR1-3), but more durable in chronic disease. Futibatinib (anti-FGFR1-4) under clinical trial evaluation.
JAK2	t(8;9)(p22;p24.1)/ *PCM1::JAK2*	[b]*ETV6* and *BCR*	Male-to-female ratio: 5.5:1; median age in the late 40s; PB eosinophilia in about 70%-80%. Commonly presenting as MPN or MDN/MPN-like BM with eosinophilia. Some in accelerated or blast phase of MPN or with extramedullary disease (B- and T-ALL/LBL, myeloid).	14%-50%, including *ASXL1, BCOR, BCORL1, CD36, EP300, ETV6, RUNX1, SRSF2, TET2, TP53*	Some achieve hematologic and cytogenetic responses to ruxolitinib but often not durable
FLT3	t(12;13)(p13.2;q12.2)/ *ETV6::FLT3*	*BCR; CCDC88C; GOLGB1; MYO18A; SPTBN1; TRIP11; ZMYM2*	Male-to-female ratio: 3:1; median age in the mid-40s; PB eosinophilia in about 70%-80%. Commonly presenting with T-ALL/LBL or myeloid sarcoma with CEL-, MPN- or MDS/MPN-like BM features.	Around 50%, including *ASXL1, RUNX1, STAT5B, SRSF2, TET2, TP53, U2AF1*	Hematologic and cytogenetic responses to FLT3 inhibitors (eg, sorafenib, sunitinib, midostaurin, gilteritinib), but the response may not be durable.
ETV6::ABL1	t(9;12)(q34.1;p13.2)/ *ETV6::ABL1*	Unknown	Male-to-female ratio: 3:1; median age in the late 40s. PB eosinophilia in about 90%-100%. Commonly presenting as CML-like with eosinophilia in chronic phase. Some in blast phase or with extramedullary T-ALL/LBL.	40%-50%, including *ARID2, CDKN1B, TP53, SMC1A*	More durable responses to second-generation ABL1-targeting TKI (eg, dasatinib, nilotinib).

PB eosinophilia is defined as eosinophils >6% and an absolute eosinophil count $>0.5 \times 10^9$/L.

aCML, atypical chronic myeloid leukemia; ALL/LBL, acute lymphoblastic leukemia/lymphoblastic lymphoma; AML, acute myeloid leukemia; BM, bone marrow; CEL, chronic eosinophilic leukemia; CML, chronic myeloid leukemia; CMML, chronic myelomonocytic leukemia; CMN, chronic myeloid neoplasm; MDS/MPN: myelodysplastic syndrome/myeloproliferative neoplasm; MPN, myeloproliferative neoplasm; PB, peripheral blood; SM, systemic mastocytosis; TK/TKI, tyrosine kinase/inhibitor.

Modified from Wang SA, Orazi A, Gotlib J, et al. The international consensus classification of eosinophilic disorders and systemic mastocytosis. *Am J Hematol.* 2023;98(8):1286-1306. doi:10.1002/ajh.26966

[a]Cases with activating point mutations of *PDGFRA* have been reported and should, as an exception with the family of M/LN-eo-TK, be considered within the spectrum of M/LN-eo-TK.

[b]Other rarely reported partner genes are *RPN1, NF-E2, RUNX1, PEX14*; however, the information is very limited.

variants are usually not cryptic, but to demonstrate the fusion involving *PDGFRA* is essential. One example is that some AMLs with t(4;12)(q12;p13) have been reported to carry a *PDGFRA* rearrangement by FISH but are insensitive to imatinib. An RNAseq study[15] demonstrated *ETV6* fusions with *SCFD2, CHIC2,* and *GSX2* at 4q12, which are too close to *PDGFRA* to be resolved by chromosomal analysis or FISH analysis (false-positive FISH). Note is made that t(4;12)(q12;p13) with true *ETV6::PDGFRA* fusion is typically presenting as CMN with eosinophilia while t(4;12)(q12;p13) involving genes other than *PDGFRA* at 4q12 partners often have no eosinophilia. False-negative FISH may also occur, indicating the need to pursue RNAseq or other diagnostic modalities in highly suspected cases. Mutations are reported in 20% to 50% of cases of M/LN-eo with *PDGFRA*[6,16] including *ASXL1, BCOR, DNMT3A, ETV6, SRSF2, PTPN11,* and *RUNX1.* The significance of these additional mutations is largely unknown.

Prognosis and Clinical Comment

Almost all patients with a *PDGFRA* fusion are sensitive to low-dose (100 mg/d) imatinib.[4,5,17] Recent data have shown that a treatment-free remission can be maintained in a proportion of patients after imatinib discontinuation and a rapid second remission can be achieved after restart of imatinib in relapsed patients.[4,17] Primary or secondary resistance is unusual, but if it occurs, it is linked to the T674I or D842V mutation within the ATP-binding domain of *PDGFRA* and associated with a poor prognosis. Such patients have shown some but not durable response to second- or third-generation TKIs[18]; therefore, rapid bridging to allogeneic hematopoietic stem cell transplantation (HSCT) is strongly encouraged.

MYELOID/LYMPHOID NEOPLASMS WITH EOSINOPHILIA AND REARRANGEMENT OF *PDGFRB*

Definition

A myeloid and/or lymphoid neoplasm derived from a pluripotent (lymphoid/myeloid) stem cell bearing a rearrangement of the *PDGFRB* leading to constitutive activation of the TK. Most cases present as chronic myeloid neoplasm (CMN), and some as acute leukemia, frequently, but not invariably, associated with eosinophilia.

Synonyms

None.

Epidemiology

Patients show a slight male predominance with a male:female ratio of 2:1. The age range of presentation is quite broad, from children to the elderly, with the median age of onset in the 40s.

General Clinical Features

Diseases mainly present as a CMN with frequent eosinophilia, rarely AML, B-ALL/LBL, or T-ALL/LBL. In cases presenting as CMN, constitutional symptoms and symptoms related with anemia are common.[19] Splenomegaly is seen in 40% to 50% of patients, and hepatomegaly is much less common. Eosinophilia-associated end-organ damage may occur, causing intermittent pain (low back, head, chest, or abdomen), skin rash, and respiratory symptoms. Serum tryptase is frequently increased, and LDH is elevated in a subset of patients.

Morphology and Immunophenotype

Leukocytosis is common, seen in 60% to 70%, and peripheral blood eosinophilia in around 70% to 80% of patients[6,9,19] and hypereosinophilia in around 50%.[4] Owing to a high white blood cell count, more than 30% of patients[4] have ≥1.0 × 10^9/L monocytes but only around 15% to 20% of patients have both relative (≥10%) and absolute monocytosis.[6,19] Anemia is common, but thrombocytopenia is less frequent. Like M/LN-eo-TK *PDGFRA*, blood eosinophil morphologic abnormalities can be observed in around half of the cases (Figure 6.2).

The bone marrow is hypercellular with an increase in eosinophils, granulocytes, and monocytes (in some cases) (see Figure 6.2). Megakaryocytes may be increased, decreased, or adequate in number, with unremarkable, dysplastic features or occasionally myeloproliferative-type large forms. Like M/LN-eo-TK with *PDGFRA*, the bone marrow may show increased, individually distributed spindled mast cells with aberrant expression of CD25, which can be highlighted by immunohistochemical stains such as CD117 and tryptase (see Figure 6.2). Rarely, focal compact dense clusters of mast cells may be seen, resembling systemic mastocytosis (SM). Significant myelofibrosis (MF-2 or MF-3) may be seen in one-third of cases. Depending on the peripheral blood and bone marrow features, these CMNs have been described resembling CEL, NOS; CMML with eosinophilia; MDS; aCML; MDS/MPN, NOS; MPN-U; or SM. In some cases, patients may present with acute leukemia, lymphoblastic leukemia, and/or extramedullary diseases (EMDs).

Genetics

PDGFRB is located at 5q32 and so far has more than 30 partner fusion genes,[3] with t(5;12)(q32;p13.2)/*ETV6::PDGFRB* being the most common (around 50%), followed by *CCDC88C::PDGFRB* and the rest mostly reported in individual cases. It was believed previously that *PDGFRB*-rearranged M/LN-eo should demonstrate a 5q31-33 abnormality on an adequate conventional karyotype. However, recent studies have shown that cryptic *PDGFRB* rearrangements are common[6,19] and frequently occur with partner genes other than *ETV6*, such as *DIAPH1*, *BCR*,[19] *AFAP1L1*, *SART3*, and *GBP1*. Cryptic fusions likely occur as a result of small deletions, inversions, or obscurity within a complex karyotype. Furthermore, some of the fusions may not even be detected by *PDGFRB* break-apart FISH probes. Therefore, if karyotype and FISH are negative, and there is suspicion for a tyrosine kinase fusion based on clinicopathological features, additional genetic testing (eg, RNAseq, optical genomic mapping) should be pursued. *PDGFRB* rearrangements with the partner genes *EBF1, SSBP2, TNIP1, ZEB2,* and *ATF7IP* are nearly exclusively detected in de novo *BCR::ABL1*-like B-ALL and not M/LN-eo-TK, whereas other partners can occur in both. Next-generation sequencing (NGS) reveals mutations in 30% to 50% cases involving *ASXL1, TET2, BCOR, ETV6, STAG2,* and *RUNX1*.[6,16,19] The prognostic impact of mutations is largely unknown.

Prognosis and Clinical Comment

Like *PDGRFA*-rearranged cases, M/LN-eo-TK with *PDGFRB* rearrangement demonstrates an excellent response to imatinib[20] with long-term complete hematologic and molecular responses. In cases presenting in blast phase of CMN or undergoing disease progression from an initial chronic phase, induction chemotherapy and/or allogenic hematopoietic cell transplantation is typically administered in addition to imatinib. However, studies have shown durable complete hematologic and molecular remissions with imatinib monotherapy even in patients in blast phase or with myeloid sarcoma.[4]

MYELOID/LYMPHOID NEOPLASMS WITH EOSINOPHILIA AND REARRANGEMENT OF *FGFR1*

Definition

A myeloid and/or lymphoid neoplasm derived from a pluripotent (lymphoid/myeloid) stem cell bears a rearrangement of the *FGFR1* leading to a heterogenous and often complex disease phenotype.

Synonyms

None.

Epidemiology

There is a slight male predominance with a male:female ratio of approximately 1.5:1. The disease often presents in the late 40 to 50s.[5,21]

General Clinical Features

A substantial subset of cases (60%-70%) presents in blast phase[21] as lymphoblastic lymphoma either with increased bone marrow blasts or as extramedullary diseases (EMD), or myeloid sarcoma that involves lymph nodes, the mediastinum, or cutaneous tissue. Around one-third of patients present with concomitant lymphoblastic lymphoma in lymph nodes and a chronic myeloid neoplasm (CMN) in bone marrow (Figure 6.3). Only 30% to 40% of cases present in chronic phase. Patients often have systemic symptoms such as fever, weight loss, and night sweats. Splenomegaly is common. Eosinophilia is variably present (70%); however, hypereosinophilia is only seen in one-third of the patients.[4]

Morphology and Immunophenotype

For cases presenting as CMN, the peripheral blood and bone marrow show features that may resemble MPN-U, CEL, NOS, MDS/MPN including CMML, aCML, and MDS/MPN, NOS. For cases with acute leukemia or EMD presentation, the blasts may be B lymphoblasts, myeloblasts, mixed phenotype, or T lymphoblasts. Cases associated with t(8;13)(p11;q12)/*ZMYM2::FGFR1* frequently present with nodal (or extranodal) T-LBL admixed with scattered or perivascular myeloid blasts, historically labeled as "bilineal lymphoma" (Figure 6.3). Cases presenting in chronic phase may subsequently progress to acute leukemia either in the bone marrow

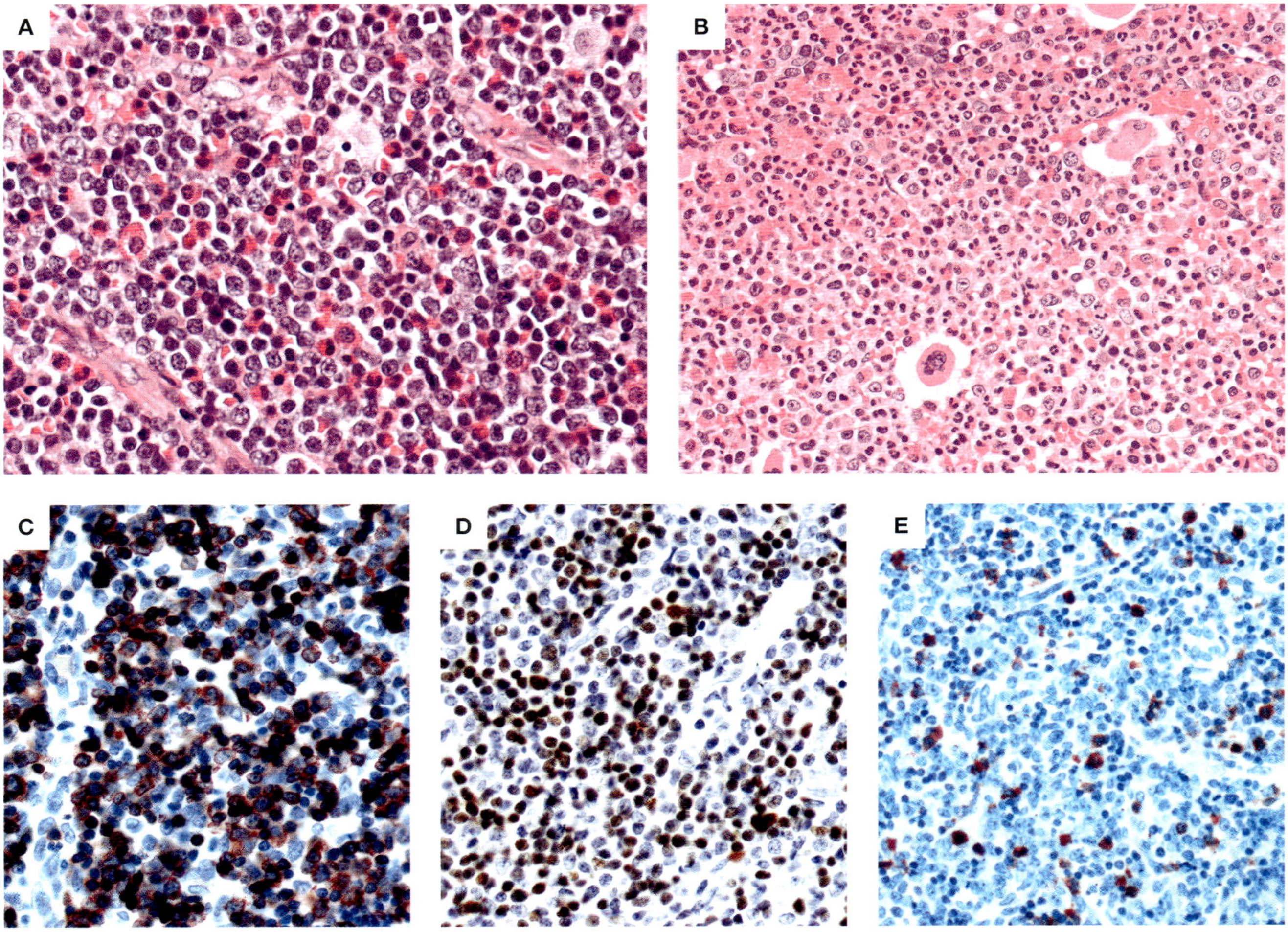

FIGURE 6.3 Common clinical presentations and histopathological findings in M/LN-eo-TK with t(8;13)(p11;q12)/*ZMYM2::FGFR1* rearrangement. Lymph node biopsy shows a blast proliferation with a significant eosinophilic infiltrate (**A**); the blasts are predominantly of T lymphoblasts, as demonstrated by CD3 (**C**) and TDT (**D**). There are scattered immature myeloid cells, demonstrated by myeloperoxidase (**E**). The bone marrow shows a myeloproliferative neoplasm with marked eosinophilia (**B**). (**A** and **B:** hematoxylin and eosin; **C:** CD3; **D:** TdT; **E:** myeloperoxidase; **A-E:** 40×).

or extramedullary locations. Conversely, patients with an initial presentation of acute leukemia or EMD may continue to show abnormal blood counts and abnormal bone marrow after achieving remission, with *FGFR1* fusion signals being demonstrated in mature hematopoietic cells. If there is an increase in blasts or a proliferation of immature cells in tissue, immunophenotypic analysis covering myeloid and lymphoid lineages is required to characterize the blast phenotype. Like *PDGFRA*- and *PDGFRB*-rearranged cases, scattered spindle mast cells (CD117 and tryptase) with aberrant CD25 expression are frequent, but only rarely forming mast cell aggregates that resemble systemic mastocytosis (SM).

The disease phenotype may differ with different partner genes. t(8;22)(p11.2;q11.2)/*BCR::FGFR1* often presents with CML-like CMN or B-ALL (B-lymphoblastic phase of M/LN-eo-TK) without significant eosinophilia,[22] while approximately half of t(8;9)(p12;q33)/*CEP110::FGFR1* show monocytosis and tonsil hypertrophy,[23] likely due to leukemia involvement. *FGFR1OP1::FGFR1* frequently presents with erythrocytosis.

Genetics

FGFR1 is located on 8p11.2. To date, there are at least 16 gene partners reported to fuse with *FGFR1* (Table 6.1). The most common partners include *ZMYM2*(13q12) followed by *BCR* (22q11). *FGFR1* rearrangements are usually not cytogenetically cryptic; however, the reported bands may range from 8p11.2 to 8p21, due to the small size of band 8p11. Confirmation of *FGFR1* gene involvement using FISH or RNAseq techniques is essential to establish a diagnosis. Targeted NGS studies show somatic mutations in 70% to 80% of cases with around 70% to 80% of them involving *RUNX1*.[16,21] *RUNX1* mutations have been associated with an acute leukemic presentation or disease progression.[21]

Prognosis and Clinical Comment

Many cases follow an aggressive course with an overall survival of <3 years. *FGFR1*-rearranged neoplasms do not respond to first-generation TKI (imatinib) therapy and only show modest activity to the third-generation TKI ponatinib. Based on a high rate of clinical and complete cytogenetic responses,[24] the *FGFR1-3* inhibitor pemigatinib was approved by the US Food and Drug Administration in August 2022 for adult patients with *FGFR1*-rearranged M/LN-eo-TK treated with at least one prior therapy. A clinical trial with futibatinib (anti-FGFR1-4) is ongoing. Allogenic HSCT is considered the best curative option,[25] and agents such as pemigatinib may be particularly useful as a bridging therapy for suitable transplant candidates.

MYELOID/LYMPHOID NEOPLASMS WITH EOSINOPHILIA AND *PCM1::JAK2* AND GENETIC VARIANTS *ETV6::JAK2* AND *BCR::JAK2*

Definition

A myeloid and/or lymphoid neoplasm derived from a pluripotent (lymphoid/myeloid) stem cell bearing a *PCM1::JAK2* gene fusion. Additional well-recognized partner genes are t(9;12)(p24.1;p13.2)/*ETV6::JAK2* and t(9;22)(p24.1;q11.2)/*BCR::JAK2*. Individual cases with other partner genes have been reported,[26] including *RPN1*/t(3;9)(q21;p24), *NF-E2*/t(9;12)(p24;q13), *RUNX1*/t(9;21)(p24·2;q22.1), and *PEX14*/t(1;9)(p36;p24.1), with clinical presentations resembling myelodysplastic syndromes (MDSs) or myeloproliferative neoplasms such as primary myelofibrosis or polycythemia vera, respectively. Although these rare rearrangements may belong to the same category, information so far is very limited. *JAK2* with partner genes such as *ATF7IP, EBF1, GOLGA5, HMBOX1, OFD1, PAX5, PPFIBP1, RFX3, SMU1, SNX29, SSBP2, STRN3, TERF2, TPR, USP25, ZBTB46, ZNF274,* and *ZNF340* are mostly reported in *BCR::ABL1*-like B-ALL. It must be noted that *PCM::JAK2* can be acquired at disease progression, or at AML relapse, which should not be considered as M/LN-eo-TK. Some cases of mature T-cell lymphoma,[27,28] including anaplastic large cell lymphoma and mycosis fungoides, have been found carrying a *PCM1::JAK2* fusion. These cases do not belong to M/LN-eo-TK if a myeloid involvement is absent.

Synonyms

None.

Epidemiology

The median age of patients with *PCM1::JAK2* at presentation is 50 years with a wide age range, and there is a male predominance (5.5:1 male:female ratio). The other two genetic variants share similar demographic features based on limited number of cases.[6,29-31]

General Clinical Features

Around half of the patients present in chronic phase, often as CEL, NOS; MPN-U; and MDS/MPN and another half in accelerated phase or blast phase, or with extramedullary disease (EMD) presentation. The blasts are often myeloid; some may be B-lymphoblastic; while T-lymphoblastic blast phase is extremely infrequent. Organomegaly (hepatosplenomegaly) and/or lymphadenopathy are very common.

Morphology and Immunophenotype

Peripheral blood eosinophilia is common in patients presenting with CMNs, ranging from mild to marked. Eosinophil morphology is variable ranging from unremarkable to abnormal with dysplastic-appearing forms as described earlier. The bone marrow of *PCM1::JAK2* often shows the typical histopathologic “triad” (Figure 6.4), which includes hypercellularity with an eosinophilic infiltrate, large aggregates of immature erythroid precursors (pronormoblasts), and myelofibrosis. The immature erythroid aggregates can be a very striking feature, referred to as “erythroid microtumors.” In some cases, erythroid hyperplasia as well as dysplasia in the erythroid, granulocytic, and/or megakaryocytic lineage may be seen. In contrast, the genetic variants of t(9;12)(p24.1;p13.2)/*ETV6::JAK2* and t(9;22)(p24.1;q11.2)/*BCR::JAK2*[6,8,30,31] often do not demonstrate the characteristic “triad.” *BCR::JAK2* may resemble CML with eosinophilia.

The features of an eosinophilic infiltrate and large aggregates of immature erythroid precursors may be seen in EMD. If the pronormoblasts form large sheets and efface the extramedullary tissue architecture, a diagnosis of myeloid sarcoma, erythroblastic, is appropriate.[6,30] Erythroid microtumors or extramedullary erythroid nodules can be confirmed by immunohistochemistry with CD71, LMO2, and/or E-cadherin (Figure 6.4). For cases with increased blasts, flow cytometry immunophenotyping and immunohistochemistry will help to characterize the blast phenotype.

Genetics

JAK2 is located at the terminal band of the short arm of chromosome 9. The vast majority of *PCM::JAK2* cases are not cryptic and demonstrate t(8;9)(p22;p24.1) if sufficient metaphases are obtained. It is generally accepted that the presence of t(8;9)(p22;p24) in the right clinical context is presumptive evidence of *PCM1::JAK2*, but FISH, at least with a probe to *JAK2*, is highly recommended for confirmation. t(9;12)(p24.1;p13.2)/*ETV6::JAK2* and t(9;22)(p24.1;q11.2)/*BCR::JAK2* are generally not cryptic. For EMD, for which karyotyping is often not available, the presence of eosinophilia and erythroid microtumor should raise a high index of suspicion for *PCM1::JAK2*. Importantly, all these genetic abnormalities (*PCM1::JAK2* and variants) can be seen in *BCR::ABL1*-like B-ALL and de novo T-ALL; therefore, demonstrating involvement of underlying myeloid element is key in making a diagnosis of M/LN-eo-TK. In *PCM1::JAK2* M/LN-eo-TK, mutations are reported in 14% to 50% of cases,[6,16,30] involving *ASXL1, TET2, BCOR, RUNX1, SRSF2, ETV6, TP53*, and *EP300*. Mutation data are scarce for t(9;12)(p24.1;p13.2)/*ETV6::JAK2* and t(9;22)(p24.1;q11.2)/*BCR::JAK2*.

Prognosis and Clinical Comment

In patients presenting with CMN, the disease may be indolent with a 5-year survival up to 80%.[29,30,32] On the other hand, in patients who present or progress to acute leukemia, the prognosis is dismal. Targeted therapy with *JAK2* inhibitors such as ruxolitinib may offer some but limited benefit[8] and may be used to bridge patients to allogeneic HSCT, which can lead to durable disease-free survival.

MYELOID/LYMPHOID NEOPLASMS WITH EOSINOPHILIA AND *FLT3* REARRANGEMENT

Definition

A myeloid and/or lymphoid neoplasm derived from a pluripotent (lymphoid/myeloid) stem cell bearing a rearrangement of *FLT3* leading to constitutive activation of the TK. The most common fusion is t(12;13)(p13;q12)/*ETV6::FLT3*, and around eight partner genes have been reported (Table 6.1).

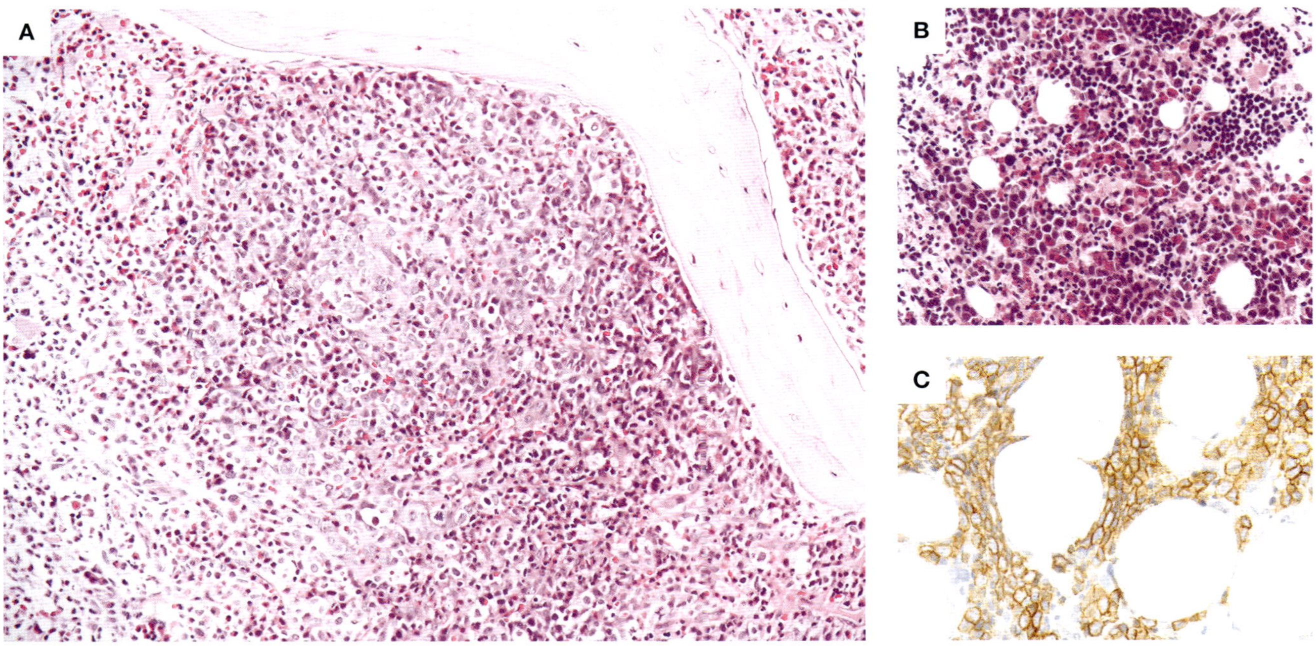

FIGURE 6.4 Characteristic bone marrow findings of M/LN-eo-TK- with *PCM1::JAK2*. The bone marrow is hypercellular, with a large nodular proliferation of immature erythroid precursors (mostly pronormoblasts), increased eosinophils, and often with fibrosis (**A**). In some cases, the immature erythroid precursors are present in multiple large aggregates or intrasinusoids (**B**), as highlighted by E-cadherin immunohistochemistry (**C**). (**A** and **B:** hematoxylin and eosin; **C**: E-cadherin; **A** and **B:** 20×; **C:** 40×).

Synonyms

None.

Epidemiology

The disease appears to be slightly more common in men with a male:female ratio of approximately 2:1. There is a broad age of presentation with the median age being in the 40s to 50s.

General Clinical Features

Patients typically present with peripheral blood abnormalities including leukocytosis, monocytosis, and cytopenia(s). Eosinophilia is common, occurring in about two-thirds of patients, but may be mild. Lymphadenopathy and splenomegaly or extramedullary disease (EMD) presentation are common, presenting in >50% of cases.[33] Clinical features may include fatigue, easy bruising, rash, or symptoms related to extramedullary involvement.

Morphology and Immunophenotype

The peripheral blood shows frequent eosinophilia, with or without eosinophilic morphologic abnormalities. Some cases may have monocytosis, resulting in a diagnosis of CMML. The bone marrow frequently shows a chronic myeloid neoplasm (CMN) that may resemble myeloproliferative neoplasms, unclassifiable, MDS/MPN such as CMML, or aCML, chronic eosinophilic leukemia, or systemic mastocytosis (SM) with associated myeloid neoplasm. Blasts can be increased. Some cases present as an acute leukemia (AML, T-ALL, or mixed phenotype acute leukemia [MPAL], rarely B-ALL) or EMD (Figure 6.5) such as T-ALL/LBL, myeloid sarcoma, MPAL, and occasionally mature T-cell lymphoma. The mature T-cell lymphoma cases have been reported to have a concomitant bone marrow CMN. Flow cytometric immunophenotyping and/or immunohistochemistry are needed to characterize blasts or lymphoma phenotype. In some cases, the bone marrow shows minimal changes (Figure 6.5), especially in patients who only present with EMD, but carry the same *FLT3* rearrangement. Extramedullary lesions often show increased eosinophils and/or mast cells associated with the blast infiltrate. Mast cell workup may identify increased spindle mast cells with aberrant CD25 expression.

Genetics

The *FLT3* gene is located on chromosome 13q12, and the most common partner gene is *ETV6* located at 12p13.2, accounting for around half of the reported cases. *ETV6::FLT3*/t(12;13)(p13;q12) is typically not cryptic. Other partner genes reported are *ZMYM2*/13q12,[34] *TRIP11*/14q32, *SPTBN1*/2p16, *GOLGB1*/3q13, *CCDC88C*/14q32, *MYO18A*/17q12, and *BCR*/22q11. In addition, there are a few cases reported in which *FLT3* appears to be rearranged with yet uncharacterized partner genes at 3q27, 5q15, 5q35, 7q36, and 13q22.[33] Some of the fusions are cryptic, such as *ZMYM2::FLT3*,[34] and require FISH or RNAseq for identification. Mutations are present in around 50% cases including variants of *ASXL1, PTPN11, RUNX1, SETBP1, SRSF2, STAT5B, TET2, TP53,* and *U2AF1*. The prognostic effect of these mutations is not known.

Prognosis and Clinical Comment

The disease tends to have an aggressive clinical course and early disease progression if untreated. FLT3 inhibitors such as sunitinib, midostaurin, sorafenib, or gilteritinib monotherapy exert anti-FLT3 activity, and some of these agents have been reported to induce hematological responses with or without complete cytogenetic response.[33,34] Some patients may achieve a sustained remission or remain in stable disease on FLT3 inhibitor monotherapy, but in some, the responses may be short-lived. Resistance may be due to an acquired *FLT3* N841K mutation in the activation loop of the TK domain.[35] Nonetheless, FLT3 inhibitors can help to bridge patients to allogeneic HSCT.

MYELOID LYMPHOID NEOPLASMS WITH EOSINOPHILIA AND *ETV6::ABL1*

Definition

A myeloid and/or lymphoid neoplasm derived from a pluripotent (lymphoid/myeloid) stem cell bears *ETV6::ABL1* fusion leading to constitutive activation of the TK. *ABL1* has been reported to fuse with other partners[36]; however, most of those cases present as *BCR::ABL1*-like B-ALL or de novo T-ALL. Therefore caution is needed not to call these cases as M/LN-eo-TK. However, rare cases with alternative partner genes such as *PRRC2B::ABL1*, have been reported to present as a

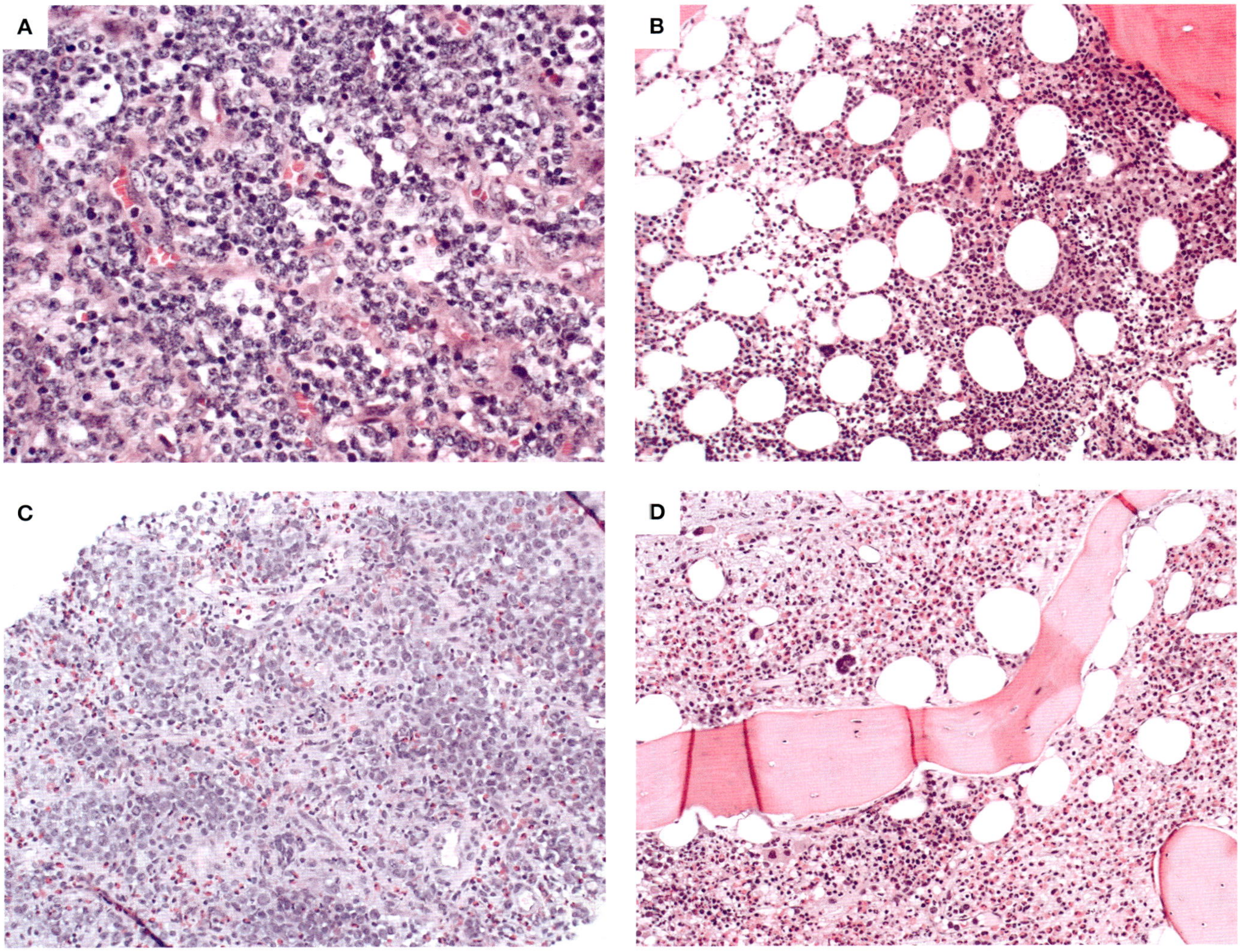

FIGURE 6.5 Representative case examples of M/LN-eo-TK with *FLT3* rearrangement. Case 1: Lymph node biopsy **(A)** shows a T-lymphoblastic lymphoma, in this case, with minimal eosinophils; bone marrow shows mild changes with a few dysplastic megakaryocytes **(B)**. *FLT3* rearrangement is demonstrated in granulocytes by FISH. Case 2: Another case shows a myeloid sarcoma in soft tissue with significant numbers of eosinophils **(C)**, and bone marrow shows a hypercellularity, dysplastic megakaryocytes, an eosinophilic infiltrate, and fibrosis, resembling chronic eosinophilic leukemia **(D)**.

chronic myeloid neoplasm or mixed phenotype leukemia with eosinophilia. Such cases would be appropriately considered as genetic variants of *ETV6::ABL1* under M/LN-eo-TK.

Synonyms

None.

Epidemiology

This is a disease predominantly of adults with a male predominance (3:1).[9] The median age of presentation is in the fourth to fifth decade of life. Pediatric cases have mostly been de novo T-ALL or *BCR::ABL1*-like B-ALL, not M/LN-eo-TK.

General Clinical Features

Patients often present with leukocytosis, eosinophilia (>90% cases, many with hypereosinophilia),[4] neutrophilia, monocytosis, and some also with increased (>1%) basophils.[4,37,38] These cases are often diagnosed as MPN with marked eosinophilia, or CEL, NOS, occasionally blast phase of MPN. Concomitant disease with a chronic myeloid neoplasm (CMN) in the bone marrow and T-LBL in lymph nodes are also reported. Most patients have splenomegaly.

Morphology and Immunophenotype

Peripheral blood often shows marked eosinophilia, with or without abnormality as described earlier. Bone marrow usually shows a marked hypercellularity, with eosinophilia. Cases have been described resembling CML with eosinophilia; CEL, NOS; Ph-negative MPN with eosinophilia, aCML, MDS/MPN, NOS, and essential thrombocythemia. Increased spindle mast cells can be encountered. Extramedullary diseases (EMDs) are mostly reported as T-ALL/LBL. Flow cytometry and immunohistochemistry are needed to characterize cases with increased blasts.

Genetics

The *ABL1* gene is located on chromosome 9q34.12, and the partner gene *ETV6* is located at 12p13.2. *ETV6::ABL1* fusion often results from a complex rearrangement involving a translocation and inversion or an insertion of *ETV6* in 9q34 or *ABL1* in 12p13. The fusion is often cryptic, and thus FISH analysis using *ETV6* and *ABL1* break-apart probes, RNAseq technology, or RT-PCR is needed for detection. The alternative splicing generates two fusion transcripts, type A (without *ETV6* exon 5) and type B (with exon 5), with type B significantly more common than type A.[39] Rarely, other partner genes, such as *PRRC2B*, have been reported to show disease features of M/LN-eo-TK and responses to TKI, and may be considered as genetic variant of *ETV6::ABL1*. Mutations involving *ARID2, TP53, SETD2, CDKN1B, PTPN11,* and *SMC1A* genes have been reported in approximately 50% of cases.[37,38]

Prognosis and Clinical Comment

Most patients present in chronic phase; however, disease progression to blast phase or EMD may occur in 30% of cases that can be AML, B-ALL, T-ALL, or myeloid sarcoma. Patients with *ETV6::ABL1* have shown variable responses to TKI targeted therapy.[37,38,40] Second- or third-generation TKIs[8] appear to be superior to imatinib in inducing responses. Durable hematological and molecular remissions have been observed in a significant number of patients presenting in chronic phase but not patients in blast phase. The prognosis is dismal in patients with disease progression despite the addition of TKI to standard chemotherapy.

References

1. Arber DA, Orazi A, Hasserjian RP, et al. International consensus classification of myeloid neoplasms and acute leukemias: integrating morphologic, clinical, and genomic data. *Blood.* 2022;140(11):1200-1228. doi:10.1182/blood.2022015850
2. Reiter A, Gotlib J. Myeloid neoplasms with eosinophilia. *Blood.* 2017;129(6):704-714. doi:10.1182/blood-2016-10-695973
3. Shomali W, Gotlib J. World Health Organization-defined eosinophilic disorders: 2022 update on diagnosis, risk stratification, and management. *Am J Hematol.* 2022;97(1):129-148. doi:10.1002/ajh.26352
4. Metzgeroth G, Steiner L, Naumann N, et al. Myeloid/lymphoid neoplasms with eosinophilia and tyrosine kinase gene fusions: reevaluation of the defining characteristics in a registry-based cohort. *Leukemia.* 2023;37(9):1860-1867. doi:10.1038/s41375-023-01958-1
5. Zhang Y, Nguyen L, Lu CM, et al. Clinical response to upfront targeted tyrosine kinase inhibitors among patients with myeloid/lymphoid neoplasms with eosinophilia and tyrosine kinase gene fusion. *Clin Lymphoma Myeloma Leuk.* 2023;23(3):e150-e163. doi:10.1016/j.clml.2022.12.008
6. Pozdnyakova O, Orazi A, Kelemen K, et al. Myeloid/lymphoid neoplasms associated with eosinophilia and rearrangements of PDGFRA, PDGFRB, or FGFR1 or with PCM1-JAK2. *Am J Clin Pathol.* 2021;155(2):160-178. doi:10.1093/ajcp/aqaa208
7. Roberts KG, Reshmi SC, Harvey RC, et al. Genomic and outcome analyses of Ph-like ALL in NCI standard-risk patients: a report from the Children's Oncology Group. *Blood.* 2018;132(8):815-824. doi:10.1182/blood-2018-04-841676
8. Schwaab J, Naumann N, Luebke J, et al. Response to tyrosine kinase inhibitors in myeloid neoplasms associated with PCM1-JAK2, BCR-JAK2 and ETV6-ABL1 fusion genes. *Am J Hematol.* 2020;95(7):824-833. doi:10.1002/ajh.25825
9. Saft L, Kvasnicka HM, Boudova L, Gianelli U, Lazzi S, Rozman M. Myeloid/lymphoid neoplasms with eosinophilia and tyrosine kinase fusion genes: a workshop report with focus on novel entities and a literature review including paediatric cases. *Histopathology.* 2023;83(6):829-849. doi:10.1111/his.15021
10. Wang SA, Orazi A, Gotlib J, et al. The international consensus classification of eosinophilic disorders and systemic mastocytosis. *Am J Hematol.* 2023;98(8):1286-1306. doi:10.1002/ajh.26966
11. Pardanani A, Brockman SR, Paternoster SF, et al. FIP1L1-PDGFRA fusion: prevalence and clinicopathologic correlates in 89 consecutive patients with moderate to severe eosinophilia. *Blood.* 2004;104(10):3038-3045. doi:10.1182/blood-2004-03-0787

12. Tzankov A, Reichard KK, Hasserjian RP, Arber DA, Orazi A, Wang SA. Updates on eosinophilic disorders. *Virchows Arch*. 2023;482(1):85-97. doi:10.1007/s00428-022-03402-8
13. Vandenberghe P, Wlodarska I, Michaux L, et al. Clinical and molecular features of FIP1L1-PDFGRA (+) chronic eosinophilic leukemias. *Leukemia*. 2004;18(4):734-742. doi:10.1038/sj.leu.2403313
14. Cools J, DeAngelo DJ, Gotlib J, et al. A tyrosine kinase created by fusion of the PDGFRA and FIP1L1 genes as a therapeutic target of imatinib in idiopathic hypereosinophilic syndrome. *N Engl J Med*. 2003;348(13):1201-1214. doi:10.1056/NEJMoa025217
15. Mueller SB, Dal Cin P, Le LP, et al. t(4;12)(q12;p13) ETV6-rearranged AML without eosinophilia does not involve PDGFRA: relevance for imatinib insensitivity. *Blood Adv*. 2022;6(3):818-827. doi:10.1182/bloodadvances.2021005280
16. Baer C, Muehlbacher V, Kern W, Haferlach C, Haferlach T. Molecular genetic characterization of myeloid/lymphoid neoplasms associated with eosinophilia and rearrangement of PDGFRA, PDGFRB, FGFR1 or PCM1-JAK2. *Haematologica*. 2018;103(8):e348-e350. doi:10.3324/haematol.2017.187302
17. Metzgeroth G, Schwaab J, Naumann N, et al. Treatment-free remission in FIP1L1-PDGFRA-positive myeloid/lymphoid neoplasms with eosinophilia after imatinib discontinuation. *Blood Adv*. 2020;4(3):440-443. doi:10.1182/bloodadvances.2019001111
18. Sadovnik I, Lierman E, Peter B, et al. Identification of Ponatinib as a potent inhibitor of growth, migration, and activation of neoplastic eosinophils carrying FIP1L1-PDGFRA. *Exp Hematol*. 2014;42(4):282-293 e4. doi:10.1016/j.exphem.2013.12.007
19. Fang H, Tang G, Loghavi S, et al. Systematic use of fluorescence in-situ hybridisation and clinicopathological features in the screening of PDGFRB rearrangements of patients with myeloid/lymphoid neoplasms. *Histopathology*. 2020;76(7):1042-1054. doi:10.1111/his.14097
20. Gotlib J. Tyrosine kinase inhibitors in the treatment of eosinophilic neoplasms and systemic mastocytosis. *Hematol Oncol Clin North Am*. 2017;31(4):643-661. doi:10.1016/j.hoc.2017.04.009
21. Strati P, Tang G, Duose DY, et al. Myeloid/lymphoid neoplasms with FGFR1 rearrangement. *Leuk Lymphoma*. 2018;59(7):1672-1676. doi:10.1080/10428194.2017.1397663
22. Montenegro-Garreaud X, Miranda RN, Reynolds A, et al. Myeloproliferative neoplasms with t(8;22)(p11.2;q11.2)/BCR-FGFR1: a meta-analysis of 20 cases shows cytogenetic progression with B-lymphoid blast phase. *Hum Pathol*. 2017;65:147-156. doi:10.1016/j.humpath.2017.05.008
23. Chen M, Wang K, Cai X, et al. Myeloid/lymphoid neoplasm with CEP110-FGFR1 fusion: an analysis of 16 cases show common features and poor prognosis. *Hematology*. 2021;26(1):153-159. doi:10.1080/16078454.2020.1854493
24. Gotlib J, Kiladjian JJ, Vannucchi A, et al. A phase 2 study of pemigatinib (FIGHT-203; INCB054828) in patients with Myeloid/Lymphoid Neoplasms (MLNs) with Fibroblast Growth Factor Receptor 1 (FGFR1) rearrangement (MLN FGFR1). *Blood*. 2021;138(suppl 1):385. doi:10.1182/blood-2021-148103
25. Hernandez-Boluda JC, Pereira A, Zinger N, et al. Allogeneic hematopoietic cell transplantation in patients with myeloid/lymphoid neoplasm with FGFR1-rearrangement: a study of the Chronic Malignancies Working Party of EBMT. *Bone Marrow Transplant*. 2022;57(3):416-422. doi:10.1038/s41409-021-01553-x
26. Levavi H, Tripodi J, Marcellino B, et al. A novel t(1;9)(p36;p24.1) JAK2 translocation and review of the literature. *Acta Haematol*. 2019;142(2):105-112. doi:10.1159/000498945
27. Fernandez-Pol S, Neishaboori N, Chapman CM, et al. Two cases of mycosis fungoides with PCM1-JAK2 fusion. *JCO Precis Oncol*. 2021;5:646-652. doi:10.1200/PO.20.00366
28. Fitzpatrick MJ, Massoth LR, Marcus C, et al. JAK2 rearrangements are a recurrent alteration in CD30+ systemic T-cell lymphomas with anaplastic morphology. *Am J Surg Pathol*. 1, 2021;45(7):895-904. doi:10.1097/PAS.0000000000001708
29. Bain BJ, Ahmad S. Should myeloid and lymphoid neoplasms with PCM1-JAK2 and other rearrangements of JAK2 be recognized as specific entities? *Br J Haematol*. 2014;166(6):809-817. doi:10.1111/bjh.12963
30. Tang G, Sydney Sir Philip JK, Weinberg O, et al. Hematopoietic neoplasms with 9p24/JAK2 rearrangement: a multicenter study. *Mod Pathol*. 2019;32(4):490-498. doi:10.1038/s41379-018-0165-9
31. Chen JA, Hou Y, Roskin KM, et al. Lymphoid blast transformation in an MPN with BCR-JAK2 treated with ruxolitinib: putative mechanisms of resistance. *Blood Adv*. 2021;5(17):3492-3496. doi:10.1182/bloodadvances.2020004174
32. Kaplan HG, Jin R, Bifulco CB, Scanlan JM, Corwin DR. PCM1-JAK2 fusion tyrosine kinase gene-related neoplasia: a systematic review of the clinical literature. *Oncologist*. 2022;27(8):e661-e670. doi:10.1093/oncolo/oyac072
33. Tang G, Tam W, Short NJ, et al. Myeloid/lymphoid neoplasms with FLT3 rearrangement. *Mod Pathol*. 2021;34(9):1673-1685. doi:10.1038/s41379-021-00817-7
34. Jawhar M, Naumann N, Knut M, et al. Cytogenetically cryptic ZMYM2-FLT3 and DIAPH1-PDGFRB gene fusions in myeloid neoplasms with eosinophilia. *Leukemia*. October 2017;31(10):2271-2273. doi:10.1038/leu.2017.240
35. Walz C, Erben P, Ritter M, et al. Response of ETV6-FLT3-positive myeloid/lymphoid neoplasm with

eosinophilia to inhibitors of FMS-like tyrosine kinase 3. *Blood*. 2011;118(8):2239-2242. doi:10.1182/blood-2011-03-343426

36. Ernst T, Score J, Deininger M, et al. Identification of FOXP1 and SNX2 as novel ABL1 fusion partners in acute lymphoblastic leukaemia. *Br J Haematol*. 2011;153(1):43-46. doi:10.1111/j.1365-2141.2010.08457.x

37. Yao J, Xu L, Aypar U, et al. Myeloid/lymphoid neoplasms with eosinophilia/basophilia and ETV6-ABL1 fusion: cell-of-origin and response to tyrosine kinase inhibition. *Haematologica*. 2021;106(2):614-618. doi:10.3324/haematol.2020.249649

38. Xie W, Wang SA, Hu S, Xu J, Medeiros LJ, Tang G. Myeloproliferative neoplasm with ABL1/ETV6 rearrangement mimics chronic myeloid leukemia and responds to tyrosine kinase inhibitors. *Cancer Genet*. 2018;228-229:41-46. doi:10.1016/j.cancergen.2018.08.002

39. Million RP, Harakawa N, Roumiantsev S, Varticovski L, Van Etten RA. A direct binding site for Grb2 contributes to transformation and leukemogenesis by the Tel-Abl (ETV6-Abl) tyrosine kinase. *Mol Cell Biol*. 2004;24(11):4685-4695. doi:10.1128/MCB.24.11.4685-4695.2004

40. Zaliova M, Moorman AV, Cazzaniga G, et al. Characterization of leukemias with ETV6-ABL1 fusion. *Haematologica*. 2016;101(9):1082-1093. doi:10.3324/haematol.2016.144345

SECTION 3

Mastocytosis

Chapter 7
Mastocytosis

Kaaren Reichard, Tracy I. George, Roos Leguit, Attilio Orazi, Andreas Reiter, Ayalew Tefferi, Alexandar Tzankov, and Sa A. Wang

Mastocytosis: General Features

Definition

Mastocytosis is a neoplastic disorder of clonal mast cells (MCs) manifested by their abnormal accumulation in one or more organ systems.[1-4]

Diagnosis and classification

Mastocytosis is separated into three disease categories: (i) cutaneous mastocytosis (CM) with only skin involvement; (ii) systemic mastocytosis (SM), with or without skin involvement; and (iii) mast cell sarcoma (MCS) (Table 7.1). The diagnostic criteria for SM are listed in Table 7.2. SM is further subtyped into indolent SM (ISM), smoldering SM (SSM), aggressive SM (ASM), mast cell leukemia (MCL), and SM with an associated myeloid neoplasm (SM-AMN) (Tables 7.3 and 7.4). Advanced SM (AdvSM) is the umbrella term used to refer to the three most aggressive forms of the disease, namely, ASM, MCL, and SM-AMN.

The subtypes of mastocytosis are diagnosed with an integrated assessment of the clinical, laboratory, pathologic, and genetic findings (Tables 7.3 and 7.4). The factors to be considered include clinical presentation, site(s) of disease involvement, burden of disease and organomegaly, presence of organ dysfunction due to MC infiltration, cytologic appearance of the MCs, percent abnormal MCs in the aspirate smear, immunohistochemical confirmation of MCs, presence of an AMN in bone marrow (BM) and involved organ systems, presence of an activating *KIT* mutation, and exclusion of a myeloid/lymphoid neoplasm with eosinophilia and tyrosine kinase gene fusion (M/LN-eo-TK).

TABLE 7.1 Mastocytosis subtypes (variants)

Cutaneous mastocytosis
Urticaria pigmentosa/maculopapular cutaneous mastocytosis
Diffuse cutaneous mastocytosis
Mastocytoma of skin
Systemic mastocytosis
Indolent systemic mastocytosis (includes bone marrow mastocytosis)[a]
Smoldering systemic mastocytosis[a]
Aggressive systemic mastocytosis[a]
Mast cell leukemia
Systemic mastocytosis with an associated myeloid neoplasm
Mast cell sarcoma

[a]The diagnosis of these variants of systemic mastocytosis requires correlation with B- and C-findings.

Synonyms

Mast cell disease.

Epidemiology

Mastocytosis has an estimated prevalence of 1 in 10,000 individuals.[5] AdvSM is much rarer with an incidence and prevalence of 0.8 and 5.2 per 1 million individuals inhabitants, respectively, in a focused region in Germany.[6] CM is largely a disease of children, whereas

TABLE 7.2 Systemic mastocytosis: diagnostic criteria

Major criterion
- Multifocal dense infiltrates of tryptase- and/or CD117-positive mast cells (≥15 mast cells in aggregates) detected in sections of bone marrow and/or other extracutaneous organ(s)[a]

In the absence of the major criterion, at least three of the following four minor criteria must be present

Minor criteria
- In sections of the bone marrow biopsy or other extracutaneous organs, >25% of mast cells are spindle shaped or have an atypical immature morphology[b]
- Mast cells in bone marrow, peripheral blood, or other extracutaneous organs express CD25, CD2, and/or CD30, in addition to mast cell markers
- *KIT* D816V mutation or other activating *KIT* mutation detected in bone marrow, peripheral blood, or other extracutaneous organs[a,c]
- Elevated serum tryptase level, persistently >20 ng/mL. In cases of systemic mastocytosis with an associated myeloid neoplasm, an elevated tryptase does not count as a systemic mastocytosis minor criterion

[a]In the absence of a *KIT* mutation, particularly in cases with eosinophilia, the presence of tyrosine kinase gene fusions associated with myeloid/lymphoid neoplasms with eosinophilia and tyrosine kinase gene fusion must be excluded.
[b]Round-cell well-differentiated morphology can occur in a small subset of cases. In these cases, it is recommended to perform both CD117 and tryptase. In addition, the mast cells are often negative for CD25 and CD2 but positive for CD30.
[c]To avoid false-negative results, use of a high-sensitivity PCR assay for detection of *KIT* D816V mutation is recommended. If negative, exclusion of *KIT* mutation variants is strongly suggested in suspected systemic mastocytosis.

TABLE 7.3 Diagnostic criteria for the various subtypes of systemic mastocytosis

Diagnostic category	Diagnostic criteria
Indolent systemic mastocytosis (ISM)	<2 B-findings and no C-findings (Table 7.4)
ISM variant:	
Bone marrow mastocytosis	Isolated and limited bone marrow involvement by ISM; tryptase level <125 ng/mL; no B- or C-findings (Table 7.4)
Smoldering systemic mastocytosis	≥2 B-findings and no C-findings (Table 7.4)
Aggressive systemic mastocytosis	≥1 C-finding (Table 7.4)
Mast cell leukemia	≥20% atypical immature mast cells[a,b]
Systemic mastocytosis with an associated myeloid neoplasm (SM-AMN)	Meets the criteria for an associated myeloid neoplasm (eg, CMML or other MDS/MPN, MDS, MPN, AML, or other myeloid neoplasm)[c] The AMN should be fully classified according to established criteria[d]

AML, acute myeloid leukemia; CMML, chronic myelomonocytic leukemia; MDS/MPN; myelodysplastic syndrome/myeloproliferative neoplasm.

[a]Atypical immature mast cells include promastocytes, metachromatic blast-like forms, and multinucleated or highly pleomorphic mast cells.

[b]In the presence of a suboptimal aspirate (dry tap), a bone marrow biopsy showing a dense, diffuse mast cell infiltration of atypical immature mast cells is sufficient to support the diagnosis of mast cell leukemia.

[c]High degree of suspicion can be raised by the presence of monocytosis, eosinophilia, splenomegaly, elevated lactate dehydrogenase, high *KIT* D816V variant allele frequency, and additional somatic mutations in genes associated with myeloid malignancies (particularly if occurring in combination) as they could be signs of an AMN.

[d]If eosinophilia is present, the presence of tyrosine kinase gene fusions associated with a myeloid/lymphoid neoplasm with eosinophilia (M/LN-eo) should be excluded. Although usually mutually exclusive, rare cases with both a *KIT* mutation and a gene fusion associated with M/LN-eo have been reported. In these rare instances, the M/LN-eo would represent the SM-associated AMN, but it is recommended assigning such cases only in instances in which both a *KIT* mutation and an M/LN-eo gene fusion are present.

SM is largely a disease of adults. SM is extraordinarily unlikely to occur in childhood, while most adult patients who have cutaneous lesions suffer from SM and not CM. The majority of SM are biologically indolent and include the ISM and SSM subtypes. Progression from ISM to AdvSM is uncommon. On the other hand, progression within AdvSM frequently occurs, eg, from SM-AMN (nonacute) to SM–acute myeloid leukemia (AML) or from ASM to MCL. MC sarcoma is a very rare, aggressive, initially localized, tissue- or bone-based disease that often progresses to secondary MCL.

General clinical features

Clinical symptoms are heterogeneous and depend on the organ system(s) involved and the degree of BM failure. Physical findings at SM diagnosis are also variable and may include skin lesions and/or organomegaly. The

TABLE 7.4 Systemic mastocytosis: B-findings and C-findings

B-Findings:

- High mast cell burden; >30% of bone marrow cellularity by mast cell aggregates (assessed on bone marrow biopsy) and serum total tryptase >200 ng/mL.
- Cytopenia (not meeting criteria for C-findings) or cytosis. Reactive causes are excluded, and criteria for other myeloid neoplasms are not met.
- Hepatomegaly without impairment of liver function, or splenomegaly without features of hypersplenism including thrombocytopenia, and/or lymphadenopathy (>1 cm size) on palpation or imaging.

C-Findings:

- Bone marrow dysfunction caused by neoplastic mast cell infiltration, manifested by ≥ 1 cytopenia: absolute neutrophil count $<1.0 \times 10^9$/L, hemoglobin level <10 g/dL, and/or platelet count $<100 \times 10^9$/L
- Palpable hepatomegaly with impairment of liver function, ascites, and/or portal hypertension
- Skeletal involvement, with large osteolytic lesions with or without pathologic fractures (pathological fractures caused by osteoporosis do not qualify as a C-finding)
- Palpable splenomegaly with hypersplenism
- Malabsorption with weight loss due to gastrointestinal tract mast cell infiltrates

latter is usually more prominent in AdvSM. Most children with CM and many adults, especially with ISM (not bone marrow mastocytosis [BMM]), show maculopapular skin lesions, whereas they may be seen in up to 50% in AdvSM.

Patients have symptoms related to the release of MC mediators in a variety of organ systems including the skin, vasculature, lungs, gastrointestinal tract, and cardiovascular system. The predominant symptoms of ISM include anaphylaxis, vomiting, syncope, angioedema, abdominal pain, diarrhea, headache, blistering, flushing, pruritus, urticaria, respiratory issues (wheezing, dyspnea), and fainting. Patients with mastocytosis report that these symptoms are disruptive and negatively impact their quality of life.[7] Osteoporosis/osteopenia is often seen and may be a presenting feature of the disease.[8] In AdvSM, the most important symptoms include fatigue, bone pain, and problems caused by organ dysfunction, which may also serve as C-findings, eg, ascites, malabsorption, and weight loss. AdvSM is frequently associated with osteosclerosis.

Peripheral blood abnormalities in SM include anemia and eosinophilia. The presence of circulating MCs is rare with the exception of some MCL cases. In patients with AdvSM in general and AMN in particular, dysplastic features, cytopenia(s), leukocytosis, circulating blasts, and/or monocytosis may be noted.[9] If leukocytosis and thrombocytosis are observed, concurrent *JAK2* V617F may occur.

Morphology

Cytology

In all forms of mastocytosis, the MCs exhibit cytologic and/or architectural atypical features. Normal MCs are round with round/oval nuclei displaying dense clumped chromatin and cytoplasm that is densely packed with deeply basophilic granules (Figure 7.1A). In contrast, in mastocytosis, MCs deviate from their normal cytologic appearance by showing atypical features. The atypical MCs may exhibit mature or immature morphology. Atypical mature MCs are characterized by enlarged size (often 3× the size of a normal MC) with a spindle-shaped, oval/elongated nucleus and hypogranular cytoplasm (Figure 7.1B and C). However, in about 10% of SM cases, the majority of MCs are round shaped (Figure 7.1D). In rare SM cases, the round-shaped MCs may exhibit a well-differentiated morphology (ie, are slightly enlarged in size with a round central nucleus and abundantly granulated cytoplasm). While this appearance may resemble normal MCs, they are distinguished by their size (larger) and clustering. The lack of CD25 expression distinguishes them from "common" round-shaped MCs seen in SM.

Atypical immature MCs consist of promastocytes, metachromatic blasts, and multinucleated/highly pleomorphic MCs. Promastocytes, despite being highly cytologically atypical, can be recognized as MCs and are typically slightly to moderately enlarged with bi- or multilobated nuclei, round shape, reticulated chromatin, and variably hypogranular cytoplasm and/or show enlarged, chunky granules (Figure 7.1E). Metachromatic blasts are intermediate to large size with round nuclear contours, dispersed chromatin, and abundant cytoplasmic granules (Figure 7.1F).

There may be a disproportionately low number of MCs on BM aspirate smears due to the fibrosis associated with the MC lesions in the core biopsy. However, a direct examination within and around the BM particles usually reveals the atypical MCs. In contrast, higher frequencies of atypical immature MCs in the aspirate smear are characteristic of MCL.

Histology

In BM biopsy sections, MC lesions are often morphologically distinctive and exhibit a focal or less commonly diffuse infiltration pattern (Figure 7.2). Focal lesions are commonly paratrabecular and/or perivascular. Paratrabecular lesions are generally accompanied by fibrosis and at least focal bone remodeling. Perivascular lesions may show hypertrophy of the media of the vessels that are often encircled by multiple layers of MCs. A diffuse MC infiltrate significantly effaces normal hematopoiesis (Figure 7.2C and D). In cases with diffuse involvement, additional findings may include osteosclerosis with thickened and remodeled bone. The MC lesions often contain an admixture of eosinophils, histiocytes, and mature small lymphocytes, which may form "target" lesions characterized by a central core of lymphocytes encircled by MCs and a layer of eosinophils at its periphery (Figure 7.2A and B). In some instances, the MCs may form the core with the lymphocytes forming the second layer.

In some instances, the MC infiltrates may be subtle or morphologically "occult" and require immunohistochemical techniques to identify the increased MCs, particularly if they are not in aggregates but individually distributed interstitially throughout the BM (Figure 7.3). In these situations, the initial impetus for the pathologist to evaluate for MCs typically stems from allergic manifestations suggestive of MC activation syndrome or by the presence of a *KIT* mutation, eg, in a patient with a myeloid neoplasm. These cases often lack the major criterion but still meet a diagnosis of SM if three minor criteria are present.

Morphologic variant

Rare cases of SM characterized by a prominent proliferation of mature, round-shaped, well-granulated MCs (a.k.a. well-differentiated) may be observed.[4,10] This type of morphology can be seen in almost all forms of mastocytosis and is therefore regarded as a morphologic variant and not a specific subtype of the disease. The MCs form clusters (Figure 7.4) and are often CD2 and CD25 negative (as opposed to other forms of mastocytosis) with CD30 positivity found in >50% of cases. Given the diagnostic significance of CD30 in this setting, it is important to note that in one study flow cytometry has been found to be more sensitive than immunohistochemistry for its detection.[11] This variant typically lacks *KIT* mutations but may carry noncanonical activating *KIT* mutations and shows a female predominance of 4:1.[1,4]

Immunophenotype

Cases with focal, compact, dense aggregates of MCs may be relatively easily appreciated on routine hematoxylin and eosin–stained sections of multiple tissue sites. However, in some cases with smaller, more occult, MC infiltrates, the MCs may be challenging to identify because of bland cytology and potential morphologic overlap with fibroblasts, histiocytes, and endothelial cells. Immunophenotypic confirmation of MCs can be performed with immunohistochemistry and/or flow cytometric techniques. Although the diagnostic utility of flow cytometry has been proposed, so far there is little or no consensus that it is clinically indicated/

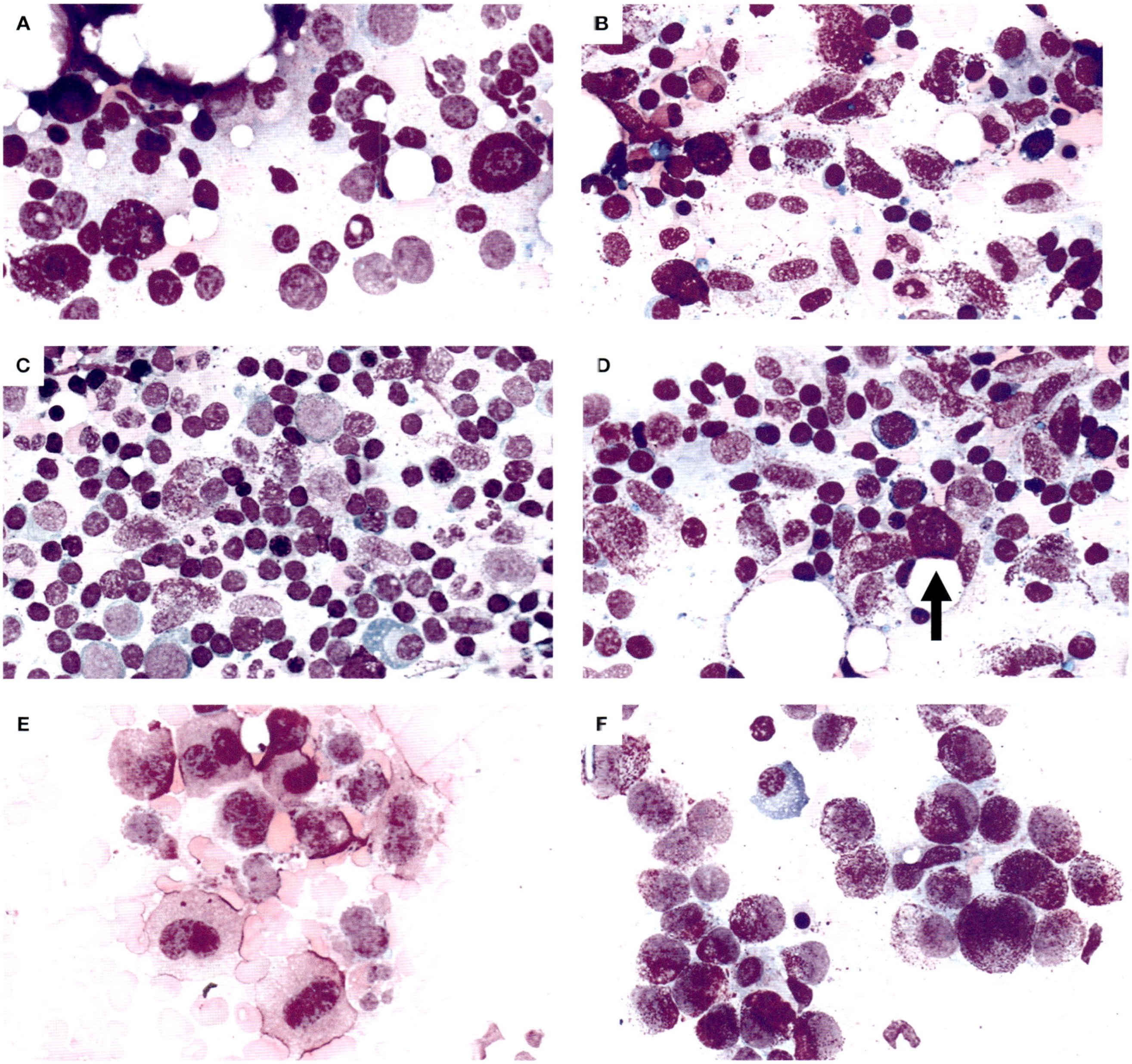

FIGURE 7.1 Mast cell morphology on bone marrow aspirate smears. **A:** Normal mast cells are round with round/oval nuclear contours, mature chromatin, and densely packed cytoplasm with deeply basophilic granules. **B-F:** Abnormal mast cells deviate from the normal appearance and may exhibit mature or immature features. **B and C:** Atypical mature mast cells are characterized by slightly enlarged size with a spindle-shaped, oval/elongated nucleus and hypogranular cytoplasm. **C:** This image demonstrates a target lesion consisting of numerous small mature lymphocytes with occasional admixed eosinophils, a rare plasma cell, and intermixed abnormal mature hypogranular and spindle-shaped mast cells. **D:** Mast cells may also exhibit a well-differentiated morphology—round shape; slightly enlarged in size; round, central nucleus; and abundantly granulated cytoplasm (arrow). **E and F:** Atypical immature mast cells consist of promastocytes, metachromatic blasts, and multinucleated/highly pleomorphic mast cells. **E:** Promastocytes, despite being highly cytologically atypical, can be recognized as mast cells and are typically slightly to moderately enlarged with bi- or multilobated nuclei, round shape, reticulated chromatin, variably hypogranular cytoplasm, and/or showing enlarged, chunky granules. **F:** Metachromatic blasts are intermediate to large with round nuclear contours, blastic-appearing chromatin, and abundant cytoplasmic granules (Wright-Giemsa stain; 1000× magnification).

necessary.[12] However, there are cases of MCL where the cells can be identified by flow cytometry in BM and peripheral blood.

MCs show metachromatic staining with Giemsa and toluidine blue stains due to the MC granule reactivity. Because neoplastic MCs are often hypogranular, these stains may appear weaker compared with the intensity observed on normal MCs. The most useful markers to identify MCs (normal and abnormal) are tryptase and CD117 (Figure 7.2E). CD117 is not specific for MCs and may be seen in a variety of other cell types; therefore, it is critical to interpret the stain in the appropriate morphologic context. Neoplastic MCs often show aberrant expression of CD25, CD2, and/or CD30 in contrast to their nonneoplastic counterparts (Figure 7.2E). Tryptase is specific for MCs but may be partial and weak in some SM cases, rarely shows weak expression in basophils, and may be expressed in myeloid blasts. Given that there may be lower sensitivity to detect MCs with tryptase, routinely performing CD117 immunohistochemistry is suggested. Basophils are, however, CD117 negative, and blasts may be CD34 positive. Dim to negative tryptase expression may be seen in SM involving the gastrointestinal tract and MC sarcoma.

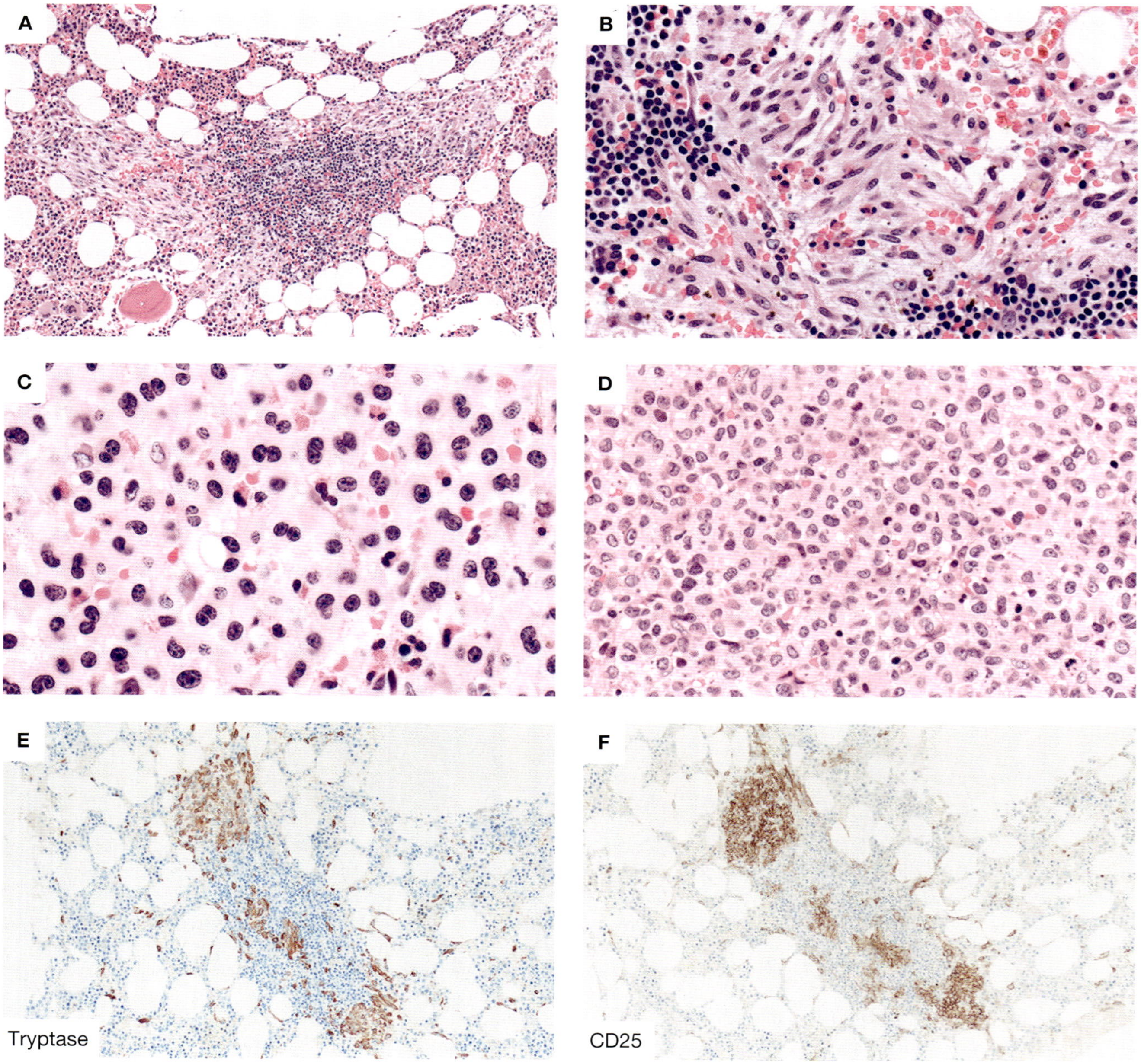

FIGURE 7.2 Mast cell morphology on bone marrow core biopsies. **A** and **B:** Mast cell lesions are often morphologically distinctive and may exhibit a focal infiltration pattern as shown here. **A:** Focal compact aggregate of mast cells with a central core of lymphocytes and admixed eosinophils forming a target lesion. **B:** Mast cells are often spindle shaped with bland nuclear features and variable numbers of admixed mature eosinophils and lymphocytes. **C:** Mast cell leukemia composed of numerous bilobed promastocytes in a diffuse infiltration pattern. **D:** Mast cell leukemia composed of sheets of metachromatic blasts with round to slightly irregular nuclear contours. **E** and **F:** Immunohistochemical studies confirm a diagnosis of systemic mastocytosis with **E** tryptase-positive mast cells in focal compact dense clusters and **F** aberrant coexpression of CD25. **A-D:** hematoxylin and eosin; **E:** immunohistochemistry for tryptase; **F:** immunohistochemistry for CD25; 400×, 1000×, 1000×, 1000×, 200×, 200× magnification, respectively.

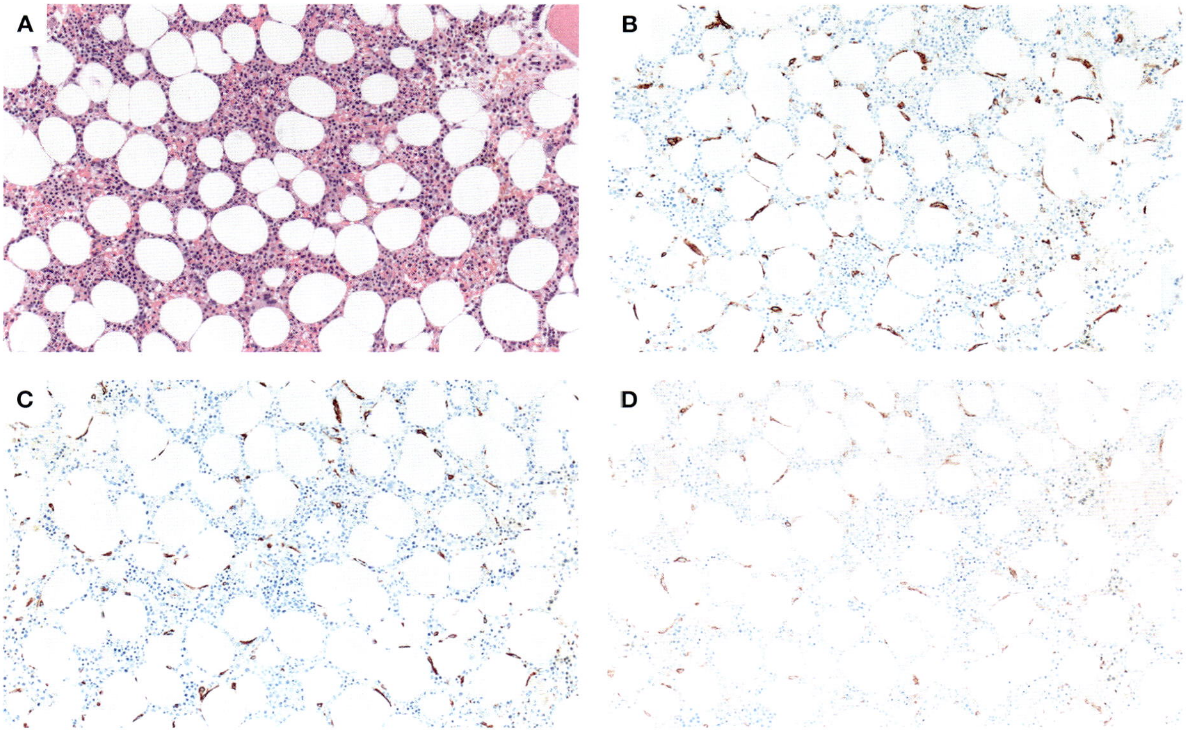

FIGURE 7.3 Morphologically occult bone marrow involvement by systemic mastocytosis. Occasionally mast cell infiltrates are morphologically occult and require immunohistochemical techniques to identify the increased mast cells, which are not in aggregates but individually distributed through the interstitium. In clinically suspicious situations, generous use of mast cell stains is needed. **B** and **C:** CD117 and tryptase highlight increased mast cells, respectively, which are predominantly spindle shaped; **D** and show aberrant coexpression of CD25. **A:** hematoxylin and eosin; **B:** immunohistochemistry for CD117; **C:** immunohistochemistry for tryptase; **D:** immunohistochemistry for CD25: 400× magnification.

MCs also express CD68, CD33, and CD45 and are negative for myeloperoxidase and CD14. CD123 may stain aberrant MCs.

Genetics

KIT gene mutations are common in SM (nearly 95% of cases).[13,14] They typically result in constitutive activation of the KIT tyrosine kinase with resultant unopposed signaling and cell proliferation.[15] The Asp816Val (D816V) mutation is most frequent (located in the activation loop of exon 17), while mutations in exon 8 to 11 or other exon 17 variants are less common.[14-16] In cases of SM that are negative for D816V, assessment for the other *KIT* variants is warranted as well as excluding tyrosine kinase gene fusions that may be seen in M/LN-eo-TK (*PDGFRA, PDGFRB, FGFR1, JAK2, FLT3, ABL1*). These latter cases often show increased, spindled, and phenotypically aberrant (eg, positive for CD25) MCs. To ensure that there are not false-negative results for the *KIT* D816V, a highly sensitive molecular assay should be utilized such as allele-specific oligonucleotide-quantitative polymerase chain reaction (PCR) or digital droplet PCR.[1]

Conventional cytogenetics of the BM aspirate is helpful when there is clinical and/or pathologic concern for an AMN. The presence of an unfavorable karyotype (eg, complex karyotype, monosomy 7) may portend a worse prognosis.

Next-generation sequencing for myeloid neoplasm-associated genetic abnormalities may also be useful in further evaluation of mastocytosis. In AdvSM, particularly SM-AMN, additional somatic mutations in genes such as *SRSF2, JAK2, RUNX1, ASXL1, TET2,* and *NRAS* may provide prognostic and diagnostic information.[17]

Prognosis and clinical comment

The outcome of patients with mastocytosis is largely predicated on the disease subtype. Those with isolated CM, typically children, and those with ISM most often do well and have a normal lifespan. The clinical course for those patients with AdvSM tends to be aggressive. Finally, MCL (immature MC morphology) and MC sarcoma have the worst prognosis.

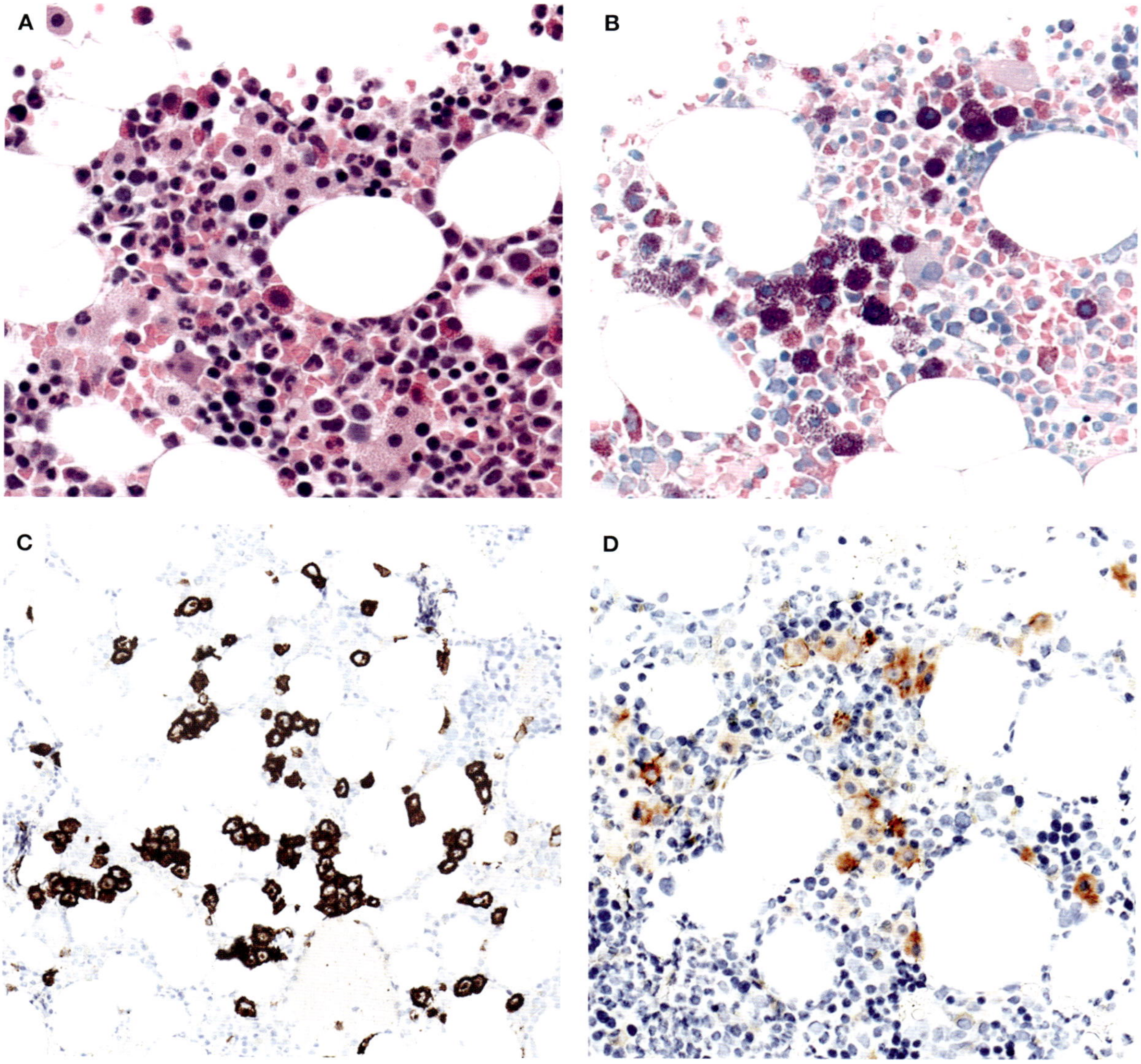

FIGURE 7.4 Well-differentiated mast cell morphology in a case of bone marrow mastocytosis. **A** and **B:** Mast cells with round shape and adequate granularity form occasional small loose clusters. **C:** Mast cells are highlighted by CD117 and show aberrant coexpression of CD30 **(D)**. (**A:** hematoxylin eosin; **B:** Giemsa; **C:** immunohistochemistry for CD117; **D:** immunohistochemistry for CD30; **A** and **B:** 800× magnification; **C** and **D:** 400× magnification).

With regard to management and risk stratification in SM, the approach to AdvSM is different from that of non-AdvSM. The latter includes CM, ISM and its variants, and SSM. Overall prognosis is excellent in non-AdvSM, and survival is near normal.[18] Accordingly, treatment in non-AdvSM is often symptomatic and includes alleviation of mast cell mediator symptoms (MCMS), cosmetically unacceptable skin lesions urticaria pigmentosa, and osteopenia that does not qualify as a "C"-finding but requires treatment to prevent osteoporosis and fractures.[14] In general, patients with non-AdvSM are advised to avoid being exposed to drugs or other situations that could trigger MC degranulation and in some instances to carry an EpiPen (epinephrine) in case of anaphylaxis.[14] Drugs that are often used to target MCMS include histamine H1 and H2 blockers, leukotriene antagonists, sodium cromolyn, corticosteroids, and epinephrine.[14] MC-directed therapy for treatment in the setting of non-AdvSM includes cladribine, midostaurin, and avapritinib, all of which are variably effective.[14]

Prognosis in AdvSM is significantly worse than that of non-AdvSM, and median survival estimates were 1, 20, and 72 months in International Consensus Classification (ICC)-defined MCL, SM-AMN, and ASM, respectively, and 19, 21, and 72 months in World Health Organization (WHO)-defined MCL, SM-associated hematologic neoplasm (AHN), and ASM.[19] Further scrutiny of survival estimates suggested significant differences between WHO-defined MCL with mature cytomorphology (median 33 months) and ICC-defined MCL (median 1 month), as well as between ICC-defined SM-AMN (median 20 months) and WHO-defined SM-AHN not classified as SM-AMN (median 85 months).[19] In a recent study of 329 patients with AdvSM, multivariable analysis that included the Mayo alliance risk factors for survival in SM (age >60 years, anemia, thrombocytopenia, increased alkaline phosphatase) confirmed more accurate survival prediction with the ICC versus WHO classification and the independent prognostic contribution of both the ICC classification for AdvSM and the Mayo alliance risk factors for survival in SM.[19] The latter also identified *ASXL1*, *RUNX1*, and *NRAS* mutations as additional risk factors for survival.[20] These observations were confirmed by other studies, which also identified splenomegaly and mutations of *SRSF2* and *CBL* as additional risk factors.[21,22] Current therapy for AdvSM includes cladribine, midostaurin, avapritinib, and allogenic hematopoietic stem cell transplantation.[14] These treatment modalities are variably effective, but their impact on survival remains uncertain.

Cutaneous Mastocytosis: General Features

Definition

Clonal/abnormal MC proliferation limited to the skin. There is no systemic involvement by MC disease (eg, no involvement of the BM and/or any other organ), and the diagnostic criteria for SM are not met. The three major variants of CM are listed in Table 7.1.[23]

Epidemiology

CM is most common in children and can be present at birth. About 50% of affected children develop skin lesions before the age of 6 months.

General Clinical Features

While some patients may be asymptomatic, systemic symptoms are encountered upon tissue release of MC mediators (histamine, cytokines, etc.) and include flushing, nausea/vomiting, anaphylaxis, "allergic" symptoms, bloating, abdominal pain, and diarrhea. A clinical feature common to all forms of CM is a positive Darier sign, which occurs when stroking of a lesion leads to localized swelling. Skin blistering and erosion may occur.

Diagnosis

In most cases, CM in children is diagnosed upon skin inspection; therefore, a skin biopsy may not be essential. If however, the diagnosis is uncertain and/or the skin manifestation occurs in an adult, a punch biopsy of an involved site should be considered.

Immunophenotype

The MCs show expression of markers that are typically present in normal MCs, ie, CD117, tryptase, CD33, and CD68. CD25, CD2, and CD30 may be variably expressed, although the frequency is lower than in adult SM with cutaneous involvement.

Genetics

Several studies have found a high rate (up to 80%) of *KIT* mutations in lesional skin samples obtained from children with CM. The *KIT* D816V mutation is found in approximately 35% of pediatric CM cases (in contrast with an almost 95% frequency in adult SM). *KIT* mutations in other exons (8, 9, 11) have been reported in 40%, and in up to 25% of cases *KIT* is wild type.[23-25]

Prognosis and clinical comment

The prognosis is excellent. While the MC lesions may occasionally spontaneously resolve within 4 to 10 years, they rather show major or partial regression by adolescence.[1,25] Most patients do not require treatment if significant systemic symptomatology is absent.

Urticaria Pigmentosa/Maculopapular CM

Definition

Clonal/abnormal MC proliferation restricted to the skin accompanied by more than three typically brown or yellow brown macules and/or papules.

Epidemiology

This CM subtype accounts for 70% to 90% of CM pediatric cases.[1]

General clinical features

Tan macules/papules often mimicking freckles involve the trunk, face, limbs, scalp, or neck. Involvement of the palms of the hands may occur but is unusual.

Maculopapular cutaneous mastocytosis (MPCM) is generally divided into two types, polymorphic and monomorphic. Polymorphic is by far the most common and is characterized by lesions that vary in size and shape. The monomorphic presentation consists of small 1- to 3-mm lesions. The polymorphic variant usually manifests in the first few weeks to 6 months of life, whereas the monomorphic variant tends to arise at toddler/school age. The monomorphic type has been reported to resemble what is seen in adults and may be associated with an increased risk of developing SM in adulthood.

Morphology

The MCs may distribute more in the papillary dermis and/or in a perivascular pattern, or form a small more band-like compact infiltrate in the upper dermis. There is often only a subtle increase in MCs (especially perivascular) in the reticular dermis, which may be difficult to detect without immunohistochemistry. A control biopsy of nonlesional skin is helpful to objectively determine the increase in MCs (Figure 7.5).

Genetics

Limited information is available. One study found *KIT* mutations in 28/31 cases—14 that harbored *KIT* D816V mutation, the remaining cases with other rare *KIT* alterations, and 3 cases wild type.[26]

Diffuse Cutaneous Mastocytosis

Definition

Abnormal MCs that infiltrate the entire skin in a generalized (not focal or nodular) pattern.

Epidemiology

This is a rare form of CM comprising 0.6% to 8% of CM cases and is the most severe because of the diffuse involvement of the skin.[27] Many patients present in infancy.

General clinical features

Extensive bullous lesions appear to predominate at the outset, whereas diffuse infiltration of the skin develops later. Because of the generalized involvement of the skin and often associated dermal edema, the skin becomes thickened and leather-like with accentuation of the skin folds resulting in a peau d'orange appearance. Because of the generalized skin involvement, patients are at high risk for more life-threatening symptoms including anaphylactic shock. As such, it is important to avoid Darier sign.

Morphology

MCs are typical including ovoid shape, abundant cytoplasm, and inconspicuous nucleoli. The MCs infiltrate the dermis in a diffuse pattern.

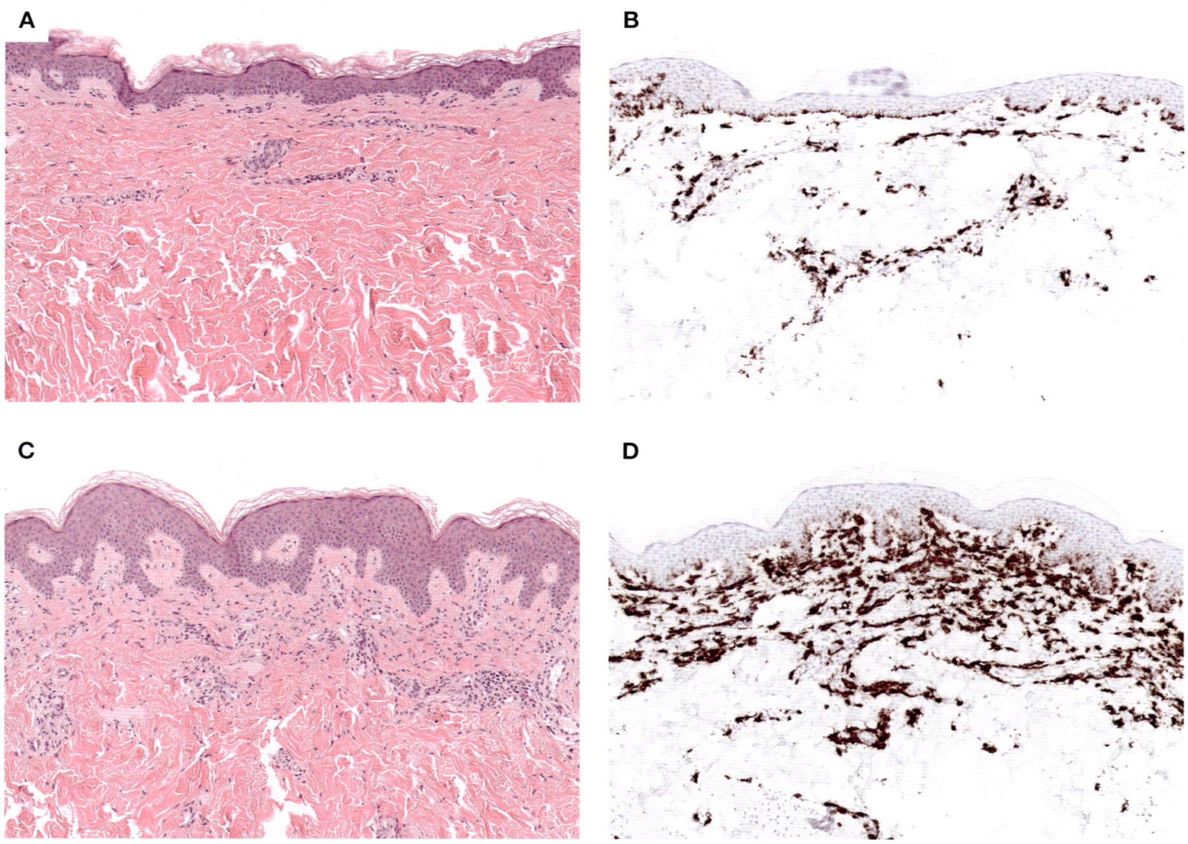

FIGURE 7.5 Maculopapular cutaneous mastocytosis (MPCM). **A** and **B:** Normal skin: As there may be subtle involvement in MPCM, a control biopsy of nonlesional skin is helpful to objectively determine the increase in mast cells. **B:** CD117-positive mast cells reveal the background expected normal number of mast cells. **C** and **D:** MPCM: Mast cells in MPCM may distribute more in the papillary dermis and form small or band-like compact infiltrates in the upper dermis. (**A:** hematoxylin and eosin; **B:** immunohistochemistry for CD117; **C:** hematoxylin and eosin; **D:** immunohistochemistry for CD117; 400× magnification).

Genetics

Limited information is available; one study found *KIT* D816 mutations in three of five cases.[26]

Prognosis and clinical comment

The disease appears to be particularly high risk in the first 2 years due to the extensive blistering and risk of life-threatening events.[27] However, these patients have an excellent chance for remission provided that the mortality from systemic mediator release is controlled.

Mastocytoma of the Skin

Definition

Abnormal nodular proliferation of MCs in the skin that typically occurs as a single lesion. In the clinical setting of >3 lesions, this is favored to be diagnosed as MPCM.

Epidemiology

Approximately 10% to 20% of CM cases in children present as mastocytoma of the skin. It typically presents at birth/infancy or early childhood, the majority developing within 3 months of life.[28]

General clinical features

Mastocytoma is an often pruritic, red-brown or yellow plaque or nodule and may urticate spontaneously or after trauma (Darier sign). It may occur anywhere on the body excluding the palms and soles.

Morphology

Mastocytoma manifests as a dense, nodular aggregate of MCs within the dermis. On occasion, the MC infiltrate may extend into the deeper dermis and subcutaneous tissue (Figure 7.6).

Genetics

One study found *KIT* alterations in three of four sequenced cases consisting of replacement of Thr417Tyr418Asp419 with Tyr, Cys443Tyr, and duplication of Asn505PheAlaPhe.[26]

Prognosis and clinical comment

Prognosis is typically indolent with involution of most lesions prior to puberty.

Systemic Mastocytosis

Indolent systemic mastocytosis

Definition

Clonal MC proliferation that meets the diagnostic criteria for SM, has <2 B-findings, lacks C-findings, and MCL and SM-AMN are excluded (Tables 7.2-7.4).

Epidemiology

ISM comprises 50% to more than 70% of all SM cases in different series.[1,29] The median age at presentation is approximately 50 years.

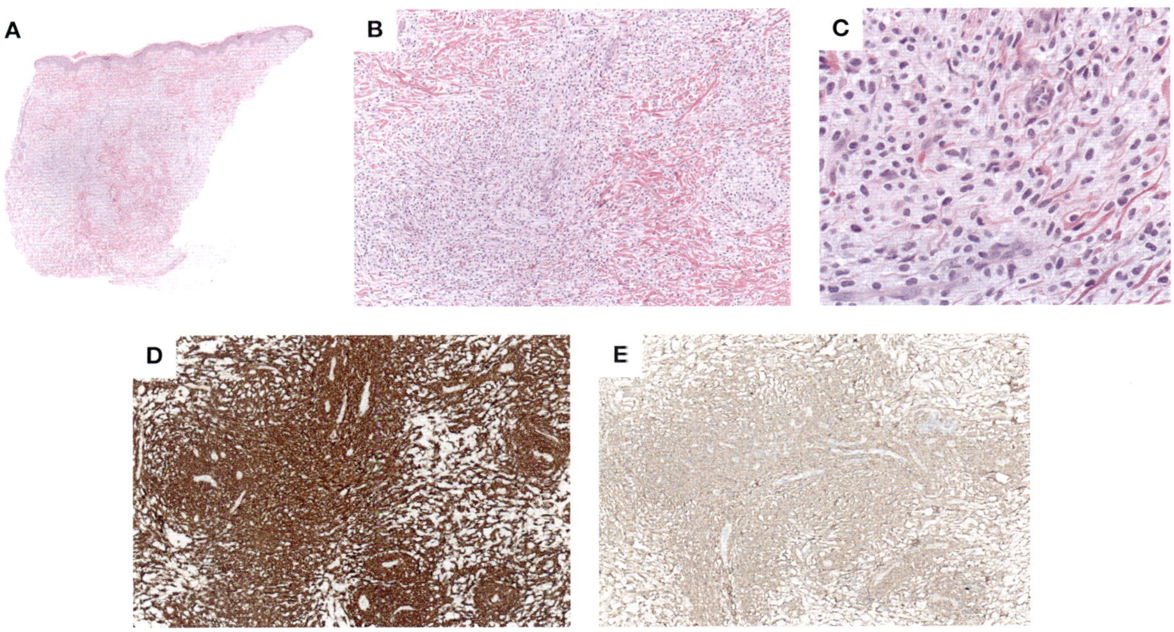

FIGURE 7.6 Mastocytoma of skin. **A-C:** Mastocytoma characterized by a nodular dermal infiltration by mast cells with abundant granular cytoplasm and bland round to oval nuclei. **Eand F:** Mast cell lineage is confirmed by immunoreactivity with CD117 **(E)** and tryptase **(F)**.

General clinical features

Approximately 75% of patients present with MPCM-like skin lesions, gastrointestinal symptoms, and MCMS. Osteopenia/osteoporosis may be a leading symptom. Constitutional symptoms and hepatosplenomegaly are not typical presenting symptoms (less than 20%) and should raise consideration of AdvSM.

Morphology

The atypical MCs are mature with hypogranular and spindled cytoplasm. Round, well-differentiated morphology may also be seen. The MCs are found in aggregates associated with variable combinations of eosinophils, lymphocytes, fibroblasts, and histiocytes (Figure 7.2). In BM, the aggregates are typically paratrabecular and perivascular and associated with fibrosis, which is often significant, and varying degrees of osteosclerosis. A small proportion of patients with ISM lack MC clusters in the BM. In the latter setting, a more generous use of immunohistochemical stains may be needed to confirm a diagnosis of SM.

Genetics

Nearly 95% of patients will harbor the *KIT* D816V mutation with the use of high-sensitivity assays. Additional mutations or cytogenetic abnormalities are usually absent. If present, this should raise the possibility of SM-AMN.

Prognosis and clinical comment

The median overall survival of patients with ISM in one study is 301 months.[29] In another study there was no significant difference in survival between ISM, SSM, and BMM groups.[30] Progression to SSM occurs in approximately 2% of patients and to ASM in 1% to 3%.[30,31]

ISM morphologic subtype: bone marrow mastocytosis

Definition

BMM is an ISM variant with isolated and limited BM involvement, absence of skin lesions, absence of B-findings, and a tryptase level of <125 ng/mL (Tables 7.3 and 7.4).

Epidemiology

About 23% to 60% of patients with ISM may be categorized as BMM.[29,32]

General clinical features

Patients tend to be older with a male predominance.[32] Approximately 86% present with MCMS including anaphylaxis (78%). Patients may present with osteoporosis. Also noted is a strong association with severe allergic reactions to a Hymenoptera sting in 62% of patients.[32]

Morphology

The BM infiltrate is similar to ISM (Figure 7.4), but a significant higher proportion (30%) of cases lack dense MC aggregates.

Genetics

Ninety-two percent of patients will demonstrate the *KIT* D816V mutation.[29]

Prognosis and clinical comment

The prognosis is typically excellent with a median overall survival not being reached in one study.[29] A recent study showed a 1.7% rate of disease progression.[30]

Smoldering systemic mastocytosis

Definition

Clonal MC proliferation that meets the diagnostic criteria for SM, has ≥2 B-findings, absence of C-findings, and MCL and SM-AMN are excluded (Tables 7.3 and 7.4).

Epidemiology

In one study of non-AdvSM excluding cutaneous forms, SSM comprised approximately 4% of patients.[30]

General clinical features

Patients are almost always adults presenting in most cases with skin lesions, hepatomegaly, splenomegaly, and lymphadenopathy. The tryptase levels are usually high.

Morphology

MCs are typically hypogranular and spindled and may demonstrate less dense infiltration pattern compared with the compact aggregates of ISM. The degree of overall MC tumor burden is typically higher in SSM than in ISM.

Genetics

In one study with <10 cases, 100% showed the *KIT* D816V mutation.[29]

Prognosis

The median survival in one study is 120 months. There is a 9% to 15% rate of progression to ASM.[27,33]

Aggressive systemic mastocytosis

Definition

Clonal MC proliferation that meets criteria for SM, has ≥1 C-finding, and MCL and SM-AMN are excluded (Tables 7.3 and 7.4).

Epidemiology

ASM is uncommon, may arise de novo or as progression from underlying ISM/SSM, and may progress to MCL.[34] The male:female ratio is approximately 1:1. The average age at diagnosis is 65 years.

General clinical features

Skin lesions are less frequent than in ISM. Patients frequently display constitutional symptoms (60%), splenomegaly (50%), and lymphadenopathy (30%).[24] The tryptase levels are usually high.

Morphology

ASM shows a proliferation of atypical mature and immature MCs that account for <20% of total nucleated cells on a BM aspirate smear. BM cores show focal or diffuse dense aggregates of MCs with varying degrees of background residual trilineage hematopoiesis. Peripheral blood smears corroborate the cytopenias demonstrated by the complete blood cell count including severe anemia (hemoglobin <10 g/dL) and thrombocytopenia (platelets <100 × 10^9/L).

Genetics

The *KIT* D816V mutation is seen in approximately 80% of patients. An abnormal karyotype is seen in approximately 20% of cases; in such instances, a diagnosis of SM-AMN should be suspected.[14] Additional (other than *KIT*) gene mutations such as *TET2* and *ASXL1* may occur and are usually diagnostic of SM-AMN (see Systemic Mastocytosis with an Associated Myeloid Neoplasm).

Prognosis and clinical comment

The prognosis is unfavorable with an overall median survival of 41 months.[14] In addition, if promastocytes and metachromatic blasts in the BM aspirate comprise ≥5% of total nucleated cells, this is associated with a significantly shorter survival[35]; therefore, it may be prudent to mention this in the BM report.

Mast cell leukemia

Definition

MCL consists of atypical immature MCs (promastocytes, metachromatic blasts, or, rarely, pleomorphic, anaplastic, multinucleated forms) that comprise ≥20% of the BM aspirate smear nucleated cells (Table 7.3) (Figure 7.1). In the presence of a suboptimal aspirate (dry tap), a good-quality BM biopsy showing diffuse infiltration by immature atypical MCs can support a diagnosis of MCL (Figure 7.2). In prior classifications, MCL was annotated as leukemic or aleukemic depending on the presence of ≥10% or <10% circulating, respectively. While this annotation is no longer necessary, it may be important to mention circulating MCs, if present, as this may be associated with more aggressive disease.[33]

Synonyms

Systemic tissue mast cell disease (not recommended).

Epidemiology

MCL is largely a disease of adults and is remarkably rare (<5% of SM cases).[19,36] In one study, the median age at presentation is 65 years.[19] MCL may arise de novo or secondary as a form of disease progression from a prior MC disease.[37] An associated myeloid neoplasm (ie, MCL-AMN) has been reported in approximately 35% of all patients with MCL.[33]

General clinical features

Patients frequently exhibit constitutional symptoms—fever, night sweats, and weight loss. C-findings are prevalent (Table 7.4) with multiple organ involvement.[37] Skin lesions are uncommon. Tryptase levels are generally increased with a median of 520 ng/mL.[36,37]

Morphology

The MCs in the BM aspirate smear usually consist of ≥20% atypical immature MCs with high-grade cytological features, including promastocytes (Figures 7.1 and 7.2) and/or metachromatic blasts (Figure 7.1), and pleomorphic, multinucleated, or anaplastic forms. On BM core biopsies, the MCs usually diffusely efface normal hematopoiesis and mostly retain a round, monocytoid appearance with bilobated, multilobated, or blast-like forms (Figure 7.2). Cases with ≥20% MCs, but in which the MCs are mature, such as well-differentiated forms, should not be labeled as MCL. These cases should lack C-findings and, for the most part, behave in a much more indolent manner than those with immature morphology[19,33,36,38]; thus, using the term "chronic MCL" seems unwarranted. The peripheral blood typically exhibits anemia and thrombocytopenia, and there may be circulating MCs. Review of the feathered edge of the smear or a buffy coat preparation is critical to identify cases with few numbers of circulating MCs.

Immunophenotype

The immunophenotypic features of MCL are similar to other variants of SM. However, hypogranulated promastocytes may show weaker tryptase staining. Therefore, CD117 immunohistochemistry should be generously utilized in these cases. Flow cytometry may be useful in identification of the MCs in BM and/or peripheral blood.

Genetics

A *KIT* mutation at D816 has been variably reported ranging from approximately 50% to 85%, and alternative *KIT* mutations in about 4% to 20%.[33,36,37] Cases that are D816V negative warrant complete *KIT* gene sequencing. Mutations in *TET2, SF3B1, ASXL1, KRAS, NRAS,* and *SRSF2* may occur. Their presence suggest a diagnosis of MCL-AMN.

Prognosis and clinical comment

The prognosis of MCL is poor with an overall median survival of <12 to 17 months.[19,36,37] Prognosis may also be negatively impacted by circulating MCs. While studies vary on the percent that worsens prognosis, a recent large study reported that any circulating MCs had an inferior effect on overall survival.[33] In multivariate analysis, mutations in *SRSF2, ASXL1,* and/or *RUNX1* were associated with unfavorable overall survival.[21,33] Additionally, a diagnosis of MCL-AMN and abnormal karyotype were associated with inferior overall survival, while *KIT* D816V positivity and midostaurin treatment were associated with better overall survival.[33] A study from the Mayo Clinic comprising 329 patients with AdvSM included 18 WHO-defined and 9 ICC-defined MCL; multivariable analysis disclosed independent prognostic contributions from ICC-defined but not WHO-defined MCL.[19] Prognostic distinction between MCL and SM-AMN/AHN was confirmed in the context of ICC and not WHO classification.[19]

Systemic mastocytosis with an associated myeloid neoplasm

Definition

Clonal MC proliferation meeting diagnostic criteria for SM in association with an additional myeloid neoplasm (Table 7.3). In some cases, the details of the myeloid neoplasm may be obscured due to extensive marrow involvement by the SM or, conversely, SM may be nonapparent (a.k.a. occult mastocytosis) when the AMN predominates. The AMN is usually diagnosed concurrently with the initial diagnosis of SM. Any type of myeloid neoplasm may be seen—myelodysplastic syndrome (MDS), myelodysplastic/myeloproliferative neoplasm (MDS/MPN), most commonly chronic myelomonocytic leukemia (CMML) (Figure 7.7), AML (Figure 7.8), particularly AML with *RUNX1::RUNX1T1* fusion, chronic myeloid leukemia, *BCR::ABL1* positive, and myeloproliferative neoplasm (MPN). Very rarely the AMN may be M/LN-eo-TK.

Synonym

Systemic mastocytosis with an AHN; systemic mastocytosis associated with a hematologic disorder; systemic mastocytosis with an associated clonal hematologic non-MC lineage disease (not recommended).

Epidemiology

SM-AMN is the second most common subtype of SM with a reported estimate of approximately 40% to 50%. The true incidence is unknown given that this entity may be underrecognized.

General clinical features

With the notable exception of cases of MCL associated with AMN, the clinical features are mostly driven by the non-MC myeloid neoplasm. For instance, in AML and MDS, cytopenic patients may experience infection due to neutropenia or easy bruising due to thrombocytopenia. In cases of MPN, there may be symptoms associated with splenomegaly. However, in some patients,

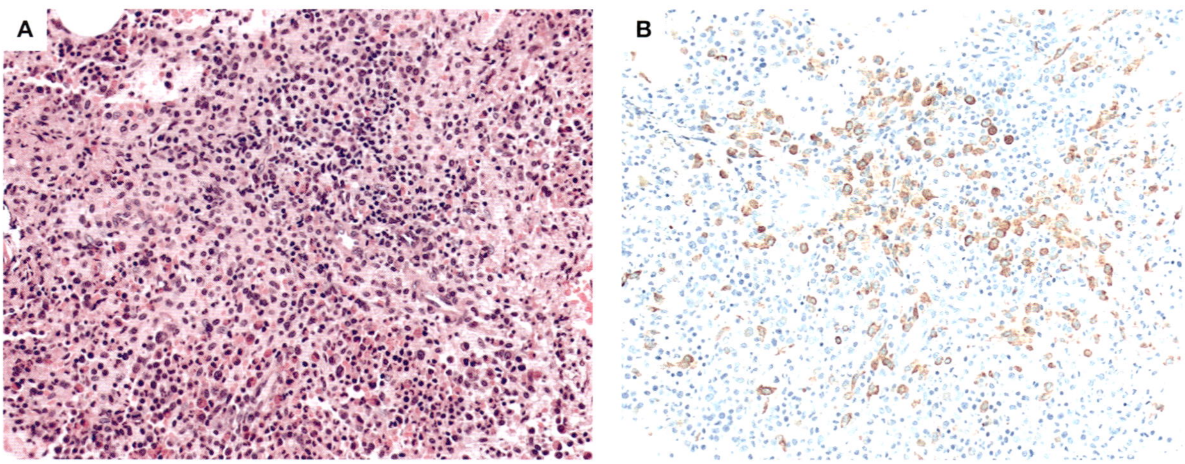

FIGURE 7.7 Systemic mastocytosis with associated myeloid neoplasm (chronic myelomonocytic leukemia [CMML]). **A:** A sneaky focus of systemic mastocytosis is seen in this case of CMML. Routinely performing a CD117 and/or tryptase immunostain in newly diagnosed cases of CMML to assess for the presence of occult systemic mastocytosis is useful. **B:** A focus of systemic mastocytosis in the setting of CMML is highlighted by tryptase immunohistochemical staining. (**A:** hematoxylin and eosin; **B:** immunohistochemistry for tryptase; 400× magnification).

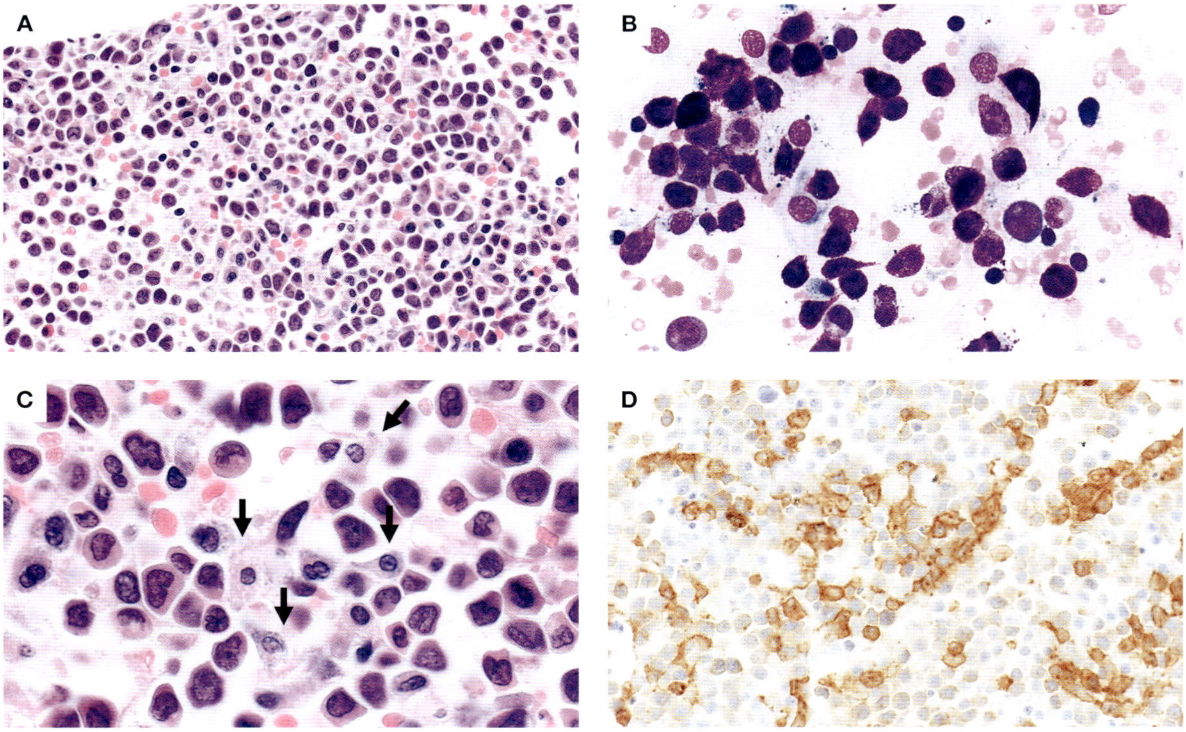

FIGURE 7.8 Systemic mastocytosis with associated myeloid neoplasm (acute myeloid leukemia with t(8;21)). **A:** Sheets of blasts at presentation with chromosomal analysis that revealed t(8:21). No overt morphologic features to suggest systemic mastocytosis. **B:** Bone marrow aspirate at 30 days postinduction chemotherapy shows a striking predominance of mast cells. **C** and **D:** Retrospective review of the original biopsy shows mast cells (**C:** arrows) that are CD117 strongly positive (**D**) admixed with the sheets of blasts. (**A:** hematoxylin and eosin; **B:** Wright-Giemsa; **C:** hematoxylin and eosin; **D:** immunohistochemistry for CD117; 400×, 1000×, 600×, 1000× magnification, respectively).

SM may cause the major issues while the AMN is relatively indolent, although in these cases the attribution of C-findings and/or observed symptomatology either to SM or AMN can be difficult.

Morphology

The pathologic picture of SM-AMN in the BM is highly variable and largely dependent on BM MC burden and the type of AMN. SM-CMML and SM-MDS/MPN, NOS are the most frequent SM-AMN combinations. In a proportion of cases, the SM component may be subtle (Figures 7.7 and 7.8); therefore, one should consider immunohistochemistry for MCs in CMML, particularly when a *KIT* mutation is found. Regardless, the BM typically exhibits marked hypercellularity due to the presence of both the AMN and the dense aggregates of MCs (Figures 7.7 and 7.8). The MCs are often spindled; however, round-shaped forms or MCs showing atypical immature morphology may also be seen. Because SM is often associated with mild to moderate eosinophilia, it is critical to assess if the BM ICC criteria are met for CEL, NOS or another MPN with accompanying eosinophilia. In cases of SM associated with eosinophilia, it is important to exclude tyrosine kinase gene fusions (*PDGFRA, PDGFRB, FGFR1, JAK2, FLT3, ABL1*) associated with M/LN-eo-TK.

Immunophenotype

In some cases the myeloid neoplasm may obscure the SM ("occult" SM); therefore, it is recommended to stain for tryptase and CD117 to highlight the MCs and to stain for CD2, CD25, and CD30 to confirm their aberrancy.[39] Conversely, in cases with a significant MC tumor burden, the AMN may be difficult to detect. Additional immunophenotypic markers, either tested by flow cytometry and/or immunohistochemistry, may clarify the specific AMN (eg, CD34, MPO, CD14, CD36, CD42b, CD56, CD61, CD64, CD71, lysozyme) and confirm the MCs (CD117, CD25, CD30). CD123, although not specific, may be helpful to identify plasmacytoid dendritic cells that may be seen in CMML. CD123 also stains myeloid blasts and sinusoidal elements and is aberrant on MCs in some cases.

Genetics

Karyotyping should be performed in each case for the AMN component. Fluorescence in situ hybridization (FISH) can also be performed, depending on the type of case. For example, if the AMN represents a monoblastic leukemia, it may be prudent to consider FISH testing for inv(16) and *KMT2A* rearrangement. In most cases, a somatic mutation in the *KIT* gene is detected. In cases of SM-CMML, the monocytes are *KIT* D816V positive in >80% of cases, indicating that they are part of the same clone (multilineage involvement). Next-generation sequencing for myeloid disorder–associated gene mutations for the AMN should be considered. The presence of such somatic mutations in genes such as *SRSF2, JAK2, RUNX1, ASXL1, TET2,* and/or *NRAS* is almost always observed in SM-AMN and helps support this diagnosis particularly if the myeloid proliferation is limited or shows equivocal morphology (eg, SM with BM neutrophilic or eosinophilic proliferation vs a concurrent MPN, MDS/MPN, or CEL, NOS). Notably, *JAK2* V617F and *KIT* D816V may be coexisting and often indicate the presence of two independent diseases, eg, ISM and essential thrombocythemia.

Prognosis

In most instances, the clinical course and prognosis are driven by the AMN and by other clinical and molecular risk factors including the Mayo alliance risk factors for survival in SM: age >60 years, anemia, thrombocytopenia, and increased alkaline phosphatase.[20] Mutations in *SRSF2, ASXL1 RUNX1,* and/or *NRAS* and an abnormal karyotype in the AMN are prognostically unfavorable.[21,22] In the cases where the SM represents ASM or MCL, the MC component may portend the worse prognosis.[19] In SM-AML, the AML may be core-binding factor positive (eg, t(8;21)(q22;q22.1)/*RUNX1::RUNX1T1*) or core-binding factor negative. In the AML *KIT* D816V–positive, core-binding factor–negative group, patients also harbor at least one somatic gene mutation (eg, *SRSF2, ASXL1, RUNX1*) and have a poor overall median survival (<6 months).[40] A study from the Mayo Clinic of 329 patients with AdvSM included 212 WHO-defined SM-AHN and 190 ICC-defined SM-AMN; multivariable analysis disclosed more accurate prognostic distinction between MCL and SM-AMN/AHN, in the context of ICC and not WHO classification.[19]

Mast Cell Sarcoma

Definition

MCS is a neoplastic, tumorous proliferation of malignant MCs.[3]

Synonyms

Malignant mast cell tumor; malignant mastocytoma (not recommended).

Epidemiology

MCS is an extraordinarily rare entity. It generally manifests in adults, although there are reports of cases in children. The male:female ratio is approximately 1:1. MCS often occurs de novo, although cases secondary to CM and SM have been reported.

General clinical features

MCS usually presents as a localized, yet significantly destructive, tumor mass involving a broad spectrum of tissue sites including bone (most common), gastrointestinal tract, soft tissue, and lymph nodes.[41] Although it most often presents as an isolated mass, within months a systemic spread may occur leading to a final phase resembling MCL. Serum tryptase level is often elevated. There may be splenomegaly and/or hepatomegaly particularly in the disseminated phase of disease.

Morphology

MCS comprises highly pleomorphic, bizarre, epithelioid, and occasionally multilobated MCs that may morphologically mimic sarcoma, carcinoma, megakaryocytes, melanoma, or even anaplastic large cell lymphoma (Figure 7.9)—the last one is further confounded by the occasional CD30 positivity. Indeed, a diagnosis of MCS can only be confirmed through the use of immunohistochemical markers (see section on immunophenotype).

Immunophenotype

MCS must be diagnosed by demonstrating immunohistochemical positivity for tryptase, although this can, in many situations, be weak and/or partial. Positivity for CD117 (Figure 7.9) is also supportive, in the appropriate overall context, but other neoplastic processes that may express CD117 such as AML, germ cell tumors (seminoma in particular), melanoma, plasma cell tumors, and gastrointestinal stromal tumors need to be excluded. MCS may also show expression of other antigens that may be seen in other morphologically mimickers; therefore, a comprehensive immunohistochemical profile is needed. For example, MCS may express CD68 (associated with histiocytic lineage); CD2, CD4, and CD25 (associated with T-cell lineage); CD30 (nonspecific) (Figure 7.9); and CD33 (myeloid/monocytic-associated marker).

Genetics

In contrast to most other subtypes of SM, which harbor a *KIT* D816V mutation in nearly 95% of cases, MCS reportedly shows this mutation in only approximately 7% to 20% of cases.[41,42] In the remaining cases, the *KIT* gene may be wild type or display other *KIT* variants. It is very important to perform the testing on the lesional tissue and not only on blood or BM.

Prognosis and clinical comment

The prognosis is typically uniformly dismal for these patients.

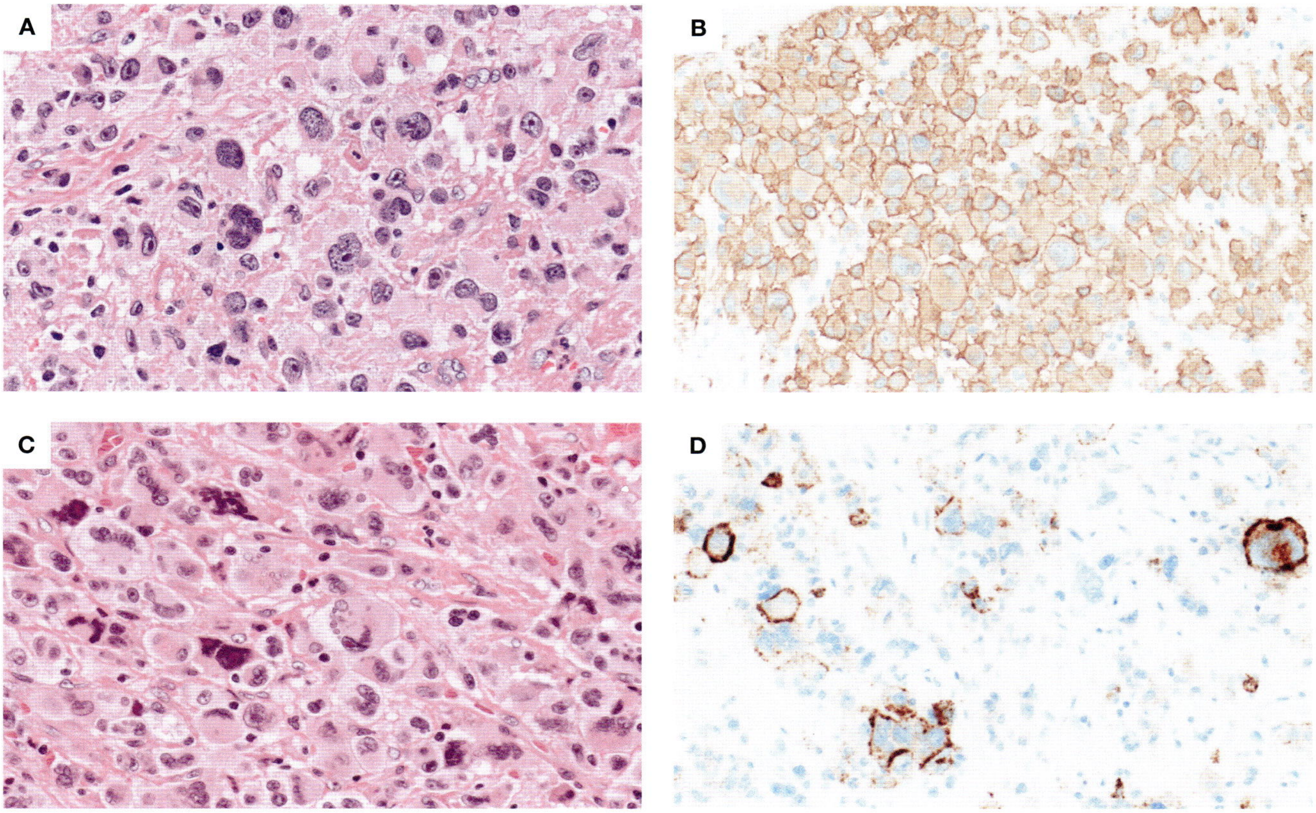

FIGURE 7.9 Mast cell sarcoma. Mast cell sarcoma comprises highly atypical, bizarre, epithelioid, occasionally multilobated, and pleomorphic mast cells **(A)** that may morphologically mimic sarcoma, carcinoma, megakaryocytes, melanoma, or even anaplastic large cell lymphoma **(C)**. Generous use of a comprehensive set of immunohistochemical stains is typically necessary to establish the diagnosis of mast cell sarcoma. In these two exemplary cases, CD117 is brightly positive **(B)**, whereas CD30 stains a subset of the abnormal atypical pleomorphic mast cells in the second **(D)**. (**A:** hematoxylin and eosin; **B:** immunohistochemistry for CD117; **C:** hematoxylin and eosin; **D:** immunohistochemistry for CD30; 1000× magnification).

References

1. Leguit RJ, Wang SA, George TI, Tzankov A, Orazi A. The international consensus classification of mastocytosis and related entities. *Virchows Arch*. 2023;482(1):99-112.
2. Wang SA, Orazi A, Gotlib J, et al. The international consensus classification of eosinophilic disorders and systemic mastocytosis. *Am J Hematol*. 2023;98(8):1286-1306.
3. Horny HP, Akin C, Arber D, et al. Mastocytosis. In: Swerdlow SH, Campo E, Harris NL, et al, eds. WHO Classification Fo Tumours of Haematopoietic and Lymphoid Tissues. IARC; 2017:62-69.
4. Tzankov A, Duncavage E, Craig FE, et al. Mastocytosis. *Am J Clin Pathol*. 2021;155(2):239-266.
5. Brockow K. Epidemiology, prognosis, and risk factors in mastocytosis. *Immunol Allergy Clin North Am*. 2014;34(2):283-295.
6. Schwaab J, Cabral do O Hartmann N, Naumann N, et al. Importance of adequate diagnostic workup for correct diagnosis of advanced systemic mastocytosis. *J Allergy Clin Immunol Pract*. 2020;8(9):3121-3127.e1.
7. Jennings SV, Slee VM, Zack RM, et al. Patient perceptions in mast cell disorders. *Immunol Allergy Clin North Am*. 2018;38(3):505-525.
8. Zanotti R, Bonifacio M, Isolan C, et al. A multidisciplinary diagnostic approach reveals a higher prevalence of indolent systemic mastocytosis: 15-years' experience of the GISM network. *Cancers*. 2021;13(24):6380. doi:10.3390/cancers13246380
9. Reiter A, George TI, Gotlib J. New developments in diagnosis, prognostication, and treatment of advanced systemic mastocytosis. *Blood*. 2020;135(16):1365-1376.
10. Álvarez-Twose I, Jara-Acevedo M, Morgado JM, et allinical, immunophenotypic, and molecular characteristics of well-differentiated systemic mastocytosis. *J Allergy Clin Immunol*. 2016;137(1):168-178.e1. doi:10.1016/j.jaci.2015.05.008
11. Morgado JM, Perbellini O, Johnson RC, et al. CD30 expression by bone marrow mast cells from different diagnostic variants of systemic mastocytosis. *Histopathology*. 2013;63(6):780-787.
12. Sánchez-Muñoz L, Teodosio C, Morgado JM, et al. Flow cytometry in mastocytosis: utility as a diagnostic and prognostic tool. *Immunol Allergy Clin North Am*. 2014;34(2):297-313.
13. Arock M, Hoermann G, Sotlar K, et al. Clinical impact and proposed application of molecular markers, genetic variants, and cytogenetic analysis in mast

cell neoplasms: status 2022. *J Allergy Clin Immunol.* 2022;149(6):1855-1865.

14. Pardanani A. Systemic mastocytosis in adults: 2023 update on diagnosis, risk stratification and management. *Am J Hematol.* 2023;98(7):1097-1116. doi:10.1002/ajh.26962
15. Orfao A, Garcia-Montero AC, Sanchez L, Escribano L; Rema. Recent advances in the understanding of mastocytosis: the role of KIT mutations. *Br J Haematol.* 2007;138(1):12-30. doi:10.1111/j.1365-2141.2007.06619.x
16. Valent P, Akin C, Sperr WR, et al. New insights into the pathogenesis of mastocytosis: emerging concepts in diagnosis and therapy. *Annu Rev Pathol.* 2023;18:361-386.
17. Jawhar M, Schwaab J, Schnittger S, et al. Additional mutations in SRSF2, ASXL1 and/or RUNX1 identify a high-risk group of patients with KIT D816V(+) advanced systemic mastocytosis. *Leukemia.* 2016;30(1):136-143.
18. Lim KH, Tefferi A, Lasho TL, et al. Systemic mastocytosis in 342 consecutive adults: survival studies and prognostic factors. *Blood.* 2009;113(23):5727-5736.
19. Tefferi A, Abdelmagid M, Al-Kali A, et al. Granularity in disease classification impacts survival prediction in advanced systemic mastocytosis: a single institution study of 329 informative cases. *Am J Hematol.* 2024;99(1):21-27.
20. Pardanani A, Shah S, Mannelli F, et al. Mayo alliance prognostic system for mastocytosis: clinical and hybrid clinical-molecular models. *Blood Adv.* 2018;2(21):2964-2972.
21. Jawhar M, Schwaab J, Hausmann D, et al. Splenomegaly, elevated alkaline phosphatase and mutations in the SRSF2/ASXL1/RUNX1 gene panel are strong adverse prognostic markers in patients with systemic mastocytosis. *Leukemia.* 2016;30(12):2342-2350.
22. Pardanani AD, Lasho TL, Finke C, et al. ASXL1 and CBL mutations are independently predictive of inferior survival in advanced systemic mastocytosis. *Br J Haematol.* 2016;175(3):534-536.
23. Schaffer JV. Pediatric mastocytosis: recognition and management. *Am J Clin Dermatol.* 2021;22(2):205-220.
24. Arase N, Wataya-Kaneda M, Murota H, et al. Genotype and phenotype analysis of patients with pediatric cutaneous mastocytosis, especially wild-type KIT patients. *J Dermatol.* 2020;47(4):426-429.
25. Polivka L, Rossignol J, Neuraz A, et al. Criteria for the regression of pediatric mastocytosis: a long-term follow-up. *J Allergy Clin Immunol Pract.* 2021;9(4):e1695-e1704.e5.
26. Bodemer C, Hermine O, Palmerini F, et al. Pediatric mastocytosis is a clonal disease associated with D816V and other activating c-KIT mutations. *J Invest Dermatol.* 2010;130(3):804-815.
27. Lange M, Niedoszytko M, Nedoszytko B, Łata J, Trzeciak M, Biernat W. Diffuse cutaneous mastocytosis: analysis of 10 cases and a brief review of the literature. *J Eur Acad Dermatol Venereol.* 2012;26(12):1565-1571.
28. Giona F. Pediatric mastocytosis: an update. *Mediterr J Hematol Infect Dis.* 2021;13(1):e2021069.
29. Pardanani A, Lim KH, Lasho TL, et al. WHO subvariants of indolent mastocytosis: clinical details and prognostic evaluation in 159 consecutive adults. *Blood.* 2010;115(1):150-151. doi:10.1182/blood-2009-10-249979
30. Trizuljak J, Sperr WR, Nekvindová L, et al. Clinical features and survival of patients with indolent systemic mastocytosis defined by the updated WHO classification. *Allergy.* 2020;75(8):1927-1938. doi:10.1111/all.14248
31. Pieri L, Bonadonna P, Elena C, et al. Clinical presentation and management practice of systemic mastocytosis. A survey on 460 Italian patients. *Am J Hematol.* 2016;91(7):692-699. doi:10.1002/ajh.24382
32. Zanotti R, Bonifacio M, Lucchini G, et al. Refined diagnostic criteria for bone marrow mastocytosis: a proposal of the European competence network on mastocytosis. *Leukemia.* 2022;36(2):516-524.
33. Kennedy VE, Perkins C, Reiter A, et al. Mast cell leukemia: clinical and molecular features and survival outcomes of patients in the ECNM Registry. *Blood Adv.* 2023;7(9):1713-1724.
34. Leguit R, Hebeda K, Kremer M, et al. The spectrum of aggressive mastocytosis: a workshop report and literature review. *Pathobiology.* 2020;87(1):2-19.
35. Sperr WR, Escribano L, Jordan JH, et al. Morphologic properties of neoplastic mast cells: delineation of stages of maturation and implication for cytological grading of mastocytosis. *Leuk Res.* 2001;25(7):529-536.
36. Pardanani A, Tefferi A, Al-Kali A, et al. Reappraisal of mast cell leukemia based on a single institution review of 16 cases: mast cell morphology determines clinical outcome. *Am J Hematol.* 2024;99(1):E1-E4.
37. Jawhar M, Schwaab J, Meggendorfer M, et al. The clinical and molecular diversity of mast cell leukemia with or without associated hematologic neoplasm. *Haematologica.* 2017;102(6):1035-1043.
38. Valent P, Sotlar K, Sperr WR, et al. Refined diagnostic criteria and classification of mast cell leukemia (MCL) and myelomastocytic leukemia (MML): a consensus proposal. *Ann Oncol.* 2014;25(9):1691-1700.
39. Johnson RC, Savage NM, Chiang T, et al. Hidden mastocytosis in acute myeloid leukemia with t(8;21)(q22;q22). *Am J Clin Pathol.* 2013;140(4):525-535.
40. Jawhar M, Döhner K, Kreil S, et al. KIT D816 mutated/CBF-negative acute myeloid leukemia: a poor-risk subtype associated with systemic mastocytosis. *Leukemia.* 2019;33(5):1124-1134.
41. Matsumoto NP, Yuan J, Wang J, et al. Mast cell sarcoma: clinicopathologic and molecular analysis of 10 new cases and review of literature. *Mod Pathol.* 2022;35(7):865-874.
42. Monnier J, Georgin-Lavialle S, Canioni D, et al. Mast cell sarcoma: new cases and literature review. *Oncotarget.* 2016;7(40):66299-66309.

SECTION 4

Myelodysplastic/ Myeloproliferative Neoplasms

Chapter 8

Chronic Myelomonocytic Leukemia

Sonam Prakash, Daniel A. Arber, Kathryn Foucar, Robert P. Hasserjian, Luca Malcovati, Attilio Orazi, and Alexa J. Siddon

Chronic Myelomonocytic Leukemia

Definition

Chronic myelomonocytic leukemia (CMML) is a clonal hematopoietic stem cell disorder characterized by peripheral blood monocytosis and features of both myelodysplastic syndrome and myeloproliferative neoplasm. As in the other types of myelodysplastic/myeloproliferative neoplasms (MDS/MPN), cytopenia is typically seen in combination with cytosis.[1]

In the presence of clonality (abnormal cytogenetics and/or at least one myeloid neoplasm-associated mutation with variant allele frequency [VAF] ≥10%), the minimal required absolute monocytosis level is $\geq 0.5 \times 10^9$/L (modified from $\geq 1 \times 10^9$/L in the 2016 revision of the 4th edition of WHO classification); however, monocytes must still comprise ≥10% of the white blood cell (WBC) count.[2] Blasts, including promonocytes, which are considered blast equivalents, account for less than 20% of the leukocytes in the peripheral blood (PB) and less than 20% of the nucleated cells in the bone marrow (BM). The diagnostic criteria for CMML are presented in Table 8.1.

Based on the WBC count, two distinct subtypes of CMML are recognized; the proliferative subtype (CMML-MP) with WBC $>13 \times 10^9$/L, and the myelodysplastic subtype (CMML-MD). Although selected mutation signatures are strongly associated with a proliferative phenotype, at present WBC count appears to be the most robust criterion to segregate these two subtypes.

Recent studies have shown that there is no clinical significance in separating out CMML-0 (<2% blasts in PB and <5% blasts in BM) from CMML-1 as in WHO 2016. Therefore, the International Consensus Classification (ICC) has reverted to a two-tier system of CMML-1 (<5% blasts in PB, <10% in BM) and CMML-2 (5%-19% blasts PB, 10%-19% in BM, or presence of Auer rods). Table 8.2 highlights the key changes to the diagnosis of CMML as compared to those in 2016 revision of the 4th edition of WHO classification.

Synonyms

None.

Epidemiology

Recent studies report an approximate incidence of CMML to be 2 to 4 cases per 100,000 persons/year. However, the incidence may be higher because of

TABLE 8.1 Diagnostic Criteria for Chronic Myelomonocytic Leukemia (CMML)[1]

- Monocytosis defined as monocytes $\geq 0.5 \times 10^9$/L and ≥10% of the WBC
- Cytopenia (thresholds same as MDS)[a]
- Blasts (including promonocytes) <20% of the cells in blood and bone marrow
- Presence of clonality: abnormal cytogenetics and/or presence of at least one myeloid neoplasm-associated mutation of at least 10% allele frequency[b]
- In cases without evidence of clonality,
    - monocytes $\geq 1.0 \times 10^9$/L and ≥10% of the WBC, and at least one of the following would be required:
        - increased blasts (including promonocytes)[c]
        - morphologic dysplasia
        - an abnormal immunophenotype consistent with CMML
- Bone marrow examination with morphologic findings consistent with CMML (hypercellularity due to a myeloid proliferation often with increased monocytes), and lacking diagnostic features of acute myeloid leukemia, myeloproliferative neoplasm, or other conditions associated with monocytosis[d]
- No *BCR::ABL1* or genetic abnormalities of myeloid/lymphoid neoplasms with eosinophilia and tyrosine kinase gene fusions

[a]Small proportion of cases may show only borderline or no cytopenia usually in early-phase disease.
[b]Based on International Consensus Group Conference, Vienna, 2018.[2]
[c]Increased blasts: ≥5% in the bone marrow and/or ≥2% in the peripheral blood.
[d]For cases lacking bone marrow findings of CMML, a diagnosis of clonal monocytosis of undetermined significance (CMUS) can be considered. If cytopenia is present, a diagnosis of clonal cytopenia and monocytosis of undetermined significance (CCMUS) could be entertained. In these diagnostic settings, however, an alternative cause for the observed monocytosis needs to be excluded on the basis of appropriate clinicopathologic correlations.
Arber DA, Orazi A, Hasserjian RP, et al. International consensus classification of myeloid neoplasms and acute leukemias: integrating morphologic, clinical, and genomic data. *Blood.* 2022;140(11):1200-1228 and Valent P, Orazi A, Savona MR, et al. Proposed diagnostic criteria for classical chronic myelomonocytic leukemia (CMML), CMML variants and pre-CMML conditions. *Haematologica.* 2019;104(10):1935-1949. doi:10.3324/haematol.2019.222059

TABLE 8.2 Summary of Key Changes to the Diagnosis of CMML in the ICC

- Threshold for absolute monocytosis is decreased to $\geq 0.5 \times 10^9/L$; monocytes should still be ≥10% of leukocytes. Demonstration of clonality is required in this "oligomonocytic" group.
- Cytopenia at diagnosis is now a required diagnostic criterion (rare exceptions are allowed).
- Bone marrow examination with findings supportive of a diagnosis of CMML is now a diagnostic criterion.
- Dysplasia is no longer a required diagnostic criterion except in cases that lack clonality, increased blasts, or an abnormal monocyte immunophenotype.
- CMML-0 is eliminated; reversion to 2-tier system with CMML-1 and CMML-2.

failure to perform BM biopsies in older individuals; moreover, the new lower threshold of absolute monocytosis defining CMML will likely increase its relative incidence among myeloid neoplasms. The etiology of CMML is unknown. Occupational exposures, environmental carcinogens, and ionizing radiation have been suggested as probable causes in some cases. CMML can be therapy-related and such cases are associated with a poor outcome.

General Clinical Features

CMML occurs commonly in older adults, with a median age at diagnosis of 65 to 75 years and a male predominance (male:female ratio of 1.5-3:1). The clinical presentation is highly variable. Patients with CMML-MD tend to present with peripheral blood cytopenias, effort intolerance, easy bruising, and transfusion dependence. Patients with CMML-MP alternatively present with leukocytosis, hepatomegaly, splenomegaly, and features of myeloproliferation, such as fatigue, symptoms from organomegaly, night sweats, weight loss, and cachexia.[3] Lymphadenopathy and leukemic skin infiltrates can be seen in CMML-MP. Approximately 30% of CMML patients can present with manifestations of antecedent or concomitant autoimmune diseases (rheumatoid arthritis, psoriasis, etc.), vasculitic syndromes, classic connective tissue diseases, and poorly defined systemic inflammatory syndromes.[4]

Morphology

Evaluation of adequate, properly stained PB and BM samples (Figure 8.1) is essential to diagnose the clinical suspicion of CMML, to rule out other differential diagnoses, and to investigate the existence of possible concurrent neoplasms. The correct identification and enumeration of monocytes, abnormal monocytes, promonocytes (monocytic blast equivalent precursors), and blasts, especially monoblasts, is essential for CMML diagnosis and grading, and distinction from acute myeloid leukemia (AML) (Figure 8.2).

Peripheral Blood

Absolute ($\geq 0.5 \times 10^9/L$) and relative (≥10% of the WBC) peripheral blood monocytosis is the hallmark of CMML. Recent data have demonstrated a similar mutational landscape between oligomonocytic CMML (cases with ≥10% circulating monocytes but an absolute monocyte count of 0.5 to $<1.0 \times 10^9/L$) and traditional CMML (absolute monocytes $\geq 1.0 \times 10^9/L$).[5] Although the diagnostic criteria do not explicitly require persistence of monocytosis in cases lacking clonality, documentation of persistent monocytosis is recommended, as is rigorous exclusion of secondary causes of monocytosis, such as infection. The monocytes in the peripheral blood are typically mature but may show morphologic abnormalities including unusual nuclear lobation and delicate nuclear chromatin (Figure 8.1).

The WBC count is increased in more than 50% of cases (CMML-MP). The remainder may show a normal or decreased WBC count (CMML-MD). However, neutropenia is rare. Eosinophilia, including eosinophils $\geq 1.5 \times 10^9/L$, can be seen in a subset of cases that in itself does not exclude a diagnosis of CMML. In these cases, it is important to demonstrate the lack of the specific gene rearrangements/fusions seen in the group of myeloid/lymphoid neoplasms with eosinophilia and tyrosine kinase (M/LN-Eo-TK) gene fusions as these would exclude a diagnosis of CMML.[1] Neutrophil precursors (promyelocytes, myelocytes, and metamyelocytes) typically account for less than 10% of the WBCs at diagnosis. Dysgranulopoiesis may be seen in a subset of cases; if a significant granulocytic left shift, granulocytic dysplasia, increased blasts, or basophilia accompanies the monocytosis, it is essential to carefully exclude an alternative diagnosis such as chronic myeloid leukemia, AML, or monocytic progression of a myeloproliferative neoplasm.

Cytopenia, as evidence of ineffective hematopoiesis, is a required diagnostic criterion for CMML. Patients often have modest thrombocytopenia (80-100 × $10^9/L$) as well as anemia, which is usually mild and may be normocytic or macrocytic. A small proportion of early-phase cases may show only borderline or no cytopenia; these cases require appropriate marrow morphology, flow cytometric immunophenotypic, and molecular data to confirm a diagnosis of CMML.

Bone Marrow

BM examination with findings supportive of CMML is required for diagnosis. The BM is typically hypercellular for age with granulocytic predominance, which can be left-shifted (Figure 8.1). Monocytes are often

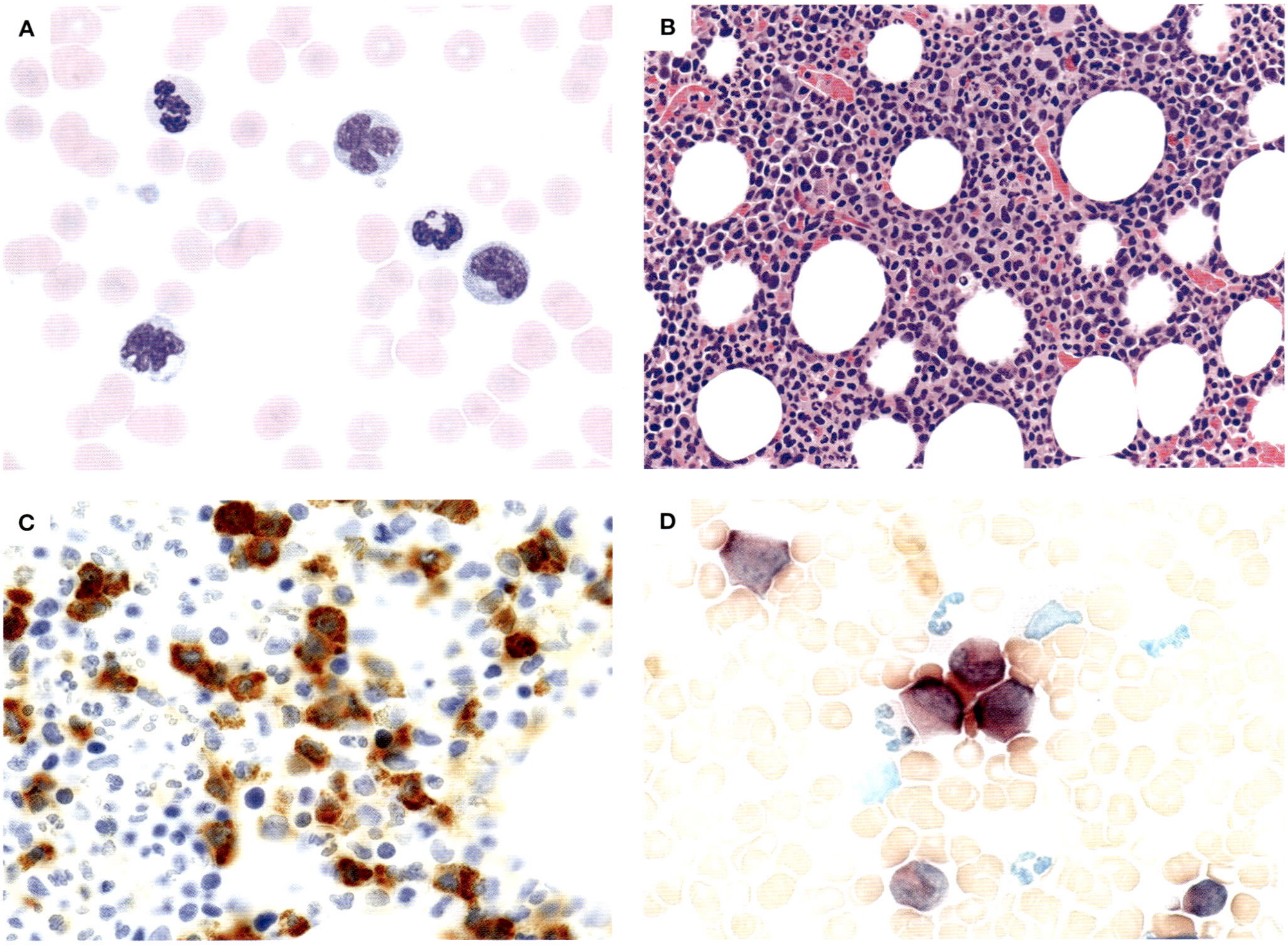

FIGURE 8.1 Morphologic features of chronic myelomonocytic leukemia. **A:** Peripheral blood with increased abnormal monocytes. **B:** Bone marrow core biopsy with granulocytic proliferation. A few dysplastic megakaryocytes are present. **C:** CD14 immunohistochemical stain highlights monocytes that were not easily identifiable on the H&E section. **D:** Nonspecific esterase cytochemical stain on the aspirate smear highlights monocytes.

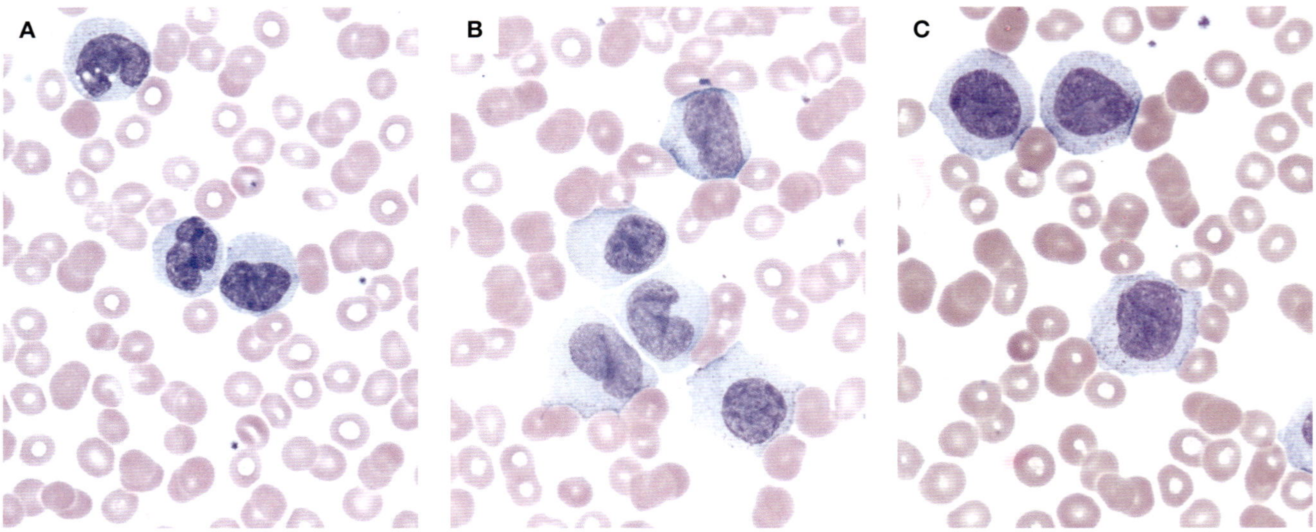

FIGURE 8.2 Morphologic distinction among abnormal monocytes, promonocytes, and monoblasts. **A:** Abnormal monocytes have convoluted or folded nuclei with condensed nuclear chromatin and no nucleoli. Cytoplasmic vacuoles and lilac-colored granules are identifiable. **B:** Promonocytes have delicately folded nuclei, fine chromatin, and overall indistinct nucleoli. **C:** Monoblasts with abundant cytoplasm, round nucleus with open chromatin, and identifiable nucleoli.

but not always increased; their identification can be difficult in Wright-Giemsa-stained smears or on H&E-stained sections. Nonspecific esterase staining on marrow aspirate smears or CD14 immunohistology may be needed to demonstrate monocytes (Figure 8.1).[6] Dysplasia in one or more hematopoietic lineages is typically seen in CMML and is particularly helpful to identify in the small subset of patients who do not have a CMML-associated mutation (Table 8.1). Evidence of dysgranulopoiesis including hyposegmented or abnormally segmented nuclei and/or abnormal cytoplasmic granulation, can be seen in a proportion of cases. Blasts and/or promonocytes may be increased; however, they must comprise <20% of nucleated cells. It is essential to distinguish abnormal monocytes from promonocytes (Figure 8.2). Promonocytes are large (20-30 μm) with convoluted/indented nuclei showing delicate/lace-like chromatin, variably prominent nucleoli, and blue-gray variably vacuolated cytoplasm. Abnormal monocytes show convoluted nuclei with more condensed chromatin, without prominent nucleoli and more cytoplasmic vacuolization and/or granularity.[7] Erythropoiesis is normal to relatively reduced, with or without dysplasia. Ring sideroblasts may be present in a subset of cases. Megakaryopoiesis is variable but usually dysplastic with micromegakaryocytes and small megakaryocytes with hypolobated nuclei seen in the majority of cases. A small percentage of CMML cases can have significant (MF ≥ 2) marrow fibrosis and its presence may be indicative of a more aggressive clinical course.[8,9]

Monocytosis can occur in *BCR::ABL1*-negative MPN such as primary myelofibrosis (PMF) and polycythemia vera (PV), where its presence is often associated with disease progression and adversely impacts survival. Marrow morphology usually allows this distinction: in CMML, the megakaryocytes are usually small and dysplastic, whereas in MPNs the megakaryocytes are more pleomorphic and often include large or giant forms. In addition, large, tight clusters of megakaryocytes are not seen in CMML.

Aggregates of mature plasmacytoid dendritic cells (PDC) can be seen in about 10% to 20% of cases of CMML. They are clonally related to the CMML and easily identified by immunohistochemistry with CD123 and other markers (see below) (Figure 8.3).[10]

The possibility of an associated systemic mastocytosis in the bone marrow, which can be subtle and hard to identify by morphology alone, would qualify the case as systemic mastocytosis with associated myeloid neoplasm (SM-AMN). This should be considered in all cases, particularly in the presence of a *KIT* mutation (see chapter on "Mastocytosis").

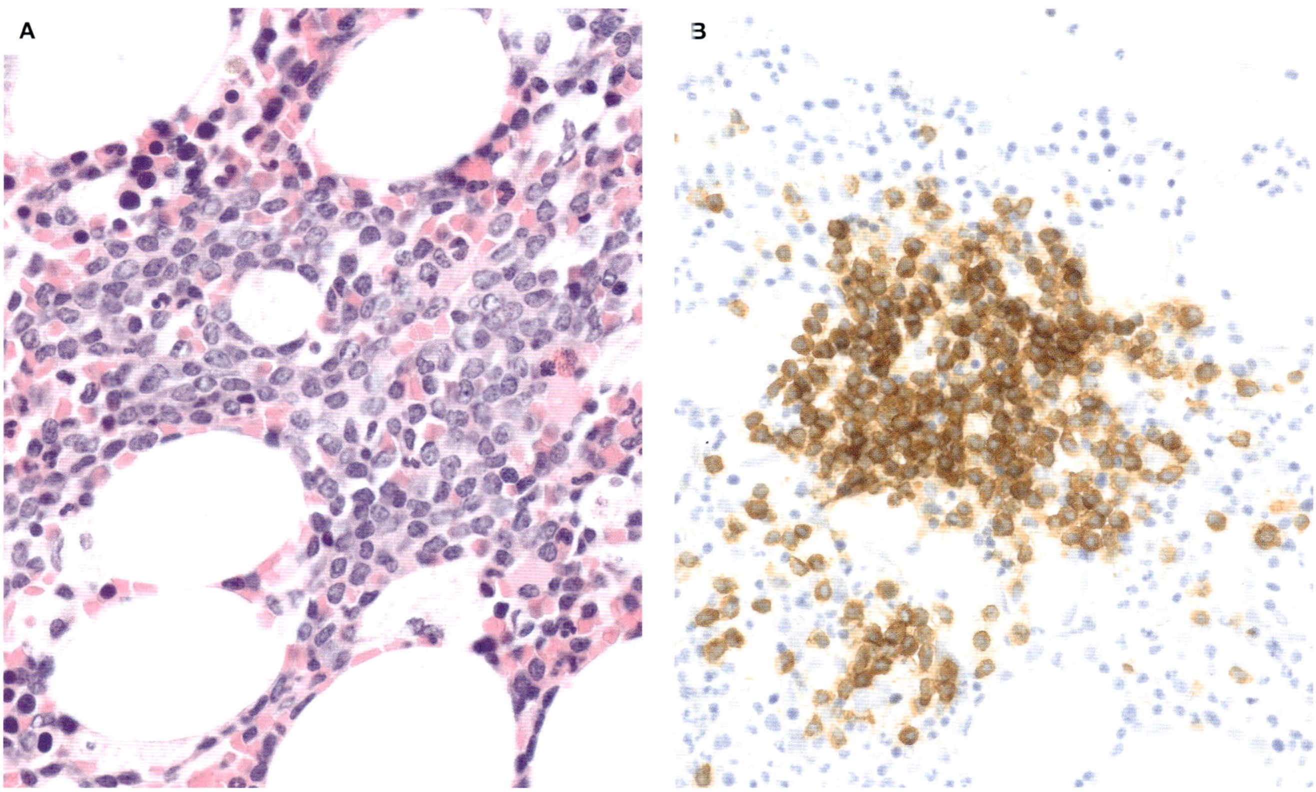

FIGURE 8.3 Aggregates of plasmacytoid dendritic cells in CMML. **A:** Nodules of mature plasmacytoid dendritic cells on the bone marrow core biopsy section. **B:** CD123 immunohistochemical stain highlights these nodules.

Extramedullary Tissues

Splenic enlargement is frequent (mainly in CMML-MP) and is due to infiltration of the red pulp by myelomonocytic cells. Lymphadenopathy due to extramedullary hematopoiesis can be seen in a minority of patients. In rare patients, tumoral proliferations of plasmacytoid dendritic cells, identical to those described in the bone marrow, may be seen in splenectomy or lymph node specimens. Cutaneous involvement in the form of mature myelomonocytic infiltrates or plasmacytoid dendritic cell proliferation can also be seen and may rarely be the initial presenting symptom.[11]

Immunophenotype

By flow cytometric immunophenotypic analysis, the blood and marrow monocytes express myelomonocytic antigens such as CD33 and CD13, with variable expressions of CD14, CD36, and CD64. The monocytes in CMML often exhibit aberrant expression of two or more antigens, including overexpression of CD56; aberrant expression of CD2; and decreased expression of HLA-DR, CD14, CD11c, CD13, CD15, CD64, or CD36.[12]

Assessment of monocyte partitioning by flow cytometric immunophenotyping (FCI) of PB can be helpful in distinguishing CMML from other monocytic neoplasms and reactive monocytosis. Based on their expression of CD14/CD16, PB monocytes can be classified into three subsets: classical MO1 ($CD14^+/CD16^-$), intermediate MO2 ($CD14^+/CD16^+$), and non-classical MO3 ($CD14^-/CD16^+$) fractions, with MO1 constituting the major monocyte population (85%) in healthy conditions.[13] An increase in classical monocytes accounting for ≥94% of the total monocyte population effectively distinguishes CMML from reactive monocytosis and clonal monocytosis associated with other myeloid neoplasms.[13] Although the sensitivity and specificity of this flow cytometric diagnostic approach is reported to be 95.1% and 90.6%, respectively, there are challenges in specific diagnostic settings such as antecedent or concomitant autoimmune diseases and poorly defined systemic inflammatory syndromes. In these cases, there is accumulation of intermediate, $CD14^+/CD16^+$ monocytes, which can interfere with flow recognition of CMML.

Plasmacytoid dendritic cells can be identified by CD123 in the BM as well as extramedullary sites. Additionally, PDC are positive for TCF4, TCL1, CD4, CD43, and CD303, and are usually negative for CD56.[10] In some cases, PDC may aberrantly express other antigens, such as CD2, CD5, CD7, CD13, or CD33.

Genetics

Cytogenetics

Clonal cytogenetic abnormalities are seen in 20% to 30% of CMML patients.[4] Common alterations include trisomy 8, abnormalities of chromosome 7, trisomy 21, deletion 20q, -Y, and complex karyotypes. Although not specific for CMML, the type of abnormality plays a role in risk stratification, with complex and monosomal karyotypes being associated with high risk.[14] Rearrangements of *KMT2A* at 11q23.3 are not typical of CMML and when present, should prompt consideration of an alternate diagnosis of AML.

Molecular Findings

Somatic mutations in at least one of the genes associated with myeloid neoplasms are identified in >90% of CMML patients.[15,16] Therefore, presence of mutations as a means to demonstrate clonality is now considered critical for confirming a diagnosis of CMML, foremost after introducing a minimum absolute monocyte count of $\geq 0.5 \times 10^9/L$. These mutations include genes involved in histone modification (*EZH2, ASXL1*), DNA methylation (*TET2, DNMT3A*), spliceosome machinery (*SRSF2, SF3B1, U2AF1*, and *ZRSR2*), regulation of cell signaling (*NRAS, KRAS, JAK2, CBL*, and *PTPN11*), and transcription factors and nucleosome assembly regulators (*RUNX1, SETBP1*). Of these, mutations involving *TET2* (60%), *SRSF2* (50%), *ASXL1* (40%), and the RAS pathway (30%) are the most frequent. *TP53* mutations are extremely infrequent in CMML (<1%). Although none of these mutations are specific for CMML, coexistence of *SRSF2* and *TET2* and biallelic *TET2* mutations are highly suggestive of CMML.[17]

The acquisition of genetic alterations in CMML remains an area of active investigation; however, it is believed that the initial driver mutation in most cases is *TET2*. Second, acquired alterations often include another *TET2* and/or *SRSF2* mutation that result in granulomonocytic expansion. *ASXL1, DNMT3A, RUNX1, SETBP1*, and *SF3B1* mutations are usually seen in CMML-MD, whereas RAS pathway and *JAK2* V617F mutations tend to occur in CMML-MP.[17]

In addition to establishing clonality, mutations in CMML have prognostic implications. Frameshift and nonsense *ASXL1* mutations are associated with adverse prognosis and a shorter overall survival, as are those in *NRAS, RUNX1*, and *SETBP1*.[16,18] *TET2*-mutated CMML is associated with a survival advantage especially in the context of multiple *TET2* and truncating mutations.[19]

NPM1 mutation is seen in a small subset of CMML (3%-5%), where it heralds a particularly aggressive clinical course with rapid progression to acute leukemia.[20] If a case qualifies as CMML and a mutation in *NPM1* is detected, it should not be reclassified as AML with mutated *NPM1*. However, since CMML with *NPM1* mutation often has an aggressive clinical course, AML-type treatment may be clinically appropriate for some patients, particularly if there are increased blasts.[20] Additionally, in a proportion of cases, *NPM1* mutation occurs as a secondary genetic abnormality (ie, not present at the time of CMML disease outset) that is acquired later, often at the time of transformation to AML, and is associated with an adverse prognosis.

JAK2 mutations can be seen in 5% to 10% of cases of CMML, commonly in CMML-MP, and can be associated with marrow fibrosis. In this latter setting, the differential diagnosis is between CMML and PMF. BM megakaryocyte morphology usually allows distinction between the two diagnoses. In addition, the mutant *JAK2* allele frequency is usually lower in CMML than in MPN.[21]

Mutations in *SF3B1* can be identified in <10% cases of CMML and may be associated with ring sideroblasts. These cases are usually CMML-MD, with a low frequency of *ASXL1* mutations, and a superior AML-free survival compared to CMML cases lacking *SF3B1* mutation.[22]

Prognosis and Clinical Comment

Numerous prognostic models that allow risk stratification as well as risk-adapted therapy have been developed for CMML that incorporate age, performance status, peripheral blood counts, blast percentage, and cytogenetic and molecular abnormalities.[4] The overall survival of CMML is variable with the median ranging from 16 to 97 months.[4] Currently, the only potentially curative therapy for CMML is allogeneic stem cell transplantation; however, given the usually advanced age at presentation, such therapy is not available for most patients. Hypomethylating agents (azacitidine and decitabine) are currently the most commonly used therapies for CMML.

Distinguishing the two variants of CMML based on leukocyte count remains important. In comparison to CMML-MD, CMML-MP is associated with an adverse prognosis as captured by various CMML-specific prognostic scoring systems.[16] The recognition of CMML-MP may also help in developing innovative therapeutic strategies specifically tailored to these patients.

Clonal Monocytosis of Undetermined Significance

Definition

Clonal monocytosis of undetermined significance (CMUS) is a recently recognized condition used to identify patients with clonal hematopoiesis and monocytosis not fulfilling criteria for CMML. It is defined as persistent monocytosis (monocytes ≥10% of the WBC and $\geq 0.5 \times 10^9$/L), unexplained by a comorbid condition, in the presence of myeloid neoplasm-associated mutation(s) without BM morphologic findings of CMML.[1] The diagnostic criteria for CMUS are listed in Table 8.3.

Synonyms

None.

Epidemiology

The incidence of CMUS is not known, as it is a recently introduced term. In one prospective study of unselected community-dwelling individuals ≥60 years old with monocytosis, clonal hematopoiesis (CH) was identified in 50.9% of individuals.[23] In patients presenting to a hematology practice for the evaluation of monocytosis, without meeting criteria for myeloid neoplasm, CH was identified in 57% of cases.[24]

TABLE 8.3 Diagnostic Criteria for *Clonal Monocytosis of Undetermined Significance* (CMUS)[1]

- Persistent monocytosis defined as monocytes $\geq 0.5 \times 10^9$/L and ≥10% of the WBC
- Absence or presence of cytopenia (thresholds same as for MDS)[a]
- Presence of at least one myeloid neoplasm-associated mutation VAF ≥ 2%[b]
- No significant dysplasia, increased blasts (including promonocytes) or morphologic findings of CMML on bone marrow examination[c]
- No criteria for a myeloid or other hematopoietic neoplasm are fulfilled
- No reactive condition that would explain a monocytosis is detected

[a]If cytopenia is present the nomenclature of *clonal cytopenia and monocytosis of undetermined significance* (CCMUS) is suggested.
[b]Variant allele frequency (VAF) threshold based on International Consensus Group Conference, Vienna, 2018.[2]
[c]Bone marrow findings of CMML include hypercellularity with myeloid predominance, often with increased monocytes and in a proportion of cases monoblasts and/or promonocytes (blast equivalents) and/or dysplasia in at least one lineage.
Arber DA, Orazi A, Hasserjian RP, et al. International consensus classification of myeloid neoplasms and acute leukemias: integrating morphologic, clinical, and genomic data. *Blood*. 2022;140(11):1200-1228 and Valent P, Orazi A, Savona MR, et al. Proposed diagnostic criteria for classical chronic myelomonocytic leukemia (CMML), CMML variants and pre-CMML conditions. *Haematologica*. 2019;104(10):1935-1949. doi:10.3324/haematol.2019.222059

General Clinical Features

In the very few studies available, CMUS affects older adults, with a median age of 73 years, similar to that seen in CMML.[24] Reactive monocytosis that can be seen in infections such as tuberculosis, chronic fungal infections, subacute bacterial endocarditis, viral, and protozoal infections (leishmaniasis), connective tissue disorders such as systemic lupus erythematosus and sarcoidosis, lipid storage disorders, recovery phase of an acute viral infection, or BM regeneration post chemotherapy, must be excluded. Anemia and thrombocytopenia can be seen in a subset of cases, and such cases are referred to as clonal cytopenia and monocytosis of undetermined significance (CCMUS).

Morphology

The peripheral smear demonstrates monocytosis. The BM findings do not meet the criteria for diagnosis of CMML or any other myeloid neoplasm. Morphologic dysplasia (≥10% of a lineage) or increased blasts/promonocytes should not be present.

Immunophenotype

Data on immunophenotype of CMUS are available from only one study of 37 patients with CMUS.[24] These patients had immunophenotypic features indistinguishable from CMML with respect to increased CD64-positive monocytes, reduced CD14 expression, and aberrant CD56 expression on monocytes. Although CD56 expression and >94% MO1 monocytes showed high specificity for the presence of CMUS (98% and 75%, respectively), the sensitivity for these findings was only 48% and 56%, respectively.

Genetics

The diagnosis of CMUS requires the presence of a gene mutation with a VAF of ≥2%. The mutations identified are similar to those seen in CMML with respect to genes mutated, number of mutations, and the VAFs.[23,24] Individuals with CMUS frequently carry either multiple gene mutations, or isolated gene mutations other than mutations seen in age-related CH. *TET2, SRSF2*, and *ASXL1* are the most frequently mutated genes in CMUS, similar to CMML.

Prognosis and Clinical Comment

Although there are only limited data, CMUS is associated with increased risk of developing cytopenia and/or an overt myeloid malignancy.[24,25] While the presence of CH in individuals with monocytosis by itself is insufficient to diagnose CMML, a mutational signature that deviates from common age-related CH, eg, coexistent *TET2* and *SRSF2* mutations, and/or the presence of cytopenias may indicate increased risk for the development of a myeloid neoplasm. While more data are needed to determine the significance of clonality including the number, type, and allele frequency of somatic mutations in CMUS, it is imperative that these patients are identified and monitored closely.

References

1. Arber DA, Orazi A, Hasserjian RP, et al. International consensus classification of myeloid neoplasms and acute leukemias: integrating morphologic, clinical, and genomic data. *Blood.* 2022;140(11):1200-1228. doi:10.1182/blood.2022015850
2. Valent P, Orazi A, Savona MR, et al. Proposed diagnostic criteria for classical chronic myelomonocytic leukemia (CMML), CMML variants and pre-CMML conditions. *Haematologica.* 2019;104(10):1935-1949. doi:10.3324/haematol.2019.222059
3. Patnaik MM, Parikh SA, Hanson CA, Tefferi A. Chronic myelomonocytic leukaemia: a concise clinical and pathophysiological review. *Br J Haematol.* 2014;165(3):273-286. doi:10.1111/bjh.12756
4. Patnaik MM, Tefferi A. Chronic myelomonocytic leukemia: 2022 update on diagnosis, risk stratification, and management. *Am J Hematol.* 2022;97(3):352-372. doi:10.1002/ajh.26455
5. Calvo X, Garcia-Gisbert N, Parraga I, et al. Oligomonocytic and overt chronic myelomonocytic leukemia show similar clinical, genomic, and immunophenotypic features. *Blood Adv.* 2020;4(20):5285-5296. doi:10.1182/bloodadvances.2020002206
6. Orazi A, Chiu R, O'Malley DP, et al. Chronic myelomonocytic leukemia: the role of bone marrow biopsy immunohistology. *Mod Pathol.* 2006;19(12):1536-1545. doi:10.1038/modpathol.3800707
7. Foucar K, Hsi ED, Wang SA, et al. Concordance among hematopathologists in classifying blasts plus promonocytes: a bone marrow pathology group study. *Int J Lab Hematol.* 2020;42(4):418-422. doi:10.1111/ijlh.13212
8. Petrova-Drus K, Chiu A, Margolskee E, et al. Bone marrow fibrosis in chronic myelomonocytic leukemia is associated with increased megakaryopoiesis, splenomegaly and with a shorter median time to disease progression. *Oncotarget.* 2017;8(61):103274-103282. doi:10.18632/oncotarget.21870
9. Gur HD, Loghavi S, Garcia-Manero G, et al. Chronic myelomonocytic leukemia with fibrosis is a distinct disease subset with myeloproliferative features and frequent JAK2 p.V617F mutations. *Am J Surg Pathol.* 2018;42(6):799-806. doi:10.1097/PAS.0000000000001058

10. Lucas N, Duchmann M, Rameau P, et al. Biology and prognostic impact of clonal plasmacytoid dendritic cells in chronic myelomonocytic leukemia. *Leukemia.* 2019;33(10):2466-2480. doi:10.1038/s41375-019-0447-3
11. Vitte F, Fabiani B, Bénet C, et al. Specific skin lesions in chronic myelomonocytic leukemia: a spectrum of myelomonocytic and dendritic cell proliferations—a study of 42 cases. *Am J Surg Pathol.* 2012;36(9):1302-1316. doi:10.1097/PAS.0b013e31825dd4de
12. Xu Y, McKenna RW, Karandikar NJ, Pildain AJ, Kroft SH. Flow cytometric analysis of monocytes as a tool for distinguishing chronic myelomonocytic leukemia from reactive monocytosis. *Am J Clin Pathol.* 2005;124(5):799-806. doi:10.1309/HRJ1-XKTD-77J1-UTFM
13. Selimoglu-Buet D, Wagner-Ballon O, Saada V, et al. Characteristic repartition of monocyte subsets as a diagnostic signature of chronic myelomonocytic leukemia. *Blood.* 2015;125(23):3618-3626. doi:10.1182/blood-2015-01-620781
14. Wassie EA, Itzykson R, Lasho TL, et al. Molecular and prognostic correlates of cytogenetic abnormalities in chronic myelomonocytic leukemia: a Mayo Clinic-French Consortium Study. *Am J Hematol.* 2014;89(12):1111-1115. doi:10.1002/ajh.23846
15. Meggendorfer M, Roller A, Haferlach T, et al. SRSF2 mutations in 275 cases with chronic myelomonocytic leukemia (CMML). *Blood.* 2012;120(15):3080-3088. doi:10.1182/blood-2012-01-404863
16. Elena C, Gallì A, Such E, et al. Integrating clinical features and genetic lesions in the risk assessment of patients with chronic myelomonocytic leukemia. *Blood.* 2016;128(10):1408-1417. doi:10.1182/blood-2016-05-714030
17. Itzykson R, Duchmann M, Lucas N, Solary E. CMML: clinical and molecular aspects. *Int J Hematol.* 2017;105(6):711-719. doi:10.1007/s12185-017-2243-z
18. Such E, Germing U, Malcovati L, et al. Development and validation of a prognostic scoring system for patients with chronic myelomonocytic leukemia. *Blood.* 2013;121(15):3005-3015. doi:10.1182/blood-2012-08-452938
19. Coltro G, Mangaonkar AA, Lasho TL, et al. Clinical, molecular, and prognostic correlates of number, type, and functional localization of TET2 mutations in chronic myelomonocytic leukemia (CMML)-a study of 1084 patients. *Leukemia.* 2020;34(5):1407-1421. doi:10.1038/s41375-019-0690-7
20. Vallapureddy R, Lasho TL, Hoversten K, et al. Nucleophosmin 1 (NPM1) mutations in chronic myelomonocytic leukemia and their prognostic relevance. *Am J Hematol.* 2017;92(10):E614-E618. doi:10.1002/ajh.24861
21. Todisco G, Creignou M, Gallì A, et al. Co-mutation pattern, clonal hierarchy, and clone size concur to determine disease phenotype of SRSF2P95-mutated neoplasms. *Leukemia.* 2021;35(8):2371-2381. doi:10.1038/s41375-020-01106-z
22. Wudhikarn K, Loghavi S, Mangaonkar AA, et al. SF3B1-mutant CMML defines a predominantly dysplastic CMML subtype with a superior acute leukemia-free survival. *Blood Adv.* 2020;4(22):5716-5721. doi:10.1182/bloodadvances.2020003345
23. van Zeventer IA, de Graaf AO, Koorenhof-Scheele TN, et al. Monocytosis and its association with clonal hematopoiesis in community-dwelling individuals. *Blood Adv.* 2022;6(14):4174-4184. doi:10.1182/bloodadvances.2021006755
24. Cargo C, Cullen M, Taylor J, et al. The use of targeted sequencing and flow cytometry to identify patients with a clinically significant monocytosis. *Blood.* 2019;133(12):1325-1334. doi:10.1182/blood-2018-08-867333
25. Gallì A, Todisco G, Catamo E, et al. Relationship between clone metrics and clinical outcome in clonal cytopenia. *Blood.* 2021;138(11):965-976. doi:10.1182/blood.2021011323

Chapter 9
Atypical Chronic Myeloid Leukemia

Marco Pizzi, Francesco Onida, Attilio Orazi, Sonam Prakash, and Sa A. Wang

Definition

Atypical chronic myeloid leukemia (aCML) is a myelodysplastic/myeloproliferative neoplasm (MDS/MPN), characterized by leukocytosis (≥13 × 10^9/L) with dysplastic neutrophilic forms, and ≥10% neutrophil precursors in the peripheral blood (PB). Anemia (Hb < 13 g/dL in males; <12 g/dL in females) and/or thrombocytopenia (<150 × 10^9/L) is also present. aCML lacks both monocytosis and hypereosinophilia. The *BCR::ABL1* fusion and genetic abnormalities associated with myeloid/lymphoid neoplasms with eosinophilia and tyrosine kinase gene fusions (M/LN-Eo-TK) are absent (Table 9.1).

Synonyms

Myelodysplastic/myeloproliferative neoplasm with neutrophilia; atypical chronic myeloid leukemia, *BCR::ABL1*-negative; aCML, Philadelphia chromosome-negative (not recommended).

TABLE 9.1 Diagnostic criteria for atypical chronic myeloid leukemia (aCML)

Leukocytosis ≥13 × 10^9/L, due to increased numbers of neutrophils and their precursors (promyelocytes, myelocytes, and metamyelocytes), the latter constituting ≥10% of PB leukocytes
Cytopenia (thresholds same as for MDS)[a]
Blasts <20% of the cells in PB and BM
Dysgranulopoiesis, including abnormal hyposegmented and/or hypersegmented neutrophils with/without abnormal chromatin clumping
No or minimal absolute monocytosis; monocytes accounting for <10% of PB leukocytes
No eosinophilia; eosinophils <10% of PB leukocytes
Hypercellular BM with granulocytic proliferation and granulocytic dysplasia, with or without dysplasia in the erythroid and megakaryocytic lineages
No *BCR::ABL1* or genetic abnormalities associated with M/LN-Eo-TK. The absence of MPN-associated driver mutations and the presence of *SETBP1* mutations in association with *ASXL1* provide additional support for a diagnosis of aCML.

BM, bone marrow; MDS, myelodysplastic syndrome; M/LN-Eo-TK, myeloid/lymphoid neoplasms with eosinophilia and tyrosine kinase gene fusions; MPN, myeloproliferative neoplasm; PB, peripheral blood.

[a]Anemia (Hb < 13 g/dL in males and <12 g/dL in females) and/or thrombocytopenia (platelets <150 × 10^9/L).

Epidemiology

aCML is a rare disease with an estimated incidence of 1 to 2 cases for every 100 cases of chronic myeloid leukemia (CML).[1] The age at diagnosis is higher than that in CML, with most patients being diagnosed in the seventh to eighth decade of life[1,2] and more than two-thirds of patients being older than 65 years.[3] Very rare cases occur in adolescents and young adults. aCML can also occur in a therapy-related setting. In most series, men are more affected than women, but the male-to-female ratio varies.

General Clinical Features

Patients with aCML have symptoms mainly related to anemia and (less frequently) thrombocytopenia.[2,4] Splenomegaly can be massive and may cause abdominal discomfort. Similar to other MDS/MPN, systemic symptoms can occur, including fatigue, weight loss, night sweats, and fever.[1,2]

Morphology

Leukocytosis (≥13 × 10^9/L) is a defining feature of aCML, with a median white blood cell count (WBC) ranging from 24 to 68 × 10^9/L. Neutrophils account for most of the circulating WBCs. They often show prominent dysplastic features, which include abnormal nuclear segmentation (pseudo-Pelger-Huët anomaly or abnormal hyperlobulation), exaggerated chromatin clumping, and cytoplasmic hypogranularity or enlarged granules (Figure 9.1).[4] Neutrophil precursors (promyelocytes, myelocytes, and metamyelocytes) account for ≥10% of the WBC, while blasts are usually <5% and always <20% of all nucleated cells. The monocyte count is either normal or slightly increased, but monocytes never exceed 10% of the WBC. By definition, eosinophils account for <1.5 × 10^9/L and <10% of WBC. The basophil count is usually normal (<2% of the WBC), but mild basophilia can occasionally be encountered. Anemia and anisopoikilocytosis are frequently documented. Platelet count is either normal or decreased.[4]

The bone marrow (BM) shows a markedly increased cellularity (usually >80%) with a high myeloid-to-erythroid ratio (typically >8:1). Granulopoiesis is left-shifted with dysplastic features similar to those seen in the PB. The erythropoiesis is usually decreased with erythroid dysplasia seen in about 40% of cases. Megakaryopoiesis can be either increased, normal or, commonly decreased. Megakaryocytic dysplasia is frequent (70%-80% of cases) and includes megakaryocytes with separated nuclei, small megakaryocytes with hypolobated nuclei, and micromegakaryocytes[2] (Figure 9.1). Blasts may be moderately increased, but account for <20% of the nucleated cells. Mild marrow fibrosis (MF-1) occurs in some cases; more severe (MF-2 or MF-3) fibrosis can be seen in 25% to 30% of cases.[2]

Immunophenotype

Despite being nonspecific to aCML, immunophenotypic and cytochemical studies may be useful by complementing the morphological evaluation. Myeloid precursors stain positive for MPO, although dysplastic neutrophils may show decreased expression of this marker. Immunostaining BM biopsies for CD34 can facilitate blast enumeration. CD117 can be used to stain early hematopoietic precursors and mast cells. CD61, CD41, and/or CD42b may facilitate the recognition of micromegakaryocytes and other dysplastic megakaryocytes (Figure 9.1), while CD14 and/or CD68-PGM1 may be useful in distinguishing monocytes from granulocytic cells. Nonspecific esterase cytochemistry may help in distinguishing neutrophilic cells from monocytes in BM aspirate smears. The presence of an increased number of monocytes should bring into question a diagnosis of aCML.

Genetics

Cytogenetic aberrations are documented in about 30% to 50% of cases. By definition, the *BCR::ABL1* fusion and genetic abnormalities associated with M/LN-Eo-TK are absent. Trisomy 8 is the most common chromosomal aberration, being documented in about 15% to 30% of cases. Other abnormalities include del(20q), −7/del(7q), and imbalances of chromosomes 9, 13, 14, 19, and 21. Fusions of *CSF3R::SPTAN1*, *NUP98::HOXA9*, *SPTBN1::FLT3* and *RYK::ATP5O* have been reported in occasional cases.[5]

The most frequently mutated genes in aCML encode epigenetic regulators (*ASXL1*, *TET2*, *SETBP1*, *EZH2*), splicing factors (*SRSF2*, *U2AF1*, *ZRSR2*), members of signaling pathways (*N/K-RAS*, *CBL*, *JAK2*), and transcription factors (*RUNX1*, *GATA2*) (Table 9.2). Although not entirely specific, some of these mutations correlate significantly with aCML and support the diagnosis.[5] Among these, *SETBP1* mutations are documented in about 25% of aCML.[6] *SETBP1* mutations are also common in chronic neutrophilic leukemia (40%), but significantly less in chronic myelomonocytic leukemia (5%-10%), and MDS/MPN not otherwise specified (10%). Other common genetic derangements of aCML include concurrent mutations in *SETBP1* and *ASXL1*, *SRSF2* and *SETBP1*, *SFSR2* and *ASXL1*, *SETBP1* and *CSF3R*, and *RUNX1* and *EZH2*.[7,8] Mutations of *ETNK1* occur in 3% to 16% of cases and foster disease progression by inducing a mutator phenotype. Although originally considered specific to aCML, they can also occur in other myeloid neoplasms.[1] Finally, *CSF3R*, *CALR*, and *MPL* mutations are very rare in strictly defined aCML (<5% of cases in most series) and their documentation should prompt careful consideration of alternative diagnoses (ie, CNL with *CSF3R* mutations; primary myelofibrosis with *CALR* or *MPL* mutations).[2,7,9]

Prognosis and Clinical Comment

aCML is an aggressive hematologic malignancy with a dismal clinical course and the outcome is not significantly affected by treatment. Life expectancy is poor with a median survival of 14 to 30 months, often because of BM failure and high rates of blast transformation.[1] At diagnosis, clinical factors independently associated with a shorter survival include age >65 years, hemoglobin (Hb) < 10 g/dL, WBC counts >50 × 10^9/L, presence of circulating immature myeloid precursors (ie, myeloblasts, promyelocytes, myelocytes, and/or metamyelocytes) and female gender.[1,3,10] *ASXL1*, *SETBP1*, *TET2*, *RUNX1*, *CUX1*, and *NRAS* mutations have also been associated with worse prognosis.[1]

Two scoring systems have been proposed to stratify patients into prognostic subgroups at diagnosis. The MD Anderson Cancer Center scoring system includes age >65 years, Hb < 10 g/dL, and WBC > 50 × 10^9/L with median survival rates of 38 months for the low-risk group (0-1 risk factors) and 9 months for the high-risk group (two to three risk factors).[10] The Mayo Clinic scoring system includes age >67 years, Hb < 10 g/dL, and the presence of *TET2* mutations, with median survival rates of 18 months for the low-risk group (0-1 risk factors) and 7 months for the high-risk group (two to three risk factors).[1]

Current therapeutic options are limited, with allogeneic hematopoietic stem cell transplantation (alloHSCT) being the only possible curative strategy. However, only a minority of patients are alloHSCT eligible.[1] Control of leukocytosis, splenomegaly,

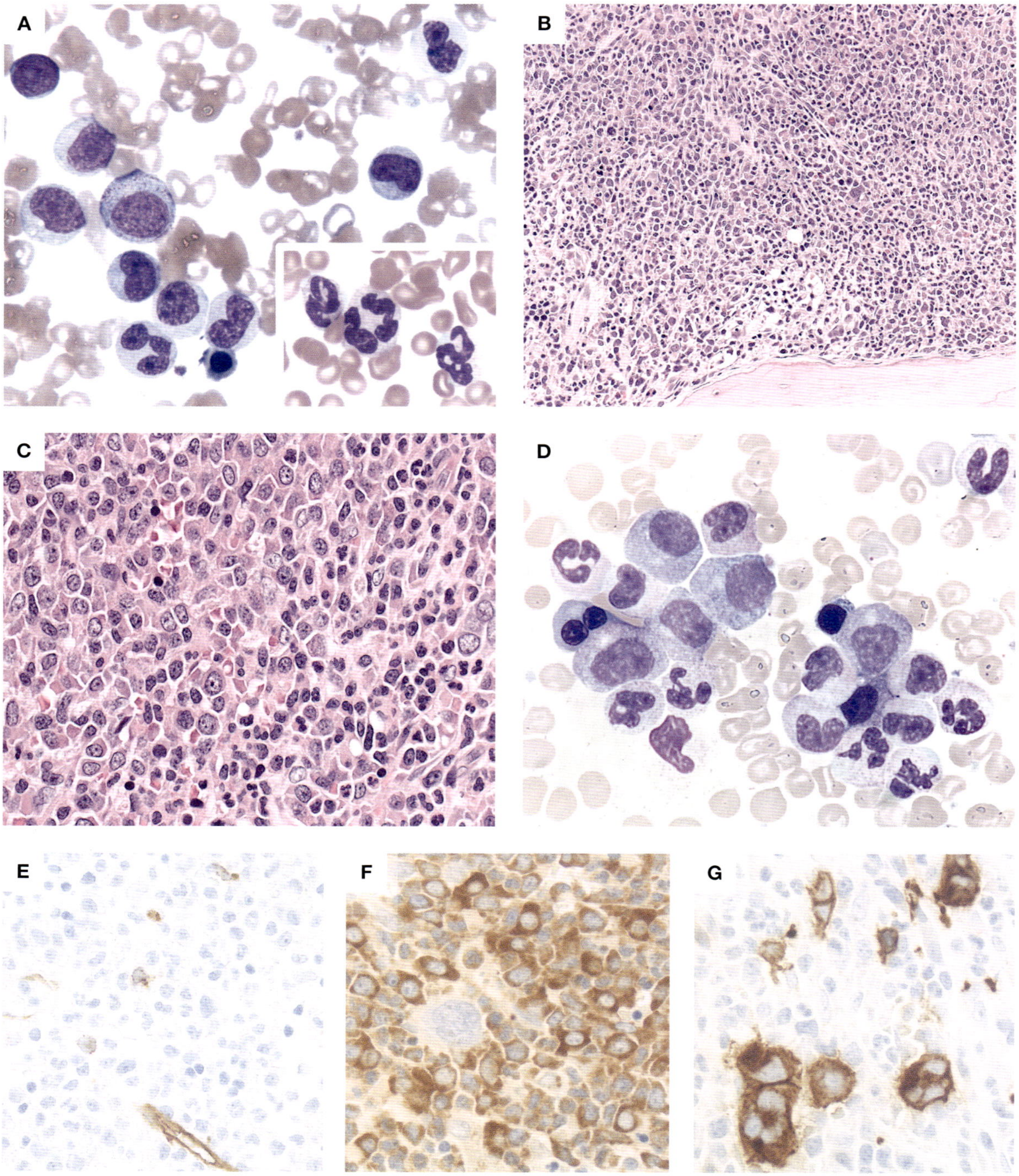

FIGURE 9.1 Morphological features of aCML in the PB and BM. Cytological examination of the PB documents circulating myeloid precursors and mature neutrophils with dysplastic features (**A**). Neutrophils can also have hyperlobulated nuclei with twisted chromatin (**A**, inset). The BM is hypercellular with increased myeloid to erythroid ratio (**B**), and left shifted granulopoiesis (**C**). Cytological examination of the BM reveals dysplastic features of both the erythroid and myeloid lineages (**D**). CD34 positive precursors (**E**), while MPO positive myeloid cells are markedly increased (**F**). CD61 immunostain highlights dysplastic megakaryocytes and micromegakaryocytes (**G**). (H&E, Wright-Giemsa and immunoperoxidase stains; original magnification: A and D, ×100; B, ×5; C, E to G, ×40).

TABLE 9.2 Recurrent gene mutations in aCML

Gene mutated	Reported frequency (%)
ASXL1	23-92
TET2	27-43
SRSF2	12-63
SETBP1	7-56
N/KRAS	10-40
EZH2	6-50
RUNX1	2-20
ETNK1	3-16
JAK2	3-12
ZRSR2	3-10
SF3B1	0-11
IDH1/IDH2	0-7
CSF3R	0-22
PTPN11	0-13
DNMT3A	0-9
U2AF1	0-15
CBL	0-21
KIT	0-7
MPL	0-3
CALR	0-4
TP53	0-9

and related symptoms may be provisionally attained with hydroxyurea or IFN-α, while anemia is generally managed with erythropoiesis-stimulating agents and red blood cell transfusions. Some efficacy of hypomethylating agents, such as 5-azacitidine (5-AZA) and decitabine, as well as that of the JAK-inhibitor ruxolitinib (as a single agent or with 5-AZA) has been reported.[1] AML-type treatment can be considered for patients with high blast counts or transforming to acute leukemia. Ideally, patients with aCML should be candidates for clinical trials evaluating novel therapies specifically targeted on the molecular profile of the disease.

References

1. Patnaik MM, Tefferi A. Atypical chronic myeloid leukemia and myelodysplastic/myeloproliferative neoplasm, not otherwise specified: 2023 update on diagnosis, risk stratification, and management. *Am J Hematol.* 2023;98(4):681-689.
2. Wang SA, Hasserjian RP, Fox PS, et al. Atypical chronic myeloid leukemia is clinically distinct from unclassifiable myelodysplastic/myeloproliferative neoplasms. *Blood.* 2014;123(17):2645-2651.
3. Ilerhunmwuwa NP, Wasifuddin M, Becerra H, Rayapureddy AK, Wang JC. Characteristics and survival outcomes of patients with atypical chronic myeloid leukemia in the United States: a SEER-based analysis. *Leuk Res Rep.* 2023;20:100383.
4. Prakash S, Arber D, Bueso-Ramos C, Hasserjian RP, Orazi A. Advances in myelodysplastic/myeloproliferative neoplasms. *Virchows Arch.* 2023;482(1):69-83.
5. Lasho T. Atypical CML-the role of morphology and precision genomics. *Best Pract Res Clin Haematol.* 2020;33(2):101133.
6. Meggendorfer M, Jeromin S, Haferlach C, Kern W, Haferlach T. The mutational landscape of 18 investigated genes clearly separates four subtypes of myelodysplastic/myeloproliferative neoplasms. *Haematologica.* 2018;103(5):e192-e195.
7. Palomo L, Meggendorfer M, Hutter S, et al. Molecular landscape and clonal architecture of adult myelodysplastic/myeloproliferative neoplasms. *Blood.* 2020;136(16):1851-1862.
8. Meggendorfer M, Haferlach T, Alpermann T, et al. Specific molecular mutation patterns delineate chronic neutrophilic leukemia, atypical chronic myeloid leukemia, and chronic myelomonocytic leukemia. *Haematologica.* 2014;99(12):e244-e246.
9. Patnaik MM, Barraco D, Lasho TL, et al. Targeted next generation sequencing and identification of risk factors in World Health Organization defined atypical chronic myeloid leukemia. *Am J Hematol.* 2017;92(6):542-548.
10. Onida F, Ball G, Kantarjian HM, et al. Characteristics and outcome of patients with Philadelphia chromosome negative, bcr/abl negative chronic myelogenous leukemia. *Cancer.* 2002;95(8):1673-1684.

Chapter 10

Myelodysplastic/Myeloproliferative Neoplasm With *SF3B1* Mutation and Thrombocytosis

Sonam Prakash, Robert P. Hasserjian, Luca Malcovati, Attilio Orazi, and Annette Schmitt-Graeff

Myelodysplastic/Myeloproliferative Neoplasm With *SF3B1* Mutation and Thrombocytosis (MDS/MPN-*SF3B1*-T)

Definition

Myelodysplastic/myeloproliferative neoplasm with *SF3B1* mutation and thrombocytosis (MDS/MPN-*SF3B1*-T) is now listed as a distinct entity in the group of MDS/MPN. It is characterized by anemia with erythroid lineage dysplasia, thrombocytosis (platelet count ≥450 × 10^9/L) with bone marrow (BM) megakaryocyte morphology similar to that seen in *BCR::ABL1*-negative MPN, and the presence of *SF3B1* mutation with a variant allele frequency (VAF) ≥10%.[1] Anemia and thrombocytosis must be present at the time of initial diagnosis.

Cases with a previous diagnosis of myelodysplastic syndrome (MDS) with mutated *SF3B1* that later develop thrombocytosis are considered to represent thrombocytotic progression of MDS. The presence of BM blasts ≥5%, peripheral blood (PB) blasts ≥1%, the cytogenetic abnormalities t(3;3)(q21.3;q26.2), inv(3)(q21.3;q26.2) or del(5q), or *BCR::ABL1* fusion, all exclude a diagnosis of MDS/MPN-*SF3B1*-T. The diagnostic criteria are summarized in Table 10.1.

Synonyms

Refractory anemia with ring sideroblasts (RS) associated with marked thrombocytosis (not recommended).

Epidemiology

The incidence of MDS/MPN-*SF3B1*-T is not known; however, it comprises >80% of cases previously categorized as MDS/MPN with RS and thrombocytosis (MDS/MPN-RS-T), which in turn represents <1% of all MDS and MDS-like entities.[2] The median age for presentation usually ranges from 71 to 75 years with a slight female predominance.[3]

General Clinical Features

Patients may present with symptoms related to refractory anemia or thrombocytosis, or to both abnormalities. Presenting symptoms include fatigue, dyspnea on exertion, weight loss, dizziness, and vasomotor symptoms. The frequency of thrombotic events is thought to be similar to that of essential thrombocythemia (ET).[4] Some patients may also develop an acquired von Willebrand disease, particularly in the presence of extreme thrombocytosis. Splenomegaly can be seen in a small subset of cases.

Morphology

Peripheral Blood

The peripheral blood typically shows anemia that may be normocytic or macrocytic. The red blood cells show anisocytosis often with a dimorphic pattern. The WBC count and differential are usually normal; however,

TABLE 10.1 Diagnostic Criteria for Myelodysplastic/Myeloproliferative Neoplasm With *SF3B1* Mutation and Thrombocytosis (MDS/MPN-*SF3B1*-T)[1]

- Thrombocytosis, with platelet count ≥450 × 10^9/L
- Anemia (threshold same as for MDS)[a]
- Blasts <1% in blood and <5% in bone marrow (BM)
- Presence of *SF3B1* mutation (VAF ≥10%), isolated or associated with abnormal cytogenetics and/or other myeloid neoplasm-associated mutations
- No history of recent cytotoxic or growth factor therapy that could explain the myelodysplastic/myeloproliferative features
- No *BCR::ABL1* or genetic abnormalities of myeloid/lymphoid neoplasms with eosinophilia and tyrosine kinase gene fusions; no t(3;3)(q21.3;q26.2), inv(3)(q21.3q26.2), or del(5q)[b]
- No history of myeloproliferative neoplasm, myelodysplastic syndrome, or other myelodysplastic/myeloproliferative neoplasm

[a]Hb < 13 g/L in males; <12 g/L in females.
[b]In a case that otherwise meets the diagnostic criteria for myelodysplastic syndrome with del(5q).
Arber DA, Orazi A, Hasserjian RP, et al. International consensus classification of myeloid neoplasms and acute leukemias: integrating morphologic, clinical, and genomic data. *Blood.* 2022;140(11):1200-1228. doi:10.1182/blood.2022015850

leukocytosis can occasionally be seen.[5] Circulating blasts are absent or rare, accounting for <1% of leukocytes. Platelets, by definition, are at least 450×10^9/L and often show anisocytosis ranging from small forms to large or giant platelets. The thrombocytosis should be sustained, particularly since some cases of MDS with mutated *SF3B1* may exhibit borderline elevated platelet counts, transiently increased above the diagnostic threshold of 450×10^9/L.

Bone Marrow

The BM is hypercellular and shows increased erythropoiesis with features of ineffective erythropoiesis, including megaloblastoid changes and other dyserythropoietic abnormalities. While most cases show increased RS, they are no longer required for the diagnosis. Megakaryocytes are increased and are morphologically similar to those seen in ET or primary myelofibrosis, a feature particularly helpful in the distinction from cases of MDS with mutated *SF3B1* that may show mild thrombocytosis (Figure 10.1). Varying degrees of granulocytic and megakaryocytic dysplasia may be seen in some cases. A subset of patients may show marrow fibrosis.[5] Any increase in blasts (≥1% in PB or ≥5% in BM) should prompt an alternative diagnosis of MDS/MPN, NOS.

Genetics

Cytogenetics

Cytogenetic abnormalities are seen in approximately 15% of patients. The most frequent ones include +8, 20q, 7q, and complex karyotype.[6]

Molecular Findings

By definition, there is an *SF3B1* mutation at VAF ≥ 10%; the most common variant is K700E.[6] Cases with features similar to MDS/MPN-*SF3B1*-T and with ≥15% RS, but lacking *SF3B1* mutation at ≥10% VAF, are classified as MDS/MPN-RS-T, NOS (discussed below). There is an associated *JAK2* V617F mutation in approximately 50% of cases, and much less frequently *CALR* or *MPL* W515 mutations (each in <10% of cases).[7] Mutations in other genes including *TET2* (25%), *DNMT3A* (15%), *ASXL1* (15%), and *SETBP1* (15%) can be seen in a smaller subset of cases.

Prognosis and Clinical Comment

Given the rarity of this entity, there are no specific evidence-based guidelines for treatment and the current management is extrapolated from related diseases such as lower risk MDS-RS and MPN. Recently, luspatercept

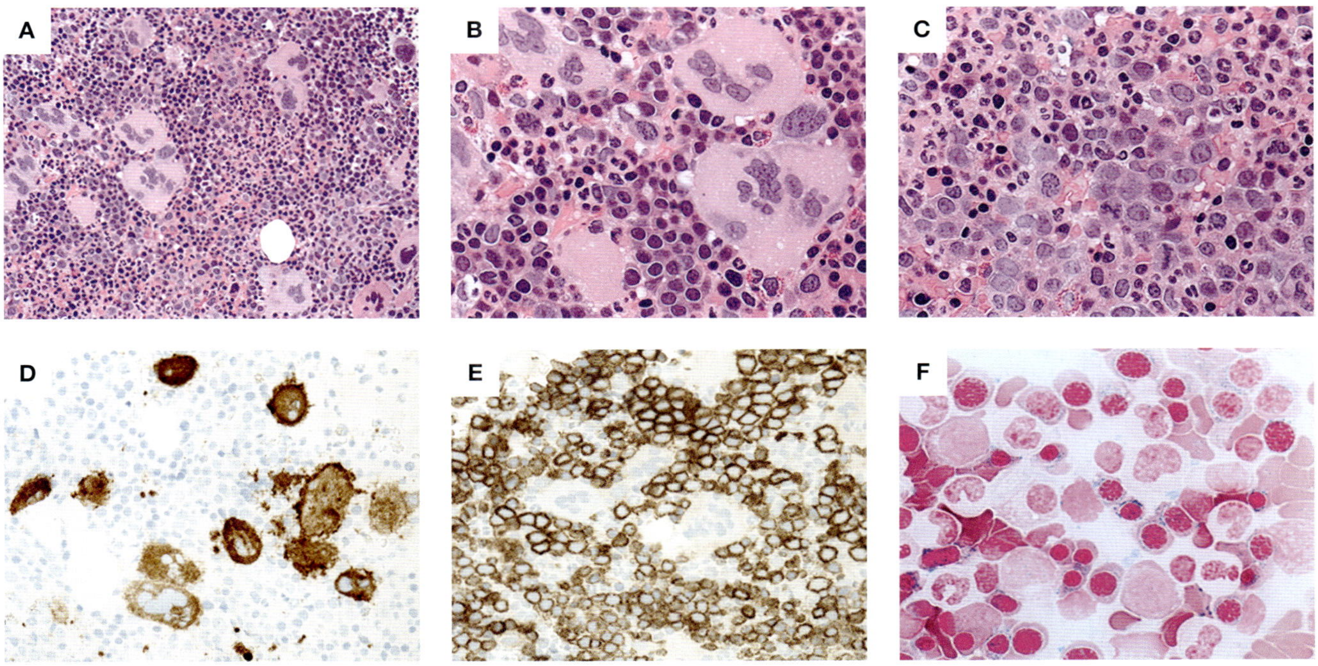

FIGURE 10.1 Morphologic features of MDS/MPN with *SF3B1* mutation and thrombocytosis. Bone marrow (BM) trephine biopsy specimen (**A-E**) and aspirate smear (**F**) from a patient presenting with macrocytic anemia, marked thrombocytosis and *SF3B1* and *JAK2* V617F co-mutation. **A-C:** H&E-stained BM sections show increased cellularity (**A**), numerous predominantly loosely clustered megakaryocytes with irregular nuclear lobation (**B**) and megaloblastoid erythropoiesis (**C**). Immunohistochemical stain for CD61 highlights megakaryocytes with pleomorphism in size (**D**). Erythropoiesis is characterized by enlarged CD71-positive islands forming confluent sheets (**E**). On aspirate smears, numerous ring sideroblasts are identified (**F,** Prussian blue stain). Original magnification: A, D, E. ×40; B, C. ×60; F. ×100.

was approved for treating lower-risk transfusion-dependent MDS/MPN-RS-T.[8] Patients with MDS/MPN-*SF3B1*-T have a higher incidence of thrombosis than MDS/MPN-RS-T, NOS and often need antiplatelet and/or cytoreductive therapy.[3]

Overall, patients with MDS/MPN-*SF3B1*-T and MDS/MPN-RS-T, NOS (the WHO revised 4th edition entity MDS/MPN-RS-T) were found to have a better median overall survival (OS) than MDS with RS and single lineage dysplasia (MDS-RS-SLD) (76 vs 63 months), and an inferior OS in comparison to patients with ET (76 vs 117 months). The leukemic transformation rate per 100 years in MDS/MPN-RS-T (1.8) is low and similar to MDS-RS-SLD (2.4) and higher than ET (0.7). Several prognostic scoring systems have been proposed. While anemia and abnormal karyotype have been shown to be associated with shorter OS,[6,9] data on the prognostic significance of somatic mutations are not consistent. In one study, age >80 years, *SF3B1* wildtype and *JAK2* wildtype were associated with lower OS.[10] Another study demonstrated abnormal karyotype, presence of *SETBP1* or *ASXL1* mutations, and anemia but not *SF3B1* wildtype or *JAK2* wildtype as adverse prognostic factors.[9] A more recent study of WHO 2016 defined MDS/MPN-RS-T demonstrated that only hemoglobin ≤10 g/dL and abnormal karyotype were associated with shorter OS in a multivariate analysis.[6] In the same study, frameshift and nonsense *ASXL1* mutations predicted an adverse OS in a univariate analysis but not in a multivariate model.

Myelodysplastic/Myeloproliferative Neoplasm With Ring Sideroblasts and Thrombocytosis, Not Otherwise Specified (MDS/MPN-RS-T, NOS)

Cases of MDS/MPN with anemia and ≥15% RS as well as thrombocytosis with megakaryocyte morphology similar to that seen in ET or PMF, which lack *SF3B1* mutation with VAF ≥ 10%, are designated as MDS/MPN-RS-T, NOS. Both the thrombocytosis and anemia must be present at the time of initial diagnosis. The diagnostic criteria are shown in Table 10.2.

The morphologic and clinical features are largely similar to those seen in MDS/MPN-*SF3B1*-T, except for the presence of ≥15% RS and absence of *SF3B1* mutation at ≥10% VAF, features required for diagnosis. These cases may show mutations in other genes involved in RNA splicing such as *SRSF2* or *U2AF1*, as well as co-occurrence of *JAK2* V617F and *ASXL1* mutations.[3,6,7] While data for comparison with MDS/MPN-*SF3B1*-T are limited, the risk of thrombosis appears to be lower[3] and the median overall survival shorter (3.3 years) as compared to MDS/MPN-*SF3B1*-T (6.9 years).[10] The clinical management is similar to MDS/MPN-*SF3B*1-T.

TABLE 10.2 Diagnostic Criteria for Myelodysplastic/Myeloproliferative Neoplasm With Ring Sideroblasts and Thrombocytosis, NOS (MDS/MPN-RS-T, NOS)[1]

- Thrombocytosis, with platelet count ≥450 × 10^9/L
- Anemia associated with erythroid-lineage dysplasia, with or without multilineage dysplasia, and ≥15% ring sideroblasts
- Blasts <1% in blood and <5% in BM
- Presence of clonality: demonstration of a clonal cytogenetic abnormality and/or somatic mutation(s). In their absence, no history of recent cytotoxic or growth factor therapy that could explain the myelodysplastic/myeloproliferative features
- Absence of *SF3B1* mutation at VAF ≥ 10%); no *BCR*::*ABL1* or genetic abnormalities of myeloid/lymphoid neoplasms with eosinophilia and tyrosine kinase gene fusions; no t(3;3)(q21.3;q26.2), inv(3)(q21.3q26.2), or del(5q)[a]
- No history of myeloproliferative neoplasm, myelodysplastic syndrome, or other myelodysplastic/myeloproliferative neoplasm

[a]In a case that otherwise meets the diagnostic criteria for myelodysplastic syndrome with del(5q).

Arber DA, Orazi A, Hasserjian RP, et al. International consensus classification of myeloid neoplasms and acute leukemias: integrating morphologic, clinical, and genomic data. *Blood.* 2022;140(11):1200-1228. doi:10.1182/blood.2022015850

References

1. Arber DA, Orazi A, Hasserjian RP, et al. International consensus classification of myeloid neoplasms and acute leukemias: integrating morphologic, clinical, and genomic data. *Blood.* 2022;140(11):1200-1228. doi:10.1182/blood.2022015850
2. Kuendgen A, Kasprzak A, Germing U. Hybrid or mixed myelodysplastic/myeloproliferative disorders - epidemiological features and overview. *Front Oncol.* 2021;11:778741. doi:10.3389/fonc.2021.778741
3. Patnaik MM, Tefferi A. Myelodysplastic syndromes with ring sideroblasts (MDS-RS) and MDS/myeloproliferative neoplasm with RS and thrombocytosis (MDS/MPN-RS-T) - "2021 update on diagnosis, risk-stratification, and management." *Am J Hematol.* 2021;96(3):379-394. doi:10.1002/ajh.26090
4. Broseus J, Florensa L, Zipperer E, et al. Clinical features and course of refractory anemia with ring sideroblasts associated with marked thrombocytosis. *Haematologica.* 2012;97(7):1036-1041. doi:10.3324/haematol.2011.053918
5. Malcovati L, Della Porta MG, Pietra D, et al. Molecular and clinical features of refractory anemia with ringed sideroblasts associated with marked thrombocytosis. *Blood.* 2009;114(17):3538-3545. doi:10.1182/blood-2009-05-222331

6. Mangaonkar AA, Lasho TL, Ketterling RP, et al. Myelodysplastic/myeloproliferative neoplasms with ring sideroblasts and thrombocytosis (MDS/MPN-RS-T): Mayo-Moffitt collaborative study of 158 patients. *Blood Cancer J.* 2022;12(2):26. doi:10.1038/s41408-022-00622-8
7. Jeromin S, Haferlach T, Weissmann S, et al. Refractory anemia with ring sideroblasts and marked thrombocytosis cases harbor mutations in SF3B1 or other spliceosome genes accompanied by JAK2V617F and ASXL1 mutations. *Haematologica.* 2015;100(4):e125-e127. doi:10.3324/haematol.2014.119032
8. Komrokji RS, Platzbecker U, Fenaux P, et al. Luspatercept for myelodysplastic syndromes/myeloproliferative neoplasm with ring sideroblasts and thrombocytosis. *Leukemia.* 2022;36(5):1432-1435. doi:10.1038/s41375-022-01521-4
9. Patnaik MM, Lasho TL, Finke CM, et al. Predictors of survival in refractory anemia with ring sideroblasts and thrombocytosis (RARS-T) and the role of next-generation sequencing. *Am J Hematol.* 2016;91(5):492-498. doi:10.1002/ajh.24332
10. Broséus J, Alpermann T, Wulfert M, et al. Age, JAK2(V617F) and SF3B1 mutations are the main predicting factors for survival in refractory anaemia with ring sideroblasts and marked thrombocytosis. *Leukemia.* 2013;27(9):1826-1831. doi:10.1038/leu.2013.120

Chapter 11

Myelodysplastic/Myeloproliferative Neoplasm, Not Otherwise Specified

Carlos E. Bueso-Ramos, Rashmi Kanagal-Shamanna, and Attilio Orazi

Definition

Myelodysplastic/myeloproliferative neoplasm not otherwise specified is a myeloid neoplasm with mixed clinical and pathological features of both MDS and MPNs, not meeting the ICC criteria for any other myeloid neoplasms.

At the time of its initial presentation MDS/MPN, NOS is characterized by the presence of cytopenia in association with myeloproliferative features. The diagnostic criteria for other MDS/MPN subtypes (chronic myelomonocytic leukemia, atypical chronic myeloid leukemia, or MDS/MPN with thrombocytosis and *SF3B1* mutation and MDS/MPN with ring sideroblasts and thrombocytosis), MDS, MPN, and M/L-Eo with tyrosine kinase gene fusions must not be fulfilled.

Establishment of clonality is expected although the diagnosis can be made in its absence (see the following).

MDS/MPN, NOS is a specific disease category and this category should not be used to diagnose advanced stage MDS, MPN, and/or triple negative MPN cases. The diagnostic criteria for MDS/MPN, NOS are summarized in Table 11.1.

MDS/MPN with i(17q)

To develop a genetic-based homogenous diagnostic classification system, MDS/MPN with isolated isochromosome (17q) (MDS/MPN with i[17q]) has been added as a new provisional subentity under the diagnostic umbrella of MDS/MPN, NOS. This subentity has an adverse prognosis and its recognition may facilitate the development of targeted therapeutic approaches. At present, it is not clear whether this is a biologically distinct entity or a variant within the spectrum of aCML as it shares with the latter a similar genomic signature. To this end, the designation under the category of MDS/MPN, NOS seems appropriate until future studies may provide a more defensive characterization. The diagnostic criteria for MDS/MPN with i(17q) are summarized in Table 11.2.

Synonyms

- Myelodysplastic/myeloproliferative neoplasm, unclassifiable (not recommended)
- Mixed myeloproliferative/myelodysplastic syndrome, unclassifiable (not recommended)

Epidemiology

Epidemiological studies on MDS/MPN, NOS are scarce, and only vague estimation exists.[1]

General Clinical Features

The clinical features of MDS/MNP, NOS overlap with those entities in the MDS and MPN categories.[2,3] By definition, peripheral blood cytopenia must be present in at least 1 lineage in addition to myeloproliferative features.

MDS/MPN with i(17q)

These cases also present with mixed myelodysplastic and myeloproliferative features with a median age of 67 years at presentation. More than half the cases have splenomegaly.[4] Progression of an underlying MPN must be excluded.

Morphology

MDS/MPN, NOS is characterized by ineffective and/or dysplastic proliferation of one or more myeloid lineages and simultaneously by effective proliferation (with or without dysplasia) of another myeloid lineage or lineages. Laboratory features usually include anemia of variable severity, with or without macrocytosis.

TABLE 11.1 Diagnostic criteria for myelodysplastic/myeloproliferative neoplasm, not otherwise specified (MDS/MPN, NOS)

Myeloid neoplasm with mixed myeloproliferative and myelodysplastic features, not meeting the WHO criteria for any other MDS/MPN, MDS, MPN[a]
- Cytopenia (thresholds same as those for MDS)[b]
- Blasts <20% of the cells in blood or bone marrow
- Clinical and morphological myeloproliferative features manifesting as a platelet count of ≥450 × 10^9/L and/or a white blood cell count of ≥13 × 10^9/L
- Presence of clonality: abnormal cytogenetics and/or presence of at least one myeloid neoplasm-associated mutation. If clonality cannot be determined, the findings have persisted and all other causes (eg, history of cytotoxic or growth factor therapy or other primary cause that could explain the myelodysplastic/myeloproliferative features) have been excluded.
- No *BCR::ABL1*; no *PDGFRA*, *PDGFRB*, *FGFR1*, or other specific rearrangement found in the group of M/LN-Eo; no *PCM1::JAK2*; no del(5q)[c]

[a]Myeloproliferative neoplasms (MPNs), those in accelerated phase and/or in post–polycythemia vera or post–essential thrombocythemia myelofibrosis, may simulate MDS/MPN, NOS. A history of MPN and/or the presence of MPN-associated mutations (in *JAK2*, *CALR*, or *MPL*) tend to exclude a diagnosis of MDS/MPN-U.
[b]Greenberg PL, et al. *Blood.* 2016;128:2096-2097.
[c]In a case that otherwise meets the diagnostic criteria for MDS syndrome with isolated del(5q).

There is evidence of effective proliferation in one or more lineages: either thrombocytosis (platelet count ≥450 × 10^9/L) or leukocytosis (white blood cell count ≥13 × 10^9/L). The median white blood cell count is usually lower in MDS/MPN, NOS (19.4 × 10^9/L) than in atypical chronic myeloid leukemia (40.8 × 10^9/L).[5] Neutrophils may show dysplastic features, but dysgranulopoiesis is seen in only about 50% of cases. There may be giant or hypogranular platelets. The bone marrow biopsy specimen is hypercellular and show proliferation in any or all the myeloid lineages. Dyserythropoiesis may be seen. Dysmegakaryopoiesis with megakaryocytes resembling those seen in MDS is found in more than half of the cases. In the remaining cases, there is a mixture of MDS- and MPN-like megakaryocytes or (rarely) a predominance of MPN-like megakaryocytes. Blasts account for <20% of leukocytes in the peripheral blood and <20% of nucleated cells in the bone marrow.[5] Although cases of MDS/MPN-SF3B1-T and MDS/MPN- RS-T are classified separately, rare cases of MDS/MPN with *SF3B1* mutation or ≥15% ring sideroblasts and ≥1% peripheral blood blasts or ≥5% bone marrow blasts belong in the MDS/MPN, NOS group.

TABLE 11.2 Diagnostic criteria for myelodysplastic/myeloproliferative neoplasm with isolated isochromosome (17q) (MDS/MPN with i(17q)

-Leukocytosis of ≥13 × 10^9/L
-Cytopenia (thresholds same those as for MDS)[a]
- Blasts <20% of the cells in blood or bone marrow
- Dysgranulopoiesis with nonsegmented or Pseudo-Pelger-Hüet neutrophils
- An i(17q), either isolated or occurring with one other additional abnormality (other than del[7q]/-7)
- Lack of *TP53* mutation
- No *BCR::ABL1* fusion; no *PDGFRA, PDGFRB, FGFR1*, or other specific rearrangements found in the group of M/LN-Eo; no *PCM1::JAK2*. Absence of MPN-associated mutations (*JAK2, CALR*, and *MPL*)[b]
- No history of recent cytotoxic or growth factor therapy that could explain the MDS/MPN features
- Diagnostic criteria for *BCR::ABL1*–positive chronic myeloid leukemia or other type of myeloproliferative or MDS/MPN are not met[b]

[a]Greenberg PL, et al. *Blood.* 2016;128:2096-2097.
[b]Presence of MPN features in the bone marrow, and/or MPN-associated mutations (in *JAK2, CALR*, or *MPL*) suggests the progression of an underlying MPN that was not diagnosed, and should be excluded; conversely, in the appropriate clinical context, mutations particularly co-mutations in *SRSF2* and *SETBP1* genes further support this diagnosis.

MDS/MPN with i(17q)

In addition to hypercellularity of the bone marrow, the typical morphological features include the following: (1) neutrophilic dysplasia characterized by marked nuclear chromatin condensation with monolobed or bilobed nuclear lobes (pseudo-Pelger-Hüet neutrophils) (Figure 11.1A) often better appreciated on peripheral blood smears (Figure 11.1B) and (2) dysplastic megakaryopoiesis (Figure 11.1C) with a predominance of small hypolobated forms (Figure 11.1D). Dyserythropoiesis is less common. About 40% of cases show marrow fibrosis (MF-2 or higher) leading to diagnostic confusion with advanced-stage MPN.[4,6,7]

Immunophenotype

The immunophenotype may be like that of MDS or MPN.

Genetics

There are no specific cytogenetic or molecular genetic findings for MDS/MPN, NOS other than the presence of isolated i(17q) abnormality for the diagnosis of its provisional subentity (see below). Due to the presence of cytosis usually leukocytosis, the *BCR::ABL1* fusion needs to be excluded. Thrombocytosis seen in cases that otherwise meet the diagnostic criteria for cases of MDS associated with inv(3)(q21.3q26.2) or t(3;3)(q21.3;q26.2) or MDS with del(5q) are excluded. Cases with specific tyrosine kinase gene fusions/rearrangements

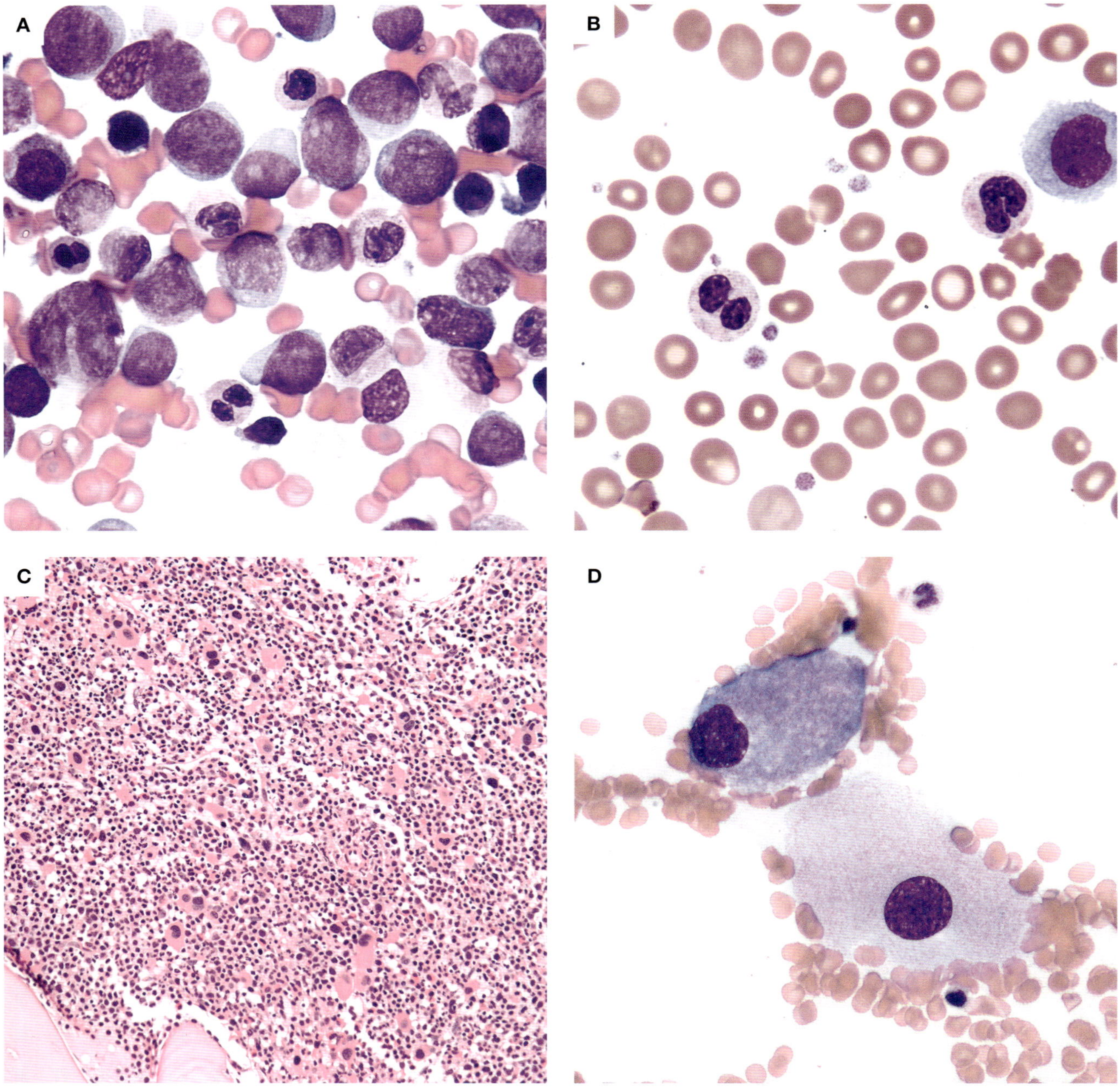

FIGURE 11.1 Bone marrow and peripheral blood morphologic features of cases of MDS/MPN with isolated i(17q): mildly increased blasts in association with neutrophilic dysplasia characterized by marked nuclear chromatin condensation with monolobed or bilobed nuclear lobes (pseudo-Pelger-Hüet neutrophils) **(A)**, that is best appreciated on peripheral blood smears **(B)**. Bone marrow biopsy shows hypercellular-for-age marrow with dysplastic megakaryocytic hyperplasia **(C)** with numerous small hypolobated forms **(D)**.

of M/LN-Eo such as *PDGFRA, PDGFRB, FGFR1, PCM1::JAK2* are excluded from this category. The presence of MPN-associated mutations (in *JAK2, CALR* and *MPL*), at high variant allele frequencies, with MPN-associated morphologic features in the bone marrow supports progression of a previously undiagnosed MPN and must be excluded.

Establishment of clonality is expected although the diagnosis can be made in the absence of clonal cytogenetic or molecular abnormalities in the following settings: (1) there is sufficient clinical and histopathologic support for MDS/MPN, (2) primary and secondary causes of MDS/MPN features, such as growth factor and/or cytotoxic therapies have been excluded, and (3) other MDS/MPN subtypes have been excluded. The presence of hypereosinophilia favors the diagnosis of CEL, NOS[8] and requires careful exclusion of an M/L-Eo associated with a tyrosine kinase gene fusion.

MDS/MPN with i(17q)

These cases have i(17q) as either the sole cytogenetic abnormality, or with one additional cytogenetic abnormality other than monosomy 7/del(7q). Cases of MDS/MPN, NOS with i(17q) show a unique somatic mutation profile.[4,9-11] Compared to MDS/MPN, NOS without i(17q), these cases have a significantly higher frequency of gene mutations involving *SRSF2* and *SETBP1* as well as concomitant (double) mutations in *SRSF2/SETBP1* genes. Additional mutations include those seen in MDS/MPN such as *ASXL1* and *TET2*, although not significantly different compared to cases lacking i(17q). The presence of co-mutations in *SRSF2* and *SETBP1* genes strongly supports this diagnosis in an appropriate clinical and morphologic context. There is notable absence of biallelic or multi-hit *TP53* mutations. The isochromosome (17q) involves deletion of 17p (encompassing *TP53* gene) and duplication of 17q segment. Therefore, these cases functionally represent monoallelic *TP53*-altered myeloid neoplasms.

Prognosis and Clinical Comment

There is very limited information available about this rare subgroup. Patients with MDS/MPN, NOS have a median overall survival (OS) of 26 months.[12] MDS/MPN with i(17q) is a prognostically aggressive condition with a median OS of 11 months.[4]

References

1. Kuendgen A, Kasprzak A, Germing U. Hybrid or mixed myelodysplastic/myeloproliferative disorders—epidemiological features and overview. *Front Oncol.* 2021;11:778741.
2. Patnaik MM, Tefferi A. Atypical chronic myeloid leukemia and myelodysplastic/myeloproliferative neoplasm, not otherwise specified: 2023 update on diagnosis, risk stratification, and management. *Am J Hematol.* 2023;98(4):681-689.
3. Shallis RM, Zeidan AM. Myelodysplastic/myeloproliferative neoplasm, unclassifiable (MDS/MPN-U): more than just a "catch-all" term? *Best Pract Res Clin Haematol.* 2020;33(2):101132.
4. Kanagal-Shamanna R, Orazi A, Hasserjian RP, et al. Myelodysplastic/myeloproliferative neoplasms-unclassifiable with isolated isochromosome 17q represents a distinct clinico-biologic subset: a multi-institutional collaborative study from the Bone Marrow Pathology Group. *Mod Pathol.* 2022;35(4):470-479.
5. Wang SA, Hasserjian RP, Fox PS, et al. Atypical chronic myeloid leukemia is clinically distinct from unclassifiable myelodysplastic/myeloproliferative neoplasms. *Blood.* 2014;123(17):2645-2651.
6. Kanagal-Shamanna R, Bueso-Ramos CE, Barkoh B, et al. Myeloid neoplasms with isolated isochromosome 17q represent a clinicopathologic entity associated with myelodysplastic/myeloproliferative features, a high risk of leukemic transformation, and wild-type TP53. *Cancer.* 2012;118(11):2879-2888.
7. McClure RF, Dewald GW, Hoyer JD, Hanson CA. Isolated isochromosome 17q: a distinct type of mixed myeloproliferative disorder/myelodysplastic syndrome with an aggressive clinical course. *Br J Haematol.* 1999;106(2):445-454.
8. Palomo L, Meggendorfer M, Hutter S, et al. Molecular landscape and clonal architecture of adult myelodysplastic/myeloproliferative neoplasms. *Blood.* 2020;136(16):1851-1862.
9. Kanagal-Shamanna R, Luthra R, Yin CC, et al. Myeloid neoplasms with isolated isochromosome 17q demonstrate a high frequency of mutations in SETBP1, SRSF2, ASXL1 and NRAS. *Oncotarget.* 2016;7(12):14251-14258.
10. Meggendorfer M, Bacher U, Alpermann T, et al. SETBP1 mutations occur in 9% of MDS/MPN and in 4% of MPN cases and are strongly associated with atypical CML, monosomy 7, isochromosome i(17)(q10), ASXL1 and CBL mutations. *Leukemia.* 2013;27(9):1852-1860.
11. Meggendorfer M, Haferlach C, Zenger M, Macijewski K, Kern W, Haferlach T. The landscape of myeloid neoplasms with isochromosome 17q discloses a specific mutation profile and is characterized by an accumulation of prognostically adverse molecular markers. *Leukemia.* 2016;30(7):1624-1627.
12. Mangaonkar AA, Swoboda DM, Coltro G, et al. Clinicopathologic characteristics, prognostication and treatment outcomes for myelodysplastic/myeloproliferative neoplasm, unclassifiable (MDS/MPN-U): Mayo Clinic-Moffitt Cancer Center study of 135 consecutive patients. *Leukemia.* 2020;34(2):656-661.

SECTION 5

Premalignant Clonal Cytopenias and Myelodysplastic Syndromes

Introduction to Premalignant Clonal Cytopenias and Myelodysplastic Syndromes

Robert P. Hasserjian

Myelodysplastic syndrome (MDS) is a hematologic malignancy that manifests clinically by cytopenias and pathologically by the presence of morphologic dysplasia in maturing hematopoietic elements. All MDSs are thought to arise from a precursor state of clonal hematopoiesis, due to expansion within the bone marrow of a clonal population originating from a mutated hematopoietic stem cell. The International Consensus Classification recognizes these clonal precursor states that do not meet formal criteria for MDS, and they are defined and discussed in Chapter 12.

A critical defining feature of MDS is the presence of at least one cytopenia, which is not otherwise clinically explained by a transient or secondary cause. The cytopenia can be an anemia (hemoglobin <13 g/dL in males, <12 g/dL in females), neutropenia (absolute neutrophil count $<1.8 \times 10^9$/L), and/or a thrombocytopenia (platelet count $<150 \times 10^9$/L). While not a formal requirement, the chronicity of cytopenias in asymptomatic patients is usually greater than 4 months. Secondary causes of cytopenia (such as a toxin, drug, infection, peripheral cell destruction, or metabolic deficiency) should be excluded. Sustained leukocytosis (white blood cell [WBC] $\geq 13.0 \times 10^9$/L) or monocytosis (monocytes $\geq 0.5 \times 10^9$/L and ≥10% of leukocytes) not explained by infection, inflammatory state, or other comorbid condition at the time of initial diagnosis excludes MDS and warrants classification as MDS/myeloproliferative neoplasm (MDS/MPN) or MPN. Persistent unexplained eosinophilia (eosinophils ≥10% of WBC and $\geq 1.5 \times 10^9$/L) tends to exclude MDS and raises concern for an eosinophilic myeloid proliferation.

Bone marrow examination is required to identify the morphologic dysplasia of myeloid, erythroid, and/or megakaryocytic elements that distinguishes clonal cytopenias from MDS. The detailed criteria for dysplasia and illustrations of dysplastic cells in each lineage are shown in Chapter 16. Conventional cytogenetics on bone marrow aspirate material is also an integral part of the workup for putative MDS and should be performed in all cases.[1] Interphase fluorescence in situ hybridization studies to assess for cytogenetic aberrations involving MDS—typically del(5q), −7/del(7q), del(20q), +8, and −17/del(17p)—may be performed if the karyotype is unsuccessful but are generally not indicated if the karyotype is adequate.[2] Next-generation sequencing (NGS) using panels that assess for mutations commonly present in MDS are part of the standard of care for suspected or newly diagnosed MDS; although NGS is typically performed on a bone marrow aspirate specimen, similar results are usually obtained if NGS is performed on a concurrent blood sample.[3] *TP53* and *SF3B1* mutations define specific MDS subtypes, and other mutations have important prognostic value that help guide patient management together with the MDS subtype, blood counts, and karyotype findings. The recommended list of mutations to be performed to diagnose and classify MDS is shown in Table 5 in the Introduction to the International Consensus Classification of Myeloid Disorders.

Flow cytometric (FCM) immunophenotyping analysis is a useful modality in supporting or helping exclude a diagnosis of MDS. Over the past 15 years, the European LeukemiaNet has developed standard guidelines that include the following: (1) methods for sample handling and processing, (2) the panel of antibodies, and (3) criteria for interpretation. These guidelines were most recently updated in 2023.[4] An evaluation of at least three to four phenotypic alterations in two different cell compartments, which include $CD34^+$ myeloblasts, granulocytic lineage, monocytes, and erythroid precursors, is recommended. A simplified FCM approach, often referred to as the Ogata score[5] may be used in resource-limited practice settings. A positive Ogata score supporting a diagnosis of MDS includes two of the four criteria: (1) ≥2% myeloblasts; (2) absence of $CD34^+$ B-cell progenitors (hematogones); (3) abnormal clustering of $CD34^+$ myeloblasts on the plot of CD45/side scatters; (4) significantly decreased granulocyte side scatter (hypogranularity). However, due to the heterogeneity of MDS and lower sensitivity of the Ogata score in MDS subtypes lacking excess blasts, a more extended panel is optimal. In hypoplastic bone marrow assessment, the detection of a

TABLE 1 The International Consensus Classification of Myelodysplastic Syndromes and Clonal Cytopenia of Undetermined Significance

Entity	Blasts	Other morphology	Cytogenetics	Mutations
Clonal cytopenia of undetermined significance (CCUS)	<5% BM, <2% PB[a]	<10% dysplasia in all lineages	Abnormality may be present. No complex karyotype,[b] −7/del(7q), or del(5q)	One or more, present at VAF ≥ 2% No multihit[c] *TP53* or *SF3B1* (VAF ≥ 10%)
MDS with del(5q) (MDS-del5q)	<5% BM, <2% PB[a]	No Auer rods in blasts	Del(5q), with up to one other abnormality except −7/del(7q)	No multihit[c] *TP53* (VAF ≥ 10%)
MDS with mutated *SF3B1* (MDS-SF3B1)	<5% BM, <2% PB[a]	No Auer rods in blasts	No del(5q), −7/del(7q), abnormal 3q26.2, or complex karyotype[b]	*SF3B1* (VAF ≥ 10%) No multihit[c] *TP53* (VAF ≥ 10%) or *RUNX1*
MDS with mutated *TP53* (MDS-TP53)	<10% BM, <10% PB		Usually complex karyotype[b]	Multihit[c] *TP53* (VAF ≥ 10%)
MDS-NOS				
- without dysplasia	<5% BM, <2% PB[a]	<10% dysplasia in all lineages	−7/del(7q) or complex karyotype[b] Not MDS-del5q[e]	Not MDS-SF3B1,[d] no multihit[c] *TP53* (VAF ≥ 10%)
- with SLD	<5% BM, <2% PB[a]	≥10% dysplasia in 1 lineage	Not MDS-del5q[e]	Not MDS-SF3B1,[d] no multihit[c] *TP53* (VAF ≥ 10%)
- with MLD	<5% BM, <2% PB[a]	≥10% dysplasia in 2-3 lineages	Not MDS-del5q[e]	Not MDS-SF3B1,[d] no multihit[c] *TP53* (VAF ≥ 10%)
MDS with excess blasts (MDS-EB)	5%-9% BM or 2%-9% PB[a]	Auer rods in blasts (if <5% BM, <2% PB blasts)	Any	No multihit[c] *TP53* (VAF ≥ 10%)
MDS/AML				
- with mutated *TP53* (MDS/AML-TP53)	10%-19% BM or 10%-19% PB	Dysplasia usually present	Usually complex karyotype[b]	*TP53* (monoallelic or multihit,[c] VAF ≥ 10%)
- with MDS-related gene mutations	10%-19% BM or 10%-19% PB	Dysplasia usually present	Any	*SRSF2, SF3B1, U2AF1, ZRSR2, ASXL1, EZH2, BCOR, STAG2,* or *RUNX1* No *TP53* (VAF ≥ 10%)
- with MDS-related cytogenetic abnormalities	10%-19% BM or 10%-19% PB	Dysplasia usually present	Complex karyotype,[f] del(5q)/t(5q)/add(5q), -7/del(7q), +8, del(12p)/t(12p)/add(12p), i(17q)/-17/add(17p)/del(17p), del(20q), or idic(X)(q13)	No *SRSF2, SF3B1, U2AF1, ZRSR2, ASXL1, EZH2, BCOR, STAG2,* or *RUNX1* No *TP53* (VAF ≥ 10%)
- NOS	10%-19% BM or 10%-19% PB	Dysplasia usually present	No MDS-related cytogenetic abnormalities, as defined above	No MDS-related gene mutations, no *TP53* (VAF ≥ 10%)

BM, bone marrow; NOS, not otherwise specified; PB, peripheral blood; VAF, variant allele frequency.

[a]One percent PB blasts confirmed on two separate occasions is considered equivalent to 2% blasts for classification purposes.

[b]Complex karyotype is defined as at least three independent cytogenetic abnormalities (excluding -Y)

[c]Multihit *TP53* mutation is defined as any of the following: (1) two distinct *TP53* mutations each with VAF ≥ 10%), (2) a single *TP53* mutation with 17p deletion on karyotype or FISH, (3) a single *TP53* mutation with VAF of >50%, or (4) a single *TP53* mutation with copy-neutral loss of heterozygosity (LOH) at the 17p *TP53* locus; if *TP53* LOH information is not available, a complex karyotype is considered equivalent.

[d]Does not fulfill all diagnostic features of MDS-SF3B1.

[e]Does not fulfill all diagnostic features of MDS-del5q.

[f]For the purposes of defining MDS-related cytogenetic abnormalities in MDS/AML, complex karyotype excludes hyperdiploid karyotypes with three or more polysomies that lack structural abnormalities.

paroxysmal nocturnal hemoglobinuria (PNH) clone by flow cytometry may support an alternate diagnosis of PNH (if a major clone) or aplastic anemia (if a smaller clone). However, a PNH clone at a very low level may also be rarely detected in some MDS cases.[6] FCM is also essential in working up patients suspected of having MDS by evaluating for other hematopoietic disorders, particularly large granular lymphocytic leukemia and B-cell lymphomas, that may present with unexplained cytopenias.

Clinical management of patients with MDS is guided by both the specific MDS subtype (Table 1) and evaluation of the prognostic risk (survival and likelihood of transformation to acute myeloid leukemia). The International Prognostic Scoring System–Revised (IPSS-R) is a five-tiered system (ranging from very-low- to very-high-risk groups) that is based on the degree of cytopenias, bone marrow blast percentage, and cytogenetic findings.[7] The more recent IPSS-molecular (IPSS-M) is a six-tiered system that incorporates the mutations of 31 genes that impact MDS prognosis.[8] The IPPS-M allows for a more accurate risk stratification, especially in lower-grade MDS. The main genes that are associated with an adverse prognosis in the IPSS-M are *ASXL1, CBL, DNMT3A, ETV6, EZH2, FLT3, IDH2, KRAS, NPM1, NRAS, RUNX1, SRSF2, TP53, U2AF1,* and *KMT2A(MLL)*-PTD, while *SF3B1* is associated with a favorable prognosis. Of note, the prognostic impact of *TP53* mutation depends on its monoallelic versus multihit status (defined in Chapter 15), while the prognostic impact of *SF3B1* depends on its co-occurrence with other mutations or del(5q) cytogenetic abnormality.

In cases where prior cytotoxic therapies may have predisposed the patient to the myeloid neoplasm, a "therapy-related" qualifier should be applied to the MDS diagnosis. Similarly, patients with a known germline predisposition should have qualification following the pathologic diagnosis, for example "MDS with excess blasts, with germline *GATA2* mutation." These qualifiers are important to include in the diagnostic field, as they help further refine prognosis and guide management beyond the MDS disease subtype and IPSS-M/IPSS-R scores.

References

1. Duncavage EJ, Bagg A, Hasserjian RP, et al. Genomic profiling for clinical decision making in myeloid neoplasms and acute leukemia. *Blood*. 2022;140(21):2228-2247.
2. Seegmiller AC, Wasserman A, Kim AS, et al. Limited utility of fluorescence in situ hybridization for common abnormalities of myelodysplastic syndrome at first presentation and follow-up of myeloid neoplasms. *Leuk Lymphoma*. 2014;55(3):601-605.
3. Lucas F, Michaels PD, Wang D, Kim AS. Mutational analysis of hematologic neoplasms in 164 paired peripheral blood and bone marrow samples by next-generation sequencing. *Blood Adv*. 2020;4(18):4362-4365.
4. van de Loosdrecht AA, Kern W, Porwit A, et al. Clinical application of flow cytometry in patients with unexplained cytopenia and suspected myelodysplastic syndrome: a report of the European LeukemiaNet International MDS-Flow Cytometry Working Group. *Cytometry B Clin Cytom*. 2023;104(1):77-86.
5. Della Porta MG, Picone C, Pascutto C, et al. Multicenter validation of a reproducible flow cytometric score for the diagnosis of low-grade myelodysplastic syndromes: results of a European LeukemiaNET study. *Haematologica*. 2012;97(8):1209-1217.
6. Wang SA, Pozdnyakova O, Jorgensen JL, et al. Detection of paroxysmal nocturnal hemoglobinuria clones in patients with myelodysplastic syndromes and related bone marrow diseases, with emphasis on diagnostic pitfalls and caveats. *Haematologica*. 2009;94(1):29-37.
7. Greenberg PL, Tuechler H, Schanz J, et al. Revised international prognostic scoring system for myelodysplastic syndromes. *Blood*. 2012;120(12):2454-2465.
8. Bernard E, Tuechler H, Greenberg P, et al. Molecular International Prognostic Scoring System for Myelodysplastic Syndromes. *NEJM Evid*. 2022;1(7):EVIDoa2200008.

Chapter 12

Clonal Cytopenia of Undetermined Significance and Other Clonal Cytopenias

Jay L. Patel, Benjamin L. Ebert, Siddhartha Jaiswal, and Luca Malcovati

Definition

Clonal cytopenia of undetermined significance (CCUS) is defined by expansion of a population of hematopoietic cells derived from a single clone, as demonstrated by the detection of non–myelodysplastic syndrome (MDS)-defining somatic mutation (at a variant allele fraction [VAF] of ≥2%) or clonal cytogenetic aberration (ie, clonal hematopoiesis) in association with sustained (at least 4 months) cytopenia that is otherwise clinically unexplained. Importantly, criteria for a diagnosis of MDS or other hematologic disorder are not met and there is no prior history of MDS or other myeloid neoplasm. The thresholds for cytopenia in this context are as follows: anemia (hemoglobin <12 g/dL in females and <13 g/dL in males), neutropenia (absolute neutrophil count $<1.8 \times 10^9$/L), and/or thrombocytopenia (platelets $<150 \times 10^9$/L). Clonal hematopoiesis of indeterminate potential (CHIP) represents a related entity defined by clonal hematopoiesis (VAF ≥ 2%) in the absence of an unexplained cytopenia or current or prior myeloid neoplasm. Clonal cytopenias associated with unique clinical syndromes include paroxysmal nocturnal hemoglobinuria (PNH) and VEXAS (vacuoles, E1 enzyme, X-linked, autoinflammation, somatic) syndrome, which also may present in association with MDS or other hematologic neoplasms.

Synonyms

None.

Epidemiology

CHIP and CCUS are rare in children and young adults, whereas they are relatively common in order adults. Few data are available about the prevalence of CCUS, as it is a recently introduced concept and requires bone marrow examination to exclude a myeloid neoplasm. Population-based studies suggest that CHIP prevalence increases steadily with age, reflecting the stochastic nature of accumulation of gene mutations in hematopoietic stem cells over time, and is influenced significantly by the sensitivity of the DNA sequencing methodology employed for detection.[1,2] At an analytical sensitivity of 2% VAF, at least 10% of individuals 70 years or older harbor one or more mutations associated with CHIP. When higher sensitivity techniques such as target-enriched or error-corrected sequencing are employed, smaller clones of unknown biological and clinical relevance are detectable in nearly all adults over the age of 50 years. Exposure to chemotherapy, smoking, and advanced age are major risk factors for development of CHIP.

General Clinical Features

CCUS may be encountered as an incidental finding in a patient with unexplained asymptomatic cytopenia leading to further hematologic and molecular genetic evaluation (Table 12.1). Individuals may also present with symptoms related to cytopenia but not meet diagnostic criteria for an overt hematologic neoplasm. The risk of progression to a myeloid neoplasm is heavily influenced by several genetic factors, including the number of gene mutations and mutation VAFs, as well as the specific biologic pathways impaired.[3] Cytopenias in CCUS must be persistent for at least 4 months and are not attributable to another underlying medical condition. A bone marrow examination is required to evaluate for diagnostic criteria for MDS or other hematologic neoplasm. Individuals with clonal cytopenia and monocytosis are separately defined as clonal cytopenia and monocytosis of undetermined significance in light of the distinct pattern of progression to chronic myelomonocytic leukemia (see Chapter 8).

Substantial data link CHIP to increased all-cause mortality primarily attributable to cardiovascular

TABLE 12.1 Summary of clinicopathologic findings in clonal cytopenia of undetermined significance and other clonal cytopenias

Type of clonal cytopenia	Clinical features	Morphology and immunophenotype	Genetics
CCUS	Clinically unexplained cytopenia, without history of hematologic neoplasm	Dysplasia is absent (<10% of cells in each hematopoietic lineage) and blasts are not increased (bone marrow examination required)	Loss-of-function mutation in epigenetic (eg, *DNMT3A*, *TET2*, or *ASXL1*), splicing, or tumor suppressor genes, or activating mutations of cell signaling genes. MDS-defining genetic abnormalities[a] are absent.
PNH	Episodic hemolytic anemia, venous thrombosis	Red cell findings related to hemolysis. Loss of GPI-associated antigens (eg, CD55, CD59, CD157, FLAER) on hematopoietic cells detected by flow cytometry. Variable bone marrow cellularity with erythroid hyperplasia or aplasia.	Loss-of-function *PIGA* mutation
VEXAS	Autoimmune manifestations, mild cytopenia	Vacuolization of erythroid and myeloid precursors	*UBA1* mutation, commonly loss of Met41 start codon

CCUS, clonal cytopenia of undetermined significance; PNH, paroxysmal nocturnal hemoglobinuria; VEXAS, vacuoles, E1 enzyme, X-linked, autoinflammation, somatic.
[a]MDS-defining genetic abnormalities are complex karyotype, del(5q), −7/del(7q), multi-hit *TP53* mutation (VAF ≥ 10%), and *SF3B1* mutation (VAF ≥ 10%).

disease such as myocardial infarction, ischemic stroke, and venous thrombosis, although direct data connecting these associations with CCUS are not available.[4] *JAK2*-mutated clones connote a particularly high risk of thrombosis and coronary artery disease but are rarely detected in individuals with cytopenia. Clonal hematopoiesis is also broadly associated with various other multisystemic inflammatory disease states including inflammatory bowel disease, chronic obstructive pulmonary disease, and vasculitis. Implicated nonhematological disease risk varies by mutated gene.[5] The principal feature underlying these nonhematologic disease associations is a proinflammatory state, fostered by clonal hematopoiesis gene mutations and mediated by higher expression of chemokines and other inflammatory mediators including IL6, IL-1β, IFNγ, and TNF.[6] Notably, a higher prevalence of clonal hematopoiesis has been reported in community-dwelling individuals with anemia of chronic disease.[7]

Morphology and Immunophenotype

Specific morphologic or immunophenotypic abnormalities are not observed in patients with CCUS. Normal trilineage hematopoiesis is present in the bone marrow, and blood and bone marrow blast counts are not elevated. Distinction of CCUS from MDS (in the absence of an MDS-defining genetic abnormality) relies on careful morphologic assessment for dysplasia, which requires procurement of adequate blood and bone marrow samples. It must be acknowledged that the combination of clonal hematopoiesis and unexplained cytopenia in the absence of bone marrow investigation does not qualify as CCUS, since an underlying myeloid neoplasm cannot be excluded.

Genetics

CCUS and MDS originate from mutations in hematopoietic stems cells that confer a fitness advantage at the cellular level resulting in clonal expansion and ineffective hematopoiesis. The range of mutation classes that may be observed has warranted deployment of multiple testing techniques (ie, conventional karyotype in conjunction with a targeted high-throughput sequencing panel) and may be increasingly more amenable to comprehensive evaluation by massively parallel sequencing.[8] The most commonly mutated genes in CCUS (*DNMT3A*, *TET2*, and *ASXL1*) are involved in epigenetic regulation and account for over two-thirds of cases. Mutations in splicing factors (*SF3B1*, *SRSF2*, *U2AF1*, *ZRSR2*) are also relatively common. Mutations in prototypical tumor suppressors (*TP53*) and oncogenes (*JAK2*) also occur but are less frequent. A minimum mutation VAF threshold of 2% is recommended for diagnosis of CCUS. CCUS also encompasses cases with cytogenetic abnormalities detected by conventional karyotype. As compared with CHIP, CCUS cases are enriched for non *DNMT3A* mutations and tend to demonstrate higher mutation VAF(s). Comutation patterns involving splicing factors and epigenetic regulators are very highly correlated with the presence of a myeloid neoplasm and when encountered clinically should prompt thorough appraisal for a myeloid malignancy. Importantly, *SF3B1* mutation (VAF ≥ 10%), multi-hit *TP53* mutation (VAF ≥ 10%), and complex karyotype, −7, del(7q), or del(5q) are considered to be MDS defining in a patient with unexplained, sustained cytopenia, even in the absence of dysplasia; the presence of any of these genetic abnormalities thus excludes CCUS. Molecular genetic features as well as laboratory testing results inform the risk of subsequent development of a myeloid neoplasm in patients with CCUS, and further study is warranted to better define higher-risk CCUS and its relationship to MDS. Careful consideration should be given to exclusion of a germline predisposition syndrome in patients with CCUS.

Prognosis and Clinical Comment

The rate of progression from CCUS to a hematologic neoplasm is augmented by mutational dynamics. The presence of two or more somatic gene mutations, high VAF (>10%), or involvement of specific genes or comutation patterns considerably escalates the risk of subsequent development of hematologic malignancy and may inform clinical management. Predictive models have been proposed, which may allow for more precise risk assessment in individual patients.[9] No specific treatment exists for patients with CCUS. The majority of patients present with mild cytopenia and do not require active treatment. Routine clinical monitoring of patients with CCUS at appropriate intervals may allow for early intervention in patients progressing to overt hematologic malignancy as well as facilitate regular assessment and potential risk mitigation of cardiovascular or other associated disease states. Clonal hematopoiesis (preexisting or donor derived) and persistent cytopenias are also encountered in patients with history of hematologic malignancy post therapy or hematopoietic stem cell transplantation, and accurate distinction from persistent or recurrent primary neoplasm is required in this setting; by convention, such cases are not considered within the spectrum of CCUS.[10]

Other Clonal Cytopenias

The specific disease entities PNH and VEXAS are characterized by peripheral blood cytopenia and clonal hematopoiesis and are associated with a variable propensity to progress to myeloid neoplasms. Clonal hematopoiesis can also be detected in the context of severe or nonsevere aplastic anemia, prompting careful appraisal of diagnostic criteria to distinguish these cases from hypoplastic MDS.

Paroxysmal nocturnal hemoglobinuria

PNH may occur at any age but is classically diagnosed in adults with recurrent episodic intravascular hemolysis leading to severe anemia as well as venous thrombosis. Patients often present with nonspecific findings including fatigue, pain, hemoglobinuria, or renal insufficiency. Patients may also present with or progress to aplastic anemia (bone marrow failure). Small PNH clones can be also detected in the context of typical MDS, but their clinical relevance remains uncertain. PNH is a rare disease with estimated global prevalence of 1.6 in 100,000 individuals. While there are no characteristic morphologic findings in PNH, blood smears from these patients frequently show red cell changes related to hemolysis, including polychromasia, reticulocytosis, and anisopoikilocytosis. Bone marrow cellularity may range from hypocellular or aplastic to normal or hypercellular and is frequently accompanied by compensatory erythroid hyperplasia with variable dyserythropoiesis (Figure 12.1A). When PNH is suspected in the setting of hemolytic anemia, high-sensitivity flow cytometry is the preferred diagnostic testing modality to evaluate for deficiency or loss of glycosylphosphatidylinositol (GPI)-linked antigens (eg, CD55, CD59, CD157, FLAER) on the surface of blood cells.[11] Red and white blood cells are both analyzed to maximize diagnostic yield. Clone size is quantified by flow cytometry and can be followed to monitor treatment efficacy and to assess for disease progression. The protein PIGA is crucial for biosynthesis of the GPI anchor, and somatic loss-of-function *PIGA* mutation constitutes the genetic basis of PNH.[12] A subset of patients with PNH may progress to overt MDS or other myeloid neoplasms. Complement inhibitor therapy in PNH has demonstrated efficacy and markedly reduces the risk of thrombotic events and hemolysis thereby improving anemia-related symptoms.

VEXAS syndrome

VEXAS syndrome is a multisystemic disease characterized by inflammatory and hematologic manifestations with underlying somatic mutation of E1 ubiquitin activating enzyme (*UBA1*). Initial observational studies suggest that pathogenic *UBA1* variants causing VEXAS are detected in approximately 1 in 13,500 individuals.[13]

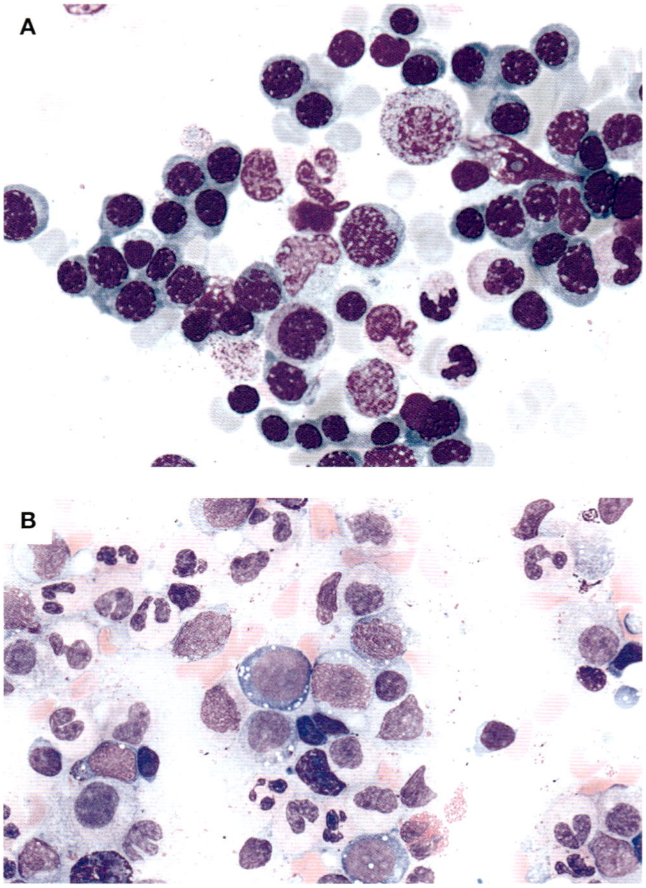

FIGURE 12.1 Bone marrow images from patients with clonal cytopenias. **A:** Bone marrow aspirate smear showing marked erythroid hyperplasia in patient with PNH; although significant dysplasia is lacking in this case, some cases may show variable dysplastic changes reflecting stress erythropoiesis in the setting of hemolysis (Wright stain). **B:** Bone marrow aspirate smear showing cytoplasmic vacuolization of myeloid and erythroid precursors in a patient with VEXAS syndrome (Wright stain).

VEXAS occurs predominantly in males with adult-onset symptoms related to autoinflammation, including fever and fatigue.[14] Other clinical manifestations may include dermatoses, vasculitis, and polyarthritis. Cytopenia is often present but is typically mild and usually manifests as macrocytic anemia. VEXAS syndrome shows vacuolization of erythroid and myeloid precursors best demonstrated on bone marrow aspirate smear (Figure 12.1B). Normally functioning UBA1 protein initiates ubiquitinylation, which is essential for maturation of autophagic vacuoles. Dysplasia is typically absent but can be challenging to assess in the context of general autoinflammation and the presence of vacuolated precursors, a finding that in isolation should not be used to support a concomitant diagnosis of MDS. Loss of the *UBA1* start codon Met41 (the initiation site of the cytoplasmic isoform of the UBA1 protein) is the canonical mutation, and additional pathogenic variants are described. Comutations are common in VEXAS, with *DNMT3A* and *TET2* being the most frequently mutated genes.[15] Mutation of high-risk myeloid disease-related genes may provide supportive evidence of coexisting MDS in VEXAS. Given the nonspecific clinical phenotype of both PNH and VEXAS, which often includes anemia and may prompt workup for a hematologic neoplasm, inclusion of *PIGA* and *UBA1* in targeted NGS panels intended for evaluation of myeloid neoplasms will likely increase the diagnostic yield. Patients with VEXAS may respond to immunosuppression and supportive care directed at specific symptomology. The potential role of hypomethylating agents and hematopoietic stem cell transplantation is under investigation.

References

1. Genovese G, Kahler AK, Handsaker RE, et al. Clonal hematopoiesis and blood-cancer risk inferred from blood DNA sequence. *N Engl J Med*. 2014;371(26):2477-2487.
2. Jaiswal S, Fontanillas P, Flannick J, et al. Age-related clonal hematopoiesis associated with adverse outcomes. *N Engl J Med*. 2014;371(26):2488-2498.
3. Steensma DP, Bejar R, Jaiswal S, et al. Clonal hematopoiesis of indeterminate potential and its distinction from myelodysplastic syndromes. *Blood*. 2015;126(1):9-16.
4. Jaiswal S, Natarajan P, Silver AJ, et al. Clonal hematopoiesis and risk of atherosclerotic cardiovascular disease. *N Engl J Med*. 2017;377(2):111-121.
5. Kessler MD, Damask A, O'Keeffe S, et al. Common and rare variant associations with clonal haematopoiesis phenotypes. *Nature*. 2022;612(7939):301-309.
6. Belizaire R, Wong WJ, Robinette ML, Ebert BL. Clonal haematopoiesis and dysregulation of the immune system. *Nat Rev Immunol*. 2023;23(9):595-610.
7. van Zeventer IA, de Graaf AO, Wouters H, et al. Mutational spectrum and dynamics of clonal hematopoiesis in anemia of older individuals. *Blood*. 2020;135(14):1161-1170.
8. Kwok B, Hall JM, Witte JS, et al. MDS-associated somatic mutations and clonal hematopoiesis are common in idiopathic cytopenias of undetermined significance. *Blood*. 2015;126(21):2355-2361.
9. Weeks LD, Niroula A, Neuberg D, et al. Prediction of risk for myeloid malignancy in clonal hematopoiesis. *NEJM Evid*. 2023;2(5):10.1056/evidoa2200310.
10. Frick M, Chan W, Arends CM, et al. Role of donor clonal hematopoiesis in allogeneic hematopoietic stem-cell transplantation. *J Clin Oncol*. 2019;37(5):375-385.
11. Dezern AE, Borowitz MJ. ICCS/ESCCA consensus guidelines to detect GPI-deficient cells in paroxysmal nocturnal hemoglobinuria (PNH) and related

disorders part 1—clinical utility. *Cytometry B Clin Cytom*. 2018;94(1):16-22.

12. Yoshizato T, Dumitriu B, Hosokawa K, et al. Somatic mutations and clonal hematopoiesis in aplastic anemia. *N Engl J Med*. 2015;373(1):35-47.
13. Beck DB, Bodian DL, Shah V, et al. Estimated prevalence and clinical manifestations of UBA1 variants associated with VEXAS syndrome in a clinical population. *JAMA*. 2023;329(4):318-324.
14. Beck DB, Ferrada MA, Sikora KA, et al. Somatic mutations in UBA1 and severe adult-onset autoinflammatory disease. *N Engl J Med*. 2020;383(27):2628-2638.
15. Gutierrez-Rodrigues F, Kusne Y, Fernandez J, et al. Spectrum of clonal hematopoiesis in VEXAS syndrome. *Blood*. 2023;142(3):244-259.

Chapter 13

Myelodysplastic Syndrome With Mutated *SF3B1*

Alexa J. Siddon, Eva Hellström-Lindberg, and Luca Malcovati

Definition

Myelodysplastic syndrome with mutated *SF3B1* (MDS-SF3B1) is a myeloid neoplasm characterized by persistent peripheral cytopenia(s), typically associated with morphologic dysplasia and ring sideroblasts, and a pathogenic *SF3B1* mutation.[1,2] Recent research has shown that ring sideroblasts do not have prognostic significance independent of the *SF3B1* mutation.[3] Therefore, the prior World Health Organization (WHO) revised fourth edition classification entity of MDS with ring sideroblasts (MDS-RS) has been eliminated: MDS-SF3B1 encompasses the majority (but not all) of cases that were previously classified as MDS-RS.[1-4]

Synonyms

MDS with low blasts and *SF3B1* mutation (not recommended).

Epidemiology

Data on the epidemiology of MDS-SF3B1 are lacking due to the new introduction of this entity, which compasses most but not all of prior MDS-RS cases. The available recent studies have shown that MDS-SF3B1 accounts for approximately 17% of MDS cases, with a slight predominance of male patients.

General Clinical Features

Symptoms of MDS-SF3B1 are similar to other types of MDS: symptomatology is typically related to cytopenias, most commonly macrocytic or normocytic anemia, less commonly thrombocytopenia, and rarely neutropenia. Some patients with MDS-SF3B1 may exhibit transiently increased or persistent borderline elevated platelet counts above the diagnostic threshold, requiring careful differentiation from myelodysplastic/myeloproliferative neoplasm with mutated *SF3B1* and thrombocytosis (MDS/MPN-SF3B1-T, see Chapter 10). Patients with MDS-SF3B1 often have mild to moderate iron overload even without receiving red cell transfusions, as a consequence of a high degree of ineffective erythropoiesis resulting in a suppression of hepcidin and an increased intestinal iron absorption. In patients receiving chronic red cell transfusions and developing severe iron overload, late symptoms of parenchymal iron loading may include arthritis, diabetes, liver failure, and arrhythmias.

Morphology

The peripheral blood may exhibit a spectrum of morphologies, ranging from normal to dysplastic features typically associated with MDS; however, dysgranulopoiesis is rare. A peripheral blood smear may show macrocytic red cells, normocytic red cells, or a dimorphic population with a subpopulation showing hypochromia. Even rare circulating blasts in peripheral blood are unusual and should prompt consideration of an alternate diagnosis of MDS-EB.[3] The bone marrow core biopsy and aspirate are typically hypercellular and erythroid predominant. Blasts are not elevated (<5% of nucleated cells), and Auer rods are absent. Erythroid dysplasia, manifesting as megaloblastoid change, irregular nuclear segmentation, and/or binucleation, is usually present but may be subtle; dysmegakaryopoiesis and dysgranulopoiesis are less frequent. Although the specific dysplastic lineages may be noted, specification of single lineage dysplasia versus multilineage dysplasia (MLD) is no longer required as this does not have prognostic impact in MDS-SF3B1[3] (Table 13.1). While ring sideroblasts are no longer required to make a diagnosis of MDS-SF3B1, it is still recommended to perform an iron stain on a cellular bone marrow aspirate being evaluated for MDS (Figure 13.1). Ring sideroblasts are defined as an erythroid precursor containing ≥5 perinuclear iron granules encircling one-third or more of the nucleus.[5] Regardless of the MDS subtype, ring sideroblasts define a type of dyserythropoiesis and can help

TABLE 13.1 Diagnostic criteria for MDS with mutated *SF3B1*

Feature	Requirements	Exclusions
Blood counts	At least one cytopenia	Sustained/unexplained leukocytosis (WBC ≥13 × 10^9/L) Sustained/unexplained monocytosis (monocytes ≥0.5 × 10^9/L and ≥10% of WBCs) Sustained/unexplained thrombocytosis (platelets ≥450 × 10^9/L)
Blast percentages	NA	≥5% in bone marrow or ≥2% in blood
Morphology	Dysplasia and ring sideroblasts are typically present but are not required	Auer rods
Cytogenetics	NA	Del(5q), −7, del(7q), abnormal 3q26, or complex karyotype[a]
Molecular genetics	*SF3B1* mutation (VAF ≥10%)	Multi-hit *TP53* mutation[b] *RUNX1* mutation
Other features	NA	NA

[a]Complex karyotype defined as ≥3 independent cytogenetic abnormalities (except -Y).
[b]See chapter 15 for definition of multi-hit *TP53* mutation.
NA, not applicable; VAF, variant allele fraction; WBC, white blood count.

establish an MDS diagnosis, in the absence of non-neoplastic causes of ring sideroblasts such as alcohol, toxins/drugs, copper deficiency, and inherited sideroblastic anemias. Additionally, finding ring sideroblasts increases the pretest probability that an *SF3B1* mutation will be detected once molecular analyses are performed. In MDS cases lacking excess blasts or a defining genetic feature, and where ring sideroblasts are identified but no *SF3B1* mutation is identified, a diagnosis of MDS, not otherwise specified (MDS, NOS) is rendered irrespective of the percentage of ring sideroblasts. In MDS cases lacking *SF3B1* mutation, MLD is associated with an inferior prognosis, while ring sideroblasts appear to have no prognostic relevance.[4,6,7]

MDS-SF3B1 does not have dysplasia as an essential requirement: cases with pathogenic *SF3B1* mutation at variant allele fraction (VAF) ≥10% in the setting of cytopenia share clinical and biologic features with dysplastic MDS-SF3B1 cases.[8] However, in cytopenic patients with an *SF3B1* mutation VAF of <10% and lacking significant dysplasia, a diagnosis of clonal cytopenia of uncertain significance is warranted. In such cases, regular clinical and hematologic follow-up, including periodic bone marrow evaluations, is recommended to monitor for development of overt MDS.

Immunophenotype

CD71 or Glycophorin A can be used to highlight the erythroid lineage, which is usually increased, and CD117 and E-cadherin help identify left-shifted erythroid precursors. CD34 immunohistochemistry on the biopsy specimen can be considered to confirm a lack of increased (≥5%) bone marrow blasts, which would exclude a diagnosis of MDS-SF3B1.

Genetics

SF3B1 is the most commonly mutated spliceosome gene in MDS and has been shown to be an initiating genetic abnormality,[9] a major determinant of clinical and morphologic phenotype, and a prognostically relevant finding. In fact, it is the only MDS-related gene that portends a favorable prognosis.[10] These key features

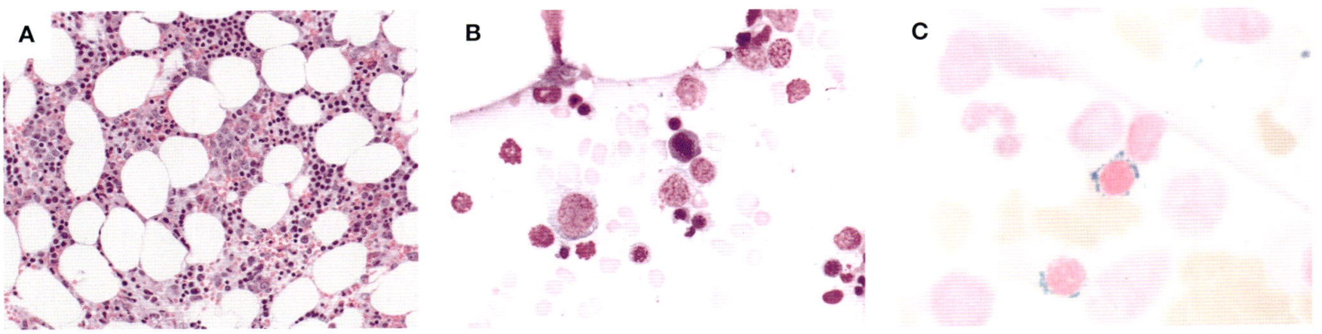

FIGURE 13.1 **A:** Bone marrow core biopsy showing an erythroid predominant marrow. **B:** Aspirate showing a dysplastic erythroid precursor with irregular nuclear contours. **C:** An iron stain of an aspirate with ring sideroblasts, identified by the presence of iron granules closely apposed to the nuclear membrane and encircling at least one-third of the nuclear circumference.

together qualify *SF3B1* mutation as a disease-defining abnormality in MDS. The *SF3B1* mutations are heterozygous, with a hotspot found at codon 700. Other frequent *SF3B1* mutations are found at codons 622, 625, 666, and 662. The mutation is typically at high VAF by definition ≥10%.

Recent studies have shown that, in cases of MDS without excess blasts, identification of an *SF3B1* variant defines a more homogenous group than those defined by ring sideroblasts.[3] Cases of MDS with ring sideroblasts comprise three mutation clusters: mutated *SF3B1, SRSF2,* or multihit *TP53,* each associated with distinct gene expression profiles, alternative splicing profiles, and clinical outcomes.[4] Cases of MDS with ring sideroblasts (irrespective of the number) that lack the *SF3B1* mutation have clinical features and outcomes similar to MDS, NOS (see Chapter 16). Moreover, the *SF3B1* mutation has been shown to outweigh any effect of single versus multilineage dysplasia on the prognosis of lower-risk MDS.[3]

Several genetic features negate the favorable prognosis associated with *SF3B1* mutations and thus preclude classification as MDS-SF3B1 if present. These include del(5q), −7/del(7q), inv(3), other abnormal 3q26, or complex karyotype (defined as ≥3 cytogenetic abnormalities, excluding -Y), as well as *RUNX1* or multihit *TP53* mutation.[3] Various other comutations, including epigenetic regulators such at *DNMT3A*, *TET2*, and *ASXL1,* can accompany the *SF3B1* mutation and have not been shown to affect the overall survival of patients with MDS-SF3B1. However, the outcomes of MDS-SF3B1 are adversely impacted by *BCOR, BCORL1, NRAS, SRSF2,* and *STAG2* mutations.[11] Finally, comutation of *JAK2* (V617F), *CALR*, or *MPL* in the setting of thrombocytosis suggests an alternate diagnosis of MDS/MPN-SF3B1-T.

Prognosis and Clinical Comment

MDS-SF3B1 has a favorable outcome among MDS subtypes, with a median overall survival of 72 to 114 months and 5-year acute myeloid leukemia transformation rate of only 5%.[10-12] Once the *SF3B1* mutation has been accounted for, ring sideroblasts appear to have no prognostic significance and are therefore no longer a requirement for the diagnosis of MDS-SF3B1.[3,13] Most patients are stratified into lower-risk Revised and Molecular International Prognostic Scoring System (IPSS-R and IPSS-M) categories, as they only rarely have adverse cytogenetic abnormalities, by definition lack the adverse mutations *RUNX1* and multihit *TP53,* and have no increase in blasts.[12,14]

Patients with MDS-SF3B1 mostly have symptomatic normo- or macrocytic anemia and may benefit from treatment with erythropoiesis-stimulating agents. More recently, luspatercept has been approved for use in patients receiving regular red cell transfusions who were refractory to or unlikely to respond to erythropoiesis-stimulating agents.[15] In those patients developing regular red cell transfusion dependency, increased levels of toxic iron species have been demonstrated[16] and iron chelation should be considered.[17]

References

1. Arber DA, Orazi A, Hasserjian RP, et al. International consensus classification of myeloid neoplasms and acute leukemias: integrating morphologic, clinical, and genomic data. *Blood.* 2022;140(11):1200-1228.
2. Hasserjian RP, Orazi A, Orfao A, Rozman M, Wang SA. The International Consensus Classification of myelodysplastic syndromes and related entities. *Virchows Arch.* 2023;482(1):39-51.
3. Malcovati L, Stevenson K, Papaemmanuil E, et al. SF3B1-mutant MDS as a distinct disease subtype: a proposal from the International Working Group for the Prognosis of MDS. *Blood.* 2020;136(2):157-170.
4. Todisco G, Creignou M, Bernard E, et al. Integrated genomic and transcriptomic analysis improves disease classification and risk stratification of MDS with ring sideroblasts. *Clin Cancer Res.* 2023;23. online ahead of print.
5. Mufti GJ, Bennett JM, Goasguen J, et al. Diagnosis and classification of myelodysplastic syndrome: international Working Group on morphology of myelodysplastic syndrome (IWGM-MDS) consensus proposals for the definition and enumeration of myeloblasts and ring sideroblasts. *Haematologica.* 2008;93(11):1712-1717.
6. Verburgh E, Achten R, Louw VJ, et al. A new disease categorization of low-grade myelodysplastic syndromes based on the expression of cytopenia and dysplasia in one versus more than one lineage improves on the WHO classification. *Leukemia.* 2007;21(4):668-677.
7. Nazha A, Komrokji R, Meggendorfer M et al Personalized prediction model to risk stratify patients with myelodysplastic syndromes. *J Clin Oncol* 2021;39(33):3737-3746.
8. Galli A, Todisco G, Catamo E, et al. Relationship between clone metrics and clinical outcome in clonal cytopenia. *Blood.* 2021;138(11):965-976.
9. Papaemmanuil E, Cazzola M, Boultwood J, et al. Somatic SF3B1 mutation in myelodysplasia with ring sideroblasts. *N Engl J Med.* 2011;365(15):1384-1395.
10. Malcovati L, Karimi M, Papaemmanuil E, et al. SF3B1mutation identifies a distinct subset of myelodysplastic syndrome with ring sideroblasts. *Blood.* 2015;126(2):233-241.

11. Lee WH, Lin CC, Tsai CH, et al. Clinico-genetic and prognostic analyses of 716 patients with primary myelodysplastic syndrome and myelodysplastic syndrome/acute myeloid leukemia based on the 2022 International Consensus Classification. *Am J Hematol.* 2023;98(3):398-407.
12. Bernard E, Tuechler H, Greenberg PL, et al. Molecular international prognostic scoring system for myelodysplastic syndromes. *NEJM Evid.* 2022;1(7):EVIDoa2200008.
13. Xiong B, Xue M, Yu Y, Wu S, Zuo X. SF3B1 mutation but not ring sideroblasts identifies a specific group of myelodysplastic syndrome-refractory cytopenia with multilineage dysplasia. *Clin Lymphoma, Myeloma & Leukemia.* 2020;20(5):329-339.e3.
14. Greenberg PL, Tuechler H, Schanz J, et al. Revised international prognostic scoring system for myelodysplastic syndromes. *Blood.* 2012;120(12):2454-2465.
15. Fenaux P, Platzbecker U, Mufti G, et al. Luspatercept in patients with lower-risk myelodysplastic syndromes. *N Engl J Med.* 2020;382(2):140-151.
16. Hoeks M, Bagguley T, van Marrewijk C, et al. Toxic iron species in lower-risk myelodysplastic syndrome patients: course of disease and effects on outcome. *Leukemia.* 2021;35(6):1745-1750.
17. Malcovati L, Hellstrom-Lindberg E, Bowen D, et al. Diagnosis and treatment of primary myelodysplastic syndromes in adults: recommendations from the European LeukemiaNet. *Blood.* 2013;122(17):2943-2964.

Chapter 14
Myelodysplastic Syndrome With del(5q)

Leonie Saft and Rami Komrokji

Definition

Myelodysplastic syndrome with del(5q) (MDS-del5q) is defined by the presence of a del(5q) cytogenetic abnormality in isolation or accompanied by one other cytogenetic abnormality, except monosomy 7 or del(7q). Most patients present with anemia with or without other cytopenia(s) and/or thrombocytosis. Dysplasia is almost always present, particularly in the megakaryocytic lineage, but rarely may be mild or absent. Myeloblasts constitute <5% of all nucleated bone marrow cells and <2% of the peripheral blood leukocytes; the presence of 1% blasts in the peripheral blood is allowed if only detected on one occasion. Auer rods are absent.

Synonyms

Myelodysplastic neoplasm with isolated deletion(5q) (not recommended); Myelodysplastic syndrome with isolated del(5q); 5q minus syndrome (not recommended).

Epidemiology

MDS-del5q accounts for approximately 8% of all cases of MDS. It is more common in women (male-to-female ratio: 1:3), with a median age of 73 years.[1]

General Clinical Features

The most common symptoms are related to anemia, which is often moderate to severe and usually macrocytic. Thrombocytosis is present in approximately one-third of cases, whereas thrombocytopenia is uncommon; rarely, patients present with pancytopenia.[2,3] Recent data from the European MDS registry showed that patients with MDS-del5q tend to have lower hemoglobin levels and higher platelet counts in comparison with other patients with MDS and were more likely to have received blood transfusions.[1]

Morphology

The bone marrow is usually hypercellular or normocellular for age. Dysplasia is not required for diagnosis but is almost always present, particularly in the megakaryocytic lineage and also not infrequently in erythroids (Table 14.1). Megakaryocytes are often increased in number and are normal to slightly decreased in size, with nonlobated or hypolobated nuclei (Figure 14.1). Megakaryocyte immunohistochemical markers (eg, CD42 and CD61) can facilitate the identification of these dysplastic megakaryocytes. Erythropoiesis may be decreased and often shows megaloblastoid changes, whereas erythroid nuclear abnormalities are usually

TABLE 14.1 Diagnostic criteria for MDS with del(5q)

Feature	Requirements	Exclusions
Blood counts	At least one cytopenia	Sustained/unexplained leukocytosis (WBC ≥ 13 × 10^9/L)Sustained/unexplained monocytosis (monocytes ≥0.5 × 10^9/L and ≥10% of WBCs)
Blast percentages	NA	≥5% in bone marrow or ≥2% in peripheral blood[a]
Morphology	Dysplasia (megakaryocytic) typically present, but not required	Auer rods
Cytogenetics	del(5q) with up to 1 additional abnormality	−7 or del(7q)
Molecular genetics	NA	Multi-hit *TP53* mutation[b]
Clinical features	NA	NA

MDS, myelodysplastic syndrome; NA, not applicable; VAF, variant allele fraction; WBC, white blood count.
[a]The presence of 1% peripheral blood blasts confirmed on 2 separate occasions qualifies for MDS with excess blasts.
[b]See Chapter 15 for definition of multi-hit TP53.

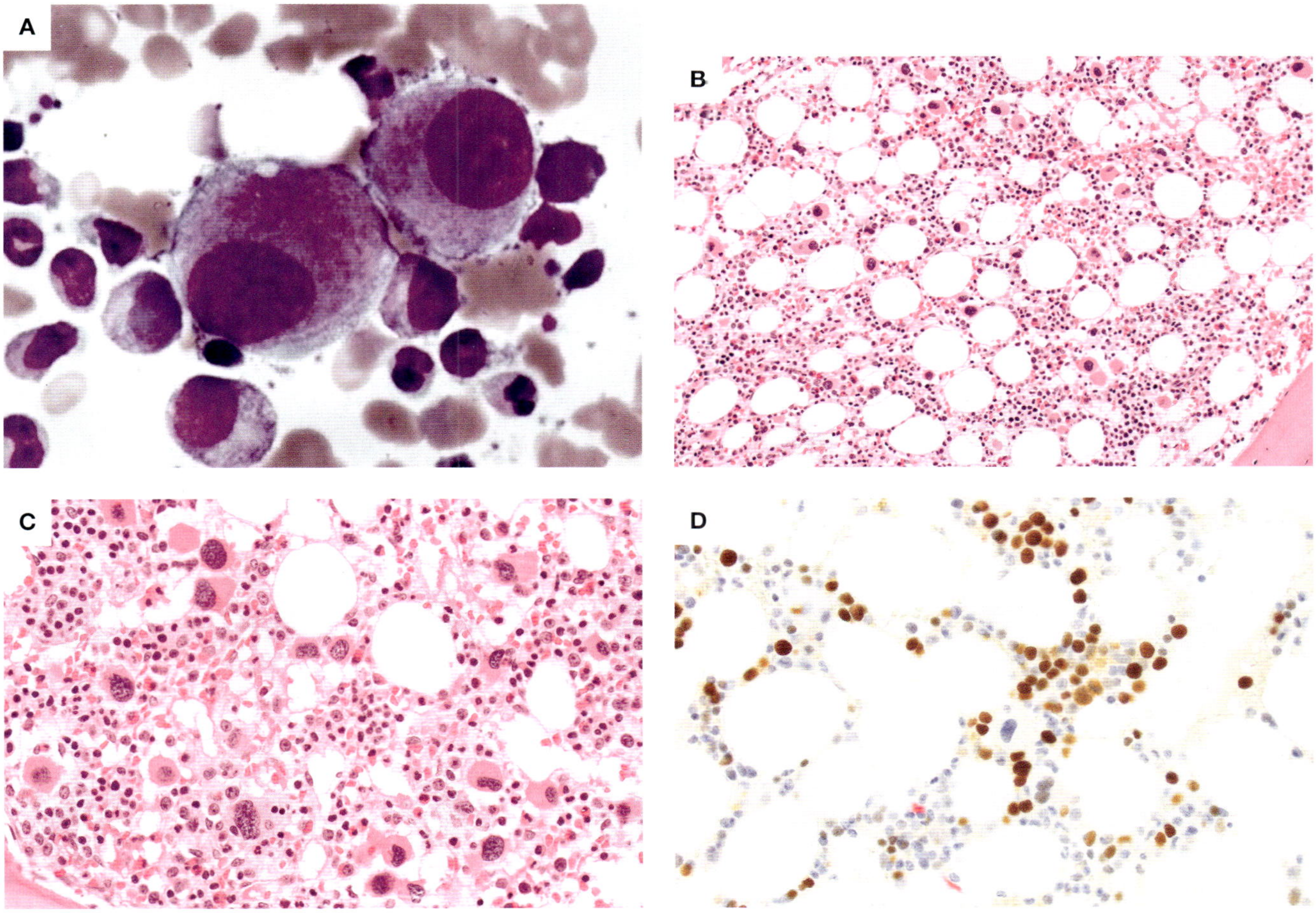

FIGURE 14.1 Myelodysplastic syndrome with del(5q). Bone marrow aspirate smear **(A)** showing two megakaryocytes with nonlobated, rounded nuclei. Bone marrow section (hematoxylin and eosin stain) at lower and higher **(B** and **C)** magnification with an increased number of megakaryocytes with small hypo- and nonlobated nuclei. P53 immunostaining shows an increased number of hematopoietic cells with strong nuclear staining in a patient with monoallelic *TP53* mutation **(D)**.

less pronounced as compared with MDS, not otherwise specified with multilineage dysplasia and higher-risk MDS. Ring sideroblasts may be present and do not exclude the diagnosis of MDS-del5q. Significant granulocytic dysplasia is uncommon and has been associated with an adverse prognosis.[4] The blast percentage is <5% in the bone marrow and <2% in the peripheral blood; 1% blasts in the peripheral blood detected on more than one occasion or the presence of any blasts with Auer rods excludes MDS-del5q and mandates a diagnosis of MDS with excess blasts. Clustering of megakaryocytes and increased reticulin fibrosis (grade 2 or 3) is usually not seen at initial diagnosis but can be a feature of disease progression. P53 immunohistochemical staining is a useful diagnostic marker since strong nuclear p53 staining, even when present at low frequency (<5%), is usually not seen in normal hematopoietic cells and may be associated with *TP53* mutation (see Genetics section).[5]

Immunophenotype

Patients with MDS-del5q tend to have a higher percentage of myeloid progenitors as compared with other lower-risk MDS subtypes and nonclonal cytopenias,[6] and aberrant CD5 and CD7 expression within the myeloid progenitor compartment is seen in a subset of MDS-del5q with high clonal disease burden.[7] A flow cytometry–based 5-parameter-del(5q) score has been proposed, including characteristics of myeloid progenitor cells (percentage and CD45-mean-fluorescence-intensity ratio) and granulocytes (side-scatter ratio and CD71 expression), that predicts for the presence of del(5q).[6]

Genetics

The defining cytogenetic abnormality is an interstitial deletion of chromosome 5 involving bands q31-q33, with or without one additional cytogenetic abnormality, except monosomy 7 or del(7q). An additional cytogenetic aberration is detected in approximately 10% to 15% of MDS-del5q, commonly +8, del(20q), del(1p), del(13q), del(9q), or -Y.[3,8] Recurrently mutated genes in newly diagnosed MDS-del5q are comparable with other MDS subtypes and include *SF3B1*, *DNMT3A*, *TP53*, *ASXL1*, and *JAK2* (Table 14.2); some cases may lack any accompanying mutations. *TP53* mutations have been reported in 15% to 20% of MDS-del5q[3,9]; while the presence of a *SF3B1* or monoallelic *TP53* mutation does not per se override the diagnosis of MDS-del5q, a multi-hit *TP53* mutation (with variant allele fraction [VAF] at least 10%) excludes MDS-del5q and mandates classification as MDS with mutated *TP53*. About 6% of MDS-del5q show concomitant *JAK2* V617F mutation, which has been associated with higher platelet counts as compared with *JAK2* wildtype cases[3] and bone marrow megakaryocyte morphology reminiscent of myeloproliferative neoplasms.[4] Owing to the limited data available, it remains uncertain if co-occurrent *JAK2* V617F affects MDS-del5q prognosis. Until further data are accumulated, it is recommended to classify such cases as MDS-del5q if other features are fulfilled.

Prognosis and Clinical Comment

MDS-del5q is clinically and cytogenetically heterogenous, with diverse individual disease courses influenced by clonal hierarchy and the succession of molecular events. The reported overall median survival ranges between 66 and 145 months, and the risk of acute myeloid leukemia progression is <10% within the first 2 years and 15% to 20% after 5 years.[4,10] *TP53* mutations (which by definition must be monoallelic) have been identified as driving force for clonal evolution, leukemic progression, and treatment resistance.[11] Recently, *TP53* mutation with VAF of ≥22% has been associated with poorer prognosis in MDS-del5q.[12] Unlike in most other MDS, *SF3B1* mutation has shown in some studies to confer adverse prognosis in MDS-del5q.[13,14]

Lenalidomide is the first-line treatment for transfusion-dependent MDS-del(5q), resulting in durable transfusion independency in the majority of patients.[15] Lenalidomide also may benefit patients with MDS-del5q who are not transfusion-dependent.[17] Despite

TABLE 14.2 Recurrently mutated genes in MDS del(5q)

Gene	Pathway/function	Frequency	Clinical and biological correlations
SF3B1	Splicing factor	18%-20%	• Associated with ring sideroblasts • May confer adverse prognosis
DNMT3A	DNA methylation	11%-18%	• Early genetic event; recurrent founder lesion in MDS • May confer adverse prognosis
***TP53* (monoallelic)**	Checkpoint/cell cycle	~18%	• More frequent in MDS-del5q as compared with other lower risk MDS subtypes (<5% blasts)[16] • Associated with increased AML risk, shorter OS, and therapy resistance • Small subclones may be present at an early disease stage
TET2	DNA methylation	~12%	• Early genetic event • May confer adverse prognosis
CSNK1A1	Proliferation, apoptosis, DNA damage response	7%-10%	• Tumor suppressor gene, located in the common deleted region at 5q32 • Associated with older age • Co-occur with *SF3B1* mutations
ASXL1	Chromatin modification	6%-10%	• Mainly frameshift mutations • Associated with disease progression and poor outcome
JAK2	Tyrosine kinase	~6%	• Associated with myeloproliferative features in the BM and elevated platelet counts

AML, acute myeloid leukemia; BM, bone marrow; MDS, myelodysplastic syndrome; OS, overall survival.
Modified from Acha P, Mallo M, Solé F. Myelodysplastic syndromes with isolated del(5q): value of molecular alterations for diagnostic and prognostic assessment. *Cancers (Basel).* 2022;14(22):5531.

this, most patients develop drug resistance after 2 to 3 years of treatment, and neoplastic stem and progenitor cells have shown to persist in the bone marrow of lenalidomide-treated patients in clinical and cytogenetic remission.[18] There is no universally accepted second-line treatment of patients experiencing lenalidomide failure, and only a limited number of patients undergo allogeneic transplantation.[13]

References

1. Bowen D, Taylor A, Fenaux P, et al. Management of MDS with isolated Del(5q) patients in the European MDS (EUMDS) registry, a unique prospective real-world dataset. *Blood.* 2021;138(suppl 1):4671.
2. Gurnari C, Piciocchi A, Soddu S, et al. Myelodysplastic syndromes with del(5q): a real-life study of determinants of long-term outcomes and response to lenalidomide. *Blood Cancer J.* 2022;12(9):132.
3. Meggendorfer M, Haferlach C, Kern W, Haferlach T. Molecular analysis of myelodysplastic syndrome with isolated deletion of the long arm of chromosome 5 reveals a specific spectrum of molecular mutations with prognostic impact: a study on 123 patients and 27 genes. *Haematologica.* 2017;102(9):1502-1510.
4. Patnaik MM, Lasho TL, Finke CM, et al. WHO-defined 'myelodysplastic syndrome with isolated del(5q)' in 88 consecutive patients: survival data, leukemic transformation rates and prevalence of JAK2, MPL and IDH mutations. *Leukemia.* 2010;24(7):1283-1289.
5. Saft L, Karimi M, Ghaderi M, et al. p53 protein expression independently predicts outcome in patients with lower-risk myelodysplastic syndromes with del(5q). *Haematologica.* 2014;99(6):1041-1049.
6. Oelschlaegel U, Westers TM, Mohr B, et al. Myelodysplastic syndromes with a deletion 5q display a characteristic immunophenotypic profile suitable for diagnostics and response monitoring. *Haematologica.* 2015;100(3):e93-e96.
7. Oelschlaegel U, Alexander Röhnert M, Mohr B, et al. Clonal architecture of del(5q) myelodysplastic syndromes: aberrant CD5 or CD7 expression within the myeloid progenitor compartment defines a subset with high clonal burden. *Leukemia.* 2016;30(2):517-520.
8. Gurney M, Patnaik MM, Hanson CA, et al. The 2016 revised World Health Organization definition of "myelodysplastic syndrome with isolated del(5q)"; prognostic implications of single versus double cytogenetic abnormalities. *Br J Haematol.* 2017;178(1): 57-60.
9. Fleti F, Chan O, Singh A, et al. TP53 mutations and variant allele frequency in myelodysplastic syndromes with del(5q): A Mayo-Moffitt study of 156 informative cases. *Am J Hematol.* 2023;98(4):E76-e79.
10. Germing U, Lauseker M, Hildebrandt B, et al. Survival, prognostic factors and rates of leukemic transformation in 381 untreated patients with MDS and del(5q): a multicenter study. *Leukemia.* 2012;26(6):1286-1292.
11. Jadersten M, Saft L, Smith A, et al. TP53 mutations in low-risk myelodysplastic syndromes with del(5q) predict disease progression. *J Clin Oncol.* 2011;29(15): 1971-1979.
12. Tefferi A, Fleti F, Chan O, et al. TP53 variant allele frequency and therapy-related setting independently predict survival in myelodysplastic syndromes with del(5q). *Br J Haematol.* 2024;204(4):1243-1248.
13. Chan O, Ali NA, Sallman D, Padron E, Lancet J, Komrokji R. Therapeutic outcomes and prognostic impact of gene mutations including TP53 and SF3B1 in patients with del(5q) myelodysplastic syndromes (MDS). *Clin Lymphoma Myeloma Leuk.* 2022;22(7):e467-e476.
14. Bernard E, Tuechler H, Greenberg PL, et al. Molecular international prognostic scoring system for myelodysplastic syndromes. *N Engl J Med Evid.* 2022;1(7).
15. List A, Dewald G, Bennett J, et al. Lenalidomide in the myelodysplastic syndrome with chromosome 5q deletion. *N Engl J Med.* 2006;355(14):1456-1465.
16. Stengel A, Meggendorfer M, Walter W, et al. Interplay of TP53 allelic state, blast count, and complex karyotype on survival of patients with AML and MDS. *Blood Adv.* 2023;7(18):5540-5548.
17. Lopez Cadenas F, Lumreras E, Xicoy B, et al. Phase 3 study of lenalidomide (LEN) vs placebo in non-transfusion dependent (TD) low risk del(5q) MDS patients - interim analysis of the European Sintra-REV trial. *Blood.* 2020;136(suppl 1):28-29.
18. Tehranchi R, Woll PS, Anderson K, et al. Persistent malignant stem cells in del(5q) myelodysplasia in remission. *N Engl J Med.* 2010;363(11):1025-1037.

Chapter 15

Myelodysplastic Syndrome With Mutated *TP53*

Mariko Yabe, Robert P. Hasserjian, David A. Sallman, and Olga K. Weinberg

Definition

Myelodysplastic syndrome with mutated *TP53* (MDS-TP53) is defined as a myeloid neoplasm in a cytopenic patient with up to 9% blasts and presence of multi-hit (bi-allelic) *TP53* alteration. MDS-TP53 is considered in an overarching *TP53*-mutated myeloid neoplasm group together with MDS/AML with mutated *TP53* and AML with mutated *TP53* due to their poor outcomes irrespective of the blast percentage. However, for classification purposes, these cases continue to be separately designated as MDS (0%-9% blasts), MDS/AML (10%-19% blasts), or AML (≥20% blasts) with mutated *TP53*, based on the blast percentage thresholds defining these three diseases.

Synonyms

Myelodysplastic neoplasm with biallelic *TP53* inactivation (not recommended).

Epidemiology

Mutations of *TP53* (including both monoallelic and multi-hit) are observed in 5% to 10% of patients with MDS overall, and both alleles of *TP53* are affected by mutation and/or deletion (multi-hit or biallelic state) in about two-thirds of *TP53*-mutated MDS cases.[1-3] Multi-hit *TP53* mutations are more common in therapy-related MDS (about 40% of cases).[2,3] In some settings, such as tertiary academic centers and prospective phase 3 trials, *TP53* mutant disease can represent upto 30% of MDS patient cohorts.

General Clinical Features

Patients with MDS-TP53, like other MDS patients, usually exhibit symptoms related to cytopenia, most frequently fatigue, shortness of breath, and decreased functional status as well as signs and symptoms related to bleeding and infections. Importantly, rates of neutropenic fever and early mortality are higher in MDS-TP53 compared to other MDS patients, potentially related to the adverse effect of this mutation on the underling immune microenvironment.[4] Some patients may be asymptomatic at initial presentation.

Morphology

MDS-TP53 typically shows significant dysplasia in multiple hematopoietic lineages; however, the presence of dysplasia is not required for the diagnosis in a cytopenic patient. In peripheral blood, the red blood cells are often macrocytic. The bone marrow biopsy is typically hypercellular (Figure 15.1A). Over one-half of cases lack excess blasts (<5% blasts) and the majority of these show multilineage dysplasia.[2,5] Prominent dyserythropoiesis is often present, including nuclear budding, karyorrhexis, multinuclearity, and megaloblastoid changes, and marrow is often erythroid-rich with decreased M:E ratio (Figure 15.1B). Erythroid precursors frequently show left-shifted maturation; however, they exhibit full maturation to the stage of mature nucleated erythroid cells, in contrast to the sheets of malignant pronormoblasts that characterize pure erythroid leukemia (a morphologic subtype of AML with mutated *TP53*). Ring sideroblasts may be present, and if they occur in the setting of increased blasts and/or chromosome 5 aberrations, can suggest the presence of a *TP53* mutation.[6] Dysgranulopoiesis and prominent dysmegakaryopoiesis are also often associated with MDS-TP53. A significant degree of reticulin fibrosis (grade 2 or 3 according to the WHO grading system) can be seen.

TP53 immunohistochemistry to evaluate mutant p53 protein accumulation within neoplastic cells can aid in screening for *TP53* mutation: *TP53* mutation is suspected in MDS when strong nuclear staining is observed in at least 2% of cells in the bone marrow biopsy (Figure 15.1C).[7,8] However, cases with truncating *TP53* mutations may exhibit negative p53 immunohistochemistry throughout the biopsy. These p53

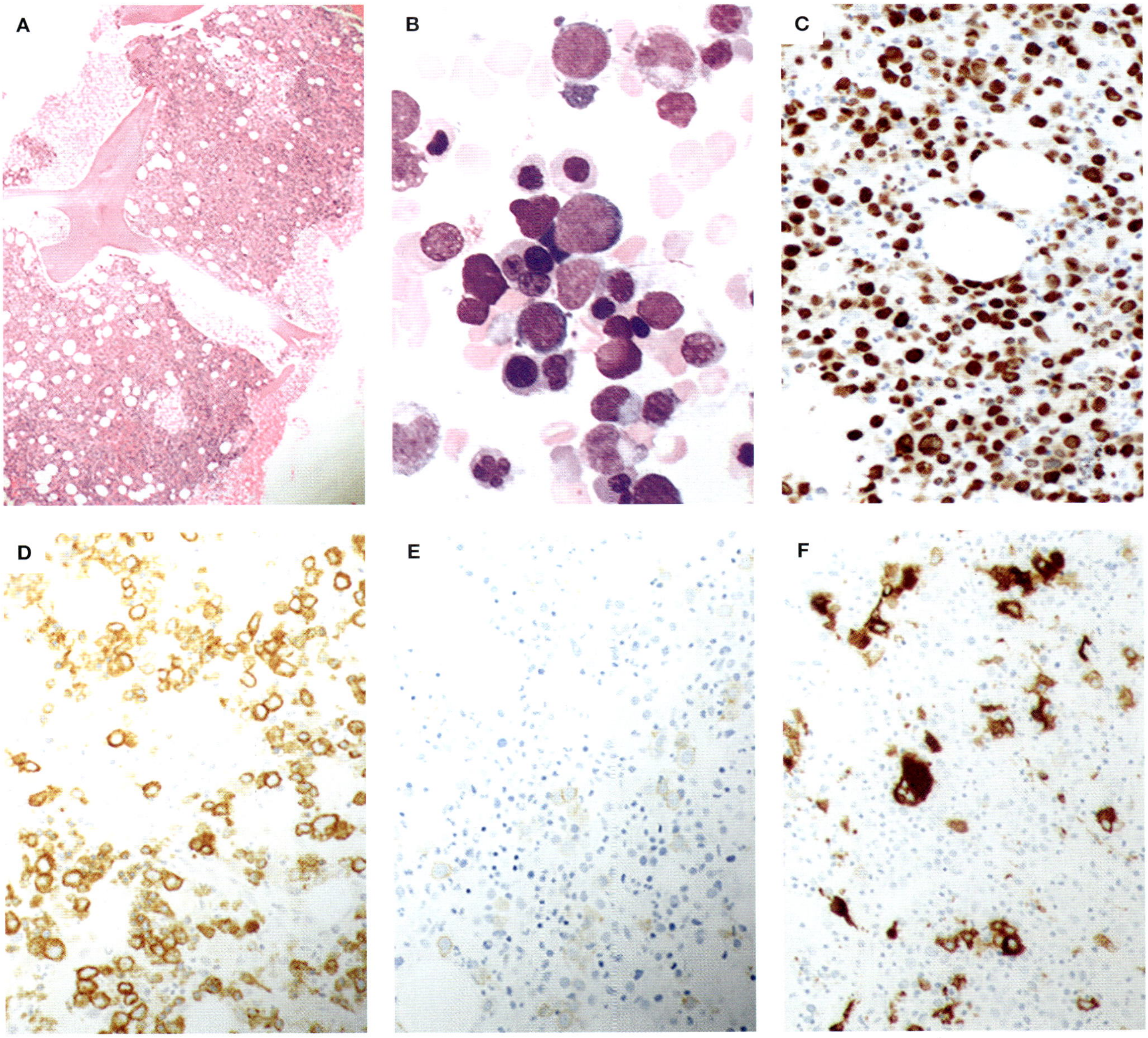

FIGURE 15.1 Myelodysplastic syndrome with mutated *TP53* (MDS-TP53). **A:** Marrow is typically hypercellular for age. **B:** Aspirate smear shows prominent dyserythropoiesis (multinucleation, nuclear budding, nuclear-cytoplasmic desynchrony). **C:** p53 immunohistochemistry shows strong nuclear stain in all three lineages. This case has *TP53* p.R248Q mutation with VAF of 64.3%, fulfilling criteria for multi-hit state (VAF > 50%). **D:** Immunohistochemistry for CD71 shows erythroid-predominant hematopoiesis. **E:** E-cadherin immunohistochemistry shows that only a small subset of erythroid precursors are early-stage erythroid cells, indicating intact maturation of erythroid lineage. **F:** CD61 immunohistochemistry highlights many dysplastic megakaryocytes.

immunohistochemistry results should always be confirmed with genetic testing, and p53 staining does not distinguish between monoallelic and multi-hit *TP53* lesions. Markers of erythroid precursors (eg, E-cadherin and CD71) may be helpful to estimate the number of primitive erythroblasts to differentiate MDS-TP53 from pure erythroid leukemia (Figure 15.1D and E). CD61 immunohistochemistry is also helpful to evaluate for the presence of dysplastic megakaryocytes, especially micromegakaryocytes or other abnormally small forms with hypolobated nuclei, which are frequently seen in MDS-TP53 (Figure 15.1F).

Immunophenotype

Flow cytometry usually reveals immunophenotypic abnormalities in various cell populations including aberrant immunophenotypes of myeloblasts and abnormal maturation patterns in granulocytes and erythroid cells. Increased numbers of blasts positive for CD34 and CD117 can be seen. However, the bone marrow blast count obtained by flow cytometry immunophenotyping is not recommended to substitute for the morphologic blast count, as it is often influenced by the dilution of the marrow aspirate by peripheral blood and loss of erythroid cells after erythrolysis; the latter can be significant in MDS-TP53, which frequently shows erythroid-predominant hematopoiesis.

Genetics

MDS-TP53 requires biallelic hits to the *TP53* gene (multi-hit or biallelic status). As *TP53* functions as a tumor suppressor gene, both copies of the gene must be inactivated by mutation and/or deletion to fully realize the loss of its tumor suppressor function. Since small, stable *TP53* clones can occur in clonal hematopoiesis of undetermined significance (CCUS), a minimal *TP53* mutation variant allele frequency (VAF) of 10% is required for the diagnosis of MDS-TP53. Multi-hit *TP53* status in MDS can be confirmed by the presence of any of the following: (1) two or more distinct *TP53* mutations (each at VAF ≥ 10%); (2) a single *TP53* mutation with VAF of >50%; or (3) a single *TP53* mutation (VAF ≥ 10%) associated with either: (a) deletion involving the *TP53* locus at 17p13.1 detected by cytogenetics or FISH; or (b) copy number-neutral loss of heterozygosity (LOH) at the 17p *TP53* locus (Table 15.1; Figure 15.2).[2,9,10] In the absence of LOH information (which is not available in many laboratories), the presence of a single *TP53* mutation at VAF ≥ 10% in the context of any complex karyotype is considered equivalent to a multi-hit *TP53* status. This is based on evidence that multi-hit *TP53* is strongly associated with complex karyotype, whereas a true monoallelic *TP53* mutation usually displays a noncomplex karyotype.[2,9] Recent data suggest differences in the pathogenicity and effect on disease outcome of specific *TP53* mutations, but it remains to be determined if different types of mutations or mutation phenotype scores should be incorporated into risk stratification of *TP53*-mutated cases.[5] It should be noted that the diagnosis of MDS-TP53 requires the presence of at least one mutated *TP53* gene: complex karyotype alone without a *TP53* mutation, even with 17p deletion, does not qualify for this category, as these cases have a better prognosis compared to MDS-TP53.[11,12]

Monoallelic *TP53* mutations in MDS have different biology from cases with multi-hit *TP53* mutation and are not included within the MDS-TP53 category. For example, overall genetic profile differs among the *TP53* allelic states, in that patients with monoallelic mutations frequently have several co-mutations and usually lack complex karyotypes, while patients with multi-hit *TP53* alterations have fewer co-mutations and nearly always have complex karyotypes. However, monoallelic *TP53* mutation appears to confer a similarly poor prognosis to cases with multi-hit mutation in patients with ≥10%, and thus monoallelic *TP53* mutations are allowed in MDS/AML with mutated *TP53* (Table 15.2).[9]

The pathogenesis of MDS-TP53 is still unclear. MDS-TP53 is frequently associated with complex karyotype, aneuploidy, and chromothripsis.[13] Unlike most

TABLE 15.1 Diagnostic criteria for MDS with mutated *TP53*

Feature	Requirements	Exclusions
Blood counts	At least one cytopenia	Sustained/unexplained leukocytosis (WBC ≥ 13 × 10^9/L) Sustained/unexplained monocytosis (monocytes ≥ 0.5 × 10^9/L and ≥10% of WBCs) Sustained/unexplained thrombocytosis (platelets ≥ 450 × 10^9/L)
Blast percentages	NA	≥10% in bone marrow or ≥10% in blood
Morphology	Dysplasia typically present, but not required	NA
Cytogenetics	Usually complex,[a] but not required	NA
Molecular genetics	Multi-hit TP53 mutation: (1) One *TP53* mutation with VAF ≥ 10% and del(17p), or (2) Two or more *TP53* mutations each with VAF ≥ 10%, or (3) Single *TP53* mutation with VAF >50%, or (4) Single *TP53* mutation with LOH at the 17p *TP53* locus[b]	NA
Other features	NA	NA

[a]Complex karyotype defined as three or more independent cytogenetic aberrations (excluding -Y).
[b]Single *TP53* mutation with VAF ≥10% and unknown LOH status allowed in the setting of complex karyotype.

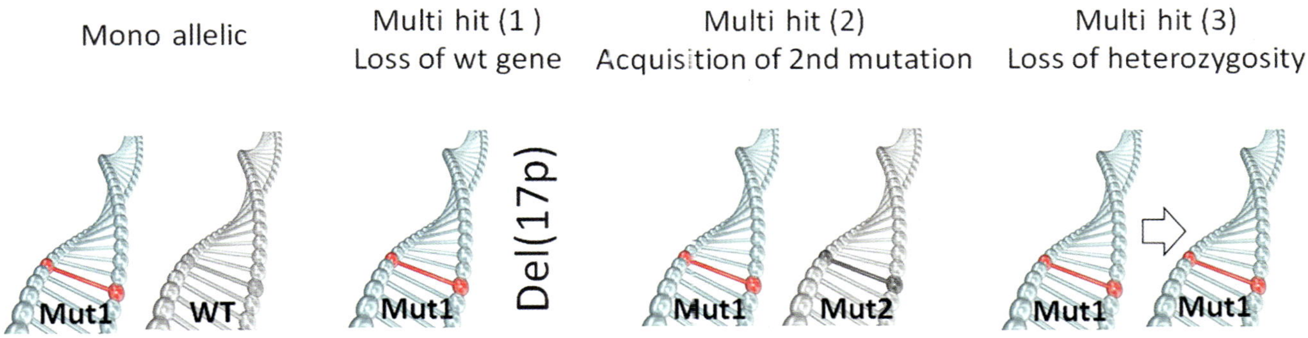

FIGURE 15.2 *TP53* allelic status. Multi-hit mutation can be defined by (1) Single *TP53* mutation (VAF ≥ 10%) + del (17p) on karyotype or FISH, (2) Two or more distinct *TP53* mutations (each at VAF ≥ 10%), (3) A single *TP53* mutation (VAF ≥ 10%) with copy-neutral loss of heterozygosity (LOH) at the 17p *TP53* locus, VAF of >50%, or complex karyotype if LOH status is unknown.

other MDS, mutations in epigenetic modifiers (*DNMT3A*, *TET2*, or *ASXL1*) or spliceosome genes (*U2AF1*, *SF3B1*, *SRSF2*, or *ZRSR2*) are relatively uncommon.[13] ETV6 expression is reduced in nearly all cases, either through gene deletion or presumed epigenetic silencing and telomere content is increased compared to other myeloid malignancies, implicating altered telomere maintenance for pathogenesis.[13] These observations suggest a distinct mechanism of disease progression and leukemic transformation in MDS-TP53 compared to other MDS cases.

Prognosis and Clinical Comment

Overall, MDS-TP53, with or without excess blasts, represents a homogeneous entity with poor outcomes (median OS ~ 1 year); the vast majority of patients fall into higher risk categories of IPSS-R and IPSS-M schemes. Some studies have suggested that a *TP53* mutation VAF >23% may more optimally reflect a multi-hit *TP53* status than the current VAF threshold of >50%.[2,9,14] There also remains some controversy over possible influence of blast percentage on patient outcome. Several recent large cohorts of patients suggest that cases with >5% have a more uniformly poor prognosis.[9,12,15] Importantly, in two of these studies, the allelic status of *TP53* did not add further prognostic discrimination in patients with >5% blasts. Thus, in the future, the definition of MDS-TP53 may evolve with accumulation of additional data.

From a treatment perspective, both MDS and AML with mutated *TP53* have had poor responses to all standard-of-care therapies and generally short survivals.[4] Thus, all patients are highly recommended for clinical trial for first-line therapy with the goal of achieving complete remission, ideally with clearance of the *TP53* mutation, and ultimately bridged to allogeneic stem cell transplantation. Outside of clinical trials, hypomethylating agents with or without venetoclax represent the most commonly used frontline therapies, although median overall survivals remain at only 6 to 12 months. Thus, novel clinical trials and hope for a new standard of care are urgently needed for this molecular group.

TABLE 15.2 Myeloid neoplasms with mutated *TP53*

Type	Cytopenia	Blasts	Genetics
MDS with mutated *TP53*	At least one lineage, no unexplained and sustained cytosis[a]	0%-9% in bone marrow and blood	Multi-hit *TP53* mutation[b] or One *TP53* mutation (VAF ≥10%) and complex karyotype[c]
MDS/AML with mutated *TP53*	At least one lineage, no unexplained and sustained cytosis[a]	10%-19% in bone marrow or blood	Any somatic *TP53* mutation (VAF ≥10%)
AML with mutated *TP53*	Not required	≥20% in bone marrow or blood, or meets the criteria for pure erythroid leukemia	Any somatic *TP53* mutation (VAF ≥10%)

[a]Cytopenia: anemia, Hb < 13 g/dL [males], <12 g/dL [females]; neutropenia, ANC < 1.8 × 10^9/L; thrombocytopenia, platelets < 150 × 10^9/L. Cytosis: sustained WBC count ≥ 13 × 10^9/L, monocytosis (≥0.5 × 10^9/L and ≥10% of leukocytes), or platelets ≥450 × 10^9/L.

[b]Defined as per Table 15.1.

[c]If *TP53* locus LOH information is not available. Complex karyotype is defined as three independent cytogenetic aberrations (excluding -Y).

References

1. Papaemmanuil E, Gerstung M, Malcovati L, et al. Clinical and biological implications of driver mutations in myelodysplastic syndromes. *Blood*. 2013;122(22):3616-3699. quiz 3699.
2. Bernard E, Nannya Y, Hasserjian RP, et al. Implications of TP53 allelic state for genome stability, clinical presentation and outcomes in myelodysplastic syndromes. *Nat Med*. 2020;26(10):1549-1556.
3. Singhal D, Wee LYA, Kutyna MM, et al. The mutational burden of therapy-related myeloid neoplasms is similar to primary myelodysplastic syndrome but has a distinctive distribution. *Leukemia*. 2019;33(12):2842-2853.
4. Daver NG, Maiti A, Kadia TM, et al. TP53-Mutated myelodysplastic syndrome and acute myeloid leukemia: biology, current therapy, and future directions. *Cancer Discov*. 2022;12(11):2516-2529.
5. Yabe M, Omarbekova AZ, Hsu M, et al. TP53 combined phenotype score is associated with the clinical outcome of TP53-mutated myelodysplastic syndromes. *Cancers*. 2021;13(21):5502.
6. Swoboda DM, Kanagal-Shamanna R, Brunner AM, et al. Marrow ring sideroblasts are highly predictive for TP53 mutation in MDS with excess blasts. *Leukemia*. 2022;36(4):1189-1192.
7. Oliva EN, Latagliata R, Sabattini E, et al. Accuracy of bone marrow histochemical TP53 expression compared to the detection of TP53 somatic mutations in patients with myelodysplastic syndromes harbouring a del5q cytogenetic abnormality. *Am J Blood Res*. 2021;11(4):417-426.
8. Cleven AH, Nardi V, Ok CY, et al. High p53 protein expression in therapy-related myeloid neoplasms is associated with adverse karyotype and poor outcome. *Mod Pathol*. 2015;28(4):552-563.
9. Grob T, Al Hinai ASA, Sanders MA, et al. Molecular characterization of mutant TP53 acute myeloid leukemia and high-risk myelodysplastic syndrome. *Blood*. 2022;139(15):2347-2354.
10. Sallman DA, Komrokji R, Vaupel C, et al. Impact of TP53 mutation variant allele frequency on phenotype and outcomes in myelodysplastic syndromes. *Leukemia*. 2016;30(3):666-673.
11. Haase D, Stevenson KE, Neuberg D, et al. TP53 mutation status divides myelodysplastic syndromes with complex karyotypes into distinct prognostic subgroups. *Leukemia*. 2019;33(7):1747-1758.
12. Weinberg OK, Siddon A, Madanat YF, et al. TP53 mutation defines a unique subgroup within complex karyotype de novo and therapy-related MDS/AML. *Blood Adv*. 2022;6(9):2847-2853.
13. Abel HJ, Oetjen KA, Miller CA, et al. Genomic landscape of TP53-mutated myeloid malignancies. *Blood Adv*. 2023;7(16):4586-4598.
14. Bahaj W, Kewan T, Gurnari C, et al. Novel scheme for defining the clinical implications of TP53 mutations in myeloid neoplasia. *J Hematol Oncol*. 2023;16(1):91.
15. Stengel A, Meggendorfer M, Walter W, et al. Interplay of TP53 allelic state, blast count and complex karyotype on survival of patients with AML and MDS. *Blood Adv*. 2023;7(18):5540-5548.

Chapter 16

Myelodysplastic Syndrome, Not Otherwise Specified

Olga Pozdnyakova, John M. Bennett, Amy E. DeZern, and Sa A. Wang

Definition

Myelodysplastic syndrome, not otherwise specified (MDS, NOS) includes three morphologic subtypes: MDS, NOS without dysplasia, MDS, NOS with single lineage dysplasia (MDS-NOS-SLD), and MDS, NOS with multilineage dysplasia (MDS-NOS-MLD). All MDS, NOS subtypes are characterized by the presence of one or more cytopenia(s), the absence of increased blasts in blood or bone marrow, and failure to meet the criteria for the genetically defined MDS subtypes MDS-SF3B1, MDS-del5q, and MDS-TP53.[1] Most MDS, NOS fall in lower-risk categories by current MDS prognostic scoring systems.[2]

Synonyms

MDS with single lineage dysplasia (SLD); MDS with multilineage dysplasia (MLD); MDS, unclassifiable (subtype defined by MDS-defining cytogenetic abnormality without dysplasia)[3]; MDS with low blasts; MDS, hypoplastic; MDS with low blasts and ring sideroblasts (not recommended).[4]

Epidemiology

MDS, NOS is a newly categorized group of MDS that is similar to the WHO-revised fourth edition entities of MDS-SLD and MDS-MLD; however, it now excludes cases of MDS-TP53 and includes cases previously classified as MDS with ring sideroblasts that are not MDS-SF3B1 (Table 16.1). Given the novelty of this morphologically defined MDS category, its precise incidence is not known. Three recent studies found that MDS, NOS comprised 37% to 46% of all MDS cases, with 22% to 39% MDS-NOS-MLD, 7% to 15% MDS-NOS-SLD, and <1% MDS, NOS, without dysplasia.[5,6] Similar to the other MDS categories, the incidence of

TABLE 16.1 Diagnostic criteria for the MDS, NOS category

Feature	Requirements	Exclusions
Blood counts	At least one cytopenia	Sustained/unexplained leukocytosis (WBC ≥ 13 × 10^9/L) Sustained/unexplained monocytosis (monocytes ≥ 0.5 × 10^9/L and ≥10% of WBCs) Sustained/unexplained thrombocytosis (platelets ≥ 450 × 10^9/L
Blast percentages	NA	≥5% in bone marrow or ≥2% in blood[a]
Morphology	MDS-NOS-SLD: dysplasia[b] in one lineage MDS-NOS-MLD: dysplasia[b] in two lineages MDS, NOS, without dysplasia: No significant dysplasia[b] in any lineage	Auer rods
Cytogenetics	MDS, NOS, without dysplasia:−7, del(7q), or complex karyotype[c]	Isolated del(5q) or del(5q) with 1 additional abnormality other than −7/del(7q)
Molecular genetics	NA	Multi-hit *TP53* mutation[d]
Other features	NA	Meeting criteria for MDS with mutated *SF3B1*

[a]The presence of 1% PB blasts confirmed on 2 separate occasions qualifies for MDS with excess blasts.
[b]Morphologic dysplasia is defined as ≥10% dysplastic forms in one or more lineages.
[c]Complex karyotype defined as at least 3 independent cytogenetic abnormalities (excluding -Y).
[d]See chapter 15 for definition of multi-hit TP53.
Chiravuri S, De Jesus O. Pancytopenia. In: *StatPearls*. StatPearls Publisiong; 2023. Accessed February 12, 2023. https://www.ncbi.nlm.nih.gov/books/NBK563146/

MDS, NOS increases with age and is more common in men than in women.[7]

General Clinical Features

Patients with MDS, NOS most often present with clinical findings related to their cytopenia(s), such as fatigue, weakness, exercise intolerance, bleeding, bruising, or infections; some patients are completely asymptomatic and come to medical attention solely due to an abnormal complete blood cell count discovered during a routine examination.

Anemia is the most common presenting cytopenia and usually macrocytic (MCV > 100 fL) and accompanied by an elevated red cell distribution width (usually > 14.5%, depending on the laboratory reference ranges). However, the global frequency of anemia in people >65 years of age is approximately 17%, reaching nearly 50% in individuals over 80 years of age, far greater than the prevalence of MDS.[8] As a result, patients presenting with anemia require an extensive work-up to exclude nonclonal causes, such as nutritional deficiency, blood loss, chronic inflammation, or chronic kidney disease. MDS may coexist with other factors contributing to anemia; therefore, a thorough diagnostic approach is needed. The diagnosis is established in a patient with persistent unexplained cytopenia by demonstrating requisite dysplasia and/or genetic aberrations on a bone marrow biopsy.

Morphology

The dysplastic morphologic features are summarized in Table 16.2.

The peripheral blood smear often shows the presence of normochromic, macrocytic RBCs, often with a dimorphic pattern. White blood cells vary in number and proportions. Mature granulocytes may demonstrate dysplastic morphology in the form of cytoplasmic hypogranulation, or rarely hypergranulation, and/or hyposegmentation (nonlobated or bilobed, pseudo-Pelger-Huët cells) (Figure 16.1A-D). Rare blasts may be present, but not reaching 2% of WBC. However, a finding of 1% blasts confirmed on two separate occasions in the absence of any secondary cause for increased blasts (such as infection, growth factor, or recovery from treatment), qualifies for MDS with excess blasts.[9] Platelet count may be normal or decreased; large platelets may be seen due to abnormal megakaryopoiesis.

The bone marrow biopsy usually shows increased overall cellularity; however, 10% to 15% of cases may show marrow hypocellularity relative to the patient's age. There is often a disturbed distribution of hematopoietic cells. Based on comprehensive review of each cell lineage in the bone marrow biopsy, aspirate smear, and peripheral blood smear, MDS, NOS is subdivided into MDS-NOS-SLD (if dysplasia ≥10% is limited to one hematopoietic lineage), MDS-NOS-MLD (if dysplasia ≥10% is seen in two or all three hematopoietic lineages), or MDS, NOS without dysplasia (if dysplasia <10% in any lineage). It is important to note that the lineage(s) manifesting dysplasia may not correspond to the actual cytopenic linage(s).

Dyserythropoiesis manifests as nuclear budding, internuclear chromatin bridging, multinucleation, karyorrhexis, basophilic stippling, and poor hemoglobinization visualized in the aspirate smear, and ring sideroblasts visualized on an iron-stained smear

TABLE 16.2 Range of morphologic abnormalities in MDS, NOS

Lineage	Erythroid	Granulocytic[a]	Megakaryocytic
Blood	Basophilic stippling Howell-Jolly bodies Nucleated RBC	Unilobed nuclei Bilobed nuclei (pseudo-Pelger-Huët cells) Hypogranulation Hypergranulation Uneven granulation Abnormal chromatin clumping	Giant platelets Hypogranular platelets Agranular platelets
Bone marrow	Multinucleation Nuclear budding Internuclear chromatin bridging Karyorrhexis Megaloblastoid changes Cytoplasmic vacuolization Ring sideroblasts	Abnormal granulation Left-shifted myelopoiesis clusters of 2-3 blasts	Hypolobated nuclei Multiple separated nuclei Micromegakaryocytes.

[a]Auer rods in blasts are excluded from this diagnostic category.

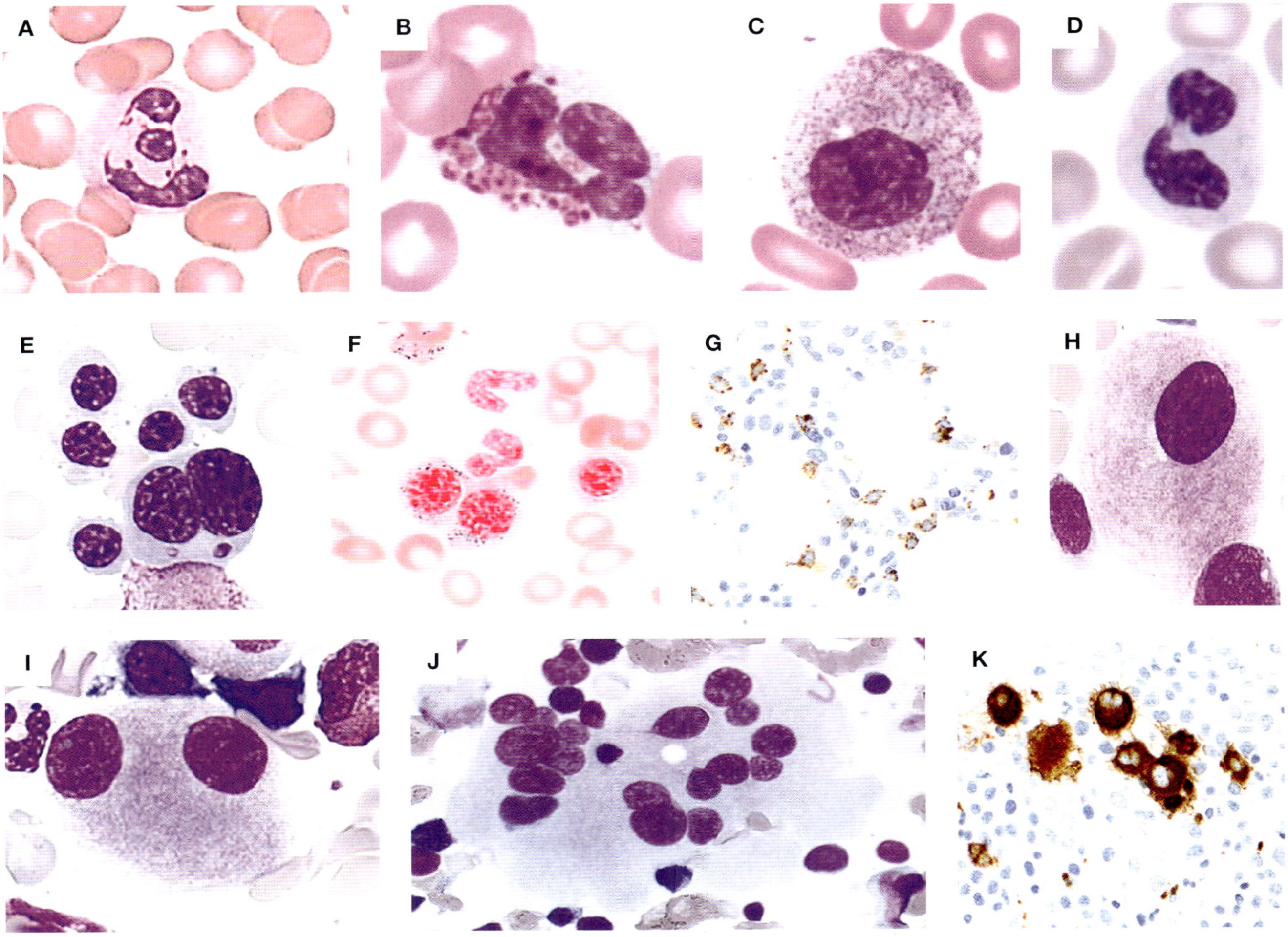

FIGURE 16.1 Spectrum of morphologic changes in myelodysplastic syndrome. **A:** Dysplastic neutrophil with abnormal nuclear lobation. **B:** Dysplastic neutrophil with uneven granulation with large granules. **C:** Dysplastic neutrophil with non-lobated nucleus with hypergranulation. **D:** Dysplastic neutrophil with bilobed (pseudo-Pelger-Huët nucleus) with hypogranulation. **E:** Dysplastic erythroid precursors with bilobed nuclei, nuclear fragments, and nuclear to cytoplasmic dyssynchrony. **F:** Ring sideroblasts on iron stain. **G:** Small clusters of blasts on CD34 stain. **H:** Dysplastic megakaryocyte with one round nucleus. **I:** Dysplastic megakaryocyte with two separated nuclei. **J:** Dysplastic megakaryocytes with multiple separated nuclei. **K:** Small megakaryocytes on CD61 stain.

(Figure 16.1E and F). Megaloblastoid changes associated with erythroid nuclear to cytoplasmic (N:C) dyssynchrony (immature nucleus and more mature cytoplasm) can be a manifestation of dysplasia, but should not be considered as dysplasia by itself. Cytoplasmic vacuolization can be seen in dysplastic early erythroid forms; however, the finding of cytoplasmic vacuolization both in the erythroid and myeloid lineages, especially in male patients, should alert to the possibility of VEXAS syndrome, a rare congenital severe inflammatory disorder associated with variants in the *UBA1* gene; importantly, VEXAS syndrome can coexist with MDS if there is qualifying dysplasia (excluding vacuolation), and most such cases fall into the MDS, NOS category.[10] An iron stain may show the presence of ring sideroblasts (Figure 16.1F), a finding that should prompt molecular testing to evaluate for the presence of an *SF3B1* pathogenic variant, which would warrant a diagnosis of MDS-SF3B1 if the allele frequency is ≥10% and other features are fulfilled. [see Chapter 13]. In the absence of *SF3B1* pathogenic variant, the percentage of ring sideroblasts should be noted in the report; however, such cases do not represent a specific MDS, NOS subtype and should be subclassified based on the number of dysplastic lineages; a recent study has shown that in the absence of defining features of MDS-SF3B1, ring sideroblasts do not bear prognostic significance in MDS, NOS.[11]

Granulocytic dysplasia in bone marrow aspirate smears shows features similar to the peripheral blood and includes hypo- or hypergranularity, uneven granulation, mono- or binucleation, dense chromatin, and small cell size. Dysplastic changes may also be observed in granulocytic precursors, such as hypogranulation, irregularly shaped and distributed granules, and small myelocytes. Dysgranulopoiesis may be limited to peripheral blood or bone marrow; therefore, it is essential to assess both. Auer rods represent a type of granulocytic dysplasia and are pathognomonic of myeloid neoplasia; if present in blasts, they exclude a diagnosis of MDS, NOS and warrant a diagnosis of MDS with excess blasts.

A well-prepared bone marrow aspirate smear is essential for accurate blast enumeration. The blast count should be less than 5% in the bone marrow. It is important to note that myeloblasts in MDS may be small and primitive-appearing, and may be difficult to distinguish from mature lymphocytes in thick areas of the smears. Additional immunophenotypic evaluation by immunohistochemistry for CD34 on the bone marrow may be required to corroborate the aspirate blast count, especially when the aspirate smear is suboptimal (Figure 16.1G).

Megakaryocytes may be increased, decreased, or normal in numbers. If present, megakaryocytic dysplasia manifests in the form of hypolobated or non-lobated, round nuclei, multiple separated nuclei, or micromegakaryocytes (small forms approximately the size of a promyelocyte). The assessment of megakaryocytic dysplasia should be based on the evaluation of at least 30 megakaryocytes when feasible, and should also be carefully evaluated in the aspirate smear in addition to the biopsy (Figure 16.1H-J). Megakaryocyte immunohistochemical stains (such as CD42 or CD61) or periodic acid-Schiff (PAS) stains can be helpful in highlighting the overall number as well as the morphology of megakaryocytes on the biopsy (Figure 16.1K). The normal "young" (early regenerating) megakaryocytes often have monolobated nuclei but abundant cytoplasmic granules; it is important not to misidentify them as dysplastic megakaryocytes. Although dysplastic morphologic changes seen in 10% or greater cells are considered dysplasia of that lineage, this cutoff may not be sufficient for dysmegakaryopoiesis in MDS when including dysplastic forms other than micromegakaryocytes. When including normal-sized forms with hypolobated nuclei or multiple separated nuclear lobes, or megakaryocytes with "naked" nuclei, a higher threshold (30% or 40%) may be more appropriate.

Some MDS, NOS cases present with hypocellular bone marrow, which raises the differential diagnosis of aplastic anemia (AA), paroxysmal nocturnal hemoglobinuria (PNH), or a congenital bone marrow failure syndrome. The distinction relies on careful morphologic evaluation to document significant dysplasia and exclusion of germline mutations as well as *PIGA* mutation that would suggest an alternate diagnosis of PNH. Currently, the ICC does not recognize a specific entity of hypoplastic MDS.

Immunophenotype

The blasts in MDS express CD34 in over 95% of cases in addition to typical myeloid markers, facilitating their enumeration in the bone marrow biopsy.[12] A finding of 2-3-cell CD34$^+$ blasts clusters in the bone marrow biopsy is abnormal and confers adverse prognosis in MDS, NOS (Figure 16.1G). CD71 (transferrin receptor) and E-cadherin help differentiate immature erythroid precursors from myeloid precursors. CD41 (platelet glycoprotein IIb) and CD61 (platelet glycoprotein IIIa) (Figure 16.1K) help highlight small dysplastic megakaryocytes that may not be easily identifiable on an H&E stain.

Genetics

Clonal cytogenetic abnormalities are present in 20% to 50% of MDS, NOS cases, while somatic pathogenic gene mutations are present in >90% of cases.[13,14] Genes that are most commonly mutated in MDS, NOS include *TET2, ASXL1, DNMT3A, SRSF2,* and *RUNX1*.[14] In most cases, more than one pathogenic variant is present. MDS with monoallelic *TP53* mutation or multiple *TP53* pathogenic variants each with <10% VAF are encompassed within MDS, NOS. Furthermore, in the presence of −7/del(7q), inv(3) or abnormal 3q26, complex karyotype, or a *RUNX1* mutation, MDS with an *SF3B1* mutation at a VAF of ≥10% (but lacking multi-hit *TP53* or excess blasts) is classified as MDS, NOS.[1] In the presence of −7/del(7q) or a complex karyotype, a diagnosis of MDS, NOS, without dysplasia, may be made in the absence of morphologic dysplasia (Table 16.1). On the contrary, cases presenting with unexplained cytopenia and non-MDS-defining genetic abnormalities in the absence of morphologic dysplasia do not qualify for an MDS-NOS diagnosis and such cases should be classified as clonal cytopenia of undetermined significance. [see Chapter 12].

Prognosis and Clinical Comment

Similar to other MDS categories, outcomes in MDS, NOS are associated with clinical features (age, performance status, and number and degree of cytopenia), morphologic findings (blast count and number of dysplastic lineages), and both cytogenetic and molecular abnormalities. The new IPSS-M prognostic scoring system in particular provides important risk stratification of MDS, NOS through the addition of mutations to the prognostic model and can be informative in guiding treatment, as outcome of patients with MDS, NOS is highly heterogeneous. Although the number of morphologically dysplastic lineages is not included in any of the prognostic scoring systems and the distinction between SLD and MLD is subject to some interobserver reproducibility, multiple studies have shown that MDS cases with MLD have an inferior prognosis and different genetic profiles compared to cases with SLD. In one recent study, MDS-NOS-MLD had 5-year survival rate of 57% compared to 71% for MDS-NOS-SLD,[5] and in another recent study of 7017 MDS patients from two institutions, MDS-NOS-MLD had median overall survivals of 49 to 56 months compared to 72 to 79 months for MDS-NOS-SLD.[11] As a result, the ICC recommends delineating MDS-SLD and MDS-MLD subtypes within the MDS, NOS category.

References

1. Hasserjian RP, Orazi A, Orfao A, Rozman M, Wang SA. The International Consensus Classification of myelodysplastic syndromes and related entities. *Virchows Arch*. 2023;482(1):39-51.
2. Greenberg PL, Tuechler H, Schanz J, et al. Revised international prognostic scoring system for myelodysplastic syndromes. *Blood*. 2012;120(12):2454-2465.
3. Swerdlow SH, Campo E, Harris NL, et al. WHO Classifications of Tumours of Haematopoietic and Lymphoid Tissues. Revised 4th ed. IARC Press; 2017.
4. Khoury JD, Solary E, Abla O, et al. The 5th edition of the World Health Organization classification of haematolymphoid tumours: myeloid and histiocytic/dendritic neoplasms. *Leukemia*. 2022;36(7):1703-1719.
5. Zhang Y, Wu J, Xu Z, et al. Impact of the international consensus classification of myelodysplastic syndromes. *Br J Haematol*. 2023;201(3):443-448.
6. Lee WH, Lin CC, Tsai CH, et al. Clinico-genetic and prognostic analyses of 716 patients with primary myelodysplastic syndrome and myelodysplastic syndrome/acute myeloid leukemia based on the 2022 International Consensus Classification. *Am J Hematol*. 2023;98(3):398-407.
7. Swerdlow SH, Campo E, Pileri SA, et al. The 2016 revision of the World Health Organization classification of lymphoid neoplasms. *Blood*. 2016;127(20):2375-2390.
8. Stauder R, Valent P, Theurl I. Anemia at older age: etiologies, clinical implications, and management. *Blood*. 2018;131(5):505-514.
9. Arber DA, Orazi A, Hasserjian RP, et al. International consensus classification of myeloid neoplasms and acute leukemias: integrating morphologic, clinical, and genomic data. *Blood*. 2022;140(11):1200-1228.
10. Beck DB, Ferrada MA, Sikora KA, et al. Somatic mutations in UBA1 and severe adult-onset autoinflammatory disease. *N Engl J Med*. 2020;383(27):2628-2638.
11. Komrokji RS, Ball S, Maggioni G, et al. S170: myelodysplastic neoplasms (MDS) classification from whom 2017 to WHO 2022 and ICC 2022)—an expanded analysis of 7017 patients on behalf of the international consortium for MDS (ICMDS). *HemaSphere*. 2023;7(S3):e616260d.
12. Della Porta MG, Lanza F, Del Vecchio L; Italian Society of Cytometry GIC. Flow cytometry immunophenotyping for the evaluation of bone marrow dysplasia. *Cytometry B Clin Cytom*. 2011;80(4):201-211.
13. Schanz J, Tuchler H, Sole F, et al. New comprehensive cytogenetic scoring system for primary myelodysplastic syndromes (MDS) and oligoblastic acute myeloid leukemia after MDS derived from an international database merge. *J Clin Oncol*. 2012;30(8):820-829.
14. Haferlach T, Nagata Y, Grossmann V, et al. Landscape of genetic lesions in 944 patients with myelodysplastic syndromes. *Leukemia*. 2014;28(2):241-247.

Chapter 17
Myelodysplastic Syndrome With Excess Blasts

Mina L. Xu, Rena Buckstein, and Robert P. Hasserjian

Definition

Excess blasts in the setting of a myelodysplastic syndrome (MDS) is defined by 5% to 9% blasts in bone marrow or 2% to 9% blasts in peripheral blood, or any Auer rods in blasts (Table 17.1). The presence of 1% circulating blasts that is confirmed on two separate occasions also meets criteria for MDS-EB.

Synonym

Myelodysplastic syndrome with excess blasts-1 (not recommended), Myelodysplastic neoplasm with increased blasts-1 (not recommended).

Epidemiology

The median age of diagnosis for all MDS is 76[1] and the 5-year age-adjusted incidence rate per 100,000 people is 28.6 for people over 65 years (https://seer.cancer.gov/explorer/.) MDS-EB comprises 15% to 23% of all MDS[2,3].

General Clinical Features

Patients typically present with symptoms and signs reflective of cytopenias such as anemia (fatigue, dyspnea on exertion, angina), thrombocytopenia (bleeding, bruising), and neutropenia (infections), although some patients may have asymptomatic disease first detected on routine blood count evaluation.

Morphology

The peripheral blood often shows dysplasia in the form of abnormal granulopoiesis and abnormal neutrophil segmentation, red cell anisopoikilocytosis, macrocytosis, and giant platelets. Circulating blasts are often seen and may contain Auer rods. The bone marrow is usually hypercellular for the patient's age, but may be hypocellular in a subset of cases. The vast majority of MDS-EB exhibits dysplasia in one or more lineages; a lack of dysplasia in the setting of increased blasts should question the diagnosis of MDS-EB and raises the differential diagnosis of early or evolving AML, other myeloid neoplasms (such as a myeloproliferative neoplasm), or transient blast elevation due to growth factors or early marrow regeneration after injury. Lack of morphologic dysplasia may also be due to poor aspiration, sample preparation or staining, which can limit evaluation for morphologic dysplasia.

There may be erythroid predominance in marrow, with erythroid elements showing megaloblastoid changes, budding, and internuclear bridging (Figure 17.1). Myeloid dysplasia manifests as nuclear hyposegmentation (pseudo-Pelger-Huët nuclei), and hypogranulation of maturing myeloid forms. The granulocytic lineage is often left shifted, with a paucity of mature forms accompanied by increased blasts, but some MDS-EB cases show increased blasts in the blood without an increase in marrow blasts. Megakaryocytic dysplasia is best visualized on core biopsy, where they are often clustered and, along with erythroid elements, dislocated toward paratrabecular regions. Dysplastic megakaryocytes are small and hypolobated or display separated rounded nuclear lobes.

MDS-EB is now one single disease category, corresponding to MDS-EB1 in the WHO revised 4th edition. The equivalent of MDS-EB2 (10%-19% blasts in bone marrow or peripheral blood) is now MDS/AML (next section); of note, MDS-EB does include some cases previously classified as MDS-EB2 due to Auer rods and/or 5% to 9% blasts in the blood but <10% blasts in the bone marrow. Pediatric patients (patients <18 years of age) are considered to have MDS-EB if blasts are 5% to 19% in bone marrow and/or 2% to 19% in peripheral blood since they demonstrate clinical features that are different from those of adult patients with MDS/AML. Additionally, there does not appear to be a significant prognostic or biologic difference between pediatric MDS with 5% to 9% versus 10% to 19% bone marrow blasts.

TABLE 17.1 Diagnostic Criteria for MDS-EB (Adult Patients Age ≥18 y)

Feature	Requirements	Exclusions
Blood counts	At least one cytopenia	Sustained/unexplained leukocytosis (WBC ≥13 × 10^9/L) Sustained/unexplained monocytosis (monocytes ≥0.5 × 10^9/L and ≥10% of WBCs) Sustained/unexplained thrombocytosis (platelets ≥450 × 10^9/L)
Blast percentages	5%-9% in bone marrow or 2%-9% in blood[a] (or Auer rods)	NA
Morphology	Dysplasia typically present, but not required Auer rods in blasts if <5% bone marrow and <2% blood blasts	NA
Cytogenetics	NA	NA
Molecular genetics	NA	Multi-hit *TP53* mutation[b]
Other features	NA	NA

[a]The finding of 1% PB blasts on at least two separate occasions also qualifies for excess blasts.
[b]See chapter 15 for definition of multi-hit *TP53* mutation.

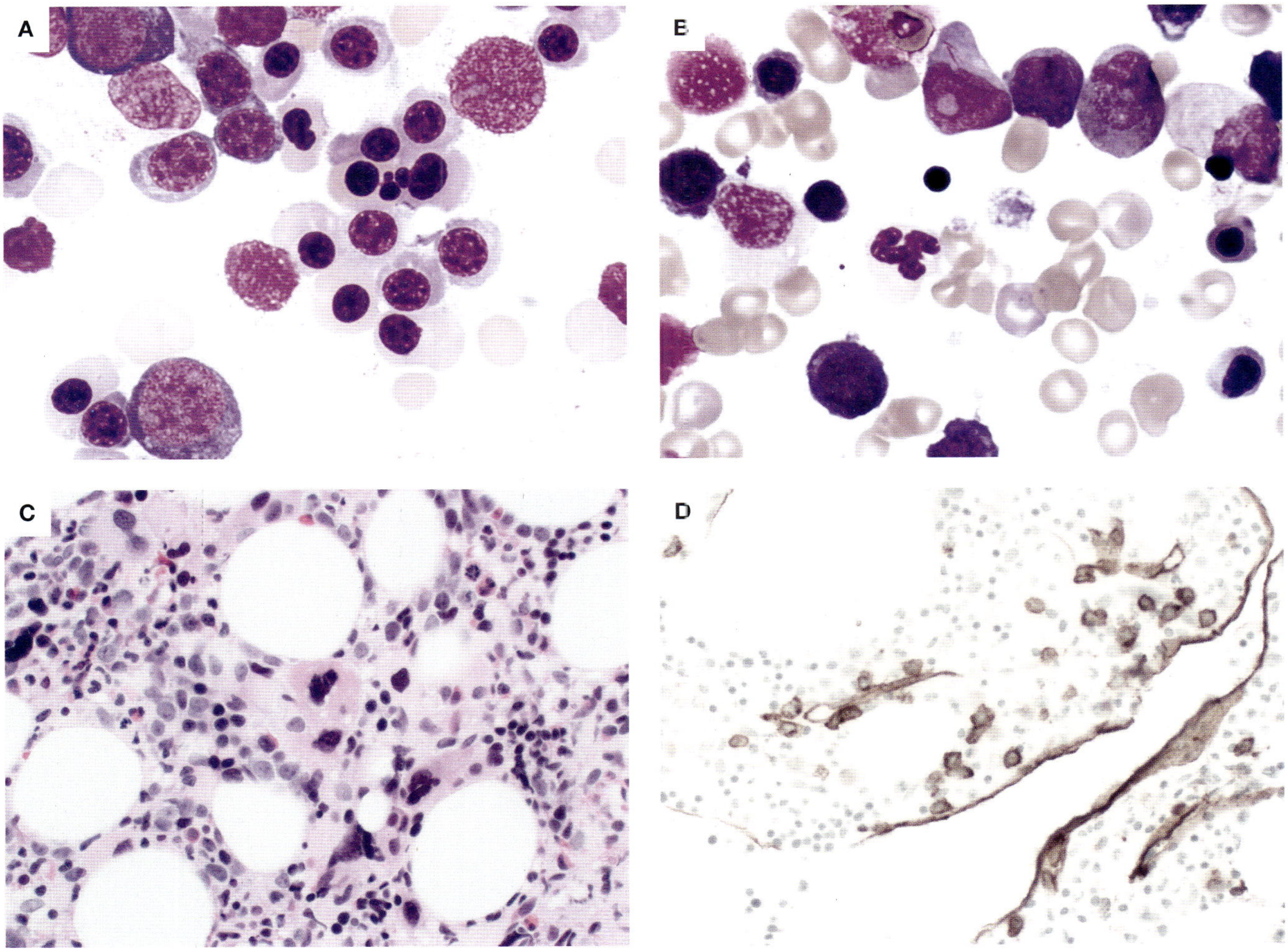

FIGURE 17.1 Aspirate showing **(A)** erythroid dysplasia **(B)** granulocytic dysplasia and blast with Auer rods **(C)** Core biopsy showing megakaryocytic dysplasia and increased early myeloid forms and **(D)** CD34[+] blasts at 5% to 10% and focally clustered.

Immunophenotype

CD34 immunostaining is useful in blast quantitation, particularly when the aspirate is suboptimal; CD34 can reveal clusters of blasts atypically located away from the paratrabecular areas. Increased (grade 2-3 of 3) marrow fibrosis is associated with worse prognosis in MDS and is seen in about 10% of MDS-EB cases.[4] The presence of increased fibrosis should be mentioned in the bone marrow report, as it may explain discordance in blast estimation between biopsy and aspirate/flow cytometry. Due to frequent CD34 positivity in dysplastic megakaryocytes, only CD34$^+$ blasts, not CD34$^+$ micromegakaryocytes (which are slightly larger than blasts) should be included in overall blast count.

Genetics

MDS-EB can present with any combination of cytogenetic and molecular abnormalities, with the exception of multihit *TP53* mutation, which supercedes MDS-EB. Blast percentage does not appear to influence the clinical behavior of MDS with biallelic loss of *TP53* activity[5] (see Chapter 15). Myeloid neoplasms with *NPM1* or *CEBPA* mutations or AML-defining translocations (see Chapters 22-32) may rarely present with less than 10% blasts and these rare cases should be carefully monitored for progression to AML (requiring a minimal blast percentage in PB or BM of 10%).[6]

Prognosis and Clinical Comment

MDS-EB may be the initial presenting diagnosis of an MDS patient first coming to clinical attention, or may occur as a progression from any other MDS subtype (except for MDS with mutated *TP53*). Conversely, MDS-EB may progress to MDS/AML or frank AML if blasts cross the applicable thresholds. Compared to MDS, NOS, the risk of transformation to AML is higher and overall survival shorter with MDS-EB, with a median overall survival of approximately 28 months.[2,3]

Clinical behavior is heterogeneous within this group, given that the blast count is only one variable that influences prognosis, currently calculated by the Revised or Molecular International Prognostic Scoring System (IPSS-R[7] or IPSS-M[3]) schemes[8] (see Chapter 16). Treatment for MDS-EB is guided by symptoms and refined by the predicted prognosis based on IPSS-R or IPSS-M. Treatments could include erythropoiesis-stimulating agents or hypomethylating agents, but allogeneic stem cell transplant is the only curative modality; it is typically offered based on disease's clinical behavior and risk score, and patient factors. The percentage of blasts pretransplantation has been shown to be an independent prognostic risk factor in terms of long-term survival after allogeneic transplant,[9] but the need for pretransplant cytoreduction is controversial.[10]

References

1. Zeidan AM, Shallis RM, Wang R, Davidoff A, Ma X. Epidemiology of myelodysplastic syndromes: why characterizing the beast is a prerequisite to taming it. *Blood Rev.* 2019;34:1-15.
2. Haase D, Germing U, Schanz J, et al. New insights into the prognostic impact of the karyotype in MDS and correlation with subtypes: evidence from a core dataset of 2124 patients. *Blood.* 2007;110(13):4385-4395.
3. Lee WH, Tsai MT, Tsai CH, et al. Validation of the molecular international prognostic scoring system in patients with myelodysplastic syndromes defined by international consensus classification. *Blood Cancer J.* 2023;13(1):120.
4. Della Porta MG, Malcovati L, Boveri E, et al. Clinical relevance of bone marrow fibrosis and CD34-positive cell clusters in primary myelodysplastic syndromes. *J Clin Oncol.* 2009;27(5):754-762.
5. Bernard E, Nannya Y, Hasserjian RP, et al. Implications of TP53 allelic state for genome stability, clinical presentation and outcomes in myelodysplastic syndromes. *Nat Med.* 2020;26(10):1549-1556. [published correction appears in *Nat Med.* 2021;27(3):562] [published correction appears in *Nat Med.* 2021;27(5):927].
6. Patel SS, Ho C, Ptashkin RN, et al. Clinicopathologic and genetic characterization of nonacute NPM1-mutated myeloid neoplasms. *Blood Adv.* 2019;3(9):1540-1545.
7. Greenberg PL, Tuechler H, Schanz J, et al. Revised international prognostic scoring system for myelodysplastic syndromes. *Blood.* 2012;120(12):2454-2465.
8. DeZern A, Greenberg PL. The trajectory of prognostication and risk stratification for patients with myelodysplastic syndromes. *Blood.* 2023;142(26):2258-2267.
9. Ma YY, Wei ZL, Xu YJ, et al. Poor pretransplantation minimal residual disease clearance as an independent prognostic risk factor for survival in myelodysplastic syndrome with excess blasts: a multicenter, retrospective cohort study. *Cancer.* 2023;129(13):2013-2022.
10. Schroeder T, Wegener N, Lauseker M, et al. Comparison between upfront transplantation and different pretransplant cytoreductive treatment approaches in patients with high-risk myelodysplastic syndrome and secondary acute myelogenous leukemia. *Biol Blood Marrow Transplant.* 2019;25(8):1550-1559.

Chapter 18

Myelodysplastic Syndrome/Acute Myeloid Leukemia

Robert P. Hasserjian and Hartmut Döhner

Definition

Myelodysplastic syndrome/acute myeloid leukemia (MDS/AML) is a myeloid neoplasm in adult patients (age ≥18 years) characterized by cytopenia(s) and 10% to 19% blasts in bone marrow and/or peripheral blood. Cases with AML-defining recurrent genetic abnormalities are excluded and are diagnosed instead as AML with the specific genetic aberration. MDS/AML may be diagnosed in patients presenting de novo or as a progression from prior MDS with <10% blasts. The diagnostic criteria for MDS/AML are shown in Table 18.1. MDS/AML is similar to the WHO revised fourth edition MDS with excess blasts-2 (MDS-EB2), except for exclusion of cases with 5% to 9% peripheral blood blasts or Auer rods and <10% blasts (which are now classified as MDS-EB) and cases with AML-defining recurrent genetic abnormalities (which are classified as AML).

Synonyms

MDS with excess blasts-2 (MDS-EB2), MDS with increased blasts-2 (MDS-IB2) (not recommended).

Epidemiology

MDS/AML is only applied to adult patients (≥18 years of age).[1] Patients have a median age of 65 to 70 years and a male predominance, similar to MDS.[2] Pediatric patients (<18 years of age) diagnosed with MDS with 10% to 19% blasts in bone marrow and/or blood are considered to have MDS-EB, since these patients demonstrate clinical features and treatment approaches different from adult MDS/AML.[3,4] MDS/AML comprises approximately 19% to 25% of all MDS cases,[2,5] similar in frequency to MDS-EB2 in the WHO revised fourth edition.

General Clinical Features

Patients typically present with symptoms related to progressive cytopenias. Some patients have history of prior cytotoxic therapies, and in such cases, the qualifier "therapy-related" should be appended to the diagnosis. Cases with known or newly discovered germline predisposition conditions should also be designated with a qualifier indicating the germline mutation or syndrome; in particular, adult patients with germline

TABLE 18.1 Diagnostic criteria for MDS/AML

Feature	Requirements	Exclusions
Blood counts	At least one cytopenia[a]	Sustained/unexplained leukocytosis (WBCs ≥ 13 × 10^9/L), monocytosis (monocytes ≥ 0.5 × 10^9/L and ≥10% of WBCs) or thrombocytosis (platelets ≥450 × 10^9/L)
Blast percentages	10%-19% in BM or 10%-19% in PB	NA
Morphology	Dysplasia typically present, but not required	NA
Cytogenetics	NA	AML-defining recurring cytogenetic abnormality
Molecular genetics	NA	*NPM1* mutation or *CEBPA* inframe bZIP mutation
Other features	NA	Age <18 y

BM, bone marrow; MDS/AML, myelodysplastic syndrome/acute myeloid leukemia; PB, peripheral blood; WBCs, white blood cells.
[a]It may be appropriate to also classify cases with 10% to 19% blasts and lacking any cytopenias as MDS/AML, but such cases are expected to be very rare and require exclusion of AML with recurrent genetic abnormalities.

DDX41 mutation can present with MDS/AML without any prior history of cytopenias.[6]

Morphology

The peripheral blood often shows circulating blasts, which can establish a diagnosis of MDS/AML if they comprise ≥10% of circulating leukocytes, even if bone marrow blasts are <10%. The vast majority of MDS/AML shows dysplasia in one or more hematopoietic lineage; if dysplasia is not seen, an evolving AML with a defining recurrent genetic abnormality should be considered. Blasts should be carefully enumerated in both the bone marrow aspirate (from at least 500 leukocytes) and peripheral blood (from at least 200 leukocytes): blast equivalents include myeloblasts, monoblasts, promonocytes, and megakaryoblasts (Figure 18.1A). A diagnosis of MDS/AML cannot be made in the context of recent granulocyte colony-stimulating factor therapy, which may transiently elevate blasts in the bone marrow or blood. Some cases of MDS/AML (particularly **MDS/AML with mutated *TP53***) exhibit an erythroid-rich background and increased pronormoblasts, including cases resembling pure erythroid leukemia but with concomitantly increased myeloblasts (Figure 18.2).

Immunophenotype

Flow cytometry immunophenotyping typically shows increased myeloblasts; however, the myeloblast percentage derived by flow cytometry should not be used

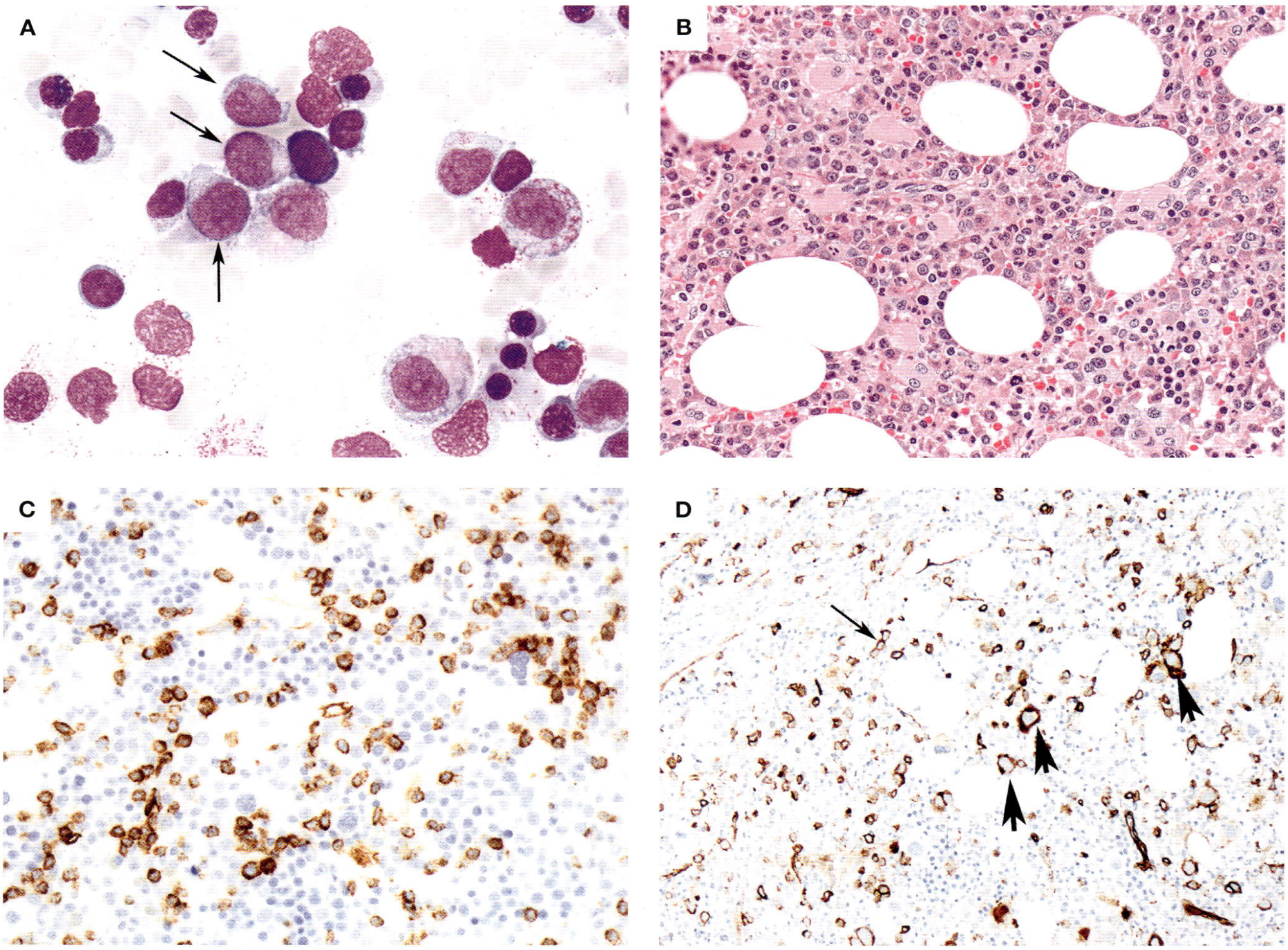

FIGURE 18.1 Myelodysplastic syndrome/acute myeloid leukemia bone marrow findings. **A:** Bone marrow aspirate showing increased myeloid blasts (arrows). **B:** Bone marrow biopsy showing architectural disorganization of hematopoiesis, limited myeloid maturation, and small, dysplastic megakaryocytes; blasts are difficult to enumerate in the bone marrow biopsy on hematoxylin and eosin stain. **C:** Bone marrow biopsy CD34 immunostain showing approximately 15% blasts, with clustering of blasts. **D:** Bone marrow biopsy CD34 immunostain showing staining of small blasts (thin arrow) as well as micromegakaryocytes (thick arrows), which are not regarded as blast equivalents.

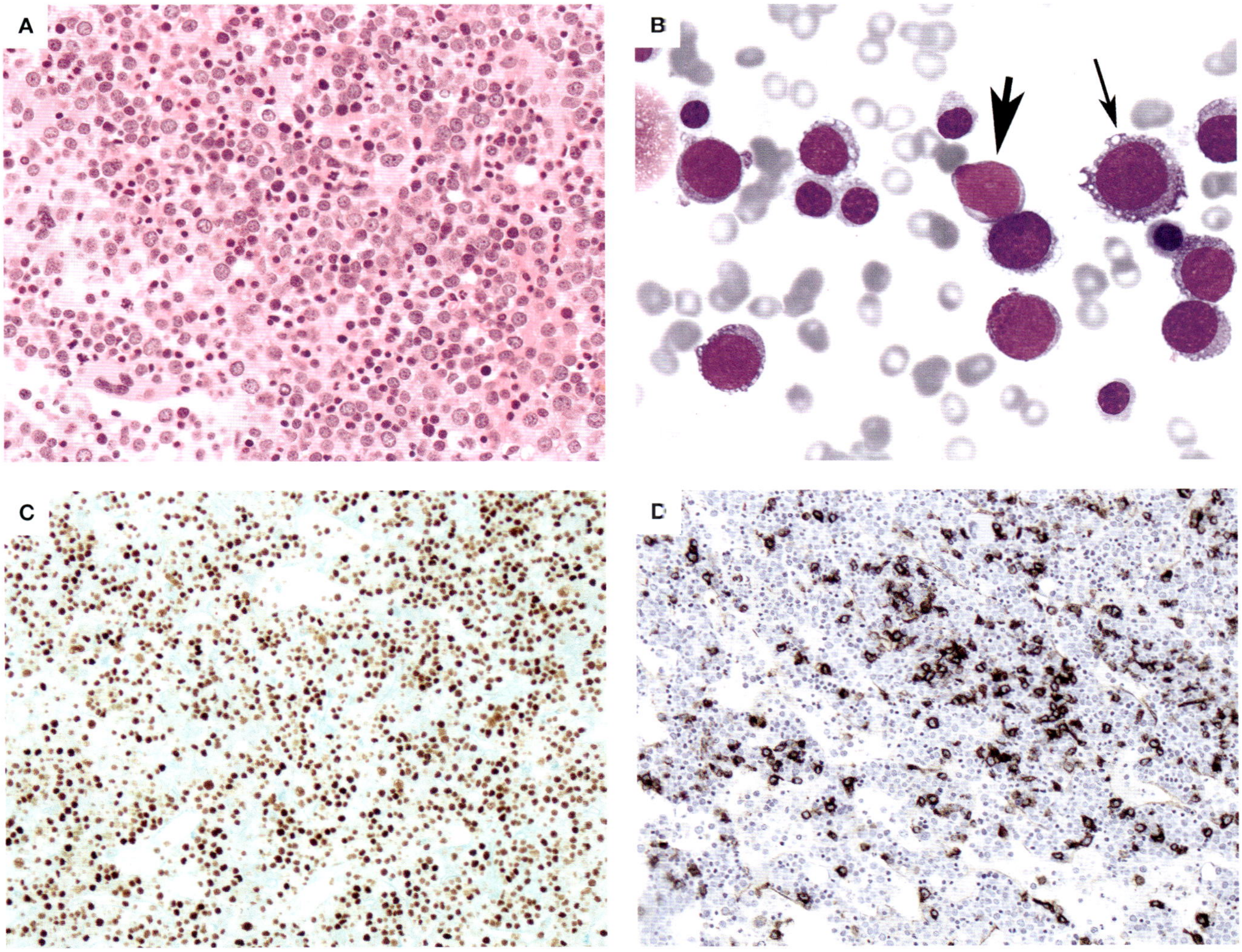

FIGURE 18.2 Myelodysplastic syndrome/acute myeloid leukemia (MDS/AML) with mutated *TP53* and erythroid predominance. **A:** Bone marrow biopsy showing expanded erythropoiesis with marked left shift and frequent large, round pronormoblasts. **B:** Bone marrow aspirate showing vacuolated pronormoblasts (thin arrow) as well as smaller myeloblasts (thick arrow). **C:** p53 immunostain showing strong, diffuse staining, indicative of mutated *TP53*. **D:** CD34 highlights increased myeloblasts (10% of the biopsy cellularity), confirming a diagnosis of MDS/AML and excluding a diagnosis of pure erythroid leukemia.

in lieu of the morphologic blast count in establishing a diagnosis of MDS/AML. Since blasts cannot be reliably enumerated in routine histologic stains of the bone marrow biopsy (Figure 18.1B), CD34 immunohistochemistry is useful in blast quantification, particularly in the event of suboptimal or otherwise nonrepresentative aspirate smears. If CD34$^+$ blasts comprise 10% or more of the bone marrow biopsy cells, a diagnosis of MDS/AML can be made even if the bone marrow aspirate smear blast count is <10% (Figure 18.1C). However, CD34 may also stain dysplastic megakaryocytes, and care must be taken to avoid counting CD34$^+$ micromegakaryocytes together with the blasts (Figure 18.1D).

Genetics

MDS/AML is heterogeneous in terms of its cytogenetics and molecular genetic abnormalities. Rare cases may show normal karyotype and lack mutations detected on standard NGS panels.[7] Cases with AML-defining recurrent genetic abnormalities are excluded. MDS/AML is subclassified similar to AML based on the presence of **myelodysplasia-related gene mutations**, **myelodysplasia-related cytogenetic abnormalities**, or **mutated *TP53*** (variant allele fraction ≥10%); cases lacking any of these genetic abnormalities are subclassified as **MDS/AML, NOS** (Table 18.2). Unlike MDS with <10% blasts (and similar to AML), data from

TABLE 18.2 Criteria for MDS/AML subtypes

Subtype	Criteria	Proportion of MDS/AML[a]
MDS/AML with myelodysplasia-related gene mutations	• Presence of one or more of the following mutations: *ASXL1, BCOR, EZH2, RUNX1, SF3B1, SRSF2, STAG2, U2AF1*, or *ZRSR2* • Absence of somatic *TP53* mutation with VAF ≥ 10%	52%-55%

MDS/AML with myelodysplasia-related cytogenetic abnormalities	• Presence of any of the following cytogenetic aberrations:
	  • Complex karyotype: ≥3 unrelated clonal chromosomal abnormalities, excluding hyperdiploid karyotypes with three or more trisomies/polysomies that lack structural abnormalities
	  • del(5q)/t(5q)/add(5q)
	  • −7/del(7q)
	  • +8
	  • del(12p)/t(12p)/add(12p)
	  • i(17q)/−17/add(17p)/del(17p)
	  • del(20q)
	  • idic(X)(q13)
	• Absence of *ASXL1, BCOR, EZH2, RUNX1, SF3B1, SRSF2, STAG2, U2AF1*, and *ZRSR2* mutations
	• Absence of somatic *TP53* mutation with VAF ≥ 10%
		7%-10%

MDS/AML with mutated *TP53*	• Presence of somatic *TP53* mutation with VAF ≥ 10%	18%-24%
MDS/AML, NOS	• Absence of myelodysplasia-related gene mutations, myelodysplasia-related cytogenetic abnormalities, or any somatic *TP53* mutation with VAF ≥ 10%	13%-20%

MDS/AML, myelodysplastic syndrome/acute myeloid leukemia; NOS, not otherwise specified; VAF, variant allele fraction.
[a]Based on data from Lee WH, Lin CC, Tsai CH, et al. Clinico-genetic and prognostic analyses of 716 patients with primary myelodysplastic syndrome and myelodysplastic syndrome/acute myeloid leukemia based on the 2022 International Consensus Classification. *Am J Hematol.* 2023;98(3):398-407 and Zhang Y, Wu J, Xu Z, et al. Impact of the international consensus classification of myelodysplastic syndromes. *Br J Haematol.* 2023;201(3):443-448.

recent studies have shown that both monoallelic and multihit *TP53* aberrations confer poor prognosis to myeloid neoplasms with ≥10% blasts, including MDS/AML and AML.[8-10] Thus, in contrast to **MDS with mutated *TP53*** (which requires multihit *TP53* lesions), a single somatic *TP53* mutation is considered sufficient for **MDS/AML with mutated *TP53***. However, the majority of **MDS/AML with mutated *TP53*** has multihit *TP53* lesions.[9,11] MDS/AML patients have mutation profiles more similar to AML than to MDS, including frequent mutations in pro-proliferative signaling genes (such as RAS pathway mutations), *IDH1* and *IDH2*.[12,13]

Prognosis and Clinical Comment

The prognosis of MDS/AML depends on the genetic subtype. Reported median survivals range from 5 to 9 months for **MDS/AML with mutated *TP53*** to 10 to 13 months for **MDS/AML with myelodysplasia-related cytogenetics abnormalities** to 16 to 23 months for **MDS/AML with myelodysplasia-related gene mutations** and **MDS/AML, NOS**.[2,5] Excluding the **MDS/AML with mutated *TP53* subgroup**, MDS/AML patients have shorter survival compared to MDS-EB patients.[2,5] However, outcome is dependent on age and therapies: younger patients who are eligible for intensive therapy and allogeneic stem cell transplant have longer survival than older patients receiving less intensive therapy.[14-16] Determining the most clinically meaningful risk stratification scheme for MDS/AML remains uncertain. While the 2022 European LeukemiaNet (ELN) AML recommendations use the MDS/AML designation to categorize patients meeting the aforementioned diagnostic criteria, data on the applicability of ELN AML risk stratification to MDS/AML are limited, particularly for patients treated with nonintensive therapies.[17] Thus, it is recommended to use revised International Prognostic Scoring System (IPSS-R) or molecular IPSS (IPSS-M) for prognosticating MDS/AML at the current time.[17,18] However, it may be appropriate to apply 2022 ELN AML risk stratification to patients treated with AML-type intensive chemotherapy in the setting of clinical trials that include both AML and MDS/AML patients. Since by definition cases in the 2022 ELN favorable risk category have AML-defining genetic abnormalities, all MDS/AML cases fall into ELN intermediate or adverse risk groups.

MDS/AML lies on the continuum between MDS and AML with respect to progressively increasing blast proliferation and impaired maturation of the neoplastic clone. Accordingly, the optimal treatment of this heterogenous group of patients is yet to be determined. While some may be treated effectively with intensive AML-type chemotherapy similar to overt AML,[10,14,19,20] less intensive MDS-type therapies (such as hypomethylating agents) may be more appropriate for other patients. In the future, treatment of individual patients in this group will likely be influenced by specific genetic characteristics and patient-related factors rather than a specific blast percentage cutoff.[14,21,22] Rapidly increasing versus stable blasts counts also may help guide treatment decisions of patients with MDS/AML. In the meantime, MDS/AML patients should be considered for eligibility for both MDS and AML trials, which will provide data to inform their optimal management in the future.[17]

References

1. Hasserjian RP, Orazi A, Orfao A, Rozman M, Wang SA. The International Consensus Classification of myelodysplastic syndromes and related entities. *Virchows Arch*. 2023;482(1):39-51.
2. Lee WH, Lin CC, Tsai CH, et al. Clinico-genetic and prognostic analyses of 716 patients with primary myelodysplastic syndrome and myelodysplastic syndrome/acute myeloid leukemia based on the 2022 International Consensus Classification. *Am J Hematol*. 2023;98(3):398-407.
3. Locatelli F, Strahm B. How I treat myelodysplastic syndromes of childhood. *Blood*. 2018;131(13):1406-1414
4. Rudelius M, Weinberg OK, Niemeyer CM, Shimamura A, Calvo KR. The International Consensus Classification (ICC) of hematologic neoplasms with germline predisposition, pediatric myelodysplastic syndrome, and juvenile myelomonocytic leukemia. *Virchows Arch*. 2023;482(1):113-130.
5. Zhang Y, Wu J, Xu Z, et al. Impact of the international consensus classification of myelodysplastic syndromes. *Br J Haematol*. 2023;201(3):443-448.
6. Makishima H, Saiki R, Nannya Y, et al. Germ line DDX41 mutations define a unique subtype of myeloid neoplasms. *Blood*. 2023;141(5):534-549.
7. Wang SA, Ok CY, Kim AS, et al. Myelodysplastic syndromes with no somatic mutations detected by next-generation sequencing display similar features to myelodysplastic syndromes with detectable mutations. *Am J Hematol*. 2021;96(11):E420-E423.
8. Stengel A, Meggendorfer M, Walter W, et al. Interplay of TP53 allelic state, blast count, and complex karyotype on survival of patients with AML and MDS. *Blood Adv*. 2023;7(18):5540-5548.
9. Stengel A, Haferlach T, Baer C, et al. Specific subtype distribution with impact on prognosis of TP53 single-hit and double-hit events in AML and MDS. *Blood Adv*. 2023;7(13):2952-2956.
10. Grob T, Al Hinai AS, Sanders MA, et al. Molecular characterization of mutant TP53 acute myeloid leukemia and high-risk myelodysplastic syndrome. *Blood*. 2022;139(15):2347-2354.
11. Bernard E, Nannya Y, Hasserjian RP, et al. Implications of TP53 allelic state for genome stability, clinical presentation and outcomes in myelodysplastic syndromes. *Nat Med*. 2020;26(10):1549-1556.
12. Chen X, Othus M, Wood BL, et al. Comparison of myeloid blast counts and variant allele frequencies of gene mutations in myelodysplastic syndrome with excess blasts and secondary acute myeloid leukemia. *Leuk Lymphoma*. 2021;62(5):1226-1233.
13. Menssen AJ, Khanna A, Miller CA, et al. Convergent clonal evolution of signaling gene mutations is a hallmark of myelodysplastic syndrome progression. *Blood Cancer Discov*. 2022;3(4):330-345.
14. Estey E, Hasserjian RP, Dohner H. Distinguishing AML from MDS: a fixed blast percentage may no longer be optimal. *Blood*. 2022;139(3):323-332.
15. Lowenberg B, Pabst T, Maertens J, et al. Therapeutic value of clofarabine in younger and middle-aged (18-65 years) adults with newly diagnosed AML. *Blood*. 2017;129(12):1636-1645.
16. Lowenberg B, Pabst T, Maertens J, et al. Addition of lenalidomide to intensive treatment in younger and middle-aged adults with newly diagnosed AML: the HOVON-SAKK-132 trial. *Blood Adv*. 2021;5(4):1110-1121.
17. Dohner H, Wei AH, Appelbaum FR, et al. Diagnosis and management of AML in adults: 2022 recommendations from an international expert panel on behalf of the ELN. *Blood*. 2022;140(12):1345-1377.
18. Huber S, Baer C, Hutter S, et al. Risk assessment according to IPSS-M is superior to AML ELN risk classification in MDS/AML overlap patients defined by ICC. *Leukemia*. 2023;37(10):2138-2141.
19. DiNardo CD, Garcia-Manero G, Pierce S, et al. Interactions and relevance of blast percentage and treatment strategy among younger and older patients with acute myeloid leukemia (AML) and myelodysplastic syndrome (MDS). *Am J Hematol*. 2016;91(2):227-232.
20. Strati P, Garcia-Manero G, Zhao C, et al. Intensive chemotherapy is more effective than hypomethylating agents for the treatment of younger patients with myelodysplastic syndrome and elevated bone marrow blasts. *Am J Hematol*. 2019;94(7):E188-E190.
21. Bacher U, Kern W, Alpermann T, et al. Prognosis in patients with MDS or AML and bone marrow blasts between 10% and 30% is not associated with blast counts but depends on cytogenetic and molecular genetic characteristics. *Leukemia*. 2011;25(8):1361-1364.
22. DiNardo CD, Garcia-Manero G, Kantarjian HM. Time to blur the blast boundaries. *Cancer*. 2022;128(8):1568-1570.

SECTION 6

Pediatric and/or Germline Disorders

Chapter 19
Juvenile Myelomonocytic Leukemia

Martina Rudelius, Katherine R. Calvo, Charlotte M. Niemeyer, Elliot Stieglitz, and Olga K. Weinberg

Definition

Juvenile myelomonocytic leukemia (JMML) is a clonal hematopoietic neoplasm of early childhood with features of both myeloproliferative neoplasm (MPN) and myelodysplastic syndrome (MDS). The primary proliferative components are monocytes and granulocytes. Megakaryocytes are typically reduced, and dysplasia of the erythroid and megakaryocytic lineages can often be observed. The percentage of blasts and promonocytes is less than 20% in the peripheral blood and bone marrow. JMML is driven by abnormal RAS signaling, and the diagnosis of JMML requires the presence of mutations in genes of the RAS pathway. Neoplasms that mimic JMML but lack RAS pathway mutations are classified as JMML-like. Noonan syndrome (NS)-associated myeloproliferation is a distinct entity from JMML and is classified separately.

Synonym

Juvenile chronic myelomonocytic leukemia. (not recommended)

Epidemiology

JMML is a rare disease with an annual incidence of about 0.13 cases per 100,000. It accounts for 1% of all cases of childhood leukemia but for 20% to 40% of childhood MDS and MPN. JMML typically presents in early childhood with a median age of 2 years. There is a male predominance with a male to female ratio of 2.5.[1,2] Neurofibromatosis type 1 (NF1) is a predisposing condition for JMML, and approximately 10% of JMML cases occur in children with NF1.[3,4] CBL syndrome is another developmental disorder caused by a germline mutation in the RAS pathway that predisposes to JMML.[5,6] Some patients with NS experience a transient myeloproliferative disorder resembling JMML in the first year of life.[7]

General Clinical Features

Splenomegaly is the most consistent clinical finding, with only a small subset of patients (<3%) having a normal spleen size at initial presentation.[8] Leukemic infiltrates of other organs results in hepatomegaly, interstitial lung disease, lymphadenopathy, enlarged tonsils, diarrhea, and gastrointestinal infections.[8,9] Pleomorphic leukemic skin infiltrates are noted in approximately 25% of patients. The presence of café-au-lait spots may indicate an underlying RASopathy such as NF1 or CBL syndrome. The central nervous system is generally spared, although ocular infiltrates and myeloid sarcoma have been described in rare instances. Elevated hemoglobin F levels support the diagnosis. The majority of children with JMML have a polyclonal hypergammaglobulinemia and autoantibodies can be present, but they rarely give rise to clinical symptoms.[1] It is important to distinguish JMML from nonmalignant conditions such as viral infections, leukocyte adhesion deficiency, Wiskott-Aldrich syndrome, and infantile malignant osteopetrosis. In these cases, JMML can be distinguished by the absence of RAS pathway mutations.

Morphology

The defining feature of JMML is leukocytosis, typically falling within the median range of 25 to 30 × 10^9/L, associated with monocytosis (>1 × 10^9/L).[10] However, it is important to note that the white blood cell count can be within the normal range and the monocyte count is <1 × 10^9/L in 7% of patients. Blood smears may show atypical monocytes with a higher nuclear to cytoplasmic ratio and abnormal nuclear shapes (Figure 19.1). Leukoerythroblastosis is a consistent feature present in >90% of cases, while blasts (including promonocytes) usually account for less than 5% and always less than 20%. Although platelet counts are variable, thrombocytopenia is common and may be severe. Macrocytic anemia may be observed especially in cases involving monosomy 7, but normocytic anemia is more frequent. In some patients, red cells appear microcytic in the absence of iron deficiency.[1]

Bone marrow findings can be variable and need to be put into a molecular and clinical context for diagnostic purposes. The bone marrow is hypercellular and most commonly hyperplastic granulopoiesis predominates, although in rare cases an expansion

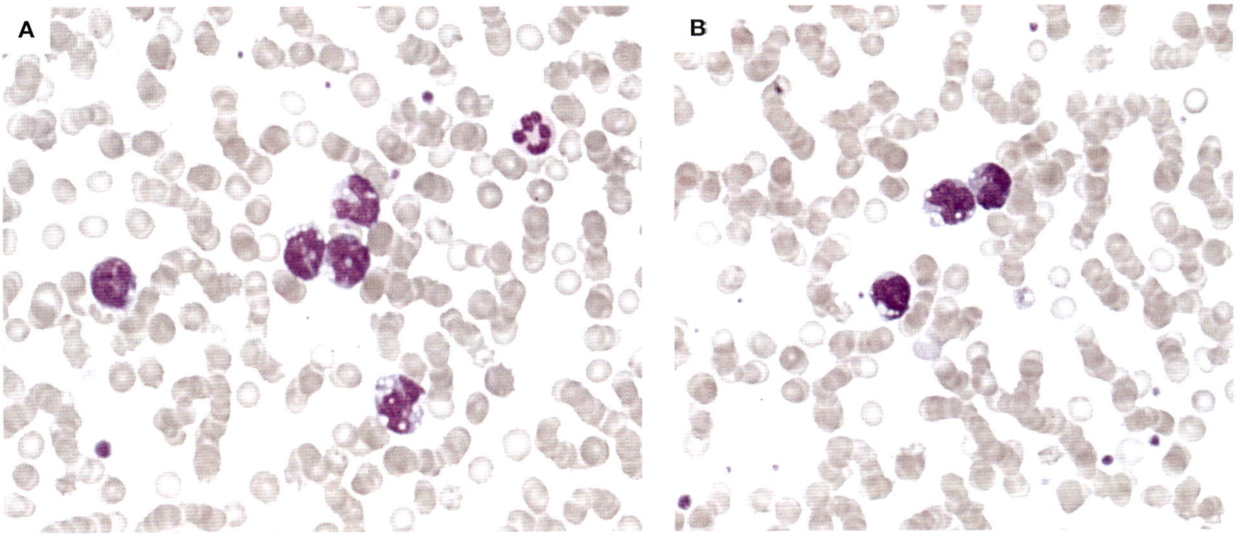

FIGURE 19.1 Juvenile myelomonocytic leukemia: Blood smears (**A** and **B**) showing abnormal monocytes, promonocytes, and few blasts with vacuolated cytoplasm.

of erythroid precursors (especially in patients with monosomy 7) may be observed. The increase in monocytes may be moderate and is usually less prominent than in the peripheral blood. Cytochemical stains such as alpha-naphthyl butyrate esterase may be helpful in highlighting the presence of monocytic cells (Figure 19.2). Blasts (including promonocytes) make up for less than 20% of bone marrow cells, and Auer rods are not present[11] (Figure 19.2). Megakaryopoiesis is typically reduced, and dysplasia of granulopoiesis (pseudo-Pelger-Huët cells; hypogranularity) and erythropoiesis is often noted (Figure 19.3). Reticulin fibrosis is occasionally present.

As outlined earlier, a leukemic course with infiltration of the spleen, liver, lung, and skin is common. The involvement is predominantly found in the splenic red pulp where splenic cords and perivascular areas show a myelomonocytic infiltrate (Figure 19.4) and in the sinusoids and portal tracts of the liver.

Immunophenotype

Bone marrow smears should be carefully evaluated to determine the number of blasts and promonocytes. CD34 immunohistochemistry on the biopsy is useful to identify myeloblasts. Monocytes can be highlighted

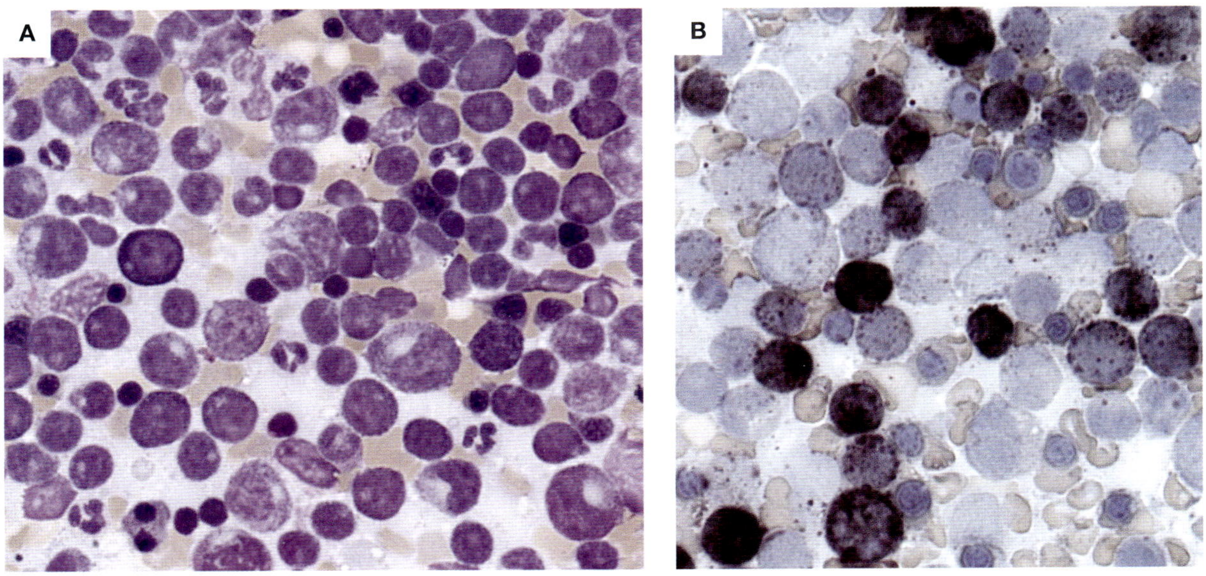

FIGURE 19.2 Juvenile myelomonocytic leukemia: Bone marrow aspirate smear (**A**) shows an increase in monocytic cells and dysplastic features of the erythropoiesis. Butyrate esterase staining (**B**) highlights monocytic cells in brown.

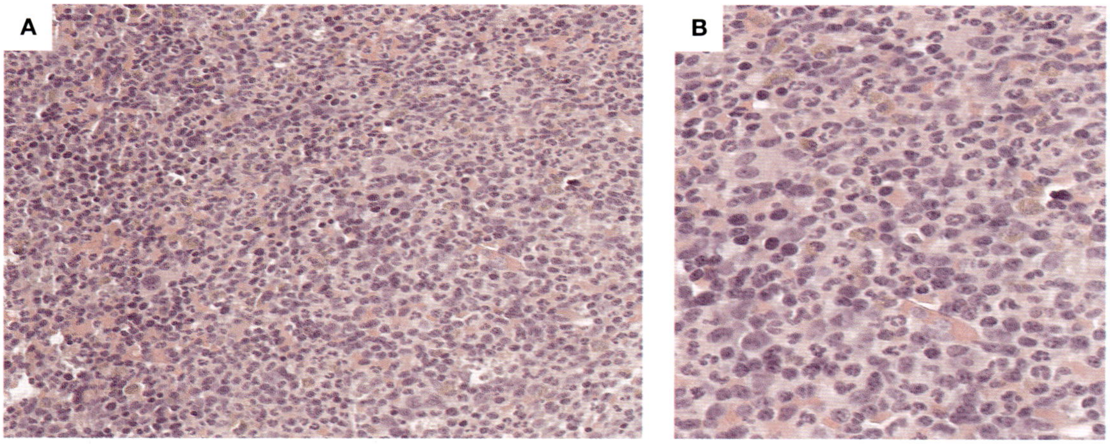

FIGURE 19.3 Juvenile myelomonocytic leukemia: Bone marrow core biopsy (**A**) shows hypercellular bone marrow with granulocytic proliferation and a slight increase in monocytic cells. **B:** Bone marrow core biopsy with reduced megakaryopoiesis. There is no excess of blasts.

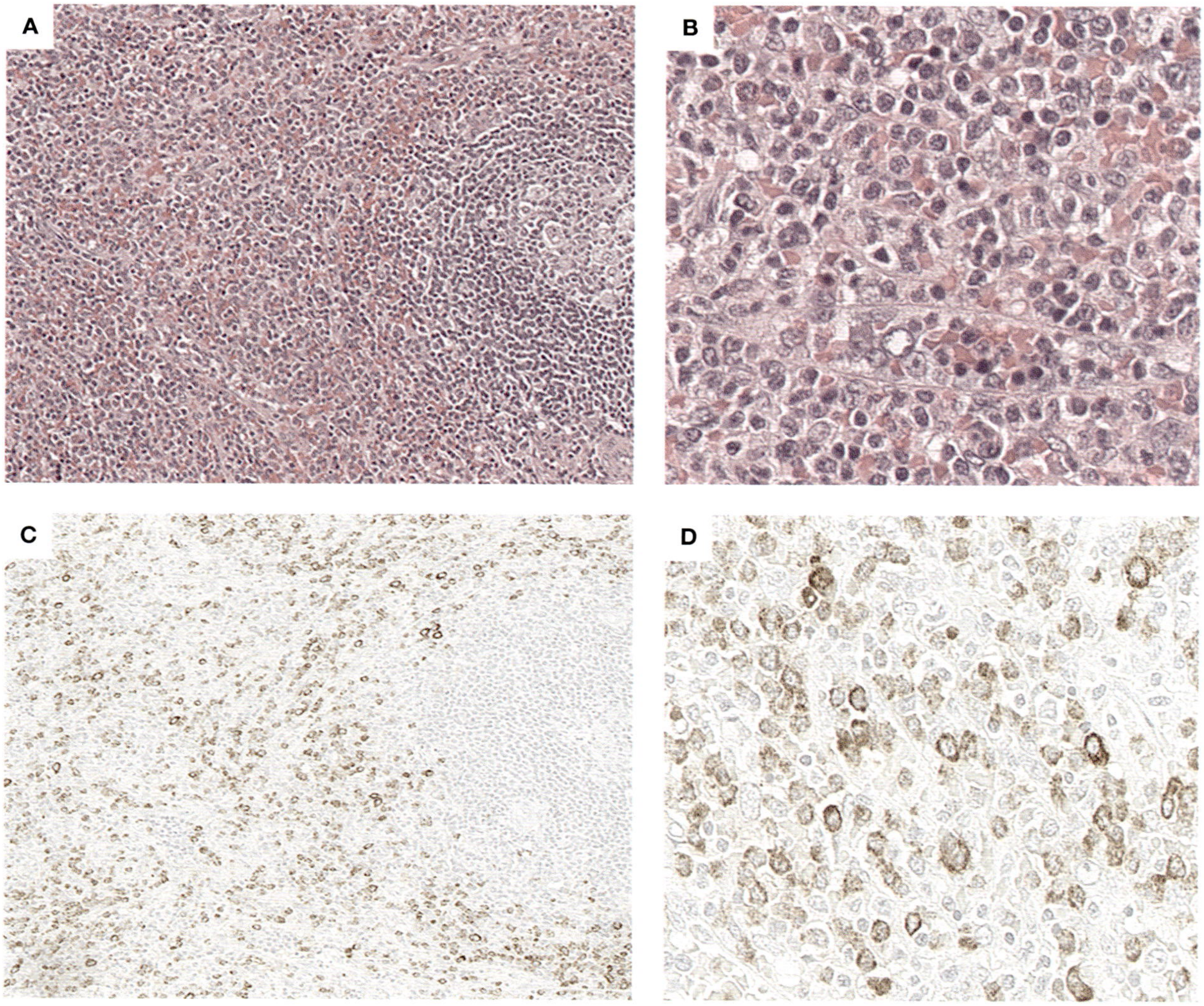

FIGURE 19.4 Leukemic infiltrate of juvenile myelomonocytic leukemia in the spleen: hematoxylin and eosin sections of the spleen (**A** and **B**) show a dense infiltrate of immature granulocytic cells in the red pulp. Myeloperoxidase immunostaining (**C** and **D**) highlights the granulocytic precursors.

by CD14 in bone marrow biopsies. In addition, CD68, CD11b, and MPO (myeloperoxidase) may be helpful in assessing extramedullary infiltrates, as granulocytic precursors may predominate (Figure 19.4). Flow cytometry shows an increased frequency of CD34+ cells with a markedly reduced percentage of both B-cell precursors and erythroid precursors, in parallel with a marked expansion of monocytic and CD7^{+} lymphoid precursors.[12]

Genetics

RAS pathway mutations in the genes *PTPN11, NRAS, KRAS, NF1, CBL*, or rarely *RRAS* or *RRAS2* are present in leukemic cells of more than 95% of patients and define genetically and clinically distinct subtypes (Table 19.1).[1,2] Two of these subtypes are defined by germline events in either *NF1* or *CBL* that progress to malignancy with acquired biallelic inactivation of the respective genes in hematopoietic cells. The other subtypes, *PTPN11, NRAS*, and *KRAS*-mutated JMML, are characterized by heterozygous, somatic gain-of-function mutations in children without germline disease. Heterozygous somatic mutations in *PTNP11* are the most common genetic alterations in JMML and can be detected in about 40% of cases. All *PTPN11* mutations are missense mutations in the repressive N-terminal SH-2 domain or in the PTP-interacting surface. Heterozygous somatic *NRAS* and *KRAS* mutations are present in approximately 15% of JMML cases each. They are classic oncogenic missense variants located in codons 12, 13, and 61. *NF1*-mutated disease accounts for 5% to 12% of JMML cases.[1] While in most of these patients biallelic *NF1* gene inactivation in hematopoietic cells is due to uniparental disomy, compound heterozygous *NF1*-inactivating mutations and somatic interstitial deletions account for up to one-third of cases.[4] Clinical signs of NF1 with at least six café-au-lait macules larger than 0.5 mm in diameter or a family history are present in the majority but not all children with NF-mutated JMML. Germline mutations in *CBL*-mutated JMML are located throughout the linker and RING finger domain of the *CBL* gene. Most patients with *CBL*-mutated JMML have 11q isodisomy in hematopoietic cells, but heterozygous mutations have been reported in a few cases.

Recurrent secondary genetic alterations in hematopoietic cells are noted in up to 50% of patients. These include mutations in RAS pathway genes (RAS double mutations), polycomb repressive complex 2 components (such as *EZH2, ASXL1*, and *DNMT3A*), and *SETBP1, JAK3, SH2B3*, and *RUNX1* genes.[13-15]

Epigenetic regulation in JMML has received considerable attention in recent years. Hypermethylation is a common feature in JMML and characterizes an aggressive course of disease.[16-18] An international consensus definition for DNA methylation in JMML subgroups allows clinical implementation and risk stratification in clinical trials.[19]

Monosomy 7 is present in about 25% of all patients with JMML, and other cytogenetic alterations in 10% of patients. The *BCR::ABL1* fusion gene is absent.

TABLE 19.1 Diagnostic criteria for Juvenile myelomonocytic leukemia

I. Clinical and hematologic criteria (the first two criteria are present in most cases; the last two are required)
• Peripheral blood monocyte count ≥1 × 10^9/L[a]
• Splenomegaly[b]
• Blast percentage in peripheral blood and bone marrow <20%
• No *BCR::ABL1* fusion
II. Genetic criteria (one criterion required)
• Somatic mutation in *PTPN11*[c] or *KRAS*[c] or *NRAS*[c] or *RRAS*[c]
• Clinical diagnosis of neurofibromatosis type 1 or germline *NF1* mutation and biallelic inactivation of NF1[d]
• Germline *CBL* mutation and loss of heterozygosity of *CBL*[e]
• Germline or somatic mutations in *RRAS2*

[a]In 7% of cases monocyte count is less than 1 × 10^9/L.
[b]Splenomegaly is absent in 3% of cases at initial diagnosis.
[c]Germline mutations need to be excluded.
[d]Rare cases of somatic biallelic *NF1* mutations cannot be excluded.
[e]Occasional heterozygous splice site mutations are observed.

Prognosis and Clinical Comment

JMML is a highly heterogeneous clinical entity. Risk factors associated with an adverse outcome include older age at diagnosis (>2 years), elevated hemoglobin F levels (>15%), presence of secondary mutations, and DNA hypermethylation.[1,2] Most patients with JMML require allogenic stem cell transplantation to achieve long-term survival. However, children with *CBL*-mutated JMML generally have a self-limiting disease with persistence of clonal hematopoiesis. Similarly, some children with *NRAS*-mutated JMML, absence of secondary mutations, normal or only slightly elevated hemoglobin F, and low methylation pattern experience spontaneous clinical regression without therapeutic intervention.[20] In addition, there is an overlap between *KRAS*- and *NRAS*-mutated JMML and a rare condition called RAS-associated autoimmune lymphoproliferative disorder, which also displays a more indolent clinical course.[21] On the other end of the spectrum, most

TABLE 19.2 Genetic features of Juvenile myelomonocytic leukemia (JMML), JMML-like neoplasms, and Noonan syndrome–associated myeloproliferative disorder (MPD)

	Mutation	Secondary mutations	Karyotype
JMML	*PTPN11, NRAS, KRAS, NF1,*[a] *CBL,*[b] rarely *RRAS, RRAS2*	Any	Any[d]
JMML-like neoplasms	Absence of RAS pathway mutation	Any	Any
Noonan syndrome–associated MPD	*PTPN11,*[c] *NRAS,*[c] *KRAS*[c] *RIT1*[c]	None	Normal[e]

[a]Germline mutation with additional aberration resulting in biallelic inactivation of the *NF1* gene.
[b]Germline mutation with additional aberration resulting in biallelic inactivation of the *CBL* gene; some cases with heterozygous germline mutation only.
[c]Germline mutation.
[d]Monosomy 7 in 25% of cases.
[e]In rare instances monosomy 7 can develop.[22]
Hofmans M, Schröder R, Lammens T, et al. Noonan syndrome-associated myeloproliferative disorder with somatically acquired monosomy 7: impact on clinical decision making. *Br J Haematol.* 2019;187(4):E83-E86.

but not all patients with *PTPN11*- and *NF1*-mutated JMML have high-risk features and a rapidly fatal course unless an allograft can successfully be performed.

Juvenile Myelomonocytic Leukemia-Like Neoplasms

Neoplasms phenotypically resembling JMML but lacking mutations encoding RAS pathway proteins are referred to as JMML-like (Table 19.2). This group includes rare disorders characterized by rearrangements of *ALK* or *ROS1*,[18] as well as *FIP1L1::RARA*[23] and *CCDC88C::FLT3142* fusions.[24]

Neoplasms with *KMT2A* or *NUP98* aberrations mimicking JMML are classified as acute myeloid leukemia and neoplasms with eosinophilia and *PDGFRA*, *PBGFRB*, or *FGFR1* rearrangements as myeloid neoplasm with eosinophilia and tyrosine kinase gene fusion. Of note, therapy-related MDS/MPN or MDS/MPN in the setting of myeloid malignancy predisposition syndromes can occasionally present with RAS pathway mutations and clinical features similar to JMML.[25]

Noonan Syndrome-Associated Myeloproliferative Disorder

NS is a clinically heterogeneous spectrum of genetic multisystem disorders caused by mutations in genes of the RAS/MAP kinase pathway. Neonates and young infants with NS and germline mutations in *PTPN11* or rarely *KRAS*, *NRAS*, and *RIT1* can develop an MPD, which in its severe form can be indistinguishable from JMML.[7] Somatic mutations are absent, and the disorder is thought to be of polyclonal origin (Table 19.2). While the myeloid proliferation generally resolves spontaneously within months, some severely affected children succumb to syndrome-related organ malformation and MPD. There is a significant overlap between germline *PTPN11* mutations observed in NS with associated MPD and somatic *PTPN11* variants noted in JMML. Analysis of nonhematopoietic tissue is required to distinguish these two disorders genetically.

The pathobiology of myeloid proliferation in NS is unknown. Recently, another presumably polyclonal transient MPD reminiscent of JMML has been described in neonates with biallelic germline mutations in *SH2B3*, the gene encoding LNK, a negative regulator of the JAK/STAT pathway.[26]

References

1. Niemeyer CM, Flotho C. Juvenile myelomonocytic leukemia: who's the driver at the wheel? *Blood.* 2019;133(10):1060-1070.
2. Wintering A, Dvorak CC, Stieglitz E, Loh ML. Juvenile myelomonocytic leukemia in the molecular era: a clinician's guide to diagnosis, risk stratification, and treatment. *Blood Adv.* 2021;5:4785-4793.
3. Shannon KM, O'Connell P, Martin GA, et al. Loss of the normal NF1 allele from the bone marrow of children with type 1 neurofibromatosis and malignant myeloid disorders. *N Engl J Med.* 1994;330(9):597-601.
4. Steinemann D, Arning L, Praulich I, et al. Mitotic recombination and compound-heterozygous mutations are predominant NF1-inactivating mechanisms in children with juvenile myelomonocytic leukemia and neurofibromatosis type 1. *Haematologica.* 2010;95(2):320-323.
5. Niemeyer CM, Kang MW, Shin DH, et al. Germline CBL mutations cause developmental abnormalities and predispose to juvenile myelomonocytic leukemia. *Nat Genet.* 2010;42(9):794-800.
6. Pérez B, Mechinaud F, Galambrun C, et al. Germline mutations of the CBL gene define a new genetic syndrome with predisposition to juvenile myelomonocytic leukaemia. *J Med Genet.* 2010;47(10):686-691.

7. Strullu M, Caye A, Lachenaud J, et al. Juvenile myelomonocytic leukaemia and Noonan syndrome. *J Med Genet*. 2014;51(10):689-697.
8. Niemeyer CM, Arico M, Basso G, et al. Chronic myelomonocytic leukemia in childhood: a retrospective analysis of 110 cases. European Working Group on Myelodysplastic Syndromes in Childhood (EWOG-MDS). *Blood*. 1997;89(10):3534-3543.
9. Luna-Fineman S, Shannon KM, Atwater SK, et al. Myelodysplastic and myeloproliferative disorders of childhood: a study of 167 patients. *Blood*. 1999;93(2):459-466.
10. Niemeyer C. JMML genomics and decisions. *Hematology Am Soc Hematol Educ Program*. 2018;1:301-312.
11. Hess JL, Zutter MM, Castleberry RP, Emanuel PD. Juvenile chronic myelogenous leukemia. *Am J Clin Pathol*. 1996;105(2):238-248.
12. Bugarin C, Antolini L, Buracchi C, et al. Phenotypic profiling of CD34+ cells by advanced flow cytometry improves diagnosis of Juvenile Myelomonocytic Leukemia. *Haematologica*. 2023;10:3324.
13. Sakaguchi H, Okuno Y, Muramatsu H, et al. Exome sequencing identifies secondary mutations of SETBP1 and JAK3 in juvenile myelomonocytic leukemia. *Nat Genet*. 2013;45(8):937-941.
14. Stieglitz E, Taylor-Weiner AN, Chang TY, et al. The genomic landscape of juvenile myelomonocytic leukemia. *Nat Genet*. 2015;47(11):1326-1333.
15. Caye A, Strullu M, Guidez F, et al. Juvenile myelomonocytic leukemia displays mutations in components of the RAS pathway and the PRC2 network. *Nat Genet*. 2015;47(11):1334-1340.
16. Lipka DB, Witte T, Toth R, et al. RAS-pathway mutation patterns define epigenetic subclasses in juvenile myelomonocytic leukemia. *Nat Commun*. 2017;8(1):2126.
17. Stieglitz E, Mazor T, Olshen AB, et al. Genome-wide DNA methylation is predictive of outcome in juvenile myelomonocytic leukemia. *Nat Commun*. 2017;8(1):2127.
18. Murakami N, Okuno Y, Yoshida K, et al. Integrated molecular profiling of juvenile myelomonocytic leukemia. *Blood*. 2018;131(14):1576-1586.
19. Schönung M, Meyer J, Nöllke P, et al. International consensus definition of DNA methylation subgroups in juvenile myelomonocytic leukemia. *Clin Cancer Res*. 2021;27(1):158-168.
20. Takagi M, Piao J, Lin L, et al. Autoimmunity and persistent RAS-mutated clones long after the spontaneous regression of JMML. *Leukemia*. 2013;27(9):1926-1928.
21. Calvo KR, Price S, Braylan RC, et al. JMML and RALD (Ras-associated autoimmune leukoproliferative disorder): common genetic etiology yet clinically distinct entities. *Blood*. 2015;125(18):2753-2758.
22. Hofmans M, Schröder R, Lammens T, et al. Noonan syndrome-associated myeloproliferative disorder with somatically acquired monosomy 7: impact on clinical decision making. *Br J Haematol*. 2019;187(4):E83-E86.
23. Miltiadous O, Petrova-Drus K, Kaicker S, et al. Successful treatment and integrated genomic analysis of an infant with FIP1L1-RARA fusion-associated myeloid neoplasm. *Blood Adv*. 2022;6(4):1137-1142.
24. Chao AK, Meyer JA, Lee AG, et al. Fusion driven JMML: a novel CCDC88C-FLT3 fusion responsive to sorafenib identified by RNA sequencing. *Leukemia*. 2020;34(2):662-666.
25. Wintering A, Smith S, Fuh B, et al. Therapy-related myeloid neoplasms resembling juvenile myelomonocytic leukemia: a case series and review of the literature. *Pediatr Blood Cancer*. 2022;69(5):e29499.
26. Blombery P, Pazhakh V, Albuquerque AS, et al. Biallelic deleterious germline SH2B3 variants cause a novel

Chapter 20

Refractory Cytopenia of Childhood and Pediatric Myelodysplastic Syndromes

Olga K. Weinberg, Katherine R. Calvo, Robert P. Hasserjian, Nicole E. Kucine, Charlotte M. Niemeyer, Attilio Orazi, and Martina Rudelius

Definition

Refractory cytopenia of childhood (RCC) is a well-recognized type of bone marrow failure and represents a biological spectrum of disease stages reflecting the plasticity of the bone marrow in children with various somatic genetic rescue events. In a proportion of RCC cases, acquired somatic mutations or cytogenetic abnormalities are present,[1] and in a subset, germline predisposition mutations are present as sole abnormality. Thus, not all cases of RCC can be classified as myelodysplastic syndrome (MDS). MDS is an acquired clonal hematopoietic stem cell disorder characterized by ineffective hematopoiesis, as evidenced by cytopenias, morphologic dysplasia, and risk for progression to acute myeloid leukemia. Pediatric MDS can either arise de novo or develop after antecedent or predisposing conditions, including certain germline mutations, inherited bone marrow failure syndromes, prior chemotherapy/radiation therapy (therapy-related MDS), or acquired severe aplastic anemia. In the absence of excess blasts, the histopathology of pediatric MDS often displays the characteristic histopathologic pattern defined as refractory cytopenia of childhood (RCC) (Table 20.1).

MDS cases without increased blasts that do not present with the histopathologic pattern of RCC are classified as MDS, not otherwise specified (MDS, NOS). This latter category also encompasses cases without cytopenias and/or dysplasia but harboring MDS-defining cytogenetic abnormalities such as monosomy 7 or mutations that are used to subtype adult type MDS. Pediatric MDS with peripheral blood blasts between 2% and 19% and/or bone marrow blasts between 5% and 19% is defined as MDS with excess blasts (MDS-EB).

Synonyms

Childhood MDS (not recommended).

Epidemiology

MDS is quite uncommon in children, accounting for <5% of all hematologic malignancies diagnosed in this age group.[4] The annual incidence of MDS in children aged 1 to 14 years has been calculated at one to two cases per million children. Cases without excess blasts are the most common MDS in childhood, accounting for >50% of cases.[5] Median age at diagnosis is approximately 7 to 8 years, although MDS can present in children of any age.

TABLE 20.1 Diagnostic criteria for refractory cytopenia of childhood (RCC)

1. **Persistent cytopenia**
   a. Cytopenia is defined according to age-adjusted values for hemoglobin, absolute neutrophil count, and platelets.
   b. Number of cytopenias[1-3]
2. **Presence of dysplastic changes in at least two lineages or in ≥10% in one lineage**
   a. Bone marrow aspirate:
      i. Erythroid lineage: nuclear budding, multinucleation, megaloblastoid changes
      ii. Myeloid lineage: Pseudo-Pelger-Huët cells, cytoplasmic hypogranulation
      iii. Megakaryocytic lineage: Separated nuclear lobes, round monolobated nucleus, micromegakaryocytes
   b. Bone marrow biopsy
      i. Hypocellular bone marrow with patchy pattern
      ii. Normocellular or hypercellular marrow with diffuse pattern
      iii. Erythroid lineage: patchy clusters, left shift, increased mitosis
      iv. Myeloid lineage: Decreased
      v. Megakaryocytic lineage: Decreased, separated nuclear lobes, round monolobated nucleus, micromegakaryocytes
3. **Other criteria**
   a. Blast percentage in peripheral blood <2% and bone marrow <5%
   b. No prior cytotoxic chemotherapy or radiation therapy
   c. No fibrosis

General Clinical Features

RCC and pediatric MDS are characterized by persistent cytopenia. In RCC, thrombocytopenia (<150 × 10^9/L) is the most common cytopenia, present in ~75%, followed by anemia (<10 g/dL) in ~50%, neutropenia (<1.0 × 10^9/L) in ~50%, and severe neutropenia (0.5 × 10^9/L) in ~25% of those affected.[6] The anemia is frequently macrocytic in 75% to 90% of cases. In contrast to adult MDS, isolated anemia is rare in RCC with features of MDS, NOS in children. Patients present with symptoms related to cytopenia(s) including bleeding, malaise, and infection.[6] Lymphadenopathy, secondary to local or systemic infection, is occasionally observed, but hepatosplenomegaly is generally absent. In patients with germline disorders, abnormalities in other organ systems may be due to the underlying predisposition syndrome.

Morphology

Peripheral blood smears are notable for red cell macrocytosis and thrombocytopenia. The red blood cells usually show anisopoikilocytosis with or without increased polychromasia. Neutrophils may display dysplastic features, including pseudo-Pelger-Huët nuclei, hypogranularity, and/or giant band forms. Platelets are characterized by anisocytosis, including giant forms. The proportion of blasts in peripheral blood varies, with 2% being an important threshold that defines excess blasts.

In bone marrow aspirates dyserythropoietic features are similar to those described in adults and include abnormal nuclear segmentation (budding), multinucleation, internuclear bridges, and megaloblastoid changes (Figure 20.1A). Granulocyte precursors may show nuclear hyposegmentation/pseudo-Pelger-Huët nuclei, hypo- or agranular cytoplasm, giant band forms, and nuclear-to-cytoplasmic dyssynchrony. Megakaryocytes are usually markedly decreased to absent but, when identified, are frequently small and hypolobated (micromegakaryocytes) or exhibit separated nuclear lobes. Micromegakaryocytes are noted in some cases and are supportive of the diagnosis RCC.

Core biopsies are an important and necessary component in the diagnostic workup (Table 20.1). The typically observed hypocellularity, as well as the patchy cellular distribution typical of RCC, is best appreciated in core biopsies. RCC often shows large islands of erythroid precursors with some maturational impairment and increased mitotic proliferation (Figure 20.1B and C). Granulopoiesis is typically severely reduced and left-shifted. Megakaryocytes can be absent and micromegakaryocytes are frequently detected. A small subset of RCC demonstrates hyper- or normocellular marrow, and these cases are characterized by morphologic changes similar to those of the more typical hypocellular RCC, including decreased myeloid-to-erythroid ratio. Erythroid precursors, especially proerythroblasts, are relatively increased. Megakaryocytes may be decreased, normal, or increased in number and dysplastic features are similar to hypocellular RCC, but ≥10% dysplastic forms are needed to designate megakaryocyte dysplasia. Blasts should be <5% by definition in cases of RCC.

The category of MDS, NOS is used to classify MDS without excess blasts and may lack dysplasia but often with MDS-defining genetic abnormalities (Table 20.2). Increased marrow fibrosis can be present in MDS, NOS. MDS-EB displays morphologic features similar to those of RCC, except for the presence of excess blasts (5%-19% in bone marrow or 2%-19% in blood) (Figure 20.2). There are insufficient data in the pediatric population to support making a distinction between cases with 5% to 9% bone marrow blasts and/or 2% to 4% peripheral blasts and those with 10% to 19% bone marrow blasts and/or 5% to 19% peripheral blasts. For this reason the MDS/acute myeloid leukemia classification in adult MDS is not adopted for childhood MDS.

Immunophenotype

Flow cytometry is often used to aid in the diagnosis of adult MDS by identifying abnormal maturation patterns or aberrant antigen expression that suggests dysplasia.[7] Flow cytometry–based scoring systems similar to those used in adults have been applied to pediatric MDS with variable success. Flow cytometry results are often normal in RCC and MDS, NOS, and the identification of immunophenotypic abnormalities among the myeloid cell populations can be difficult to interpret as similar abnormalities have been identified in pediatric patients with aplastic anemia or other non-MDS cytopenias. In pediatric MDS-EB, flow cytometry has been shown to have more utility.[8]

Immunohistochemical staining of bone marrow biopsies can be very helpful in diagnosing MDS. CD61 stain can assist in the identification of micromegakaryocytes, a finding that strongly favors a diagnosis of RCC over aplastic anemia (Figure 20.1D). CD34 staining may also aid in identifying an increased number of myeloblasts. However, normal early hematogones

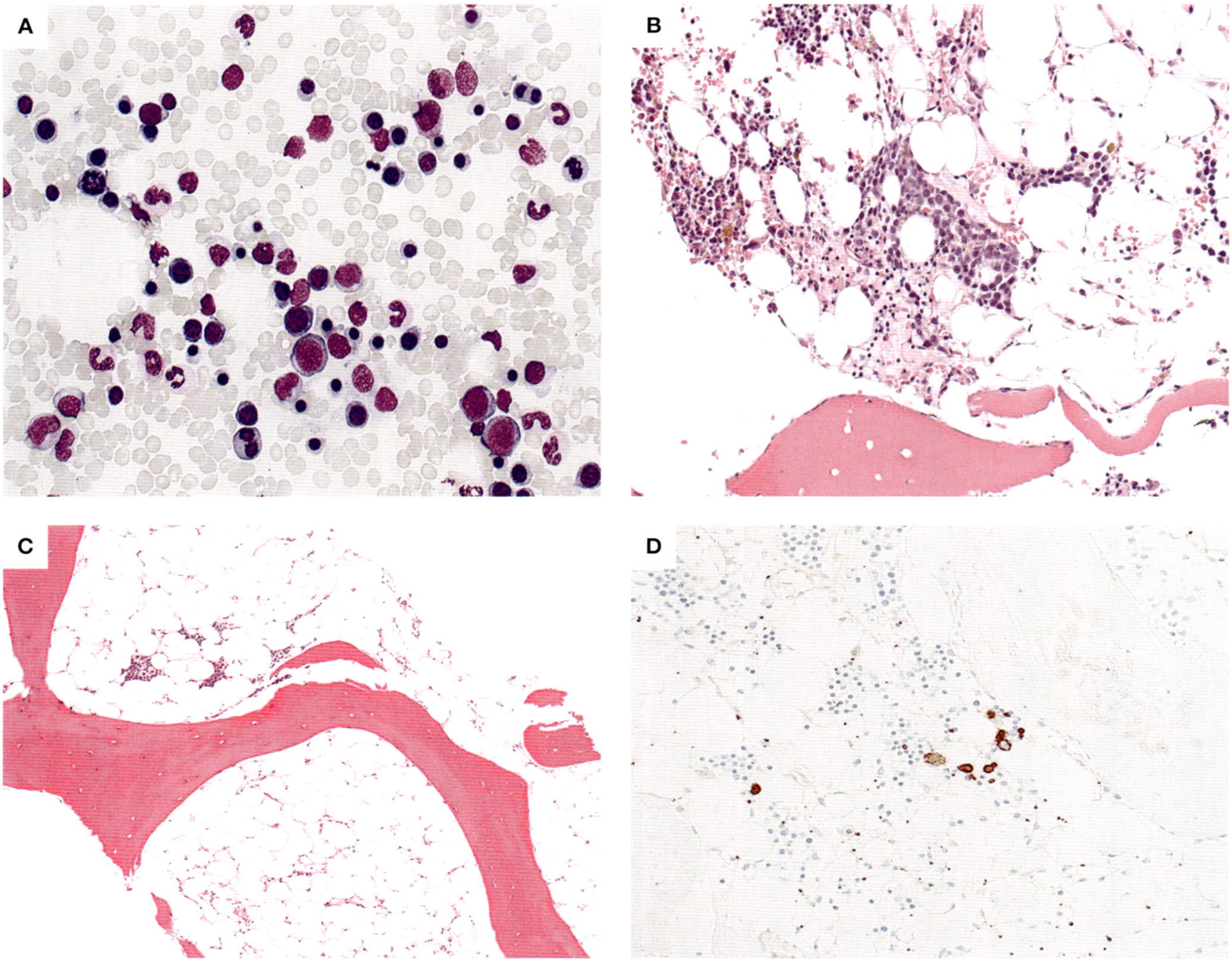

FIGURE 20.1 Refractory cytopenia of childhood. Bone marrow aspirate smear (**A**) and bone marrow core biopsy (**B**) with erythroid hyperplasia and dyserythropoiesis. Overall cellularity is usually markedly decreased (**C**). Megakaryocytes can be highlighted with CD61 immunohistochemical stain (**D**).

may also express CD34, so careful marrow evaluation is required, with possible additional staining with TdT, PAX5, and/or CD79a to identify B-cell precursors. Increased myeloblasts (≥5%) by CD34 and CD117 immunostains would support a diagnosis of MDS-EB.

Genetics

Normal karyotypes are observed in ~72% to 86% of RCC, with normal karyotypes being somewhat less common in normocellular or hypercellular cases. The

TABLE 20.2 Refractory cytopenia of childhood and pediatric myelodysplastic syndromes

	Cytopenias	Blasts	Cytogenetics	Number of dysplastic lineages
Refractory cytopenia of childhood (RCC)	≥1	<5% BM <2% PB	Any	≥1
MDS, NOS	0-3	<5% BM <2% PB	Any or MDS defining if no dysplasia or cytopenia	0-3
MDS with excess blasts	0-3	5%-19% BM 2%-19% PB	Any	0-3

BM, bone marrow; MDS, NOS, myelodysplastic syndrome, not otherwise specified; PB, peripheral blood.

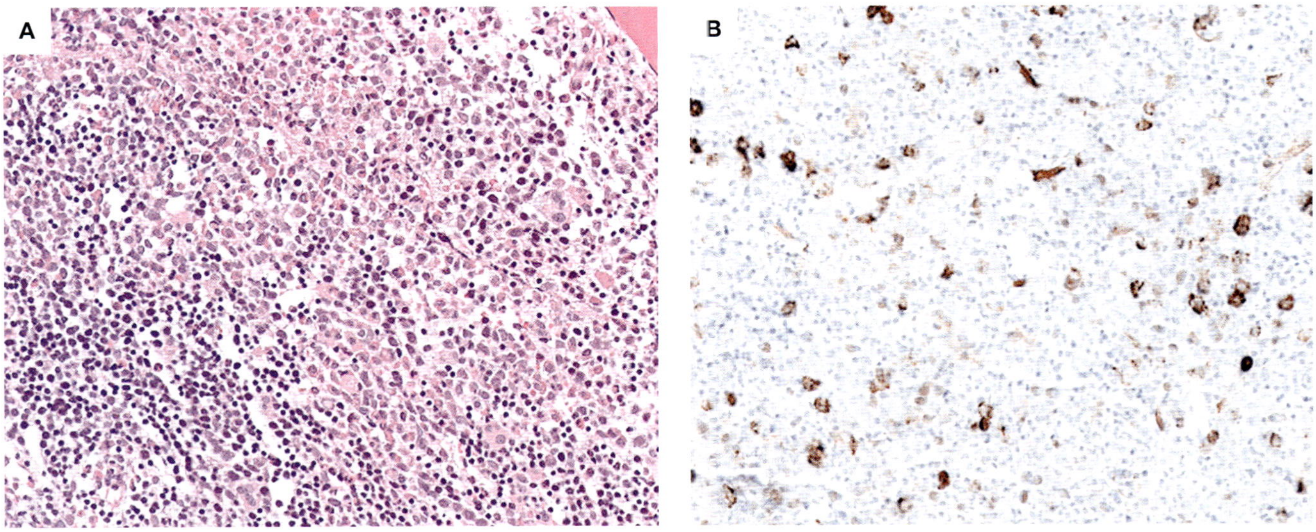

FIGURE 20.2 Myelodysplastic syndrome with excess blasts. Hematoxylin and eosin stain of bone marrow biopsy shows hypercellular bone marrow with disrupted architecture, left-shifted granulopoiesis, and monolobulated megakaryocytes (**A**). Myeloblasts are highlighted by CD34 immunohistochemistry (**B**).

most common cytogenetic abnormality is monosomy 7, identified in 20% of all cases but more frequently identified in normocellular or hypercellular RCC (~19%).[9] Other recurrent aberrations include trisomy 8 and complex karyotypes. In MDS-EB, an abnormal karyotype is more commonly identified (55%-60% of cases), with monosomy 7 being the most common abnormality (29%-32%).[10]

Approximately 20% of RCC cases have an underlying germline predisposition, including GATA2 deficiency, SAMD9/SAMD9L syndrome, Fanconi anemia, or RUNX1 deficiency.[11,12] GATA2 deficiency and SAMD9/SAMD9L germline disease account for approximately half of these monosomy 7 cases.[11,12]

Somatic mutations are variably identified in pediatric MDS (9%-34% of cases) and are more common in MDS-EB.[3] In RCC, somatic mutations are identified in 13% to 17% of cases, whereas in MDS-EB, somatic mutations are identified in 65% to 68% of cases.[13] The most commonly mutated genes include *SETBP1, ASXL1, RUNX1, PTPN11, NRAS, KRAS*, and *NF1*.[3] In total, RAS pathway mutations (most commonly in *PTPN11* and *NRAS*, and also in *KRAS, CBL*, and *NF1*) are present in 12% to 45% of cases.[3] Cases with monosomy 7 have more somatic mutations compared with those with normal karyotypes (56% vs 18%)[13] and are enriched in mutations in *SETBP1, ASXL1*, and *RUNX1*, even in cases without germline mutations in *SAMD9/9L* or *GATA2*.

Prognosis and Clinical Comment

In the absence of excess blasts, patients with RCC with normal karyotype or trisomy 8 can experience a long stable course of their disease, while patients with monosomy 7 have a median time to progression of 17 months.[6,14] Although RCC with multilineage dysplasia (MLD) is associated with more frequent abnormal karyotype and increased risk of disease progression compared with RCC with single lineage dysplasia (SLD), the International Consensus Classification does not recommend to separate SLD from MLD in either RCC or MDS, NOS.[14] Allogeneic hematopoietic stem cell transplantation (HSCT) is the treatment of choice for nearly all patients with pediatric MDS. Immunosuppressive therapy can be a therapy option for some patients with RCC and a hypocellular marrow in the absence of abnormal karyotype or germline predisposition, although a proportion of these children will subsequently need HSCT for either nonresponse or relapse.[9,15] Outcome in patients with RCC is superior to that observed in patients with MDS-EB.[16] The presence of a structurally complex (≥3 chromosomal aberrations including at least one structural alteration) karyotype implies an inferior prognosis.[17] While some of the classical inherited bone marrow failure disorders like Fanconi anemia, Shwachman-Diamond syndrome, and severe congenital neutropenia require special consideration for MDS therapy, outcome of HSCT in large pediatric series appears independent of the presence of a *GATA2* or *SAMD9/SAMD9L* germline mutation.

References

1. Hasegawa D. The current perspective of low-grade myelodysplastic syndrome in children. *Int J Hematol.* 2016;103(4):360-364.
2. Yoshimi A, Niemeyer C, Baumann I, et al. High incidence of Fanconi anaemia in patients with a morphological picture consistent with refractory cytopenia of childhood. *Br J Haematol.* 2013;160(1):109-111.
3. Wlodarski MW, Hirabayashi S, Pastor V, et al. Prevalence, clinical characteristics, and prognosis of GATA2-related myelodysplastic syndromes in children and adolescents. *Blood.* 2016;127(11):1387-1518.
4. Hasle H, Niemeyer CM, Chessells JM, et al. A pediatric approach to the WHO classification of myelodysplastic and myeloproliferative diseases. *Leukemia.* 2003;17(2):277-282.
5. Passmore SJ, Chessells JM, Kempski H, Hann IM, Brownbill PA, Stiller CA. Paediatric myelodysplastic syndromes and juvenile myelomonocytic leukaemia in the UK: a population-based study of incidence and survival. *Br J Haematol.* 2003;121(5):758-767.
6. Kardos G, Baumann I, Passmore SJ, et al. Refractory anemia in childhood: a retrospective analysis of 67 patients with particular reference to monosomy 7. *Blood.* 2003;102(6):1997-2003.
7. Westers TM, Ireland R, Kern W, et al. Standardization of flow cytometry in myelodysplastic syndromes: a report from an international consortium and the European LeukemiaNet Working Group. *Leukemia.* 2012;26(7):1730-1741.
8. Aalbers AM, van den Heuvel-Eibrink MM, de Haas V, et al. Applicability of a reproducible flow cytometry scoring system in the diagnosis of refractory cytopenia of childhood. *Leukemia.* 2013;27(9):1923-1925.
9. Yoshimi A, van den Heuvel-Eibrink MM, Baumann I, et al. Comparison of horse and rabbit antithymocyte globulin in immunosuppressive therapy for refractory cytopenia of childhood. *Haematologica.* 2014;99(4):656-663.
10. Niemeyer CM, Kratz CP. Paediatric myelodysplastic syndromes and juvenile myelomonocytic leukaemia: molecular classification and treatment options. *Br J Haematol.* 2008;140(6):610-624.
11. Sahoo SS, Pastor VB, Goodings C, et al. Clinical evolution, genetic landscape and trajectories of clonal hematopoiesis in SAMD9/SAMD9L syndromes. *Nat Med.* 2021;27(10):1806-1817.
12. Wlodarski MW, Sahoo SS, Niemeyer CM. Monosomy 7 in pediatric myelodysplastic syndromes. *Hematol Oncol Clin North Am.* 2018;32(4):729-743.
13. Pastor V, Hirabayashi S, Karow A, et al. Mutational landscape in children with myelodysplastic syndromes is distinct from adults: specific somatic drivers and novel germline variants. *Leukemia.* 2017;31(3):759-762.
14. Hasegawa D, Chen X, Hirabayashi S, et al. Clinical characteristics and treatment outcome in 65 cases with refractory cytopenia of childhood defined according to the WHO 2008 classification. *Br J Haematol.* 2014;166(5):758-766.
15. Hama A, Takahashi Y, Muramatsu H, et al. Comparison of long-term outcomes between children with aplastic anemia and refractory cytopenia of childhood who received immunosuppressive therapy with antithymocyte globulin and cyclosporine. *Haematologica.* 2015;100(11):1426-1433.
16. Bortnick R, Wlodarski M, de Haas V; for EWOG-MDS, et al. Hematopoietic stem cell transplantation in children and adolescents with GATA2-related myelodysplastic syndrome. *Bone Marrow Transplant.* 2021;56(11):2732-2741.
17. Göhring G, Michalova K, Beverloo HB, et al. Complex karyotype newly defined: the strongest prognostic factor in advanced childhood myelodysplastic syndrome. *Blood.* 2010;116(19):3766-3769.

Chapter 21

Hematologic Malignancies With Germline Predisposition

Katherine R. Calvo, Courtney D. DiNardo, Jeffery M. Klco, Charlotte M. Niemeyer, Martina Rudelius, and Akiko Shimamura

Definition

Genetic predisposition to hematologic malignancy is defined by a higher risk of hematologic malignancy in patients born with a germline pathogenic/likely pathogenic (P/LP) gene variant compared with matched populations without a P/LP variant. This category focuses on conditions associated with a high risk of primary myelodysplastic syndrome (MDS), acute myeloid leukemia (AML), and acute lymphoblastic leukemia. Genes primarily predisposing to solid tumors with subsequent hematologic malignancy following genotoxic therapy for the solid tumor are not included in this classification. Germline disorders with an increased risk of juvenile myelomonocytic leukemia are discussed in Chapter 19. Hematologic malignancies associated with Down syndrome are discussed in Chapter 37.

Germline cancer predisposition is identified in an increasing subset of patients with hematologic malignancies, with the frequency dependent on the cohort but overall estimated at around 10% to 20% of patients with hematologic malignancy, with higher frequencies in pediatric patients. Germline variants predisposing to malignancy may be familial and inherited or may arise de novo in the patient without presence in either parent. In de novo cases, the germline mutation may have originated from gonadal mosaicism in sperm, ova, or the fertilized egg. Prior to the availability of broad genetic testing, diagnosis of inherited cancer predisposition syndromes was reliant on characteristic syndromic features that often presented in childhood. It is now recognized that such syndromes have highly variable phenotypes and may present with hematologic malignancy without any overt syndromic features. Absence of syndromic features does not rule out an underlying genetic predisposition condition. An unusually young age of presentation can be an important clue to a genetic malignancy predisposition condition; however, genetic predisposition to malignancy may present at any age—there is no upper age cutoff for these conditions.

The list of genes with germline genetic alterations predisposing to hematologic malignancies is rapidly expanding. The major categories outlined herein include well-characterized conditions with substantial evidence supporting genetic predisposition to hematologic malignancy. Newer conditions or those with limited available data are categorized as provisional conditions of diagnostic importance.

The identification of hematologic neoplasms with germline P/LP variants is critical as it informs diagnosis, treatment, screening of related donors for stem cell transplantation, selection of transplant conditioning regimens, and genetic counseling for affected family members. A high index of suspicion of germline predisposition is particularly important when planning a related donor transplant. The inadvertent use of seemingly healthy related transplant donors who harbor the same germline P/LP variant as the patient has led to donor-derived MDS and AML, failed engraftment, poor graft function, or other impairment, underscoring the need for increased awareness and recognition of hematologic neoplasms with germline predisposition. Early diagnosis prior to malignancy development offers opportunities for surveillance and potential early preventive intervention. Many of these germline conditions are associated with additional comorbidities such as bone marrow failure, increased solid tumor risk, immune deficiency, or additional organ dysfunction, so timely diagnosis allows appropriate evaluation, prevention of complications, and monitoring for disease progression. Early diagnosis also allows family planning and family counseling. Diagnosis of a germline predisposition condition also informs hematopathologic diagnosis of MDS, since many of these conditions even at baseline have significant marrow dyspoiesis with features overlapping with MDS-related dysplasia, which can cause a misdiagnosis.

Synonyms

Cancer predisposition syndrome, hereditary cancer predisposition syndrome, inherited cancer syndromes, familial neoplasms, familial MDSs/familial leukemias.

Epidemiology

Genetic predisposition to hematologic malignancies affects both genders and all races. These malignancies may present at any age. Although many conditions present in childhood and early adulthood, these also present in older/elderly adults. Notably, germline mutations in *DDX41* predispose to malignancies late in life.

General Clinical Features

Although many genetic predisposition conditions may manifest specific clinical features (see following descriptions), these findings are highly variable and are often absent even in conditions commonly considered syndromic. Additionally, some genetic predisposition conditions only present with hematologic malignancy as their sole clinical manifestation. A thorough clinical history, detailed family history, complete physical examination, and screening laboratory tests can identify signs of a potential genetic predisposition condition. Particular attention should be paid to a history of longstanding cytopenia(s) even if mild or asymptomatic or history of macrocytosis prior to the onset of malignancy. Clues to a potential underlying germline predisposition are outlined in Table 21.1.

TABLE 21.1 Clues to an underlying genetic predisposition condition

- Presentation with cancer at an unusually young age or lack of risk factors. Note: advanced age does not rule out genetic predisposition
- A personal history of multiple cancers
- Antecedent history of cytopenia(s), bone marrow failure, or unexplained macrocytosis
- First- or second-degree relative with a hematologic malignancy or a solid tumor suggestive of a genetic predisposition condition. Note: a negative family history does not rule out a genetic predisposition condition.
- Comorbidities associated with genetic predisposition conditions, such as congenital anomalies, idiopathic pulmonary fibrosis, liver abnormalities, immune deficiencies, atypical infections, lymphedema, hypogonadism, short stature, bleeding propensity.
- For somatic mutation panel: persistence even in remission of a mutation in a gene known to cause germline genetic predisposition, especially if the variant allele frequency is suggestive of germline origin. The germline origin of the variant may be confirmed by testing a nonhematopoietic tissue such as cultured skin fibroblasts or identification of the same mutation in parents or siblings.
- Related donor with poor stem cell mobilization or cytopenias/marrow abnormalities
- Chromosomal abnormalities commonly associated with specific germline predisposition to hematologic malignancy conditions:
  - Monosomy 7/deletion of 7q: GATA2, SAMD9/L, inherited bone marrow failure conditions
  - Del(20q) or i7q: Shwachman-Diamond syndrome
  - Gains of chromosome 1q or 3q: Fanconi anemia
  - Trisomy 8: GATA2
  - Hypodiploid ALL: TP53/Li-Fraumeni syndrome
- Characteristic patterns of somatic mutations, particularly in childhood/young adulthood (see text for discussion of individual conditions)

ALL, acute lymphoblastic leukemia.

Morphology

The detection of a germline mutation predisposing to hematologic malignancy does not equate with having a hematologic malignancy. In general, the same criteria used for diagnosis of hematologic malignancy in sporadic disease apply to patients with germline predisposition with some important caveats. As outlined in the MDS chapter, morphologic dysplasia in myeloid, erythroid, or megakaryocytic lineages is defined by equal or greater than 10% of the cells in the lineage demonstrating dysplastic features. Importantly, bone marrow morphology of patients with germline predisposition may show evidence of hypocellularity for age with intrinsic mild to moderate dyspoiesis resembling dysplasia at baseline prior to the development of malignancy, and some of these patients may have stable cytopenia and dyspoiesis over time without developing myeloid malignancy. Pathologists and hematologists are cautioned not to overdiagnose MDS in patients with germline predisposition based solely on mild to moderate morphologic dyspoiesis without additional supporting evidence of progression to MDS. The development of myeloid malignancy is typically associated with frank multilineage dysplasia, increased blasts, and/or acquired high-risk clonal cytogenetic or genetic abnormalities often in the setting of worsening cytopenia and increased marrow cellularity (Table 21.2). The interpretation of MDS diagnosis must be made in the context of the specific germline predisposition syndrome. Patients with germline mutations associated with thrombocytopenia, including mutations in *RUNX1, ANKRD26,* and *ETV6*, may have at baseline small hypolobated megakaryocytes or megakaryocytes with separated nuclear lobes associated with impaired maturation (Figure 21.1). These patients may have stable isolated

TABLE 21.2 Features associated with progression to myelodysplastic syndrome in patients with germline predisposition[a]

Two of three of the following:
• Acquired pathogenic genetic alteration.   • Monosomy 7, monosomy 5, del(7q), del(5q), multihit *TP53* mutations (defined as 2 or more distinct *TP53* mutations each with VAF ≥10%, or a single *TP53* mutation with (1) 17p deletion on cytogenetics, (2) VAF of ≥50%, or 3) copy neutral LOH at the 17p*TP53* locus), *TP53* mutation (VAF ≥ 10%) and complex karyotype (often with loss of 17p), or *SF3B1* mutation (VAF ≥ 10%) are considered MDS defining[b] • Cytopenia in a new lineage(s) or progressive cytopenia,[c] particularly in the context of increasing marrow cellularity • Multilineage dysplasia[d]
Or:
Increased blasts • ≥5% in marrow; ≥2% in peripheral blood

LOH, loss of heterozygosity; MDS, myelodysplastic syndrome; VAF, variant allele frequency.

[a]These are guidelines and are not intended as absolute criteria; clinical judgment must be applied in each case.

[b]Genetic alterations should be interpreted in the context of the specific germline condition.

[c]In adults, cytopenias are defined as hemoglobin <12 g/dL in females and <13 g/dL in males, absolute neutrophil count $<1.8 \times 10^9$/L, and/or platelets $<150 \times 10^9$/L. In children, cytopenia is defined according to age-adjusted values for hemoglobin, absolute neutrophil count, and platelet count.

[d]Baseline marrows in patients with germline mutations may show evidence of dyspoiesis; hence, care must be taken not to overinterpret dysmorphology as criteria for MDS in the absence of additional supporting evidence. Patients with germline mutations in *RUNX1*, *ANKRD26*, and *ETV6* with isolated thrombocytopenia commonly show megakaryocytic atypia at baseline, and as a sole finding this is not sufficient for a diagnosis of MDS. Dysplasia is defined as dysplastic cytologic changes in ≥10% of erythroid cells, ≥10% of granulocytic cells, and/or ≥10% of megakaryocytes.

thrombocytopenia with dysmegakaryopoiesis for many years without developing MDS. Clonal hematopoiesis is not uncommon in patients with germline predisposition and must be considered within the context of the specific germline predisposition syndrome, as well as associated blood and bone marrow findings.

Immunophenotype

Flow cytometry analysis of marrow and/or blood may be helpful in identifying abnormal immunophenotypic expression patterns in malignant blasts, cells, or dysplastic cells. The immunophenotype of myeloid blasts in patients with germline predisposition and MDS or AML may display abnormal expression of CD7, CD2, or CD123 or lack expression of CD38. Flow cytometry analysis of blasts in acute lymphoblastic leukemia is critical for establishing blast lineage and identification of aberrant expression patterns. Additionally, flow cytometry may be critical in the identification of underlying immunodeficiency that is associated with some of the germline predisposition syndromes including marked decrease to absence of monocytes, B cells, B-cell precursors, dendritic cells, and NK cells in GATA2 deficiency. Immunohistochemistry performed on the bone marrow core biopsy or clot section is often critical for enabling proper diagnosis particularly in cases with poor or hemodiluted aspirates. CD34 is helpful in identifying increased blasts for cases in which the blasts are CD34 positive. CD42b and CD61 can aid in recognition of megakaryocytic dysplasia by highlighting micromegakaryocytes and small monolobated megakaryocytes that are missed on the hematoxylin and eosin stain. Myeloperoxidase and CD71 or glycophorin can be of help in confirming the M:E ratio.

Genetics

Owing to the high variability of clinical presentation, broad testing of multiple genes is now recommended as an integral part of the diagnostic evaluation for genetic predisposition to hematologic malignancy. The genetic patterns (dominant, recessive, X-linked) for each condition are summarized in Tables 21.3-21.9. A single heterozygous P/LP variant in a gene causing recessive (biallelic) germline genetic predisposition should not be assumed to be causative merely based on its presence in a patient(s) with a hematologic malignancy. Since genetic testing requires several weeks and results may require additional evaluation, this is best initiated early to avoid delaying urgent therapies such as transplant. Variants of unknown clinical significance may require further evaluation beyond the scope of this chapter; so, consultation with an expert is recommended. Since many genes may be mutated in either the germline or somatic context, mutations identified on somatic panels, particularly those at near-heterozygous frequency, may require further evaluation using a nonhematopoietic DNA source (such as skin fibroblast cultures) to distinguish somatic from germline mutations. For germline genetic diagnosis, it is best practice to utilize panels designed for detection of germline mutations since the panel composition, regions covered within a given gene, as well as required extragenic regions (ie, promoter mutations in *ANKRD26*, intronic mutations in *GATA2*), copy number variant detection, and variant filtering may differ from that of somatic mutation panels; whole exome or genome sequencing may also be appropriate.

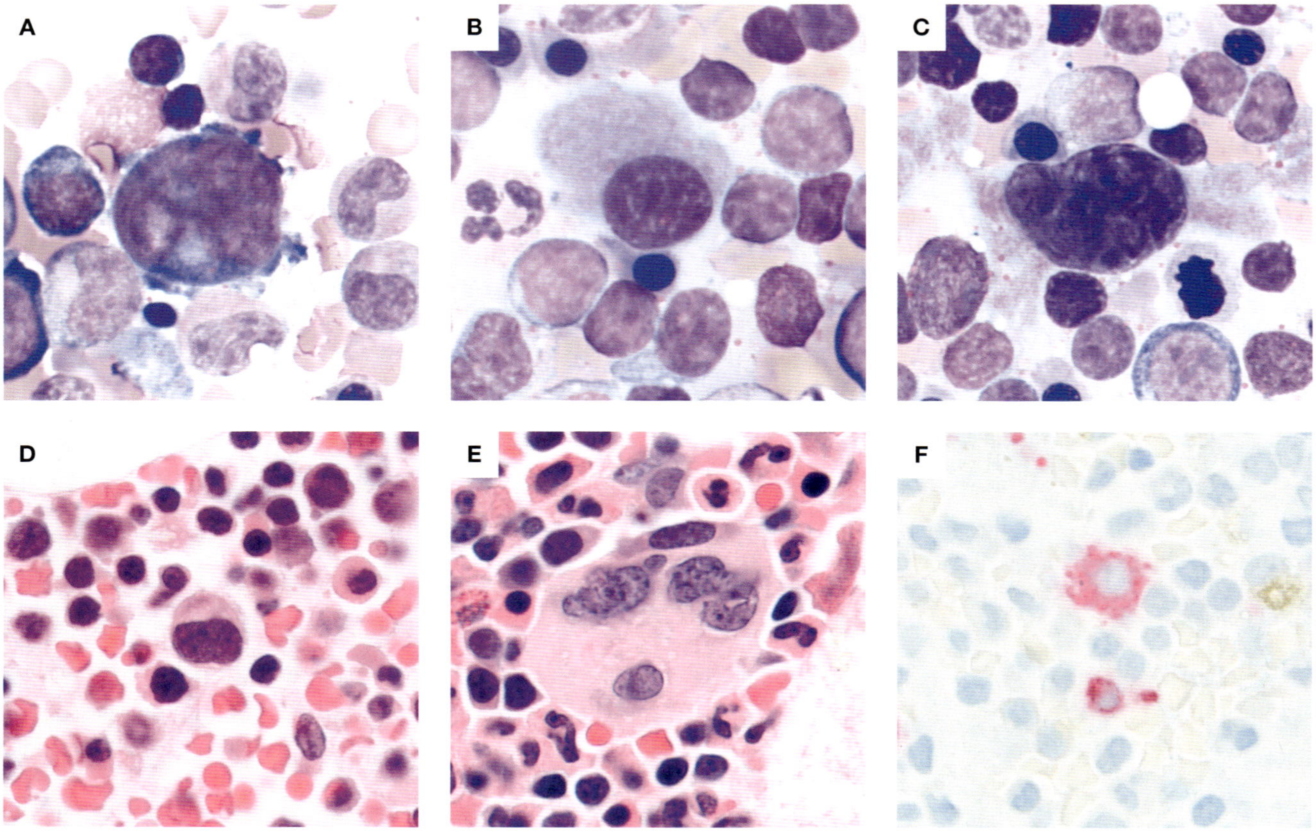

FIGURE 21.1 Baseline dysmegakaryopoiesis associated with germline mutations in *RUNX1*. Patients with RUNX1 familial platelet disorder and isolated thrombocytopenia often show baseline dysmegakaryopoiesis composed of small abnormal monolobated megakaryocytes that can be seen on aspirate smears **(A-C)** or trephine core biopsies **(D)**; megakaryocytes with separated nuclear lobes may also be present **(E)**. CD61 immunohistochemistry performed on the biopsy may be helpful in identifying small forms **(F)**. Pathologists are cautioned not to overinterpret dysmegakaryopoiesis in patients with platelet disorders as evidence of myelodysplastic syndrome (MDS) in the absence of other MDS-defining abnormalities.

Hematologic neoplasms with germline predisposition without a constitutional disorder

These conditions typically present with malignancy without other organ system dysfunction.

Myeloid neoplasms with germline *CEBPA* mutation

Heterozygous germline P/LP variants in *CEBPA*, which encodes CCAAT/enhancer binding protein alpha, are associated with familial AML with autosomal dominant inheritance.[1] The development of AML is associated with an acquired mutation in the second *CEBPA* allele, typically within the C terminus, plus additional variable somatic mutations, and is associated with an overall favorable prognosis (10-year overall survival of 67%).[2] Patients with biallelic *CEBPA*-mutated AML should be evaluated further for a potential germline *CEBPA* condition. The germline *CEBPA* P/LP variants are typically frameshift or nonsense mutations near the amino terminus of the protein. Germline P/LP variants in the C terminus have also been reported. The second somatic mutation is typically a missense or in-frame indel within the C-terminal bZIP domain. Although patient numbers are limited, the AML penetrance associated with N-terminal germline *CEBPA* P/LP variants appears particularly high (>80%) compared with that with C-terminal germline *CEBPA* P/LP variants (around 50%). Following chemotherapy, these patients are prone to developing subsequent new distinct primary leukemia clones that are still sensitive to chemotherapy, in contrast to relapsed disease from a resistant primary clone. The myeloblast immunophenotype often demonstrates aberrant expression of CD7.

Myeloid or lymphoid neoplasms with germline *DDX41* mutation

Germline *DDX41* P/LP variants are often truncating and are among the most common predisposing to myeloid malignancy with an estimated prevalence of 3% of myeloid malignancies.[3] The development of myeloid malignancy is associated with a second acquired *DDX41* mutation, most commonly R525H, in about half of cases.[4] *DDX41* is located on chromosome

TABLE 21.3 Hematologic neoplasms with germline predisposition without a constitutional disorder affecting multiple organ systems

Gene(s)	Disease	Inheritance pattern	MDS, AML, ALL	Other malignancies	Other phenotypic findings (variable, may be absent)	Additional lab tests
CEBPA		AD	AML			AML may harbor additional somatic *CEBPA*
DDX41		AD	MDS, AML > ALL	CMML, CML, MPN, lymphoma (NHL, HL), CLL, MM	Malignancies typically present at older age	Malignancy may harbor somatic *DDX41*
TP53	Li-Fraumeni syndrome	AD	B-ALL (de novo low hypodiploid), MDS, AML (typically therapy-related myeloid malignancy)	Solid tumors (adrenocorticocarcinoma, brain tumor [especially choroid plexus carcinoma], premenopausal breast cancer, osteosarcoma, soft tissue sarcomas, GI tumors, melanoma, lung cancer, other), lymphoma.		
MLH1, MSH2, MSH6, PMS2, EPCAM	Congenital mismatch repair disorders (CMMRDs)	AR	ALL, AML	Lymphomas, solid tumors (GI (colorectal and small bowel, gastric, pancreatic), endometrial, urinary tract, CNS tumors, sebaceous adenomas, other	Hyper/hypopigmented spots on skin (café au lait macules), polyposis, immunoglobulin deficiencies (rare), hypermutated cancers	
MBD4		AR	AML	Colonic polyposis, uveal melanoma, nervous system tumors, other solid tumors	Hypermutated AML	

AD, autosomal dominant; ALL, acute lymphoblastic leukemia; AML, acute myeloid leukemia; AR, autosomal recessive; CLL, chronic lymphocytic leukemia; CML, chronic myeloid leukemia; CMML, chronic myelomonocytic leukemia; GI, gastrointestinal; HL, hodgkin lymphoma; MM, multiple myeloma; MDS, myelodysplastic syndrome; MPN, myeloproliferative neoplasm; NHL, non-hodgkin lymphoma.

5 and is one of the DEAD-box helicase family of genes. In contrast to many other germline predisposition syndromes, patients with germline *DDX41* P/LP variants typically present with myeloid malignancy at an older age in the sixth decade or later, overlapping with the age presentation of sporadic MDS and AML. Patients may present with cytopenia, macrocytosis, and normocellular or hypocellular marrow with erythroid dysplasia with or without increased blasts in the setting of a normal karyotype and normal immunophenotype. In some cases, years of mild cytopenia may precede the development of MDS. Lymphoid neoplasms have also been described in families with germline *DDX41* mutations.[5]

TABLE 21.4 Hematologic neoplasms with germline predisposition associated with a constitutional platelet disorder

Gene	Disease	Inheritance patterns	MDS, AML, ALL	Other malignancies	Other phenotypic findings (variable, may be absent)	Additional lab tests
ANKRD26	Thrombocytopenia-2 (THC2)	AD	MDS, AML	CML	Thrombocytopenia and qualitative platelet dysfunction (mild)	
ETV6	Thrombocytopenia-5 (THC5)	AD	B-ALL > MDS, AML	MPN, MPAL, MM	Thrombocytopenia, bleeding, rare reports of solid tumors	
RUNX1	Familial platelet disorder with associated myeloid malignancy (FPDMM)	AD	MDS, AML, T-ALL > B-ALL	Lymphoma, CMML, myeloma	Thrombocytopenia, bleeding, platelet functional abnormalities (aspirin-like abnormalities, alpha and/or delta granule abnormalities), eczema, asthma, allergies, GI abnormalities, abnormal pulmonary function test	Platelet aggregation

AD, autosomal dominant; ALL, acute lymphoblastic leukemia; AML acute myeloid leukemia; CML, chronic myeloid leukemia; CMML, chronic myelomonocytic leukemia; GI, gastrointestinal; MM, multiple myeloma; MDS, myelodysplastic syndrome; MPAL, mixed-phenotype acute leukemia; MPN, myeloproliferative neoplasm.

TABLE 21.5 Hematologic neoplasms with germline predisposition associated with a constitutional disorder affecting multiple organ systems

Gene(s)	Disease	Inheritance pattern	MDS, AML, ALL	Other malignancies	Other phenotypic findings (variable, may be absent)
ERCC6L2		AR	MDS, AML, T-ALL		Bone marrow failure, neurologic abnormalities
GATA2	GATA2 deficiency, Emberger, MonoMac, DCML	AD	MDS, AML, ALL, MDS/MPN	Lymphoma	Bone marrow failure/cytopenias, immunodeficiency, viral infections (eg, warts), atypical mycobacterial infections, low dendritic cell/monocyte/B cell/NK cell, lymphedema, pulmonary alveolar proteinosis, sensorineural hearing loss
SAMD9	MIRAGE	AD	MDS, AML		Bone marrow failure/cytopenias, infection, immunodeficiency, skin, growth restriction, skeletal, adrenal hypoplasia, endocrine, genital anomalies, enteropathy, cardiopulmonary, craniofacial, neurocognitive
SAMD9L	Ataxia-pancytopenia	AD	MDS, AML		Bone marrow failure, growth retardation, ataxia/CNS, neurocognitive, endocrine, skin, skeletal, urogenital, GI, craniofacial, cardiopulmonary

AD, autosomal dominant; ALL, acute lymphoblastic leukemia; AML, acute myeloid leukemia; AR, autosomal recessive; CNS, central nervous system; DCML, dendritic cell, monocyte, lymphocyte deficiency; GI, gastrointestinal; MDS, myelodysplastic syndrome; MIRAGE, myelodysplasia, infection, restriction of growth, adrenal hypoplasia, genital phenotypes, enteropathy syndrome; MPN, myeloproliferative neoplasm.

Myeloid or lymphoid neoplasms with germline *TP53* mutation/Li-Fraumeni syndrome

Li-Fraumeni syndrome is a cancer predisposition syndrome caused by autosomal dominant germline heterozygous P/LP variants in *TP53*, which encodes a key checkpoint regulator of the cell cycle, DNA repair, and apoptosis.[6,7] Approximately 7% to 20% of germline *TP53* P/LP variants arise de novo, so family history may be negative. The most common malignancies in individuals with germline P/LP variants *TP53* mutations are listed in Table 21.3. Hematologic malignancies, particularly hypodiploid acute lymphoblastic leukemia (ALL), account for approximately 4% of Li-Fraumeni-associated neoplasms. Germline *TP53* P/LP variants are present in over half of pediatric low-hypodiploid acute lymphoblastic leukemia and are associated with poor outcome. Myeloid malignancies such as MDS or AML in patients with Li-Fraumeni syndrome typically occur following treatment of a primary neoplasm, ie, they are therapy related. Given the implications for additional cancer development, it is critical to distinguish germline from somatic *TP53* P/LP variants by testing a nonhematopoietic tissue such as cultured skin fibroblasts. Identification of a germline *TP53* P/LP variant informs clinical decisions, such as minimizing exposure to ionizing radiation, and allows implementation of recommended cancer surveillance. The marrow is typically normocellular at baseline.

Myeloid and lymphoid neoplasms with constitutional mismatch repair deficiency

Constitutional mismatch repair deficiency (CMMRD) syndrome is caused by biallelic germline P/LP variants in the mismatch repair genes. Clinical manifestations are variable (see Table 21.3). The cancer risk phenotype overlaps with but is distinct from that of Lynch syndrome, which is caused by heterozygous P/LP variants in the mismatch repair genes. The incidence of primary hematologic malignancy appears to be much lower in Lynch syndrome (caused by heterozygous mutations in the mismatch repair genes) than with CMMRD.

Myeloid neoplasms with germline *MBD4* mutation

MBD4 encodes a base excision repair gene that functions to prevent DNA damage from methylation on cytosine resides resulting in spontaneous deamination to thymidine. Cases of early-onset AML, including familial cases, with biallelic germline loss-of-function P/LP variants in the *MBD4* gene were identified with a unique mutational signature where >95% of mutations exhibited the methylation damage signature CG > TC.[8] Acquisition of somatic P/LP variants in additional myeloid malignancy genes, particularly biallelic CG > TA mutations in *DNMT3A* and *IDH1/IDH2* hot spot mutations, was identified. Solid tumors, adenomatous colorectal polyposis, and uveal melanoma have also been described among the *MBD4*-associated neoplasms.

Hematologic neoplasms with germline predisposition associated with a constitutional platelet disorder

Germline P/LP variants in *RUNX1*, *ANKRD26*, and *ETV6* are associated with lifelong thrombocytopenia and/or platelet dysfunction with increased risk of developing myeloid and/or lymphoid neoplasia depending on the gene. Some patients are misdiagnosed with

TABLE 21.6 Hematologic neoplasms with germline predisposition associated with a constitutional disorder affecting multiple organ systems: Bone Marrow Failure Syndromes

Genes	Disease	Inheritance pattern	MDS, AML, ALL	Other malignancies	Other phenotypic findings (variable, may be absent)	Additional lab tests
AD: *RPL5, RPL9, RPL11, RPL15, RPL18, RPL26, RPL27, RPL31, RPL35, RPL35A, RPS7, RPS10, RPS15A, RPS17, RPS19, RPS24, RPS26, RPS27. RPS28. RPS29* **XLR:** *GATA1, TSR2*	Diamond-Blackfan anemia	AD/XLR	MDS, AML	Solid tumors: osteosarcoma, colorectal cancer, soft tissue sarcoma, other	Macrocytic anemia with red cell aplasia, short stature, congenital anomalies (thumbs, cardiac, craniofacial, cleft lip/cleft palate, kidney). *RPL35A* deletions associated with severe neutropenia and immunodeficiency.	Elevated erythrocyte adenosine deaminase
AR: *FANCA, FANCC, FANCD1 (BRCA2), FANCD2, FANCE, FANCF, FANCG (XRCC9), FANCI, FANCJ (BRIP1), FANCL, FANCM, FANCN (PALB2), FANCO (RAD51C), FANCP (SLX4), FANCQ (ERCC4), FANCS (BRCA1), FANCT (UBE2T), FANCU (XRCC2), FANCV (REV7/MAD2L2), FANCW (RFWD3), FANCY (FAAP100)* **AD:** *FANCR (RAD51)***XLR:** *FANCB*	Fanconi anemia	AD/AR/XLR	MDS, AML, T-ALL (FANCD1/BRCA2)	Solid tumors: head and neck/GI squamous cell carcinomas, liver tumors, vaginal/vulvar squamous cell carcinomas. FANCD1/BRCA2 subtypes: brain tumors, Wilms tumors, other.	Bone marrow failure/aplastic anemia, short stature, skin hyper/hypopigmentation, craniofacial dysmorphologies, endocrinopathies, skeletal anomalies, genitourinary abnormalities, congenital hearing loss, external/internal ear dysmorphologies, eye abnormalities, CNS abnormalities, VACTERL-H (vertebral anomalies, anal atresia, congenital heart disease, tracheoesophageal =fistula, esophageal atresia, renal, limb anomalies, hydrocephalus)	Increased chromosomal breakage with mitomycin C or diepoxybutane
AD: ELANE, GFI1, TCIRG1**AR:** *HAX1, G6PC3, JAGN1, CSF3R, VPS45***XLR:** *WAS***AD:** *CLPB*	Severe congenital neutropenia	AD/AR/XLR	MDS, AML		**CLPB**: developmental delay, 3-methylglutaconic aciduria, cataracts, congenital anomalies; **G6PC3:** cardiac, superficial veins, genitourinary anomalies, endocrinopathies, skin hyperelasticity; **HAX1**: neurodevelopmental; **JAGN1**: developmental delay, skeletal anomalies; **WAS**: monocytopenia, immunologic abnormalities	
AR: *SBDS, DNAJC21,* EFL1* **AD**: SRP54* *Phenotype can resemble SDS or SCN	Shwachman-Diamond syndrome and related disorders	AR	MDS, AML		Bone marrow failure/aplastic anemia, exocrine pancreatic dysfunction, short stature, skeletal anomalies (including metaphyseal dysostosis and thoracic dystrophy), osteopenia, transient liver transaminitis/hepatomegaly in early childhood, endocrinopathies, immunologic abnormalities, inflammatory conditions, neurocognitive/CNS abnormalities	Low pancreatic isoamylase (age >3 y); low fecal elastase
AD: *TERC, TINF2, ZCCHC8, NAF1, RPA1* **AR:** *NOP10, NHP10, WRAP53, CTC1, STN1, DCLRE1B* **AD/AR:** *TERT, RTEL1, PARN, ACD* **XLR:** *DKC1*	Telomere biology disorder/dyskeratosis congenita	AD/AR/XLR	MDS, AML	Lymphoma, solid tumors (head and neck squamous cell carcinomas).	Hoyeraal-Hreidarsson syndrome, nail dystrophy, skin pigmentation, leukoplakia, pulmonary fibrosis/abnormalities, liver cirrhosis/abnormalities, arteriovenous malformations, premature greying or alopecia, GI abnormalities, renal/genitourinary abnormalities, skeletal anomalies, retinal/eye anomalies, immunologic abnormalities, poor growth/short stature, bone marrow failure/aplastic anemia, cytopenias, red cell macrocytosis	Short telomere length (variable)

AD, autosomal dominant; ALL, acute lymphoblastic leukemia; AML, acute myeloid leukemia; AR, autosomal recessive; CNS, central nervous system; GI, gastrointestinal; MDS, myelodysplastic syndrome; SCN, severe congenital neutropenia; SDS, Shwachman-Diamond syndrome; XLR, X-linked recessive.

TABLE 21.7 Acute lymphoblastic leukemia with germline predisposition

Gene(s)	Inheritance pattern	MDS, AML, ALL	Other malignancies	Other phenotypic findings (variable, may be absent)
IKZF1	AD	B-ALL, possibly also T-ALL	Lymphoma	Immunodeficiency (CVID, B-cell deficiency), autoimmune cytopenias, autoimmune conditions
PAX5	AD	B-ALL		Developmental delay, intellectual disability, autism spectrum disorder

AD, autosomal dominant; ALL, acute lymphoblastic leukemia; AML, acute myeloid leukemia; CVID, common variable immunodeficiency; MDS, myelodysplastic syndrome.

TABLE 21.8 Additional conditions with germline predisposition to hematologic malignancy

Gene(s)	Disease	Inheritance pattern	MDS, AML, ALL	Other malignancies	Other phenotypic findings (variable, may be absent)
BLM	Bloom syndrome	AR	MDS, AML, ALL	Lymphomas (B-, T-, Burkitt), solid tumors (adenocarcinomas, head and neck squamous cell carcinomas, other)	IUGR/short stature, craniofacial anomalies, photosensitivity, malar rash, UV-induced erythematous rash, telangiectasias and poikiloderma, café-au-lait macules, oral fissures, hypogonadism, early gonadal failure, immunodeficiency, type 2 diabetes, chronic lung disease. Increased sister chromatid exchange.
XPC: specific founder mutation in North African patients	Xeroderma pigmentosa, subtype C	AR	MDS, AML, T-ALL	Skin cancers (melanoma)	Photosensitivity, dry skin, freckling, hearing loss, ataxia, cognitive impairment, seizures.

ALL, acute lymphoblastic leukemia; AML, acute myeloid leukemia; AR, autosomal recessive; IUGR, intrauterine growth restriction; MDS, myelodysplastic syndrome.

TABLE 21.9 Provisional germline genetic predisposition to hematologic malignancy

Genes	Disease	Inheritance pattern	MDS, AML, ALL	Other malignancies	Other phenotypic findings (variable, may be absent)
MPL	Congenital amegakaryocytic thrombocytopenia (CAMT)	AR	MDS	Pre-B-ALL	Thrombocytopenia typically in infancy/early childhood, often progressing to severe aplastic anemia, CNS anomalies, ocular/orbital anomalies
CSF3R		AD	MDS, AML		Neutrophilia
DNMT3A	Tatton-Brown-Rahman syndrome	AD	AML		Overgrowth, intellectual disability
MECOM	Thrombocytopenia radioulnar synostosis	AD	MDS		Radioulnar synostosis/limb malformation, immunologic, congenital anomalies, hearing impairment
TET2		AD	AML	CMML, lymphoma	

AD, autosomal dominant; ALL, acute lymphoblastic leukemia; AML acute myeloid leukemia; AR, autosomal recessive; CNS, central nervous system; CMML, chronic myelomonocytic leukemia; MDS, myelodysplastic syndrome.

immune thrombocytopenia purpura (ITP) and are properly diagnosed after they develop myeloid malignancy and undergo molecular testing. Importantly, each of these entities is associated with intrinsic baseline dysmegakaryopoiesis in the bone marrow (see Figure 21.1) that should not be considered as MDS defining in the setting of isolated thrombocytopenia without additional supporting criteria. Progression to MDS is associated with multilineage cytopenias (in addition to thrombocytopenia), multilineage dysplasia, high-risk cytogenetic or acquired somatic mutations, and/or increased blasts (see Table 21.2).

Myeloid or lymphoid neoplasms with germline *RUNX1* mutation

RUNX1 (aka *AML1* and *CBFA2*) is located on chromosome 21 and encodes a subunit of the core binding transcription factor that is necessary for hematopoiesis including megakaryopoiesis and proplatelet formation. *RUNX1* is one of the most commonly targeted genes in chromosomal translocations associated with acute leukemia. Germline heterozygous P/LP variants in *RUNX1* lead to thrombocytopenia and platelet dysfunction with an increased risk of hematologic malignancies, most commonly myeloid including MDS, AML, and chronic myelomonocytic leukemia (CMML) and also involving lymphoid neoplasia (eg, T-ALL or B-ALL). Approximately 40% of patients with germline *RUNX1* P/LP variants develop hematologic malignancy that typically occurs in young adulthood with an average age of 34 years and a wide range from pediatric to elderly ages.[9] Baseline bone marrow findings include hypocellularity with normal numbers of megakaryocytes and frequent small hypolobated forms or frank megakaryocytic dysplasia.[10] There may be increased eosinophils. The marrow features can morphologically resemble ITP in some cases. Development of myeloid malignancy is associated with new onset of cytopenia and/or cytoses, multilineage dysplasia, cytogenetic abnormalities, acquired genetic mutations including a second somatic *RUNX1* mutation, and/or increased blasts often in association with increased bone marrow cellularity.[11] Clonal hematopoiesis with P/LP variants in *BCOR* is common.[12] Platelet aggregation studies are abnormal, typically demonstrating impaired aggregation to collagen, arachidonic acid, adenosine diphosphate, and dense granule storage deficiency. Some patients are misdiagnosed with ITP for many years before they develop myeloid malignancy and undergo genetic testing.

Myeloid neoplasms with germline *ANKRD26* mutation

ANKRD26 is located on chromosome 10p12.1. Germline heterozygous P/LP variants in *ANKRD26* involve the 5′ untranslated region disrupting the binding of corepressors FLI1 and RUNX1 leading to increased *ANKRD26* expression and signaling in the MPL pathway resulting in impaired proplatelet formation. Patients have mild to moderate thrombocytopenia and increased risk of myeloid malignancy with typical onset ranging from 35 to 70 years of age.[13] The most common myeloid malignancies reported are MDS and AML; CMML and chronic lymphocytic leukemia are also reported. Dysmegakaryopoiesis is a common bone marrow feature found in patients with stable disease and no malignancy. Progression to MDS/AML has been associated with additional cytopenia/cytoses, multilineage dysplasia, increased blasts, and/or cytogenetic/molecular abnormalities.[13]

Myeloid or lymphoid neoplasms with germline *ETV6* mutation

ETV6 is a member of the ETS family of transcription factors and is located on chromosome 12p13. Germline heterozygous P/LP variants in *ETV6* primarily involve the ETS DNA-binding domain and are associated with mild to moderate thrombocytopenia. There is an increased incidence of hematologic malignancies including B lymphoblastic leukemia (most common), MDS, AML, CMML, and myeloma.[14,15] Platelet size is normal, and the bone marrow at baseline may show an increase in small hypolobated megakaryocytes with or without associated dyserythropoiesis.[16] Approximately 30% of carriers develop hematologic malignancies. Solid tumors are also reported less frequently.

Hematologic neoplasms with germline predisposition associated with a constitutional disorder affecting multiple organ systems

These conditions may be associated with comorbidities affecting other organ systems; however, the clinical phenotypic spectrum is broad and patients with these conditions may present with a hematologic malignancy as their sole manifestation of their condition (see Table 21.5). Knowledge of associated comorbidities informs clinical evaluation, monitoring, and care decisions to reduce complications.

Myeloid neoplasms with germline *GATA2* mutations

GATA2 is located on chromosome 3 and encodes a transcription factor that is required for hematopoiesis. Germline heterozygous P/LP variants in *GATA2* are associated with immunodeficiency, lymphedema, warts, and high incidence of myeloid malignancy.[17-20] However, a subset of patients present with myeloid malignancy without recognition of preceding or concomitant syndromic features. The age at which myeloid malignancy develops is broad ranging from pediatric patients to older adults, with a median age of 12 to 35 years depending on the study.[21,22] De novo germline *GATA2* P/LP variants are common; hence, a family history of myeloid malignancy may be lacking. The most common myeloid malignancies are hypocellular MDS, AML, and CMML. A subset of patients present with bone marrow failure and hypocellular marrows that may morphologically overlap with idiopathic aplastic anemia. These patients are at high risk of transformation to MDS and AML.[23] Flow cytometric analysis of the marrow may be helpful in identifying the underlying immunodeficiency demonstrating markedly decreased to absent monocytes, B cells, B-cell precursors, NK cells, and/or dendritic cells.[24] Most cases of MDS demonstrate hypocellular marrow with dysmegakaryocytic dysplasia with micromegakaryocytes and characteristic megakaryocytes with separated nuclear lobes (Figure 21.2). Myeloid dysplasia is common with hyposegmented and hypogranular forms. Monosomy 7, trisomy 8, and der(1;7) (q10p10) are the most common cytogenetic abnormalities. The somatic mutational landscape of myeloid malignancy is characterized by acquired mutations in *ASXL1* and *STAG2;* lack of mutations in *SF3B1* in contrast to sporadic MDS; and emergence of *RUNX1*, *SETBP1*, or *RAS* mutations associated with leukemic transformation.[25,26]

Myeloid neoplasms with germline *SAMD9* or *SAMD9L* mutations[27]

SAMD9 (sterile alpha motif domain-containing protein 9) and its paralogue *SAMD9L* are located adjacent to each other on chromosome 7q21. These genes encode IFN- and TNF-a-responsive proteins that have been implicated in a variety of processes including viral defense responses, growth suppression, inflammation, endosomal fusion, and development. Heterozygous germline disease-causing variants in *SAMD9* are associated with MIRAGE syndrome (myelodysplasia, infections, restriction of growth, adrenal hypoplasia, genital phenotypes, and enteropathy). Heterozygous germline disease-causing variants in *SAMD9L* are associated with ataxia-pancytopenia syndrome characterized by cerebellar ataxia, pancytopenia/bone marrow failure, and predisposition to myeloid malignancy. *SAMD9/SAMD9L* function as growth suppressors, and the germline mutations are typically heterozygous missense mutations resulting in gain of function and further growth suppression leading to cytopenia. De novo heterozygous frameshift mutations in the P-loop NTPase domain of *SAMD9L* have been reported in an autoinflammatory condition SAMD9L-SAAD

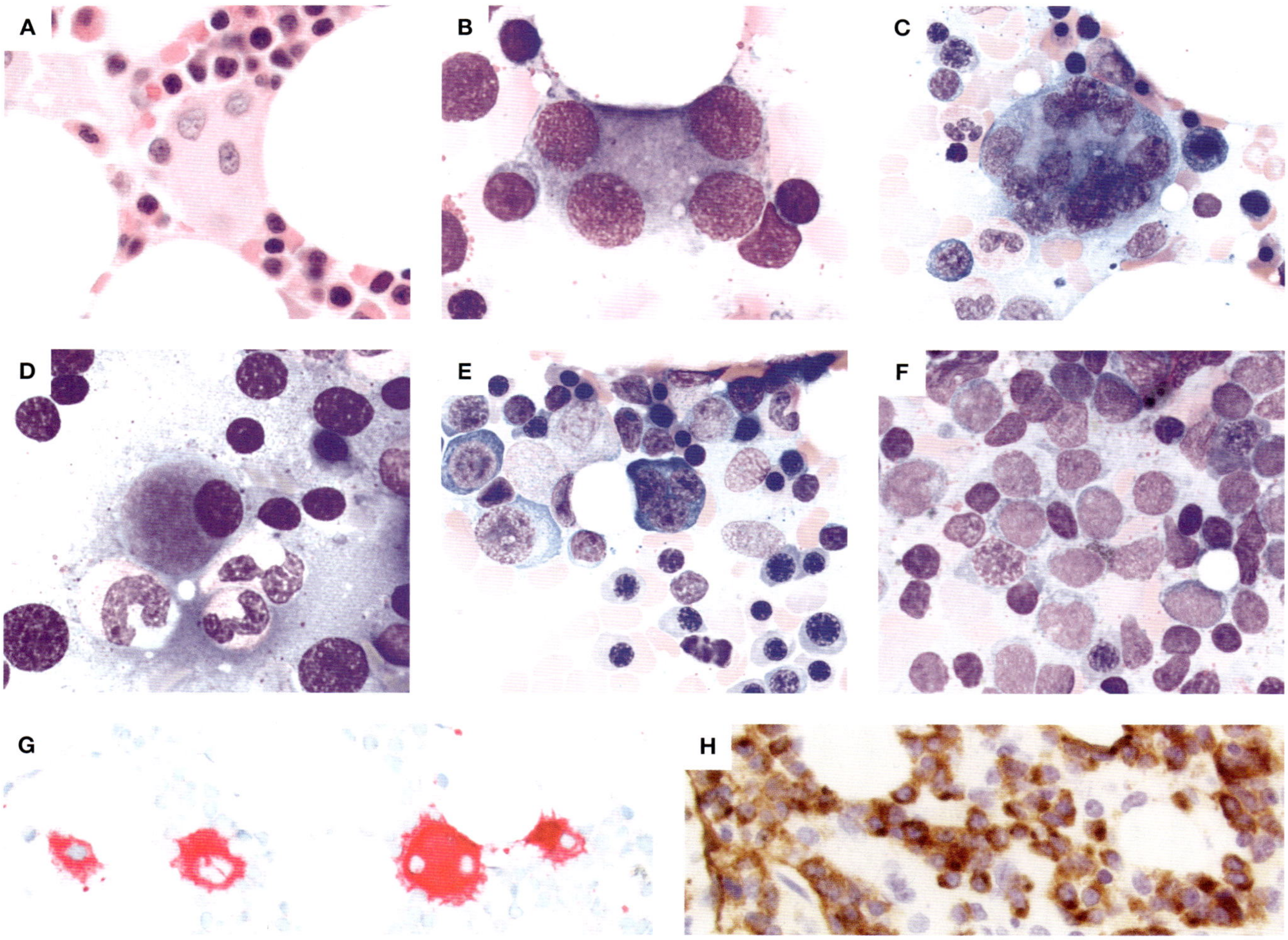

FIGURE 21.2 Features of myeloid malignancy in GATA2 deficiency. Myelodysplastic syndrome in patients with germline mutations in GATA2 is often associated with hypocellularity and markedly dysplastic megakaryocytes with separated nuclear lobes, mononuclear forms, and micromegakaryocytes **(A-D)**. Erythroid predominance is common with some degree of dyserythropoiesis **(E)** and/or dysmyelopoiesis with abnormal granulation and hyposegmentation. Progression to acute myeloid leukemia **(F)** is not uncommon. CD61 immunohistochemistry is helpful in identifying dysplastic megakaryocytes **(G)**. CD34 immunohistochemistry is useful for detection of increased blasts on marrow biopsies **(H)** in cases where the blasts express CD34.

(SAMD9L-associated autoinflammatory disease).[28] Clinical features of these syndromes can vary widely, and syndromic features may be absent in patients with germline disease-causing variants in these genes. Both *SAMD9* and *SAMD9L* gain-of-function mutations are characterized by a propensity to acquire monosomy 7 due to loss of the chromosome carrying the mutated *SAMD9/SAMD9L* allele (adaptation by aneuploidy). *SAMD9* mutations often arise de novo, and penetrance has been reported to be high. *SAMD9*, *SAMD9L*, and *GATA2* germline P/LP variants are among the most common germline mutations in pediatric MDS and refractory cytopenia of childhood and often present without syndromic features.[29] Cytopenias due to bone marrow failure outside the context of malignancy are common and may involve a single lineage, typically thrombocytopenia, or multiple lineages. Some clinical features of *SAMD9/SAMD9L* are listed in Table 21.5.

Genetic diagnosis may be hampered by somatic loss of the mutant *SAMD9/SAMD9L* allele, typically by elimination of chromosome 7 carrying the mutant allele, or somatic reversion via uniparental disomy with subsequent expansion of the revertant clone, so a strong level of suspicion and genetic analysis of nonhematopoietic tissue may be needed. Acquisition of a loss-of-function mutation in *cis* with the mutant allele allows escape from the growth-suppressive effects of the original mutation and provides an additional diagnostic clue. Blood counts and marrow cellularity may improve following somatic reversion, although monosomy 7/del7q increases the risk of clonal evolution to monosomy 7 MDS. Loss of monosomy 7/del7q accompanied by spontaneous hematologic recovery has been observed in some young children.

The marrow is typically hypocellular. The marrow may exhibit megakaryocyte dysplasia reminiscent of germline *GATA2* conditions (Figure 21.3); however,

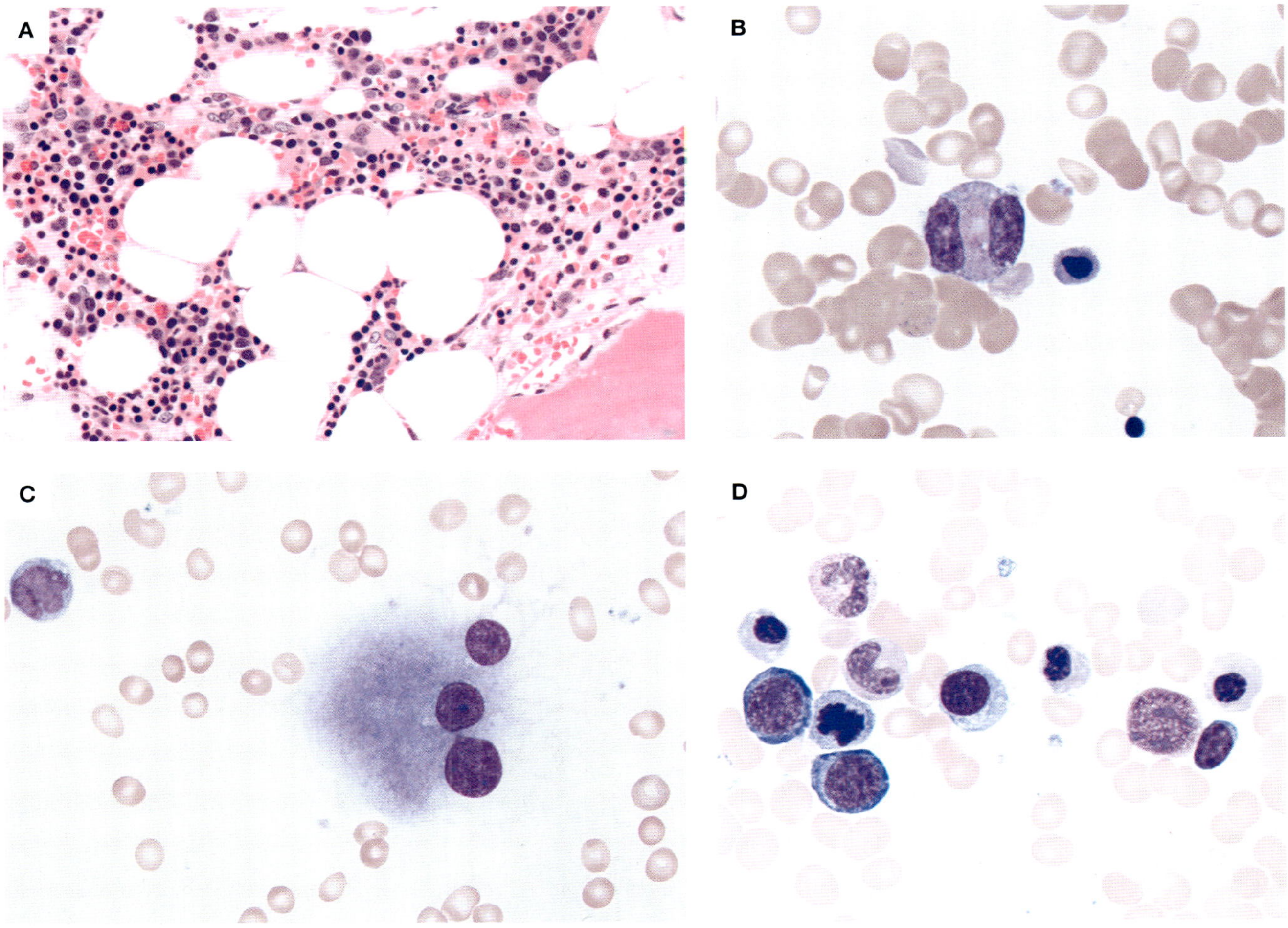

FIGURE 21.3 Refractory cytopenia of childhood associated with germline mutations in *SAMD9* or *SAMD9L* and monosomy 7. Marrow is typically hypocellular (**A**) with evidence of dysplasia that may be subtle or mild to moderate with dysmyelopoiesis (**B**), dysmegakaryopoiesis (**C**), and/or dyserythropoiesis (**D**).

dysplasia is variable and may be mild or absent. As noted earlier, monosomy 7/del7q is common.

Myeloid neoplasms with germline *ERCC6L2* mutation

Autosomal recessive P/LP variants in the *ERCC6L2* gene are associated with a hypocellular marrow, variable cytopenia, and progression to myeloid malignancies.[30,31] The reported median age of hematologic malignancy onset is 37 years with a range of 12 to 65 years.[31] One case of T-ALL has been reported. Some patients had neurologic or neuropsychiatric conditions. Dysplasia in the erythroid and megakaryocytic lineages and a few cases with reticulin fibrosis have been reported. The myeloid malignancies were typically erythroleukemias, and prognosis is poor. The *ERCC6L2*-associated MDS or AML harbors somatic *TP53* mutations, and clonal hematopoiesis with *TP53* mutations is common prior to malignancy development.

Myeloid neoplasms associated with bone marrow failure syndromes

The inherited marrow failure syndromes (see Table 21.6) are a heterogenous category of conditions that are characterized by bone marrow failure involving one or more blood lineages with varying additional clinical manifestations. Importantly, patients may lack syndromic features and present only with hematologic malignancy. In some instances, the marrow hypocellularity may be disproportionately severe compared with the blood counts and marrow hypocellularity alone is not an indication for transplant but must be interpreted within the context of the blood counts.

Fanconi anemia

Fanconi anemia (FA) is caused by P/LP variants in any of 23 genes functioning in DNA repair (see Table 21.6). Most genetic subtypes of FA follow a recessive pattern of inheritance with the exception of *FANCB* (X-linked) and *FANCR/RAD51* (autosomal dominant). The gold standard for diagnosis is increased chromosomal breakage with mitomycin C or diepoxybutane. Somatic mosaicism resulting from reversion of the Fanconi anemia mutation in lymphocytes may yield a negative chromosomal breakage test, so diagnosis may require testing cultured skin fibroblasts and genetic testing. For the recessive genes, diagnosis with genetic testing requires demonstration of biallelic P/LP variants in *trans*.

Clinical presentation is highly variable. Patients may present with marrow failure or malignancy at any age, although patients with congenital anomalies are typically diagnosed in childhood. For AML, the estimated cumulative incidence at age 40 years is 15% to 20%, while estimated cumulative incidence of MDS at age 50 years is 40%.[32] AML risk is particularly high in the *FANCD1/BRCA2* subtype, with a cumulative incidence of 80% at age 10 years. Patients with Fanconi anemia may also present with T-ALL, typically in the *FANCD1/BRCA2* subtype. Risk of solid tumors, including squamous cell carcinomas of the oral/gastrointestinal tract/vulva, and hepatocellular carcinomas is also elevated with Fanconi anemia. Patients with Fanconi anemia are highly sensitive to the genotoxic effects of chemotherapy and radiation used for cancer therapy and hematopoietic stem cell transplant, so diagnosis of Fanconi anemia informs tailored dose reduction.

Heterozygous P/LP variants in Fanconi anemia genes are common in the general population and have not been associated with adverse outcomes following stem cell transplantation for idiopathic severe aplastic anemia,[33] nor have heterozygous P/LP variants in *FANCA* or *FANCC* been associated with increased risk of malignancy in a family study of Fanconi anemia.[34] Overall, heterozygous P/LP variants in recessive Fanconi anemia genes have not been associated with increased risk of hematologic malignancy.[35]

The bone marrow at baseline is typically hypocellular, and mild baseline dysmorphologies are commonly present and must be distinguished from MDS. Progression to MDS is often associated with acquisition of monosomy 7.

Telomere biology disorders

Telomere biology disorders (TBDs), also called dyskeratosis congenita, are disorders caused by impaired telomere maintenance resulting in premature telomere shortening.[36] Diagnostic evaluation includes flow–fluorescence in situ hybridization FISH for telomere length and genetic testing (see Table 21.6). Children with TBD typically have telomere length below the first percentile for age in multiple lymphocyte subsets. In addition, diagnostic genetic testing is also recommended since short telomeres in lymphocytes may also be seen secondary to other conditions such as immunologic disorders and adults with TBD frequently do not exhibit the characteristic patterns of telomere length below the first percentile for age. Somatic reversions have been described with TBD either directly involving the causative gene or indirectly through other pathways.

Although TBD was originally described with the clinical triad of leukoplakia, nail dysplasia, and reticular or mottled skin pigmentation in dyskeratosis congenita, the majority of patients lack these findings. Some of the additional clinical features are listed in

Table 21.6. Of note, patients may present with malignancy without any additional clinical findings. The cumulative incidence of hematologic malignancy is 2% by age 50 years and is now recognized in MDS presenting in older adults and 11% by age 50 years for solid cancers.[37] Patients with autosomal dominant P/LP variants in *TERT* or *TERC* may display variable penetrance and present in adulthood with pulmonary fibrosis, hepatic cirrhosis, or MDS.

The bone marrow is typically hypocellular and may have features of mild dyspoiesis at baseline. Hematopoietic stem cell transplant must be tailored to minimize exposure to genotoxic agents that may exacerbate comorbidities such as pulmonary or liver dysfunction or arteriovenous malformations.

Shwachman-Diamond syndrome

The majority of cases of Shwachman-Diamond syndrome (SDS) are caused by biallelic loss-of-function P/LP variants in the *SBDS* gene, which functions in ribosome biogenesis.[38,39] Overlapping clinical features of SDS have been described in patients with P/LP variants in *SRP54*, *DNAJC21*, or *EFL1*; however, current data indicate that *SRP54* and *DNAJC21* appear clinically and biologically more similar to severe congenital neutropenia, and progression to myeloid malignancies has been reported. Leukemia risk with *EFL1* germline P/LP variants is currently unknown.

SDS was originally described in patients with neutropenia and exocrine pancreatic dysfunction, but these may be absent (see clinical features in Table 21.6). Patients may also present with isolated thrombocytopenia or anemia or may show bicytopenia or pancytopenia. Exocrine pancreatic dysfunction may be asymptomatic, but pancreatic isoamylase typically remains low after the age of 3 years. Patients with SDS are at increased risk for MDS and AML. Prognosis of MDS and AML is poor. The risk of worsening cytopenia(s), clonal myeloid evolution, or AML is estimated at 20% by age 18 years. The Severe Chronic Neutropenia International Registry reported a 1% per year progression rate to MDS/AML in patients with SDS, with a cumulative risk of MDS/AML reaching 36% by 30 years of age.

The bone marrow is typically hypocellular even if cytopenia is mild. Myeloid dysplasia such as nuclear hyposegmentation and cytoplasmic hypogranularity are common, and mild megakaryocytic dysplasia may be present in a small subset of cells. Erythroid dysplasia is uncommon at baseline. Clonal cytogenic abnormalities involving i(7q) and del(20q) are common but are not associated with progression to malignancy in patients with SDS. Small stable clones with heterozygous *TP53* mutations are common in patients with SDS from an early age; however, myeloid malignancies were observed to carry biallelic *TP53* mutations.

Severe congenital neutropenia

Severe congenital neutropenias (SCNs) describe a category of genetic conditions characterized by severe neutropenia from an early age and an increased risk of severe bacterial infections[40,41] (see Table 21.6). The most common genetic cause of SCN is autosomal dominant P/LP variants in the *ELANE* gene, which encodes neutrophil elastase. The *ELANE* P/LP variants, typically missense or truncating mutations affecting the more distal protein regions, trigger the unfolded protein response upon *ELANE* expression during myelopoiesis and results in apoptosis. Patients with *ELANE* P/LP variants have a high risk of developing MDS or AML. For SCN the median incidence of AML has been estimated at 21% 15 years following initiation of granulocyte colony-stimulating factor treatment. The majority of leukemias in patients with *ELANE* P/LP variants harbor somatic mutations in *CSF3R*, resulting in a truncation of CSF3R protein with defective internalization and aberrant signaling and often also acquire *RUNX1* or *RAS* pathway mutations. Clonal hematopoiesis with *CSF3R* clones in the absence of additional associated mutations or other high-risk features may persist for years without progression to malignancy so are not necessarily an indication for hematopoietic stem cell transplant in isolation.

At baseline, the marrow for SCN typically manifests promyelocyte arrest with normocellularity, although some cases only manifest a myeloid left-shift without maturation arrest. Increased eosinophils, which may be mildly dysplastic, are also commonly observed in the marrow.

Diamond-Blackfan anemia

Diamond-Blackfan anemia (DBA) is primarily caused by pathogenic autosomal dominant loss-of-function P/LP variants in genes encoding ribosomal proteins[42,43] (see Table 21.6). X-linked P/LP variants in *GATA1* or *TSR2* also cause a DBA phenotype. Erythrocyte adenosine deaminase levels are frequently elevated.

DBA is typically characterized by severe reticulocytopenic macrocytic anemia, with red blood cell aplasia in the marrow. DBA typically presents in infancy, although presentation well into adulthood has been reported. As with the other marrow failure syndromes, patients may lack anemia or other clinical features (see Table 21.6). Patients with large deletions involving the *RPL35A* gene may also develop severe neutropenia and immunodeficiencies. The anemia improves with corticosteroid therapy for the majority of patients. Around 20% of patients require red cell transfusions. A subset of patients can spontaneously improve their hemoglobin levels, although this may be transient and malignancy risk remains even in patients in remission for anemia.

The bone marrow at baseline shows red cell aplasia with occasional erythroblasts and early erythroid progenitors. The lymphoid, granulocytic, and megakaryocytic lineages are typically normal. Although marrow cellularity may initially be normal, the marrow can become increasingly hypocellular with age. Marrow hypoplasia often correlates with the development of neutropenia and/or thrombocytopenia.

Juvenile myelomonocytic leukemia associated with neurofibromatosis, Noonan syndrome, or Noonan syndrome–like disorders

This is discussed in Chapter 19.

Hematologic neoplasms associated with Down Syndrome

This is discussed in Chapter 37.

Acute lymphoblastic leukemia with germline predisposition

Germline P/LP variants in *PAX5* and *IKZF1* have been associated with predisposition to B lymphoblastic leukemia (see Table 21.7). Predisposition to lymphoid malignancies is also associated with immunodeficiency syndromes such as ataxia telangiectasia, Nijmegen breakage syndrome, or inborn errors of immunity.[44-46] Genes predisposing to both myeloid and acute lymphoblastic malignancies (eg, *TP53*, *ETV6*, and others) were described previously.

Acute lymphoblastic leukemia with germline *PAX5* mutation[44,47]

PAX5 encodes a DNA-binding transcription factor that regulates B-cell development. Family studies identified autosomal dominant P/LP variants in *PAX5* associated with an increased incidence of B-ALL with variable penetrance. B-ALL with germline *PAX5* P/LP variants is associated with chromosomal loss of 9p containing the wild-type copy of PAX5 and retention of the mutated copy in the leukemic cells. The immunophenotype and morphology of the blasts is similar to that of sporadic B-ALL. *PAX5* is also frequently mutated somatically in B-ALL.

Acute lymphoblastic leukemia with germline *IKZF1* mutation

IKZF1 encodes IKAROS, a zinc finger transcription factor critical for lymphoid development. Several kindreds and individuals have been reported with germline P/LP variants in *IKZF1* associated with impaired B-cell maturation, common variable immunodeficiency with B-cell lymphopenia, B-ALL, and possibly T-ALL.[45,48,49] Somatic mutations in *IKZF1* are also common in de novo B-ALL or lymphoid blast crisis in chronic myeloid leukemia.

Additional conditions with germline predisposition to hematologic malignancy

Additional rare germline P/LP variants predisposing to the development of primary MDS, AML, or ALL include Bloom syndrome (*BLM*) and xeroderma pigmentosum type C (*XPC*)[50,51] (see Table 21.8).

Bloom syndrome

Bloom syndrome, also called Bloom-Torre-Machacek syndrome or congenital telangiectatic erythema, is caused by autosomal recessive P/LP variants in the *BLM* gene encoding the RecQ helicase RECQL3.[52] BLM P/LP variants result in genomic instability characterized by increased sister chromatid exchanges.

Bloom syndrome is most commonly reported in the Ashkenazi Jewish population. Some clinical features are summarized in Table 21.8. Although cases of AML (mean age of diagnosis: 18 years) are more common than those of acute lymphoblastic leukemia (mean age of diagnosis: 20 years), the majority of myeloid malignancies in these patients have been reported following chemotherapy for a prior primary malignancy.[52]

Xeroderma pigmentosa, type C[50,53]

Xeroderma pigmentosa is an autosomal recessive condition caused by P/LP variants in the nucleotide excision repair genes. Some clinical features are listed in Table 21.8. Individuals from North Africa homozygous for the xeroderma pigmentosa type C gene *XPC* c.1643_1644 delTG; p.Val548AlafsX572 (delTG) mutation were found to have an increased risk for developing MDS and AML in childhood or young adulthood. T-ALL was also observed. Anemia often preceded the development of myeloid malignancy. These myeloid malignancies were characterized by complex karyotypes and *TP53* mutations. The risk of patients with other *XPC* mutations or from other ethnicities remains to be ascertained.

Provisional germline genetic predisposition to hematologic malignancy

Limited cases of hematologic malignancy have been reported with germline mutations in *DNMT3A* (Tatton-Brown-Rahman syndrome),[54,55] *CSF3R*,[56] *CAMT*,[57,58] *MECOM*,[59] *SRP72*,[60] and *TET2*[61,62] (see Table 21.9). Further data will clarify hematologic malignancy risk with these germline mutations. Newly discovered genes with germline genetic alterations that predispose to hematologic malignancies will be added to the ICC as sufficient data emerges.

References

1. Tawana K, Fitzgibbon J. CEBPA-associated familial acute myeloid leukemia (AML). In: Adam MP, Feldman J, Mirzaa GM, eds., GeneReviews((R)). 1993.
2. Tawana K, Wang J, Renneville A, et al. Disease evolution and outcomes in familial AML with germline CEBPA mutations. *Blood*. 2015;126(10):1214-1223.
3. Makishima H, Bowman TV, Godley LA. DDX41-associated susceptibility to myeloid neoplasms. *Blood*. 2023;141(13):1544-1552.
4. Polprasert C, Schulze I, Sekeres MA, et al. Inherited and somatic defects in DDX41 in myeloid neoplasms. *Cancer Cell*. 2015;27(5):658-670.
5. Lewinsohn M, Brown AL, Weinel LM, et al. Novel germ line DDX41 mutations define families with a lower age of MDS/AML onset and lymphoid malignancies. *Blood*. 2016;127(8):1017-1023.
6. Guha T, Malkin D. Inherited TP53 mutations and the Li-Fraumeni syndrome. *Cold Spring Harb Perspect Med*. 2017;7(4):a026187.
7. Schneider K, Zelley K, Nichols KE, Garber J. Li-fraumeni syndrome. In: Adam MP, Feldman J, Mirzaa GM, eds., GeneReviews((R)). 1993..
8. Palles C, West HD, Chew E.; Genomics England Research Consortium, CORGI Consortium, WGS500 Consortium, et al. Germline MBD4 deficiency causes a multi-tumor predisposition syndrome. *Am J Hum Genet*. 2022;109(5):953-960.
9. Schlegelberger B, Heller PG. RUNX1 deficiency (familial platelet disorder with predisposition to myeloid leukemia, FPDMM). *Semin Hematol*. 2017;54(2):75-80.
10. Cunningham L, Merguerian M, Calvo KR, et al. Natural history study of patients with familial platelet disorder with associated myeloid malignancy. *Blood*. 2023;142(25):2146-2158.
11. Kanagal-Shamanna R, Loghavi S, DiNardo CD, et al. Bone marrow pathologic abnormalities in familial platelet disorder with propensity for myeloid malignancy and germline RUNX1 mutation. *Haematologica*. 2017;102(10):1661-1670.
12. Homan CC, Drazer MW, Yu K; NISC Comparative Sequencing Program, et al. Somatic mutational landscape of hereditary hematopoietic malignancies caused by germline variants in RUNX1, GATA2, and DDX41. *Blood Adv*. 2023;7(20):6092-6107.
13. Noris P, Favier R, Alessi MC, et al. ANKRD26-related thrombocytopenia and myeloid malignancies. *Blood*. 2013;122(11):1987-1989.
14. Zhang MY, Churpek JE, Keel SB, et al. Germline ETV6 mutations in familial thrombocytopenia and hematologic malignancy. *Nat Genet*. 2015;47(2):180-185.
15. Noetzli L, Lo RW, Lee-Sherick AB, et al. Germline mutations in ETV6 are associated with thrombocytopenia, red cell macrocytosis and predisposition to lymphoblastic leukemia. *Nat Genet*. 2015;47(5):535-538.
16. Poggi M, Canault M, Favier M, et al. Germline variants in ETV6 underlie reduced platelet formation, platelet dysfunction and increased levels of circulating CD34+ progenitors. *Haematologica*. 2017;102(2):282-294.
17. Hahn CN, Chong CE, Carmichael CL, et al. Heritable GATA2 mutations associated with familial myelodysplastic syndrome and acute myeloid leukemia. *Nat Genet*. 2011;43(10):1012-1017.
18. Hsu AP, Sampaio EP, Khan J, et al. Mutations in GATA2 are associated with the autosomal dominant and sporadic monocytopenia and mycobacterial infection (MonoMAC) syndrome. *Blood*. 2011;118(10):2653-2655.
19. Dickinson RE, Griffin H, Bigley V, et al. Exome sequencing identifies GATA-2 mutation as the cause of dendritic cell, monocyte, B and NK lymphoid deficiency. *Blood*. 2011;118(10):2656-2658.
20. Ostergaard P, Simpson MA, Connell FC, et al. Mutations in GATA2 cause primary lymphedema associated with a predisposition to acute myeloid leukemia (Emberger syndrome). *Nat Genet*. 2011;43(10):929-931.
21. Spinner MA, Sanchez LA, Hsu AP, et al. GATA2 deficiency: a protean disorder of hematopoiesis, lymphatics, and immunity. *Blood*. 2014;123(6):809-821.
22. Wlodarski MW, Hirabayashi S, Pastor V, et al. Prevalence, clinical characteristics, and prognosis of GATA2-related myelodysplastic syndromes in children and adolescents. *Blood*. 2016;127(11):1387-1397.
23. Calvo KR, Hickstein DD. The spectrum of GATA2 deficiency syndrome. *Blood*. 2023;141(13):1524-1532.
24. Ganapathi KA, Townsley DM, Hsu AP, et al. GATA2 deficiency-associated bone marrow disorder differs from idiopathic aplastic anemia. *Blood*. 2015;125(1):56-70.
25. West RR, Calvo KR, Embree LJ, et al. ASXL1 and STAG2 are common mutations in GATA2 deficiency patients with bone marrow disease and myelodysplastic syndrome. *Blood Adv*. 2022;6(3):793-807.
26. Largeaud L, Collin M, Monselet N, et al. Somatic genetic alterations predict hematological progression in GATA2 deficiency. *Haematologica*. 2023;108(6):1515-1529.

27. Sahoo SS, Kozyra EJ, Wlodarski MW. Germline predisposition in myeloid neoplasms: unique genetic and clinical features of GATA2 deficiency and SAMD9/SAMD9L syndromes. *Best Pract Res Clin Haematol.* 2020;33(3):101197.
28. de Jesus AA, Hou Y, Brooks S, et al. Distinct interferon signatures and cytokine patterns define additional systemic autoinflammatory diseases. *J Clin Invest.* 2020;130(4):1669-1682.
29. Sahoo SS, Pastor VB, Goodings C; European Working Group of MDS in Children EWOG-MDS, et al. Clinical evolution, genetic landscape and trajectories of clonal hematopoiesis in SAMD9/SAMD9L syndromes. *Nat Med.* 2021;27(10):1806-1817.
30. Douglas SPM, Siipola P, Kovanen PE, et al. ERCC6L2 defines a novel entity within inherited acute myeloid leukemia. *Blood.* 2019;133(25):2724-2728.
31. Hakkarainen M, Kaaja I, Douglas SPM, et al. The clinical picture of ERCC6L2 disease: from bone marrow failure to acute leukemia. *Blood.* 2023;141(23):2853-2866.
32. Alter BP, Giri N, Savage SA, et al. Malignancies and survival patterns in the National Cancer Institute inherited bone marrow failure syndromes cohort study. *Br J Haematol.* 2010;150(2):179-188.
33. McReynolds LJ, Wang Y, Thompson AS, et al. Population frequency of Fanconi pathway gene variants and their association with survival after hematopoietic cell transplantation for severe aplastic anemia. *Biol Blood Marrow Transplant.* 2020;26(5):817-822.
34. McReynolds LJ, Giri N, Leathwood L, Risch MO, Carr AG, Alter BP. Risk of cancer in heterozygous relatives of patients with Fanconi anemia. *Genet Med.* 2022;24(1):245-250.
35. Deng J, Altintas B, Haley JS, et al. Most Fanconi anemia heterozygotes are not at increased cancer risk: a genome-first DiscovEHR cohort population study. *Genet Med.* 2024;26(3):101042.
36. Revy P, Kannengiesser C, Bertuch AA. Genetics of human telomere biology disorders. *Nat Rev Genet.* 2023;24(2):86-108.
37. Alter BP, Giri N, Savage SA, Rosenberg PS. Cancer in the National Cancer Institute inherited bone marrow failure syndrome cohort after fifteen years of follow-up. *Haematologica.* 2018;103(1):30-39.
38. Warren AJ. Molecular basis of the human ribosomopathy Shwachman-Diamond syndrome. *Adv Biol Regul.* 2018;67:109-127.
39. Reilly CR, Shimamura A. Predisposition to myeloid malignancies in Shwachman-Diamond syndrome: biological insights and clinical advances. *Blood.* 2023;141(13):1513-1523.
40. Rosenberg PS, Zeidler C, Bolyard AA, et al. Stable long-term risk of leukaemia in patients with severe congenital neutropenia maintained on G-CSF therapy. *Br J Haematol.* 2010;150(2):196-199.
41. Touw IP. Game of clones: the genomic evolution of severe congenital neutropenia. *Hematology Am Soc Hematol Educ Program.* 2015;2015:1-7.
42. Da Costa L, Leblanc T, Mohandas N. Diamond-Blackfan anemia. *Blood.* 2020;136(11):1262-1273.
43. Vlachos A, Rosenberg PS, Atsidaftos E, Alter BP, Lipton JM. Incidence of neoplasia in Diamond Blackfan anemia: a report from the Diamond Blackfan anemia Registry. *Blood.* 2012;119(16):3815-3819.
44. Shah S, Schrader KA, Waanders E, et al. A recurrent germline PAX5 mutation confers susceptibility to pre-B cell acute lymphoblastic leukemia. *Nat Genet.* 2013;45(10):1226-1231.
45. Churchman ML, Qian M, Te Kronnie G, et al. Germline genetic IKZF1 variation and predisposition to childhood acute lymphoblastic leukemia. *Cancer Cell.* 2018;33(5):937-948 e8.
46. Schutte P, Moricke A, Zimmermann M, et al. Preexisting conditions in pediatric ALL patients: spectrum, frequency and clinical impact. *Eur J Med Genet.* 2016;59(3):143-151.
47. Auer F, Ruschendorf F, Gombert M, et al. Inherited susceptibility to pre B-ALL caused by germline transmission of PAX5 c.547G>A. *Leukemia.* 2014;28(5):1136-1138.
48. Kuehn HS, Boisson B, Cunningham-Rundles C, et al. Loss of B Cells in patients with heterozygous mutations in IKAROS. *N Engl J Med.* 2016;374(11):1032-1043.
49. Boutboul D, Kuehn HS, Van de Wyngaert Z, et al. Dominant-negative IKZF1 mutations cause a T, B, and myeloid cell combined immunodeficiency. *J Clin Invest.* 2018;128(7):3071-3087.
50. Sarasin A, Quentin S, Droin N, et al. Familial predisposition to TP53/complex karyotype MDS and leukemia in DNA repair-deficient xeroderma pigmentosum. *Blood.* 2019;133(25):2718-2724.
51. Oetjen KA, Levoska MA, Tamura D, et al. Predisposition to hematologic malignancies in patients with xeroderma pigmentosum. *Haematologica.* 2020;105(4):e144-e146.
52. Cunniff C, Bassetti JA, Ellis NA. Bloom's syndrome: clinical spectrum, molecular pathogenesis, and cancer predisposition. *Mol Syndromol.* 2017;8(1):4-23.
53. Nikolaev S, Yurchenko AA, Sarasin A. Increased risk of internal tumors in DNA repair-deficient xeroderma pigmentosum patients: analysis of four international cohorts. *Orphanet J Rare Dis.* 2022;17(1):104.
54. Tatton-Brown K, Zachariou A; Clinical Assessment of the Utility of Sequencing and Evaluation as a Service CAUSES Research Study, Deciphering Developmental Disorders DDD Study, et al. The Tatton-Brown-Rahman syndrome: A clinical study of 55 individuals with de novo constitutive DNMT3A variants. *Wellcome Open Res.* 2018;3:46.
55. DiNardo CD, Beird HC, Estecio M, et al. Germline DNMT3A mutation in familial acute myeloid leukaemia. *Epigenetics.* 2021;16(5):567-576.

56. Trottier AM, Druhan LJ, Kraft IL, et al. Heterozygous germ line CSF3R variants as risk alleles for development of hematologic malignancies. *Blood Adv.* 2020;4(20):5269-5284.

57. Ballmaier M, Germeshausen M. Congenital amegakaryocytic thrombocytopenia: clinical presentation, diagnosis, and treatment. *Semin Thromb Hemost.* 2011;37(6):673-681.

58. Germeshausen M, Ballmaier M. CAMT-MPL: congenital amegakaryocytic thrombocytopenia caused by MPL mutations—heterogeneity of a monogenic disorder—a comprehensive analysis of 56 patients. *Haematologica.* 2021;106(9):2439-2448.

59. Ripperger T, Hofmann W, Koch JC, et al. MDS1 and EVI1 complex locus (MECOM): a novel candidate gene for hereditary hematological malignancies. *Haematologica.* 2018;103(2):e55-e58.

60. Kirwan M, Walne AJ, Plagnol V, et al. Exome sequencing identifies autosomal-dominant SRP72 mutations associated with familial aplasia and myelodysplasia. *Am J Hum Genet.* 2012;90(5):888-892.

61. Duployez N, Goursaud L, Fenwarth L, et al. Familial myeloid malignancies with germline TET2 mutation. *Leukemia.* 2020;34(5):1450-1453.

62. Kaasinen E, Kuismin O, Rajamaki K, et al. Impact of constitutional TET2 haploinsufficiency on molecular and clinical phenotype in humans. *Nat Commun.* 2019;10(1):1252.

SECTION 7

Acute Myeloid Leukemias

Chapter 22

Acute Promyelocytic Leukemia With t(15;17)(q24.1;q21.2)/*PML::RARA* and Acute Promyelocytic Leukemia With Other *RARA* Rearrangements

Kathryn Foucar, Devon Chabot-Richards, Jeffery M. Klco, and Martin S. Tallman

Definition

Acute promyelocytic leukemia (APL) is a subtype of AML defined by t(15;17)(q24.1;q21.2)/*PML::RARA* and is characterized by a predominance of morphologically distinctive promyelocytes that are most frequently hypergranular (typical) type, or less often micro/hypogranular type, usually manifesting with coagulopathy that is associated with risk of early death from hemorrhage or, less commonly, thrombosis.

Synonym

M3 AML, French-American-British (FAB) classification (not recommended).

Epidemiology

APL can occur at any age but predominates in young to middle-aged adults and accounts for about 5% to 13% of AML cases.[1] The median age of APL in adults is ~50 years. APL accounts for about 5% to 10% of pediatric AML with a median age of onset of 9 to 12 years.[2]

General Clinical Features

The predominant distinctive clinical features of patients with APL are those linked to disseminated intravascular coagulation and increased plasmin-dependent fibrinolysis, but a small proportion of patients with APL may manifest with striking thrombophilia. There is significant risk of early death from coagulopathy (usually within the first week after diagnosis) in patients with APL that persists for days, even after initiation of all-trans retinoic acid (ATRA) differentiation therapy. Consequently, rapid diagnosis of APL is essential along with aggressive management of coagulopathy.

Morphology

Blast and blast equivalents (abnormal promyelocytes) should account for ≥10% of cells in blood or bone marrow. In some cases of APL there may be partial bone marrow effacement; in these rare cases the 10% blast/promyelocyte threshold may not be met. Although a range in promyelocytic morphology is common in cases of APL, the most prototypic promyelocytes are large with generally round or kidney bean–shaped nuclei and moderate to abundant cytoplasm, which is hypergranular with variable stacked Auer rods in typical APL. The intense cytoplasmic granulation may obscure the nucleus (Figure 22.1A). Owing to the profound pancytopenia that is characteristic of typical, hypergranular APL, the diagnostician must search the feather edge, sides, and thick areas of the blood smear to identify rare circulating hypergranular promyelocytes. Leukocytosis is common in micro/hypogranular APL, and the leukemia cells often have large bilobed nuclei (sliding plates) with moderate to abundant hypogranular cytoplasm due to the submicroscopic size of the granules (Figure 22.1B). Morphologically these bilobed, hypogranular promyelocytes can mimic acute monocytic leukemia. A rare hyperbasophilic variant of APL has been described in which the leukemic promyelocytes have deeply basophilic cytoplasm with cytoplasmic blebbing. The rapid identification of abnormal promyelocytes, including in all cases of leukemia with monocytic features, with myeloperoxidase (MPO) cytochemical stain is needed to avoid delay in the diagnosis of APL. By MPO cytochemical stain intense positive staining in all promyelocytes is

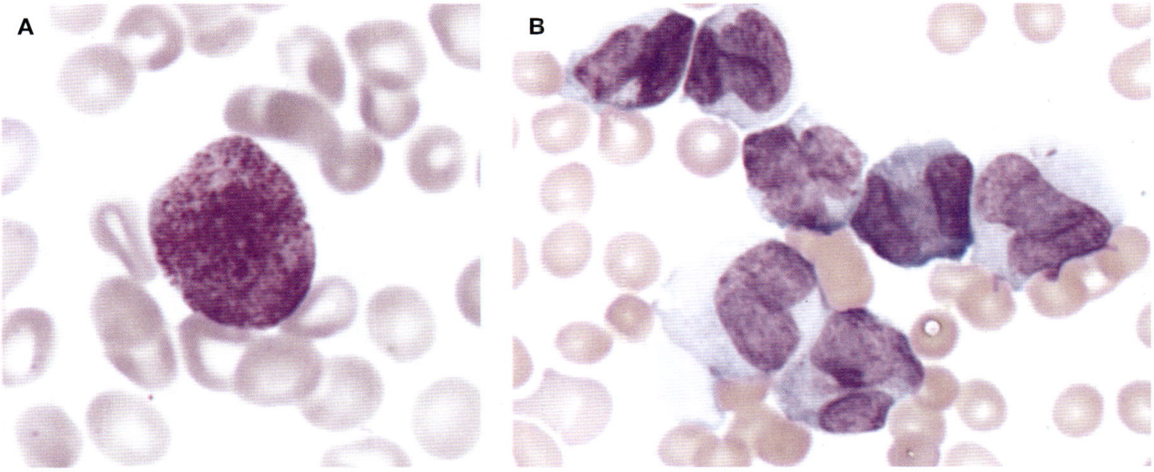

FIGURE 22.1 **A:** This blood smear from an 18-year-old man with profound pancytopenia shows rare circulating hypergranular promyelocytes (Wright). **B:** This blood smear is from a 64-year-old man who presented with marked leukocytosis (WBC 208.8 × 10^9/L) and severe thrombocytopenia. A monocytic leukemia was suspected initially, but FISH detected *PML::RARA* confirming a diagnosis of micro/hypogranular acute promyelocytic leukemia (Wright).

characteristic regardless of whether granules are visible on Wright stain. This should be coupled with rapid molecular genetic testing by FISH (fluorescence in situ hybridization) or PCR (polymerase chain reaction) for *PML::RARA* on all cases of possible, suspected, and even morphologically obvious APL, for rapid definitive diagnosis. (See genetics section.)

Other less common findings in APL cases include associated absolute basophilia in blood and markedly increased basophils in bone marrow, as well as cases of APL with prominent bone marrow fibrosis.[3]

Immunophenotype

APL cases exhibit a characteristic immunophenotypic profile that can support a presumptive diagnosis of this leukemia, especially when markedly increased side scatter, due to cytoplasmic granulation of the leukemia cells, is also evident on flow histograms. Antigens that are typically expressed in APL include CD117, CD33, CD13, and MPO. Antigens that are usually negative include CD34, HLA-DR, CD15, CD11a/b, and CD18. Some cases of micro/hypogranular APL can show a spectrum of CD34 expression; similarly, cases of APL with bcr3 transcript (short form) may be CD34 positive. About 20% of cases of APL express CD56, which has been linked to relapse in some studies.[4]

Genetics

The translocation (15;17)(q24.1;q21.2) fuses the *PML* tumor suppressor gene with the *RARA* transcription regulator gene, leading to uncontrolled proliferation and block of cell differentiation. Three different lengths of fusion transcripts, the bcr1 (long form), bcr2 (variable form), and bcr3 (short form), are described, fusing a consistent breakpoint in intron 2 of *RARA* with heterogeneous breakpoints in *PML*. Identification of the specific transcript type is necessary for selection and interpretation of measurable residual disease testing.

In new cases of suspected APL, rapid identification of the *PML::RARA* transcript, most often by FISH, is required. Rare cases may be cryptic by either conventional karyotyping or FISH; molecular testing such as reverse transcription PCR is required for definitive diagnosis in these cases. Additional cytogenetic abnormalities, including complex karyotype, are seen in some cases. Molecular studies reveal a mutational landscape distinct from other types of myeloid leukemia, including increased rates of *WT1, KRAS,* and *NRAS* mutations with lower incidence of mutations in other myeloid neoplasm-associated genes including *TP53, DNMT3A, TET2,* and *ASXL1*. *FLT3*-ITD and TKD mutations are also identified in a significant number of cases.[5,6] In some studies, concurrent *FLT3* mutations are linked to the bcr3 isoform, micro/hypogranular subtype, higher white blood cell (WBC) count, and higher risk of relapse. Complex karyotype has also been linked to adverse outcome in limited studies.[7]

APL With Other *RARA* Translocations

Variant *RARA* translocations are reported in <10% of patients with APL[8] (Table 22.1). These cases typically involve *RARA* translocations with a number of alternate translocation partners; however, rare cases involving other retinoic acid receptor family genes have been

TABLE 22.1 Recurrent variant translocations seen in APL, with morphologic correlations and treatment response

Variant translocation	Morphologic correlation	Other findings	Treatment response
ZBTB16 11q23.2	Numerous fine granules Absence of Auer rods Pelgeroid neutrophils	Often CD56 positive	Resistant to ATRA and ATO
NPM1 5q35.1	Numerous granules Absence of Auer rods Occasional hypogranular forms	Diminished CD13 expression	Responsive to ATRA, ATO response unclear
STAT5B 17q21.2	Typical APL morphology	Typical immunophenotype Often cryptic on karyotype, RNA-seq may be required	Resistant to ATRA and ATO
IRF2BP2 1q42	Typical APL morphology	May express CD34 and HLA-DR	Responsive to ATRA and ATO
TBL1XR1 3q26	Hypogranular morphology	Typical immunophenotype May be cryptic on karyotype, RNA-seq may be required	Resistant to ATRA, responsive to ATO
STAT3 17q21	Typical APL morphology	Typical immunophenotype Often cryptic on karyotype, RNA-seq may be required	May be resistant to ATRA and ATO
FIP1L1 4q12	Typical APL morphology	May express HLA-DR	Responsive to ATRA, ATO response unclear
BCOR Xp11.4	Typical APL morphology, reports of atypical cytoplasmic inclusions	Typical immunophenotype	Responsive to ATRA, may be resistant to ATO

APL, acute promyelocytic leukemia; ATO, arsenic trioxide; ATRA, all-trans retinoic acid; RNA-seq, RNA sequencing.
Coffman B, Chabot-Richards D. Diagnosis of variant translocations in acute promyelocytic leukemia. *Adv Mol Pathol.* 2021;4:37-48. doi:10.1016/j.yamp.2021.06.002

reported.[8,9] It is important to identify these uncommon cases because cases with other *RARA* translocations are often ATRA resistant. Cases with t(11;17)(q23.2;q21.2)/*ZBTB16::RARA* are the most common and exhibit some morphologic similarities to APL with *PML::RARA*, but Auer rods are rare and neutrophils can show pseudo-Pelger-Huet changes (Figure 22.2).

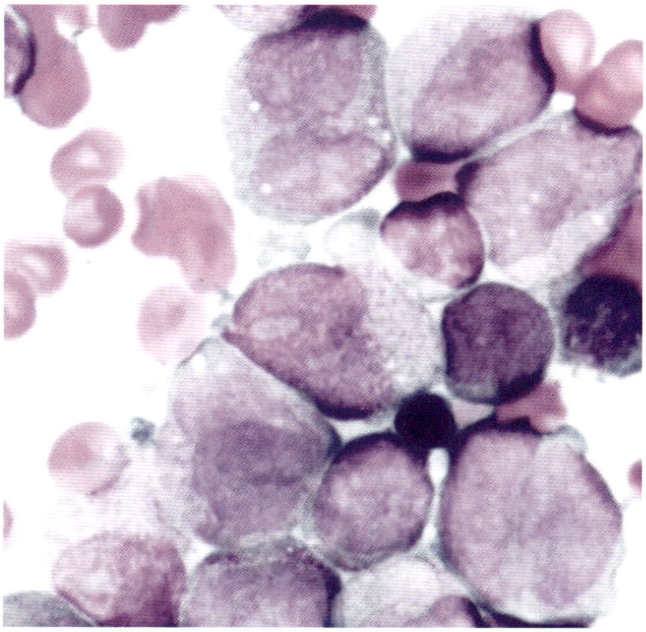

FIGURE 22.2 This bone marrow aspirate smear shows some features suggestive of micro/hypogranular acute promyelocytic leukemia (APL), in this case of APL with a variant RARA translocation (*ZBTB16::RARA*) (Wright).

Prognosis and Clinical Comment

Degradation of the PML::RARA fusion protein is a key goal in APL therapy, not only to gradually eradicate leukemia cells but also to reduce the risk of early death from coagulopathy. The two agents that synergistically degrade PML::RARA protein are ATRA and arsenic trioxide (ATO) resulting in induction of terminal maturation and apoptosis of the leukemic cells[10] (Figure 22.3).

Treatment protocols for APL include differentiation-inducing agents (ATRA or ATO) alone (for low-risk patients) or with concurrent single-agent chemotherapy; remission rates are very high, and relapses are uncommon.[11] Chemotherapy-free treatment protocols for children have also been described. Factors linked to less favorable long-term outcome include complex karyotype and CD56 expression.[7] Development of differentiation syndrome, the likely consequence of ATRA-induced effects on differentiating promyelocytes that result in increased leukemia cell adhesiveness and release of proinflammatory cytokines triggering both hemostasis and a systemic inflammatory response, is an adverse event that occurs in a

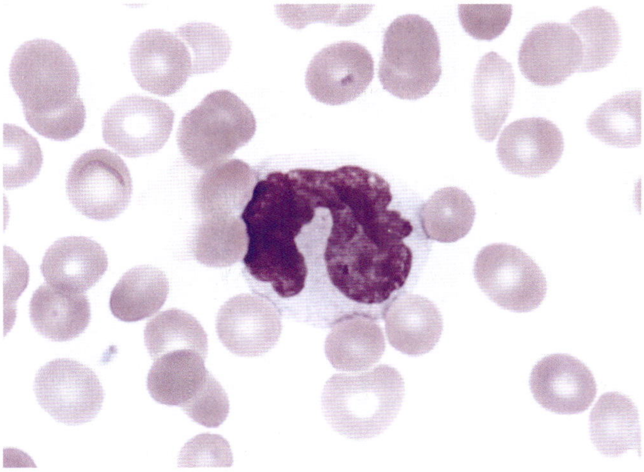

FIGURE 22.3 This blood smear is from a 16-year-old boy on all-trans retinoic acid (ATRA) therapy for acute promyelocytic leukemia (APL), which shows the atypical, monocytic appearance of ATRA-induced maturation of APL cells.

proportion of patients with APL requiring rapid and aggressive clinical management.[12]

References

1. Österroos A, Maia T, Eriksson A, et al. A risk score based on real-world data to predict early death in acute promyelocytic leukemia. *Haematologica*. 2022;107(7):1528-1537. doi:10.3324/haematol.2021.280093
2. Gurnari C, Voso MT, Girardi K, Mastronuzzi A, Strocchio L. Acute promyelocytic leukemia in children: a model of precision medicine and chemotherapy-free therapy. *Int J Mol Sci*. 2021;22(2):642. doi:10.3390/ijms22020642
3. Rieu JB, Canali A, Thene E, Tavitian S, Bertoli S. Acute promyelocytic leukaemia associated with atypical basophilia. *Br J Haematol*. 2023;201(6):1017. doi:10.1111/bjh.18793
4. Maenhout TM, Moreau E, Van Haute I, Desmet S, Deeren D. Minimal coexpression of CD34+/CD56+ in acute promyelocytic leukemia is associated with relapse. *Am J Clin Pathol*. 2015;144(2):347-351. doi:10.1309/AJCPBS3W1RJDGPZU
5. Noguera NI, Catalano G, Banella C, et al. Acute promyelocytic leukemia: update on the mechanisms of leukemogenesis, resistance and on innovative treatment strategies. *Cancers*. 2019;11(10):1591. doi:10.3390/cancers11101591
6. Liquori A, Ibañez M, Sargas C, Sanz MÁ, Barragán E, Cervera J. Acute promyelocytic leukemia: a constellation of molecular events around a single PML-RARA fusion gene. *Cancers*. 2020;12(3):624. doi:10.3390/cancers12030624
7. Epstein-Peterson ZD, Derkach A, Geyer S, et al. Effect of additional cytogenetic abnormalities on survival in arsenic trioxide-treated acute promyelocytic leukemia. *Blood Adv*. 2022;6(11):3433-3439. doi:10.1182/bloodadvances.2021006682
8. Coffman B, Chabot-Richards D. Diagnosis of variant translocations in acute promyelocytic leukemia. *Adv Mol Pathol*. 2021;4:37-48. doi:10.1016/j.yamp.2021.06.002
9. Zhao J, Liang JW, Xue HL, et al. The genetics and clinical characteristics of children morphologically diagnosed as acute promyelocytic leukemia. *Leukemia*. 2019;33(6):1387-1399. doi:10.1038/s41375-018-0338-z
10. Miller KP, Venkataraman G, Gocke CD, et al. Bone marrow findings in patients with acute promyelocytic leukemia treated with arsenic trioxide. *Am J Clin Pathol*. 2019;152(5):675-685. doi:10.1093/ajcp/aqz087
11. Sanz MA, Fenaux P, Tallman MS, et al. Management of acute promyelocytic leukemia: updated recommendations from an expert panel of the European LeukemiaNet. *Blood*. 2019;133(15):1630-1643. doi:10.1182/blood-2019-01-894980
12. Stahl M, Tallman MS. Differentiation syndrome in acute promyelocytic leukaemia. *Br J Haematol*. 2019;187(2):157-162. doi:10.1111/bjh.16151

Chapter 23

Acute Myeloid Leukemia With t(8;21)(q22;q22.1)/*RUNX1::RUNX1T1*

Sandeep Gurbuxani, Tracy I. George, Angela M. Lager, and Olatoyosi M. Odenike

Definition

Acute myeloid leukemia (AML) with t(8;21)(q22;q22)/*RUNX1::RUNX1T1* is an acute myeloid leukemia showing neutrophilic maturation.

Synonyms

Acute myeloid leukemia, t(8;21)(q22;q22.1); acute myeloid leukemia *CBF-alpha/ETO, RUNX1::RUNX1T1*. (not recommended)

Epidemiology

The t(8;21)(q22;q22) is found in approximately 8% to 12% of cases of AML and is the most common cytogenetic abnormality in pediatric patients with AML.[1,2]

General Clinical Features

Clinical presentation is nonspecific and related to the proliferation of blasts and subsequent bone marrow failure with consequences of anemia, neutropenia, and thrombocytopenia. The white blood cell count is lower in cases with t(8;21)(q22;q22.1) when compared with patients with inv(16)(p13.1q22) or t(16;16)(p13.1;q22)/*CBFB::MYH11*.[3] Patients may present with extramedullary disease or myeloid sarcoma as an initial presentation.

Morphology

The common morphological features include the presence of large blasts with abundant basophilic cytoplasm, often containing numerous azurophilic granules and perinuclear clearing or hofs (Figure 23.1A). A few blasts in many cases show very large granules (pseudo-Chédiak-Higashi granules), suggesting abnormal fusion. Auer rods are frequently found and appear as a single long and sharp rod with tapered ends (Figure 23.1B); they may be detected in mature neutrophils. In addition to the large blast cells, some smaller blasts, predominantly in the peripheral blood, may be found. Promyelocytes, myelocytes, and mature neutrophils with variable dysplasia are present in the bone marrow. These cells may show abnormal nuclear segmentation (eg, pseudo-Pelger-Huët nuclei) and/or cytoplasmic staining abnormalities, including homogeneous pink-colored cytoplasm in neutrophils. Dysplasia of other cell lines, however, is uncommon. Eosinophil precursors are frequently increased but they do not exhibit the cytological or cytochemical abnormalities characteristic of AML associated with abnormalities of chromosome 16; basophils and/or mast cells are sometimes present in excess. A monocytic component is usually minimal or absent. Erythroblasts and megakaryocytes are morphologically normal. Ten percent blasts in bone marrow or blood are required for a diagnosis of AML; rare cases may present with a blast count of less than 10% but should be diagnosed as AML when t(8;21) is present. An increased frequency of systemic mastocytosis has been detected in bone marrows from patients with AML with t(8;21)(q22;q22)/*RUNX1::RUNX1T1*; immunohistochemistry with antibody against tryptase can be useful in detecting mastocytosis.[4]

Immunophenotype

Most cases of AML with the t(8;21)/*RUNX1::RUNX1T1* display a characteristic immunophenotype with a subpopulation of blast cells showing high-intensity expression of CD34, together with myeloperoxidase and CD13 but relatively weak expression of CD33 (Figure 23.2). There are usually signs of granulocytic differentiation with subpopulations of cells showing granulocytic maturation demonstrated by CD15 and/or CD65 expression. Sometimes populations of blasts showing maturation asynchrony are present (eg, coexpressing CD34 and CD15). These leukemias frequently express the lymphoid markers CD19 and PAX5 and may express cytoplasmic CD79a. Some cases are

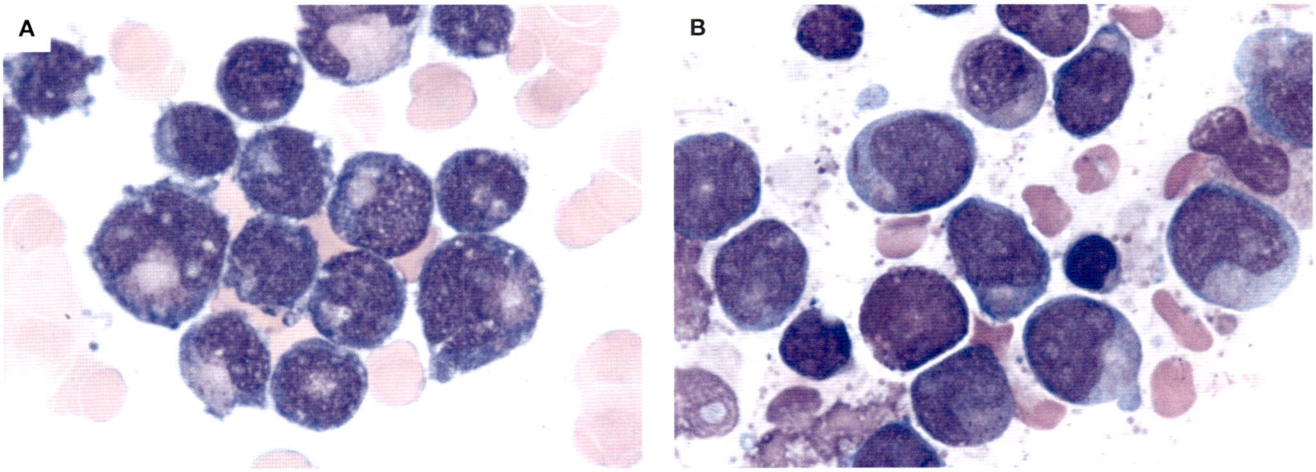

FIGURE 23.1 Acute myeloid leukemia with t(8;21)(q22;q22.1). **A:** Blasts show abundance of basophilic granules, perinuclear clearing with salmon-pink cytoplasm. **B:** Blasts may contain fine Auer rods with pointed ends.

terminal deoxynucleotidyl transferase (TdT) positive; however, TdT expression is generally weak.[5] CD56 is expressed in a fraction of cases and may have adverse prognostic significance likely due to association with *KIT* mutations.[6]

Genetics

The t(8;21)(q22;q22) (Figure 23.3) involves the *RUNX1* gene, which encodes the alpha subunit of core binding factor (*CBFA*, also called *AML1*) on chromosome 21 and the *RUNX1T1* (*ETO* or *MTG8*) gene on chromosome 8.[7] Based on chromosome band resolution the cytogenetic breakpoints of the *RUNX1::RUNX1T1* translocation map to chromosomes 21q22 and 8q22. However, on the molecular level the *RUNX1T1* gene maps to chromosome 8q21.3. The molecular consequence of the t(8;21) is the generation of the *RUNX1::RUNX1T1* fusion transcript. The most common fusion transcript involves the juxtaposition of exon 5 of the *RUNX1* (*AML1*) gene and exon 2 of the *RUNX1T1* (*ETO*) gene. The abnormal fusion transcript is expressed from the abnormal chromosome 8 [der(8)t(8;21)] while a reciprocal fusion is not expressed. Over 70% of patients show additional chromosome abnormalities: eg, loss of a sex chromosome or del(9q) with loss of 9q22, trisomy 4, and trisomy 8.[8] In addition, high-throughput sequencing studies have shown somatic mutations in signaling pathways (*KIT, FLT3*-ITD, *RAS, JAK2, CBL,* and *PTPN11*), epigenetic regulators (*ASXL1, ASXL2, EZH2*), and cohesion complex (*RAD21, STAG2, SMC1a*) in more than 90% of the cases.[9] Furthermore, in contrast to AML with *CBFB::MYH11*, the spectrum of mutations is more complex and mutations in MYC signaling pathways (*MGA, CCND2*) occur at a higher frequency.[10]

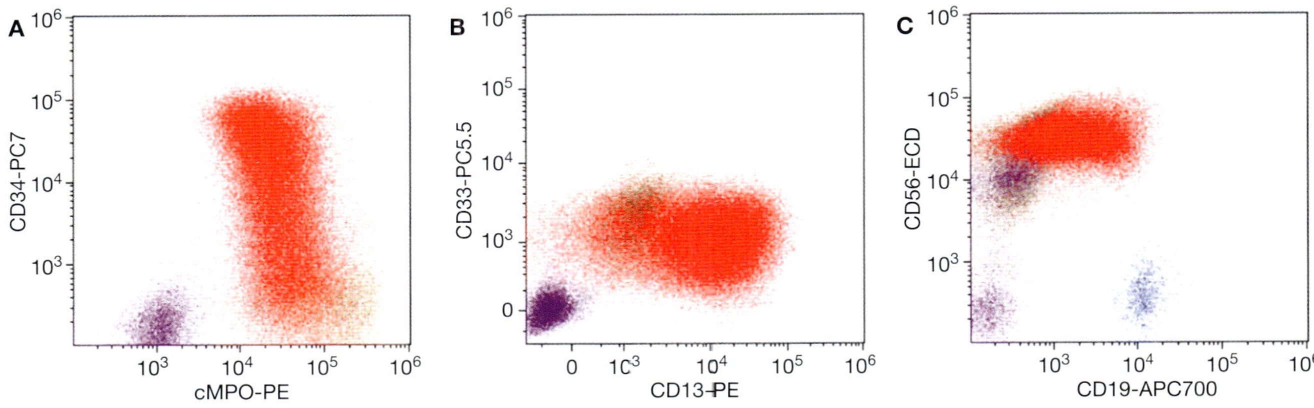

FIGURE 23.2 Flow cytometry shows brighter than normal expression of CD34 in myeloperoxidase-positive blasts (**A**). Blasts are CD13 positive but typically show dim or no CD33 expression (**B**). Aberrant expression of B-cell antigen CD19 is frequently observed, and blasts may express CD56 (**C**).

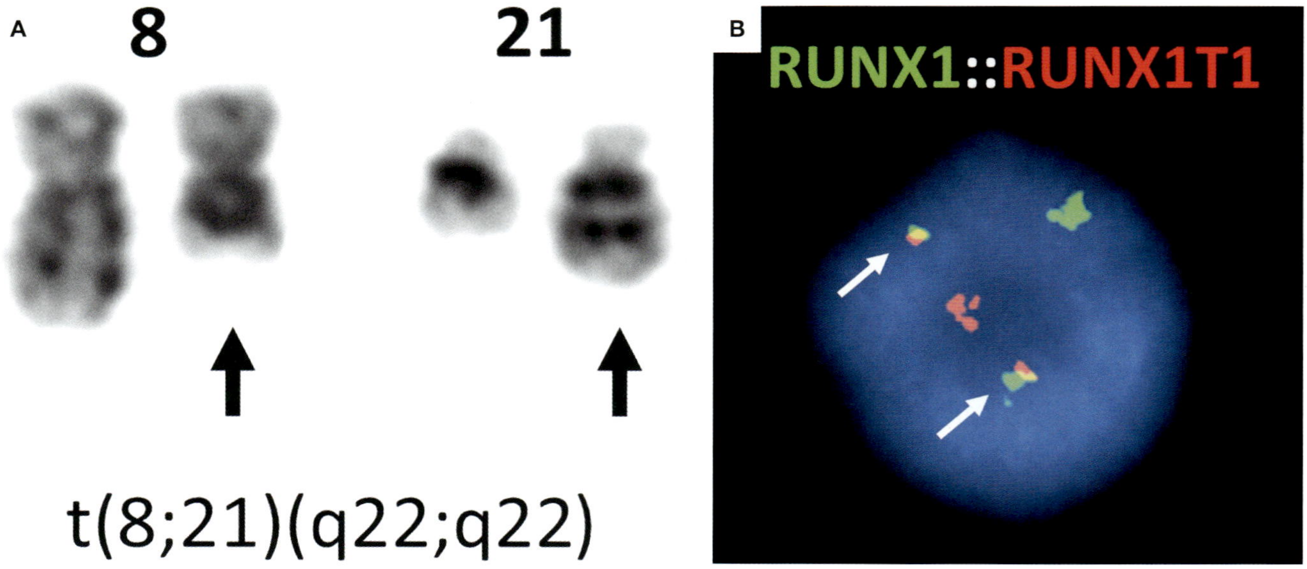

FIGURE 23.3 Acute myeloid leukemia with t(8;21)(q22;q22.1)/*RUNX1::RUNX1T1*. **A:** G-banding shows a reciprocal translocation between the long arm of chromosome 8 and the long arm of chromosome 21. **B:** Dual-color, dual-fusion fluorescence in situ hybridization with *RUNX1* probe labeled in green and *RUNX1T1* probe labeled in red. The separate green and red signals represent the normal configuration of *RUNX1* and *RUNX1T1*, respectively. The yellow fusion signals represent the *RUNX1::RUNX1T1* fusion on the abnormal chromosome 8 [der(8)t(8;21)] and the *RUNX1T1::RUNX1* fusion on the abnormal chromosome 21 [der(22)t(8;21)].

Prognosis and Clinical Comment

Contemporary regimens that incorporate gemtuzumab ozogamicin have been associated with a significant improvement in outcome.[11] Acute myeloid leukemia with t(8;21)(q22;q22)/*RUNX1::RUNX1T1* is classified as a favorable risk group in the 2022 European LeukemiaNet risk stratification.[12] However, the overall survival and survival after relapse is lower when compared with AML with *CBFB::MYH11*. Earlier retrospective studies showed the presence of *KIT* mutations to be associated with higher incidence of relapse in adult[3] but not in pediatric patients.[13] However, more recent studies have shown that measurement of *RUNX1::RUNXIT1* transcripts by quantitative reverse transcription polymerase chain reaction (qRT-PCR)-based assay provides better prognostic information: >2.5 log reduction after cycle 1, >3 log after cycle 2, and achievement of minimal residual disease (MRD) negativity after therapy outweigh the prognostic importance of *KIT* mutations.[14] Prospective monitoring of MRD by qPCR-based assay is recommended for appropriate risk stratification and for decision regarding hematopoietic stem cell transplant.[15]

References

1. Grimwade D, Walker H, Oliver F, et al. The importance of diagnostic cytogenetics on outcome in AML: analysis of 1,612 patients entered into the MRC AML 10 trial. The Medical Research Council Adult and Children's Leukaemia Working Parties. *Blood*. 1998;92(7):2322-2333. doi:10.1182/blood.V92.7.2322
2. Byrd JC, Mrózek K, Dodge RK, et al. Pretreatment cytogenetic abnormalities are predictive of induction success, cumulative incidence of relapse, and overall survival in adult patients with de novo acute myeloid leukemia: results from Cancer and Leukemia Group B (CALGB 8461). *Blood*. 2002;100(13):4325-4336. doi:10.1182/blood-2002-03-0772
3. Paschka P, Marcucci G, Ruppert AS, et al. Adverse prognostic significance of KIT mutations in adult acute myeloid leukemia with inv(16) and t(8;21): a Cancer and Leukemia Group B Study. *J Clin Oncol*. 2006;24(24):3904-3911. doi:10.1200/jco.2006.06.9500
4. Johnson RC, Savage NM, Chiang T, et al. Hidden mastocytosis in acute myeloid leukemia with t(8;21)(q22;q22). *Am J Clin Pathol*. 2013;140(4):525-535. doi:10.1309/ajcp1q0ysxeahnkk
5. Porwit-MacDonald A, Janossy G, Ivory K, et al. Leukemia-associated changes identified by quantitative flow cytometry. IV. CD34 overexpression in acute myelogenous leukemia M2 with t(8;21). *Blood*. 1996;87(3):1162-1169. doi:10.1182/blood.V87.3.1162.bloodjournal8731162
6. Baer MR, Stewart CC, Lawrence D, et al. Expression of the neural cell adhesion molecule CD56 is associated with short remission duration and survival in acute myeloid leukemia with t(8;21)(q22;q22). *Blood*. 1997;90(4):1643-1648.
7. Downing JR. The AML1-ETO chimaeric transcription factor in acute myeloid leukaemia: biology and clinical significance. *Br J Haematol*. 1999;106(2):296-308. doi:10.1046/j.1365-2141.1999.01377.x

8. Peterson LF, Boyapati A, Ahn E-Y, et al. Acute myeloid leukemia with the 8q22;21q22 translocation: secondary mutational events and alternative t(8;21) transcripts. *Blood*. 2007;110(3):799-805. doi:10.1182/blood-2006-11-019265
9. Al-Harbi S, Aljurf M, Mohty M, Almohareb F, Ahmed SOA. An update on the molecular pathogenesis and potential therapeutic targeting of AML with t(8;21)(q22;q22.1);RUNX1-RUNX1T1. *Blood Adv*. 2020;4(1):229-238. doi:10.1182/bloodadvances.2019000168
10. Faber ZJ, Chen X, Gedman AL, et al. The genomic landscape of core-binding factor acute myeloid leukemias. *Nat Genet*. 2016;48(12):1551-1556. doi:10.1038/ng.3709
11. Hills RK, Castaigne S, Appelbaum FR, et al. Addition of gemtuzumab ozogamicin to induction chemotherapy in adult patients with acute myeloid leukaemia: a meta-analysis of individual patient data from randomised controlled trials. *Lancet Oncol*. 2014;15(9):986-996. doi::10.1016/S1470-2045(14)70281-5
12. Döhner H, Wei AH, Appelbaum FR, et al. Diagnosis and management of AML in adults: 2022 recommendations from an international expert panel on behalf of the ELN. *Blood*. 2022;140(12):1345-1377. doi:10.1182/blood.2022016867
13. Pollard JA, Alonzo TA, Gerbing RB, et al. Prevalence and prognostic significance of KIT mutations in pediatric patients with core binding factor AML enrolled on serial pediatric cooperative trials for de novo AML. *Blood*. 2010;115(12):2372-2379. doi:10.1182/blood-2009-09-241075
14. Rücker FG, Agrawal M, Corbacioglu A, et al. Measurable residual disease monitoring in acute myeloid leukemia with t(8;21)(q22;q22.1): results from the AML Study Group. *Blood*. 2019;134(19):1608-1618. doi:10.1182/blood.2019001425
15. Heuser M, Freeman SD, Ossenkoppele GJ, et al. 2021 Update on MRD in acute myeloid leukemia: a consensus document from the European LeukemiaNet MRD Working Party. *Blood*. 2021;138(26):2753-2767. doi:10.1182/blood.2021013626

Chapter 24

Acute Myeloid Leukemia With inv(16)(p13.1q22) or t(16;16)(p13.1;q22)/*CBFB::MYH11*

Sandeep Gurbuxani, Tracy I. George, Angela M. Lager, and Olatoyosi M. Odenike

Definition

Acute myeloid leukemia (AML) with inv(16)(p13.1q22) or t(16;16)(p13.1;q22)/*CBFB::MYH11* is an acute myeloid leukemia that usually shows monocytic and granulocytic differentiation and the presence of a characteristically abnormal eosinophil component in the marrow.[1]

Synonyms

Acute myeloid leukemia, *CBF-beta::MYH11*, acute myeloid leukemia, inv(16)(p13.1q22), acute myeloid leukemia, t(16;16)(p13.1;q22), acute myeloid leukemia with abnormal marrow eosinophils (includes all variants), acute myelomonocytic leukemia with abnormal eosinophils, FAB M4Eo. (not recommended)

Epidemiology

AML with inv(16)(p13.1q22) or t(16;16)(p13.1;q22) accounts for 10% of adult and 6% of childhood AML.[2]

General Clinical Features

Clinical presentation is nonspecific and related to the proliferation of blasts and subsequent bone marrow failure with consequences of anemia, neutropenia, and thrombocytopenia. The white blood cell count is higher in AML with inv(16)(p13.1q22) or t(16;16)(p13.1;q22)/*CBFB::MYH11* than in cases with t(8;21)(q22;q22).[3] Extramedullary disease is more common when compared with most AML, and patients may present with lymphadenopathy and organomegaly. Myeloid sarcoma may be present at initial diagnosis or at relapse and may be the only evidence for involvement by AML.

Morphology

A diagnosis of AML can be made with a blast count of ≥10%. There is evidence for monocytic differentiation, and monoblasts, promonocytes, immature monocytes can be present in addition to myeloid blasts. Bone marrow eosinophils may be increased, and the hallmark of this type of AML is the presence of eosinophils with large, abnormal, purple-violet granules (Figure 24.1A). While the majority of cases of inv(16)(p13.1q22)/t(16;16)(p13.1;q22)/*CBFB::MYH11* have been identified as having abnormal eosinophils, in some cases they are rare and difficult to find. Occasional cases with this genetic abnormality have been reported to lack eosinophilia or to show only granulocytic maturation without a monocytic component or demonstrate only monocytic differentiation. The marrow trephine biopsy is usually hypercellular but may occasionally be normocellular. Residual normal hematopoiesis is reduced.

Immunophenotype

Most of these leukemias are characterized by the presence of a blast population expressing bright CD34 and CD117 (Figure 24.1B), along with populations differentiating toward granulocytic (CD13, CD33, CD15, CD65, MPO positive) and monocytic (CD14, CD4, CD11b, CD11c, CD64, CD36, and lysozyme positive) lineages. Maturation asynchrony is often seen. Coexpression of CD2 with granulocytic markers is frequent but not specific for this diagnosis.

Genetics

The inv(16)(p13.1q22) (Figure 24.2), found in the vast majority of this subtype, and the less common t(16;16)(p13.1;q22) both result in the fusion of the *CBFB* gene

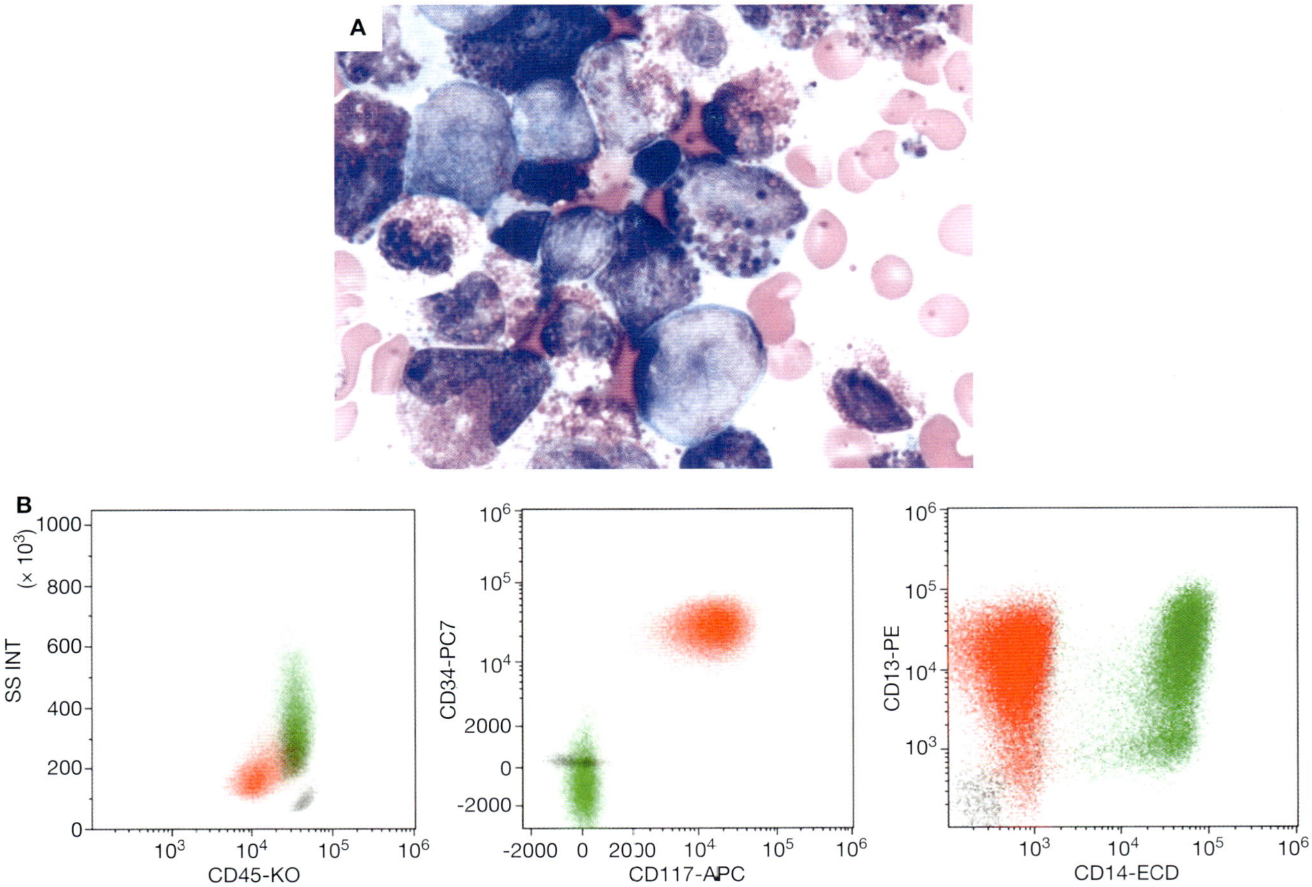

FIGURE 24.1 **A:** Acute myeloid leukemia with inv(16)(p13.1q22) showing an abnormal eosinophil with prominent basophilic granule. **B:** Flow cytometry shows mixed population of blasts (red) and monocytes (green). Blasts show bright coexpression of CD34 and CD117, and monocytes show expected pattern of CD13 and CD14 expression.

at 16q22 to the *MYH11* gene at 16p13.1.[1,4] The *CBFB* gene codes for the core binding factor (CBF) beta subunit, which heterodimerizes with CBFA, which is also known as runt-related transcription factor 1, RUNX1, encoded by the *RUNX1* gene. The *RUNX1* gene is also involved in AML with t(8;21)(q22;q22)/*RUNX1::RUNX1T1*. By conventional cytogenetic analysis, the inv(16)(p13.1q22)/t(16;16)(p13.1;q22) is a subtle rearrangement that may be overlooked when metaphase preparations are suboptimal. Thus, at diagnosis, the use of fluorescence in situ hybridization (FISH) and/or reverse transcription polymerase chain reaction (RT-PCR) methods may be necessary to document the genetic alteration. There have been over 10 reported *CBFB::MYH11* fusion transcripts in patients with *CBFB::MYH11*-positive AML. However, the most common *CBFB::MYH11* fusion transcript involves the juxtaposition of exon 5 of *CBFB* to exon 34 of *MYH11* (type A fusion), which accounts for up to 90% of cases.[5] Secondary cytogenetic abnormalities occur in approximately 40% of cases, with +22, +8, del(7q) or +21, and hyperdiploidy most commonly observed.[6,7] Trisomy 22 is fairly specific for patients with inv(16)(p13.1q22), being very rarely detected with other primary aberrations in AML, whereas +8 is commonly seen in patients with other primary aberrations. Rare cases of AML and chronic myeloid leukemia with both inv(16)(p13.1q22) and t(9;22)(q34;q11.2) have been reported, and this finding in chronic myeloid leukemia is usually associated with accelerated or blast phases of the disease.[8] Submicroscopic alterations in additional genes have been described in more than 90% of patients and include mutations in *KIT* (exons 8 and 17, 30%-40% patients), *NRAS* (45%), *KRAS* (13%), and *FLT3* (14%).[6,9]

Prognosis and Clinical Comment

European Leukemia Network risk classification for AML with inv(16)(p13.1q22) or t(16;16)(p13.1;q22) is favorable.[10] Treatment regimens including intensive consolidation are associated with a high rate of complete remission.[11] Overall survival is further improved

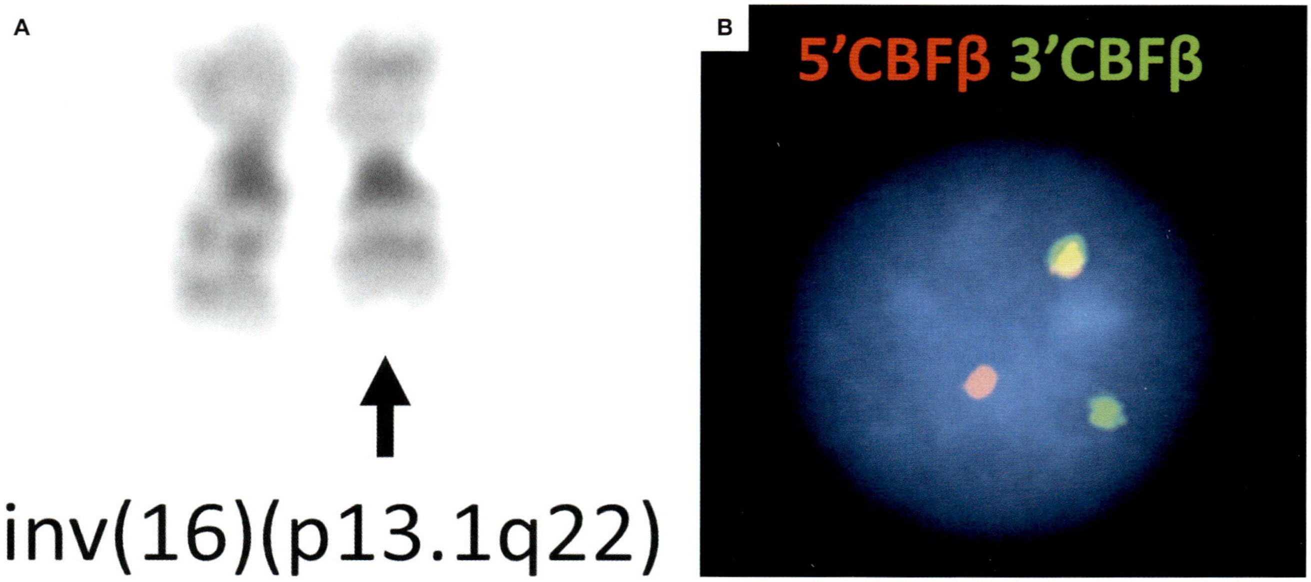

FIGURE 24.2 Acute myeloid leukemia with inv(16)(p13.1q22). **A:** G-banding shows rejoining of bands 16p13.1 and 16q22 resulting from the inversion (solid arrow) along with the normal chromosome 16. **B:** Dual-color, break-apart FISH with the 5′ region of *CBFB* labeled in red and the 3′ region labeled in green. The yellow fusion signal represents the normal configuration of *CBFB*, while the separate red and green signals represent the rearranged copy of *CBFB*, which is consistent with either inv(16)(p13.1q22) or t(16;16)(p13.1;q22).

by addition of gemtuzumab ozogamicin.[12] Older age, elevated white blood cell count, and *FLT3* tyrosine kinase domain mutations are associated with an unfavorable outcome. Role of secondary genetic abnormalities including gain of chromosome 22, trisomy 8, and presence of *KIT* mutations is variable and likely influenced by the age of patient population and therapy. Inability to achieve 3- to 4-log reduction in measurable residual disease monitored by quantitative RT-PCR at the end of consolidation is considered a more robust predictor of adverse outcome and maybe used for risk stratification and decisions regarding subsequent therapy.[13,14]

References

1. Le Beau MM, Larson RA, Bitter MA, Vardiman JW, Golomb HM, Rowley JD. Association of an inversion of chromosome 16 with abnormal marrow eosinophils in acute myelomonocytic leukemia. A unique cytogenetic-clinicopathological association. *N Engl J Med*. 1983;309(11):630-636. doi:10.1056/nejm198309153091103
2. Grimwade D, Walker H, Oliver F, et al. The importance of diagnostic cytogenetics on outcome in AML: analysis of 1,612 patients entered into the MRC AML 10 trial. The Medical Research Council Adult and Children's Leukaemia Working Parties. *Blood*. 1998;92(7):2322-2333. doi:10.1182/blood.V92.7.2322
3. Paschka P, Marcucci G, Ruppert AS, et al. Adverse prognostic significance of KIT mutations in adult acute myeloid leukemia with inv(16) and t(8;21): a Cancer and Leukemia Group B Study. *J Clin Oncol*. 2006;24(24):3904-3911. doi:10.1200/jco.2006.06.9500
4. Liu P, Tarlé SA, Hajra A, et al. Fusion between transcription factor CBF beta/PEBP2 beta and a myosin heavy chain in acute myeloid leukemia. *Science*. 1993;261(5124):1041-1044.
5. Kadkol SS, Bruno A, Dodge C, Lindgren V, Ravandi F. Comprehensive analysis of CBFbeta-MYH11 fusion transcripts in acute myeloid leukemia by RT-PCR analysis. *J Mol Diagn*. 2004;6(1):22-27. doi:10.1016/s1525-1578(10)60487-4
6. Paschka P, Du J, Schlenk RF, et al. Secondary genetic lesions in acute myeloid leukemia with inv(16) or t(16;16): a study of the German-Austrian AML Study Group (AMLSG). *Blood*. 2013;121(1):170-177. doi:10.1182/blood-2012-05-431486
7. Han SY, Mrózek K, Voutsinas J, et al. Secondary cytogenetic abnormalities in core-binding factor AML harboring inv(16) vs t(8;21). *Blood Adv*. 2021;5(10):2481-2489. doi:10.1182/bloodadvances.2020003605
8. Wu Y, Slovak ML, Snyder DS, Arber DA. Coexistence of inversion 16 and the Philadelphia chromosome in acute and chronic myeloid leukemias: report of six cases and review of literature. *Am J Clin Pathol*. 2006;125(2):260-266. doi:10.1309/f0mx-5cl8-cedy-3w86
9. Opatz S, Bamopoulos SA, Metzeler KH, et al. The clinical mutatome of core binding factor leukemia. *Leukemia*. 2020;34(6):1553-1562. doi:10.1038/s41375-019-0697-0
10. Döhner H, Wei AH, Appelbaum FR, et al. Diagnosis and management of AML in adults: 2022 recommendations from an international expert panel on behalf of the ELN. *Blood*. 2022;140(12):1345-1377. doi:10.1182/blood.2022016867

11. Grimwade D, Hills RK, Moorman AV, et al. Refinement of cytogenetic classification in acute myeloid leukemia: determination of prognostic significance of rare recurring chromosomal abnormalities among 5876 younger adult patients treated in the United Kingdom Medical Research Council trials. *Blood.* 2010;116(3):354-365. doi:10.1182/blood-2009-11-254441
12. Hills RK, Castaigne S, Appelbaum FR, et al. Addition of gemtuzumab ozogamicin to induction chemotherapy in adult patients with acute myeloid leukaemia: a meta-analysis of individual patient data from randomised controlled trials. *Lancet Oncol.* 2014;15(9):986-996. doi:10.1016/S1470-2045(14)70281-5
13. Yin JAL, O'Brien MA, Hills RK, Daly SB, Wheatley K, Burnett AK. Minimal residual disease monitoring by quantitative RT-PCR in core binding factor AML allows risk stratification and predicts relapse: results of the United Kingdom MRC AML-15 trial. *Blood.* 2012;120(14):2826-2835. doi:10.1182/blood-2012-06-435669
14. Heuser M, Freeman SD, Ossenkoppele GJ, et al. 2021 Update on MRD in acute myeloid leukemia: a consensus document from the European LeukemiaNet MRD Working Party. *Blood.* 2021;138(26):2753-2767. doi:10.1182/blood.2021013626

Chapter 25

Acute Myeloid Leukemia With t(9;11)(p21.3;q23.3)/*KMT2A::MLLT3* and Other *KMT2A* Rearrangements

Wayne Tam, Harry Paul Erba, and Yen-Chun Liu

Definition

Acute myeloid leukemia with t(9;11)(p21.3;q23.3)/*KMT2A::MLLT3*

This acute myeloid leukemia (AML) entity is characterized by a t(9;11)(p21.3;q23.3) that results in an in-frame *KMT2A::MLLT3* fusion. The peripheral blood or bone marrow blast percentage cutoff for this diagnosis has decreased from 20% in the revised fourth edition World Health Organization (WHO) classification to the current 10%.

Synonyms

AML with t(9;11)(p22;q23); *MLLT3-MLL* (not recommended).

Epidemiology

AMLs with *KMT2A::MLLT3* can be seen in all ages, but their frequencies vary by age. AMLs with *KMT2A::MLLT3*, the most common *KMT2A* rearrangement, account for 1% to 2% of the de novo AMLs in adults and 5% to 10% of the pediatric AMLs (Table 25.1).[1,2] *KMT2A* rearrangement, of which about 25% to 30% is *KMT2A::MLLT3*, is the most common driver alteration in infant AML, present in >50% of cases.

In secondary AMLs occurring in patients after cytotoxic treatments, *KMT2A* rearrangement is also a common driver; a qualifier "therapy-related" following the diagnosis should be used for cases with such history (eg, AML with t(9;11)(p21.3;q23.3)/*KMT2A::MLLT3*, therapy-related). This subset of therapy-related AMLs with *KMT2A* rearrangements are associated with exposure to topoisomerase II inhibitors (eg, doxorubicin and etoposide) and account for roughly 30% of the therapy-related myeloid neoplasms.[3] They tend to occur with a shorter latency (1-5 years) compared with those therapy-related myeloid neoplasms associated with monosomies, complex karyotype, and *TP53* aberrations occurring 5 to 10 years after exposure to alkylating agents and/or radiation therapy.[3]

General Clinical Features

The clinical presentation, including variable degree of cytopenia and leukocytosis, may overlap with other AML entities. Extramedullary involvement in both adults and pediatric patients has been reported. When compared with patients with AML with normal karyotype, patients with AML with *KMT2A* rearrangements showed increased early mortality (within 60 days) associated with an increased risk of bleeding, as well as clinical and laboratory features of disseminated intravascular coagulation. Pediatric patients with AML with *KMT2A* rearrangements are more likely to show hyperleukocytosis.

Morphology

Blasts in AML with *KMT2A* rearrangements usually demonstrate myelomonocytic or monocytic/monoblastic differentiation (Figure 25.1). In cases with monocytic/monoblastic differentiation, promonocytes and monoblasts are considered as blast equivalents for blast enumeration. Blasts in this entity may demonstrate variable degree of myeloid differentiation or megakaryoblastic differentiation, the latter seen preferentially in the pediatric population and less frequently in adults. In cases with monocytic/monoblastic differentiation, blasts are usually large in size with abundant cytoplasm. MPO (myeloperoxidase) and NSE (nonspecific esterase) cytochemical stain can be used to confirm myeloid as well as monocytic/monoblastic differentiation. Blast count in the bone marrow involved by AML with *KMT2A* rearrangements is usually high and appears higher than that in AML with normal karyotype.

TABLE 25.1 The most common translocation partner genes in acute myeloid leukemia with *KMT2A* rearrangements

		Frequencies (%)			
Chromosome/ Cytoband	**Gene**	**Overall**	**Infant**	**Pediatric**	**Adult**
9p22	*MLLT3 (AF9)*	34-35	26-29	38-41	33-34
10p12	*MLLT10 (AF10)*	19-21	27-28	20-24	12-14
19p13.1	*ELL*	11-12	15-16	7-8	16-17
6q27	*AFDN (MLLT4, AF6)*	9-10	1-2	8-9	13-14
19p13.3	*MLLT1 (ENL)*	4-5	1-2	6-7	4-5
4q21.3	*AFF1 (AF4)*	1-2	2-3	0-1	1-2
10q21.3	*TET1*	0-1	0	0-1	0-1

Adapted from Meyer C, Burmeister T, Groger D, et al. The MLL recombinome of acute leukemias in 2017. *Leukemia.* 2018;32(2):273-284. and Meyer C, Larghero P, Almeida Lopes B, et al. The KMT2A recombinome of acute leukemias in 2023. *Leukemia.* 2023;37(5):988-1005.

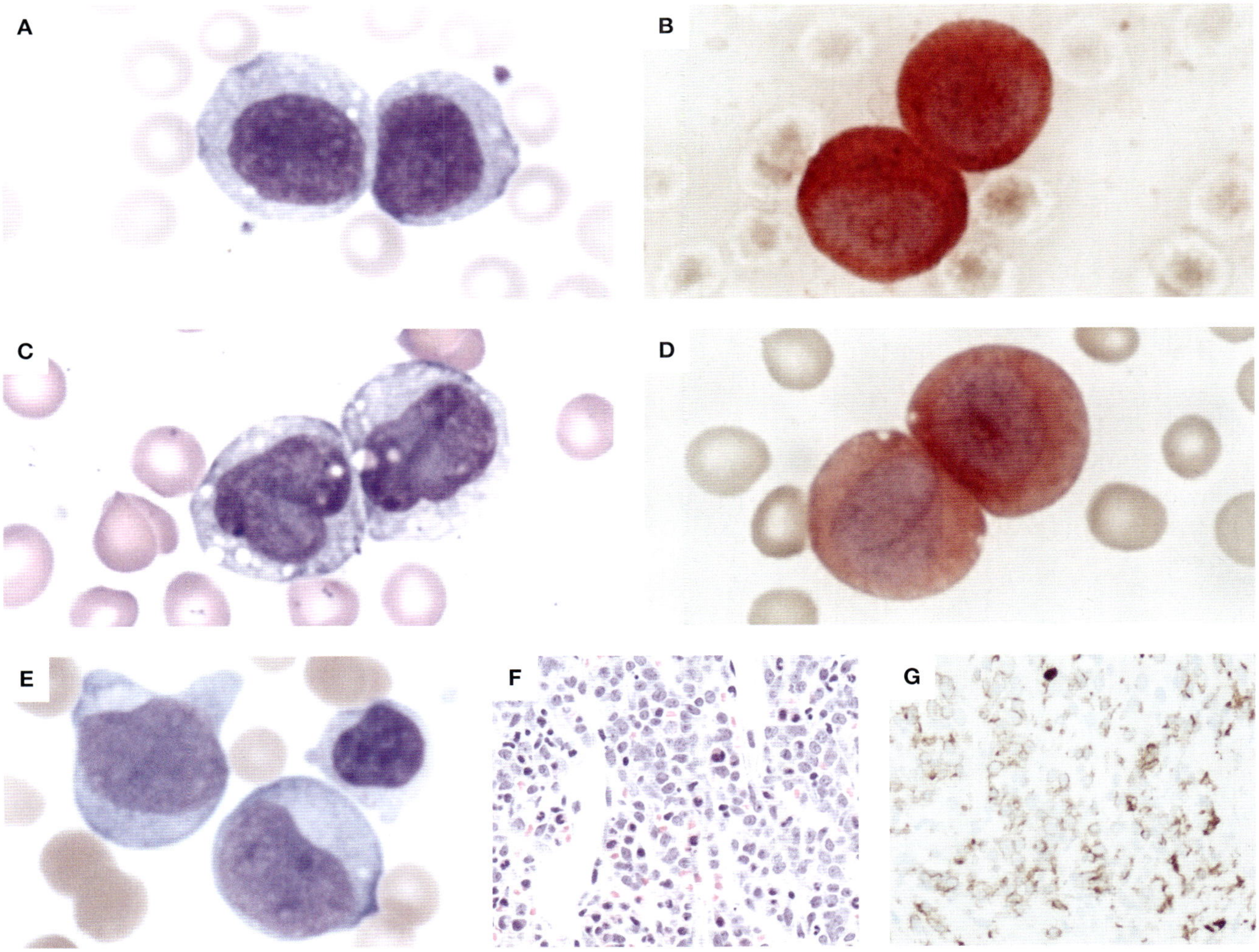

FIGURE 25.1 **A** and **B:** Acute myeloid leukemia (AML) with t(9;11)(p21.3;q23.3)/*KMT2A::MLLT3* showing monoblasts **(A)** positive for NSE cytochemical stain **(B)**. **C** and **D:** AML with *KMT2A* rearrangement showing promonocytes **(C)** positive for NSE stain **(D)**. This is a case of t(10;11)(p12;q23.3)/*KMT2A::MLLT10*. **E-G:** AML with *KMT2A* rearrangement showing blasts with megakaryoblastic differentiation (**E:** aspirate smear; **F:** biopsy section) highlighted by the CD42b immunostain **(G)**. This is a case of t(10;11)(p12;q23.3)/*KMT2A::MLLT10*.

Immunophenotype

The blasts in this entity demonstrate a broad spectrum of immunophenotypic features depending on the lineage differentiation. Blasts can demonstrate an immunophenotype of mature monocytes (positive for CD64, CD14, CD36, and dim CD15; negative for CD34 and CD117) or immature monocytic cells (positive for CD64; loss of CD14, CD13, or CD36; increased CD34, CD117, or CD15).[4] Blasts can also demonstrate a typical myeloid blast immunophenotype (positive for CD34, CD117, CD13, CD33, HLA-DR, and variable MPO) or an immunophenotype reminiscent of acute promyelocytic leukemia (positive for CD117, CD13, and CD33; negative for CD34 and HLA-DR). Cases with myelomonocytic differentiation can present with two blast populations showing myeloid and monocytic differentiation, respectively.[4] Lesions with megakaryoblastic differentiation may demonstrate expression of CD41, CD61, or CD42b by flow cytometry, but immunostains for megakaryocytic markers in the trephine biopsy section are usually recommended for further evaluation. Lysozyme and MPO immunostains can be used to evaluate the extramedullary involvement. By flow cytometry, AML with *KMT2A* rearrangements may show aberrant, usually heterogeneous, expression of NG2, a member of the chondroitin sulfate proteoglycan family.

AML With Other *KMT2A* Rearrangements

This AML entity is characterized by in-frame *KMT2A* fusions in which 5′ *KMT2A* is fused with the 3′ partner gene other than *MLLT3*. The diagnosis requires a blast percentage ≥10%. These AMLs were previously classified as AML, not otherwise specified in the revised fourth edition WHO classification. The establishment of this new entity expands the umbrella group of AML with recurrent genetic abnormalities. This entity does not include cases with *KMT2A* partial tandem duplication.

Synonyms

AML with 11q23 (*MLL*) abnormalities (not recommended).

Epidemiology

AML with other *KMT2A* rearrangements account for 1% to 2% of the de novo AMLs in adults and 10% to 15% of the pediatric AML. The frequencies of the most common partner genes for *KMT2A* rearrangements in AML are listed in Table 25.1.[1,2]

General clinical features, morphology, and immunophenotype

The clinical, morphologic, and immunophenotypic findings of AML with other *KMT2A* rearrangements are similar to those of AML with *KMT2A::MLLT3*, as described earlier.

Genetics

KMT2A gene, previously named *mixed-lineage leukemia* (*MLL*), *MLL1*, *ALL1*, and *HRX*, encodes a transcriptional coactivator regulating the expression of target genes. AML with *KMT2A* rearrangements, irrespective of the translocation partners, demonstrates a gene expression signature distinct from other AMLs. *HOX* cluster genes (especially *HOXA7-HOXA10*) and the *HOX* cofactor *MEIS1* are generally overexpressed in AML with *KMT2A* rearrangements. *HOX* genes are implicated to contribute to the stem cell–like characteristics of acute leukemia with *KMT2A* rearrangements.

KMT2A protein contains multiple functional domains including the Menin-binding motif in the N-terminus and the PHD/BD domains in the midportion (Figure 25.2A). Since *KMT2A* rearrangements involve fusion of the 5′ *KMT2A* with the 3′ partner gene, the domains within the N terminus of KMT2A protein are preserved, whereas the domains in the midportion and C terminus of KMT2A are frequently lost (Figure 25.2B). The mechanisms of leukemogenesis caused by *KMT2A* fusions have not been completely delineated but apparently involve gene regulation. The retained Menin-binding motif in the KMT2A fusion protein enables complex formation with cofactors including Menin. The complex binds to the *HOXA* promoter and upregulates *HOXA* gene expression.[5] Fusion proteins containing the C terminus of AFF1 or MLLT1 (AF4 and ENL family protein) can lead to constitutive transcriptional activation through formation of the AEP complex containing AF4/ENL family protein and recruitment of histone methyltransferase DOT1L that induce transcriptional activation and maintenance.[6] Rare translocation with the 5′ partner gene fused with the 3′ *KMT2A*, such as the *NUP98::KMT2A* fusion, shows a distinctly different gene expression pattern[7] and is not considered as part of the entity.

Although AML with *KMT2A* rearrangements demonstrate diverse partner genes (>80 described), the majority involve one of the seven common

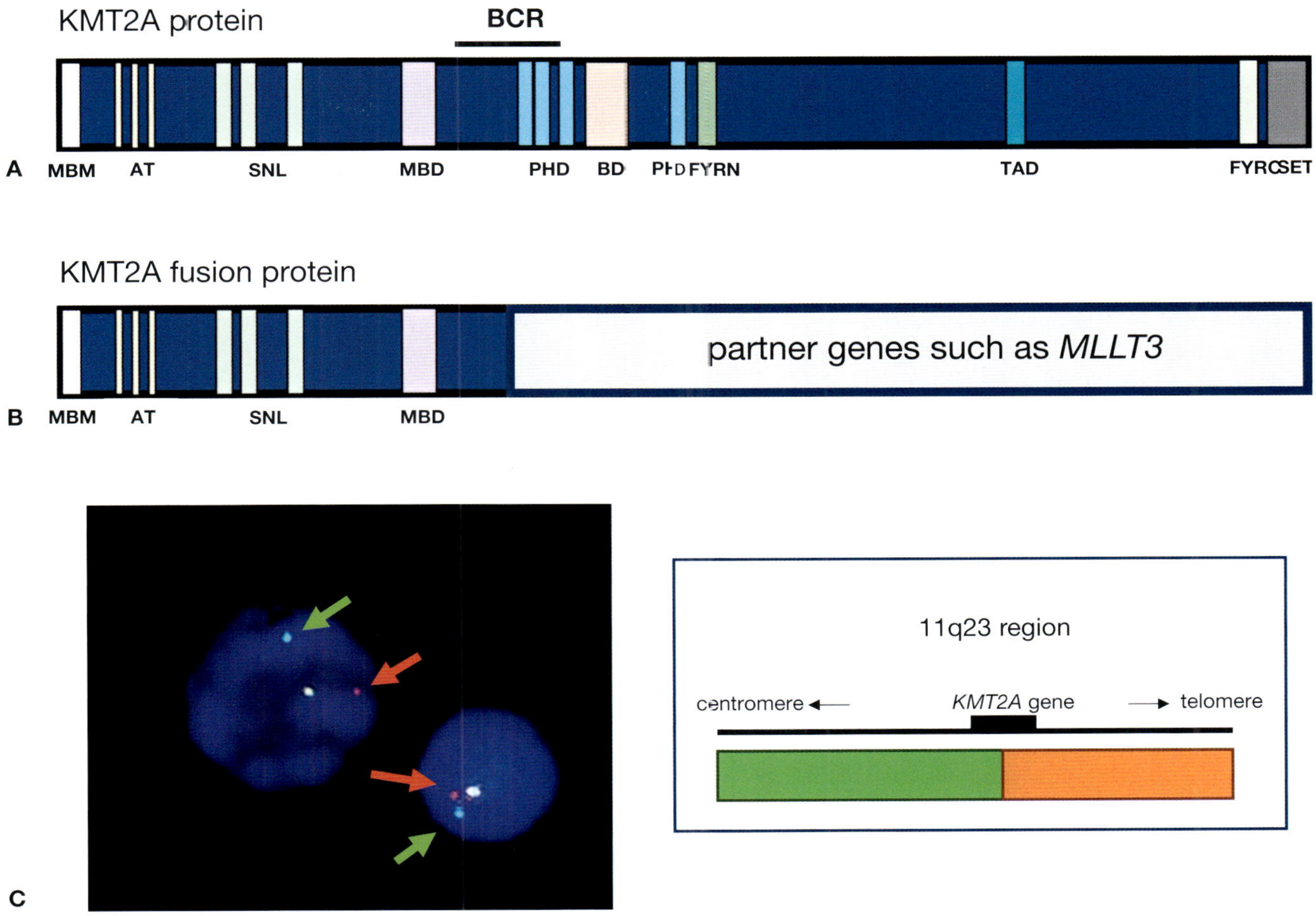

FIGURE 25.2 **A** and **B:** The structure of the wildtype KMT2A protein and the KMT2A fusion proteins. AT, hooks (DNA binding); BCR, breakpoint cluster region; BD, bromodomain (histone binding); FYRN and FYRC, phenylalanine/tyrosine-rich N- and C-terminal domains (dimerization domains after Taspase1 cleavage to assemble the KMT2A backbone); MBM, Menin-binding motif; MBD, methyl DNA-binding domain; PHD, plant homeodomain finger domain (PHD1, PHD2, PHD3, and PHD4; mediating protein interaction); SET, H3K4 histone methyltransferase domain; SNL, Speckled nuclear localization domains; TAD, transactivation domain. **(C)** Interphase FISH showing *KMT2A* rearrangement using break-apart *KMT2A* probe. 5′*KMT2A* is green and 3′*KMT2A* is red. Arrows indicate separation of the 5′*KMT2A* and 3′*KMT2A* signals.

partner genes in Table 25.1. The t(11;16)(q23;p13)/*KMT2A::CREBBP* fusion is enriched in therapy-related lesion.[8] In addition, there have been occasional reports of AML with *KMT2A* rearrangements, which occurred as lineage switching at relapse after target therapy, such as anti-CD19 CAR T-cell or blinatumomab, in patients with B-lymphoblastic leukemia/lymphoma harboring the same *KMT2A* rearrangements. There are likely some differences in the biology of these cases compared with other de novo or therapy-related AMLs with *KMT2A* rearrangements; disruption of the epigenetic regulation has been implicated to change the transcriptional program and lead to the ultimate lineage switching.[9]

The breakpoints for the *KMT2A* rearrangements in AML occur within the major breakpoint cluster region (BCR) between intron 7 and exon 13 of *KMT2A*.[1,2] The breakpoints of *KMT2A* fusions are unlikely to be random since certain *KMT2A* partner genes show preference for certain breakpoints.[2] AML with *KMT2A* rearrangements associated with exposure to topoisomerase II inhibitors tend to have breakpoints within intron 11 probably due to the distribution of topoisomerase cleavage sites. The preference for the BCR may have a pathogenic implication since it overlaps with the PHD/BD domains encoded by *KMT2A* exons 11 to 18, which have been shown to be a functional platform connecting histone targeting and transcriptional regulation.[10]

While karyotyping may fail to identify cryptic *KMT2A* rearrangements, the vast majority of the *KMT2A* rearrangements can be identified by fluorescence in situ hybridization (FISH) studies (Figure 25.2C). RNA sequencing (unbiased or targeted) has facilitated the discovery of novel *KMT2A* rearrangement cryptic to FISH such as the *KMT2A::USP2* fusion. On rare occasions, RNA sequencing also helps distinguish the out-of-frame *KMT2A* rearrangements identified by FISH without functional in-frame fusion transcript. Karyotyping and RNA sequencing can help identify the translocation partner genes that may have clinical impact regarding prognosis and molecular-based measurable residual disease (MRD) monitoring. Studies using quantitative reverse transcription polymerase chain reaction for *KMT2A::MLLT3* fusion transcripts demonstrated that MRD positivity is highly predictive of relapse.

AML cases with *KMT2A* rearrangements usually demonstrate low number of comutations.[11] The most common comutations involve the RAS pathway (such as *KRAS, NRAS,* and *PTPN11*) occurring in roughly one-third of the patients. *FLT3* mutations (TKD more common than ITD) can also be identified. The comutations mentioned previously tend to be subclonal and are likely acquired later in the disease process.[11]

Prognosis and Clinical Comment

The translocation partner genes have been implicated to impact the prognosis of AML with *KMT2A* rearrangements, but the relationship may also be influenced by other factors such as age and treatment. AML with t(9;11)(p21.3;q23.3)/*KMT2A::MLLT3* was found to have better prognosis when compared with AMLs with other *KMT2A* rearrangements. AML with t(9;11)(p21.3;q23.3)/*KMT2A::MLLT3* is thus considered as intermediate risk by the 2022 European LeukemiaNet (ELN) risk classification, whereas AMLs with other *KMT2A* rearrangements are considered as adverse risk.[12] However, this advantageous prognostic impact of *KMT2A::MLLT3* fusion was only seen in younger adults (<60 years old) in some study.[11] In a meta-analysis of pediatric AML cases, patients with t(9;11)(p21.3;q23.3)/*KMT2A::MLLT3* did not show significant better outcome; instead, t(1;11)(q21;q23)/*KMT2A::MLLT11* fusion was reported to have superior prognosis, whereas cases with t(6;11)(q27;q23)/*KMT2A::AFDN* fusions, t(10;11)(p11.2;q23)/*KMT2A::ABI1* fusions, as well as t(10;11)(p12;q23)/*KMT2A::NEBL* fusions were noted to have inferior outcome in the same cohort.[13] *EVI1* overexpression has been found in patients with AML with *KMT2A* rearrangements and was associated with inferior outcome. Therapy-related lesions with *KMT2A* rearrangements tend to demonstrate inferior prognosis when compared with de novo cases. Menin inhibitors have demonstrated promising results in patients with relapsed/refractory AML with *KMT2A* rearrangements. For example, revumenib (SNDX-5613) monotherapy was associated with a 56% overall response rate in this patient population (20% complete remission). There was clinical evidence of differentiation leading to these responses; differentiation syndrome was observed as a treatment-related adverse event. Pharmacodynamic studies demonstrated decreased expression of *HOXA9* and *MEIS1* during the first cycle of therapy in most subjects. Mechanisms of resistance are being elucidated and include the emergence of *MEN1* mutations.[14] The impact of these novel therapies on the prognosis of AML with *KMT2A* rearrangements with different translocation partners is not entirely clear at the current time.

References

1. Meyer C, Burmeister T, Groger D, et al. The MLL recombinome of acute leukemias in 2017. *Leukemia.* 2018;32(2):273-284.
2. Meyer C, Larghero P, Almeida Lopes B, et al. The KMT2A recombinome of acute leukemias in 2023. *Leukemia.* 2023;37(5):988-1005.
3. McNerney ME, Godley LA, Le Beau MM. Therapy-related myeloid neoplasms: when genetics and environment collide. *Nat Rev Cancer.* 2017;17(9):513-527.
4. Konoplev S, Wang X, Tang G, et al. Comprehensive immunophenotypic study of acute myeloid leukemia with KMT2A (MLL) rearrangement in adults: a single-institution experience. *Cytometry B Clin Cytom.* 2022;102(2):123-133.
5. Krivtsov AV, Armstrong SA. MLL translocations, histone modifications and leukaemia stem-cell development. *Nat Rev Cancer.* 2007;7(11):823-833.
6. Okuda H, Stanojevic B, Kanai A, et al. Cooperative gene activation by AF4 and DOT1L drives MLL-rearranged leukemia. *J Clin Invest.* 2017;127(5):1918-1931.
7. Fisher JN, Thanasopoulou A, Juge S, et al. Transforming activities of the NUP98-KMT2A fusion gene associated with myelodysplasia and acute myeloid leukemia. *Haematologica.* 2020;105(7):1857-1867.
8. Xie W, Tang G, Wang E, et al. t(11;16)(q23;p13)/KMT2A-CREBBP in hematologic malignancies: presumptive evidence of myelodysplasia or therapy-related neoplasm? *Ann Hematol.* 2020;99(3):487-500.
9. Tirtakusuma R, Szoltysek K, Milne P, et al. Epigenetic regulator genes direct lineage switching in MLL/AF4 leukemia. *Blood.* 2022;140(17):1875-1890.
10. Wang Z, Song J, Milne TA, et al. Pro isomerization in MLL1 PHD3-bromo cassette connects H3K4me readout to CyP33 and HDAC-mediated repression. *Cell.* 2010;141(7):1183-1194.

11. Bill M, Mrozek K, Kohlschmidt J, et al. Mutational landscape and clinical outcome of patients with de novo acute myeloid leukemia and rearrangements involving 11q23/KMT2A. *Proc Natl Acad Sci U S A*. 2020;117(42):26340-26346.
12. Dohner H, Wei AH, Appelbaum FR, et al. Diagnosis and management of AML in adults: 2022 recommendations from an international expert panel on behalf of the ELN. *Blood*. 2022;140(12):1345-1377.
13. Balgobind BV, Raimondi SC, Harbott J, et al. Novel prognostic subgroups in childhood 11q23/MLL-rearranged acute myeloid leukemia: results of an international retrospective study. *Blood*. 2009;114(12):2489-2496.
14. Issa GC, Aldoss I, DiPersio J, et al. The menin inhibitor revumenib in KMT2A-rearranged or NPM1-mutant leukaemia. *Nature*. 2023;615(7954):920-924.

Chapter 26

Acute Myeloid Leukemia With t(6;9)(p22.3;q34.1)/*DEK::NUP214*

Genevieve M. Crane, Heesun J. Rogers, and Martin S. Tallman

Definition

Acute myeloid leukemia (AML) with t(6;9)(p22.3;q34.1)/*DEK::NUP214* is a rare AML subtype more often seen in young adults and children, associated with frequent bone marrow dysplasia, blood or bone marrow basophilia in a subset, and adverse prognosis. It is included in the group of AML with recurrent genetic abnormalities demonstrating the t(6;9)(p22.3;q34.1) rearrangement and having ≥10% peripheral blood or bone marrow blasts.[1-3]

Synonyms

AML with t(6;9)(p22.3;q34.1);*DEK-CAN* (not recommended).

Epidemiology

AML with t(6;9)(p22.3;q34.1)/*DEK::NUP214* is a rare subtype of AML comprising 0.7% to 1.8%[4,5] of AML cases and up to 1.4% of pediatric AML.[5,6] In the pediatric population, there is a relative male predominance (male:female of 1.76) but without definite sex predilection in the adult population.[2,7] This AML occurs in both children and adults with a younger median age compared with most other forms of AML.[5] The adult median age is reported as 38 to 46 years[2,4,7] with a pediatric median age of 10 to 13 years.[4,6,8] It is rare at the extremes of age. The *DEK::NUP214* rearrangement is also seen in a subset of myelodysplastic syndromes (MDSs) or other myeloid neoplasms.[2,9]

General Clinical Features

Patients typically present with moderate to severe anemia and thrombocytopenia or pancytopenia. Pediatric patients tend to show lower hemoglobin levels than adults.[5] Overall, patients tend to present with a lower white blood cell count than seen in other subtypes of AML (median WBC of 12×10^9/L),[5,9] but median white blood cell count is higher in patients with concurrent *FLT3* internal tandem duplication (ITD) mutation.[7] Most cases represent de novo AML (66%-88% of adults, 97% of children) with a smaller fraction evolving from an underlying myeloid neoplasm or being therapy-related.[5,7]

Rarely, t(6;9)(p22.3;q34.1)/*DEK::NUP214* is associated with MDS but shows a high risk of progression to AML. Morphologic and clinical features appeared similar to cases presenting as AML in a pediatric series.[6] In adult patients, MDS with t(6;9)(p22.3;q34.1) was associated with lower white blood cell count, lower blast count, and higher platelet count, and patients tended to be older at presentation as compared with patients with AML with the same translocation.[2] However, approximately 50% of patients with MDS and t(6;9)(p22.3;q34.1) had reported a morphologic diagnosis of MDS with excess blasts-2 (blasts 10%-19%) and would fall under the current definition of AML.

Morphology

The blasts are myeloid, but morphologic features and phenotype are not specific and overlap with other AML subtypes other than acute promyelocytic leukemia or acute megakaryocytic leukemia.[5] AML with maturation and acute myelomonocytic leukemia are commonly reported.[6,8,9] The blasts typically show round to irregular or folded nuclei and may show azurophilic granules, cytoplasmic vacuoles, or Auer rods (25%-36%) (Figure 26.1).[2,5,9] By cytochemistry, they are positive for myeloperoxidase. Nonspecific esterase may be positive in a subset of cases.

Mild basophilia, defined as ≥2% basophils in the peripheral blood or bone marrow, has been variably associated with this AML subtype[5,8,9] but was not consistently observed in all cohorts[2,4] or in a pediatric series.[6]

Dysplasia is reported in almost all cases, most commonly in erythroid and granulocytic lineages, but multilineage dysplasia is also frequent[4,5,9] (Figures 26.2 and 26.3). Dysmegakaryopoiesis was reported in 33%

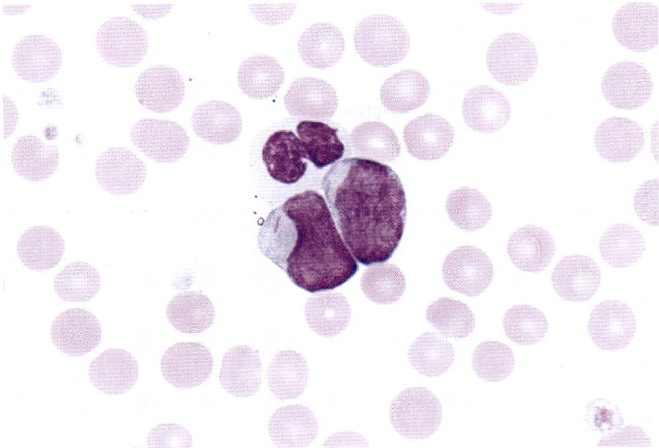

FIGURE 26.1 A peripheral blood smear with circulating blasts with an Auer rod and dysplastic neutrophil with cytoplasmic hypogranulation. (1000×, Wright-Giemsa).

to 56% of cases.[2,4] Mild to moderate bilineal dysplasia was also reported in all cases of a pediatric series.[6] Multilineage dysplasia is more common in cases initially categorized as MDS, which tends to show a higher frequency of megakaryocytic dysplasia.[2] Ring sideroblasts are reported in a subset.[8] In evaluation of the core biopsy, the bone marrow is typically hypercellular,[4] often with increased reticulin fibrosis to various degrees.[9]

Immunophenotype

The blasts typically show a nonspecific myeloid phenotype and express CD13, CD33, CD38, CD117, CD123, HLA-DR, and myeloperoxidase and are positive for CD34, CD117, CD15, CD52, and CD9 in the majority of cases.[2,4,5,9] Blasts in at least a subset of cases are positive for CD9 or TdT[8,9] and/or monocyte-associated antigens such as CD4, CD14, CD36, and CD64.[2] A subset of cases may show expression of aberrant lymphoid markers such as CD2, CD7,[4] and/or CD19 but are negative for CD3 (surface and cytoplasmic), CD5, and PAX5 without evidence of mixed phenotype acute leukemia.[2] Expression of CD10, CD41, and/or CD56 appears rare.

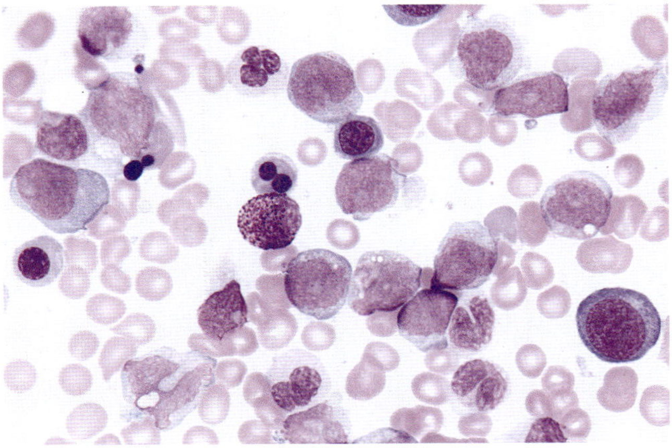

FIGURE 26.2 A bone marrow aspirate smear showing increased blasts with dysplastic erythroid precursors and granulocytes and slightly increased basophils. (1000×, Wright-Giemsa).

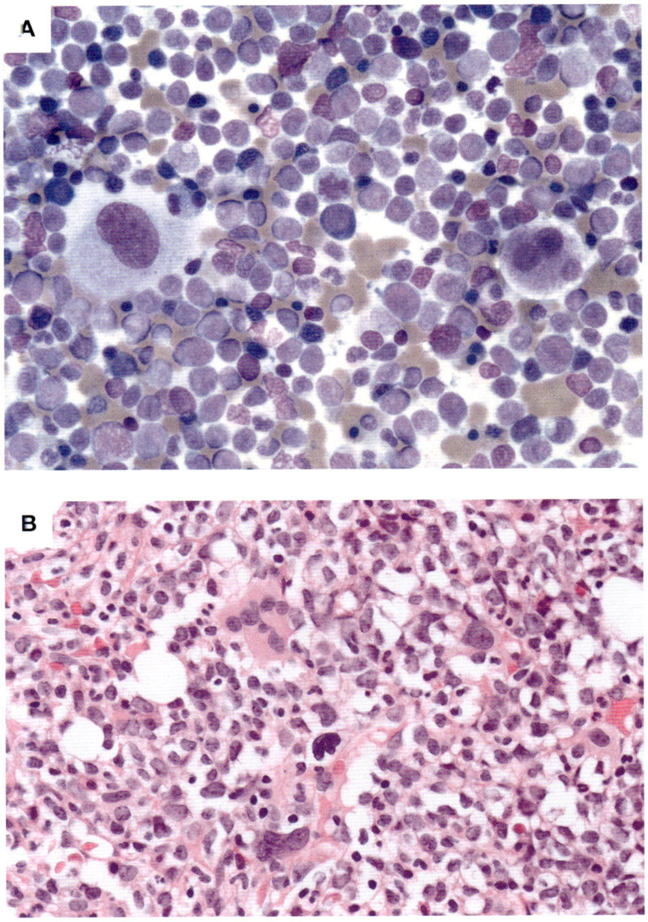

FIGURE 26.3 **A:** A bone marrow aspirate smear demonstrating dysplastic megakaryocytes and increased blasts and dysplastic erythroid precursors and granulocytic cells in the background. (500×, Wright-Giemsa) **B:** A core biopsy demonstrating hypercellularity with increased blasts, disordered maturation, and dysplastic megakaryocytes (500×, H&E).

Genetics

The characteristic t(6;9)(p22.3;q34.1), first recognized in 1976, results in the rearrangement between the *DEK* gene at 6p22.3 (role in chromatin remodeling) and the *NUP214* gene (a component of the nuclear pore complex, formerly known as *CAN*) at 9q34.[2,6] Breakpoints occur within introns and result in a *DEK::NUP214* chimeric fusion gene and a novel 165-kd protein, which functions as an aberrant transcription factor, alters nuclear transport, and may increase protein synthesis.[7] The effects of this fusion gene product appear relatively restricted by cellular subtype for leukemic initiation.[10] The t(6;9) can be detected by conventional karyotype and/or fluorescence in situ hybridization, and *DEK::NUP214* fusion transcripts can be detected by reverse transcription polymerase chain reaction, with detection of the *DEK::NUP214* rearrangement being useful for monitoring molecular measurable residual disease.[3]

The t(6;9)(p22.3;q34.1) is often present as the sole chromosomal abnormality (58%-88% of patients)[2,5,7,9] but may be seen as part of a complex karyotype (10%) or in conjunction with other cytogenetic abnormalities, most commonly trisomy 8 and/or trisomy 13.[2,6-8] Clonal evolution is also reported at relapse.[9]

The majority of AML with t(6;9)(p22.3;q34.1) show at least one somatic mutation (~80%).[4] *FLT3*-ITD mutations are common in both pediatric (42%-69%) and adult (73%-88%) patients.[2,4-7,9,11] *FLT3* tyrosine kinase domain mutations are less common, but *FLT3* D835 mutations have been reported in both AML and MDS cases with t(6;9)(p22.3;q34.1).[2] Overall, AML with t(6;9)(p22.3;q34.1) is notable for being associated with only a small number of concurrent mutations, which do not appear to be essential for initiation or maintenance of the leukemia.[10,11] Recurrent mutations are detected in *DNMT3A, IDH1, IDH2, PTPN11, TET2, WT1*, and RAS genes *(HRAS, KRAS*, and *NRAS)*, with *NRAS*[2,4] and *KRAS*[11] being the most frequent recurrent mutations in reported series. RAS pathway mutations are also common in MDS with t(6;9)(p22.3;q34.1), reported in 50% of cases.[2] The t(6;9)(p22.3;q34.1)/*DEK::NUP214* rearrangement is associated with a unique gene expression profile including *HOXA* and *HOXB* gene overexpression.[6]

Prognosis and Clinical Comment

AML with t(6;9)(p22.3;q34.1) is a distinct clinical entity with a poor prognosis in adult or pediatric patients.[5,12] Concurrent *FLT3*-ITD mutation is common and may be associated with higher white blood cell count and/or bone marrow blast percentage. It has been associated with an adverse effect on survival in some studies but not others.[2,6] As patients with the t(6;9)(p22.3;q34.1) are often young adults or pediatric population, many patients will be candidates for allogeneic stem cell transplantation (allo-SCT).[2] Patients who undergo allo-SCT in the first complete response (CR) had a 5-year overall survival of 53% compared with 23% for patients treated with consolidation chemotherapy as postremission therapy.[7] Most clinicians would recommend allo-SCT in first CR (CR1) as the preferred therapeutic approach as does the National Comprehensive Cancer Network.

References

1. Arber DA, Orazi A, Hasserjian RP, et al. International consensus classification of myeloid neoplasms and acute leukemias: integrating morphologic, clinical, and genomic data. *Blood*. 2022;140(11):1200-1228.
2. Fang H, Yabe M, Zhang X, et al. Myelodysplastic syndrome with t(6;9)(p22;q34.1)/DEK-NUP214 better classified as acute myeloid leukemia? A multicenter study of 107 cases. *Mod Pathol*. 2021;34(6):1143-1152.
3. Dohner H, Wei AH, Appelbaum FR, et al. Diagnosis and management of AML in adults: 2022 recommendations from an international expert panel on behalf of the ELN. *Blood*. 2022;140(12):1345-1377.
4. Visconte V, Shetty S, Przychodzen B, et al. Clinicopathologic and molecular characterization of myeloid neoplasms with isolated t(6;9)(p23;q34). *Int J Lab Hematol*. 2017;39(4):409-417.
5. Slovak ML, Gundacker H, Bloomfield CD, et al. A retrospective study of 69 patients with t(6;9)(p23;q34) AML emphasizes the need for a prospective, multicenter initiative for rare 'poor prognosis' myeloid malignancies. *Leukemia*. 2006;20(7):1295-1297.
6. Sandahl JD, Coenen EA, Forestier E, et al. t(6;9)(p22;q34)/DEK-NUP214-rearranged pediatric myeloid leukemia: an international study of 62 patients. *Haematologica*. 2014;99(5):865-872.
7. Kayser S, Hills RK, Luskin MR, et al. Allogeneic hematopoietic cell transplantation improves outcome of adults with t(6;9) acute myeloid leukemia: results from an international collaborative study. *Haematologica*. 2020;105(1):161-169.
8. Alsabeh R, Brynes RK, Slovak ML, Arber DA. Acute myeloid leukemia with t(6;9) (p23;q34): association with myelodysplasia, basophilia, and initial CD34 negative immunophenotype. *Am J Clin Pathol*. 1997;107(4):430-437.
9. Oyarzo MP, Lin P, Glassman A, Bueso-Ramos CE, Luthra R, Medeiros LJ. Acute myeloid leukemia with t(6;9)(p23;q34) is associated with dysplasia and a high frequency of flt3 gene mutations. *Am J Clin Pathol*. 2004;122(3):348-358.
10. Chiriches C, Khan D, Wieske M, et al. Activation of signaling pathways in models of t(6;9)-acute myeloid leukemia. *Ann Hematol*. 2022;101(10):2179-2193.
11. Papaemmanuil E, Gerstung M, Bullinger L, et al. Genomic classification and prognosis in acute myeloid leukemia. *N Engl J Med*. 2016;374(23):2209-2221.
12. Tarlock K, Alonzo TA, Moraleda PP, et al. Acute myeloid leukaemia (AML) with t(6;9)(p23;q34) is associated with poor outcome in childhood AML regardless of FLT3-ITD status: a report from the Children's Oncology Group. *Br J Haematol*. 2014;166(2):254-259.

Chapter 27

Acute Myeloid Leukemia With inv(3)(q21.3q26.2) or t(3;3)(q21.3;q26.2)/*GATA2*; *MECOM*(*EVI1*) and Acute Myeloid Leukemia With Other *MECOM* Rearrangements

Genevieve M. Crane, Hartmut Döhner, and Heesun J. Rogers

Definition

Acute myeloid leukemia (AML) with inv(3)(q21.3q26.2) or t(3;3)(q21.3;q26.2)/*GATA2*; *MECOM(EVI1)* is associated with adverse prognosis, increased expression of *EVI1*, haploinsufficiency of *GATA2*, and frequent additional genetic alterations including RAS/MAPK pathway mutations, monosomy 7, and/or complex karyotype.[1,2] Normal or elevated platelet counts may be seen, and multilineage dysplasia is common with characteristic nonlobated or bilobated dysplastic megakaryocytes in bone marrow. This entity is defined as a myeloid neoplasm with ≥10% blasts in peripheral blood or bone marrow and evidence of inv(3)(q21.3q26.2) or t(3;3)(q21.3;q26.2) rearrangements of the *MDS1/EVI1* complex (*MECOM*) on chromosome 3q26.2.[3,4] AML with other *MECOM* rearrangements, as detailed later, are also recognized when ≥10% blasts in peripheral blood or bone marrow are present.

Synonyms

AML with inv(3)(q21q26.2) or t(3;3)(q21;q26.2); *RPN1-EVI1* (not recommended).

Epidemiology

AML with inv(3)(q21.3q26.2) or t(3;3)(q21.3;q26.2) [inv(3)/t(3;3)] is a rare subtype of AML comprising 1% to 2.5% of newly diagnosed AML with no gender predilection.[1,2,5-8] A broad median age range at diagnosis has been reported, 48 to 63 years in larger series, which is slightly younger than average for other types of AML.[1,2,6] A significant subset of cases are therapy-related (17%-32%) or progress from a prior myelodysplastic syndrome (MDS) or myeloproliferative neoplasm, which are overrepresented compared with the frequency in unselected AML.[1] MDS cases with inv(3)/t(3;3) are rare (<1% of MDS) and show a high risk of progression to AML.[2]

General Clinical Features

Patients typically present with anemia. Platelet counts tend to be higher on average than other AML subtypes, and a subset show thrombocytosis, but platelet counts are variable (median platelet counts of 80-107 × 10^9/L) with thrombocytopenia often present.[1,2,6-8] Normal to slightly elevated leukocyte counts are common, but a wide range is reported.[6,9] Elevated leukocyte counts ≥20 × 10^9/L have been associated with inv(3)(q21.3q26.2) and *NRAS* mutation in some series without other differences in clinical presentation.[1] Hepatosplenomegaly is seen in a subset, but lymphadenopathy is rare.[2] The clinical course is generally aggressive and associated with chemoresistance and markedly adverse outcomes.[1]

Morphology

The blast morphologic features are not specific, including blast features seen in AML with or without maturation, acute myelomonocytic leukemia, or less commonly acute megakaryoblastic leukemia.[7] The peripheral blood may show dysplastic granulocytes, giant or hypogranular platelets with or without circulating blasts. In the bone marrow, multilineage dysplasia is frequent, seen in more than half of cases. Megakaryocytes are normal to slightly increased in numbers. Dysplastic megakaryocytes are the most

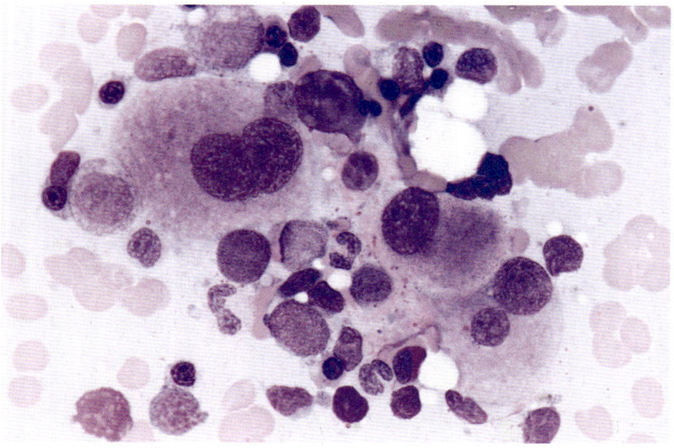

FIGURE 27.1 A bone marrow aspirate smear showing increased blasts and characteristic dysplastic small megakaryocytes with nonlobated and bilobated nuclei. (1000×, Wright-Giemsa).

frequent and have characteristic morphologic features (present in >80% of cases)[2,8] with small forms with nonlobated or bilobated nuclei (Figures 27.1 and 27.2). Immunohistochemistry for megakaryocytes such as CD41, CD42b, CD61, CD62P, and factor VIII-related antigen may further highlight the small dysplastic forms. Other dysplastic megakaryocytic features may include widely separated, small nuclei or micromegakaryocytes. Dyserythropoiesis (irregular nuclear contours, budding nuclei, multinucleation, megaloblastoid change, or ring sideroblasts) and dysgranulopoiesis (hyposegmented or hypersegmented forms, pseudo-Pelger-Huet nuclear abnormalities, cytoplasmic hypogranulation, or abnormal granules) are also common (46% and 32% of AML cases, respectively)[2,9] (Figure 27.3). There is variable bone marrow cellularity and reticulin fibrosis.[6]

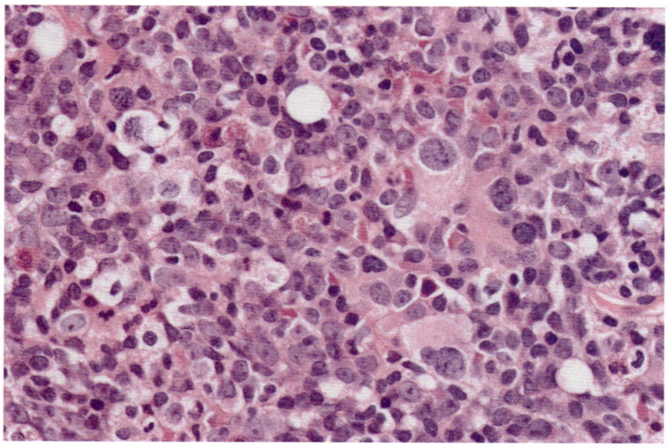

FIGURE 27.2 A bone marrow core biopsy showing hypercellularity with increased blasts and dysplastic small, hypolobated megakaryocytes. (500×, H&E).

Immunophenotype

The blasts typically express myeloid antigens including CD13, CD15, CD33, CD34, CD38, CD117, myeloperoxidase (subset), and HLA-DR. Aberrant expression of CD56 or CD7 is frequent. Megakaryocytic markers such as CD41 and CD61 can be used to identify megakaryocytic differentiation, seen in a subset of cases.

Genetics

Cytogenetic analysis with conventional karyotype is the gold standard for diagnosis of AML with inv(3)/t(3;3) with the majority of patients showing inv(3)(q21.3q26.2) (58%-81%).[1,10] Fluorescence in situ hybridization (FISH) can be confirmatory for *MECOM* rearrangement and has good sensitivity and specificity with the ability to detect a wide range of breakpoints, including cytogenetically cryptic rearrangements.[7] Single nucleotide polymorphism microarrays and comparative genomic hybridization may be complementary.

In contrast to many oncogenic rearrangements, inv(3)/t(3;3) does not result in a fusion transcript. Instead, the rearrangement results in enhancer hijacking by placing the distal *GATA2* enhancer from 3q21.3 in the proximity of the promoter of *EVI1,* resulting in overexpression of the *MECOM* isoform of *EVI1*, loss of expression of *MDS1-EVI1* transcripts from the alternative *MECOM* promoter, and haploinsufficiency of *GATA2.*[11,12] Aberrant expression of *EVI1* is noted in almost all AML cases with inv3/t(3;3) and in 5% to 10% of other newly diagnosed AML subsets. *EVI1* expression is implicated in the pathogenesis of AML with effects on hematopoietic stem cell self-renewal, impairment of differentiation in erythroid and myeloid cells, and multilineage dysplasia. Disruption of normal *GATA2* expression is also likely contributory to leukemogenesis as it is a transcription factor essential for normal hematopoietic development, with haploinsufficiency associated with range of cytopenias and germline predisposition to myeloid disorders including MDS and AML.[3,11] Overall, AML with inv(3)/t(3;3) appears to result from a global distortion of hematopoiesis.

Additional cytogenetic abnormalities are common (55%-75% of cases), with increased frequency at relapse (82%) and with acquisition of additional abnormalities during disease progression (37%).[1,2] A complex karyotype is reported in 18% to 25% of newly diagnosed cases[1,2,6,7] and 35% of recurrent/refractory cases.[1] Monosomy 7 is the most frequent concurrent abnormality (40%-76% of cases) with other

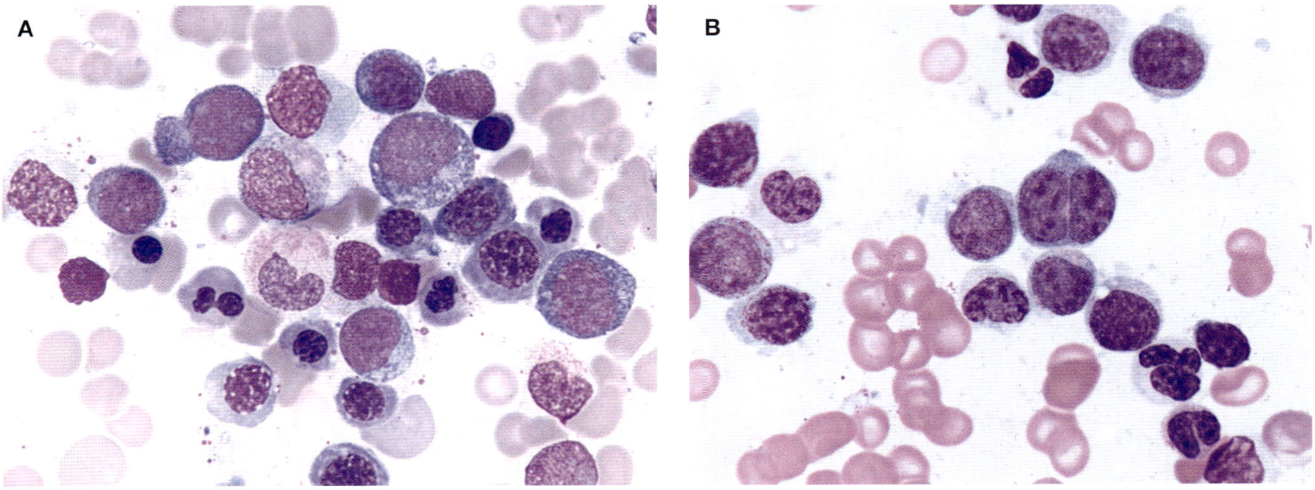

FIGURE 27.3 **A** and **B:** Bone marrow aspirate smears showing increased blasts and dysplastic erythroid precursors **(A)** and dysplastic granulocytes **(B)**. (1000×, Wright-Giemsa).

cytogenetic abnormalities including del(7q) in 3% to 11% of cases and del(5q) in 6% to 16% of cases.[1,2,5-7,9] A subset of cases of de novo AML with inv(3)/t(3;3) have been reported to show concurrent or subclonal t(9;22)/*BCR::ABL1* rearrangements.[2] Acquisition of inv(3)/t(3;3) in *BCR::ABL1*-positive chronic myeloid leukemia cases in transformation to blast phase is also reported.[12] They appear to show a similar mutational and gene expression profile as compared with other AML with inv(3)/t(3;3), although the data for these cases are limited.[12]

Concurrent mutations frequently involve the RAS-MAPK signaling pathway (71%-98% of cases) with mutations in *NRAS* (24%-28%), *KRAS* (11%-14%), *PTPN11* (20%-27%), *NF1* (4%-9%), and *CBL* (2%-9%) described.[1,5,6,12] Other recurrent mutations have been identified in splicing factors (*SF3B1* [most common], *ZRSR2, SRSF2, PRPF8, PHF6,*[5] and *U2AF1*), transcription factors (*GATA2, RUNX1, ETV6, CEBPA*, and *FOXP1*), and factors involved in DNA methylation and chromatin remodeling (*DNMT3A, IDH1, IDH2, TET2, ASXL1, NCOR, BCOR*, and *NPM1*).[1,5,9,12] *FLT3*-ITD and *FLT3*-TKD mutations are found in a subset, 13% and 7% of patients, respectively.[6,12] Mutations in tumor suppressor genes (*TP53, WT1*) are reported, but cases with *TP53* mutations appear to comprise a minor subset (5%-10%).[9,10,12] *NRAS* and *KRAS* mutations have been associated with higher leukocyte and peripheral blood blast counts, respectively.[1] *ASXL1* mutation may independently associate with poor overall survival, and *NRAS* and *ASXL1* mutations have been associated with secondary AML with inv(3)/t(3;3).[1] Concurrent *NPM1* mutations appear rare, but the presence of inv(3)/t(3;3) would take precedence for diagnostic categorization.[3]

Prognosis and Clinical Comment

AML with inv(3)/t(3;3) is associated with a very poor outcome, both after high-intensity and lower-intensity regimens.[1,5,6,8,13] The outcomes are similarly poor for patients regardless of the blast count.[2] Secondary cytogenetic abnormalities such as complex karyotype and monosomy 7 appear to be associated with an even worse outcome.[2,6,8] Remissions are achieved in 30% to 50%, both after intensive chemotherapy and hypomethylating agent-based therapy; however, remissions are very short-lived. Median overall survival times are between 6 and 10 months.[1,5,6] Allogeneic hematopoietic cell transplantation (HCT) currently is the only potentially curative treatment option for patients with inv(3)/t(3;3); however, outcome after allogeneic HCT also remains poor, with only about 25% of patients achieving long-term remission.[1,14] Achievement of a complete remission prior to allogeneic HCT is a major determinant of outcome after transplantation. In the 2022 AML European LeukemiaNet genetic risk classification, AML with inv(3)/t(3;3) as well as AML with other *MECOM* rearrangements are categorized in the adverse-risk group.[4]

AML With Other *MECOM* Rearrangements

Balanced translocations involving 3q26.2 with more than 30 partner genes have been reported with some being cytogenetically cryptic.[9] Additional 3q26.2 rearrangements recognized as recurrent genetic events diagnostic of AML in the setting of ≥10% peripheral blood or bone marrow blasts include the following[3,4]: t(2;3)(p11~23;q26.2)/*MECOM::?*; t(3;8)(q26.2;q24.2)/

MYC, *MECOM*; t(3;12)(q26.2;p13.2)/*ETV6*::*MECOM*; t(3;21)(q26.2;q22.1)/*MECOM*::*RUNX1*.

Similar to AML with inv(3)/t(3;3), patients typically present at a relatively younger age compared with overall AML without sex predilection.[9] Morphologic features, including prominent dysplasia and blast phenotype, do not differ significantly from AML with inv(3)/t(3;3).[9,11] However, median platelet count and white blood cell count at presentation may be slightly lower with median platelets of 55 × 10^9/L compared with 144 × 10^9/L in AML with inv(3)/t(3;3) in one series.[6] The genetic landscape also appears similar with frequent monosomy 7 (31%) or loss of 7q, complex karyotype (21%-43%), and mutations in the RAS-MAPK pathway and splicing complex genes.[6,9] Rearrangement involving the *MECOM* locus in cytogenetically cryptic cases can be detected and followed by FISH analysis or by molecular methods.

While not specific, increased *EVI1* expression is also seen in the majority of AML with 3q26.2 abnormalities due to rearrangement often involving superenhancers of genes important in myeloid development such as *MYC* and *RUNX1* and is associated with poor therapy response and outcome.[7,11] There is also loss or absence of normal *MDS1-EVI1* transcripts.[11] Dysregulation of *EVI1* appears to be the primary driving event of leukemogenesis,[2,6] but altered *GATA2* expression with allelic loss or skewed expression at this locus has also been observed in many of these cases, even though the distal *GATA2* enhancer at 3q21 is not directly involved in the rearrangement.[11] Data on AML with *MECOM* rearrangements other than the classical inv(3)/t(3;3) are scarce. One study showed that AML with other *MECOM* rearrangements may have a somewhat better outcome, but they are still associated with poor outcome.[6]

References

1. Richard-Carpentier G, Rausch CR, Sasaki K, et al. Characteristics and clinical outcomes of patients with acute myeloid leukemia with inv(3)(q21q26.2) or t(3;3)(q21;q26.2). *Haematologica*. 2023;108(9):2331-2342.
2. Rogers HJ, Vardiman JW, Anastasi J, et al. Complex or monosomal karyotype and not blast percentage is associated with poor survival in acute myeloid leukemia and myelodysplastic syndrome patients with inv(3)(q21q26.2)/t(3;3)(q21;q26.2): a Bone Marrow Pathology Group study. *Haematologica*. 2014;99(5):821-829.
3. Arber DA, Orazi A, Hasserjian RP, et al. International consensus classification of myeloid neoplasms and acute leukemias: integrating morphologic, clinical, and genomic data. *Blood*. 2022;140(11):1200-1228.
4. Dohner H, Wei AH, Appelbaum FR, et al. Diagnosis and management of AML in adults: 2022 recommendations from an international expert panel on behalf of the ELN. *Blood*. 2022;140(12):1345-1377.
5. Papaemmanuil E, Gerstung M, Bullinger L, et al. Genomic classification and prognosis in acute myeloid leukemia. *N Engl J Med*. 2016;374(23):2209-2221.
6. Lugthart S, Groschel S, Beverloo HB, et al. Clinical, molecular, and prognostic significance of WHO type inv(3)(q21q26.2)/t(3;3)(q21;q26.2) and various other 3q abnormalities in acute myeloid leukemia. *J Clin Oncol*. 2010;28(24):3890-3898.
7. Baldazzi C, Luatti S, Zuffa E, et al. Complex chromosomal rearrangements leading to MECOM overexpression are recurrent in myeloid malignancies with various 3q abnormalities. *Genes Chromosomes Cancer*. 2016;55(4):375-388.
8. Sitges M, Boluda B, Garrido A, et al. Acute myeloid leukemia with inv(3)(q21.3q26.2)/t(3;3)(q21.3;q26.2): study of 61 patients treated with intensive protocols. *Eur J Haematol*. 2020;105(2):138-147.
9. Gao J, Gurbuxani S, Zak T, et al. Comparison of myeloid neoplasms with nonclassic 3q26.2/MECOM versus classic inv(3)/t(3;3) rearrangements reveals diverse clinicopathologic features, genetic profiles, and molecular mechanisms of MECOM activation. *Genes Chromosomes Cancer*. 2022;61(2):71-80.
10. Summerer I, Haferlach C, Meggendorfer M, Kern W, Haferlach T, Stengel A. Prognosis of MECOM (EVI1)-rearranged MDS and AML patients rather depends on accompanying molecular mutations than on blast count. *Leuk Lymphoma*. 2020;61(7):1756-1759.
11. Ottema S, Mulet-Lazaro R, Beverloo HB, et al. Atypical 3q26/MECOM rearrangements genocopy inv(3)/t(3;3) in acute myeloid leukemia. *Blood*. 2020;136(2):224-234.
12. Groschel S, Sanders MA, Hoogenboezem R, et al. Mutational spectrum of myeloid malignancies with inv(3)/t(3;3) reveals a predominant involvement of RAS/RTK signaling pathways. *Blood*. 2015;125(1):133-139.
13. Tazi Y, Arango-Ossa JE, Zhou Y, et al. Unified classification and risk-stratification in acute myeloid leukemia. *Nat Commun*. 2022;13(1):4622.
14. Halaburda K, Labopin M, Houhou M, et al. AlloHSCT for inv(3)(q21;q26)/t(3;3)(q21;q26) AML: a report from the acute leukemia working party of the European society for blood and marrow transplantation. *Bone Marrow Transplant*. 2018;53(6):683-691.

Chapter 28

Acute Myeloid Leukemia With Other Rare Recurring Translocations

Jeffery M. Klco and Daniel A. Arber

Definition

Acute myeloid leukemias (AMLs) with other rare recurring translocations encompass a broad range of AML subtypes (Table 28.1) across the age spectrum that lack other defining AML-associated molecular or cytogenetic alterations. These AMLs can be diagnosed with ≥10% blasts and arise de novo or secondary, requiring the appropriate diagnostic qualifiers.

Epidemiology

A common theme of oncogenic fusions in acute leukemias is the deregulation of transcription factors or epigenetic modifiers.[1] These can converge on key pathways that influence hematopoietic cell renewal, such as the HOX gene deregulation that is observed in AMLs with *NUP98* fusions, *PICALM::MLLT10* and *KAT6A::CREBBP*.

General Clinical Features

The molecular subtypes associated with non-Down syndrome megakaryoblastic leukemias, such as *RBM15::MRTFA*, *NUP98::KDM5A*, and *CBFA2T3::GLIS2*, are almost exclusively found in the pediatric age group and typically present with thrombocytopenia.[2] Likewise, *ETV6::MNX1* is also highly enriched in young children.[3] Leukemia cutis, clinical features of hemophagocytosis, and coagulopathies have been reported in patients with AML with *KAT6A::CREBBP*.[4] *KAT6A::CREBBP*, *PRDM16::RPN1*, and *RUNX1::CBFA2T3* AMLs can arise de novo or secondary. Patients with AML with *NUP98::NSD1* commonly present with high white blood cell count.

Morphology

These AMLs can be diagnosed with ≥10% blasts. Depending on the morphologic or clinical associations, the blasts and background hematopoietic elements will have variable morphologies. AMLs associated with megakaryoblastic morphology will have medium to large blasts with basophilic cytoplasm lacking granules that may also have cytoplasmic blebs. Marrow fibrosis is common, which may compromise the ability to effectively sample the bone marrow via aspirate, and bone marrow core biopsy with immunohistochemistry is recommended. Many of the included categories are also associated with morphologic dysplasia and can be observed after cytotoxic treatments and thus require the appropriate qualifier. This includes AMLs with some of the rare *NUP98* fusion partners, *PRDM16::RPN1*, *KAT6A::CREBBP*, and *RUNX1::CBFA2T3*, in adults.[5-7] Overall, *NUP98*-rearranged AMLs have variable morphology depending on the fusion partner. *NUP98::KDM5A* AMLs are predominantly megakaryoblastic or erythroblastic, but monocytic AMLs have also been reported.[8,9] AMLs with *NUP98::NSD1* are myelomonocytic or monocytic/monoblastic. Notably, NUP98 leukemias can also present as T lymphoblastic leukemia/lymphoma, with *RAP1GDS1* being a common fusion partner; this is also true for *PICALM::MLLT10* leukemias. *KAT6A::CREBBP* AMLs commonly have a monocytic morphology and can also present with hemophagocytosis.

Immunophenotype

Megakaryoblastic leukemias express platelet glycoproteins, such as CD42b, CD41, or CD61. Detection by flow cytometry can be challenging due to high background, and intracellular staining can be beneficial. Immunohistochemistry for CD42b is useful in a bone marrow core biopsy, especially for fibrotic samples with poor aspirates. In general, megakaryoblasts are commonly negative for CD34, CD45, and myeloperoxidase but may be positive for other myeloid markers, such as CD13 or CD33. *CBFA2T3::GLIS2* AMLs typically have the RAM phenotype, characterized by CD56 expression and a lack of HLA-DR, decreased CD38, and dim to negative CD45 expression. Leukemias with monocytic

TABLE 28.1 Categories of AML with other rare recurring translocations

Translocation	Age	Unique pathologic or clinical features	Known cooperating mutations	Cytogenetics
AML with t(1;3)(p36.3;q21.3)/*PRDM16::RPN1*	Older adults	Can occur after MDS or therapy with variable morphologies	None	Commonly is the sole abnormality detected by cytogenetics
AML with t(3;5)(q25.3;q35.1)/*NPM1::MLF1*	Variable, with peak incidence in 4th decade of life	None, but may occur after MDS	None	Commonly is the sole abnormality detected by cytogenetics
AML with t(8;16)(p11.2;p13.3)/*KAT6A::CREBBP*	Variable	Commonly monocytic with hemophagocytosis; congenital cases can resolve spontaneously	None	Detected by conventional cytogenetics; can be complex
AML (megakaryoblastic) with t(1;22)(p13.3;q13.1)/*RBM15::MRTFA*	Infants	Megakaryoblastic with marrow fibrosis	None	Commonly is the sole abnormality detected by cytogenetics
AML with t(5;11)(q35.2;p15.4)/*NUP98::NSD1*	Children	Myelomonocytic or monocytic; commonly with high WBC count	*FLT3*-ITD and *WT1*	Commonly cryptic
AML with t(11;12)(p15.4;p13.3)/*NUP98::KDM5A*	Infants	Typically megakaryoblastic or erythroblastic, but monocytic differentiation has also been reported	*RB1* loss	Commonly cryptic
AML with *NUP98* and other partners	Children	Variable features	Variable	Commonly cryptic
AML with t(7;12)(q36.3;p13.2)/*ETV6::MNX1*	Infants	Variety of morphologies are observed, including megakaryoblastic	None	Commonly cryptic; +19 is a common secondary event
AML with t(10;11)(p12.3;q14.2)/*PICALM::MLLT10*	Variable	Can also present as T-ALL	*PHF6* and *TP53*	Detected by conventional cytogenetics
AML with t(16;21)(p11.2;q22.2)/*FUS::ERG*	Variable	Variable	None	Complex cytogenetics can also be observed. Fusion is sometimes cryptic.
AML with t(16;21)(q24.3;q22.1)/*RUNX1::CBFA2T3*	Variable	Can occur after therapy	None	Additional cytogenetic alterations are noted, including +8 or complex cytogenetics
AML with inv(16)(p13.3q24.3)/*CBFA2T3::GLIS2*	Infants	Megakaryoblastic, commonly with RAM immunophenotype	Rare	Cryptic

AML, acute myeloid leukemia; MDS, myelodysplastic syndrome; WBC, white blood cell.

morphology, such as those with *KAT6A::CREBBP*, express characteristic markers (CD33, CD13, CD4, CD15, and HLA-DR) and typically lack CD34 or CD117. Consistent unique immunophenotypic changes are not routinely observed for *FUS::ERG*, *NPM1::MLF1*, *PRDM16::RPN1*, or *RUNX1::CBFA2T3* AMLs, but many of these fusions are rare.

Genetics

Over 40 different fusion partners have been described for NUP98 leukemias, with *NUP98::NSD1* being the most common. These AMLs are frequently associated with *FLT3*-ITD and *WT1* mutations and typically have normal karyotype or trisomy 8. In contrast, *NUP98::KDM5A* AMLs commonly have loss of *RB1* or chromosome 13 structural variations. A variety of other recurrent alterations are observed in the other NUP98 rearranged leukemias.[8,9] Trisomy 19, which is overall rare in AML, is enriched in *ETV6::MNX1* cases.[3] Not all t(7;12) cases have a defined chimeric *ETV6::MNX1* fusion detected as some of the breakpoints include regulatory elements of *ETV6*. Similarly, regulatory elements adjacent to *RPN1* enhance expression of *PRDM16* in the t(1;3)(p36.3;q21.3). Other partners with *PRDM16* have also been described, including *ETV6*.[6] *CCDC28A* and *SETBP1* fusions to *NPM1* have also been reported, which likely have similar overall clinicopathologic features to *NPM1::MLF1* AML.[10,11] Likewise, *RUNX1::CBFA2T2* fusions have also been identified, which are presumably similar to *RUNX1::CBFA2T3* fusions.

Prognosis and Clinical Comment

With the exception of *RBM15::MRTFA*, AMLs with megakaryoblastic features typically have an inferior outcome. This is especially true for *CBFA2T3::GLIS2* AML, although recently these patients have been found to be responsive to FOLR1 inhibitors.[12] Spontaneous remission in congenital AMLs with *KAT6A::CREBBP* has been observed but is inconsistent.[4] *NUP98* fusions and potentially other fusions that result in similar expression profiles potentially respond to menin inhibitors. Patients with AML with *RUNX1::CBFA2T3* have similar outcomes to other core-binding factor AMLs. *FUS::ERG* and *PRDM16* fusions are associated with inferior outcome.

References

1. Umeda M, Ma J, Westover T, et al. A new genomic framework to categorize pediatric acute myeloid leukemia. *Nat Genet*. (2024);56(2):281-293.
2. de Rooij JD, Branstetter C, Ma J, et al. Pediatric non-Down syndrome acute megakaryoblastic leukemia is characterized by distinct genomic subsets with varying outcomes. *Nat Genet*. 2017;49(3):451-456. doi:10.1038/ng.3772
3. Espersen ADL, Noren-Nystrom U, Abrahamsson J, et al. Acute myeloid leukemia (AML) with t(7;12)(q36;p13) is associated with infancy and trisomy 19: data from Nordic Society for Pediatric Hematology and Oncology (NOPHO-AML) and review of the literature. *Genes Chromosomes Cancer*. 2018;57(7):359-365. doi:10.1002/gcc.22538
4. Coenen EA, Zwaan CM, Reinhardt D, et al. Pediatric acute myeloid leukemia with t(8;16)(p11;p13), a distinct clinical and biological entity: a collaborative study by the International-Berlin-Frankfurt-Munster AML-study group. *Blood*. 2013;122(15):2704-2713. doi:10.1182/blood-2013-02-485524
5. Xie W, Hu S, Xu J, Chen Z, Medeiros LJ, Tang G. Acute myeloid leukemia with t(8;16)(p11.2;p13.3)/KAT6A-CREBBP in adults. *Ann Hematol*. 2019;98(5):1149-1157. doi:10.1007/s00277-019-03637-7
6. Duhoux FP, Ameye G, Montano-Almendras CP, et al. PRDM16 (1p36) translocations define a distinct entity of myeloid malignancies with poor prognosis but may also occur in lymphoid malignancies. *Br J Haematol*. 2012;156(1):76-88. doi: 10.1111/j.1365-2141.2011.08918.x
7. Noort S, Zimmermann M, Reinhardt D, et al. Prognostic impact of t(16;21)(p11;q22) and t(16;21)(q24;q22) in pediatric AML: a retrospective study by the I-BFM Study Group. *Blood*. 2018;132(15):1584-1592. doi:10.1182/blood-2018-05-849059
8. Iacobucci I, Wen J, Meggendorfer M, et al. Genomic subtyping and therapeutic targeting of acute erythroleukemia. *Nat Genet*. 2019;51(4):694-704. doi:10.1038/s41588-019-0375-1
9. Bertrums EJM, Smith JL, Harmon L, et al. Comprehensive molecular and clinical characterization of NUP98 fusions in pediatric acute myeloid leukemia. *Haematologica*. 2023;108(8):2044-2058. doi:10.3324/haematol.2022.281653
10. Martelli MP, Rossi R, Venanzi A, et al. Novel NPM1 exon 5 mutations and gene fusions leading to aberrant cytoplasmic nucleophosmin in AML. *Blood*. 2021;138(25):2696-2701. doi:10.1182/blood.2021012732
11. Raimondi SC, Dube ID, Valentine MB, et al. Clinicopathologic manifestations and breakpoints of the t(3;5) in patients with acute nonlymphocytic leukemia. *Leukemia*. 1989;3(1):42-47.
12. Le Q, Hadland B, Smith JL, et al. CBFA2T3-GLIS2 model of pediatric acute megakaryoblastic leukemia identifies FOLR1 as a CAR T cell target. *J Clin Invest*. 2022;132(22):e157101. doi:10.1172/JCI157101

Chapter 29

Acute Myeloid Leukemia With t(9;22)(q34.1;q11.2)/*BCR::ABL1*

Adam Bagg, Sandeep Gurbuxani, and Selina Luger

Definition

Acute myeloid leukemia (AML) with t(9;22)(q34.1;q11.2)/*BCR::ABL1* is a de novo AML in which patients show no evidence (either before or after therapy) of chronic myeloid leukemia (CML). Cases that meet the criteria for mixed-phenotype acute leukemia are excluded from this category.

Synonyms

Ph+ acute myeloid leukemia (not recommended).

Epidemiology

AML with *BCR::ABL1* accounts for <1% of all AMLs and occurs primarily in adults, with a male predominance.[1,2]

General Clinical Features

Patients most commonly present with leukocytosis with an expansion of blasts and variable presence of anemia and thrombocytopenia. AML with *BCR::ABL1* that is by definition de novo may be difficult to distinguish from CML presenting in myeloid blast transformation. However, a number of variables may help distinguish the two from one another (Table 29.1). From a clinical perspective, as compared with patients with CML in blast phase, those with de novo AML with *BCR::ABL1* are less likely to present with splenomegaly. Medical history of previous leukocytosis suggests underlying CML.

Morphology

The morphological features of AML with *BCR::ABL1* are nonspecific; they demonstrate the presence of bone marrow and peripheral blood myeloblasts, with features ranging from those of minimal differentiation to those of granulocytic maturation. Importantly, unlike all other AMLs with recurrent cytogenetic abnormalities that require only ≥10% blasts, AML with *BCR::ABL1* requires ≥20% blasts to avoid potential overlap with CML in accelerated phase. AML with *BCR::ABL1* may be associated with hemophagocytosis. As compared with patients with CML in blast phase, those with de novo AML with *BCR::ABL1* may show less basophilia (<2%), lower bone marrow cellularity (80% vs 95%-100%), a lower nonblast myeloid:erythroid ratio, fewer "dwarf" megakaryocytes, and no evidence of CML after induction chemotherapy.[1,2]

Immunophenotype

AML with *BCR::ABL1* demonstrates expression of myeloid antigens (CD13 and CD33) and CD34. Aberrant expression of CD19, CD7, and TdT appears to be common, as compared with CML in myeloid blast phase. However, cases meeting the specific criteria for a mixed phenotype should be diagnosed as mixed-phenotype acute leukemia with *BCR::ABL1*.[1,2]

Genetics

All cases demonstrate t(9;22)(q34.1;q11.2) or molecular genetic evidence of *BCR::ABL1* fusion by fluorescence in situ hybridization or reverse transcription polymerase chain reaction. Both e13a2/e14a2 (p210) and e1a2 (p190) fusion transcripts may occur.[3] Patients with CML in blast phase will have the t(9;22)(q34.1;q11.2) in 100% of metaphases while those with AML with Ph chromosome may not. Furthermore, once in remission post induction therapy, persistence of the t(9;22)(q34.1;q11.2) suggests underlying CML. In most cases, cytogenetic abnormalities, such as loss of chromosome 7, gain of chromosome 8, and complex karyotypes, are present in addition to t(9;22)(q34.1;q11.2) but do not help in distinguishing CML in myeloid blast phase from de novo AML with *BCR::ABL1* fusion.[1,2] *RUNX1* appears to be the most commonly mutated gene in AML with *BCR::ABL1*, occurring more frequently in

TABLE 29.1 Features that may help distinguish de novo *BCR::ABL1*+ AML from CML presenting in myeloid blast phase

Feature	Favors de novo *BCR::ABL1*+ AML	Favors CML presenting in myeloid blast phase
Splenomegaly	No	Yes
Basophilia	No	Yes
Increased marrow cellularity	No	Yes
Increased M:E ratio	No	Yes
"Dwarf" megakaryocytes	No	Yes
Evidence of CML after induction	No	Yes
Lymphoid antigens on myeloblasts	Yes	No
<100% t(9;22)-positive metaphases	Yes	No
P190 (e1) breakpoint	Yes	No
NPM1 or *FLT3* mutations	Yes	No
Loss of *IKZF1*, *CDKN2A*, IGH, or TR genes	Yes	No

AML, acute myeloid leukemia; CML, chronic myeloid leukemia; M:E, myeloid:erythroid.

this setting (38%) as compared with AML in general (~10%).[4] However, this heightened frequency is similarly seen in CML in myeloid blast phase. Mutations in *NPM1* and *FLT3* internal tandem duplications (ITDs) are infrequent. However, when present, *NPM1* mutations have been reported more frequently in AML with *BCR::ABL1* and *FLT3*-ITDs and are restricted to AML with *BCR::ABL1*, while not occurring in blast transformation of CML.[1,5] When both an *NPM1* mutation and *BCR::ABL1* are present, the *NPM1* mutation supersedes the *BCR::ABL1* and is considered as a favorable risk category. Loss of *IKZF1* and *CDKN2A* in AML with *BCR::ABL1*, as well as cryptic deletions within the IGH and TRG genes, has been reported in a single older study. These deletions are also reported in B-lymphoblastic leukemia with *BCR::ABL1*, but they do not appear to occur in myeloid blast transformation of CML; if these results are confirmed, such testing may be a useful means of distinguishing between these disorders.[6] Differential expression of *CD25* and *ID4* mRNA might also help to distinguish the two considerations,[7] but this too needs to be validated in larger studies. Late acquisition of a *BCR::ABL1* fusion in a preexisting AML or other hematologic neoplasm has also been reported but is not considered sufficient for a diagnosis of AML with *BCR::ABL1*.[8] This phenomenon also occurs in the setting of patients with *FLT3*-mutated AML who are treated with FLT3 inhibitors, with this fusion (and activating mutations in the RAS signaling pathway) developing as mechanism of resistance to the targeted therapy,[9] and has also been described in the setting of treatment with a BCL2 inhibitor.[10] Notwithstanding the ultimate classification of the AML and the timing of acquisition of the *BCR::ABL1*, therapy targeting the BCR::ABL1 oncoprotein is indicated in cases with this acquired abnormality.

Prognosis and Clinical Comments

AML with *BCR::ABL1* appears to be an aggressive disease, with poor response to traditional AML therapy or tyrosine kinase inhibitor (TKI) therapy alone.[2] This may not be due to *BCR::ABL1* itself but rather from other high-risk genetic abnormalities that are present in most cases.[11] The use of TKIs in combination with standard AML chemotherapy has been shown to be feasible, and improved survival may be obtained with allogeneic hematopoietic cell transplantation (HSCT) in first remission.[12] However, the benefit of TKI + chemotherapy versus TKI or chemotherapy alone is uncertain, and indication for allogeneic HSCT in first CR should be a matter of discussion, particularly in the presence of favorable genetic aberrations and/or the absence of high-risk features.[11]

References

1. Konoplev S, Yin CC, Kornblau SM, et al. Molecular characterization of de novo Philadelphia chromosome-positive acute myeloid leukemia. *Leuk Lymphoma*. 2013;54(1):138-144. doi:10.3109/10428194.2012.701739
2. Soupir CP, Vergilio JA, Dal Cin P, et al. Philadelphia chromosome-positive acute myeloid leukemia: a rare aggressive leukemia with clinicopathologic features distinct from chronic myeloid leukemia in myeloid blast crisis. *Am J Clin Pathol*. 2007;127(4):642-650. doi:10.1309/B4NVER1AJJ84CTUU

3. Piedimonte M, Ottone T, Alfonso V, et al. A rare BCR-ABL1 transcript in Philadelphia-positive acute myeloid leukemia: case report and literature review. *BMC Cancer*. 2019;19:50.
4. Orsmark-Pietras C, Landberg N, Lorenz F, et al. Clinical and genomic characterization of patients diagnosed with the provisional entity acute myeloid leukemia with BCR-ABL1, a Swedish population-based study. *Genes Chromosomes Cancer*. 2021;60(6):426-433. doi:10.1002/gcc.22936
5. Neuendorff NR, Burmeister T, Dörken B, Westermann J. BCR-ABL-positive acute myeloid leukemia: a new entity? Analysis of clinical and molecular features. *Ann Hematol*. 2016;95(8):1211-1221. doi:10.1007/s00277-016-2721-z
6. Nacheva EP, Grace CD, Brazma D, et al. Does BCR/ABL1 positive acute myeloid leukaemia exist? *Br J Haematol*. 2013;161(4):541-550. doi:10.1111/bjh.12301
7. Boucher L, Sorel N, Desterke C, et al. Deciphering potential molecular signatures to differentiate Acute Myeloid Leukemia (AML) with *BCR::ABL1* from Chronic Myeloid Leukemia (CML) in blast crisis. *Int J Mol Sci*. 2023;24(20):15441. doi:10.3390/ijms242015441
8. Kurt H, Zheng L, Kantarjian HM, et al. Secondary Philadelphia chromosome acquired during therapy of acute leukemia and myelodysplastic syndrome. *Mod Pathol*. 2018;31(7):1141-1154. doi:10.1038/s41379-018-0014-x
9. McMahon CM, Ferng T, Canaani J, et al. Clonal selection with RAS pathway activation mediates secondary clinical resistance to selective FLT3 inhibition in acute myeloid leukemia. *Cancer Discov*. 2019;9(8):1050-1063. doi:10.1158/2159-8290.CD-18-1453
10. Adrianzen-Herrera D, Jordan-Bruno X, Devitt KA, Conant JL, Gardner JA. Acquired BCR-ABL1 fusion and IDH1 clonal evolution following BCL2 inhibitor treatment in refractory acute myeloid leukemia. *Leuk Res*. 2021;100:106494. doi:10.1016/j.leukres.2020.106494
11. Neuendorff NR, Hemmati P, Arnold R, et al. BCR-ABL+ acute myeloid leukemia: are we always dealing with a high-risk disease? *Blood Adv*. 2018;2(12):1409-1411. doi:10.1182/bloodadvances.2018015594
12. Cai W, He X, Chen S, et al. Clinical and laboratory characteristics of 12 Ph/BCR-ABL positive acute myeloid leukemia patients. *Zhonghua Xue Ye Xue Za Zhi*. 2015;36(5):398-402. doi:10.3760/cma.j.issn.0253-2727.2015.05.010

Chapter 30

Acute Myeloid Leukemia With Mutated *NPM1*

Sanjay S. Patel, Andrew H. Wei, and Olga K. Weinberg

Definition

Acute myeloid leukemia (AML) with mutated *NPM1* is most frequently associated with a 4-bp frameshift insertion in exon 12. This results in loss of W288 and W290 (or W290 alone) and acquisition of a new C-terminal nuclear export signal (NES). The net effect is aberrant localization of cytoplasmic (mutant), rather than nucleolar (wild-type), NPM1.[1] A blast count of ≥10% in either peripheral blood or bone marrow is required to establish the diagnosis. This AML subtype is often associated with myelomonocytic or monocytic features, a normal karyotype, and favorable prognosis in the absence of concomitant adverse-risk cytogenetic lesions.

Synonyms

Acute myeloid leukemia with cytoplasmic nucleophosmin (not recommended).

Epidemiology

NPM1 mutation is one of the most common recurrent somatic lesions in AML. Mutations in *NPM1* are relatively specific for AML, found in approximately 30% of all cases (60% with a normal karyotype). *NPM1* mutation is less common in children, comprising 6% of pediatric AML cases.[2]

General Clinical Features

AML with mutated *NPM1* is more common in females and may present with an elevated white blood cell count, especially if *FLT3*-ITD is also present. Most cases are de novo, with a prior history of myelodysplastic syndrome (~7%) or prior cytotoxic therapy (~1%) uncommon.[3] Features of disseminated intravascular coagulation may be present at diagnosis, reminiscent of acute promyelocytic leukemia. Although *NPM1* mutation is rarely identified among patients with myeloid neoplasia and <20% blasts, such cases likely represent AML with mutated *NPM1* in evolution.[4]

Morphology

The morphology of AML with mutated *NPM1* is most commonly monocytic or myelomonocytic (Figure 30.1). *NPM1* mutation is associated with the presence of "cup-shaped" blasts characterized by peripheral nuclear invaginations/depressions (Figure 30.1). Multilineage dysplasia is present in approximately 25% cases but lacks prognostic significance.

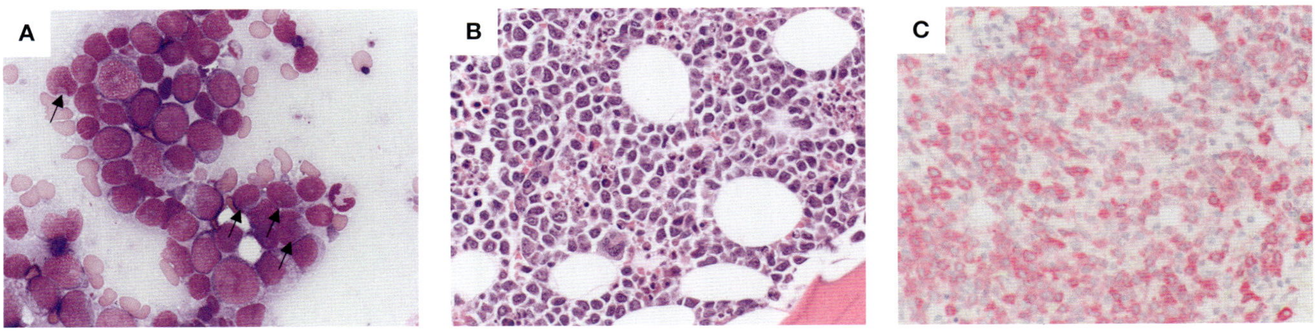

FIGURE 30.1 Representative morphology and immunohistochemistry findings in a patient with acute myeloid leukemia with mutated *NPM1*. **A:** Bone marrow aspirate smear shows numerous myeloid blasts with "cup-like" nuclear invaginations (arrows) (Wright-Giemsa, 1000×). **B:** Bone marrow biopsy shows replacement by myeloid blasts with monocytoid features; rare megakaryocytes and erythroid progenitors are also present (hematoxylin-eosin, 600×). **C:** Leukemic cells show cytoplasmic expression of mutant NPM1 protein (NPM1c) (fast red, antibody clone: PA1-46356 [ThermoFisher], 600×).

Immunophenotype

AML with mutated *NPM1* is frequently positive for KIT (CD117), CD33 (high), CD13 (often low), and CD123, with absence of CD34 and/or HLA-DR.[5] A small population of *NPM1*-mutated cells with a leukemic stem cell phenotype ($CD34^+$, $CD38^-$, $CD123^+$) may be present.[6] In addition to CD34/HLA-DR-negative cases, two other major phenotypic groups have been identified: one exhibiting an immature myeloid phenotypic and another with monocytic antigen expression (eg, CD14, CD36, CD64).[5,7,8] Immunohistochemical (IHC) detection of cytoplasmic NPM1 may be used as a surrogate for *NPM1* mutation in cases of extramedullary AML (myeloid sarcoma), most commonly involving the skin, gingiva, or lymph nodes if mutation analysis is not feasible (Figure 30.1).[1] IHC detection of cytoplasmic NPM1 may also play a role in identifying rare exon 5, 9, or 11 variants linked to generation of novel NES sequences.[9]

Genetics

Approximately 80% of AML cases with mutated *NPM1* have normal karyotype; abnormal karyotypes in the remaining cases are predominantly associated with intermediate risk. Common chromosomal abnormalities include trisomy 8 and/or del(9q), which, although commonly associated with myelodysplasia, do not alter classification or prognosis in this context. *NPM1* mutations are usually mutually exclusive with recurrent AML-defining cytogenetic abnormalities (eg, t(8;21), inv(16)/t(16;16), t(15;17)). Rare co-occurrence of *NPM1* mutation and t(9;22) associated with chronic myeloid leukemia (CML) has been described; the diagnosis of AML with mutated *NPM1* should be retained in the absence of evidence of CML.

Prognosis and Clinical Comment

The European LeukemiaNet 2022 classification categorizes AML with mutated *NPM1* treated with intensive chemotherapy in the absence of concomitant *FLT3*-ITD as clinically favorable, whereas concomitant presence of *FLT3*-ITD is associated with intermediate risk.[10] Copresence of poor-risk karyotypic abnormalities results in adverse prognosis.[10] Other co-occurring gene variants reported to have a modifying effect on *NPM1*-mutant AML include *NRAS*, *RAD21*, or *FLT3*-TKD, which are reported to enhance prognosis, whereas *NPM1* co-occurring with *WT1* or *FLT3*-ITD

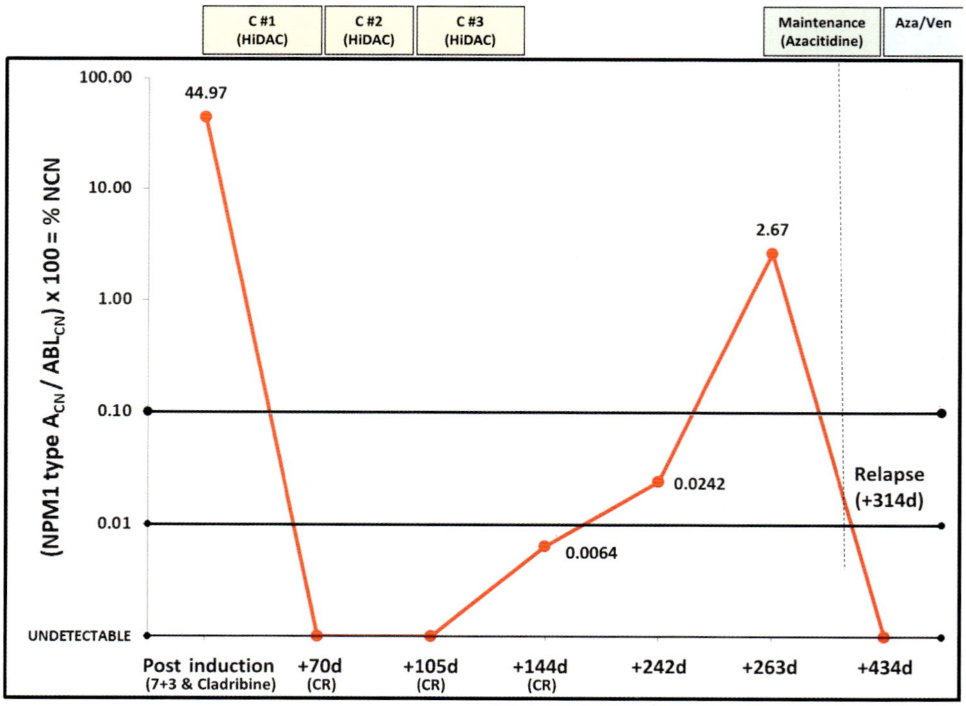

FIGURE 30.2 Longitudinal assessment for minimal/measurable residual disease (MRD) in a patient with acute myeloid leukemia with mutated *NPM1* using RT-qPCR detection of type A mutant transcript in bone marrow samples. Serial measurement showed MRD post-induction chemotherapy with 7 + 3 and cladribine (NCN 44.97%) followed by an initial period of molecular remission during high-dose Ara-C (HiDAC) consolidative therapy. Subsequent measurements showed a rising transcript level (beginning at day 144 post induction, NCN 0.0064%, then NCN 2.67% at day 263); maintenance therapy with azacitidine was initiated but discontinued given persistent increase in transcript levels on peripheral blood testing. Eventual overt relapse was documented on bone marrow evaluation at day 314 post induction but followed by molecular remission status-post additional therapy with decitabine and venetoclax.

plus *DNMT3A* mutations is associated with adverse outcomes.[11] In contrast, secondary-type AML mutations do not appear to negatively impact the prognosis of *NPM1*-mutated AML.[12]

Detection of minimal/measurable residual disease (MRD) following intensive chemotherapy by reverse transcriptase quantitative polymerase chain reaction (RT-qPCR) has been shown to be a powerful independent prognostic indicator for inferior outcome.[13] *NPM1* mutation is recurrent in 91% of cases at relapse, making it a stable marker of MRD after intensive chemotherapy.[14] Persistence of *NPM1*-mutant MRD by RT-qPCR is associated with increased risk of relapse after intensive chemotherapy and has greater prognostic relevance than baseline genetic risk profiling.[13] Guidelines for monitoring *NPM1*-mutant MRD have been updated by the European LeukemiaNet in 2021 and provide a structured approach for early detection of AML relapse.[15] The most common *NPM1* mutation (type A) accounts for 74% of possible *NPM1* variants, followed by type B (6%) and D (9%).[13] It should be noted, however, that low-level *NPM1* MRD persistence may spontaneously resolve in remission.[16] High levels of MRD are strongly associated with increased relapse risk, particularly in patients known to be *FLT3*-ITD positive at diagnosis.[16] Serial monitoring of *NPM1*-mutant MRD may identify patients with rising MRD (≥1-log interval increase) at high risk of imminent clinical relapse who may be candidates for preemptive intervention (Figure 30.2).

References

1. Falini B, Mecucci C, Tiacci E, et al. Cytoplasmic nucleophosmin in acute myelogenous leukemia with a normal karyotype. *N Engl J Med.* 2005;352(3):254-266.
2. Mullighan C, Kennedy A, Zhou X, et al. Pediatric acute myeloid leukemia with NPM1 mutations is characterized by a gene expression profile with dysregulated HOX gene expression distinct from MLL-rearranged leukemias. *Leukemia.* 2007;21(9):2000-2009.
3. Thiede C, Koch S, Creutzig E, et al. Prevalence and prognostic impact of NPM1 mutations in 1485 adult patients with acute myeloid leukemia (AML). *Blood.* 2006;107(10):4011-4020.
4. Patel SS, Ho C, Ptashkin RN, et al. Clinicopathologic and genetic characterization of nonacute NPM1-mutated myeloid neoplasms. *Blood Adv.* 2019;3(9):1540-1545.
5. Liu Y-R, Zhu H-H, Ruan G-R, et al. NPM1-mutated acute myeloid leukemia of monocytic or myeloid origin exhibit distinct immunophenotypes. *Leuk Res.* 2013;37(7):737-741.
6. Martelli MP, Pettirossi V, Thiede C, et al. CD34+ cells from AML with mutated NPM1 harbor cytoplasmic mutated nucleophosmin and generate leukemia in immunocompromised mice. *Blood.* 2010;116(19):3907-3922.
7. Mason EF, Kuo FC, Hasserjian RP, Seegmiller AC, Pozdnyakova O. A distinct immunophenotype identifies a subset of NPM1-mutated AML with TET2 or IDH1/2 mutations and improved outcome. *Am J Hematol.* 2018;93(4):504-510.
8. Perriello VM, Gionfriddo I, Rossi R, et al. CD123 is consistently expressed on NPM1-mutated AML cells. *Cancers.* 2021;13(3):496.
9. Martelli MP, Rossi R, Venanzi A, et al. Novel NPM1 exon 5 mutations and gene fusions leading to aberrant cytoplasmic nucleophosmin in AML. *Blood.* 2021;138(25):2696-2701.
10. Döhner H, Wei AH, Appelbaum FR, et al. Diagnosis and management of AML in adults: 2022 recommendations from an international expert panel on behalf of the ELN. *Blood.* 2022;140(12):1345-1377.
11. Papaemmanuil E, Gerstung M, Bullinger L, et al. Genomic classification and prognosis in acute myeloid leukemia. *N Engl J Med.* 2016;374(23):2209-2221.
12. Eckardt J-N, Bill M, Rausch C, et al. Secondary-type mutations do not impact outcome in NPM1-mutated acute myeloid leukemia–implications for the European leukemia net risk classification. *Leukemia.* 2023;37:1-4.
13. Ivey A, Hills RK, Simpson MA, et al. Assessment of minimal residual disease in standard-risk AML. *N Engl J Med.* 2016;374(5):422-433.
14. Krönke J, Bullinger L, Teleanu V, et al. Clonal evolution in relapsed NPM1-mutated acute myeloid leukemia. *Blood.* 2013;122(1):100-108.
15. Heuser M, Freeman SD, Ossenkoppele GJ, et al. 2021 Update on MRD in acute myeloid leukemia: a consensus document from the European LeukemiaNet MRD Working Party. *Blood.* 2021;138(26):2753-2767.
16. Tiong IS, Dillon R, Ivey A, et al. Clinical impact of NPM1-mutant molecular persistence after chemotherapy for acute myeloid leukemia. *Blood Adv.* 2021;5(23):5107-5111.

Chapter 31

Acute Myeloid Leukemia With In-Frame bZIP *CEBPA* Mutations

Alexa J. Siddon, Nikolai A. Podoltsev, Jorge Sierra, and Olga K. Weinberg

Definition

Acute myeloid leukemia (AML) with in-frame basic leucine zipper (bZIP) *CEBPA* mutations (*CEBPA*^{bZIP}) is a subgroup of AML with recurrent genetic abnormalities. It is characterized by presence of ≥10% clonal immature myeloblasts containing at least one pathogenic in-frame mutation in the bZIP region of the *CEBPA* gene (*CEBPA*^{smbZIP}). AML with in-frame *CEBPA*^{smbZIP} has a normal karyotype in 70% of cases.[1]

The prior category of AML with biallelic mutations of *CEBPA* (*CEBPA*^{bi}) has been discontinued as several studies have now shown that it is in fact the presence of a *CEBPA*^{smbZIP} that defines this as a favorable AML category.[1-3]

Synonyms

AML with mutated bZIP *CEBPA* (not recommended).

Epidemiology

About 5% to 15% of pediatric and 7% to 16% of adult patients with AML have in-frame *CEBPA*^{bZIP}. There is a higher incidence of *CEBPA* mutations observed in Asian patients. About one-third to half of *CEBPA* mutations in patients with AML are single (*CEBPA*^{sm}) and others are double, with each mutation affecting a different allele (*CEBPA*^{bi}).[1,3]

In a large retrospective analysis of 4708 patients with newly diagnosed AML,[1] the subgroups of patients with *CEBPA*^{bi} and *CEBPA*^{smbZIP} had best outcomes and were significantly younger (median age of 46 and 50 years, respectively), whereas patients with non-bZIP *CEBPA*^{sm} were significantly older (median age of 63 years) and were more comparable with the wildtype *CEBPA* group. A continuous decrease in prevalence of *CEBPA*^{bi} and *CEBPA*^{smbZIP} was seen with increasing age, whereas the prevalence of non-bZIP *CEBPA*^{sm} increased.

Most patients have somatic *CEBPA* mutations leading to sporadic AML but approximately 10% of patients with *CEBPA*^{bi} have one allele that is inherited or a de novo germline mutation. These patients have a predisposition to acquisition of second cooperating somatic *CEBPA* mutation and early development of AML.[4] This myeloid neoplasm with germline *CEBPA* mutation is classified together with other hematological neoplasms with germline predisposition, which is discussed separately in Chapter 21 (Hematologic Neoplasms with Germline Predisposition).

General Clinical Features

Signs and symptoms of AML with *CEBPA*^{smbZIP} are similar to those of other types of AML; patients often present with bone marrow failure leading to bruising, bleeding, fatigue, and infection. Patients with *CEBPA*^{smbZIP} have clinical presentations similar to those with *CEBPA*^{bi} AML, but with younger age at presentation and higher white cell counts.[1,3]

Morphology

The morphologic features of AML with *CEBPA*^{smbZIP} typically are of AML without maturation or with maturation. Less commonly seen is AML with monocytic or myelomonocytic differentiation. Multilineage dysplasia is frequently seen, most prominent in the granulocyte and megakaryocyte lineages, which does not affect the overall prognosis[5] (Figure 31.1).

The ICC has lowered the minimum blast count for AML with recurrent genetic abnormalities from ≥20% to ≥10% myeloblasts. Therefore, the diagnosis of AML with in-frame *CEBPA*^{smbZIP} can be made with a blast count of at least 10% in blood and/or bone marrow. In patients with <10% blasts and an in-frame *CEBPA*^{smbZIP}, the diagnosis should remain myelodysplastic syndrome until additional data are collected about the clinical behavior and outcomes of this rare occurrence.

Immunophenotype

The myeloblasts in AML with *CEBPA*^{smbZIP} are typically positive by flow cytometry for CD34, CD117, and HLA-DR, with atypical high expression of CD15, CD65, CD64, and MPO. Furthermore, they also frequently express aberrant CD7 and are usually negative for CD56[6] (Figure 31.1).

Genetics

CEBPA is a single-exon, intronless gene that encodes for CCAAT/enhancer-binding protein-α, which is a lineage-specific bZIP transcription factor required to form myeloid progenitors from multipotent hematopoietic stem cells, and is found on chromosome 19.q13.1.[7,8] The *CEBPA* gene contains two transactivation domains (TADs) near the N terminus and an acid-rich DNA-binding domain and leucine zipper dimerization domain at the C terminus, collectively known as bZIP (Figure 31.2).

The mRNA is translated into either a full-length 42-kDA isoform or a truncated 30-kDa isoform. In AML, *CEBPA* mutations are most commonly N-terminal frameshift mutations that result in early truncation of the p42 isoform, with preservation of the p30 isoform. Other *CEBPA* mutations are typically in-frame insertions or deletions (indels) at the bZIP close to the C-terminal region and alter DNA binding and dimerization[9] (Figure 31.3).

The laboratory diagnosis of *CEBPA* mutation can be achieved by various molecular techniques, such as Sanger sequencing, polymerase chain reaction with fragment analysis, and/or next-generation sequencing.

Prognosis and Clinical Comment

Earlier studies have shown that patients with AML and *CEBPA*^{bi} have favorable outcomes with complete remission rates after intensive chemotherapy approaching 90% and very infrequent chemoresistance to induction therapy. Leukemia relapse appears in approximately 30% of cases, and the probability of long-term survival from several series is 60% to 89% with better results in children.[1-3,10,11] In *CEBPA*^{bi} AML the presence of comutations in tyrosine kinase genes such as *FLT3, CSF3R, KIT,* and *JAK3* appear to portend a worse outcome.[12] The postremission treatment in patients with

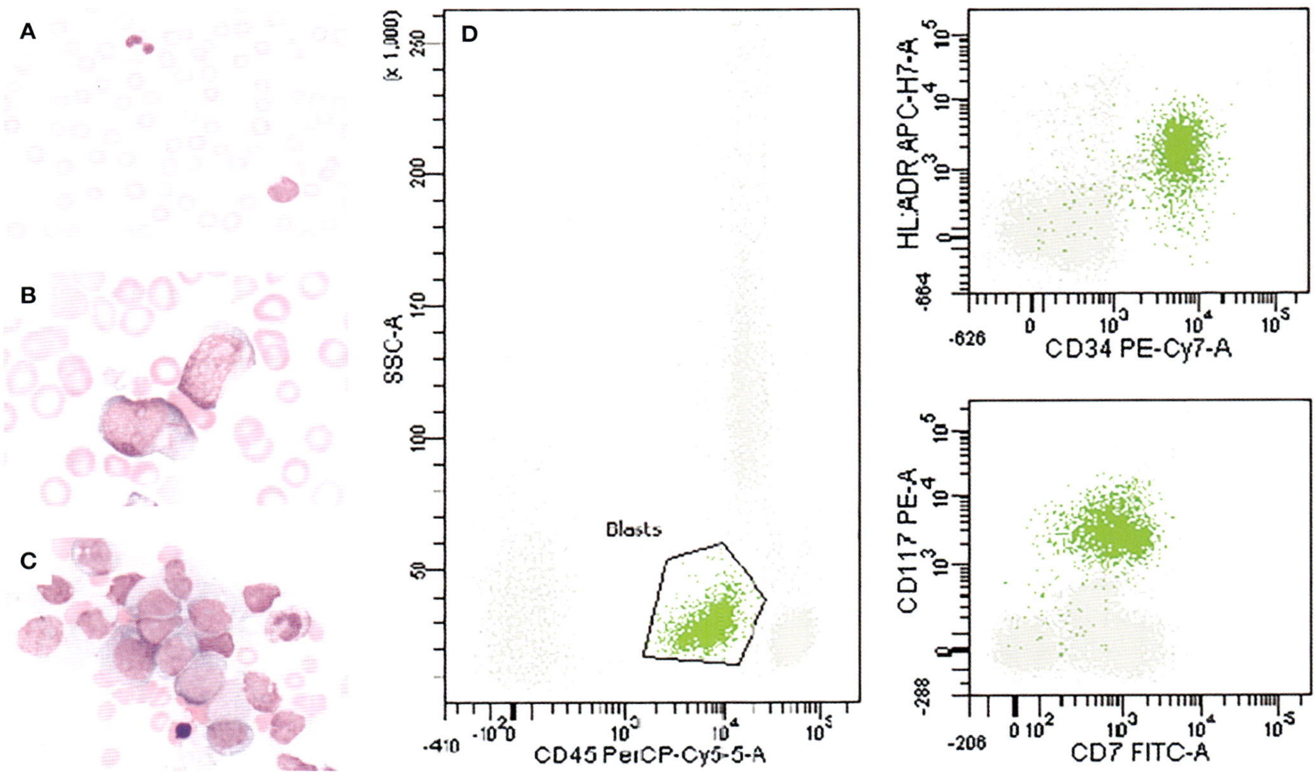

FIGURE 31.1 **A:** Peripheral blood demonstrating a dysplastic (hypogranular, pseudo-Pelger-Huet) granulocyte and a blast. **B** and **C:** Multiple myeloblasts containing Auer rods **(B)** and occasional dysplastic erythroid precursors **(C)**. **D:** Flow cytometry showing blasts (green) that are CD45(dim)+ CD34^{+} CD117^{+} HLADR+ CD7(dim)+.

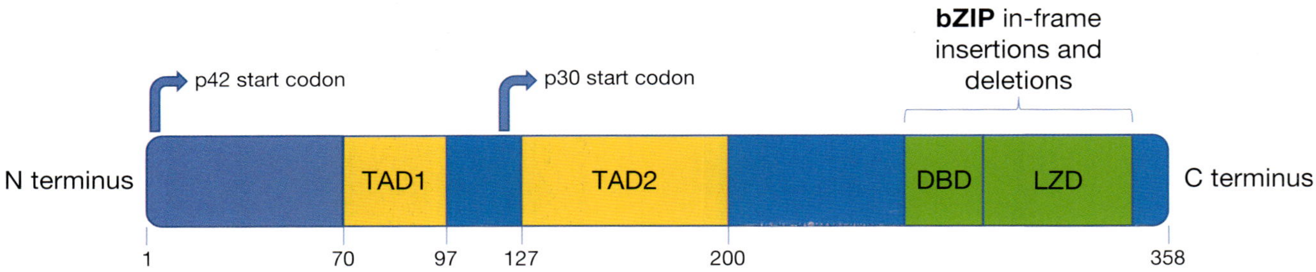

FIGURE 31.2 Schematic of the *CEBPA* gene. The N terminus starts at amino acid 1 and continues to the C terminus, ending at amino acid 358. In-frame bZIP mutations are present at the C-terminal aspect. Abbreviations: DBD, DNA-binding domain; LZD, leucine zipper domain; TAD, transactivation domain.

CEBPA^{bi} AML has typically been with intermediate- or high-dose cytarabine and/or autologous transplantation, avoiding the risk of an allogeneic procedure until relapse. Measurable residual disease studies may help to decide the best timing for allogeneic transplantation in patients in morphological remission, although the techniques need further refinement and standardization.

Until recently, the entire group of patients with AML with *CEBPA*^{sm} were considered to have prognosis comparable with those with wildtype *CEBPA*. However, more recent analyses including adult and pediatric patients with AML[2] indicate that the good prognosis is confined to patients with *CEBPA*^{bZIP} irrespective of their occurrence as single mutation (*CEBPA*^{smbZIP}) or together

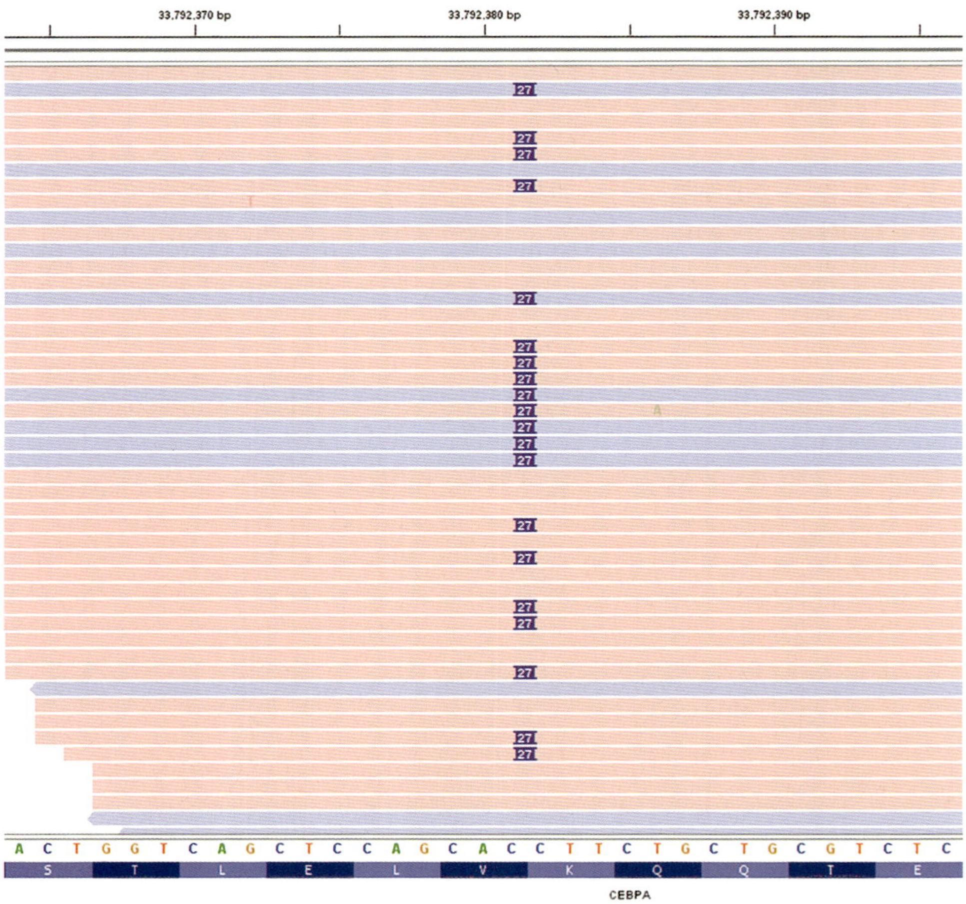

FIGURE 31.3 Example of a bZIP insertion. An integrated genome viewer[15] image of the next-generation sequencing results from DNA of a patient with *CEBPA*^{smbZIP} comprising a 27-base insertion at 34% variant allelic frequency. (Image courtesy of Dr. Karl Hager and Jennifer Adams, Yale New Haven Hospital, CT, USA and Robinson JT, Thorvaldsdóttir H, Winckler W, et al. Integrative genomics viewer. *Nat Biotechnol.* 2011;29(1):24-26.

with other *CEBPA* mutations such as *CEBPA*^{bi}. As AML with *CEBPA*^{bZIP} results in unique gene expression profile, clinical features and favorable biology leading to high complete remission rates, and long median event-free and overall survival, it is recognized as a separate entity (AML with in-frame bZIP *CEBPA* mutations). Other *CEBPA* mutations including the most common involving N-terminal transactivation domains (*CEBPA*^{smTAD}) have not been found to have favorable prognostic impact on AML outcomes when occurring without *CEBPA*^{bZIP}. Approximately 90% of *CEBPA*^{bi} mutant cases carry bZIP in-frame mutations.[1] These data are the basis for the new International Consensus Classification (ICC) category of AML with in-frame *CEBPA*^{bZIP}.

The recent European LeukemiaNet (ELN) guidelines include AML with in-frame *CEBPA*^{bZIP} in the favorable genetic risk.[13] According to these guidelines the coexistence of myelodysplasia-related mutations such as *ASXL1, BCOR, EZH2, RUNX1,SF3B1, SRSF2, STAG2, U2AF1*, and/or *ZRSR2* should not change the allocation of AML with in-frame *CEBPA*^{bZIP} to the favorable category. A recent validation of the ELN 2022 prognostic classification confirms the very good outcome of patients with AML with in-frame *CEBPA*^{bZIP} with an overall survival at 5 years close to 70%.[14]

References

1. Taube F, Georgi JA, Kramer M, et al. CEBPA mutations in 4708 patients with acute myeloid leukemia: differential impact of bZIP and TAD mutations on outcome. *Blood*. 2022;139(1):87-103.
2. Tarlock K, Lamble A, Wang J, et al. CEBPA bZip Mutations are associated with favorable prognosis in de novo AML: a report from the Children's Oncology Group. *Blood*. 2021;138(13):1137-1147.
3. Wakita S, Sakaguchi M, Oh I, et al. Prognostic impact of CEBPA bZIP domain mutation in acute myeloid leukemia. *Blood Adv*. 2022;6(1):238-247.
4. Yuan J, He R, Alkhateeb HB. Sporadic and familial acute myeloid leukemia with CEBPA mutations. *Curr Hematol Malig Rep*. 2023;18(5):121-129.
5. Bacher U, Schnittger S, Macijewski K, et al. Multilineage dysplasia does not influence prognosis in CEBPA-mutated AML, supporting the WHO proposal to classify these patients as a unique entity. *Blood*. 2012;119(20):4719-4722.
6. Mannelli F, Ponziani V, Bencini S, et al. CEBPA–double-mutated acute myeloid leukemia displays a unique phenotypic profile: a reliable screening method and insight into biological features. *Haematologica*. 2017;102(3):529-540.
7. Keeshan K, Santilli G, Corradini F, Perrotti D, Calabretta B. Transcription activation function of C/EBPalpha is required for induction of granulocytic differentiation. *Blood*. 2003;102(4):1267-1275.
8. Schmidt L, Heyes E, Grebien F. Gain-of-function effects of N-terminal CEBPA mutations in acute myeloid leukemia. *Bioessays*. 2020;42(2):e1900178.
9. Grossmann V, Schnittger S, Schindela S, et al. Strategy for robust detection of insertions, deletions, and point mutations in CEBPA, a GC-rich content gene, using 454 next-generation deep-sequencing technology. *J Mol Diagn*. 2011;13(2):129-136.
10. Marcolin R, Guolo F, Minetto P, et al. A simple cytofluorimetric score may optimize testing for biallelic CEBPA mutations in patients with acute myeloid leukemia. *Leuk Res*. 2019;86(June):106223.
11. Ningombam A, Verma D, Kumar R, et al. Prognostic relevance of NPM1, CEBPA, and FLT3 mutations in cytogenetically normal adult AML patients. *Am J Blood Res*. 2023;13(1):28-43.
12. Zhang Y, Wang F, Chen X, et al. Companion gene mutations and their clinical significance in AML with double mutant CEBPA. *Cancer Gene Ther*. 2020;27(7-8):599-606.
13. Dohner H, Wei AH, Appelbaum FR, et al. Diagnosis and management of AML in adults: 2022 recommendations from an international expert panel on behalf of the ELN. *Blood*. 2022;140(12):1345-1377.
14. Huber S, Baer C, Hutter S, et al. AML classification in the year 2023: how to avoid a Babylonian confusion of languages. *Leukemia*. 2023;37(7):1413-1420.
15. Robinson JT, Thorvaldsdóttir H, Winckler W, et al. Integrative genomics viewer. *Nat Biotechnol*. 2011;29(1):24-26.

Chapter 32

Acute Myeloid Leukemia and Myelodysplastic Syndrome/Acute Myeloid Leukemia With Mutated *TP53*

Olga K. Weinberg, Maria Rozman, and Richard M. Stone

Definition

Acute myeloid leukemia (AML) and myelodysplastic syndrome/acute myeloid leukemia (MDS/AML) with mutated *TP53* are considered as a myeloid neoplasm with *TP53* mutation (defined as any somatic *TP53* mutation with a variant allele frequency [VAF] ≥10%). *TP53*-mutated AML is considered a subset of AML with recurrent genetic abnormalities. Diagnosis of AML with *TP53* mutation requires presence of ≥20% marrow and/or peripheral blood blasts and MDS/AML with *TP53* mutation 10% to 19% blasts in marrow or blood. Pure erythroid leukemia, which is highly associated with *TP53* mutations, is now also included under AML with mutated *TP53* and is eliminated as a separate entity when this mutation is present. In cases occurring in the setting of prior chemotherapy "therapy related" should be included as a qualifier statement after the diagnosis.

Synonyms

AML with *TP53* mutation.
MDS/AML with *TP53* mutation.

Epidemiology

TP53 mutations are seen in 5% to 10% of patients with de novo MDS and AML, 25% to 40% of patients with therapy-related MDS and AML, and 50% of patients with AML with a complex karyotype (CK).[1] CKs are usually monosomal and frequently include 5q deletion and 17p deletion, the latter being sometimes difficult to detect in complex cytogenetic rearrangements. *TP53* alterations are associated with older age in AML, occurring in up to 25% of cases in elderly individuals.[1] Although *TP53* mutations occur across many morphological subtypes of AML, they are more frequently seen in pure erythroid leukemia, in therapy-related AML, and in a blast proliferation that has progressed from an underlying myeloproliferative neoplasm or MDS, found in up to a third of cases.[1] In the setting of prior therapy, *TP53* mutations are present in about 30% of patients, while in elderly patients with complex-karyotype AML, *TP53* lesions occur in up to 70% of cases.[2] The higher frequency of *TP53* mutations in therapy-related AML appears to be related to selection/expansion of preexisting chemotherapy-resistant hematopoietic stem cell clones carrying age-related *TP53* mutations rather than direct induction of *TP53* mutation by cytotoxic chemotherapy.[3]

General Clinical Features

TP53 mutations in malignant cells from patients with myeloid neoplasms is more frequently seen in older age, lower blast counts, adverse risk karyotypes, and exposure to antecedent chemotherapy. Mutant *TP53* AML and mutant *TP53* AML/MDS represent a molecular homogeneous group with distinct clinicopathologic characteristics and outcomes that vary little according to marrow blast count at diagnosis.[4] In a recent study of 717 patients with MDS and 734 patients with non-therapy-related AML, AML with mutated *TP53* comprised 52 cases, the majority of which were formerly classified as AML with myelodysplasia-related changes (48/52; 92%).[5] *TP53* germline mutations occur in patients with Li Fraumeni syndrome, an autosomal dominant familial cancer predisposition syndrome that has an 8% risk of MDS and AML.[6] *TP53* mutations are frequently associated with CK, which is present in 10% to 12% of de novo MDS and AML cases and in therapy-related or secondary diseases (25%-40%).[1] Patients with CK and

TP53 mutations, on average, have eight chromosomal aberrations with higher rates of *TP53* deletions when compared with patients with CK and *TP53* wild type.[1]

Morphology

Most cases have morphological evidence of multilineage dysplasia, which must be assessed on well-stained smears of peripheral blood and bone marrow. Dyserythropoiesis is characterized by megaloblastosis, karyorrhexis, and nuclear irregularity, fragmentation, or multinucleation. Ring sideroblasts and cytoplasmic vacuoles are additional features of dyserythropoiesis. Dysmegakaryopoiesis is characterized by micromegakaryocytes and normal-sized or large megakaryocytes with nonlobated or multiple separate nuclei. Dysgranulopoiesis is characterized by neutrophils with hypogranular cytoplasm, hyposegmented nuclei (pseudo-Pelger-Huët), or otherwise abnormally segmented nuclei, but in some cases there is insufficient granulopoiesis to assess for dysplasia.[7] Prior studies found correlation between dysplasia and AML with unfavorable cytogenetic abnormalities.[8] To fulfill pure erythroid leukemia criteria, greater than 80% of bone marrow nucleated elements must correspond to erythroid precursors, predominantly at the pronormoblast stage of maturation (Figure 32.1).

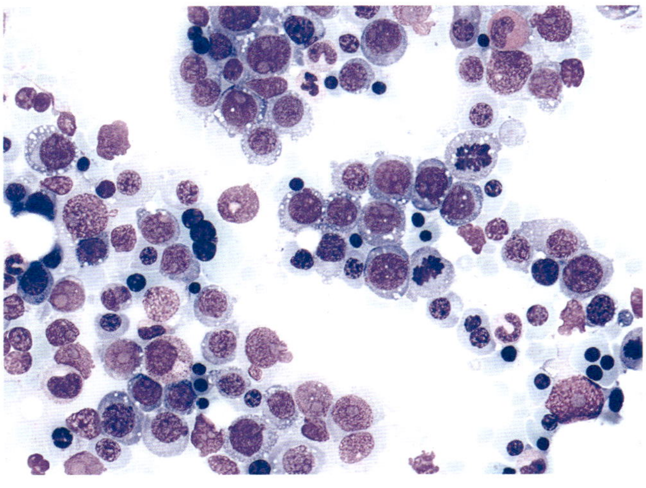

FIGURE 32.1 Acute myeloid leukemia with mutated *TP53* (pure erythroid leukemia type). Hypercellular bone marrow smear showing marked increase of the erythroid precursors, many of them being pronormoblats; severe dyserythropoiesis (cytoplasmic vacuolization, megaloblastosis, multinucleation); and few myeloid blasts.

Immunophenotype

Blast count in AML and MDS/AML with mutated *TP53* should be based on bone marrow aspirate smears but can also be aided by multiparameter flow cytometry or immunohistochemistry. Blasts often express CD34, CD117, and HLA-DR, CD13, CD33, and myeloperoxidase, and aberrancies can often be seen. Maturing monocyte, myeloid, and/or erythroid lineages can also show immunophenotypic aberrations. Small studies demonstrated brighter expression of CD34 with decreased CD33 and aberrant expression of CD5 in blasts of AML with CK, while AML with mutated *TP53* blasts exhibited brighter expression of CD13.[9] In pure erythroid leukemia, a majority of pronormoblasts expressed bright CD36, aberrant CD7, CD13, CD33 (subset), and CD117 and are typically negative for HLA-DR and CD34.[7] Mutant p53 protein expression patterns can also be assessed by immunohistochemistry, and studies suggest that it can correlate with *TP53* mutation and allelic states in patients with AML.[10]

Genetics

The presence of a CK, defined as ≥3 chromosomal abnormalities, comprises 10% to 12% of all patients with AML and constitutes the second largest cytogenetic subset of patients with AML (after those with normal karyotype). CK in both AML and MDS is frequently associated with *TP53* mutations. Assessment of co-occurring gene mutations has identified *TP53*-altered AML to cluster as a unique disease subgroup based on similar natural history despite the presence of other frequent AML-related single-nucleotide mutations such as *TET2, NPM1, FLT3, DNMT3A, IDH1,* and *IDH2*.[11] In contrast, mutations involving signaling pathways (ie, *FLT3, RAS, PTPN11, BCOR, JAK2, NF1*) and polycomb-related genes (ie, *SF3B1, KDM6A, SRSF2*) frequently occurred in subclones, indicating that these alterations may occur in *TP53*-mutated AML throughout clonal evolution. Mutations involving *ASXL1, CBL,* and *U2AF1* genes arise almost identically in subclones of *TP53*, and with *TP53* as a variant in a novel incoming subclone.[11] AML with *TP53* mutations are not specifically correlated with a unique transcriptional signature by standard RNA sequencing.

Prognosis and Clinical Comment

Patients with AML with mutated *TP53* have significantly poorer prognosis and lower overall survival as compared with patients with *TP53* wild-type AML due to resistance to standard AML therapies[12]; this is true for both intensive chemotherapy approaches and for low-intensity regimens.[13] Even with the recently approved addition of the bcl-2 inhibitor venetoclax to hypomethylating agents in patients age >74 years or in those with significant comorbidities or venetoclax-based therapies, the median overall survival (OS) remains low at only 5 to 6 months, despite encouraging complete remission rates of 40% to 60%.[14] The VAF for *TP53* mutations appears to play a role in prognosis in *TP53*-mutated AML and MDS,[4,15] as a high VAF has been demonstrated to be an independent, adverse prognostic factor for OS both in patients with *TP53*-mutant MDS and AML. Nevertheless, the adequate VAF threshold is not fully established and may depend on the treatment used. Higher *TP53* VAFs were associated with a lower OS in elderly patients treated with low-intensity therapies. In patients treated with low-dose cytarabine, a VAF > 40% was independently associated with higher rates of relapse and worse relapse-free survival and OS, which was not true for patients who were treated with a hypomethylating agent. Outcomes with high-intensity therapies appear to depend less on *TP53* VAFs, with similar OS, event-free survival, and complete remission rates even with VAF < 20%.[16] This may be the result of expanding subclones that are selected for during treatment.

References

1. Hou HA, Chou WC, Kuo YY, et al. TP53 mutations in de novo acute myeloid leukemia patients: longitudinal follow-ups show the mutation is stable during disease evolution. *Blood Cancer J*. 2015;5(7):e331.
2. Schoch C, Kern W, Kohlmann A, Hiddemann W, Schnittger S, Haferlach T. Acute myeloid leukemia with a complex aberrant karyotype is a distinct biological entity characterized by genomic imbalances and a specific gene expression profile. *Genes Chromosomes Cancer*. 2005;43(3):227-238.
3. Wong TN, Ramsingh G, Young AL, et al. Role of TP53 mutations in the origin and evolution of therapy-related acute myeloid leukaemia. *Nature*. 2015;518(7540):552-555.
4. Weinberg OK, Siddon A, Madanat YF, et al. TP53 mutation defines a unique subgroup within complex karyotype de novo and therapy-related MDS/AML. *Blood Adv*. 2022;6(9):2847-2853.
5. Huber S, Baer C, Hutter S, et al. AML classification in the year 2023: how to avoid a Babylonian confusion of languages. *Leukemia*. 2023;37(7):1413-1420.
6. Garber JE, Goldstein AM, Kantor AF, Dreyfus MG, Fraumeni JF Jr, Li FP. Follow-up study of twenty-four families with Li-Fraumeni syndrome. *Cancer Res*. 1991;51(22):6094-6097.
7. Reichard KK, Tefferi A, Abdelmagid M, et al. Pure (acute) erythroid leukemia: morphology, immunophenotype, cytogenetics, mutations, treatment details, and survival data among 41 Mayo Clinic cases. *Blood Cancer J*. 2022;12(11):147.
8. Haferlach T, Schoch C, Löffler H, et al. Morphologic dysplasia in de novo acute myeloid leukemia (AML) is related to unfavorable cytogenetics but has no independent prognostic relevance under the conditions of intensive induction therapy: results of a multiparameter analysis from the German AML Cooperative Group studies. *J Clin Oncol*. 2003;21(2):256-265.
9. Dannheim KC, Pozdnyakova O, Dal Cin P, Weinberg OK. Immunophenotypic dysplasia and aberrant T-cell antigen expression in acute myeloid leukaemia with complex karyotype and TP53 mutations. *J Clin Pathol*. 2018;71(12):1051-1059.
10. Tashakori M, Kadia T, Loghavi S, et al. TP53 copy number and protein expression inform mutation status across risk categories in acute myeloid leukemia. *Blood*. 2022;140(1):58-72.
11. Rücker FG, Schlenk RF, Bullinger L, et al. TP53 alterations in acute myeloid leukemia with complex karyotype correlate with specific copy number alterations, monosomal karyotype, and dismal outcome. *Blood*. 2012;119(9):2114-2121.
12. Prochazka KT, Pregartner G, Rücker FG, et al. Clinical implications of subclonal TP53 mutations in acute myeloid leukemia. *Haematologica*. 2019;104(3):516-523.
13. Kadia TM, Jain P, Ravandi F, et al. TP53 mutations in newly diagnosed acute myeloid leukemia: clinicomolecular characteristics, response to therapy, and outcomes. *Cancer*. 2016;122(22):3484-3491.
14. Granowicz EM, Jonas BA. Targeting TP53-mutated acute myeloid leukemia: research and clinical developments. *OncoTargets Ther*. 2022;15:423-436.
15. Sallman DA, Komrokji R, Vaupel C, et al. Impact of TP53 mutation variant allele frequency on phenotype and outcomes in myelodysplastic syndromes. *Leukemia*. 2016;30(3):666-673.
16. Deng J, Wu X, Ling Y, et al. The prognostic impact of variant allele frequency (VAF) in TP53 mutant patients with MDS: a systematic review and meta-analysis. *Eur J Haematol*. 2020;105(5):524-539. doi:10.1111/ejh.13483

Chapter 33

Acute Myeloid Leukemia and Myelodysplastic Syndrome/Acute Myeloid Leukemia With Myelodysplasia-Related Gene Mutations

Olga K. Weinberg, Courtney D. DiNardo, Hartmut Döhner, Eric Duncavage, and Elli Papaemmanuil

Definition

Acute myeloid leukemia (AML) and acute myeloid leukemia/myelodysplastic syndrome (AML/MDS) with myelodysplasia-related (MR) gene mutations is defined by the International Consensus Classification as AML harboring mutations in *ASXL1, BCOR, EZH2, RUNX1, SF3B1, SRSF2, STAG2, U2AF1,* or *ZRSR2*. This entity, in part, replaces the prior category of AML with myelodysplasia-related changes (AML-MRCs) and is applicable irrespective of any prior history of MDS or MDS/MPN and additionally incorporates the prior entity of AML with mutated *RUNX1*. Cases with other recurring genetic abnormalities in the classification, including mutations of *TP53*, take precedence over this category. This category, however, takes precedence over AML with MR cytogenetic abnormalities, or AML, not otherwise specified. The blast count requirement for AML with MR gene mutation is ≥20% in blood or bone marrow and 10% to 19% for AML/MDS with MR gene mutation. AML with MDS-related gene mutations is associated with adverse prognosis by European LeukemiaNet (ELN) guidelines in patients receiving standard intensive therapies.

Synonyms

Secondary AML (not recommended).

Epidemiology

The revised fourth edition of the World Health Organization Classification category of AML with MR changes was an attempt to identify patients with a worse prognosis; however, the challenges with standardizing the definition of morphologic dysplasia highlighted the need for an improved and genomic-driven approach to AML classification. Recent data indicate that genetic characteristics, rather than clinical history, have more prognostic relevance in classifying biologically distinct AML subgroups. Various gene mutations are commonly associated with AML arising from MDS and in the background of therapy-related disease and have been proposed alongside MDS-associated cytogenetic abnormalities as a further defining feature of AML-MRC. Lindsley et al.[1] found that the presence of a mutation in *SRSF2, SF3B1, U2AF1, ZRSR2, ASXL1, EZH2, BCOR,* or *STAG2* was >95% specific for the diagnosis of so-called secondary AML. Papaemmanuil et al.[2] furthermore confirmed lower survival rates and higher relapse rates in patients with chromatin-spliceosome gene mutations (including *ASXL1, BCOR, EZH2, MLL*-PTD, *RUNX1, SF3B1, SRSF2, STAG2, U2AF1,* or *ZRSR2*) receiving intensive chemotherapy as compared with other subgroups. Baer et al. identified a similar mutational pattern including *SRSF2, U2AF1, SF3B1, ASXL1, EZH2, BCOR,* and *STAG2* that appeared to distinguish AML-MRC from non-AML-MRC patients in terms of outcomes to standard chemotherapeutic approaches.[3]

General Clinical Features

MR gene mutations have been described as having a strong association with secondary AML transformed from MDS and chronic myelomonocytic leukemia, and patients with de novo AML carrying secondary AML-type mutations shared similar clinicopathological features with patients with clinically confirmed secondary AML. Despite the possible presence of an unrecognized antecedent MDS before AML diagnosis in patients with MR mutations, such mutations can be detected in more than 30% of patients with rigorously clinically defined de novo AML.[4] Patients with AML with MR gene mutations typically present at older age, with lower blast count, with less proliferative disease, and with higher incidence of antecedent hematologic disease when compared with AML without MR gene mutations.[5] AML with MR gene mutations is frequent, especially in older patients (>60) and in those with clinically defined secondary AML, where the majority of patients are characterized as AML with MR gene mutations.[4] Fuhrmann et al found that 67% of patients with AML, not otherwise specified showed at least 1 MR mutation and are now better classified as AML with MR gene mutations; this rate is similar to the rate of MR mutations (71%) seen in the prior category of AML-MRC with multilineage dysplasia.[6] In contrast, only 39% of patients in AML-MRC with MR cytogenetics had one or more MR mutations. Tsai *et al* found that, in younger patients, secondary mutations had significantly negative prognostic impacts on outcome, similar to the older patients.[7]

Morphology

Dysplasia in AML must be assessed on well-stained smears of peripheral blood and bone marrow. Despite the rapidly expanding knowledge of the mutations and functional pathways in AML, relatively few studies have evaluated the association of mutations with specific dysplastic features. Devillier et al. evaluated 94 patients with AML-MRC and found that *ASXL1* mutations were associated with a higher degree of dysgranulopoiesis but not dyserythropoiesis or dysmegakaryopoiesis.[8] In AML with normal karyotype, cohesin pathway mutations were found to be associated with a higher degree of megakaryocytic dysplasia and megakaryocytes with separated lobes and *STAG2* mutations were marginally associated with greater myeloid lineage dysplasia.[9]

Immunophenotype

In AML, flow cytometry is crucial for detection of leukemic blasts, blast lineage assignment, and identification of aberrant immunophenotypic features that allow distinction of abnormal blast populations from normal progenitors. Increased numbers of blasts can be identified by multiparameter flow cytometry or immunohistochemistry. Assessment of lymphoid markers should be included in the initial evaluation of AML to confirm correct lineage assignment and to evaluate for aberrant expression of a nonlineage marker on an abnormal myeloid blast population. Aberrant lymphoid markers including CD7 and CD56 are frequently seen. Expression of myeloid antigens is usually at aberrantly high or low levels. Maturing monocyte, myeloid, and/or erythroid lineages can also show immunophenotypic aberrations.

Genetics

MR mutations can be detected in more than 30% of patients with rigorously clinically defined de novo AML and have been shown to confer a negative prognostic impact in elderly patients. Tazi et al found that patients with ≤2 aneuploidies enriched for "MDS-related" cytogenetic abnormalities clustered with MR-type mutations.[5] A recent study found that older patients with MR mutations had a significantly lower frequency of unfavorable-risk cytogenetic changes.[7] Furthermore, younger patients with AML with MR mutations had lower rates of *CEBPA* double mutations and *CEBPA* bZIP in-frame mutations but a higher rate of *IDH2* and *ETV6* mutations than those without MR mutations.[7] Older patients with AML with MR mutations harbored fewer *KIT*, *TP53*, and *DNMT3A* mutations but more *TET2* mutations than those without MR mutations. Overall patients with AML with MR mutations have fewer co-occurring *NPM1* but more frequent *PHF6* mutations.[7] A recent study suggested that having two or more secondary mutations is associated with a particularly poor prognosis and is more frequently associated with antecedent hematologic disease.[5] Although a variant allele frequency (VAF) cutoff has not been established, it is recommended that a minimum VAF of 10% is used.

Prognosis and Clinical Comment

AMLs with MR gene mutations have been associated with inferior survival following intensive chemotherapy regimens[1,2,4,7] and are categorized as adverse-risk in the 2022 ELN genetic risk classification highlighting the benefit from allogeneic hematopoietic cell transplantation in first remission.[4] This diagnostic classification is also important for initial front-line treatment decision making, as the liposomal formulation of daunorubicin and cytarabine, CPX-351, is an approved frontline intensive regimen that is approved specifically for patients with newly diagnosed AML and antecedent hematologic disorder or MDS-related genomics based on an improvement in remission rate and overall survival compared with the standard 7 + 3 treatment regimen.[10]

One study suggested that more than one MDS-related gene mutation confers even more adverse prognosis.[5] Whether the presence of MR gene mutations confer inferior outcome in other disease entities, in particular favorable-risk AML such as AML with mutated *NPM1*, remains an area of active investigation.

Data on the prognostic impact of AML with MR gene mutations in older patients receiving less intense therapies are scarce, but there are increasing reports of similar outcomes in patients with/without MDS-related gene mutations suggesting the adverse risk outcomes are specific to intensive treatment approaches. In a recent study of older patients receiving monotherapy with hypomethylating agents (HMA), outcome was intermediate and similar to patients with AML with mutated *NPM1*,[11] Figure 33.1. Similarly, comparable outcomes have been seen in patients with spliceosome mutations treated with HMA + venetoclax regimen, with retrospective data highlighting favorable outcomes in patients with MDS-related gene mutations receiving HMA + venetoclax regimens (and in the absence of *TP53* and signaling mutations including *FLT3-ITD, NRAS,* and *KRAS*).[12]

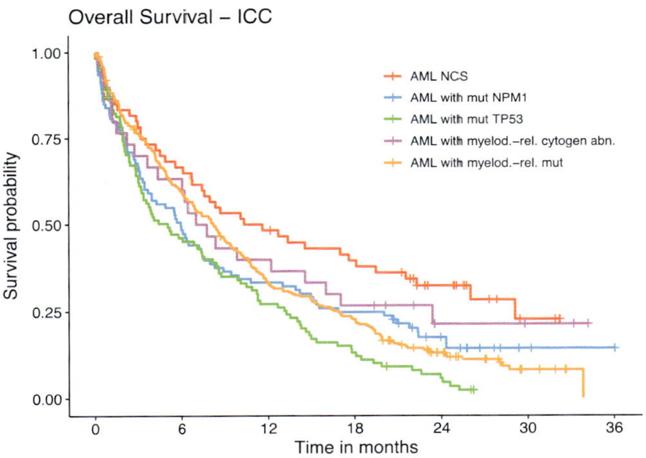

Number at risk (number of events)

	0	6	12	18	24	30	36
AML NCS	60 (0)	40 (20)	29 (31)	23 (36)	13 (40)	3 (42)	0 (42)
AML with mut NPM1	93 (0)	45 (48)	31 (62)	23 (70)	11 (76)	2 (78)	1 (78)
AML with mut TP53	102 (0)	46 (54)	27 (73)	13 (87)	5 (94)	0 (97)	0 (97)
AML with myelod.–rel. cytogen abn.	30 (0)	19 (11)	12 (18)	8 (22)	3 (23)	2 (23)	0 (23)
AML with myelod.–rel. mut	266 (0)	156 (106)	86 (175)	59 (202)	24 (226)	5 (232)	0 (233)

FIGURE 33.1 Overall survival by International Consensus Classification (ICC) categories in older patients receiving monotherapy with hypomethylating agents. (Adapted from Jahn E, Saadati M, Fenaux P, et al. Clinical impact of the genomic landscape and leukemogenic trajectories in non-intensively treated elderly acute myeloid leukemia patients. *Leukemia*. 2023;37(11):2187-2196.)

References

1. Lindsley RC, Mar BG, Mazzola E, et al. Acute myeloid leukemia ontogeny is defined by distinct somatic mutations. *Blood*. 2015;125(9):1367-1376.
2. Papaemmanuil E, Gerstung M, Bullinger L, et al. Genomic classification and prognosis in acute myeloid leukemia. *N Engl J Med*. 2016;374(23):2209-2221.
3. Baer C, Walter W, Stengel A, et al. Molecular classification of AML-MRC reveals a distinct profile and identifies MRC-like patients with poor overall survival. *Blood*. 2019;134:2735.
4. Gardin C, Pautas C, Fournier E, et al. Added prognostic value of secondary AML-like gene mutations in ELN intermediate-risk older AML: ALFA-1200 study results. *Blood Adv*. 2020;4(9):1942-1949.
5. Tazi Y, Arango-Ossa JE, Zhou Y, et al. Unified classification and risk-stratification in acute myeloid leukemia. *Nat Commun*. 2022;13(1):4622.
6. Fuhrmann I, Lenk M, Haferlach T, et al. AML, NOS and AML-MRC as defined by multilineage dysplasia share a common mutation pattern which is distinct from AML-MRC as defined by MDS-related cytogenetics. *Leukemia*. 2022;36(7):1939-1942.
7. Tsai, XCH, Sun, KJ, Lo, MY et al Poor prognostic implications of myelodysplasia-related mutations in both older and younger patients with de novo AML. *Blood Cancer J*. 13(1), 4 (2023). doi: 10.1038/s41408-022-00774-7
8. Devillier R, Mansat-De Mas V, Gelsi-Boyer V, et al. Role of ASXL1 and TP53 mutations in the molecular classification and prognosis of acute myeloid leukemias with myelodysplasia-related changes. *Oncotarget*. 2015;6(10):8388-8396.
9. Weinberg OK, Gibson CJ, Blonquist TM, et al. Association of mutations with morphological dysplasia in de novo acute myeloid leukemia without 2016 WHO Classification-defined cytogenetic abnormalities. *Haematologica*. 2018;103(4):626-633.
10. Lancet JE, Uy GL, Newell LF, et al. CPX-351 versus 7+3 cytarabine and daunorubicin chemotherapy in older adults with newly diagnosed high-risk or secondary acute myeloid leukaemia: 5-year results of a randomised, open-label, multicentre, phase 3 trial. *Lancet Haematol*. 2021;8(7):e481-e491.
11. Jahn E, Saadati M, Fenaux P, et al. Clinical impact of the genomic landscape and leukemogenic trajectories in non-intensively treated elderly acute myeloid leukemia patients. *Leukemia*. 2023;37(11):2187-2196.
12. Senapati J, Urrutia S, Loghavi S, et al. Venetoclax abrogates the prognostic impact of splicing factor gene mutations in newly diagnosed acute myeloid leukemia. *Blood*. 2023;142(19):1647-1657. doi:10.1182/blood.2023020649

Chapter 34

Acute Myeloid Leukemia and Myelodysplastic Syndrome/Acute Myeloid Leukemia With Myelodysplasia-Related Cytogenetic Abnormalities

Olga K. Weinberg, Daniel A. Arber, Paola Dal Cin, and Olatoyosi M. Odenike

Definition

Acute myeloid leukemia (AML) and myelodysplastic syndrome/acute myeloid leukemia (MDS/AML) with myelodysplasia-related (MR) cytogenetic abnormalities are defined by the presence of a complex karyotype (CK; ≥3 unrelated clonal chromosomal abnormalities in the absence of other class-defining recurring genetic abnormalities), del(5q)/−7/del(7q),+8, del(12p), del(17p), del(20q), and idic(X)(q13) (Table 34.1). The prior category of AML with myelodysplasia-related changes (MRC) is eliminated and is partially replaced with AML with MR cytogenetic abnormalities and AML with MR gene mutations. Cases of AML and MDS/AML with mutated *TP53* and AML and MDS/AML with MR gene mutations are excluded from this category. The blast count requirement for AML is ≥20% in peripheral blood and/or bone marrow and for MDS/AML is 10% to 19%.

Synonyms

Secondary AML (not recommended).

TABLE 34.1 Defining myelodysplasia-related cytogenetic abnormalities

Complex karyotype (≥3 unrelated clonal chromosomal abnormalities in the absence of other class-defining recurring genetic abnormalities)
del(5q)[a]
7/del(7q)[a]
trisomy 8
del(12p)[a]
del(17p)[a]
del(20q)
idic(X)(q13)

[a]Losses involving 5q, 7q, 12p, or 17p often arise not as simple deletions but rather as products of unbalanced rearrangements.

Epidemiology

The prior category of AML with MRC (AML-MRC) was an attempt to identify patients with a worse prognosis, but controversy over the significance of morphologic dysplasia highlighted a need for a better-defined approach to AML classification. Recent data indicate that genetic characteristics, rather than clinical history (de novo, secondary after an antecedent MDS or MDS/myeloproliferative neoplasm [MPN], or therapy-related), have most relevance in classifying biologically distinct AML subgroups. Mutations of *ASXL1, BCOR, EZH2, RUNX1, SF3B1, SRSF2, STAG2, U2AF1,* or *ZRSR2* qualify for a diagnosis of AML with MR gene mutations.[1] In the absence of a MR gene mutation, *TP53* mutation, or other recurring genetic abnormalities definitive of specific AML categories, a case is diagnosed as AML with MR cytogenetic abnormalities based on specific karyotype findings. Therapy-related AML, seen in ~75% of cases, typically presents 5 to 7 years after first exposure to alkylating agents or radiation, is often preceded by MDS, and is frequently accompanied by chromosome 5 and/or 7 abnormalities, CK, and *TP53* mutations and would now be considered as AML with mutated *TP53*.[2] Similar cases without a *TP53* mutation would be diagnosed as AML with MR cytogenetic abnormalities. Therapy-related AML is no longer considered a distinct disease entity, but the term "therapy-related" is now used as a diagnostic qualifier to the disease entities that are primarily defined by their genetic profile. Similarly, cases progressing from MDS or MDS/MPN should be designated as such in a diagnostic qualifier.

General Clinical Features

A recent study suggests that patients with AML with MR cytogenetic abnormalities presented at similar age as AML, not otherwise specified patients.[3] However, other studies find that AML patients with MR cytogenetic abnormalities typically present at older age, with lower blast count, and have a higher incidence of antecedent hematologic disease.[4] When compared with AML with normal karyotype cases and cytogenetically abnormal cases without MDS-related cytogenetic abnormalities, patients with AML with MR cytogenetic abnormalities show a significantly worse prognosis.[5] A small study suggests that there may be an additive adverse impact with the combination of MDS-related cytogenetic abnormalities and history of prior MDS or MDS/MPN.[5]

Morphology

Previous studies suggest that multilineage dysplasia is associated with unfavorable cytogenetics and secondary AML, which are poor prognostic factors; however, some reports find that multilineage alone has no independent prognostic relevance in AML.[6,7] The presence of dysplasia is not required for a diagnosis of AML with MR cytogenetic abnormalities but should be noted in a report. Multilineage dysplasia must be assessed on well-stained bone marrow smears. Dysgranulopoiesis is typically characterized by neutrophils with hypogranular cytoplasm or hyposegmented nuclei (pseudo-Pelger-Huët). Dyserythropoiesis is characterized by megaloblastosis, karyorrhexis, and nuclear irregularity, fragmentation, or multinucleation. Ring sideroblasts and cytoplasmic vacuoles are additional features of dyserythropoiesis. Dysmegakaryopoiesis is characterized by micromegakaryocytes and normal-sized or large megakaryocytes with nonlobated or separated nuclear lobes.

Immunophenotype

Increased numbers of blasts can be identified by multiparameter flow cytometry or immunohistochemistry. Blasts often express CD34, CD117, and HLA-DR, as well as myeloid markers including CD13 and CD33. Aberrant lymphoid markers including CD7 and CD56 are frequently seen. Expression of myeloid antigens is usually at aberrantly high or low levels. Maturing monocyte, myeloid, and/or erythroid lineages can also show immunophenotypic aberrations. A few studies have suggested that AML-MRC cases (as defined by the WHO fourth edition) were more likely to have granulocyte and monocyte abnormalities than AML cases without cytogenetic abnormalities.[8]

Genetics

Most cases of AML-MRC were associated with adverse genetic abnormalities, particularly −5/del(5q), −7/del(7q), and/or CK.[9] CK, defined as ≥3 chromosomal abnormalities, comprises 10% to 12% of AML patients and constitutes the second largest cytogenetic subset of AML patients (after those with normal karyotype). A CK is defined as three or more unrelated chromosomal abnormalities in the absence of other class-defining recurring genetic abnormalities. Of note, a CK excludes hyperdiploid karyotypes with three or more trisomies (or polysomies) without structural abnormalities. Recently, Tazi et al defined a novel cytogenetic subgroup by the presence of ≥1 trisomies, frequently involving +8, +11, +13, +21, and + 22 but no deletions. This group had infrequent involvement of *TP53* and was associated with more favorable disease, even when ≥3 trisomies were present.[4] In the same study, patients with MDS-related cytogenetic abnormalities clustered with secondary AML-type mutations including *SRSF2, SF3B1, U2AF1, ZRSR2, ASXL1, EZH2, BCOR, STAG2, RUNX1, SETBP1,* and *MLLPTD* mutations.[4] Additional mutations in signaling pathways (ie, *FLT3, RAS, CBL, PTPN11*), transcription factors (*RUNX1, WT1*), epigenetic regulators (*IDH1, IDH2, TET2*), and *TP53* have been implicated in the leukemogenic process. Patients with CK are associated with mutations in *TP53* (present in 65% of CK cases) but with paucity of other acquired mutations.[4] A recent study of 604 previously untreated AML patients unfit for intensive chemotherapy showed MR cytogenetic abnormalities such as trisomy 8 (17%, n = 47), −7/del(7q) (14%, n = 39), CK (9%, n = 26), del(20q) (6%, n = 16), −5/del(5q) (5%, n = 14), del(12p) (3%, n = 8), and −17/del(17p)/abn(17p) (3%, n = 7).[3]

Trisomy 8 is one of the most common cytogenetic alterations in AML, with a frequency between 10% and 15%, and is associated with mutations in DNA methylation genes, spliceosome complex genes, and myeloid transcription factor genes.[10] AML with del(20q) occurs in 2% of previously untreated AML patients, with around 63% of these patients showing CK.[9] While these cytogenetic abnormalities were not considered MDS-defining in prior WHO classifications, they are considered to be poor prognostic indicators in the setting of an increase in blasts and are included as MDS-related in the International Consensus Classification (ICC) definition of AML and MDS/AML. Prior classifications also included some balanced chromosomal abnormalities as MDS-related, but those are now eliminated from this category with many now included in the category of AML with other rare recurring translocations.

Monosomal karyotype, defined by the presence of one single autosomal monosomy (excluding isolated loss of X or Y) in association with at least one additional or one structural chromosomal abnormality, is considered by some to be an AML-MR cytogenetic abnormality[11];

however, the ICC and European LeukemiaNet (ELN) do not currently recognize this as MR-defining. A number of studies have shown that AML with monosomal karyotype presents with a significantly worse overall survival, disease-free survival, and complete response rate.[12]

As noted previously, cases with *TP53* mutations or with MR gene mutations (see prior chapters) take precedence of AML with MR cytogenetic abnormalities when both are present. In such cases, however, it is appropriate to note the presence of both findings in the diagnostic report.

Prognosis and Clinical Comment

Compared to other types of AML, AML with unfavorable cytogenetics (MR cytogenetics) has inferior outcomes, including lower remission rates ranging between 30% and 50% and shorter overall survival.[1] Patients diagnosed with AML with MR cytogenetic abnormalities are typically older and often present with a higher burden of comorbidities.[13] Due to their advanced age and associated health concerns, they are less likely to undergo curative intensive chemotherapy regimens, unlike younger patients. The presence of MR cytogenetic abnormalities is often associated with secondary AML-type mutations, lower blast counts, and a higher incidence of antecedent hematologic disease.[4] Studies utilizing the Cancer and Leukemia Group B criteria have strongly correlated relapse rates with a patient's cytogenetic risk.[1] Unfavorable cytogenetics, defining adverse ELN risk categories, offer crucial prognostic information that significantly influences treatment decisions. Specifically, genetic abnormalities such as −7, −5/del(5q), monosomal karyotypes, and complex cytogenetics involving at least three abnormalities independently carry an adverse prognosis regardless of the treatment type.

References

1. Döhner H, Wei AH, Appelbaum FR, et al. Diagnosis and management of AML in adults: 2022 recommendations from an international expert panel on behalf of the ELN. *Blood*. 2022;140(12):1345-1377.
2. Kayser S, Döhner K, Krauter J; German-Austrian AMLSG, et al. The impact of therapy-related acute myeloid leukemia (AML) on outcome in 2853 adult patients with newly diagnosed AML. *Blood*. 2011;117(7):2137-2145.
3. Fuhrmann I, Lenk M, Haferlach T, et al. AML, NOS and AML-MRC as defined by multilineage dysplasia share a common mutation pattern which is distinct from AML-MRC as defined by MDS-related cytogenetics. *Leukemia*. 2022;36(7):1939-1942.
4. Tazi Y, Arango-Ossa JE, Zhou Y, et al. Unified classification and risk-stratification in acute myeloid leukemia. *Nat Commun*. 2022;13(1):4622.
5. Fang H, He R, Chiu A, et al. Genetic factors in acute myeloid leukemia with myelodysplasia-related changes. *Am J Clin Pathol*. 2020;153(5):656-663.
6. Miesner M, Haferlach C, Bacher U, et al. Multilineage dysplasia (MLD) in acute myeloid leukemia (AML) correlates with MDS-related cytogenetic abnormalities and a prior history of MDS or MDS/MPN but has no independent prognostic relevance: a comparison of 408 cases classified as "AML not otherwise specified" (AML-NOS) or "AML with myelodysplasia-related changes" (AML-MRC). *Blood*. 2010;116(15):2742-2751.
7. Döhner H, Estey EH, Amadori S, et al. Diagnosis and management of acute myeloid leukemia in adults: recommendations from an international expert panel, on behalf of the European LeukemiaNet. *Blood*. 2010;115(3):453-474.
8. Weinberg OK, Hasserjian RP, Li B, Pozdnyakova O. Assessment of myeloid and monocytic dysplasia by flow cytometry in de novo AML helps define an AML with myelodysplasia-related changes category. *J Clin Pathol*. 2017;70(2):109-115.
9. Brezinová J, Zemanová Z, Ransdorfová S, et al. Prognostic significance of del(20q) in patients with hematological malignancies. *Cancer Genet Cytogenet*. 2005;160(2):188-192.
10. Hemsing AL, Hovland R, Tsykunova G, Reikvam H. Trisomy 8 in acute myeloid leukemia. *Expert Rev Hematol*. 2019;12(11):947-958.
11. Kayser S, Zucknick M, Döhner K; German-Austrian AML Study Group, et al. Monosomal karyotype in adult acute myeloid leukemia: prognostic impact and outcome after different treatment strategies. *Blood*. 2012;119(2):551-558.
12. Breems DA, Van Putten WL, De Greef GE, et al. Monosomal karyotype in acute myeloid leukemia: a better indicator of poor prognosis than a complex karyotype. *J Clin Oncol*. 2008;26(29):4791-4797.
13. Byrd JC, Mrózek K, Dodge RK, et al. Pretreatment cytogenetic abnormalities are predictive of induction success, cumulative incidence of relapse, and overall survival in adult patients with de novo acute myeloid leukemia: results from Cancer and Leukemia Group B (CALGB 8461). *Blood*. 2002;100(13):4325-4336.

Chapter 35

Acute Myeloid Leukemia and Myelodysplastic Syndrome/Acute Myeloid Leukemia, Not Otherwise Specified

Daniel A. Arber, John M. Bennett, Kathryn Foucar, Attilio Orazi, Roland B. Walter, and Gina Zini

Introduction and Definition

The categories of acute myeloid leukemia and myelodysplastic syndrome/acute myeloid leukemia, not otherwise specified (AML, NOS and MDS/AML, NOS) include cases that fulfill neither the criteria for inclusion in any of the previously described AML entity groups nor the criteria for blast transformation of a myeloproliferative neoplasm. These cases lack any of the entity-defining recurring cytogenetic abnormalities or gene mutations, including *TP53* mutations, the myelodysplasia-related gene mutations or myelodysplasia-related cytogenetic abnormalities, or any of the other AML defining rare recurring translocations as defined in Chapter 28. Consequently, none of the AML, NOS subtypes discussed in this chapter is an actual biologically defined disease. Instead, AML, NOS subtypes are lineage-based categories that may be helpful for communication with clinicians and patients, monitoring response to therapy, or to highlight unique clinical associations.

While the elimination of the therapy-related myeloid neoplasm category as well as the elimination of AML associated with multilineage dysplasia as a separate category or of cases occurring in patients with a prior myelodysplastic syndrome (MDS) or a prior myelodysplastic/myeloproliferative neoplasm (MDS/MPN) as disease criteria will result in most of such cases still being classified as other distinct AML entity types, a small subset of such cases will fall into AML, NOS and the use of qualifiers for prior cytotoxic therapy, prior MDS, prior MDS/MPN, and the presence of germline gene mutations not associated with other disorders should be noted in the diagnosis as described in the Introduction to Myeloid Disorders.

With this more restrictive definition, the frequency of AML, NOS appears to be decreased from prior classifications, but it is difficult to provide frequency data for the various AML, NOS subtypes. Of note, prior epidemiologic data based on the French-American-British Cooperative Group (FAB) Classification are no longer valid due to the current exclusion of many prognostically significant genetic AML entity subtypes in the ICC. Except for pure erythroid leukemia, the blast criterion, including blast equivalents, for AML, NOS remains as 20% or more in peripheral blood or bone marrow, and the criteria for MDS/AML, NOS require 10% to 19% peripheral blood or bone marrow blasts.

It is recommended that the blast percentage in the bone marrow be determined from a 500-cell differential count using an appropriate Romanowsky type stain (eg, Wright-Giemsa stain). In the peripheral blood, the differential should ideally include 200 leukocytes but may not be possible in patients with severe leukopenia. If an aspirate smear is not obtainable due to bone marrow fibrosis and if the blasts express CD34, immunohistochemical detection of CD34 on biopsy sections may enable the diagnosis of AML or MDS/AML if the respective 20% or more or 10% to 19% blast thresholds are met. The major criteria required for this diagnosis are based on examination of bone marrow aspirates, peripheral blood smear, and bone marrow biopsy sections. The recommendations for classification apply only to specimens obtained prior to chemotherapy.

The primary basis for subclassification of AML, NOS is the morphological and cytochemical/immunophenotypic features of the leukemic cells, previously defined by the FAB, which indicate the major lineages involved and their degree of maturation. Cytochemical studies are often useful in the subtyping of AML, NOS, but they are not considered essential for diagnosis, given the reduced availability in many laboratories and the lack of prognostic significance of any of the morphologic/immunophenotypic subgroups.

A diagnosis of AML or MDS/AML, NOS should not be made in the absence of appropriate cytogenetic and molecular genetic studies and should not be used as a place holder for cases pending such studies.

Additionally, while the subtypes described in the following sections apply to cases with 20% or more blasts (ie, AML, NOS), subclassification of MDS/AML, NOS is not recommended due to difficulty in applying the criteria in those samples in which morphology overlaps that of high-grade MDS.

Synonym

Acute myeloid leukemia, defined by differentiation (not recommended).

Epidemiology

Most prior epidemiology data on cases with these morphologic features were based largely on the FAB classification and did not take into account the genetic subtypes that are now removed from this category. A recent study found that the frequency of AML, NOS decreased from 38.1% in the WHO revised 4th edition to 24.1% using the ICC,[1] but that study failed to classify cases in the ICC rare recurring cytogenetic abnormality category (see Chapter 28) and therefore overestimated AML, NOS using correct ICC criteria. Therefore, there are currently insufficient studies to precisely define the incidence of AML, NOS or its subtypes.

General Clinical Features

Patients present with evidence of bone marrow failure, including neutropenia, anemia, and thrombocytopenia. Some patients will present with leukocytosis with variable numbers of circulating blast cells, but blasts may be rare in the peripheral blood. Patients with AML with monoblastic or monocytic features often present with bleeding disorders. Extramedullary masses, cutaneous and gingival infiltration, and central nervous system involvement may also be more common in that group compared to other AML types. A rare association between acute megakaryoblastic leukemia and mediastinal nonseminomatous germ cell tumors is reported in young adult males.[2]

Morphology and Immunophenotype

Morphologic and immunophenotypic features vary by category and are described here. Overall, they are largely similar to those originally described by the FAB group (see the following text and figures).[3] With the exception of pure erythroid leukemia, all demonstrate an increase in myeloblasts with variations in the cytologic and cytochemical features (see Table 35.1) that correlate with immunophenotype differences. Blasts may express early hematopoietic-associated antigens (eg, CD34, CD38, and HLA-DR), antigens associated with myeloid (CD13, CD33, CD117, MPO, HLA-DR), monocytic (CD4, CD11b, CD14, CD15, CD36, CD65, CD68, and lysozyme), and/or megakaryocytic (CD41, CD42, CD61, and von Willebrand factor) maturation. Blast cells usually express at least two myeloid-associated markers, differentiating them from acute undifferentiated leukemia. Like other AML types, a subset of cases may show TdT positivity or demonstrate aberrant lymphoid antigen expression.

Genetics

By definition, cases in this category cannot have any of the genetic abnormalities or disease defining gene mutations specific for other AML or MDS/AML types.

TABLE 35.1 Cytologic and cytochemical features of more common Acute Myeloid Leukemia, Not Otherwise Specified (AML, NOS) variants. Traditional cytochemical features are listed as well as blast features that may be determined by morphology or flow cytometry immunophenotyping

	Cytochemistry		Marrow blast features		
	MPO[a]	NSE	Granulocyte maturation ≥10%	Monocytes ≥20%	Monocytes ≥80%
AML with minimal differentiation	–[b]	–	–	–	–
AML without maturation	+	–	–	–	–
AML with maturation	+	–	+	–	–
Acute myelomonocytic leukemia	+	≥20%	+	+	–
Acute monoblastic and monocytic leukemia	±	>80%	–	+	+
Acute megakaryoblastic leukemia	–	–	±	–	–

MPO, myeloperoxidase or Sudan Black B; NSE, nonspecific esterase.

[a]+, ≥3% blasts positive.

[b]MPO may be positive by immunophenotyping methods.

Of note, cases with features of minimal differentiation often demonstrate mutations of *RUNX1*, which would now place such a case in the category of AML with myelodysplasia-associated gene mutations (see Chapter 33). The presence of associated hemophagocytosis (in particular erythrophagocytosis) in a monocytic or monoblastic AML should raise concern for AML with t(8;16)(p11.2;p13.3)/*KAT6A::CREBBP*, which is a distinct entity in the classification (see Chapter 28). Similarly, AML with inv(3)(q21.3q26.2) or t(3;3)(q21.3;q26.2)/*GATA2, MECOM* and AML with t(1;22)(p13.3;q13.1)/*RBM15::MRTFA*, or cases of blast transformation of a myeloproliferative neoplasm, may express megakaryocytic markers, but should not be diagnosed as AML, NOS (eg, acute megakaryoblastic leukemia).

Prognosis and Clinical Comment

Once the various genetic AML subtypes are excluded, there appears to be no prognostic significance for cases subclassified based on morphologic differentiation or immunophenotype. A study of 5,848 patients meeting criteria for AML, NOS using the WHO 4th edition criteria across four large databases found no prognostic difference among FAB-like subcategories of AML, NOS when cases with mutations of *CEBPA* and *NPM1* were removed from this group (mutations defining provisional entities in that classification).[4] The expansion of genetic categories of AML in subsequent classifications, including the ICC, appears to further reduce the potential for prognostic significance in subtyping these disorders. However, recognition of the various morphology blast cell types defined by the FAB remains important for diagnostic pathologists to properly identify blast cells.

The key features of most cytologic variants of AML, NOS are summarized in Table 35.1 and Figure 35.1. Three types, all of which are extremely rare, have more unique features and are described in more detail.

PURE ERYTHROID LEUKEMIA

Definition

Pure erythroid leukemia is a neoplastic proliferation of immature cells with morphologic and/or immunophenotypic features exclusive to the erythroid lineage. These immature erythroid cells should represent over 80% of the bone marrow cells, with 30% or more marrow cells being proerythroblasts. There should be no significant myeloblastic component. Pure erythroid leukemia as a subtype of AML, NOS is extremely rare as it does not fulfill the criteria for inclusion in any of the previously described AML groups, including AML with mutated *TP53*, or meet criteria for blast transformation of a myeloproliferative neoplasm.

Unique Clinical Features

In addition to typical features of AML, these patients often present with severe anemia with circulating erythroblasts. Cases lacking features of AML with mutated *TP53* may be more common in infants and children.

Morphology

Pure erythroid leukemia is characterized by the presence of medium-sized to large erythroblasts, usually with round nuclei, fine chromatin, and one or more nucleoli (proerythroblasts) (Figure 35.2). The cytoplasm is deeply basophilic and agranular and frequently contains vacuoles. Occasionally, the blasts are smaller, with scanty cytoplasm, and can resemble the lymphoblasts of acute lymphoblastic leukemia. The cells are negative for MPO and Sudan Black B staining; they show reactivity with alpha-naphthyl acetate esterase, acid phosphatase, and periodic acid–Schiff (PAS) (with PAS, usually in a block-like staining pattern corresponding the cytoplasmic vacuoles). In bone marrow biopsies, the cells appear undifferentiated and are arranged in a sheet-like pattern, but an intrasinusoidal pattern may occur.[5] Erythroblasts should constitute over 80% of marrow cells on either aspirate smears or marrow biopsy material, and proerythroblasts should constitute 30% or more of total cells.

Immunophenotype

The erythroblasts usually express glycophorin A and/or C, and hemoglobin A, as well as the less lineage-specific marker CD71. However, glycophorin and/or hemoglobin can be negative in the presence of poorly differentiated erythroblasts. E-cadherin, which stains early erythroid forms, is positive in most of such cases and is fairly specific for erythroid differentiation.[6] The blasts are often positive for CD117 and usually negative for HLA-DR and CD34. CD36 is positive in most cases but is not specific for erythroblasts and can be expressed by monocytes and megakaryocytes. Antigens associated with megakaryocytes, such as CD41 and CD61 are usually negative, but rare cases with partial expression of these markers may occur.

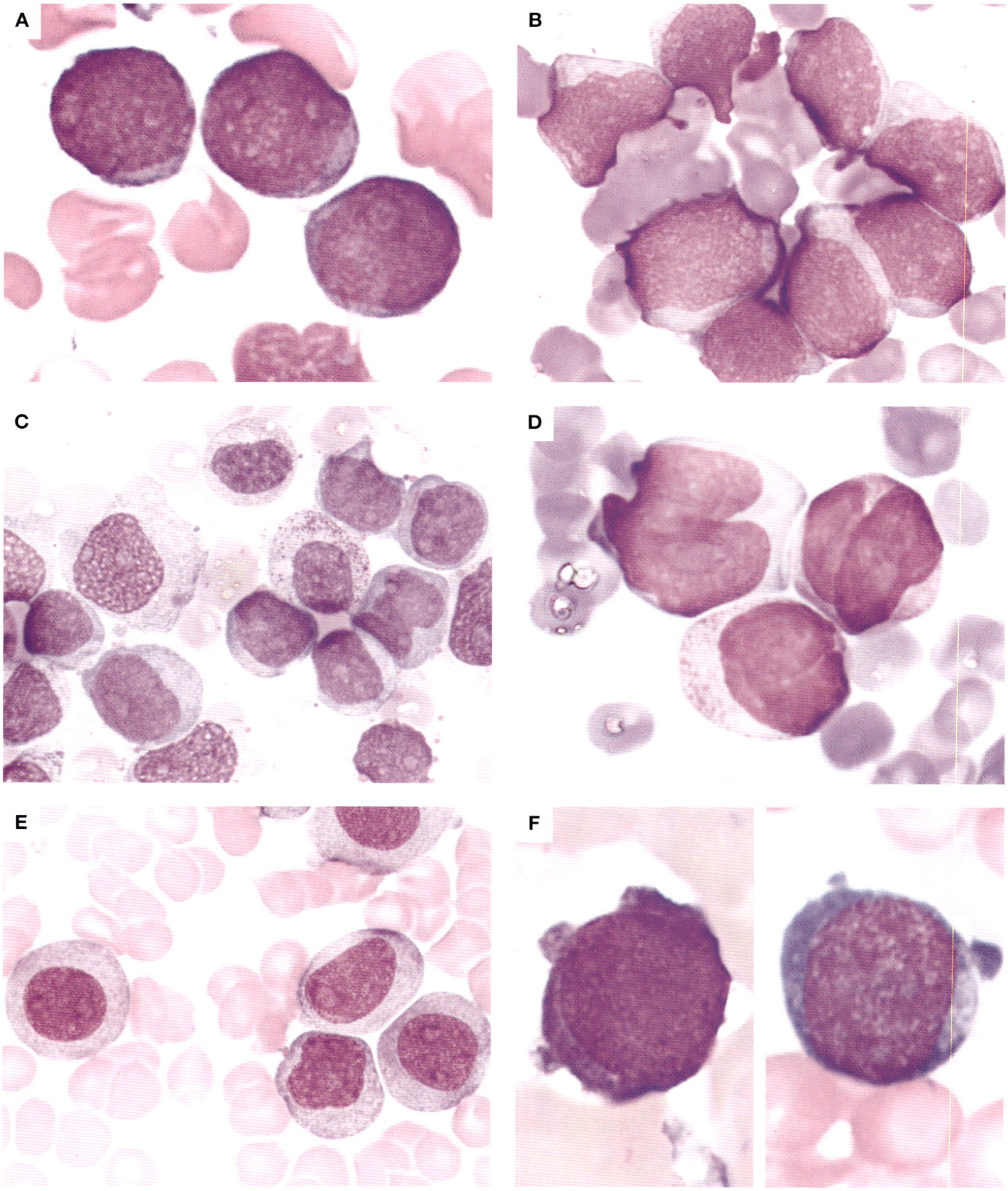

FIGURE 35.1 Common blast cell morphologic features in acute myeloid leukemia, not otherwise specified (AML, NOS). **A** and **B:** Myeloblasts without maturation showing variable amounts of cytoplasm, usually with minimal granules. The blasts in **A** were myeloperoxidase and nonspecific esterase negative, but expressed myeloid antigens by flow cytometry, consistent with minimal differentiation. The blasts in **B** were myeloperoxidase positive by cytochemistry, supporting AML without maturation, but the morphologic features may be similar between the two groups. **C:** Blasts with fine azurophilic granulation are present. Promyelocytes, myelocytes, and mature neutrophils constitute 10% or more of bone marrow cells, features of AML with maturation. Blasts may have variable granules and Auer rods. **D** and **E:** Monocytic features in AML. **D** shows monocytic cells with abundant, slightly basophilic cytoplasm and fine granules. Nuclear folds are present in two cells suggesting promonocytic differentiation. **E** shows monoblasts with more immature, round nuclei and abundant basophilic cytoplasm. Variable granulation with or without Auer rods and vacuoles may occur in these blast types. Monocytic versus myelomonocytic features may be difficult to determine without cytochemical studies. **F:** Two representative megakaryoblasts with round nuclei, deeply basophilic cytoplasm, and cytoplasmic blebbing. Cytoplasmic blebbing is often present, but is not specific for megakaryoblastic lineage, which must be confirmed by immunophenotyping. (**A-C:** Image provide by Maria Rozman, Barcelona, Spain.)

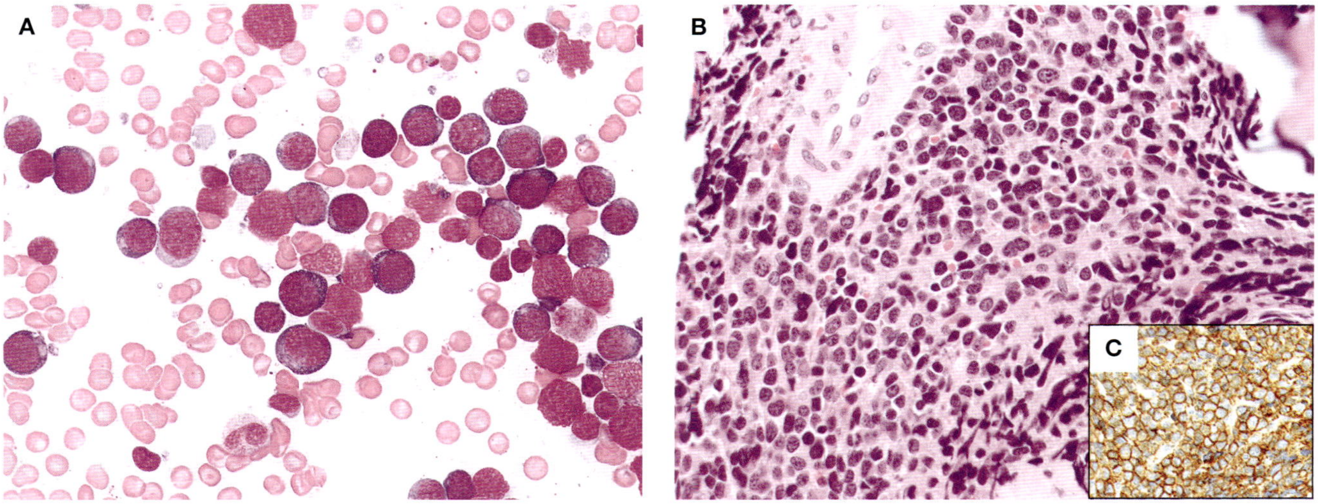

FIGURE 35.2 Pure erythroid leukemia in a 4-year-old. **A:** The marrow is composed of over 80% erythroid precursors with a predominance of proerythroblasts. **B:** The marrow biopsy contains sheets of similar cells that express glycophorin **C** (inset) confirming erythroid lineage. Genetic studies failed to identify a recurring genetic abnormality and specifically a mutation in *TP53*, making a diagnosis of pure erythroid leukemia appropriate.

Genetics

Most cases that meet criteria for pure erythroid leukemia have genetic changes that except for their low myeloblast count would place them in other AML categories in the ICC, particularly AML with mutated *TP53*, which allows for cases meeting criteria for pure erythroid leukemia with a *TP53* mutation and would trump a diagnosis of pure erythroid leukemia, and AML with myelodysplasia-related cytogenetic abnormalities in the absence of mutated *TP53* but in the presence of a complex karyotype or chromosome 5 and/or 7 abnormalities. Cases without these abnormalities appear to be more common in infants and children, some of which have cytogenetic abnormalities involving *NUP98*,[7] which are considered specific entities in the category of AML with other rare recurring translocations (see Chapter 28). Some cases with *NUP98* fusions, however, also harbor *TP53* mutations, making precise classification difficult. Rare cases without *TP53* mutations but with other genetic abnormalities, including *CIC::NUTM2A* and *NFIA::RUNX1T1*,[7,8] are described and would currently fall into this AML, NOS category.

ACUTE BASOPHILIC LEUKEMIA

Definition

Acute basophilic leukemia is an extremely rare AML type with 20% or more peripheral blood or bone marrow blasts in which the primary differentiation is to basophils. Acute basophilic leukemia does not fulfill the criteria for inclusion in any of the previously described AML groups or meet criteria for blast transformation of a myeloproliferative neoplasm.

Morphology

The circulating peripheral blood and bone marrow blasts are medium-sized, with a high N:C ratio; an oval, round, or irregular nucleus characterized by dispersed chromatin and 1 to 3 prominent nucleoli. The cytoplasm is moderately basophilic and contains a variable number of coarse basophilic granules that are positive with metachromatic staining (ie, toluidine blue). There may be vacuolation of the cytoplasm. Immature forms can be seen, but mature basophils are usually sparse (Figure 35.3). Electron microscopy shows that the granules have features characteristic of basophil precursors. They contain an electron-dense particulate substance, are internally bisected (eg, have a theta character), or contain crystalline material arranged in a pattern of scrolls or lamellae,[9] although the latter is more typical of mast cells and mast cell leukemia must be excluded. The blasts are usually negative for naphthol AS-D chloroacetate esterase (CAE), Sudan Black B staining, MPO, and nonspecific esterase. The lack of CAE reactivity is helpful in excluding mast cell leukemia, which is typically CAE positive. Although not specific, the most characteristic cytochemical reaction is metachromatic staining with toluidine blue. The blasts also usually show a diffuse pattern of staining with acid

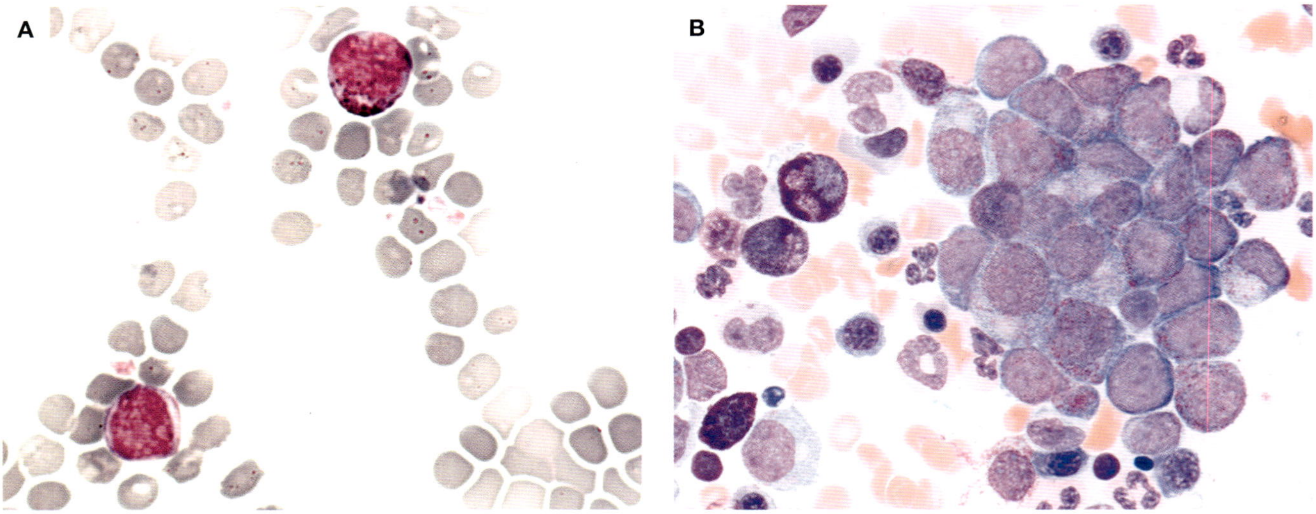

FIGURE 35.3 Acute basophilic leukemia. **A:** The peripheral blood image shows a blast in the lower left and a basophilic promyelocyte in the upper right. **B:** On a toluidine blue stain of the marrow aspirate, basophilic granules stain purple in color due to the presence of heparin and histamine. A cluster of granular blasts and basophilic promyelocytes are identified.

phosphatase, and in some cases show PAS positivity in large blocks. Bone marrow biopsy shows diffuse replacement by blast cells.

Immunophenotype

The blasts express myeloid markers such as CD13 and CD33; are usually positive for CD9 as well as for CD123, CD203c, and CD11b; and are negative for other monocytic markers, MPO and CD117. Blasts may express CD34. Unlike normal basophils, they may be positive for HLA-DR but are negative for CD117. Immunophenotypic detection of abnormal mast cells expressing CD117, tryptase, and CD25 distinguishes mast cell leukemia from acute basophilic leukemia. Cases of AML with blasts showing partial mast cell differentiation described in literature as myelomastocytic leukemia, which is not an entity in any current classification, may be confused with acute basophilic leukemia, but expression of CD117 and tryptase in such cases excludes acute basophilic leukemia. Some cases of acute basophilic leukemia are positive for membrane CD22 and/or TdT. Other membrane and cytoplasmic lymphoid-associated markers are usually negative.[10]

Genetics

A recurrent t(X;6)(p11.2;q23.3) resulting in *MYB::GATA1* appears to occur in male infants with acute basophilic leukemia.[11,12] Other cytogenetic abnormalities reported in this AML type include t(3;6)(q21;p21) and abnormalities involving 12p.[13]

ACUTE PANMYELOSIS WITH MYELOFIBROSIS

Definition

Acute panmyelosis with myelofibrosis (APMF) is an extremely rare acute-onset panmyeloid proliferation with 20% or more bone marrow or peripheral blood blasts, accompanying fibrosis of the bone marrow, and a lack of splenomegaly.[14,15] APMF does not fulfill the criteria for inclusion in any of other AML, MDS/AML, MDS, or MDS/MPN group with fibrosis. Based on these exclusions, it is not clear if APMF remains a unique disease category.

Morphology

The peripheral blood usually shows marked pancytopenia with no or minimal anisopoikilocytosis and variable macrocytosis. Rare erythroblasts can be seen, but teardrop-shaped cells (dacrocytes) are not observed. Occasional neutrophil precursors, including blasts, may be present. Abnormal platelets may be noted. Bone marrow aspiration is frequently unsuccessful. Bone marrow biopsy supplemented with immunohistochemistry is required for diagnosis.[16,17] The bone marrow is hypercellular and shows, within a diffusely fibrotic stroma, increased erythroid precursors, increased granulocyte precursors, and increased megakaryocytes (panmyelosis), with variability in terms of the relative proportion of each component. However, numerous dysplastic megakaryocytes with hyposegmented nuclei are usually seen (Figure 35.4).

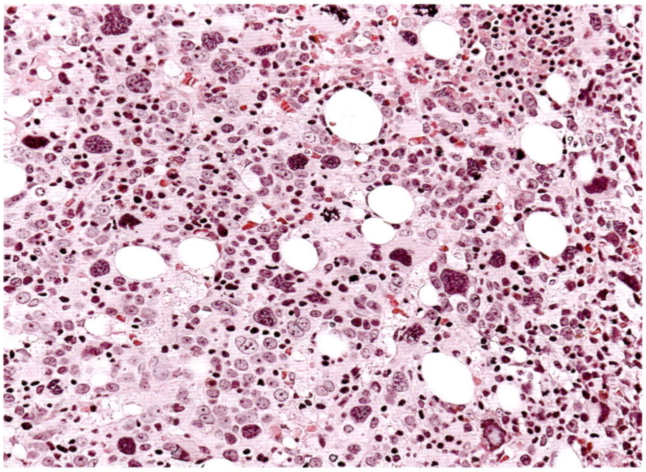

FIGURE 35.4 Acute panmyelosis with myelofibrosis. The marrow is markedly hypercellular with increased fibrosis and a mix of myeloid and erythroid precursors and dysplastic megakaryocytes.

The overall frequency of blasts in APMF marrows is variable; based on bone marrow biopsy, a median value of 22.5% was found in one study.[14] Most cases have a range of 20% to 25%. In most patients, reticulin staining shows markedly increased fibrosis often with coarse fibers (ie, MF-2 or MF-3 fibrosis); diffuse collagenous fibrosis is less common.

Immunophenotype

If the bone marrow specimen obtained for immunological markers is adequate or if circulating blasts are present, the cells show phenotypic heterogeneity, with varying degrees of expression of myeloid-associated antigens. The blasts usually express CD34 and one or more myeloid-associated antigens including CD13, CD33, and CD117,[14,16,17] but MPO is usually negative. In some cases, the immature cells express erythroid antigens. Immunohistochemistry can facilitate determination of the relative proportions of the various myeloid components in the biopsy specimen and is generally used to confirm the multilineage nature of the proliferation. These confirm the presence of panmyelosis and allow exclusion of unilineage-predominant proliferations, such as acute megakaryoblastic leukemia.

Genetics

There is no association between APMF, as currently defined, and specific recurrent genetic abnormalities. Cases with similar features to what are described here may demonstrate myelodysplasia-related gene mutations or cytogenetic abnormalities and would be classified as those types of AML rather than APMF.

References

1. Attardi E, Savi A, Borsellino B, et al. Applicability of 2022 classifications of acute myeloid leukemia in the real-world setting. *Blood Adv*. 2023;7(17):5122-5131.
2. Nichols CR, Roth BJ, Heerema N, Griep J, Tricot G. Hematologic neoplasia associated with primary mediastinal germ-cell tumors. *N Engl J Med*. 1990;322(20):1425-1429.
3. Bennett JM, Catovsky D, Daniel MT, et al. Proposed revised criteria for the classification of acute myeloid leukemia. A report of the French-American-British Cooperative Group. *Ann Intern Med*. 1985;103(4):620-625.
4. Walter RB, Othus M, Burnett AK, et al. Significance of FAB subclassification of "acute myeloid leukemia, NOS" in the 2008 WHO classification: analysis of 5848 newly diagnosed patients. *Blood*. 2013;121(13):2424-2431.
5. Wang SA, Hasserjian RP. Acute erythroleukemias, acute megakaryoblastic leukemias, and reactive mimics: a guide to a number of perplexing entities. *Am J Clin Pathol*. 2015;144(1):44-60.
6. Ohgami RS, Chisholm KM, Ma L, Arber DA. E-cadherin is a specific marker for erythroid differentiation and has utility, in combination with CD117 and CD34, for enumerating myeloblasts in hematopoietic neoplasms. *Am J Clin Pathol*. 2014;141(5):656-64.
7. Chisholm KM, Heerema-McKenney AE, Choi JK, et al. Acute erythroid leukemia is enriched in NUP98 fusions: a report from the Children's Oncology Group. *Blood Adv*. 2020;4(23):6000-6008.
8. Zhu GG, Inam Z, Calleroz A, Pillai V, Schore RJ, Cheng J. Pediatric acute erythroid leukemias with monocytic antigen expression and novel chromosomal translocations. *Pediatr Blood Cancer*. 2023;70(8):e30333.
9. Peterson LC, Parkin JL, Arthur DC, Brunning RD. Acute basophilic leukemia. A clinical, morphologic, and cytogenetic study of eight cases. *Am J Clin Pathol*. 1991;96(2):160-170.
10. Staal-Viliare A, Latger-Cannard V, Didion J, et al. CD203c /CD117—an useful phenotype profile for acute basophilic leukaemia diagnosis in cases of undifferentiated blasts. *Leuk Lymphoma*. 2007;48(2):439-441.
11. Dastugue N, Duchayne E, Kuhlein E, et al. Acute basophilic leukaemia and translocation t(X;6)(p11;q23). *Br J Haematol*. 1997;98(1):170-176.
12. Quelen C, Lippert E, Struski S, et al. Identification of a transforming MYB-GATA1 fusion gene in acute basophilic leukemia: a new entity in male infants. *Blood*. 2011;117(21):5719-5722.
13. Hoyle CF, Sherrington P, Hayhoe FG. Translocation (3;6)(q21;p21) in acute myeloid leukemia with abnormal thrombopoiesis and basophilia. *Cancer Genet Cytogenet*. 1988;30(2):261-267.

14. Orazi A, O'Malley DP, Jiang J, et al. Acute panmyelosis with myelofibrosis: an entity distinct from acute megakaryoblastic leukemia. *Mod Pathol.* 2005;18(5):603-614.
15. Sultan C, Sigaux F, Imbert M, Reyes F. Acute myelodysplasia with myelofibrosis: a report of eight cases. *Br J Haematol.* 1981;49(1):11-16.
16. Suvajdzic N, Marisavljevic D, Kraguljac N, et al. Acute panmyelosis with myelofibrosis: clinical, immunophenotypic and cytogenetic study of twelve cases. *Leuk Lymphoma.* 2004;45(9):1873-1879.
17. Thiele J, Kvasnicka HM, Zerhusen G, et al. Acute panmyelosis with myelofibrosis: a clinicopathological study on 46 patients including histochemistry of bone marrow biopsies and follow-up. *Ann Hematol.* 2004;83(8):513-521.

Chapter 36
Myeloid Sarcoma

Marco Pizzi, Richard A. Larson, Attilio Orazi, and Stefano A. Pileri

Definition

Myeloid sarcoma (MS) is an extramedullary tumor mass of myeloid blasts, with or without maturation, causing at least partial tissue effacement. Nondestructive and/or non-tumor-forming blast infiltrates outside the bone marrow (BM) belong to the spectrum of extramedullary acute myeloid leukemia (AML), eg, *leukemia cutis*, but are not included in the MS category.

Synonyms

Granulocytic sarcoma; myelosarcoma; extramedullary myeloid tumor; chloroma; myeloblastoma (not recommended).

Epidemiology

MS is a rare disorder, occurring in both adults and children, with slight male predominance (male-to-female ratio: 1.5:1-2:1). Adult cases have a median age at diagnosis of 45 to 65 years. The disease occurs in one of following settings: (i) solitary (de novo or aleukemic) MS; (ii) MS with concurrent AML; (iii) MS as initial manifestation of relapse in a previously diagnosed AML; (iv) MS following non-AML myeloid neoplasms.[1] BM evaluation, including immunophenotyping and cytogenetic and molecular analysis, is mandatory in all the cases to clarify the clinicopathologic setting.

Solitary MS accounts for about 0.8% of newly diagnosed AML. Most cases progress to overt AML, and the time to progression depends on genetic and clinical features (eg, patient age and sex; disease location). MSs with concurrent AML are clinically detected in 2% to 9% of AML, but their prevalence is as high as 20% when ^{18}F-fluorodeoxyglucose (^{18}FDG) positron emission tomography/computed tomography (PET/CT) studies are applied.[2] MSs following non-AML myeloid disorders are most frequent in blast phase myeloproliferative neoplasms (MPNs) and myelodysplastic syndromes with excess blasts. Such cases tend to have higher age at diagnosis.[1] Finally, MSs presenting as initial manifestation of relapse in a previously diagnosed AML occur most frequently in patients treated with allogeneic hematopoietic stem cell transplantation (allo-HSCT). They have been variably associated with prior graft-versus-host disease.

General Clinical Features

The signs and symptoms of MS depend on tumor size and location. Although MS can occur in virtually any organ, the most common sites include the skin (25%-30%), soft tissue and bones (30%-35%), lymph nodes (20%-25%), the gastrointestinal tract (10%-15%), the reproductive system (5%-10%), the head and neck region (5%-10%), and the central nervous system (6%-7%). Specific locations correlate with age and ethnicity and with the clinical setting. Gastrointestinal and reproductive tract involvement is more common in patients <70 years, mediastinal locations are more frequent in Asians, and testicular, soft tissue, and cutaneous involvement is enriched in MS presenting as initial manifestation of relapse in patients previously diagnosed with AML.[1,3]

MS may present as either single or multiple lesions, especially in cases with concurrent AML. In this setting, ^{18}FDG-PET/CT studies have disclosed a median of two lesions per patient (range: 1-12 lesions) with highly variable glucose uptake values.[2] MSs rarely occur also in association with lymphoid and solid tumors. Such MS may be therapy-related or derive from tumor cell progenitors, which are shared with the associated malignancy. This is most likely the case of concurrent MS and germ cell tumors of the mediastinum.[4]

Morphology

MS consists of aggregates of blasts with diffuse or interstitial growth pattern (Figure 36.1). Stromal fibrosis and necrotic areas can be seen. Rarely, discrete aggregates of mature plasmacytoid dendritic cells can also be documented. In lymph nodes, the myeloid infiltrate causes total effacement of nodal architecture or expands paracortical areas with preservation of reactive germinal centers (Figure 36.2).[5]

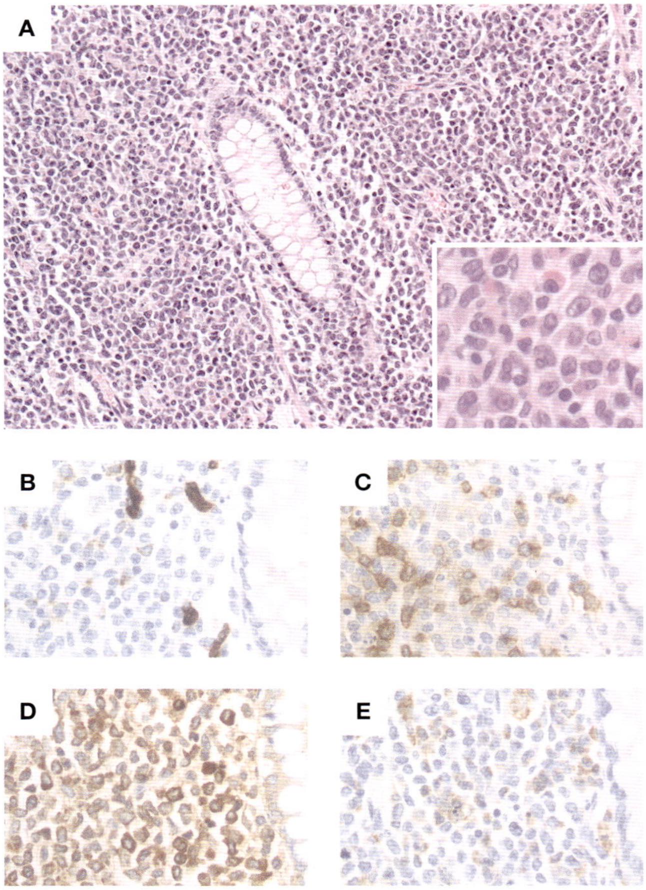

FIGURE 36.1 Myeloid sarcoma of the large bowel. The intestinal wall is effaced by confluent sheets of myeloid blasts **(A)**. Tumor cells are small to medium-sized with finely dispersed chromatin, small nucleoli and scant cytoplasm (**A,** insert). They are focally positive for CD34 **(B)** with partial expression of CD117 **(C)** and diffuse positivity for MPO **(D)**. CD68-PGM1 immunostain is positive in occasional cells **(E)**. (H&E and Immunoperoxidase stains; original magnification, A. ×10; B, C, and D. ×40).

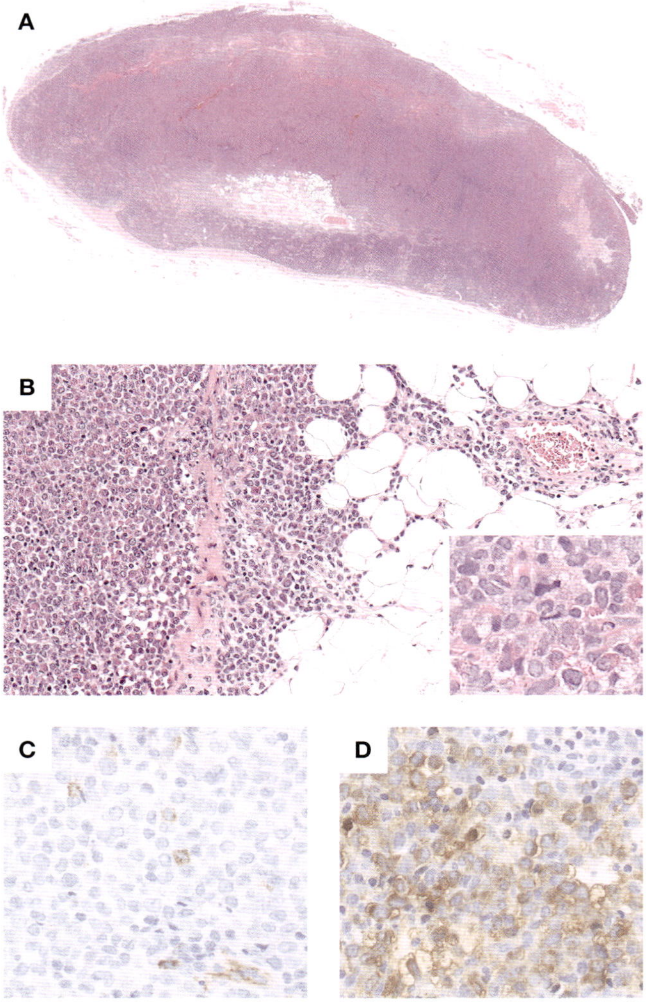

FIGURE 36.2 Nodal myeloid sarcoma in acute myeloid leukemia with inv(16)(p13.1q22)/*CBFB::MYH11*. Nodal architecture is almost completely effaced by confluent sheets of blasts admixed with eosinophilic precursors **(A)**. The neoplastic infiltrate extends beyond the nodal capsule into the perinodal fat **(B)** and consists of small myeloblasts with open chromatin and scant cytoplasm, admixed with eosinophilic precursors at different stages of maturation (**B,** insert). The blasts are almost completely negative for CD34 **(C)**, while they express MPO **(D)** and CD117 (not shown). (H&E and Immunoperoxidase stains; original magnification: A. ×1.25; B. ×10; C and D. ×40).

Most MSs have myeloblast morphology, with variable degrees of maturation toward more differentiated myeloid precursors, such as promyelocytes. A proportion of the cases shows myelomonocytic or pure monoblastic morphology with blasts displaying irregular nuclei, prominent nucleoli, and abundant, pale, or slightly basophilic cytoplasm. MSs with myelomonocytic and monoblastic morphology are particularly common in the skin.

Megakaryoblastic and erythroblastic differentiation is exceedingly rare and tends to correlate with blast transformation of MPN. Erythroblastic sarcomas are also reported in children and can mimic Ewing sarcoma or other poorly differentiated solid tumors.

Cases associated with blast phase of MPN may show myeloblasts admixed with aggregates of mature myeloid cells (eg, granulocytes) or with foci of trilineage extramedullary hematopoiesis. Such cases should not be confused with nodular extramedullary hematopoiesis (ie, accumulation of mature hematopoietic cells), which can be seen in advanced-stage MPN. These lesions are composed of myeloid, erythroid, and megakaryocytic precursors at different stages of maturation but lack a significant blast component.

Immunophenotype

The phenotype of MS varies according to blast lineage. CD34 and CD117 are positive in most MSs with myeloblastic features but may be negative (or only focally positive) in cases with myelomonocytic and monoblastic differentiation (Figure 36.1). Myeloperoxidase is expressed in most myeloblastic and in all myelomonocytic MSs but is negative in monoblastic cases. By immunohistochemistry, the latter express monocytic markers, such as CD68-PGM1, CD14, CD163, and CD4.[1,5] Negativity for TCL1, CD303, and TCF4 and positivity for lysozyme support distinction from blastic plasmacytoid dendritic cell neoplasm (BPDCN). Foci of mature plasmacytoid dendritic cells express TCL1, CD303, CD123, TCF4, and CD4 but are usually negative for BCL2, CD56, and SOX4. This helps in the differential diagnosis with BPDCN. Erythroblastic MSs are positive for CD71, glycophorin-A/C, e-cadherin, and hemoglobin, while megakaryoblastic MSs express CD41, CD42b, CD61, and LAT.[5] CD68-KP1, CD33, and CD43 are positive in the vast majority of MSs, but they are not specific. Aberrant expression of TdT, CD3, CD5, and/or cytokeratins is reported in a subset of cases.[1,5] Positivity for CD45 is usually dim, consistent with what is observed in nonneoplastic blasts. Discrepant phenotypes can be documented in clonally related lesions at different time points or anatomic sites, as a result of therapy-related or immune-mediated selective pressures.

Genetics

Cytogenetic aberrations occur in 45% to 65% of MSs and overlap with those observed in AML. The most common abnormalities include t(8;21)(q22;q22.1)/*RUNX1::RUNX1T1*, inv(16)(p13.1q22), or t(16;16)(p13.1;q22)/*CBFB::MYH11*; chromosome 11q23.3/*KMT2A* rearrangements; trisomy 8; −7/del(7q), del(5q); and trisomy 4 (Table 36.1). Of these, t(8;21)(q22;q22.1)/*RUNX1::RUNX1T1* has been associated with orbital MS in children and inv(16)(p13.1q22) or t(16;16)(p13.1;q22)/*CBFB::MYH11* with MS arising in the abdominal cavity.[6] Complex karyotypes occur in up to 39% of cases and are most common in secondary MS.[7] The *NFIA::CBFA2T3* fusion, corresponding to t(1;16)(p31;q24), has been repeatedly documented in erythroblastic sarcoma/pure erythroid leukemia of childhood and is specific to this condition.[8]

The mutational landscape of MS, although not yet fully characterized, seems to be largely similar to that of AML. Mutated genes include *NPM1*, *FLT3*-ITD, and *FLT3*-TKD; the tyrosine kinase receptor *KIT*; RAS pathway genes (*KRAS*; *NRAS*; *PTPN11*; *CBL*); the tumor suppressor *TP53*; epigenetic modifiers (*TET2*; *DNMT3A*; *IDH1*; *IDH2*; *ASXL1*); transcription factors (*RUNX1*; *WT1*); and genes encoding spliceosome proteins (*SRSF2*; *SF3B1*).[9,10] Of these, *KIT*, RAS pathway, and *NPM1* mutations are enriched in AML with

TABLE 36.1 Recurrent genetic aberrations of myeloid sarcoma

Cytogenetic abnormality	Frequency (%)
t(8;21)(q22;q22.1)/*RUNX1::RUNX1T1*	2-77
11q23.3/*KMT2A* rearrangements	0-13
inv(16)(p13.1q22) or t(16;16)(p13.1;q22)/*CBFB::MYH11*	0-11
+8	0-7
+4	0-7
−7/del(7q)	0-13
del(5q)	2-8
Complex karyotype	5-39
Gene mutated	**Frequency (%)**
NPM1	5-50
FLT3-ITD	6-15
FLT3-TKD	2-17
KIT	0-20
NRAS	10-30
KRAS	2-15
TET2	15-21
RUNX1	2-7
IDH1 or *IDH2*	2-43
PTPN11	14-17
EZH2	5-17
DNMT3A	6-28
ASXL1	4-17
TP53	0-21
CBL	2-11
SRSF2	2-21

associated MS. In such cases, genetic profiling discloses a strong relationship between paired AML and MS samples, with slight differences consistent with linear or divergent clonal evolution.[9,11]

The genetic bases of extramedullary blast seeding have been investigated by early studies, which suggested a pathogenic role for *NFE3* mutations.[11] The lack of such mutations in a subsequent series of MS[12] has challenged this hypothesis and points toward other genetic drivers for extramedullary blast colonization.

Prognosis and Clinical Comment

The survival rates of MS parallel those seen in patients with more typical presentation of blood and BM involvement by AML with similar genetic features. Many clinical, laboratory, and genetic features have been associated with prognosis, yielding to conflicting and inconclusive results. To date, response to therapy is the best determinant of overall outcome.

Although MS may occur as a solitary tumor, local therapy is not sufficient. The median time to the emergence of AML is 5 to 12 months after inadequate (local) or delayed systemic therapy.[6] Isolated MS at relapse is rare and heralds systemic relapse. ^{18}FDG-PET/CT scans may identify multiple, clinically occult tumors.[2]

Data on therapeutic regimens are only available from retrospective clinical series. The best outcomes have followed systemic chemotherapy appropriate for AML. Most recent regimens have included cytarabine and an anthracycline. Response to allo-HSCT is variable, with 5-year survival rates of 47%.[6] Case reports using venetoclax and hypomethylating agents, as used for older or less fit patients with AML, have been published.

Postremission therapy has been inadequately studied. Focal radiotherapy has been used as consolidation therapy, but it is unclear whether this modality improves outcomes over chemotherapy alone. Twenty gray is sufficient for myeloblasts, and its use is dependent in part on the radiation site. Targeted therapy with tyrosine kinase inhibitors has been used for MS with a *BCR::ABL1* or *PDGFRA* rearrangement. Tretinoin (ATRA) and arsenic trioxide should be used for extramedullary acute promyelocytic leukemia. There is limited experience with *FLT3*, *IDH1*, or *IDH2* inhibitors. At present, there are not enough data to support a risk-adjusted therapy, particularly in the setting of isolated MS. Owing to the rarity of this disorder and in order to include larger groups of patients, controlled prospective multicenter studies are necessary.[13]

References

1. Kawamoto K, Miyoshi H, Yoshida N, Takizawa J, Sone H, Ohshima K. Clinicopathological, cytogenetic, and prognostic analysis of 131 myeloid sarcoma patients. *Am J Surg Pathol.* 2016;40(11):1473-1483.
2. Stölzel F, Lüer T, Löck S, et al. The prevalence of extramedullary acute myeloid leukemia detected by (18) FDG-PET/CT: final results from the prospective PETAML trial. *Haematologica.* 2020;105(6):1552-1558.
3. Goyal G, Bartley AC, Patnaik MM, Litzow MR, Al-Kali A, Go RS. Clinical features and outcomes of extramedullary myeloid sarcoma in the United States: analysis using a national data set. *Blood Cancer J.* 2017;7(8):e592. e592–e592. doi:10.1038/bcj.2017.79
4. Taylor J, Donoghue MTA, Ho C, et al. Germ cell tumors and associated hematologic malignancies evolve from a common shared precursor. *J Clin Invest.* 2020;130(12):6668-6676.
5. Pileri SA, Ascani S, Cox MC, et al. Myeloid sarcoma: clinico-pathologic, phenotypic and cytogenetic analysis of 92 adult patients. *Leukemia.* 2007;21(2):340-350.
6. Bakst RL, Tallman MS, Douer D, Yahalom J. How I treat extramedullary acute myeloid leukemia. *Blood.* 2011;118(14):3785-3793.
7. Claerhout H, Van Aelst S, Melis C, et al. Clinicopathological characteristics of de novo and secondary myeloid sarcoma: A monocentric retrospective study. *Eur J Haematol.* 2018;100(6):603-612.
8. Linnik Y, Pastakia D, Dryden I, Head DR, Mason EF. Primary central nervous system erythroid sarcoma with NFIA-CBFA2T3 translocation: a rare but distinct clinicopathologic entity. *Am J Hematol.* 2020;95(11): E299-E301.
9. Kashofer K, Gornicec M, Lind K, et al. Detection of prognostically relevant mutations and translocations in myeloid sarcoma by next generation sequencing. *Leuk Lymphoma.* 2018;59(2):501-504.
10. Choi M, Jeon YK, Sun C-H, et al. RTK-RAS pathway mutation is enriched in myeloid sarcoma. *Blood Cancer J.* 2018;8(5):43. doi:10.1038/s41408-018-0083-6
11. Lazarevic V, Orsmark-Pietras C, Lilljebjörn H, et al. Isolated myelosarcoma is characterized by recurrent NFE2 mutations and concurrent preleukemic clones in the bone marrow. *Blood.* 2018;131(5):577-581.
12. Anekpuritanang T, Klairmont MM, Gradowski J, et al. In a multi-institutional cohort of myeloid sarcomas, NFE2 mutation prevalence is lower than previously reported. *Blood Adv.* 2021;5(23):5057-5059.
13. Shahin O, Ravandi F. Myeloid sarcoma. *Curr Opin Hematol.* 2020;27(2):88-94.

SECTION 8

Myeloid Proliferations Associated With Down Syndrome

Chapter 37

Myeloid Proliferations Associated With Down Syndrome

Michele E. Paessler, Benjamin A. Kaumeyer, and Sarah K. Tasian

TRANSIENT ABNORMAL MYELOPOIESIS OF DOWN SYNDROME

Definition

Transient abnormal myelopoiesis (TAM) is a rare, preleukemic clonal myeloproliferative disorder associated with somatic mutations of *GATA1* occurring exclusively in the neonatal period in 25% to 30% of newborns with constitutional trisomy 21.

Synonyms

Transient leukemia of Down syndrome, transient aberrant myelopoiesis in Down syndrome, fetal leukemia of Down syndrome (not recommended).

Epidemiology

Constitutional trisomy 21 (Down syndrome; DS) is the most common chromosomal abnormality, occurring in one of every 700 newborn babies (6000 cases/year) in the United States. DS in infants can be associated with a spectrum of hematologic abnormalities, ranging from neutrophilia, thrombocytopenia, macrocytosis, and polycythemia. Clinical TAM is detected in the blood of 10% to 15% of neonates with DS, while another 15% have silent TAM with no noticeable clinical features. TAM has also been reported to occur in patients with trisomy 21 mosaicism.[1]

Virtually all cases of TAM are associated with somatic mutation in *GATA1*, a transcription factor that is crucial for normal megakaryocyte and erythroid development, that is acquired prenatally in utero. These truncating mutations produce shorter-length GATA1 proteins and serve as a clonal marker in the progression to myeloid leukemia associated with DS (ML-DS). Of note, patients with DS are also at increased risk of developing B-cell acute lymphoblastic leukemia with 2.1% incidence by 10 years of age and 2.7% by 30 years of age.[2,3]

General Clinical Features

TAM can manifest in infants with DS within the first 6 months of life, but the median age of presentation typically is 3 to 7 days after birth. Neonates classically present with leukocytosis and detectable peripheral blasts, usually megakaryoblastic, and may have end-organ involvement with palpable hepatomegaly (40% of cases), splenomegaly (30%), and skin rash (~10%). Bone marrow involvement is usually minimal or absent when rarely assessed (generally not clinically indicated). Some infants also experience jaundice, ascites, and pericardial and/or pleural effusions, which can result in respiratory distress. Less common, but severe, clinical manifestations of TAM include hepatic fibrosis, hydrops fetalis, and multisystem organ dysfunction.

Importantly, neonates with DS and TAM have an increased risk (~30% of patients) of developing subsequent ML-DS during the first 5 years of life, so require close physical examination and blood count monitoring in the perinatal and early childhood period. To date, a priori predictive biomarkers of ML-DS development have not been identified.[4]

Clinical laboratory features of TAM typically demonstrate leukocytosis, even white blood cell (WBC) counts ≥100,000/μL in 20% to 30% of cases, with associated thrombocytopenia and circulating peripheral blood blasts that may raise initial suspicion for acute leukemia. It is noteworthy that approximately 15% of patients with TAM may be clinically asymptomatic. Therefore, the diagnosis may be incidental and discovered during routine laboratory assessments for other clinical purposes. Rarely, detection of TAM in peripheral blood may provide the first clinical suspicion of DS in a newborn and lead to confirmatory diagnostic constitutional trisomy 21 testing. As mentioned earlier, TAM has also been reported in patients without clinical features of DS who are subsequently determined to have trisomy 21 mosaicism in blood and bone marrow.

Morphology

TAM blasts in the peripheral blood morphologically may range from undifferentiated to large with a high nuclear to cytoplasmic ratio. Characteristic features also include round nuclei with fine, dispersed chromatin and discrete, small nucleoli with deep basophilic cytoplasm and characteristic cytoplasmic blebbing (Figure 37.1). Occasionally, megakaryocyte nuclei may be seen in peripheral blood circulation. Other blood findings include anisocytosis, thrombocytosis or thrombocytopenia, and large platelets. Of note, circulating blasts can be observed in neonates without DS and in neonates with DS without TAM and may represent benign etiologies of neonatal sepsis or stress and left shift. However, a blast percentage exceeding 10% should prompt *GATA1* mutation testing given longer-term clinical implications in infants with confirmed TAM and increased risk of subsequent ML-DS.

Immunophenotype

Immunophenotype characteristics of the blasts in TAM are similar to those of ML-DS. TAM blasts typically express panhematopoietic antigen CD45, stem cell antigens CD34 and CD117, myeloid antigens CD33 and CD13, and megakaryocytic antigens CD41, CD61, and CD42b. Additionally, non-lineage-specific antigens, such as CD7 and CD56, are commonly expressed.[5,6]

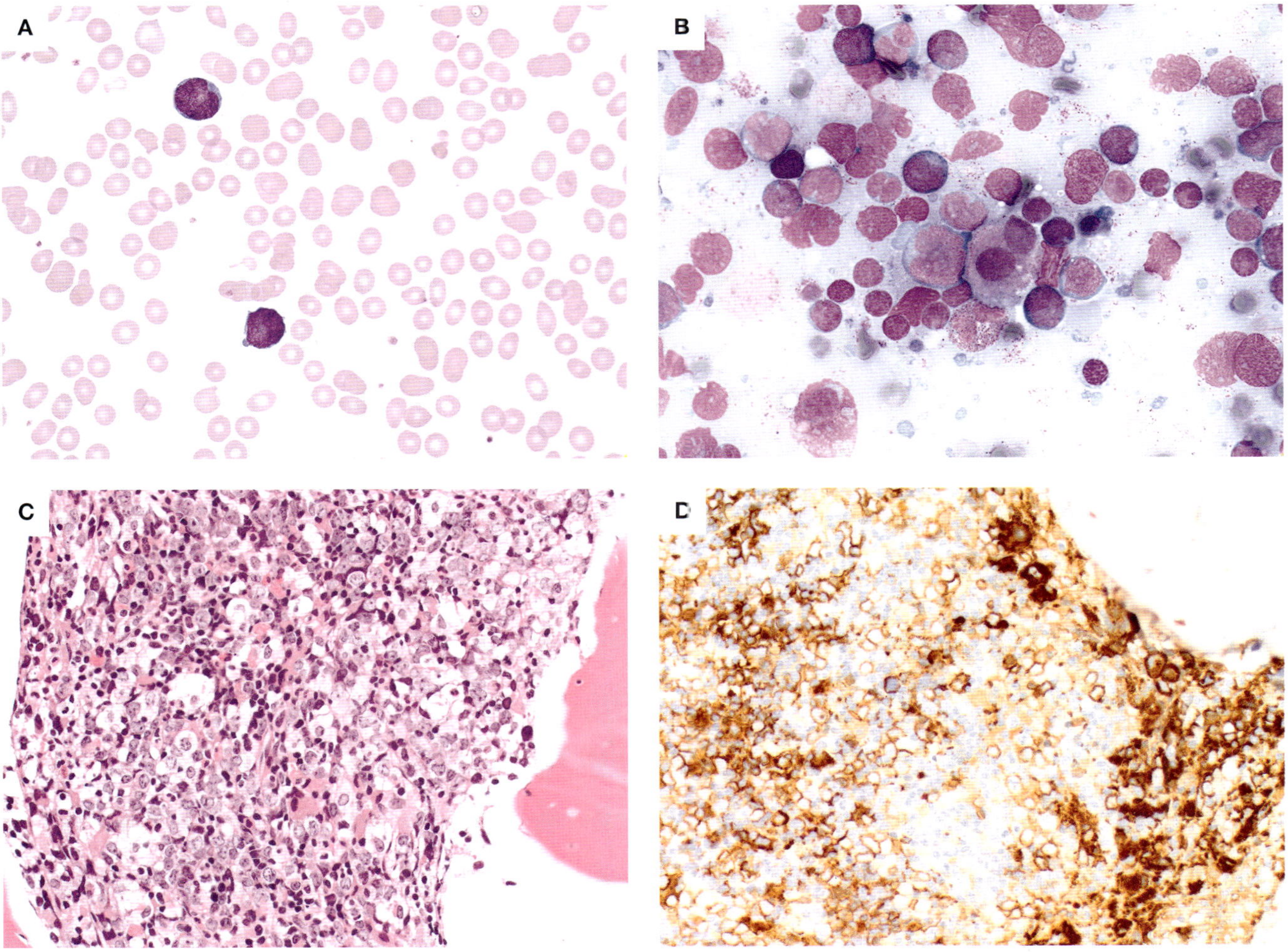

FIGURE 37.1 Myeloid leukemia associated with Down syndrome demonstrating characteristic megakaryoblastic differentiation. **A:** Peripheral blood smear showing blasts with basophilic cytoplasm and cytoplasmic blebs. **B:** Bone marrow touch imprint (Wright-Giemsa stain) showing scattered blasts and a dysplastic bilobed megakaryocyte. **C:** Bone marrow core biopsy showing a proliferation of blasts within a background of scattered megakaryocytes with dysplastic features. Moderate increased marrow fibrosis is also seen (reticulin stain showed MF 1-2). **D:** CD42b immunohistochemistry is positive in the majority of blasts and highlights background megakaryocytes.

Genetics

The diagnosis of TAM requires confirmation of constitutional trisomy 21, which may be established relatively rapidly via karyotype. As mentioned earlier, TAM and ML-DS are both associated with mutations in the *GATA1* gene in virtually all cases.[7] *GATA1* is a zinc finger transcription factor on the X chromosome. Its full-length form, termed *GATA1* long, is critical for normal erythroid and megakaryocytic differentiation. Most *GATA1* mutations, whether deletions, insertions, or point mutations, are clustered in exons 2 or 3, which leads to a truncated protein termed GATA1 short (GATA1s). *GATA1* mutations seen in TAM/ML-DS are localized at the 5′ end of the gene, resulting in the exclusive production of the variant GATA1s that lacks the N-terminal activation domain and disrupts normal hematopoiesis, thereby facilitating TAM development. *GATA1* exon 2/3 mutation analysis can be performed in patients with clinical suspicion of TAM. The presence of these mutations is a distinctive molecular marker and highlights the clonal relationship between TAM and ML-DS, as the same mutations are identified in patients with both TAM and ML-DS. Subsequent development of ML-DS in patients with history of TAM is usually driven by acquisition of additional somatic chromosomal abnormalities or genetic mutations in *GATA1*-mutant cells, such as dup (1q), del(6q), del(7p), +8,+11, and +21.[8,9]

Prognosis and Clinical Comment

The clinical course of TAM is variable; most infants experience spontaneous resolution of peripheral leukocytosis and organomegaly (if present) within 2 to 3 months without need for treatment, although mortality due to end-organ failure can occur in a minority of cases.[10] A small percentage of neonates with DS and high-risk TAM, particularly those with WBC counts ≥100,00, ascites or pleural effusions, and/or massive hepatosplenomegaly, benefit from low-dose chemotherapy for more rapid cytoreduction and improvement of end-organ dysfunction until natural resolution of TAM pathophysiology. Cytarabine 10 mg/m^2 every 12 hours intravenously or subcutaneously × 5 to 7 days is most commonly used for such patients with good effect. Occasionally, a second (or third) course of low-dose cytarabine is necessary for patients with persistent or recurrent leukocytosis. Higher-dosed chemotherapy and leukapheresis procedures are not recommended or generally necessary and may paradoxically increase morbidity and mortality.[10] Importantly, use of low-dose cytarabine in neonates with TAM has not been shown to reduce incidence of subsequent ML-DS.[11]

MYELOID LEUKEMIA ASSOCIATED WITH DOWN SYNDROME

Definition

ML-DS is a myeloid neoplasm that usually presents in children with DS before 5 years of age and has a characteristic set of clinical, morphologic, immunophenotypic, and genetic findings characterized by the presence of somatic *GATA1* mutation. Notably, myeloid neoplasms that develop in patients with DS after the age of 4 years frequently lack *GATA1* mutations and should be considered sporadic myelodysplastic syndrome (MDS) or acute myeloid leukemia (AML).[12] TAM can precede ML-DS and often present identical morphologic findings and *GATA1* mutations. However, ML-DS can be distinguished from TAM by the older age of the patients (TAM uniformly resolves by 3 months of age) and failure of the myeloid proliferation to spontaneously regress.

Cases of ML-DS most frequently present as acute megakaryoblastic leukemia, although overt AML may be preceded by an MDS-like phase.[13] Nevertheless, there are no significant biological differences between AML and MDS-like presentations in the population with DS, so a diagnosis of ML-DS does not require the presence of 20% blasts.

Synonyms

Acute myeloid leukemia associated with Down syndrome (not recommended).

Epidemiology

ML-DS almost always presents before the age of 5 years (median age 1.6 years), and approximately 1% to 2% of children with DS develop ML-DS.[14,15] Children with a history of TAM are at increased risk of ML-DS with approximately 30% eventually developing ML-DS.

Morphology

Overt leukemia may be preceded by a relatively indolent MDS-like phase, which can last for several months, and frequently presents with thrombocytopenia. During this time, the bone marrow (if assessed) may show a proliferation of small megakaryocytes without a significant increase in blasts.[13,16] Dyserythropoiesis and marrow fibrosis may also be seen.

Most cases of ML-DS present with prominent megakaryoblastic differentiation. Blasts are frequently present in the blood (Figure 37.1), although most patients do not have an elevated WBC count. Red blood cells often show anisopoikilocytosis, including dacrocytes reflecting marrow fibrosis. Thrombocytopenia and giant platelets may be present, similar to characteristics seen with TAM.

Bone marrow aspirates may be hemodilute due to marrow fibrosis. The blasts often display megakaryoblastic differentiation with round to slightly irregular nuclei, a moderate amount of basophilic cytoplasm, and occasional cytoplasmic blebs. Some cases may show a population of blasts with a more primitive, undifferentiated appearance. Micromegakaryocytes, erythroid precursors with megaloblastoid changes, and dysgranulopoiesis may be observed.

Immunophenotype

ML-DS blasts have a similar immunophenotype as the blasts identified in TAM, with evidence of megakaryoblastic differentiation.[17] They are typically positive for CD117, CD13, CD33, CD38, CD11b, CD7, CD4(dim), CD41, CD42b, CD61, CD36, and CD71, while negative for cMPO, TdT, CD14, CD15, and glycophorin A.[5,6] In contrast to TAM, the blasts in ML-DS are less likely to express CD34 while more likely to express CD11b.[5,17] Also, CD7 and CD11b are expressed more frequently in ML-DS compared with acute megakaryoblastic leukemia in patients without DS. Of note, the nonmalignant myeloblasts in the regenerating bone following chemotherapy can show aberrant expression of CD34, CD56, and heterogeneous HLA-DR; this finding should not be interpreted as evidence of residual disease in patients with ML-DS.[18] Although the blasts in ML-DS commonly demonstrate a megakaryoblastic phenotype, nonmegakaryocytic AML including AML with minimal differentiation are reported.

Genetics

The combination of germline trisomy 21 and somatic mutations in *GATA1* is specific for both TAM and ML-DS.[19] In fact, genetic profiling has demonstrated that ML-DS develops from evolution of a TAM clone after accumulating additional genetic lesions.[8,9] These additional mutations include multiple components of the cohesion complex (*STAG2, RAD21, SMC3,* and *SMC1A*), *CTCF, EZH2, KANSL1,* JAK family kinases, *MPL, SH2B3,* and multiple *RAS* pathway genes. Trisomy 8 is also a common finding.

Prognosis and Clinical Comment

Given the high incidence of future ML-DS that requires intensive chemotherapy for cure, regular clinical monitoring of children with TAM (or history of TAM) is required. Initially, all infants with TAM should be closely followed by physical examination, complete blood count (CBC) with differential, and imaging if indicated until resolution of blasts and normalization of CBC occurs. The Children's Oncology Group (COG) standards for children with DS and history of TAM then include CBC monitoring and physical examination until the second birthday and every 3 to 6 months until the fourth birthday. Routine bone marrow assessment is not required unless CBC abnormalities suspicious for ML-DS are detected.

Recent clinical trials by the COG and other pediatric oncology consortia have reported excellent clinical outcomes of children with ML-DS when treated with six cycles of multiagent chemotherapy (cytarabine, daunomycin, and thioguanine) regimens, with 5-year event-free survival and overall survival exceeding 90%. Of note, these regimens are less intensive than those used for children with non-DS-associated AML and are associated with higher survival rates.

References

1. Hitzler J, Garraus M. Myeloid leukemia associated with Down syndrome (ML-DS). UpToDate 139448. 2023. Myeloid leukemia associated with Down syndrome (ML-DS) (medilib.ir).
2. Buitenkamp TD, Izraeli S, Zimmermann M, et al. Acute lymphoblastic leukemia in children with Down syndrome: a retrospective analysis from the Ponte di Legno study group. *Blood.* 2014;123(1):70-77.
3. Li Z, Chang TC, Junco JJ, et al. Genomic landscape of Down syndrome-associated acute lymphoblastic leukemia. *Blood.* 2023;142(2):172-184.
4. Bhatnagar N, Nizery L, Tunstall O, Vyas P, Roberts I. Transient abnormal myelopoiesis and AML in Down syndrome: an update. *Curr Hematol Malig Rep.* 2016;11(5):333-341.
5. Langebrake C, Creutzig U, Reinhardt D. Immunophenotype of Down syndrome acute myeloid leukemia and transient myeloproliferative disease differs significantly from other diseases with

morphologically identical or similar blasts. *Klin Pädiatr.* 2005;217(3):126-134.

6. Wang L, Peters JM, Fuda F, et al. Acute megakaryoblastic leukemia associated with trisomy 21 demonstrates a distinct immunophenotype. *Cytometry B Clin Cytom.* 2015;88(4):244-252.
7. Hitzler JK, Cheung J, Li Y, Scherer SW, Zipursky A. GATA1 mutations in transient leukemia and acute megakaryoblastic leukemia of Down syndrome. *Blood.* 2003;101(11):4301-4304.
8. Yoshida K, Toki T, Okuno Y, et al. The landscape of somatic mutations in Down syndrome-related myeloid disorders. *Nat Genet.* 2013;45(11):1293-1299.
9. Labuhn M, Perkins K, Matzk S, et al. Mechanisms of progression of myeloid preleukemia to transformed myeloid leukemia in children with Down syndrome. *Cancer Cell.* 2019;36(3):340-138.e10.
10. Boucher AC, Caldwell KJ, Crispino JD, Flerlage JE. Clinical and biological aspects of myeloid leukemia in Down syndrome. *Leukemia.* 2021;35(12):3352-3360.
11. Flasinski M, Scheibke K, Zimmermann M, et al. Low-dose cytarabine to prevent myeloid leukemia in children with Down syndrome: TMD Prevention 2007 study. *Blood Adv.* 2018;2(13):1532-1540.
12. Hasle H, Abrahamsson J, Arola M, et al. Myeloid leukemia in children 4 years or older with Down syndrome often lacks GATA1 mutation and cytogenetics and risk of relapse are more akin to sporadic AML. *Leukemia.* 2008;22(7):1428-1430.
13. Lange BJ, Kobrinsky N, Barnard DR, et al. Distinctive demography, biology, and outcome of acute myeloid leukemia and myelodysplastic syndrome in children with Down syndrome: children's Cancer Group Studies 2861 and 2891. *Blood.* 1998;91(2):608-615.
14. Taub JW, Berman JN, Hitzler JK, et al. Improved outcomes for myeloid leukemia of Down syndrome: a report from the Children's Oncology Group AAML0431 trial. *Blood.* 2017;129(25):3304-3313.
15. Marlow EC, Ducore J, Kwan ML, et al. Leukemia risk in a cohort of 3.9 million children with and without Down syndrome. *J Pediatr.* 2021;234:172-180.e3.
16. Zipursky A, Thorner P, De Harven E, Christensen H, Doyle J. Myelodysplasia and acute megakaryoblastic leukemia in Down's syndrome. *Leuk Res.* 1994;18(3):163-171.
17. Karandikar NJ, Aquino DB, McKenna RW, Kroft SH. Transient myeloproliferative disorder and acute myeloid leukemia in Down syndrome. An immunophenotypic analysis. *Am J Clin Pathol.* 2001;116(2):204-210.
18. Hsu FC, Hudson C, Wilson ER, et al. The impact of Down syndrome-specific nonmalignant hematopoietic regeneration in the bone marrow on the detection of leukemic measurable residual disease. *Cytometry B Clin Cytom.* 2023;104(4):311-318.
19. Greene ME, Mundschau G, Wechsler J, et al. Mutations in GATA1 in both transient myeloproliferative disorder and acute megakaryoblastic leukemia of Down syndrome. *Blood Cells Mol Dis.* 2003;31(3):351-356.

SECTION 9

Blastic Plasmacytoid Dendritic Cell Neoplasm

Chapter 38
Blastic Plasmacytoid Dendritic Cell Neoplasm

Fabio Facchetti, Andrew A. Lane, Luisa Lorenzi, and Stefano A. Pileri

Definition

Blastic plasmacytoid dendritic cell neoplasm (BPDCN) is an extremely rare hematologic malignancy characterized by a proliferation of immature plasmacytoid dendritic cells (pDCs), with a high frequency of skin and bone marrow involvement and poor outcome. The term BPDCN was initially introduced in the third edition World Health Organization Classification as an acute myeloid leukemia (AML)-related neoplasm and is currently classified as a distinct myeloid neoplasm entity.[1,2]

Synonyms

None.

Epidemiology

BPDCN accounts for <0.5% of all hematological malignancies. Patients are predominantly males (M/F: 3-4/1), with a median age at diagnosis of 67 years.[2,3] Rarely BPDCN has been reported in young individuals and children (median age: 10 years), but without the gender bias seen in adults.[4] The disease does not show racial or geographic predisposition.

General Clinical Features

In 70% to 90% of cases, BPDCN manifests initially with skin lesions, either alone (approximately 50%) or associated with lymphadenopathy. In 10% to 30% of cases, skin lesions with systemic bone marrow and/or blood involvement occur from the beginning, while a leukemic presentation alone is rare (7%) and mainly reported in younger individuals (median 52 years). Notably, in 24% of pediatric BPDCN the skin is not involved.[2,3,5,6]

Skin lesions are usually asymptomatic, single, or multiple, with variable sizes and features, including erythematous to bluish plaques and nodules, often surrounded by a yellowish halo, or hematoma-like lesions[7] (Figure 38.1A-C). Frequently they initially occur on sun-exposed areas (head, neck, or upper trunk) and disseminate during disease progression.[8] In 50% to 90% of cases, the bone marrow is extensively involved at presentation, while circulating blasts are less frequent. Patients may have severe cytopenias, reflecting the bone marrow involvement. Lymph node, spleen, and liver involvement occur in 40% to 50%, 9% to 25%, and 6% to 17% of cases, respectively. Symptomatic or occult central nervous system (CNS) involvement at diagnosis has been reported in 8% to 60% of patients and frequently occurs at disease relapse.[9] Less common sites of involvement include oral mucosa, lungs, tonsils, soft tissues, and eyes. In 15% to 20% of cases, BPDCN can be preceded by, occur concurrently with, or be followed by another myeloid neoplasm, mostly chronic myelomonocytic leukemia (CMML), myelodysplastic syndrome, or AML.[2,3]

BPDCN is frequently subject to diagnostic delay (mean 6.2 months from symptom onset; range 2-18 months), due to various factors such as its rarity, unusual clinical presentation, and overall limited experience of pathologists and clinicians with this entity.

Morphology

BPDCN manifests a wide histological spectrum, with tumor cells varying from medium-sized monomorphic blasts with roundish nuclei and inconspicuous nucleoli to pleomorphic cells with irregular nuclei or lymphoblast-like or monocytoid cells; immunoblastoid cells typically occur in cases with *MYC* gene rearrangement. The cytoplasm is generally scant, eosinophilic, and devoid of granules (Figure 38.2A and B). Mitotic activity is variable, as is the Ki-67 proliferation index (20%-80%). The skin infiltrate is usually extensive, involving the dermis and the subcutaneous fat but sparing the epidermis and adnexa. In lymph nodes, BPDCN initially involves the interfollicular areas, sparing B-cell follicles.[2,3,6] Tumor cell morphology is also quite heterogeneous on blood and marrow

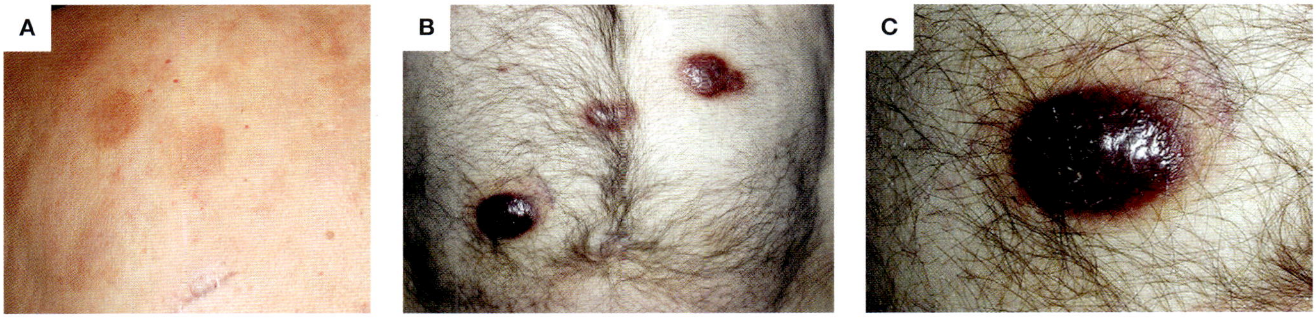

FIGURE 38.1 **A-C:** Various clinical presentation of cutaneous lesions in BPDCN: erythematous plaques (**A**) or hemorrhagic nodules (**B**), frequently surrounded by a yellowish halo (**C**).

smears.[5] Typical BPDCN blasts are medium sized with a round or irregular, often eccentric nucleus; small nucleoli; and faintly and irregularly basophilic cytoplasm. Small, clear cytoplasmic vacuoles are frequently found, and occasionally cells show a cytoplasmic protuberance ("tadpole cells") (Figure 38.2C). More rarely blasts have lymphoid-like or monoblastic-like features. Occasional cells may have azurophilic fine granules. In about one-third of cases, residual hematopoiesis shows dysplastic granulocytes and megakaryocytes, and monocytes can be increased.[5]

Immunophenotype

Immunotyping is essential for BPDCN diagnosis and is generally performed on skin or bone marrow biopsies.[2,3,5,6] When possible, flow cytometry analysis on marrow aspirates or blood samples should integrate with immunohistochemical evaluation, since some phenotypic discordances can occur. Moreover, flow cytometry is more sensitive and useful to distinguish BPDCN cells from reactive pDCs in cases of limited bone marrow involvement.[5]

The BPDCN immunophenotype includes a combination of markers regularly expressed in pDCs as well as those that are not normally expressed in pDCs (Table 38.1). Notably, the relatively common expression of TdT (30% of cases) or various combinations of non-lineage-specific myeloid, B-cell, and T-cell lymphoid antigens (eg, CD2, CD5, CD7, CD13, CD33, CD10, CD22, CD79a, BCL6, and/or CD117) can erroneously influence the diagnosis. Similar to pDCs, BPDCN blasts are negative for lineage-specific markers, such as CD3, CD19, CD20, myeloperoxidase, CD14, lysozyme, CD163, and CD11c. CD34 is only very rarely expressed in BPDCN (Table 38.2).[2,3,5,6]

TCF4, CD123, and TCL1 are typically expressed in BPDCN, while CD303 expression is more variable. CD304 is used only on flow cytometry. TCF4 is highly specific for BPDCN, being negative in other myeloid neoplasms including AML and only rarely expressed in B-lymphoblastic leukemia. In contrast, CD123 is often positive in myeloid blasts, although with dimmer expression compared with BPDCN. Coexpression of TCF4 and CD123 is highly specific for BPDCN. TCL1 is strongly expressed in most BPDCN, but it is also positive in about 20% of AML, in B-cell malignancies, and in T-cell prolymphocytic leukemia. Positivity for CD4, CD56, and CD123 occurs in more than 90% of BPDCN cases, but this combination should not be used

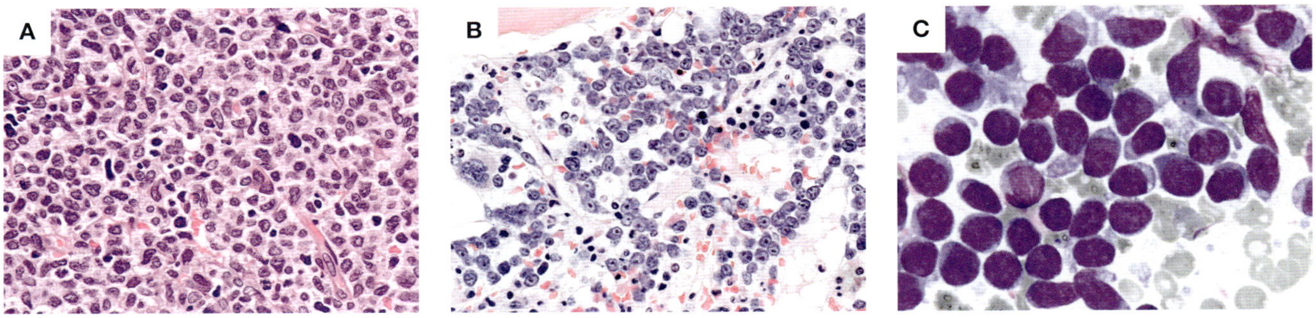

FIGURE 38.2 **A-C:** Examples of the variable morphology of tumor cells in BPDCN, varying from medium-sized pleomorphic cells with irregular elongated twisted nuclei (**A**) to immunoblast-like cells (**B**) (hematoxylin-eosin stain). In bone marrow aspirate (**C**) blasts often contain small peripheral cytoplasmic clear vacuoles and occasionally pseudopod-like extensions ("tadpole cells") (May-Grunwald-Giemsa stain).

TABLE 38.1 Immunophenotype of BPDCN tumor cells compared with reactive/normal pDCs

Positive in BPDCN and reactive pDCs	CD4, CD123, TCL1, CD303, TCF4 Additional: MX1, CD2AP, BCL11a, SPIB, CD304 (only by flow cytometry)
Positive in pDCs with loss or aberrant expression in BPDCN	CD68 (negative or paranuclear dots in BPDCN), Granzyme B (negative in BPDCN)
Positive in BPDCN and usually negative in pDCs	Consistent: CD56, BCL2, SOX4 Frequent: CD7, CD33 Occasional: CD2, CD5, CD10, CD13, CD117, CD79a, IRF4, BCL6, S100 TdT (10%-80% of tumor cells) Ki-67 (20%-80%)
Negative in BPDCN and reactive pDCs	CD3, CD19, CD20, CD11c, CD14, CD163, myeloperoxidase, lysozyme, CD34

BPDCN, blastic plasmacytoid dendritic cell neoplasm; pDC, plasmacytoid dendritic cell.

as a sole and sufficient criterion for diagnosis, since it can occur in AML and myeloid sarcomas with monocytic differentiation.

Various marker combinations have been proposed for BPDCN diagnosis and for distinguishing it from mimickers, which especially include AML and lymphoblastic leukemias presenting in the skin, and also mature B-cell lymphomas. BPDCN diagnosis should optimally be based on the expression of at least two pDCs antigens (TCF4, CD123, CD303, TCL1, and/or CD304) (Figure 38.3A-C), together with negativity for CD3, CD19, CD20, CD14, lysozyme, myeloperoxidase, and CD34 (Table 38.2).

TABLE 38.2 Diagnostic criteria for BPDCN

Sites of involvement at presentation	Skin (70%-90%) Bone marrow (50%-90%) Lymph nodes (40%-50%) Spleen (9%-25%) Liver (6%-17%) CNS (8%-60%)
Tumor cell morphology	Tissues: Mostly medium-sized monomorphic blasts with roundish nuclei, inconspicuous nucleoli, and scant eosinophilic cytoplasm. Sometimes lymphoblast-like, monocytoid, immunoblastoid, or pleomorphic blasts Blood and bone marrow smears: Medium-sized blasts with round or irregular nucleus, small nucleoli, faintly and irregularly basophilic cytoplasm. Often small clear cytoplasmic vacuoles and occasionally cytoplasmic protuberance Rarely lymphoid-like or monoblastic-like blasts
Immunoprofile	At least two of the following expressed: TCF4, CD123, CD303, TCL1, CD304 Also typically expressed: CD4, CD56
Exclusionary markers	Negative for CD3, CD19, CD20, CD14, lysozyme, myeloperoxidase, CD34

The distinction of BPDCN from pDCs hyperplasia or clonal proliferations of mature pDCs associated with CMML is mainly based on morphology (blastoid vs mature cells) and immunophenotype: in contrast to mature pDCs, BPDCN cells strongly express BCL2, CD56, and SOX4 (Table 38.1).[3,10] BPDCN must also be distinguished from AML associated with increased pDCs (AML-pDCs) in the bone marrow and peripheral blood, where pDCs can express CD34 and are typically CD56 and TCL1 negative. Notably, 75% of cases of AML-pDCs are characterized by *RUNX1* mutations, which are rarely detected in BPDCN[11] (see Genetics section).

Genetics

A complex karyotype (≥3 chromosomal aberrations) is observed in 50% to 75% of cases and is associated with inferior overall survival.[12] Chromosomes 5, 6, 9, 12, 13, and 15 are the most frequently affected and result in loss of tumor suppressor and cell-cycle regulator genes such as *CDKN1B/2A/2B*, *RB1*, *TP53*, *LATS2*, and *IKZF1*. Although none of these alterations are specific for BPDCN, the coexistence of deletions of several tumor suppressor genes represents a peculiar genomic feature of BPDCN. Inactivation of *IKZF1* and of *ETV6* are considered early events in the pathogenesis of BPDCN since they are found in morphologically uninvolved bone marrow of patients presenting with extramedullary disease. Rearrangements of the *MYB* gene are common in young and pediatric patients. *MYC* fusions are associated with immunoblastic morphology, strong and diffuse MYC protein expression, and more aggressive behavior. Notably, *MYB* and *MYC* rearrangements are mutually exclusive.

The BPDCN gene expression signature diverges from that of AML as well as lymphoid leukemias, being enriched in pDCs-related genes. It also significantly differs from normal pDCs by upregulation of cell proliferation genes and downregulation of genes encoding for type I interferons and regulation of the immune system. SOX4, a transcription factor involved in *TCF4* upregulation and pDC commitment, is upregulated in BPDCN compared with pDCs and is considered pivotal in BPDCN oncogenesis. Overexpression of genes related to Notch signaling, NF-κB activation, corticosteroid pathway, as well as BCL2 and CyclinD1 is typically found in BPDCN.[10,12]

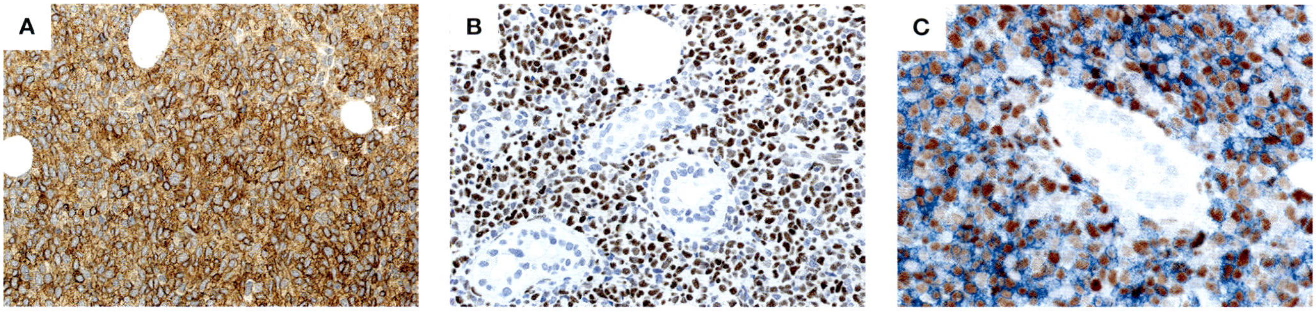

FIGURE 38.3 **A-C:** BPDCN positivity for highly specific markers including strong membranous CD123 (**A**), nuclear TCF4 (**B**), and membranous CD303 (**C**), the last shown in a double stain with TCF4 (CD303 cell membrane blue, TCF4 nuclear brown).

BPDCN is characterized by multiple but nonspecific mutations, many of which also occur in myeloid neoplasms; however, unlike AML, *FLT3*-ITD and *NPM1* mutations are rare in BPDCN. The most frequently mutated genes are *TET2* (36%-80%) and *ASXL1* (31%-44%), which are often comutated. Other genes affecting the epigenetic program (*EZH2, ATRX, IDH1, IDH2, DNMT3A, IKAROS* family, *SUZ12, ARID1A, PHF2, CHD8*) can be mutated. In addition, BPDCN often shows mutations involving the RAS pathway (*NRAS, KRAS*), splicing factors (*SF3B1, SRSF2, ZRSR2*), and tumor suppression (*TP53, RB1, ATM*).[12] No clonal rearrangements of T-cell or B-cell receptor genes are found in BPDCN, and the exceptional occurrence of *TRG* clonal rearrangements likely reflects clonal bystander T cells or T-cell clonotype expansion.[2]

Clonal hematopoiesis is highly prevalent in patients with BPDCN, suggesting that the earliest events in BPDCN pathogenesis occur in hematopoietic progenitor cells.[13] Frequent loss-of-function mutations of *ZRSR2,* located on X chromosome (Xp22.2), have been suggested to explain the striking male predominance of BPDCN. Mutations induced by ultraviolet radiation exposure, acquired by pDCs or committed precursors when circulating to the skin, can precede the acquisition of alterations associated with malignant transformation and impact the selection of neoplastic clones and disease evolution.[8] Clonal BPDCN evolution is characterized by additional mutations occurring during progression or in different sites, and BPDCN shares common mutations with co-occurring myeloid neoplasms such as CMML.[12,14]

Prognosis and Clinical Comment

Median overall survival ranges from 9 to 24 months and appears to be influenced by the pattern of organ involvement at diagnosis, with additional variation possibly related to diagnostic delay and experience of the clinical center. The general approach to treatment involves intensive induction therapy to achieve remission followed by hematopoietic stem cell transplantation (SCT). The best likelihood of long-term disease-free survival is with allogenic SCT in first complete remission, although there are some reports of favorable outcomes with autologous transplant.[2,3,5-7]

Historically, leukemia or lymphoma combination chemotherapy regimens have been given, with better outcomes using intensive therapy and acute lymphoblastic leukemia (ALL)–type regimens in retrospective analyses.[7] More recently, based on high response rates, the CD123-targeting recombinant protein drug tagraxofusp was approved in the United States and European Union for BPDCN, consisting of interleukin 3 fused to a diphtheria toxin payload.[15] Venetoclax is also active in BPDCN, consistent with its upregulated expression of BCL2 protein and functional BCL2 dependency revealed by mitochondrial apoptotic profiling.[10,16] All treatments should include CNS prophylaxis, similar to that used in high-risk ALL regimens, given the tumor's CNS tropism.[7,9]

References

1. Arber DA, Orazi A, Hasserjian RP, et al. International consensus classification of myeloid neoplasms and acute leukemias: integrating morphologic, clinical, and genomic data. *Blood.* 2022;140(11):1200-1228.
2. Facchetti F, Petrella T, Pileri SA. Blastic plasmacytoid dendritic cell neoplasm. In: Swerdlow SH, Campo E, Harri NL, et al, eds. WHO Classification of Tumors of Haematopoietic and Lymphoid Tissues. IARC; 2017:173-177.
3. Facchetti F, Cigognetti M, Fisogni S, Rossi G, Lonardi S, Vermi W. Neoplasms derived from plasmacytoid dendritic cells. *Mod Pathol.* 2016;29(2):98-111.
4. Cuglievan B, Connors J, He J, et al. Blastic plasmacytoid dendritic cell neoplasm: a comprehensive review in pediatrics, adolescents, and young adults

(AYA) and an update of novel therapies. *Leukemia.* 2023;37(9):1767-1778.

5. Garnache-Ottou F, Vidal C, Biichlé S, et al. How should we diagnose and treat blastic plasmacytoid dendritic cell neoplasm patients? *Blood Adv.* 2019;3(24):4238-4251.
6. Laribi K, Baugier de Materre A, Sobh M, et al. Blastic plasmacytoid dendritic cell neoplasms: results of an international survey on 398 adult patients. *Blood Adv.* 2020;4(19):4838-4848.
7. Pagano L, Zinzani PL, Pileri S, et al. Unmet clinical needs and management recommendations for blastic plasmacytoid dendritic cell neoplasm: a consensus-based position paper from an Ad Hoc international expert panel. *Hemasphere.* 2023;7(3):e841.
8. Griffin GK, Booth CAG, Togami K, et al. Ultraviolet radiation shapes dendritic cell leukaemia transformation in the skin. *Nature.* 2023;618(7966):834-841.
9. Pemmaraju N, Wilson NR, Khoury JD, et al. Central nervous system involvement in blastic plasmacytoid dendritic cell neoplasm. *Blood.* 2021;138(15):1373-1377.
10. Sapienza MR, Fuligni F, Agostinelli C, et al. Molecular profiling of blastic plasmacytoid dendritic cell neoplasm reveals a unique pattern and suggests selective sensitivity to NF-kB pathway inhibition. *Leukemia.* 2014;28(8):1606-1616.
11. Xiao W, Chan A, Waarts MR, et al. Plasmacytoid dendritic cell expansion defines a distinct subset of RUNX1-mutated acute myeloid leukemia. *Blood.* 2021;137(10):1377-1391.
12. Renosi F, Roggy A, Giguelay A, et al. Transcriptomic and genomic heterogeneity in blastic plasmacytoid dendritic cell neoplasms: from ontogeny to oncogenesis. *Blood Adv.* 2021;5:1540-1551.
13. Khanlari M, Yin CC, Takahashi K, et al. Bone marrow clonal hematopoiesis is highly prevalent in blastic plasmacytoid dendritic cell neoplasm and frequently sharing a clonal origin in elderly patients. *Leukemia.* 2022;36(5):1343-1350.
14. Sadigh S, DeAngelo DJ, Garcia JS, et al. Cutaneous manifestations of myeloid neoplasms exhibit broad and divergent morphologic and immunophenotypic features but share ancestral clonal mutations with bone marrow. *Mod Pathol.* 2024;37(1):100352. doi: 10.1016/j.modpat.2023.100352
15. Pemmaraju N, Lane AA, Sweet KL, et al. Tagraxofusp in blastic plasmacytoid dendritic-cell neoplasm. *N Engl J Med.* 2019;380(17):1628-1637.
16. Montero J, Stephansky J, Cai T, et al. Blastic plasmacytoid dendritic cell neoplasm is dependent on BCL2 and sensitive to venetoclax. *Cancer Discov.* 2017;7(2):156-164.

SECTION 10

Lymphoblastic Neoplasms

Introduction to Lymphoblastic Neoplasms

Amy Duffield, Michael J. Borowitz, Sindhu Cherian, Mark D. Ewalt, Elias Jabbour, Charles G. Mullighan, Leonie Saft, and David T. Teachey

Lymphoblastic Neoplasms

Since the publication of the revised 4th edition of the World Health Organization classification, our understanding of the biology and genomics of acute lymphoblastic leukemia/lymphoma (ALL) has greatly expanded and evolved. Several new translocations and other genetic alterations have been identified and included as novel entities, while some subtypes that were thought to be a single disease are now subdivided based on distinct molecular features. The specifics of this refined system are fully detailed in Chapters 40 and 41; however, this introduction is focused on the characteristics of B- and/or T-ALL that appear common across subtypes.

Definition

Lymphoblastic leukemias/lymphomas can be subdivided into neoplasms derived from precursor lymphoid cells committed to either the B- or T-cell lineage, although rare NK-cell leukemias have been described (Chapter 42). The neoplastic cells of both entities are typically small to medium-sized blasts, and immunophenotypic demonstration of lineage antigen expression is required for diagnosis.

B-lymphoblastic leukemia/lymphoma (B-ALL/B-LBL) is a neoplasm of precursor B cells that involves the bone marrow and blood or presents as a mass lesion. This neoplasm is referred to as B-lymphoblastic leukemia (B-ALL) in patients who present primarily with marrow involvement and as B-lymphoblastic lymphoma (B-LBL) in those with a mass lesion without significant marrow involvement. The distinction between leukemia and lymphoma is arbitrary in patients with both marrow involvement and a mass lesion; however, in pediatric treatment protocols, a threshold of ≥25% blasts in the bone marrow is typically used to define leukemia/B-ALL.[1] In contrast to many acute myeloid leukemias, a diagnosis of B-ALL does not require a specific percentage of blasts. The rare patients who present with low levels of lymphoid blasts should be closely followed, with cytogenetic and molecular analysis performed, as the development of overt B-ALL is likely.[2] There are, however, rare reports of patients with small populations that have the immunophenotypic or cytogenetic features of B-ALL but resolve without treatment.[3]

T-lymphoblastic leukemia/lymphoma (T-ALL/LBL) is a neoplasm of lymphoblasts committed to the T-cell lineage involving bone marrow, blood, and/or tissue. As with B-ALL, presentation with marrow involvement or mass lesions determines when the disease is termed leukemia or lymphoma, respectively. T-lymphoblastic lymphoma (T-LBL) often presents with a mediastinal mass, and may also involve lymph nodes or extranodal sites, but with <25% blasts in the bone marrow. In patients who present with both a mass lesion and marrow involvement, ≥25% blasts in the marrow is used to define leukemia/T-ALL for many treatment protocols. As with B-ALL, a diagnosis of T-ALL does not require a specific percentage of blasts in the marrow, and the identification of even rare T lymphoblasts is thought to be pathologic and should trigger further evaluation. Although the presence of expanded populations of T lymphoblasts in extrathymic tissues is typically pathologic, occasionally indolent proliferations of T-lymphoid blasts are identified, and careful morphologic, immunophenotypic, and genetic evaluation is suggested to confirm the clonal nature of such populations.[4]

Some entities other than ALL may contain B or T lymphoblasts, including chronic myeloid leukemia in lymphoid blast phase (Chapter 1) and "myeloid/lymphoid neoplasms with eosinophilia and tyrosine kinase gene fusions" (Chapter 6). Both harbor specific recurrent genetic abnormalities that often have important clinical, prognostic, and therapeutic implications, and these neoplasms should not be classified as ALL/LBL.

Epidemiology

The estimated number of new cases of ALL/LBL in the United States is approximately 6540 per year (2022), and historically approximately 75% to 85% of these cases are B-ALL/LBL.[5] The estimated annual incidence worldwide is 0.75 to 0.94 cases of ALL/LBL per 100,000 population.[6] ALL accounts for approximately 80% of childhood leukemias but only about 20% of adult acute leukemias, and 75% of cases occur in children less than 6 years of age. The incidence decreases until about 50 years of age, when it begins to climb slightly. B-ALL/LBL incidence differs based on self-identified race, affecting white and Hispanic patients more commonly than black patients, with a higher incidence in Hispanic children in the United States.[7]

T-ALL/LBL is more common in adolescents than in younger children and is more common in males than in females. T-ALL accounts for approximately 25% of cases of adult ALL. Most (85%-90%) lymphomatous presentations of precursor lymphoid neoplasms are T-LBL. When compared with B-ALL, the incidence of T-ALL/LBL is higher in the black population and lower in the Hispanic population.

Etiology

The etiology of B-ALL/LBL is unknown, although it is associated with exposure to ionizing radiation, rare germline variants (Chapter 21), and certain genetic diseases such as Down syndrome. Genome-wide association studies have shown an increased risk of B-ALL associated with certain single nucleotide polymorphisms in many genes, including *ARID5B, CDKN2A/B, CEBPE, GATA3,* and *IKZF1;* several of these variants are associated with specific subtypes of B-ALL, such as the association between the *GATA3* rs3824662A allele and B-ALL, *BCR::ABL1*-like.[8-11]

Familial ALL is rare, with some of the described kindreds having mutations in *ETV6, IKZF1, PAX5,* and *TP53.*[12] Sequencing of large ALL cohorts has demonstrated germline mutations in genes including *ETV6* and *PAX5,* often in patients with no known family history of leukemia. Low hypodiploid B-ALL/LBL in children is also associated with germline *TP53* mutations and Li Fraumeni syndrome.[13] Rare germline mutations in *BRCA1* and *BRCA2* have also been observed in patients with ALL, although it is uncertain if these mutations are the drivers of the leukemia.[14]

Some of the translocations associated with ALL have been identified in neonatal specimens months to years before the development of disease, suggesting prenatal initiation of the genetic alterations in childhood leukemia.[15] Monozygotic twins with concordant leukemia frequently share genetic abnormalities; however, these findings are thought to reflect somatic mutations occurring in one twin and shared via *in utero* circulation.[16]

Rare cases of secondary B-ALL following chemotherapy or radiation for a prior malignancy have been documented. It is unclear whether this represents an inherent predisposition to malignancies or a true therapy-related leukemia[17]; however, there is increasing evidence that some cases represent true therapy-related leukemias.[18,19] There does appear to be an increase in high-risk cytogenetic abnormalities and genetic mutations in secondary B-ALL, which is associated with poor outcomes.[20] Recently, an increased risk for secondary B-ALL has been noted in patients treated with lenalidomide, which tends to present with cytopenias and low-level marrow involvement, and may respond to withdrawal of lenalidomide.[21]

The etiology of T-ALL/LBL is also unknown. One study reported a set of T-ALL cases in monozygotic twins who shared the same T-cell receptor (TCR) gene rearrangement, suggesting an *in utero* origin of the earliest genetic lesions.[22] Individuals with ataxia telangiectasia have an increased risk of developing T-ALL.[23]

General clinical features

The bone marrow is involved in all cases classified as B-ALL, and most patients present with evidence of bone marrow failure, specifically thrombocytopenia, anemia, and/or neutropenia. The leukocyte count may be markedly elevated, normal, or decreased. Peripheral blood findings do not necessarily reflect the level of marrow involvement, and circulating blasts may be rare even in cases of B-ALL with extensive marrow involvement. Bone pain and arthralgias can be prominent symptoms, which may manifest as general irritability in young children. Extramedullary involvement is common in B-ALL; the disease shows a predilection for lymph nodes, spleen, and liver, with the associated findings of lymphadenopathy, splenomegaly, and/or hepatomegaly. Involvement of the central nervous system (CNS) or testes is seen in a small percentage of patients.

Patients presenting with B-LBL often lack systemic symptoms, and most have limited-stage disease, with no or only low-level marrow involvement. The most frequent sites of involvement in B-LBL are the skin, soft tissue, bone, and lymph nodes. Head and neck presentations of B-LBL are particularly common in children (Figure 1),[24] and B-LBL can rarely manifest as lytic bone lesions.[25] In contrast to T-LBL, mediastinal masses are uncommon in B-LBL.

T-ALL more commonly presents with a higher leukocyte count than B-ALL, and leukopenia is less common than in B-ALL. T-ALL can present with anemia and thrombocytopenia; however, even in patients with a high tumor burden, T-ALL often shows relative sparing of normal bone marrow hematopoiesis in comparison with B-ALL. Like in B-ALL, patients with T-ALL

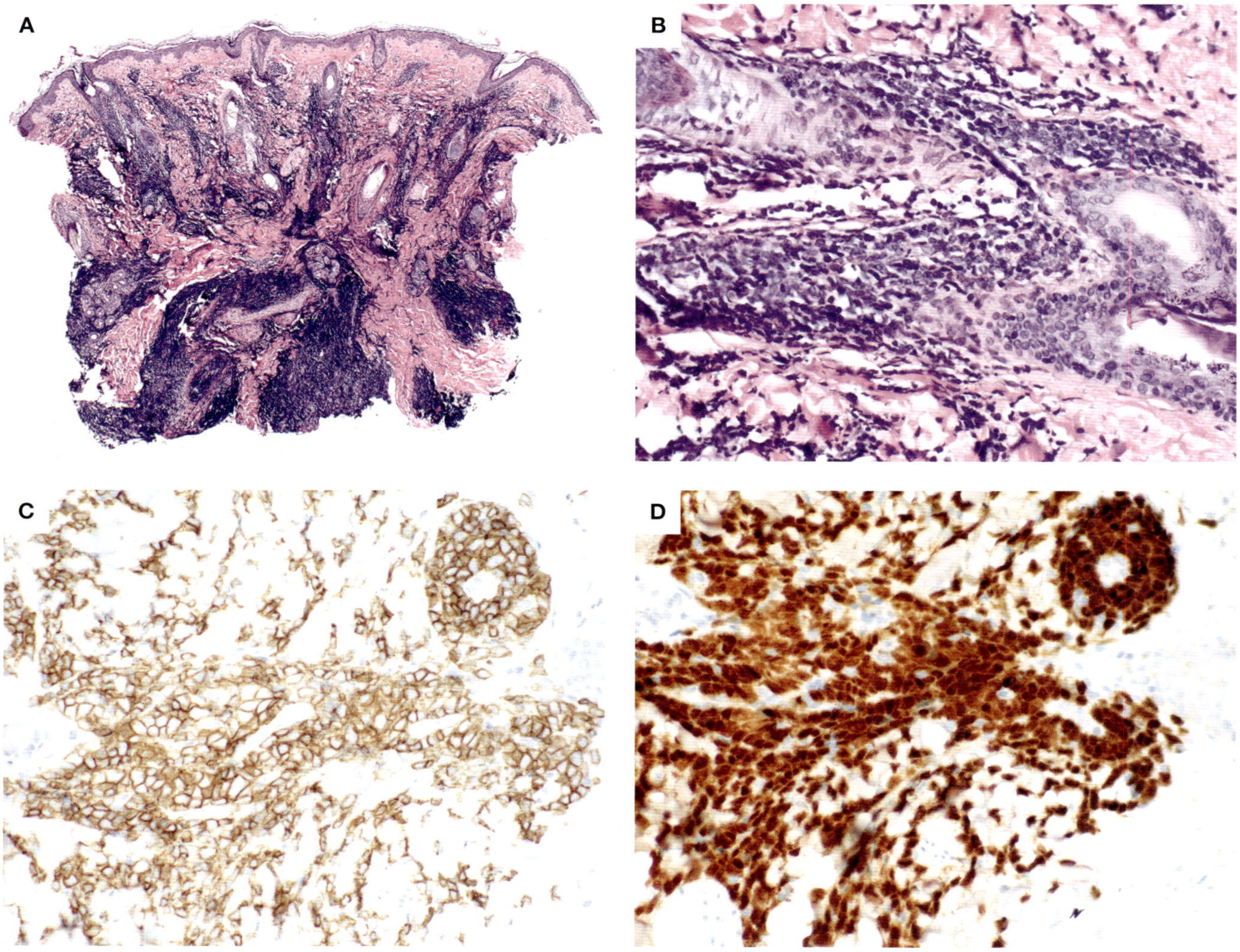

FIGURE 1 Cutaneous B-lymphoblastic lymphoma. B-lymphoblastic lymphoma presenting on the forehead of an 8-year-old child. A punch biopsy (**A:** hematoxylin and eosin [H&E]) shows a predominantly deep dermal infiltrate of lymphoblasts (**B:** H&E) that express CD19 **(C)** and TdT **(D)**.

can also present with bone pain. Patients with leukemic presentations may also have a large mediastinal or other tissue mass, and lymphadenopathy and hepatosplenomegaly are common. CNS and testicular involvement, while relatively uncommon, are seen with a higher frequency than in B-ALL. Patients with T-LBL often present at an advanced stage or with bulky disease, most often an anterior mediastinal mass. Mediastinal involvement may result in compromise of regional anatomic structures, causing dyspnea, dysphagia, and/or superior vena cava syndrome. Pleural or pericardial effusions are also common in patients with mediastinal involvement. T-LBL may involve extranodal sites, including skin, tonsils, liver, and spleen, although patients with extranodal disease typically have concurrent nodal or mediastinal involvement.

Morphology

The morphologic features of B-lymphoblastic and T-lymphoblastic proliferations are essentially indistinguishable. In smear and touch preparations, the lymphoblasts in B-ALL/LBL range from small blasts with scant cytoplasm, condensed chromatin, and indistinct nucleoli to larger cells with a moderate amount of light-blue or basophilic cytoplasm, open nuclear chromatin, and one or more prominent nucleoli (Figure 2). The lymphoblasts may exhibit various morphologic features, including cytoplasmic pseudopods ("hand-mirror cells"), vacuolated cytoplasm, or coarse azurophilic granules. The nuclei may be round or may show convolutions. Nuclear convolutions are thought to be relatively more frequent in T- than B-ALL, although this is not of diagnostic value. Lymphoblasts must be

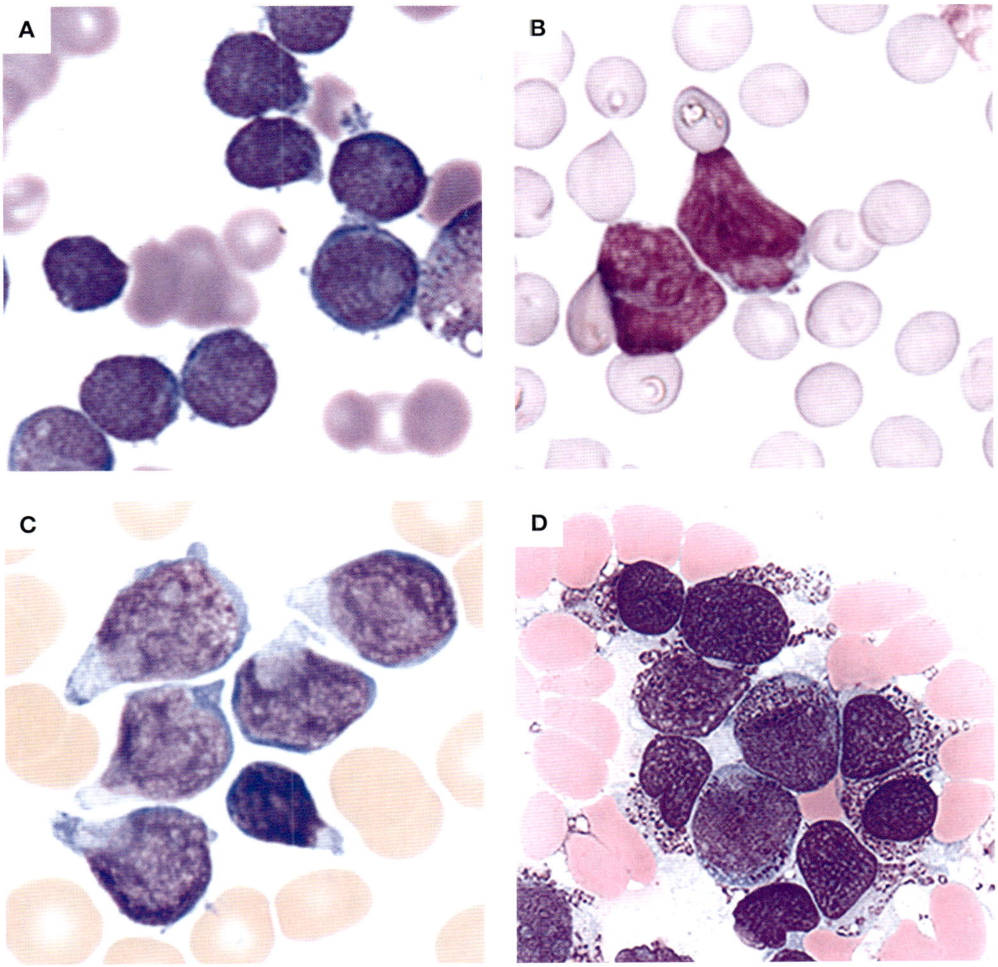

FIGURE 2 Variable blast morphology in B-lymphoblastic leukemia. **A:** Classical lymphoblasts with finely stippled chromatin, scant cytoplasm, and inconspicuous nucleoli (Wright Giemsa stain, all images). **B:** Lymphoblasts with convoluted nuclear borders. **C:** So-called hand mirror cells with most of the cytoplasm at one pole, forming a projection referred to as a uropod. **D:** "Granular" acute lymphoblastic leukemia/lymphoma with blasts containing coarse azurophilic granules. These are lysosomes that lack myeloperoxidase and other enzymes seen in myeloid granules.

distinguished from normal B-cell precursors (hematogones), which can mimic blasts in aspirate smears. Hematogones typically have higher nuclear:cytoplasmic ratios than B lymphoblasts, with homogeneous chromatin and indistinct nucleoli (Figure 3).

Most cases of B-ALL can be diagnosed by blood or a marrow aspirate, but cases with a packed marrow or marrow fibrosis at initial diagnosis may require a bone marrow biopsy. Bone marrow sections usually show very high cellularity with diffuse infiltration by lymphoblasts but often relatively well-preserved megakaryopoiesis. Significant marrow fibrosis (grades 2-3) is seen in approximately 10% of cases. While extensive marrow necrosis is rare at initial presentation, both necrosis and fibrosis have been associated with higher-risk B-ALL/LBL and inferior treatment response.[26,27] Patchy infiltration of the bone marrow can be observed at relapse. B-LBL is generally characterized by a diffuse or (less commonly) paracortical pattern of lymph node involvement. A single-file pattern of infiltration of soft tissue is often seen. There are typically frequent mitotic figures, and some cases may have scattered tingible body macrophages imparting a "starry-sky" pattern.

As noted earlier, the lymphoblasts in T-ALL/LBL are usually morphologically indistinguishable from those of B-ALL/LBL. In some cases, T lymphoblasts may resemble more mature lymphocytes and may be difficult to distinguish from a mature T-cell neoplasm without immunophenotypic studies. In T-LBL the involved lymph nodes typically demonstrate complete effacement of architecture, although some cases show a predominantly paracortical distribution (Figure 4). Mitotic figures are readily identified in most cases. In the thymus, involvement by T-LBL characteristically

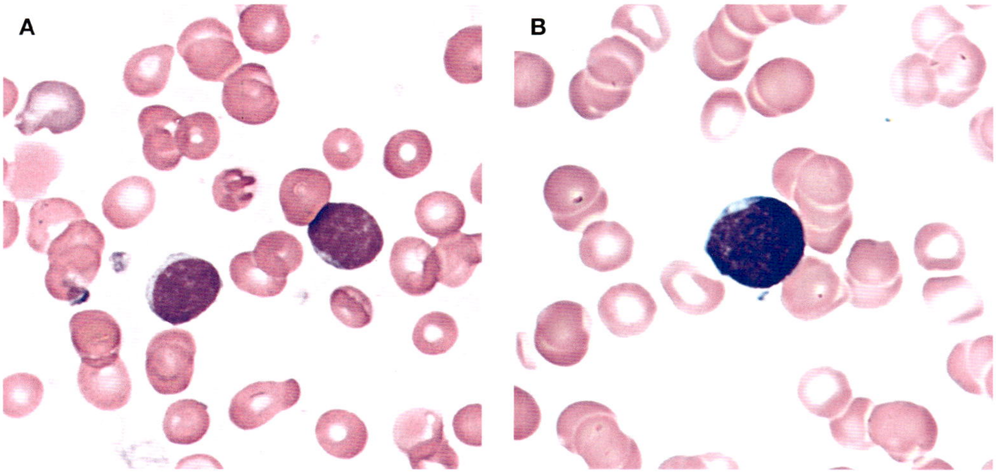

FIGURE 3 Wright-Giemsa stain appearance of hematogones compared with lymphoblasts. **A:** Hematogones have a very high nuclear:cytoplasmic ratio, with compact uniform chromatin and only a thin rim of cytoplasm (Wright-Giemsa stain, all images). **B:** A typical lymphoblast is larger with more cytoplasm, fine chromatin, and inconspicuous nucleoli.

shows extensive replacement of the thymic parenchyma with permeative infiltration of the surrounding fibroadipose tissue.

Cases with histologic findings of lymphoblasts in the setting of increased eosinophils should prompt consideration for B-ALL with t(5;14) (Chapter 40) or a "myeloid/lymphoid neoplasm with eosinophilia and tyrosine kinase gene fusion" (Chapter 6). Peripheral blood or bone marrow biopsies that contain lymphoid blasts in a setting of myeloid hyperplasia raise the

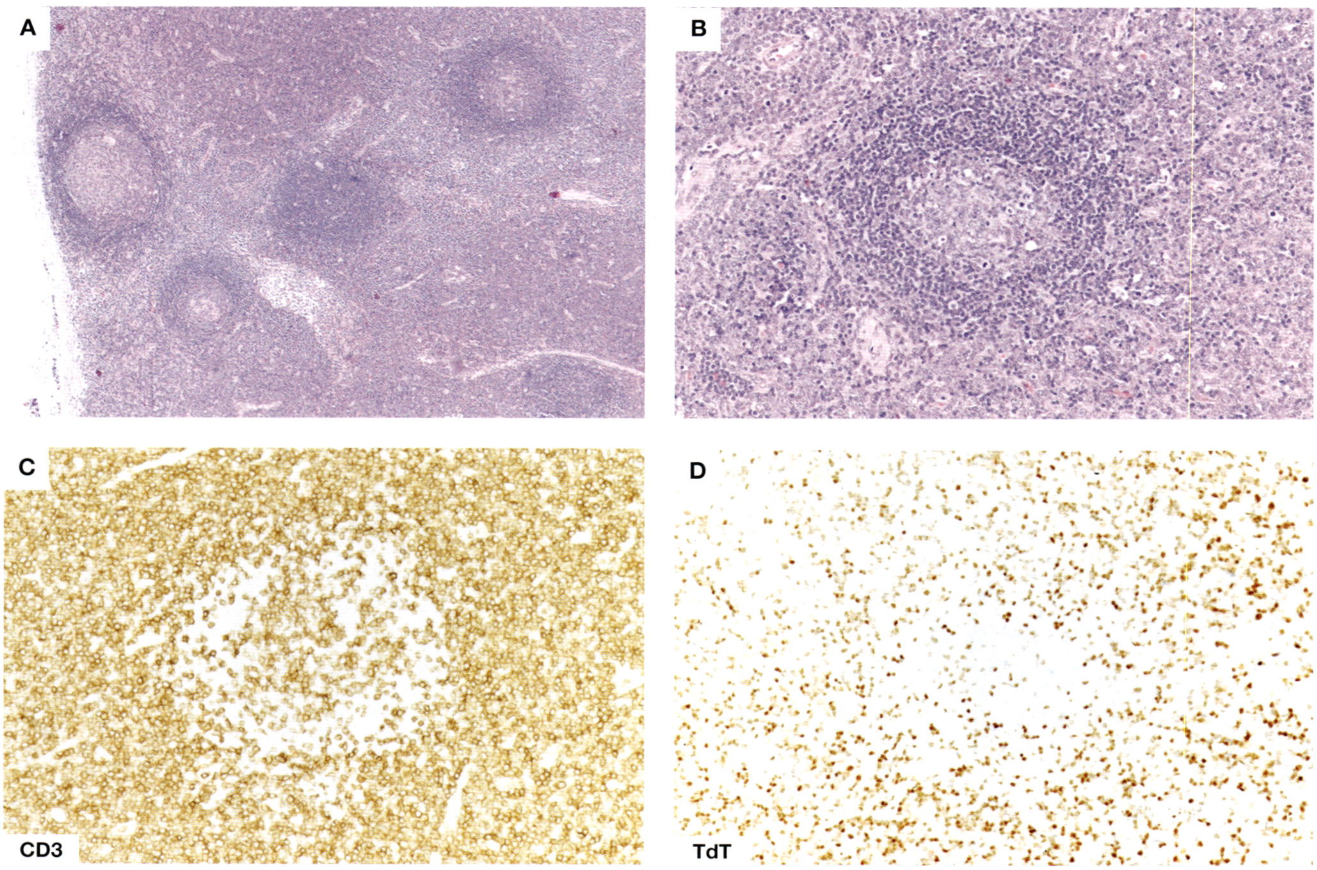

FIGURE 4 T-lymphoblastic lymphoma involving a lymph node. Although lymphoblasts most commonly efface lymph node architecture, in some cases, as in the one illustrated here, there may be only an interfollicular expansion with preservation of germinal centers (hematoxylin and eosin, **A** and **B**). The lymphoblasts are positive for CD3 **(C)** and TdT **(D)**.

possibility of chronic myeloid leukemia in lymphoid blast phase (Chapter 1).

Immunophenotype

Immunophenotypic demonstration of B- or T-cell lineage antigen expression is required for the diagnosis of ALL. Flow cytometry provides a rapid and accurate means for lineage assignment. The lymphoblasts in B-ALL/LBL are almost always positive for the B-cell markers CD19, cytoplasmic CD79a, and cytoplasmic CD22 (Figure 5). None of these B-cell markers is, by itself, specific for B-ALL/LBL, but coexpression of two or more of these markers or high-intensity expression is compatible with the diagnosis. In most cases, the lymphoblasts are dimly CD45 positive, although they may be negative for CD45. Most cases of B-ALL/LBL express CD10, and there is variable expression of CD20 and CD34 on the blasts. Strong expression of CD20 is seen in a minor subset of B-ALL cases at initial diagnosis or as a feature of upregulation during induction therapy. Clonal surface immunoglobulin light chain is characteristically absent, although low-level or partial light chain expression is seen in a minor subset of B-ALL/LBL cases.[28] The myeloid-associated antigens CD13 and CD33 may be expressed on B lymphoblasts. By contrast, expression of CD117 is very rare in B-ALL/LBL.[29] Isolated or low-level expression of myeloperoxidase is also seen in a subset of otherwise typical cases of B-ALL/LBL (Figure 6) and should not, by itself, trigger classification as mixed phenotype acute leukemia (Chapter 39).[30] Some subtypes of B-ALL show characteristic immunophenotypic features, which may facilitate identification (Chapter 40).

Although B lymphoblasts and hematogones both have immature B-precursor immunophenotypes, the pattern of antigen expression on these cell types nearly always differs on flow cytometric analysis. Hematogones display an organized pattern of acquisition and loss of normal antigens.[31] In contrast, using highly sensitive flow cytometry panels, B-ALL shows patterns that differ from normal, with either aberrant antigen expression or over- or underexpression of markers that are normally expressed on precursor B cells.[32,33]

In tissue sections, CD19, CD79a, and PAX5 are most frequently used to demonstrate B-cell differentiation in B-ALL/LBL. CD79a should not be used as a sole marker of B-cell differentiation because it can also be aberrantly expressed in T-ALL.[34] PAX5 and CD19 are sensitive and specific markers for B-cell lineage in tissue sections, but both are also characteristically positive in AML with *RUNX1::RUNX1T1*. Rarely, myeloperoxidase expression on blasts can also be detected in tissue sections by immunohistochemistry in otherwise typical cases of B-ALL/LBL (see Figure 6). TdT and CD34 are used in immunohistochemical analysis of tissue to confirm the immaturity of the B lymphoblasts, with the caveat that aggressive mature B-cell lymphomas may also express TdT in the setting of transformation or progression.[35]

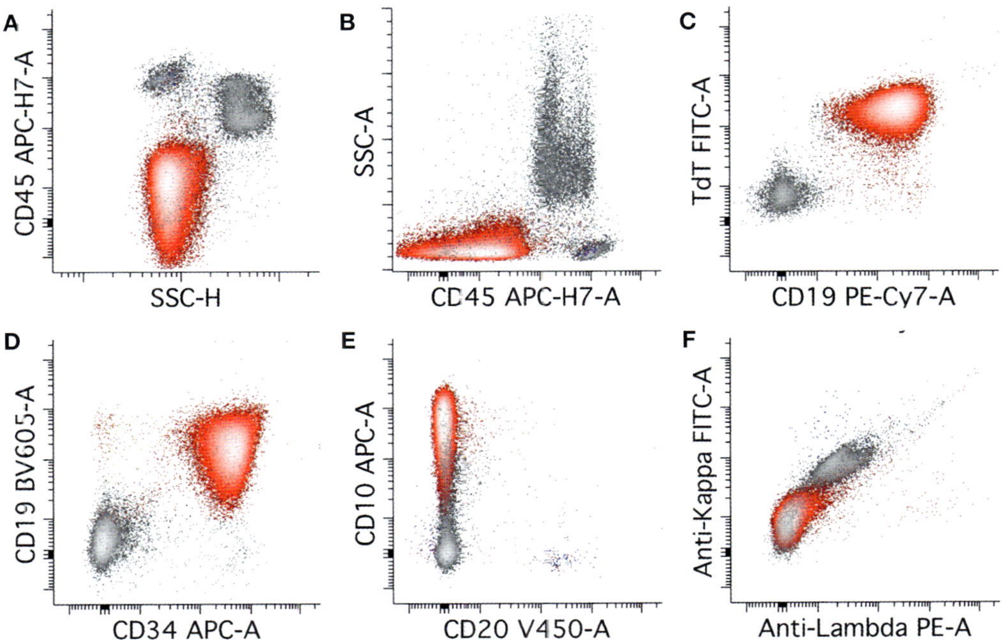

FIGURE 5 Flow cytometry analysis of a representative B-lymphoblastic leukemia. There is a distinct population of blasts (red) with dim CD45 and low right angle scatter (**A** and **B**). The blasts express CD19 and TdT (**C**), CD34 (**D**), and CD10 (**E**), but lack CD20 (**E**), and surface light chain (**F**) expression.

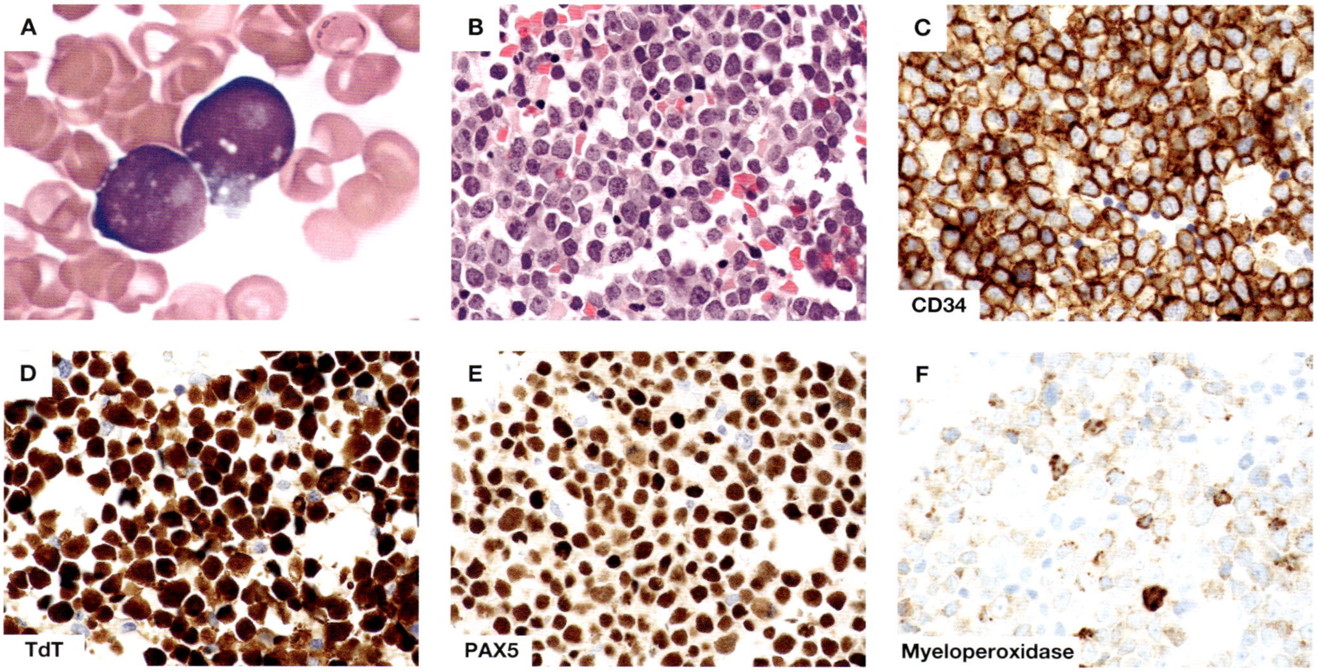

FIGURE 6 B-lymphoblastic leukemia with expression of myeloperoxidase. Blasts exhibit typical morphology in the aspirate (**A:** Wright-Giemsa stain) and bone marrow biopsy (**B:** hematoxylin and eosin). The lymphoblasts express CD34 **(C)**, TdT **(D)**, Pax-5 **(E)**, and dim myeloperoxidase **(F)** but are negative for CD117 (not shown). Optimally, flow cytometry should be performed to exclude a diagnosis of mixed-phenotype acute leukemia.

Flow cytometry also provides a rapid and accurate means for the diagnosis of T-ALL/LBL (Figure 7). The best lineage-specific marker in T-ALL/LBL is CD3, and essentially all cases of T-ALL/LBL express cytoplasmic CD3. Of note, unlike the strict criteria applied for lineage assignment in T/myeloid mixed phenotype acute leukemias, the intensity of cytoplasmic CD3 expression in T-ALL/LBL may be dim and not reach the level of the mature T cells, particularly in early T precursor (ETP) ALL. The intensity of surface CD3

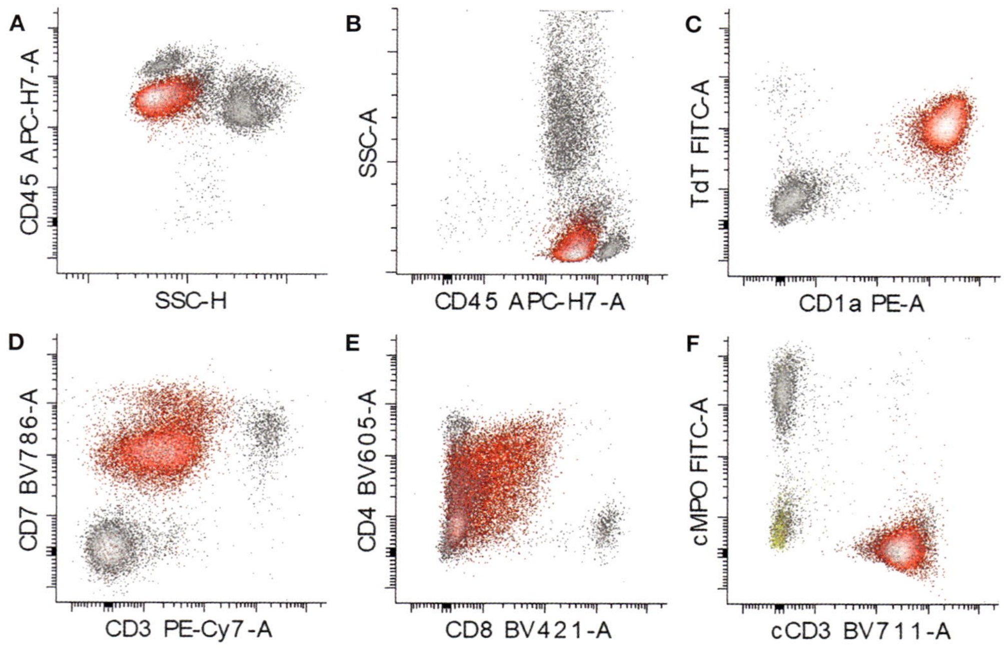

FIGURE 7 Flow cytometry analysis of a representative T-lymphoblastic leukemia. There is a distinct population of blasts (red) with dim CD45 and low right angle scatter (**A** and **B**). The blasts express TdT **(C)**, CD1a **(C)**, and CD7 **(D)**, without surface CD3 **(D)**. The blasts also express dim CD4 and CD8 **(E)**, as well as cytoplasmic CD3 **(F)**, but lack expression of myeloperoxidase **(F)**.

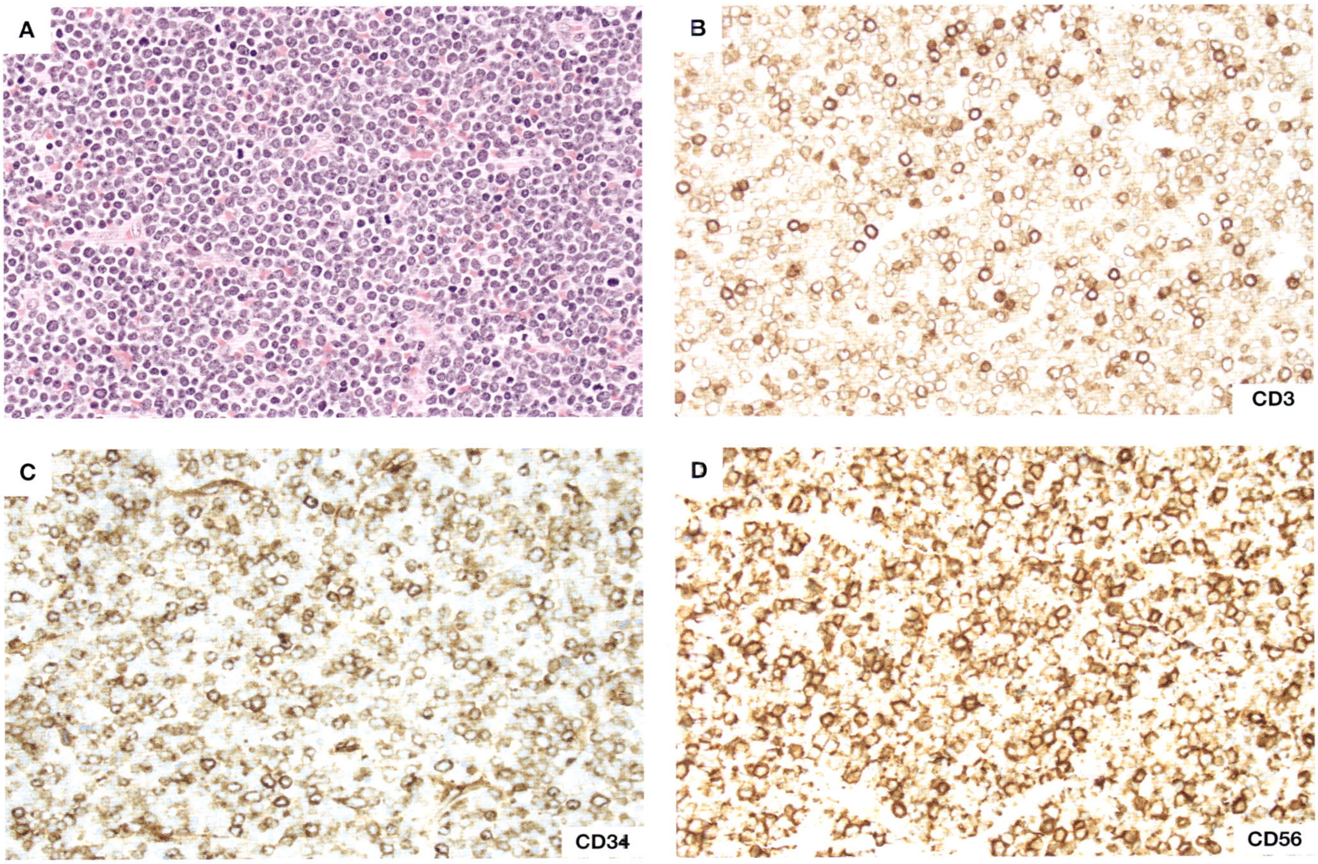

FIGURE 8 Immunohistochemistry of CD56-positive T-lymphoblastic lymphoma. **A:** Hematoxylin and eosin section showing uniform infiltrate of small blasts with scant cytoplasm. In this case, the blasts express CD3 (**B**), CD34 (**C**), and CD56 (**D**).

expression is variable in T-ALL/LBL, ranging from absent to moderately strong. In tissue sections, CD3 expression is essentially always demonstrable by immunohistochemistry, even in cases with a more immature phenotype (Figure 8). CD7 is highly expressed in a preponderance of cases of T-ALL/T-LBL, and the absence of CD7 expression in a neoplasm with T-cell differentiation should prompt consideration for a mature T-cell leukemia/lymphoma. The expression of other T-lineage antigens, including CD2, CD4, CD5, and CD8, is highly variable in T-ALL/LBL. Commonly used markers of immaturity include TdT, CD34, and CD1a, all of which are variably expressed in T-ALL/LBL, while HLA-DR is usually negative. CD99 is frequently overexpressed in T-lymphoblasts compared with mature T-cells; however, CD99 should not be used by itself to establish immaturity. Coexpression of CD4/CD8 and CD10 expression are both seen in T-ALL, but neither pattern is specific for immaturity as these immunophenotypes can also be seen in mature T-cell lymphomas. Normal cortical thymocytes also show CD4/CD8 coexpression, CD1a expression, and lack of surface membrane CD3; however, the T-cell precursors in thymoma, thymic hyperplasia, and indolent T-lymphoblastic proliferations usually show a continuous maturation pattern that includes populations of $CD4^-/CD8^-$, $CD4^+/CD8^+$, $CD4^+/CD8^-$, and $CD4^-/CD8^+$ T cells. As noted earlier, a subset of T-ALL/LBL shows aberrant expression of CD79a. The myeloid-associated antigens CD13 and/or CD33 are also aberrantly expressed in 19% to 32% of cases of T-ALL, and this feature is frequently associated with the expression of CD34.[36,37] CD117 expression is seen in approximately 15% of cases of T-ALL/LBL, most of which have an ETP immunophenotype (Chapter 41). Aberrant CD56 expression is detected in 7% to 10% of T-ALL/LBL and is commonly associated with the expression of myeloid markers and progenitor markers, as well as a lower leukocyte count at presentation[38] (see Figure 8). Phenotypically, T-LBL is more frequently characterized by a mature thymic immunophenotype and less frequent expression of myeloid antigens than T-ALL.[39]

Genetics

Nearly all cases of B-ALL/LBL have clonal rearrangements of the immunoglobulin heavy chain (IGH). In addition, TCR gene rearrangements may be seen in a substantial proportion of B-ALL/LBL cases; therefore, the demonstration of IGH and TCR gene rearrangements is not helpful for lineage assignment.[40] Cytogenetic abnormalities are seen in most cases of B-ALL/LBL. Numerous recurrent genetic alterations occur in B-ALL, including copy number alterations, translocations, other structural rearrangements, and specific mutations. In many cases these alterations are fundamental to the pathogenesis of disease and define specific entities with unique phenotypic and prognostic features (Chapter 40). Importantly, classical cytogenetic analysis fails to identify a subset of subtype-defining drivers because the alterations may be cryptic (eg, *ETV6::RUNX1*), diverse (eg, *NUTM1*, *MEF2D*, and *ZNF384*-rearranged B-ALL), or defined by focal DNA copy number alterations or sequence mutations. Additional single gene mutations are also common in B-ALL/LBL. While many of these mutations are not disease defining, some are associated with particular entities (Chapter 40). More recently, large-scale studies that use clustering algorithms to correlate RNA sequencing (RNA-seq)-based gene expression (GEX) patterns with genetic findings have enabled the identification of multiple new subtypes of B-ALL that have distinct driver mutations and GEX profiles.[41]

Most cases of T-ALL/LBL show clonal rearrangements of the TCR genes, although these are less frequent in immature subtypes such as ETP-ALL.[42] IGH gene rearrangements are also seen in approximately 20% of cases of T-ALL/LBL.[43] Karyotypic abnormalities are identified in 50% to 70% of cases of T-ALL/LBL.[44,45] Translocations are frequently seen, which often juxtapose the regulatory region of one of the TCR loci with a partner gene, leading to dysregulated transcription of the latter. Cases with some of the common translocations are subclassified as "provisional entities" (Chapter 41); however, not all of the common fusions define provisional entities, including cases with translocations involving *MYC* and the cytoplasmic tyrosine kinase *LCK*.[46] Additionally, although not formally recognized as an entity in the International Consensus Classification, rare cases of *BCR::ABL1*-positive T-ALL occur. Chromosomal deletions also occur in T-ALL/LBL. The most common deletion is del(9p), resulting in loss of the tumor suppressor gene *CDKN2A*, which is identified in over 50% of cases.[47] The most commonly mutated gene in T-ALL/LBL is *NOTCH1*, and over 60% of T-ALL/LBL cases have at least one mutation in this gene, which is responsible for gene expression changes in early T-cell development.[48] Additionally, 20% to 30% of T-ALL/LBL cases contain mutations in *FBXW7*, a negative regulator of *NOTCH1*.[49] Many other chromosomal abnormalities and mutations are also seen in T-ALL/LBL, some of which are discussed in Chapter 41.

The techniques used to identify these cytogenetic and molecular abnormalities are varied. Many entities can now be recognized using a combination of karyotype, fluorescence in situ hybridization, multiplex polymerase chain reaction, or next-generation sequencing studies, and some entities have immunohistochemical or flow cytometric surrogates. Whole transcriptome sequencing or unbiased RNA-seq is probably the single most robust method that can be used to detect most lesions. This methodology is becoming increasingly widely available.

Prognosis and clinical comment

B-ALL has a good prognosis in children but is less favorable in adults. The overall complete remission rate is >95% in children versus 60% to 85% in adults. In developed/industrialized countries, at least 90% of children with B-ALL are cured with contemporary chemotherapy protocols, compared with fewer than 50% of adults.[50,51] Children between 1 and 10 years of age and with white blood cell (WBC) counts <50,000/uL are conventionally considered standard risk and typically require less intensive therapy than those with higher-risk disease. In addition to age and WBC count, slow response to initial therapy as assessed by morphological examination of blood and/or bone marrow and the presence of minimal residual disease (MRD) after therapy are all associated with adverse prognosis in both children and adults.[52-55] The presence of CNS disease at diagnosis is also associated with adverse outcomes in pediatric patients.[56] The impact of specific genetic lesions on prognosis is discussed in Chapter 40. More intensive therapy improves cure rates for patients at higher risk for relapse, and therapy with more intensive pediatric-type regimens is associated with better outcomes in younger adults.[57,58] The prognosis of B-LBL is also relatively favorable, and, like that of B-ALL, appears to be better in children than in adults.[59] Immunotherapy directed against CD19 with either bispecific antibodies[60,61] or chimeric antigen receptor T-cells[62] has been shown to be very effective in patients with recurrent disease, and trials of the former have recently shown its effectiveness in frontline therapy.[63]

In children, T-ALL is generally considered a higher-risk disease than B-ALL. In contrast to B-ALL, WBC count and age at diagnosis do not significantly affect prognosis. In adults, the prognosis of T-ALL may be better than that of B-ALL, although this may reflect the fact that relatively few adults with B-ALL have good-risk cytogenetic features. T-ALL is associated with a higher risk of induction failure than B-ALL. The presence of MRD at the end of induction therapy is an adverse prognostic factor, but patients who are MRD positive at end induction still do very well if they become MRD negative following an additional block of therapy.[64-66] T-ALL is also associated with both a higher risk of early relapse and isolated CNS relapse.[67] Some genetic features have prognostic implications in T-ALL/LBL (Chapter 41). The *NOTCH1* mutations commonly identified in T-ALL/LBL are associated with a favorable early treatment response in pediatric and adult patients; however, this early response does not necessarily result in improved survival.[68,69] In adults, any prognostic impact of *NOTCH1/FBXW7* mutations may be overshadowed by coincident alterations in *KRAS*, *NRAS*, or *PTEN*, which appear associated with poorer prognosis.[70] The prognosis of T-LBL depends on patient age, disease stage, and lactate dehydrogenase levels.[71]

References

1. Murphy SB. Childhood non-Hodgkin's lymphoma. *N Engl J Med.* 1978;299(26):1446-1448. doi:10.1056/NEJM197812282992606
2. Kirtek T, Hamdan H, Van Arnam JS, et al. Spontaneous remission of acute lymphoblastic leukemia: a series of nine cases and a review of literature. *Int J Lab Hematol.* 2023;45(4):489-495. doi:10.1111/ijlh.14042
3. Roberts I, Fordham NJ, Rao A, Bain BJ. Neonatal leukaemia. *Br J Haematol.* 2018;182(2):170-184. doi:10.1111/bjh.15246
4. Saglam A, Singh K, Gollapudi S, et al. Indolent T-lymphoblastic proliferation: a systematic review of the literature analyzing the epidemiologic, clinical, and pathologic features of 45 cases. *Int J Lab Hematol.* 2022;44(4):700-711. doi:10.1111/ijlh.13873
5. Siegel RL, Miller KD, Wagle NS, Jemal A. Cancer statistics, 2023. *CA Cancer J Clin.* 2023;73(1):17-48. doi:10.3322/caac.21763
6. Yi M, Zhou L, Li A, Luo S, Wu K. Global burden and trend of acute lymphoblastic leukemia from 1990 to 2017. *Aging (Albany NY).* 2020;12(22):22869-22891. doi:10.18632/aging.103982
7. Feng Q, de Smith AJ, Vergara-Lluri M, et al. Trends in acute lymphoblastic leukemia incidence in the United States by race/ethnicity from 2000 to 2016. *Am J Epidemiol.* 2021;190(4):519-527. doi:10.1093/aje/kwaa215
8. Noetzli L, Lo RW, Lee-Sherick AB, et al. Germline mutations in ETV6 are associated with thrombocytopenia, red cell macrocytosis and predisposition to lymphoblastic leukemia. *Nat Genet.* 2015;47(5):535-538. doi:10.1038/ng.3253
9. Shah S, Schrader KA, Waanders E, et al. A recurrent germline PAX5 mutation confers susceptibility to pre-B cell acute lymphoblastic leukemia. *Nat Genet.* 2013;45(10):1226-1231. doi:10.1038/ng.2754
10. Walsh KM, de Smith AJ, Chokkalingam AP, et al. GATA3 risk alleles are associated with ancestral components in Hispanic children with ALL. *Blood.* 2013;122(19):3385-3387. doi:10.1182/blood-2013-08-524124
11. Koller PB, Zhang H, Kantarjian H, et al. GATA3 rs3824662A allele in B-cell acute lymphoblastic leukemia in adults, adolescents and young adults: association with CRLF2 rearrangement and poor prognosis. *Am J Hematol.* 2021;96(3):E71-E74. doi:10.1002/ajh.26065
12. Klco JM, Mullighan CG. Advances in germline predisposition to acute leukaemias and myeloid neoplasms. *Nat Rev Cancer.* 2021;21(2):122-137. doi:10.1038/s41568-020-00315-z
13. Comeaux EQ, Mullighan CG. TP53 mutations in hypodiploid acute lymphoblastic leukemia. *Cold Spring Harb Perspect Med.* 2017;7(3):a026286. doi:10.1101/cshperspect.a026286
14. Brady SW, Roberts KG, Gu Z, et al. The genomic landscape of pediatric acute lymphoblastic leukemia. *Nat Genet.* 2022;54(9):1376-1389. doi:10.1038/s41588-022-01159-z
15. Gale KB, Ford AM, Repp R, et al. Backtracking leukemia to birth: identification of clonotypic gene fusion sequences in neonatal blood spots. *Proc Natl Acad Sci U S A.* 1997;94(25):13950-13954. doi:10.1073/pnas.94.25.13950
16. Ford AM, Bennett CA, Price CM, Bruin MC, Van Wering ER, Greaves M. Fetal origins of the TEL-AML1 fusion gene in identical twins with leukemia. *Proc Natl Acad Sci U S A.* 1998;95(8):4584-4588. doi:10.1073/pnas.95.8.4584
17. Ganzel C, Devlin S, Douer D, Rowe JM, Stein EM, Tallman MS. Secondary acute lymphoblastic leukaemia is constitutional and probably not related to prior therapy. *Br J Haematol.* 2015;170(1):50-55. doi:10.1111/bjh.13386
18. Saygin C, Kishtagari A, Cassaday RD, et al. Therapy-related acute lymphoblastic leukemia is a distinct entity with adverse genetic features and clinical outcomes. *Blood Adv.* 2019;3(24):4228-4237. doi:10.1182/bloodadvances.2019000925
19. Swaika A, Frank RD, Yang D, et al. Second primary acute lymphoblastic leukemia in adults: a SEER analysis of incidence and outcomes. *Cancer Med.* 2018;7(2):499-507. doi:10.1002/cam4.1266
20. Riazat-Kesh YJRA, Mascarenhas J, Bar-Natan M. "Secondary" acute lymphoblastic/lymphocytic leukemia: done playing second fiddle? *Blood Rev.* 2023;60:101070. doi:10.1016/j.blre.2023.101070
21. Geyer MB, Shaffer BC, Bhatnagar B, et al. Lenalidomide-associated B-cell ALL: clinical and pathologic correlates

and sensitivity to lenalidomide withdrawal. *Blood Adv.* 2023;7(13):3087-3098. doi:10.1182/bloodadvances.2022009212

22. Ford AM, Pombo-de-Oliveira MS, McCarthy KP, et al. Monoclonal origin of concordant T-cell malignancy in identical twins. *Blood.* 1997;89(1):281-285.
23. Taylor AM, Metcalfe JA, Thick J, Mak YF. Leukemia and lymphoma in ataxia telangiectasia. *Blood.* 1996;87(2):423-438.
24. Lee WJ, Moon HR, Won CH, et al. Precursor B- or T-lymphoblastic lymphoma presenting with cutaneous involvement: a series of 13 cases including 7 cases of cutaneous T-lymphoblastic lymphoma. *J Am Acad Dermatol.* 2014;70(2):318-325. doi:10.1016/j.jaad.2013.10.020
25. Iravani S, Singleton TP, Ross CW, Schnitzer B. Precursor B lymphoblastic lymphoma presenting as lytic bone lesions. *Am J Clin Pathol.* 1999;112(6):836-843. doi:10.1093/ajcp/112.6.836
26. Anil J, Alnemri A, Lytle A, et al. Bone marrow fibrosis is associated with non-response to CD19 CAR T-cell therapy in B-acute lymphoblastic leukemia. *Am J Hematol.* 2023;98(12):1888-1897. doi:10.1002/ajh.27098
27. Badar T, Shetty A, Bueso-Ramos C, et al. Bone marrow necrosis in acute leukemia: Clinical characteristic and outcome. *Am J Hematol.* 2015;90(9):769-773. doi:10.1002/ajh.24074
28. Navid F, Mosijczuk AD, Head DR, et al. Acute lymphoblastic leukemia with the (8;14)(q24;q32) translocation and FAB L3 morphology associated with a B-precursor immunophenotype: the Pediatric Oncology Group experience. *Leukemia.* 1999;13(1):135-141. doi:10.1038/sj.leu.2401244
29. Suggs JL, Cruse JM, Lewis RE. Aberrant myeloid marker expression in precursor B-cell and T-cell leukemias. *Exp Mol Pathol.* 2007;83(3):471-473. doi:10.1016/j.yexmp.2007.08.012
30. McGinnis E, Yang D, Au N, et al. Clinical and laboratory features associated with myeloperoxidase expression in pediatric B-lymphoblastic leukemia. *Cytometry B Clin Cytom.* 2021;100(4):446-453. doi:10.1002/cyto.b.21966
31. McKenna RW, Washington LT, Aquino DB, Picker LJ, Kroft SH. Immunophenotypic analysis of hematogones (B-lymphocyte precursors) in 662 consecutive bone marrow specimens by 4-color flow cytometry. *Blood.* 2001;98(8):2498-2507. doi:10.1182/blood.v98.8.2498
32. Keeney M, Wood BL, Hedley BD, et al. A QA program for MRD testing demonstrates that systematic education can reduce discordance among experienced interpreters. *Cytometry B Clin Cytom.* 2018;94(2):239-249. doi:10.1002/cyto.b.21528
33. Theunissen P, Mejstrikova E, Sedek L, et al. Standardized flow cytometry for highly sensitive MRD measurements in B-cell acute lymphoblastic leukemia. *Blood.* 2017;129(3):347-357. doi:10.1182/blood-2016-07-726307
34. Hashimoto M, Yamashita Y, Mori N. Immunohistochemical detection of CD79a expression in precursor T cell lymphoblastic lymphoma/leukaemias. *J Pathol.* 2002;197(3):341-347. doi:10.1002/path.1126
35. Duffield AS, Dogan A, Amador C, et al. Progression of follicular lymphoma and related entities: Report from the 2021 SH/EAHP workshop. *Am J Clin Pathol.* 2023;159(6):572-597. doi:10.1093/ajcp/aqad042
36. Gupta R, Garg N, Kotru M, Kumar D, Pathak R. Immunophenotypic characteristics of T lineage acute lymphoblastic leukemia: absence of immaturity markers-TdT, CD34 and HLADR is not uncommon. *Am J Blood Res.* 2022;12:1-10.
37. Hoehn D, Medeiros LJ, Chen SS, et al. CD117 expression is a sensitive but nonspecific predictor of FLT3 mutation in T acute lymphoblastic leukemia and T/myeloid acute leukemia. *Am J Clin Pathol.* 2012;137(2):213-219. doi:10.1309/AJCPR3N3JMSYLPFG
38. Fischer L, Gökbuget N, Schwartz S, et al. CD56 expression in T-cell acute lymphoblastic leukemia is associated with non-thymic phenotype and resistance to induction therapy but no inferior survival after risk-adapted therapy. *Haematologica.* 2009;94(2):224-229. doi:10.3324/haematol.13543
39. Patel JL, Smith LM, Anderson J, et al. The immunophenotype of T-lymphoblastic lymphoma in children and adolescents: a Children's Oncology Group report. *Br J Haematol.* 2012;159(4):454-461. doi:10.1111/bjh.12042
40. van der Velden VHJ, Brüggemann M, Hoogeveen PG, et al. TCRB gene rearrangements in childhood and adult precursor-B-ALL: frequency, applicability as MRD-PCR target, and stability between diagnosis and relapse. *Leukemia.* 2004;18(12):1971-1980. doi:10.1038/sj.leu.2403505
41. Gu Z, Churchman ML, Roberts KG, et al. PAX5-driven subtypes of B-progenitor acute lymphoblastic leukemia. *Nat Genet.* 2019;51(2):296-307. doi:10.1038/s41588-018-0315-5
42. Zuurbier L, Gutierrez A, Mullighan CG, et al. Immature MEF2C-dysregulated T-cell leukemia patients have an early T-cell precursor acute lymphoblastic leukemia gene signature and typically have non-rearranged T-cell receptors. *Haematologica.* 2014;99(1):94-102. doi:10.3324/haematol.2013.090233
43. Szczepański T, Pongers-Willemse MJ, Langerak AW, et al. Ig heavy chain gene rearrangements in T-cell acute lymphoblastic leukemia exhibit predominant DH6-19 and DH7-27 gene usage, can result in complete V-D-J rearrangements, and are rare in T-cell receptor alpha beta lineage. *Blood.* 1999;93(12):4079-4085.
44. Han X, Bueso-Ramos CE. Precursor T-cell acute lymphoblastic leukemia/lymphoblastic lymphoma and acute biphenotypic leukemias. *Am J Clin Pathol.* 2007;127(4):528-544. doi:10.1309/2QE3A6EKQ8UYDYRC
45. Graux C, Cools J, Michaux L, Vandenberghe P, Hagemeijer A. Cytogenetics and molecular genetics of T-cell acute lymphoblastic leukemia: from thymocyte

to lymphoblast. *Leukemia.* 2006;20(9):1496-1510. doi:10.1038/sj.leu.2404302

46. Weng AP, Millholland JM, Yashiro-Ohtani Y, et al. c-Myc is an important direct target of Notch1 in T-cell acute lymphoblastic leukemia/lymphoma. *Genes Dev.* 2006;20(15):2096-2109. doi:10.1101/gad.1450406
47. Girardi T, Vicente C, Cools J, De Keersmaecker K. The genetics and molecular biology of T-ALL. *Blood.* 2017;129(9):1113-1123. doi:10.1182/blood-2016-10-706465
48. Gallo Llorente L, Luther H, Schneppenheim R, Zimmermann M, Felice M, Horstmann MA. Identification of novel NOTCH1 mutations: increasing our knowledge of the NOTCH signaling pathway. *Pediatr Blood Cancer.* 2014;61(5):788-796. doi:10.1002/pbc.24852
49. Malyukova A, Dohda T, von der Lehr N, et al. The tumor suppressor gene hCDC4 is frequently mutated in human T-cell acute lymphoblastic leukemia with functional consequences for Notch signaling. *Cancer Res.* 2007;67(12):5611-5616. doi:10.1158/0008-5472.CAN-06-4381
50. Miller KD, Nogueira L, Mariotto AB, et al. Cancer treatment and survivorship statistics, 2019. *CA Cancer J Clin.* 2019;69(5):363-385. doi:10.3322/caac.21565
51. Jeha S, Choi J, Roberts KG, et al. Clinical significance of novel subtypes of acute lymphoblastic leukemia in the context of minimal residual disease-directed therapy. *Blood Cancer Discov.* 2021;2(4):326-337. doi:10.1158/2643-3230.BCD-20-0229
52. Coustan-Smith E, Sancho J, Hancock ML, et al. Clinical importance of minimal residual disease in childhood acute lymphoblastic leukemia. *Blood.* 2000;96(8):2691-2696.
53. Schultz KR, Pullen DJ, Sather HN, et al. Risk- and response-based classification of childhood B-precursor acute lymphoblastic leukemia: a combined analysis of prognostic markers from the Pediatric Oncology Group (POG) and Children's Cancer Group (CCG). *Blood.* 2007;109(3):926-935. doi:10.1182/blood-2006-01-024729
54. Silverman LB, Sallan SE. Newly diagnosed childhood acute lymphoblastic leukemia: update on prognostic factors and treatment. *Curr Opin Hematol.* 2003;10(4):290-296. doi:10.1097/00062752-200307000-00007
55. van Dongen JJ, Seriu T, Panzer-Grümayer ER, et al. Prognostic value of minimal residual disease in acute lymphoblastic leukaemia in childhood. *Lancet.* 1998;352(9142):1731-1738. doi:10.1016/S0140-6736(98)04058-6
56. Clarke M, Gaynon P, Hann I, et al. CNS-directed therapy for childhood acute lymphoblastic leukemia: Childhood ALL Collaborative Group overview of 43 randomized trials. *J Clin Oncol.* 2003;21(9):1798-1809. doi:10.1200/JCO.2003.08.047
57. Boissel N, Auclerc M-F, Lhéritier V, et al. Should adolescents with acute lymphoblastic leukemia be treated as old children or young adults? Comparison of the French FRALLE-93 and LALA-94 trials. *J Clin Oncol.* 2003;21(5):774-780. doi:10.1200/JCO.2003.02.053
58. Hallböök H, Gustafsson G, Smedmyr B, et al. Treatment outcome in young adults and children >10 years of age with acute lymphoblastic leukemia in Sweden: a comparison between a pediatric protocol and an adult protocol. *Cancer.* 2006;107(7):1551-1561. doi:10.1002/cncr.22189
59. Maitra A, McKenna RW, Weinberg AG, Schneider NR, Kroft SH. Precursor B-cell lymphoblastic lymphoma. A study of nine cases lacking blood and bone marrow involvement and review of the literature. *Am J Clin Pathol.* 2001;115(6):868-875. doi:10.1309/Q5GV-3K00-WAC6-BBUB
60. Gökbuget N, Dombret H, Bonifacio M, et al. Blinatumomab for minimal residual disease in adults with B-cell precursor acute lymphoblastic leukemia. *Blood.* 2018;131(14):1522-1531. doi:10.1182/blood-2017-08-798322
61. Brown PA, Ji L, Xu X, et al. Effect of postreinduction therapy consolidation with blinatumomab vs chemotherapy on disease-free survival in children, adolescents, and young adults with first relapse of b-cell acute lymphoblastic leukemia: a randomized clinical trial. *JAMA.* 2021;325(9):833-842. doi:10.1001/jama.2021.0669
62. Seng MS, Meierhofer AC, Lim FL, Soh SY, Hwang WYK. A review of CAR-T therapy in pediatric and young adult b-lineage acute leukemia: clinical perspectives in singapore. *Onco Targets Ther.* 2023;16:165-176. doi:10.2147/OTT.S271373
63. Litzow MR, Sun Z, Mattison RJ, et al. Blinatumomab for MRD-negative acute lymphoblastic leukemia in adults. *N Engl J Med.* 2024;391(4):320-333. doi:10.1056/NEJMoa2312948
64. Wood B, Devidas M, Summers RJ, et al. Prognostic significance of ETP phenotype and minimal residual disease in T-ALL: a Children's Oncology Group Study. *Blood.* 2023;142(24):2069-2078. doi:10.1182/blood.2023020678
65. Willemse MJ, Seriu T, Hettinger K, et al. Detection of minimal residual disease identifies differences in treatment response between T-ALL and precursor B-ALL. *Blood.* 2002;99(12):4386-4393. doi:10.1182/blood.v99.12.4386
66. Schrappe M, Valsecchi MG, Bartram CR, et al. Late MRD response determines relapse risk overall and in subsets of childhood T-cell ALL: results of the AIEOP-BFM-ALL 2000 study. *Blood.* 2011;118(8):2077-2084. doi:10.1182/blood-2011-03-338707
67. Goldberg JM, Silverman LB, Levy DE, et al. Childhood T-cell acute lymphoblastic leukemia: the Dana-Farber Cancer Institute acute lymphoblastic leukemia consortium experience. *J Clin Oncol.* 2003;21(19):3616-3622. doi:10.1200/JCO.2003.10.116
68. Zuurbier L, Homminga I, Calvert V, et al. NOTCH1 and/or FBXW7 mutations predict for initial good prednisone response but not for improved outcome in

pediatric T-cell acute lymphoblastic leukemia patients treated on DCOG or COALL protocols. *Leukemia.* 2010;24(12):2014-2022. doi:10.1038/leu.2010.204

69. Mansour MR, Sulis ML, Duke V, et al. Prognostic implications of NOTCH1 and FBXW7 mutations in adults with T-cell acute lymphoblastic leukemia treated on the MRC UKALLXII/ECOG E2993 protocol. *J Clin Oncol.* 2009;27(26):4352-4356. doi:10.1200/JCO.2009.22.0996

70. Trinquand A, Tanguy-Schmidt A, Ben Abdelali R, et al. Toward a NOTCH1/FBXW7/RAS/PTEN-based oncogenetic risk classification of adult T-cell acute lymphoblastic leukemia: a Group for Research in Adult Acute Lymphoblastic Leukemia study. *J Clin Oncol.* 2013;31(34):4333-4342. doi:10.1200/JCO.2012.48.5292

71. Morel P, Lepage E, Brice P, et al. Prognosis and treatment of lymphoblastic lymphoma in adults: a report on 80 patients. *J Clin Oncol.* 1992;10(7):1078-1085. doi:10.1200/JCO.1992.10.7.1078.

Chapter 39
Acute Leukemias of Ambiguous Lineage

Anna Porwit, Marie C. Béné, Michael J. Borowitz, Etan Orgel, and Olga K. Weinberg

Definition

Acute leukemias of ambiguous lineage (ALALs) include biologically diverse leukemias that fail to show commitment to either the myeloid or lymphoid lineages or display evidence of commitment to more than one lineage.[1,2] Cases in the former group are referred to as acute undifferentiated leukemias (AULs), and those in the latter as mixed-phenotype acute leukemias (MPALs) (Table 39.1). MPAL cases can contain two or more completely separable single-lineage leukemia populations or have a single blast population expressing markers of more than one lineage. While the first of these is often referred to as bi- (or tri-) lineal leukemia and the latter as bi- (tri-) phenotypic leukemia, these are not different entities but rather represent different immunophenotypic patterns that can change over time, either spontaneously or under the influence of therapy. The presenting immunophenotype can be B/myeloid, T/myeloid, or very rarely B/T or B/T/myeloid.[3] In most cases, the blast population shows various subsets, some with the biphenotypic pattern and some of single-lineage immunophenotype (Figure 39.1). The different treatment regimens for acute myeloid leukemia (AML) and acute lymphoblastic leukemia (ALL) make ALAL a diagnostic and therapeutic challenge.

Some subcategories of MPAL (Table 39.1) can be defined based on genetic features. However, these characteristics are not specific, and identical genetic alterations can, under circumstances currently not well understood, produce B, T, or myeloid leukemia. Thus, distinguishing MPAL from single-lineage leukemia with the same genetic driver requires a very thorough immunophenotypic definition (Table 39.2).

Epidemiology

ALAL is uncommon, accounts for 2% to 3% of acute leukemia, ie, 0.35 cases/1,000,000 person-years, and has a male predominance (M:F1.6:1).[4] Among MPAL cases, the B/myeloid subtype accounts for 59%, whereas T/myeloid, B/T, and trilineage subtypes account for 35%, 4%, and 2%, respectively.[5] AUL cases are extremely rare.

Diagnostic Criteria

All ALAL categories require that the total number of morphologically defined blasts in blood, bone marrow, or involved tissue must be greater or equal to 20%.[1,2,6] Blasts most often have a cytologically undifferentiated appearance but sometimes blast populations with distinctive sizes and different morphological features can be seen (Figure 39.2). Extensive immunophenotyping, most often by flow cytometry (FCM) with broad panels including intracytoplasmic markers, is essential for an accurate diagnosis and classification[1,2,7] (Table 39.2).

A diagnosis of MPAL requires that lineage assignment criteria (Table 39.2) are fulfilled and that each lineage is immunophenotypically aberrant so that small populations of normal myeloid, B-, or T-cell progenitors are not misinterpreted. Typically, >5% blasts of each lineage are found. For cases with aberrant populations representing less than 5% of all cells, a diagnosis of AML (or ALL) is best rendered, supplemented by a comment describing the presence of the small population of other lineage. These are important to mention because minor populations may expand after therapy and should be followed.

Cytogenetically defined leukemias that meet the immunophenotypic criteria of MPAL but fulfill criteria of other well-defined entities[1,2] should not be considered MPAL. Specifically excluded from an MPAL diagnosis are cases of mixed blast phase developing in patients with a history of chronic myeloid leukemia, myeloid/lymphoid neoplasms with eosinophilia and tyrosine kinase mutations, and AML with t(8;21)(q22;q22.1) *RUNX::RUNX1T1;* the latter expresses many markers otherwise considered B specific. Additionally, cases that have cytogenetic or molecular alterations associated with myelodysplastic syndrome (MDS), or have *TP53* mutations, are better classified together with their AML counterparts if they have a predominantly myeloid phenotype, as they appear to behave similarly.

TABLE 39.1 Acute leukemia of ambiguous lineage

Acute undifferentiated leukemia	
MPAL with recurrent genetic abnormalities	
	MPAL with *BCR::ABL1*
	MPAL, with t(v;11q23.3); *KMT2A* rearranged
	MPAL with *ZNF384* rearrangement
	MPAL with *BCL11B* rearrangement
MPAL with defining immunophenotypic changes	
	B/myeloid MPAL, NOS
	T/myeloid MPAL, NOS
	B/T/myeloid MPAL
	B/T MPAL
ALAL, NOS	

ALAL, acute leukemia of ambiguous lineage; MPAL, mixed-phenotype acute leukemia; NOS, not otherwise specified.

Immunophenotype

Immunophenotypic criteria (Table 39.2) are used for lineage assignment of leukemic blast populations in MPAL. In general, when assessing markers to determine lineage, the more the markers of that lineage are expressed, and the closer they are in intensity to their normal counterparts, the more specific they are for that lineage. Multiparameter FCM is the preferred immunophenotyping method to allow detection of coexpression of lymphoid and myeloid differentiation antigens on the same population or to demonstrate separate leukemic populations.[7,8]

The presence of a blast population expressing various markers can be demonstrated by immunohistochemistry on tissue sections (Figure 39.3), but it is more difficult to show the diversity of a blast population and coexpression of markers using this methodology.

AUL is defined by a lack of lineage-specific markers (Table 39.2). These cases typically express a hematopoietic progenitor-associated immunophenotype with expression of CD45 and CD34, possibly with HLA-DR, CD38, and/or CD7. No more than one myeloid marker (such as CD117, CD13, CD33) should be present. There is insufficient information to know how best to classify cases of AUL that have cytogenetic abnormalities and/or molecular findings associated with MDS. Exceptional cases may not fulfill the criteria for MPAL

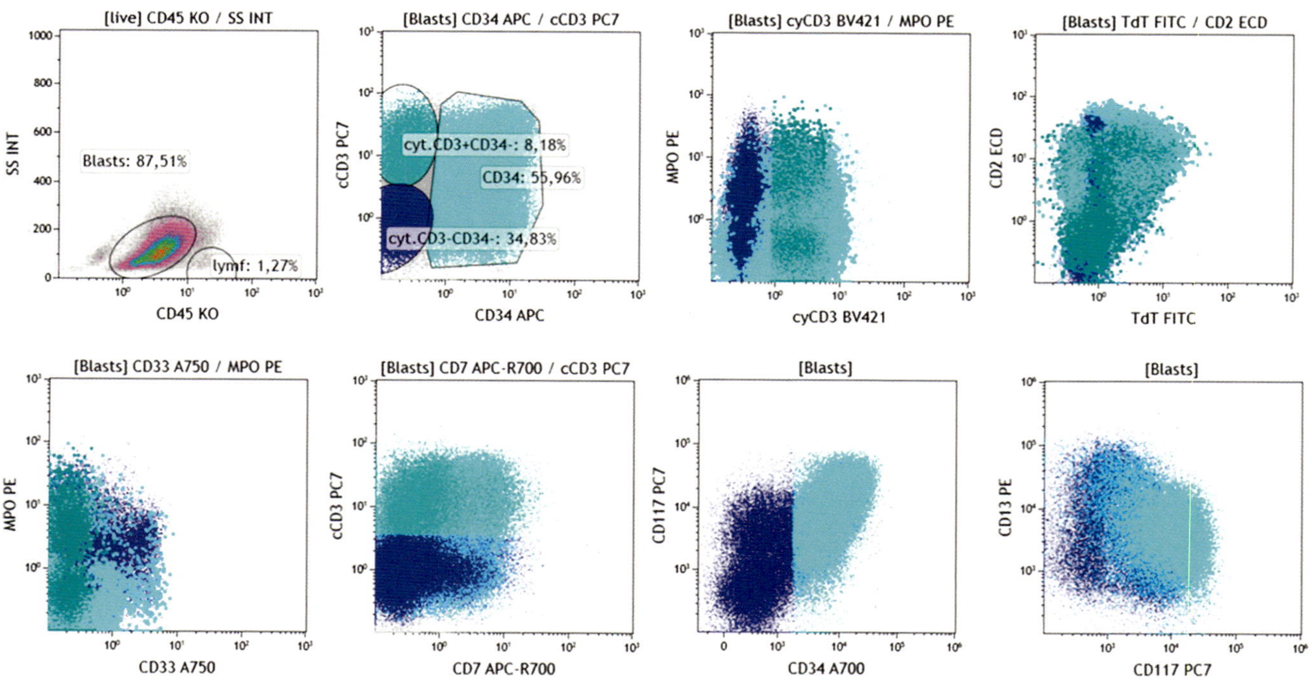

FIGURE 39.1 T-myeloid MPAL with *BCL11B* activation showing several subpopulations of blasts. The top left dot plot shows a massive infiltration of the bone marrow by blasts (87%). On the second top left dot plot, three populations are present: cyt.CD3$^-$/CD34$^-$ (dark blue); cyt.CD3$^+$/CD34$^-$ (aquamarine); and cyt.CD3$^+$ (typical smear pattern from negative to positive)/CD34$^+$ (cyan). The third plot shows frank MPO expression by the cyt.CD3$^-$/CD34$^-$ (dark blue) cells and partial expression of MPO in the cyt.CD3$^+$ (aquamarine and cyan) populations. The last plot shows minimal expression of CD2 on the T compartment lacking CD34 (aquamarine) but definitive CD2 expression on the CD34$^+$ compartment (cyan) with possibly some weak expression of TdT. The bottom panel shows that the cyt.CD3$^-$/CD34$^-$ (dark blue) cells also express CD33, partly CD117, and clearly CD13. The predominant CD34$^+$ cyan population is partly CD33, clearly CD117 and CD13, and partly CD7.

TABLE 39.2 Criteria for diagnosis of mixed phenotype acute leukemia with a biphenotypic pattern

B lineage		
	Strong CD19 *and*	1 or more marker expression of CD10, CD22, CD20, or CD79a
	Weak CD19 *and*	2 more strongly expressed: CD10, CD22, CD20, or CD79a
	Immunohistochemistry for B-lineage-associated markers	PAX5
T lineage		
	CD3 cytoplasmic or surface	Other T-lineage markers possible but not required
Myeloid lineage		
	MPO	
	Monocytic differentiation	NSE, CD64, CD11c, CD14, or lysozyme

MPO, myeloperoxidase; NSE, non-specific esterase.

or for acute leukemia of a single lineage or for AUL. Such extremely rare cases are best referred to as ALAL, not otherwise specified (NOS).

B-cell component of MPAL: Following previously published criteria,[1,2] B-lineage designation in MPAL requires CD19 expression, but CD19 alone is not a sufficient criterion for assigning B-cell lineage. In cases with strong expression of CD19 (as seen in stage I B-cell precursors or mature B cells), at least one other B-cell-associated marker should be strongly expressed (cyt.CD79a, CD10, or cyt./sCD22). If CD19 expression is weak, two other B-lineage markers are needed. Of these, cyt.CD79a is probably the most sensitive, although it may occur in T-ALL and cannot be used alone in the diagnosis of B/T leukemia. Membrane CD22 is also considered a confirmatory marker for B-lineage assignment provided basophils are excluded. CD10 may be used as confirmatory evidence of B lineage, particularly when brightly expressed, although it can be expressed in some T-ALL and more rarely AML cases. In cases where a bone marrow trephine has been performed, immunohistochemical stains for PAX5 are useful.

T-cell component of MPAL: T-lineage assignment requires that blasts show strong cyt.CD3 expression.[1,2] While this expression is usually heterogeneous (smear-like), the brightest expression should be comparable with that of background T cells present in the analyzed sample. The predictive value of only dim cyt.CD3 expression in defining T lineage is unclear as it is sometimes seen in cases otherwise consistent with AML and often disappears in residual blasts during treatment or at relapse. Cyt.CD3 expression can also be demonstrated by immunohistochemistry on tissue sections. Since some commonly applied antibodies react with the CD3 zeta chain, the presence of activated NK cells should be excluded. It is better to use antibodies directed to CD3 epsilon chain. Membrane CD3 expression is T-cell

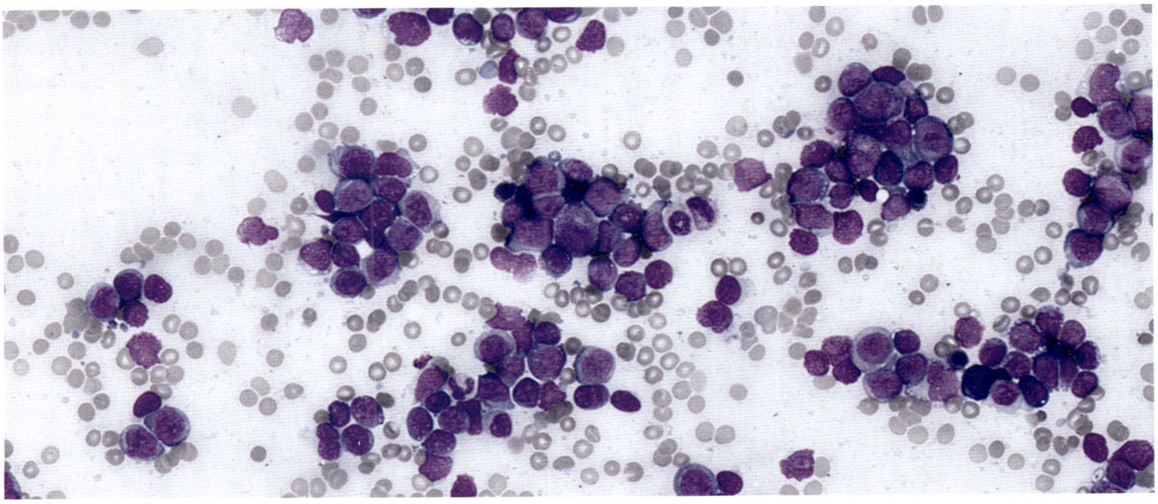

FIGURE 39.2 *KMT2A*-rearranged B/myeloid MPAL with two morphologically distinct populations. Bone marrow smear stained with May-Grünwald Giemsa showing two blast populations: medium-sized agranular blasts corresponding to those with a B-cell immunophenotype and larger, partly granular blasts that showed monocytic differentiation by flow cytometry.

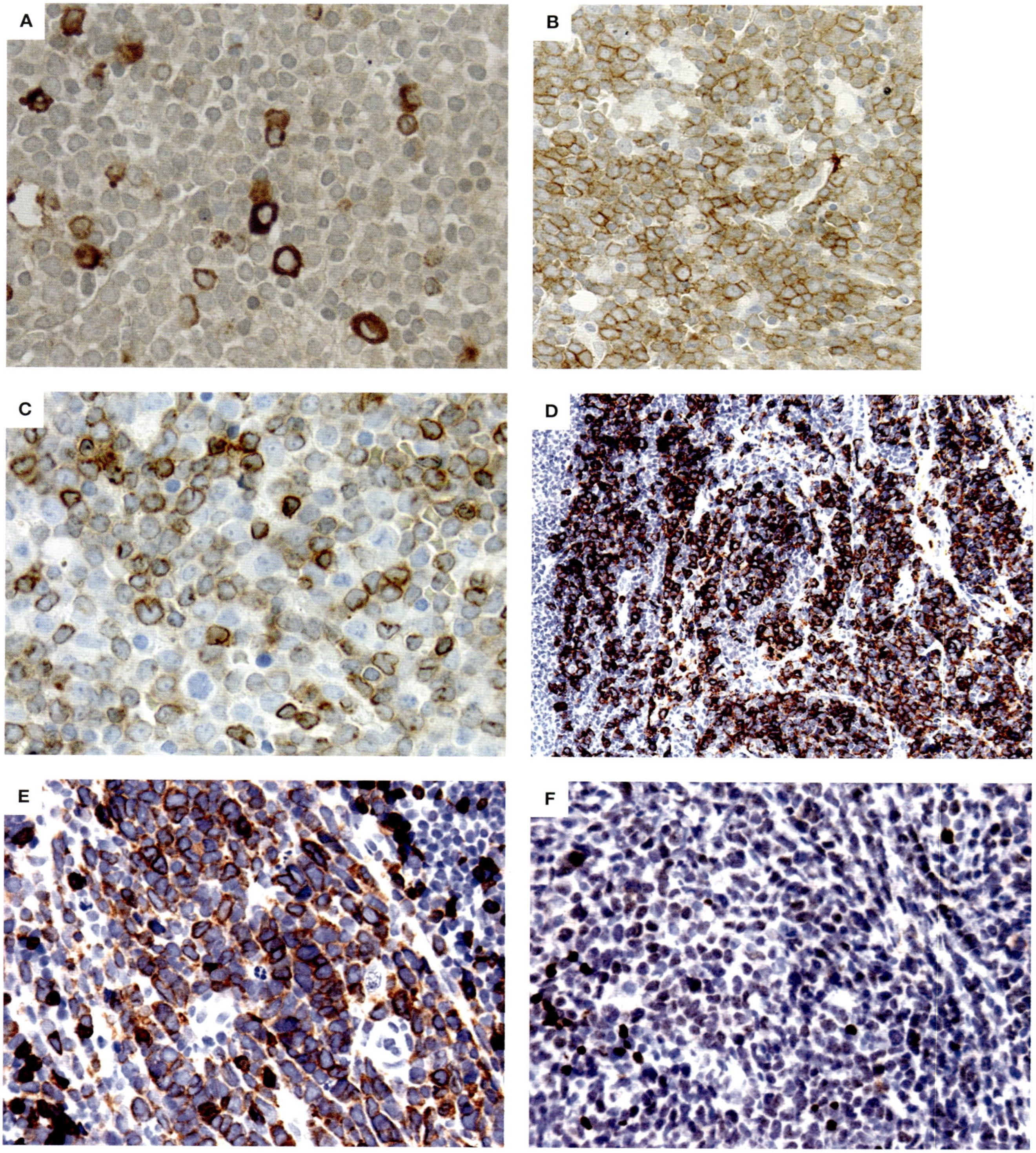

FIGURE 39.3 Immunohistochemical findings in T/myeloid MPAL (a-c, bone marrow biopsy) and B/myeloid MPAL (d-f, lymph node sections). **A:** MPO expression: Cells expressing MPO are larger and much less frequent but amount to ≥10% of blasts. **B:** CD117 immunostaining in the same case shows that all blasts are positive and **(C)** a large fraction is CD3 positive. **D:** MPO-positive blasts **(E)** CD79a and **(F)** weak expression of PAX5. (Adapted from Porwit A, Béné MC. Multiparameter flow cytometry applications in the diagnosis of mixed phenotype acute leukemia. *Cytometry B Clin Cytom*. 2019;96(3):183-194.)

specific but other T-cell-associated markers (CD2, CD4, CD5, CD7, CD8) can be seen in AML and in rare cases of B-cell ALL. However, when associated with cyt.CD3, they may support the T lineage of the blasts.

Myeloid component of MPAL: Myeloperoxidase (MPO) is considered the most specific marker for myeloid lineage. Cyt.MPO can be detected by FCM, cytochemistry, or immunohistochemistry. Published studies have recommended various cutoffs for MPO expression,[5,9,10] but currently no specific threshold is set by International Consensus Classification for MPO positivity due to lack of consistent data. Antigen expression of the blasts should be determined by assessing the fluorescence shift and distribution pattern of the leukemic population against an appropriate control of normal negative population. Extra care should be taken to discriminate small MPO+ leukemic populations (5%-10%) from background nonneoplastic myeloid blasts that express normal immunophenotypic patterns.

MPO expression, typically weak, can also be seen in otherwise typical B-ALL cases, notably those with uniform and bright expression of CD19 and CD10 or CD34 (Figure 39.4). Although such cases have been referred to in the literature as MPAL B/M^{isoMPO},[11] they are not currently considered MPAL, so it is perhaps less confusing if they are called B^{isoMPO} ALL.

In cases where MPO is negative, monocytic differentiation should be established by abnormal expression of more than one monocyte-associated antigen including CD11c, CD14, CD64, or lysozyme (Figure 39.5).

MPAL cases typically show immunophenotypic heterogeneity, including complex displays with brighter, weaker, or absent expression of lineage-specific markers on subpopulations of cells. In cases with a bilineal pattern, expression of MPO is not required. Rather, a diagnosis can be rendered based on separate populations of lymphoid and myeloid blasts that independently meet immunophenotypic criteria for ALL or AML (Figure 39.6). MPAL may have in addition "stem cell–like" populations expressing markers of neither lineage suggesting the origin of the two populations from this common stem cell (Figure 39.6).

Lineage switch: Following initial therapy, some cases of ALL or AML may persist or recur as a leukemia of another lineage. Most cases of lineage transformation involve a switch from ALL to AML after ALL-directed therapy. A retrospective review of leukemia cases with lineage switch often reveals the presence of an unrecognized or underappreciated

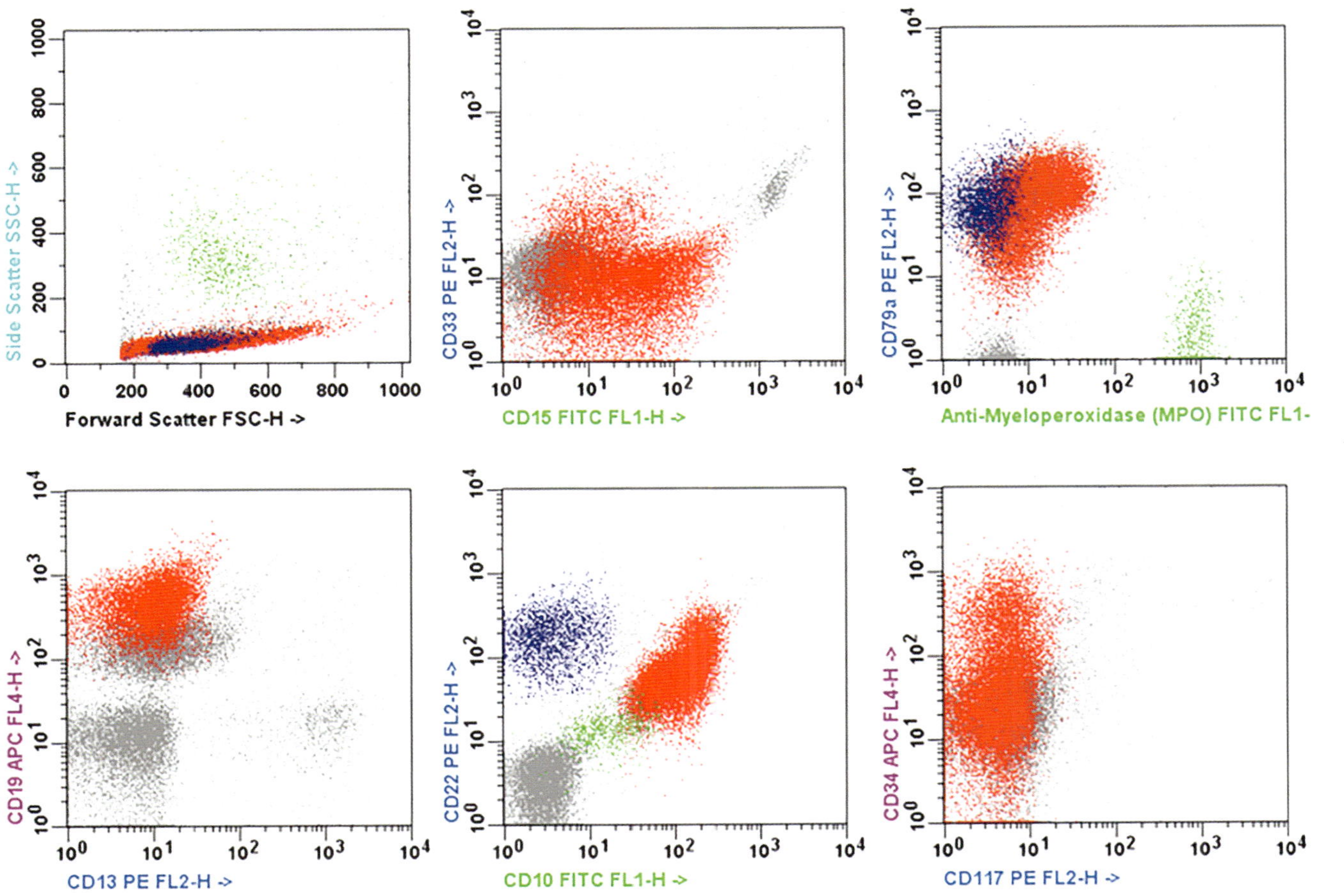

FIGURE 39.4 Flow cytometry of B^{isoMPO} ALL. Bone marrow immunophenotyping showing a population of blasts (red) positive for CD19 (bright), CD10, CD22, cyt.CD79a and with heterogenous CD34 expression. Aberrant expression of CD15 is seen in a fraction of blasts, but CD13 and CD33 are negative. Weak expression of myeloperoxidase is seen in a fraction of blasts (right upper plot). *KMT2A* rearrangement was not detected.

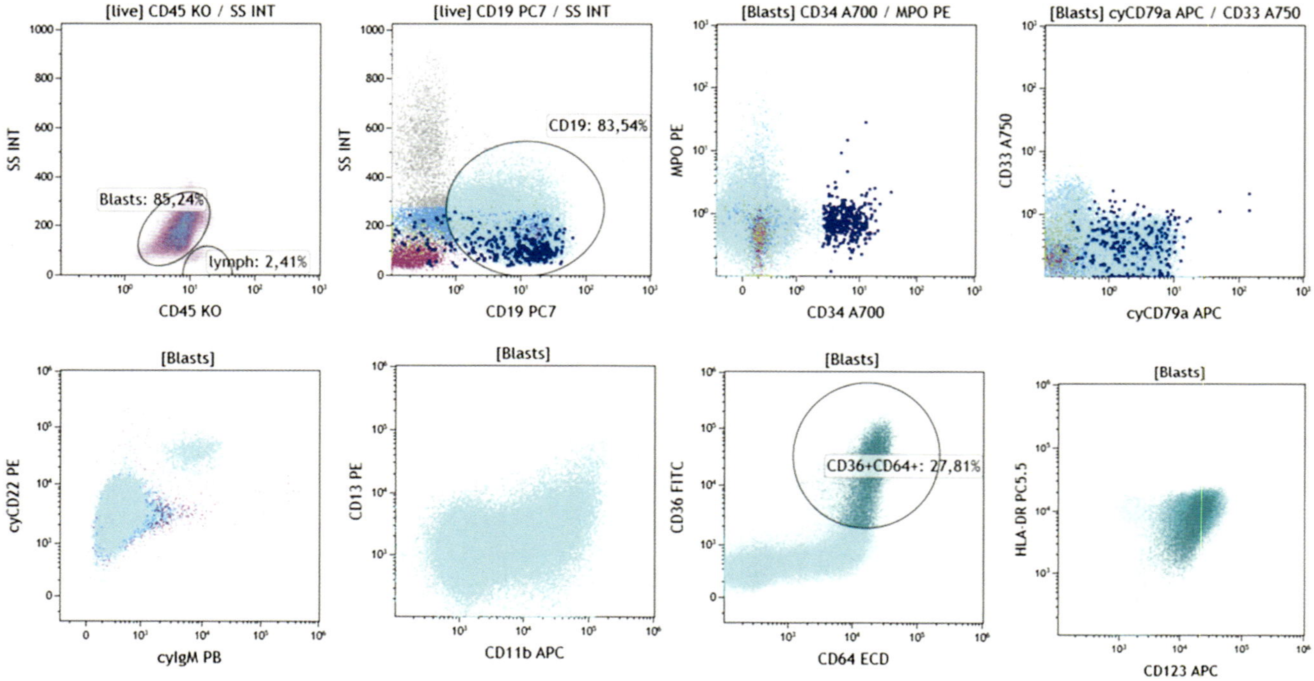

FIGURE 39.5 *KMT2A*-rearranged B/Myeloid MPAL with monocytic component (the same case as in Fig. 39.2). The top left panel shows the heavy infiltration of this bone marrow by a blastic population (85%, cyan dots). These blasts express CD19 and partial cyt.CD79a but lack CD34, MPO, and CD33 (upper panel). Of note, a minor population (dark blue) shows coexpression of CD19, CD34, and cyt.CD79. B lineage is supported by cyt.CD22 (the bottom left plot). Most of the blast cells lack CD11b, CD13, CD64, and CD36 but coexpress HLA-DR and CD123. A subset displays a monocytic immunophenotype with CD11b, partial CD13, and clear CD36 and CD64 expression together with also HLA-DR and CD123 (aquamarine dots).

malignant small population in the initial specimen diagnosed as ALL,[12] underlying the importance of identifying small myeloid populations in ALL cases, even if they are not large enough to permit a diagnosis of MPAL.

The selective pressure brought on by specific therapies can influence these transformations, especially in MPAL turning into AML after the use of B-cell-specific therapy such as blinatumomab.[13,14] However, frank ALL to AML lineage switch must be distinguished from the B-monocytic transition commonly seen early in therapy in B-ALL with *DUX4* rearrangements[15] and other B-ALL subtypes. Such changes do not affect prognosis with continued ALL therapy.

Although less common, AML to ALL transformations have been reported, and the latency interval between completion of induction and lineage switch is generally longer in these cases. It may in some cases represent a treatment-related ALL.

Genetics

As discussed in detail in the following text, subsets of MPAL can be recognized based on recurring genetic alterations. It is critical to note that these alterations are shared with ALL subsets so that immunophenotype defines the underlying diagnosis, and genetic findings identify subsets within MPAL (or ALL), potentially useful for risk stratification. Many other genetic alterations have been described that are seen across many subtypes of ALAL. The majority (64%-87%) of MPAL cases have an abnormal karyotype.[1,5] Reports include cases with MDS-related cytogenetic abnormalities including 17p deletions, and, as noted earlier, these are best considered AML. However, cases meeting criteria for MPAL with 17p deletion or a complex karyotype and a dominant lymphoid phenotype may remain in the MPAL category as it is less clear that these behave like AML. Cytogenetic abnormalities, particularly observed in the B/myeloid subtype, include del[13](p32), trisomy 4, del(6q), 12p11.2 abnormalities, and noncomplex and complex tetraploidy/near-tetraploidy.

Gene mutations found within MPAL are a mixture of those commonly seen in both AML and ALL. Assessment of the frequency of various mutations is difficult because some of the cases included in prior studies were, or should have been classified as AML. In general, the number of detected mutations in MPAL is similar to those of AML and T-ALL, with a

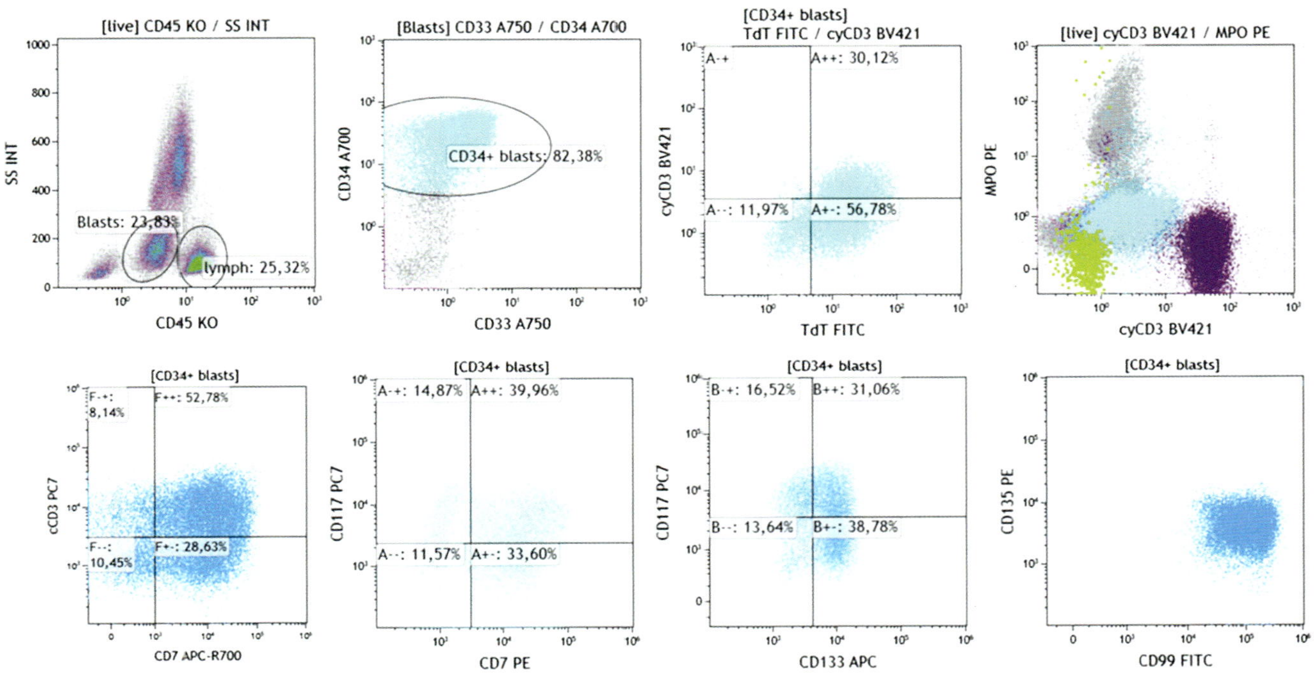

FIGURE 39.6 MPAL with MPO-negative myeloid component. The top left plot shows the blast population with low side scatter (SSC)/ intermediate CD45 (23.8%). The next plot shows CD34$^+$ blasts (cyan) with weak CD33 expression. Combined cyt.CD3 and TdT demonstrate double positivity in 30% of CD34$^+$ cells, while 57% of CD34$^+$ cells are positive for TdT but not for cyt.CD3 and 12% of CD34$^+$ cells are negative for both cyt-CD3 and TdT. The last plot on this top panel indicates that CD34$^+$ cells are negative for MPO and a fraction of CD34$^+$ cells is cyt.CD3$^+$ reaching fluorescence intensity of CD3$^+$ T cells (purple). Cyt.CD3-CD2$^+$ NK cells (green) serve as negative control. The bottom panel focuses on the CD34$^+$ blasts, showing that there is a fraction of CD34$^+$ blasts negative for CD7, CD117, CD133, and cyt. CD3. These cells were CD38+ and HLA-DR + CD33dim. The blast population was negative for CD19, CD2, CD5, CD4, CD8, membrane CD3, and CD1a but positive for cyt.CD79a. A fraction was positive for CD13 and CD10. Karyotype showed three 21-ring chromosomes.

range of 0 to 7 (median, 2), but appears to be significantly higher than in cases of B-ALL.[16] Mutated AML-associated genes include *FLT3*, *RUNX1*, and *CEBPA*, and the ALL-associated genes include *CDKN2A*, *PAX5*, and *ETV6*. *IKZF* is also commonly mutated, and many MPAL cases harbor mutually exclusive mutations of *WT1*, *ETV6*, *RUNX1*, or *CEBPA*.[17]

Prognosis and Clinical Outcome

Outcome data in ALAL are challenging to interpret due to the rarity and heterogeneity of both the disease and therapy. Changes in classification over time also make interpretation of outcome data difficult.[18,19] However, several trends are evident: adults generally fare worse than pediatric patients,[20,21] and genetic changes appear to influence MPAL outcomes and may help to identify patient subsets who will respond favorably to chemotherapy and may be spared more intensive treatment.

Therapeutic approaches to MPAL have varied over time, although all include two key decision points: (1) initial chemotherapy and (2) role of stem cell transplantation (SCT). In both pediatric and adult populations, current international consensus guidelines recommend beginning with lymphoid-directed therapy in nearly all cases,[22-25] although an international Berlin-Frankfurt-Münster consensus statement recommends myeloid therapy for infrequent, immunophenotypically defined cases lacking key lymphoid-associated antigens.[22] Most patients with MPAL will achieve a complete remission[26] with lymphoid therapy. The role for SCT in first remission remains uncertain. Recommendations for adults with MPAL generally favor SCT[24,25] if a donor is available. The benefit from SCT in pediatric patients is less clear, and early disease response may be useful to identify patients who may be cured with chemotherapy alone,[20,27] while patients with poor responses, inadequate treatment, or high-risk disease may benefit from SCT in first remission.[22,28] Future directions in MPAL research will focus on identifying and validating risk-stratified therapy based on genomics and disease response, including potential integration of molecular-targeted therapies, especially in patients with *BCR::ABL1* MPAL. Rare examples of the efficacy of CAR-T cell indicate that this could also be an option.[29]

ACUTE UNDIFFERENTIATED LEUKEMIA

Definition

AUL is an acute leukemia with ≥20% blasts in blood and/or bone marrow where an ALL, AML, or MPAL diagnosis cannot be made due to the lack of specific lymphoid and myeloid markers on blast cells. Immunophenotyping must include an adequate panel of antibodies and exclude rare entities such as blastic plasmacytoid dendritic cell neoplasm, NK-cell leukemia, or basophilic leukemia. Nonhematopoietic tumors should also be excluded.

Synonyms

Blast cell leukemia, stem cell leukemia, undifferentiated leukemia (not recommended).

Epidemiology

A survey of Surveillance, Epidemiology, and End Results database that covered 27% of the US population over the years 2000 to 2016 rendered an incidence of 1.34 per 10^6 persons/year, which is lower than the previously reported incidence of 1.6 per 10^6 persons/year.[30] Declining incidence during the studied period probably reflects more stringent criteria for AUL diagnosis.

General Clinical Features

The median age is 74 years with >70% of patients being older than 50 years.[30] Presentation characteristics are similar as in other patients with acute leukemia.

Morphology

Blasts morphology is nonspecific. MPO and esterases are negative by cytochemistry.

Immunophenotype

The blast population is usually CD45dim, CD34⁺, and HLA-DR⁺ and may express CD38, TdT, and/or CD7 (Figure 39.7). Strong expression of CD19 or positivity for cyt.CD3 and MPO excludes the AUL diagnosis. However, cases with only weak CD19, not supported by any other B-cell marker, as well as MPO-negative cases with only one myeloid marker can also be classified as AUL.[31] Other B-cell-associated markers such as cyt.CD22 or cyt.CD79a can be partly or dimly expressed in the absence of CD19, and CD4 or CD56 may also be present as they are not considered lineage specific. However, when multiple markers of different lineages are present that do not meet criteria for MPAL, a diagnosis of ALAL NOS is preferred.

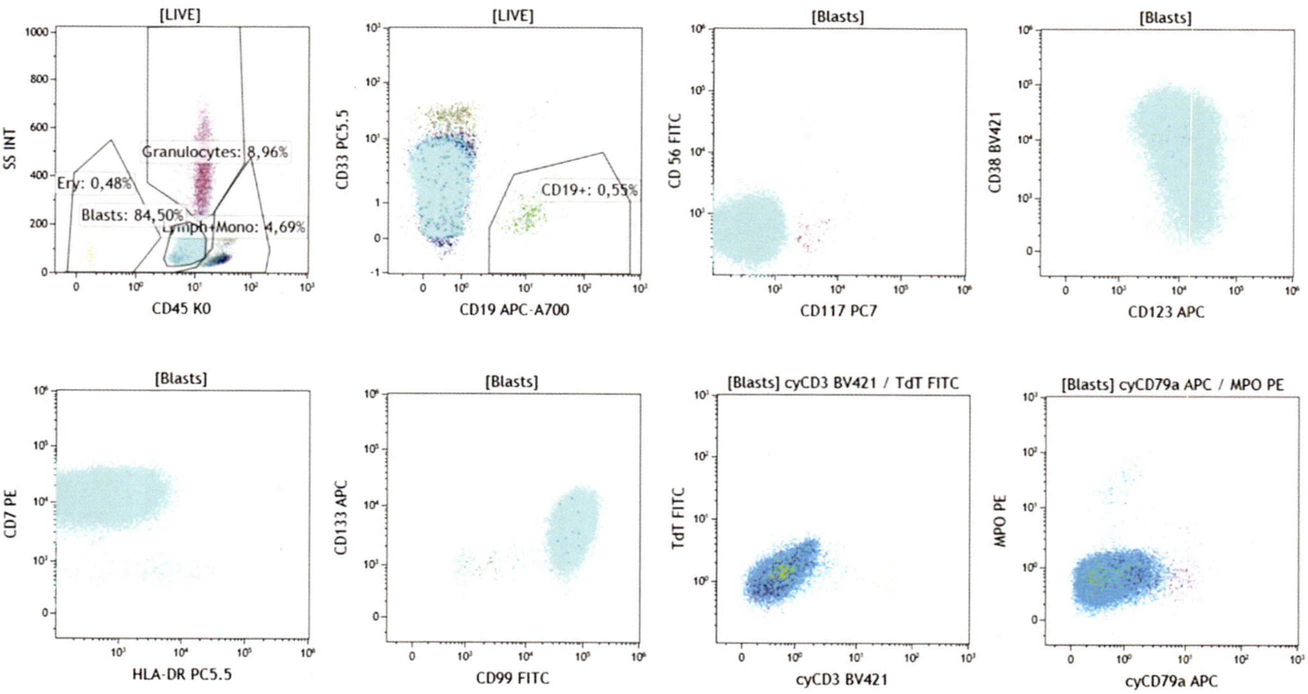

FIGURE 39.7 Acute undifferentiated leukemia. This bone marrow sample shows 84.5% cells in the blast gate (CD45dim, cyan dots). Blasts are CD33^{dim}, HLA-DR^{dim}, CD7⁺, CD99⁺⁺, and CD133⁺ but negative for CD34, CD117, CD19, CD56, cyt.CD3, MPO, TdT, and other B-cell, T-cell, and myeloid markers. Cytogenetics showed a normal karyotype, and next generation sequencing detected a *RUNX1* mutation (40%).

Genetics

In a series of 24 well-defined cases,[31] 58% of the patients had a normal karyotype, and within abnormal karyotypes, trisomy 13 was the most common. Most frequent pathogenic mutations involved *PHF6*, *SRSF2*, *RUNX1*, *ASXL1*, and *BCOR* (~30% of cases each). Some cases of AUL have been reported to carry activation of *BCL11B* (see following discussion and Chapter 41.)

Prognosis and Clinical Comment

In small published series, the prognosis of AUL is generally poor, even when excluding cases with MDS-related genetic lesions. Clinical outcome in patients who received induction chemotherapy was similar between AUL and acute myeloid leukemia with minimal differentiation, but children with AUL generally fared better with improved outcomes relative to adults.[30] There is no standard therapeutic approach to AUL. Depending on donor availability, SCT in first remission is often recommended, although the evidence for this recommendation is sparse.

MIXED-PHENOTYPE ACUTE LEUKEMIA WITH RECURRENT GENETIC ABNORMALITIES

MPAL With t(9;22)(q34.1;q11.2), *BCR::ABL1*

Definition

MPAL with t(9;22)(q34.1;q11.2), *BCR::ABL1* is an acute leukemia that fulfills criteria of MPAL and carries a *BCR::ABL1* rearrangement demonstrated by fluorescence in situ hybridization (FISH), polymerase chain reaction, or conventional cytogenetics. This diagnosis should not be rendered in patients with a previous diagnosis of chronic myeloid leukemia (CML).

Synonym

Biphenotypic acute leukemia with t(9;22)(q34.1;q11.2) (not recommended).

Epidemiology

The t(9;22)(q34.1;q11.2)/*BCR::ABL1* rearrangement occurs in approximately 8% of MPAL cases[5] and <1% of all leukemia cases. It is more common in adults.

General clinical features

Presentation is similar to patients with ALL with *BCR::ABL1*, although splenomegaly without lymphadenopathy should suggest CML in mixed blast phase.

Morphology

In many cases there are two populations of larger and smaller blasts suggesting the presence of lymphoblasts and myeloblasts. Background maturing granulocytosis and/or basophilia should not be present as these findings suggest underlying CML.

Immunophenotype

Most cases of MPAL with *BCR::ABL1* present with a B/myeloid immunophenotype; only rare cases of T/myeloid, B/T, and B/T/myeloid have been reported.[29,32] The B-cell component is most often CD19⁺CD10⁺⁺ with coexpression of CD13 and/or CD33 and/or CD66c. CD34 is variably expressed. The myeloid blast population is most often CD34⁺/CD33⁺/MPO⁺ but MPO negative B/myeloid MPALs with myeloid component similar to AML with minimal differentiation may occur.

Genetics

Complex karyotypes may be seen. The p190 fusion transcript is more common, and it is reported in approximately 60% of the cases, and various additional cytogenetic abnormalities can also be found in such cases.

Prognosis and clinical comment

Concurrent administration of first- or later-generation tyrosine kinase inhibitors, together with chemotherapy, improves the outcomes of patients with MPAL *BCR::ABL1*, and reported overall survivals are similar to those of patients with *BCR::ABL1* B-ALL.[33,34]

MPAL, With t(v;11q23.3); *KMT2A* Rearranged

Definition

MPALs with t(v;11q23.2), *KMT2A* rearrangement are acute leukemias that fulfill MPAL criteria and carry a translocation resulting in *KMT2A* rearrangement.

Synonym

Mixed-phenotype acute leukemia with *MLL* rearrangement (not recommended).

Epidemiology

KMT2A rearrangement occurs in approximately 10% of MPAL cases[5] and <1% of all leukemia cases. It is most common in infants but may occur in children and younger adults.

General Clinical Features

Presentation is similar to patients with B-ALL with *KMT2A* rearrangement. White blood counts are often very high, and central nervous system involvement is common.

Morphology

In many cases there are two populations of larger and smaller blasts, the latter suggesting lymphoblasts and the former, with abundant cytoplasm suggesting monoblasts (Figure 39.2), often esterase positive. Rarely, MPO may be detected by cytochemistry in a subset of blasts.

Immunophenotype

Most MPAL cases with a *KMT2A* rearrangement are B/myeloid. The B-cell component most often has a B-I or "pro-B" ALL phenotype, typically CD19$^+$ CD10$^-$. CD34 expression is variable, CD20 is usually negative, and other B-cell markers such as CD22, CD24, and cyt.CD79a are often weakly expressed. As in *KMT2A*-rearranged ALL, there may be weak expression of CD15, CD65, and/or CD33 while CD66 is negative. NG2 is often positive. The myeloid blast population is often of monocytic lineage and MPO negative as illustrated in Figure 39.5. Rare cases of T/myeloid and B/T KMT2A-rearranged MPAL have been reported.[35,36] Myeloid or biphenotypic populations may be very small at diagnosis and, especially in patients with high leukocytosis, masked by numerous lymphoblasts. These small populations should be followed in posttherapy samples because lineage switch is fairly common in this entity after induction therapy.

Genetics

KMT2A rearrangements are detected by break-apart FISH or karyotyping analysis. Translocation (4;11)(q21.3;q23.3), ie, *KMT2A::AFF1,* is the most common, but other fusion partners have also been reported such as t(9;11)(p21-22;q23.2);*KMT2A::MLLT3,* t(10;11)(p12;q23);*MLL::MLLT10,* and t(11;19)(q23.2;p13.1), *KMT2A::MLLT1.* Additional chromosomal changes may be present, and some may occur with lineage switch.

Prognosis and Clinical Comment

Patients with *KMT2A*-rearranged MPAL are mainly treated with ALL protocols but have a poor prognosis. *KMT2A* MPAL is often diagnosed in retrospect. AML therapy is typically used in patients who undergo lineage switch after initial treatment. As in other forms of MPAL, the role for SCT in CR1 remains uncertain for both children and adults but may improve outcome in patients with poor therapy response.

B/Myeloid MPAL With *ZNF384* Rearrangement

Definition

MPAL with t(v;12p13), rearranged *ZNF384* (*ZNF384r*) is an acute leukemia that fulfills criteria of MPAL and carries a translocation resulting in a *ZNF384* rearrangement.

Epidemiology

The *ZNF384* transcription factor gene is rearranged in approximately 10% of MPAL cases.[17,37,38] *ZNF384r* MPAL is most common in children and rarely seen in younger adults (<60 years of age). In childhood B/myeloid MPAL, fusion genes involving *ZNF384* have been identified in nearly 50% of cases.

General Clinical Features

Presentation is the same as in patients with B-ALL with *ZNF384* rearrangement. High leukocytosis is uncommon.

Morphology

The blasts are of non-specific morphology. MPO may be detected by cytochemistry in a subset of blasts.

Immunophenotype

CD19 expression is usually strong and supported by CD22 and/or cyt.CD79a expression while CD10 expression is absent or weak and typically seen only in a subset of blasts. Strong expression of CD34 and CD33 is common, while CD13, CD15, CD66c, and/or CD117 are seen in a fraction of blasts in some cases. MPO is seen in a fraction of blasts[39]; this is a particularly important distinguishing feature because *ZNF384*r B-ALL typically expresses myeloid-associated surface markers. To date, there have been no reported cases of T/myeloid, B/T, or B/T/myeloid MPAL with *ZNF384* rearrangements.

Genetics

The *ZNF384* rearrangement involves several gene partners (>10), such as *TCF3* (most common) or *EP300, TAF15* or *CREBBP.* The genomic landscape of childhood *ZNF384* is similar to that of *ZNF384*r B-ALL, except for *KDM6A* alterations, which have been observed only in MPAL.[17] Moreover, *ZNF384*r MPAL shows enrichment of stem cell pathways and genes upregulated in early T-precursor (ETP)-ALL. Additional chromosomal changes, including complex karyotype, have been reported.

Prognosis and Clinical Comment

The outcomes for *ZNF384r* MPAL do not significantly differ from other cases of B/myeloid MPAL.[17] Similar treatment principles apply for frontline therapy, beginning with ALL-directed induction chemotherapy.

T/Myeloid MPAL With *BCL11B* Alteration

Definition

MPAL with deregulated *BCL11B* gene (on chromosome 14q32) is an acute leukemia that fulfills T/myeloid MPAL criteria (Table 39.2) and is associated with an activating alteration of the *BCL11B* gene (see Chapter 42.) *BCL11B* deregulation can also be seen in ETP-ALL or AUL.

Epidemiology

This entity accounts for 10% to 15% of MPAL, and *BCL11B* deregulation is seen exclusively in T/myeloid cases.[40–42] Male predominance has been reported.

General clinical features

Presentation is similar to that of patients with ETP T-ALL.

Morphology

Blasts are morphologically nonspecific. MPO may be detected by cytochemistry in a subset of blasts.

Immunophenotype

BCL11B deregulated leukemias have usually an immature immunophenotype characterized by the presence of several blast subpopulations (Figure 39.1). Most blasts are positive for HLA-DR, CD117, and/or CD34$^+$ as well as CD2. Cyt.CD3$^+$ and CD7 are seen in a fraction of the blasts, but T-cell-associated markers such as CD5, CD4, CD8, and CD1a are negative (Figure 39.1). Given the phenotypic overlap with ETP-ALL,[43] this diagnosis virtually always requires demonstration of MPO.

Genetics

The genetic alterations that produce *BCL11B* activation are described in Chapter 42 under the category of "ETP-ALL, *BCL11B* activated." As with that entity there are also recurrent additional genetic alterations in T/myeloid MPAL especially ones involving *FLT3*, *RUNX1*, and *WT1*. To date there are too few cases studied to know if there are any significant genetic differences between ETP and T/myeloid MPAL with *BCL11B* activation.

Prognosis and clinical comment

Data describing outcomes for this newly described subgroup are not yet available, although outcome is likely to be similar to that seen in ETP-ALL with *BCL11B* activation.

MIXED-PHENOTYPE ACUTE LEUKEMIA WITH DEFINING IMMUNOPHENOTYPIC CHANGES

MPAL, B/Myeloid, Not Otherwise Specified

Definition

B/myeloid MPAL, NOS is a mixed-phenotype acute leukemia that involves B and myeloid lineage and does not fulfill criteria of an MPAL with a recurrent genetic alteration.

Epidemiology

B/myeloid MPAL, NOS comprises <1% of all leukemia cases and represent approximately 30% of MPAL cases.

General clinical features

Presentation is similar to that of patients with other acute leukemias.

Morphology

Blasts may be morphologically nonspecific, or there may be two blast populations with distinctive sizes and/or a population with some granulation or rare Auer rods. MPO or esterase may be detected by cytochemistry in a subset of blasts.

Immunophenotype

The blasts express CD19 with other B-cell markers fulfilling criteria for B-lineage assignment, although markers of mature B cells such as CD20 are rare. Myeloid antigen expression must fulfill criteria described earlier unless there is a bilineal pattern with the myeloid component fulfilling criteria for AML.

Genetics

Most cases carry an abnormal karyotype; tetraploid or near-tetraploid leukemia cases relatively often present with a B/myeloid immunophenotype, typically with a dominant B-ALL population. Mutations including *DNMT3A*, *FLT3*, *ASXL1*, *TET2*, and others seen in either ALL or AML may be detected.

T/Myeloid MPAL, Not Otherwise Specified

Definition

T/myeloid MPAL, NOS is a mixed-phenotype acute leukemia that involves T and myeloid lineages and does not fulfill criteria of MPAL with a recurrent genetic alteration. Because ETP-ALL is defined by an immature hematopoietic phenotype with nonspecific myeloid features such as CD13 or CD33 expression, the main distinction between T/myeloid MPAL and ETP-ALL is the presence of MPO in T/myeloid MPAL.

Epidemiology

T/myeloid MPAL comprises <1% of all leukemia cases and represents approximately 20% of MPAL cases.

General Clinical Features

Presentation is similar to that of other patients with acute leukemia.

Morphology

Blasts usually have a cytologically undifferentiated appearance, but sometimes there may be two blast populations with distinctive sizes and/or a population with some granulation or rare Auer rods. MPO or esterase may be detected by cytochemistry in a subset of blasts.

Immunophenotype

At least a fraction of blasts express cyt.CD3 that reaches the fluorescence intensity of normal T cells, most often together with CD7 that may also be expressed on a cyt. CD3-negative blast population. CD2 and/or CD5 may be detected, but significant expression of markers of more mature T cells including membrane CD3 or CD4 is rare. Myeloid antigen expression must fulfill criteria described earlier (Table 39.2) unless there is a bilineal pattern with the myeloid component fulfilling criteria for AML (Figure 39.8).

Genetics

T/myeloid MPAL, NOS has a mutational and gene expression profile that overlaps with that of ETP-ALL with frequent alterations in the transcription factors WT1, ETV6, or RUNX1. T/myeloid MPAL, NOS has a low mutation frequency of core T-ALL genes *CDKN2A* and *NOTCH1*or of the *KIT* gene that is frequently involved in AML.

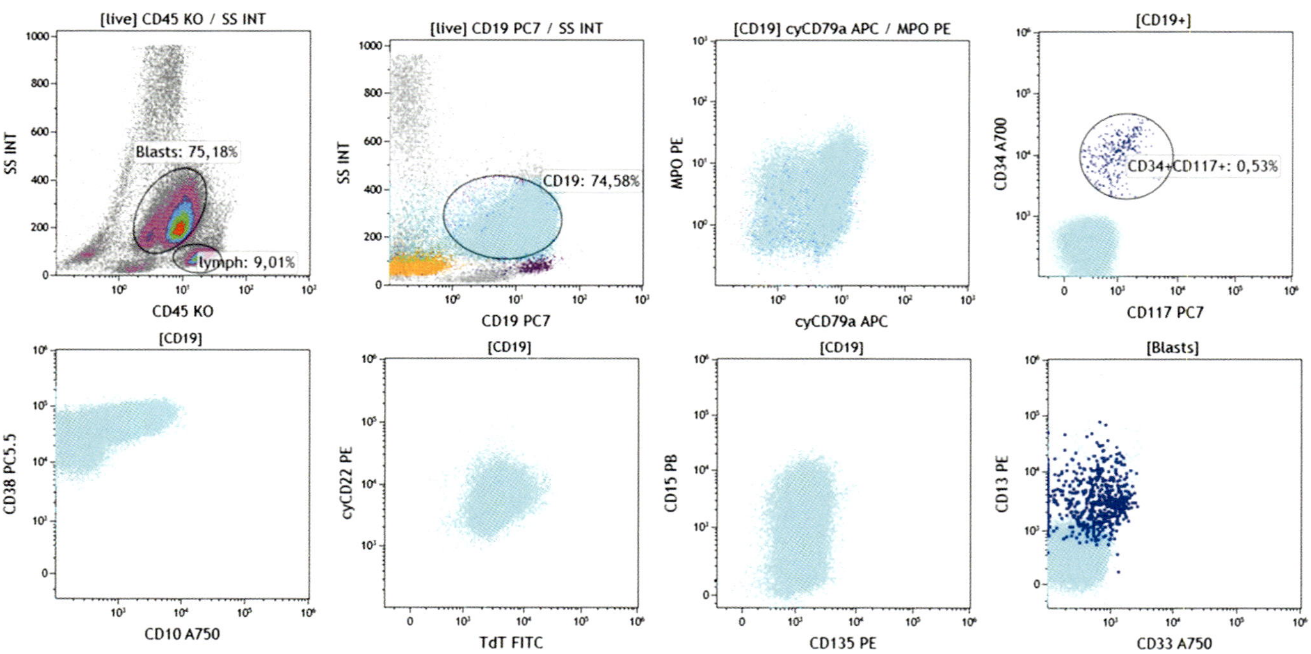

FIGURE 39.8 MPAL B/myeloid, not otherwise specified. The top left plot shows a blast population with intermediate SSC and CD45 (75%). It appears in cyan dots on the next plots indicating B lineage with CD19 and cyt.CD79a expression. These cells also display partial expression of MPO in the absence of CD117 and CD34. A minor population highlighted in dark blue coexpresses CD117 and CD34, but these cells do not express CD19 and cyt.CD79a and most probably represent rare residual immature progenitors. The bottom panel completes the B-lineage immunophenotype with cyt.CD22 and partial CD10. A bright expression of CD38 and TdT is also shown. Blasts weakly express CD135 (FLT3) and partly the myeloid antigen CD15 in the absence of CD33 and CD13. No *KMT2A* rearrangement or *BCR::ABL1* was detected.

Prognosis and clinical comment

Prognosis and clinical outcome are discussed in detail earlier. Response to therapy in T/myeloid MPAL may occur later than in B/myeloid MPAL, analogous to differences between T-ALL and B-ALL.

B/T/Myeloid MPAL and B/T MPAL

These types of MPAL have been reported very rarely,[5] and little is known of their specific clinical or genetic characteristics. They must meet the defined immunophenotypic criteria for each lineage and should not express MPAL-associated genetic features. The total blast population must be >20%, and as noted above, if <5% blasts of a one lineage are present a description of the phenotype, rather than definitive diagnosis, is recommended.

References

1. Borowitz MJ, Béné MC, Harris NJ, et al. Acute leukaemias of ambiguous origin. In: Swerdlow SH, Campo E, Harris NL, et al, eds. WHO Classification of Tumours of Haematopoietic and Lymphoid Tissues. 4th ed. IARC; 2008.
2. Borowitz MJ, Béné MC, Harris NJ, et al. Acute leukaemias of ambiguous origin. In: Swerdlow SH, Campo E, Harris NL, et al, eds. 4th ed rev. IARC; 2017.
3. Béné MC, Castoldi G, Knapp W, et al. Proposals for the immunological classification of acute leukemias. European Group for the Immunological Characterization of Leukemias (EGIL). *Leukemia.* 1995;9(10):1783-1786.
4. Aggarwal N, Weinberg OK. Update on acute leukemias of ambiguous lineage. *Clin Lab Med.* 2021;41(3):453-466.
5. Porwit A, Béné MC. Multiparameter flow cytometry applications in the diagnosis of mixed phenotype acute leukemia. *Cytometry B Clin Cytom.* 2019;96(3):183-194.
6. Weinberg OK, Arber DA, Döhner H, et al. The International Consensus Classification of acute leukemias of ambiguous lineage. *Blood.* 2023;141(18):2275-2277.
7. Béné MC, Nebe T, Bettelheim P, et al. Immunophenotyping of acute leukemia and lymphoproliferative disorders: a consensus proposal of the European LeukemiaNet Work Package 10. *Leukemia.* 2011;25(4):567-574.
8. van Dongen JJ, Lhermitte L, Böttcher S, et al. EuroFlow antibody panels for standardized n-dimensional flow cytometric immunophenotyping of normal, reactive and malignant leukocytes. *Leukemia.* 2012;26(9):1908-1975.
9. Guy J, Antony-Debré I, Benayoun E, et al. Flow cytometry thresholds of myeloperoxidase detection to discriminate between acute lymphoblastic or myeloblastic leukaemia. *Br J Haematol.* 2013;161(4):551-555.
10. Khoury JD, Solary E, Abla O, et al. The 5th edition of the World Health Organization classification of haematolymphoid tumours: myeloid and histiocytic/dendritic neoplasms. *Leukemia.* 2022;36(7):1703-1719.
11. Weinberg OK, Dennis J, Zia H, et al. Adult mixed phenotype acute leukemia (MPAL): B/myeloid MPAL^{isoMPO} is distinct from other MPAL subtypes. *Int J Lab Hematol.* 2023;45(2):170-178.
12. Chen C, Yu W, Alikarami F, et al. Single-cell multiomics reveals increased plasticity, resistant populations, and stem-cell-like blasts in *KMT2A*-rearranged leukemia. *Blood.* 2022;139(14):2198-2211.
13. Abdo Y, Gibson GD, Jain SP, Milner CP, Hilal T. Treatment of relapsed B/T-cell mixed phenotype acute leukemia with blinatumomab. *Cureus.* 2023;15(6):e40661.
14. Brethon B, Lainey E, Caye-Eude A, et al. Case report: targeting 2 antigens as a promising strategy in mixed phenotype acute leukemia—combination of blinatumomab with gemtuzumab ozogamicin in an infant with a KMT2A-rearranged leukemia. *Front Oncol.* 2021;11:637951.
15. Novakova M, Zaliova M, Fiser K, et al. DUX4r, ZNF384r and PAX5-P80R mutated B-cell precursor acute lymphoblastic leukemia frequently undergo monocytic switch. *Haematologica.* 2021;106(8):2066-2075.
16. Takahashi K, Wang F, Morita K, et al. Integrative genomic analysis of adult mixed phenotype acute leukemia delineates lineage associated molecular subtypes. *Nat Commun.* 2018;9(1):2670.
17. Alexander TB, Gu Z, Iacobucci I, et al. The genetic basis and cell of origin of mixed phenotype acute leukaemia. *Nature.* 2018;562(7727):373-379.
18. Pomerantz A, Rodriguez-Rodriguez S, Demichelis-Gomez R, et al. Mixed-phenotype acute leukemia: suboptimal treatment when the 2008/2016 WHO classification is used. *Blood Res.* 2016;51(4):233-241.
19. Weinberg OK, Seetharam M, Ren L, Alizadeh A, Arber DA. Mixed phenotype acute leukemia: a study of 61 cases using World Health Organization and European Group for the immunological classification of leukaemias criteria. *Am J Clin Pathol.* 2014;142(6):803-808.
20. Maruffi M, Sposto R, Oberley MJ, Kysh L, Orgel E. Therapy for children and adults with mixed phenotype acute leukemia: a systematic review and meta-analysis. *Leukemia.* 2018;32(7):1515-1528.
21. Shi R, Munker R. Survival of patients with mixed phenotype acute leukemias: a large population-based study. *Leuk Res.* 2015;39(6):606-616.
22. Hrusak O, de Haas V, Stancikova J, et al. International cooperative study identifies treatment strategy in childhood ambiguous lineage leukemia. *Blood.* 2018;132(3):264-276.
23. Orgel E, Alexander TB, Wood BL, et al. Mixed-phenotype acute leukemia: a cohort and consensus research strategy from the Children's Oncology Group acute leukemia of ambiguous lineage task force. *Cancer.* 2020;126(3):593-601.

24. Wolach O, Stone RM. How I treat mixed-phenotype acute leukemia. *Blood*. 2015;125(16):2477-2485.
25. Wolach O, Stone RM. Optimal therapeutic strategies for mixed phenotype acute leukemia. *Curr Opin Hematol*. 2020;27(2):95-102.
26. Li MY, Lin ZH, Hu MM, et al. Secondary donor-derived humanized CD19-modified CAR-T cells induce remission in relapsed/refractory mixed phenotype acute leukemia after allogeneic hematopoietic stem cell transplantation: a case report. *Biomark Res*. 2020;8:36.
27. Oberley MJ, Raikar SS, Wertheim GB, et al. Significance of minimal residual disease in pediatric mixed phenotype acute leukemia: a multicenter cohort study. *Leukemia*. 2020;34(7):1741-1750.
28. Munker R, Labopin M, Esteve J, Schmid C, Mohty M, Nagler A. Mixed phenotype acute leukemia: outcomes with allogeneic stem cell transplantation. A retrospective study from the Acute Leukemia Working Party of the EBMT. *Haematologica*. 2017;102(12):2134-2140.
29. Kohla SA, Sabbagh AA, Omri HE, et al. Mixed phenotype acute leukemia with two immunophenotypically distinct B and T blasts populations, double Ph (+) chromosome and complex karyotype: report of an unusual case. *Clin Med Insights Blood Disord*. 2015;8:25-31.
30. Qasrawi A, Gomes V, Chacko CA, et al. Acute undifferentiated leukemia: data on incidence and outcomes from a large population-based database. *Leuk Res*. 2020;89:106301.
31. Weinberg OK, Hasserjian RP, Baraban E, et al. Clinical, immunophenotypic, and genomic findings of acute undifferentiated leukemia and comparison to acute myeloid leukemia with minimal differentiation: a study from the bone marrow pathology group. *Mod Pathol*. 2019;32(9):1373-1385.
32. Rahman K, George S, Tewari A, Mehta A. Mixed phenotypic acute leukemia with two immunophenotypically distinct blast populations: report of an unusual case. *Cytometry B Clin Cytom*. 2013;84(3):198-201.
33. Qasrawi A, Ramlal R, Munker R, Hildebrandt GC. Prognostic impact of Philadelphia chromosome in mixed phenotype acute leukemia (MPAL): a cancer registry analysis on real-world outcome. *Am J Hematol*. 2020;95(9):1015-1021.
34. Shimizu H, Yokohama A, Hatsumi N, et al. Philadelphia chromosome-positive mixed phenotype acute leukemia in the imatinib era. *Eur J Haematol*. 2014;93(4):297-301.
35. Naghashpour M, Lancet J, Moscinski L, Zhang L. Mixed phenotype acute leukemia with t(11;19)(q23;p13.3)/MLL-MLLT1(ENL), B/T-lymphoid type: a first case report. *Am J Hematol*. 2010;85(6):451-454.
36. Syed S, Song A, Hussaini M. Expanding diagnostic criteria: multiorgan T-Cell/myeloid mixed phenotype acute leukemia with t(v;11q23) *KMT2A*-rearrangement successfully treated by allogeneic stem cell transplant. *Leuk Res Rep*. 2022;17:100306.
37. Sudutan T, Erbilgin Y, Hatirnaz Ng O, et al. Zinc finger protein 384 (*ZNF384*) impact on childhood mixed phenotype acute leukemia and B-cell precursor acute lymphoblastic leukemia. *Leuk Lymphoma*. 2022;63(12):2931-2939.
38. Wang Q, Cai WZ, Wang QR, et al. Integrative genomic and transcriptomic profiling reveals distinct molecular subsets in adult mixed phenotype acute leukemia. *Am J Hematol*. 2023;98(1):66-78.
39. Zaliova M, Winkowska L, Stuchly J, et al. A novel class of ZNF384 aberrations in acute leukemia. *Blood Adv*. 2021;5(21):4393-4397.
40. Di Giacomo D, La Starza R, Gorello P, et al. 14q32 rearrangements deregulating *BCL11B* mark a distinct subgroup of T-lymphoid and myeloid immature acute leukemia. *Blood*. 2021;138(9):773-784.
41. Montefiori LE, Bendig S, Gu Z, et al. Enhancer hijacking drives oncogenic *BCL11B* expression in lineage-ambiguous stem cell leukemia. *Cancer Discov*. 2021;11:2846-2867.
42. Montefiori LE, Mullighan CG. Redefining the biological basis of lineage-ambiguous leukemia through genomics: BCL11B deregulation in acute leukemias of ambiguous lineage. *Best Pract Res Clin Haematol*. 2021;34(4):101329.
43. Coustan-Smith E, Mullighan CG, Onciu M, et al. Early T-cell precursor leukaemia: a subtype of very high-risk acute lymphoblastic leukaemia. *Lancet Oncol*. 2009;10(2):147-156.

Chapter 40

B-Lymphoblastic Leukemias/Lymphomas

Amy Duffield, Michael J. Borowitz, Sindhu Cherian, Mark D. Ewalt, Stephen Hunger, Elias Jabbour, Charles G. Mullighan, and Leonie Saft

B-lymphoblastic leukemia/lymphoma (B-ALL/LBL) has long been recognized to comprise a heterogeneous group of diseases with distinct genetic characteristics; in the last several years many new entities with recurrent genetic abnormalities have been described, resulting in a significant expansion of the subclassification of B-ALL (Table 40.1). Most of these entities can be distinguished based on unique gene expression (GEX) profiles (Figure 40.1). Some are common and some are rare, and they show different rates of occurrence in patients of different ages (Figure 40.2).

B-ALL/LBL WITH RECURRENT GENETIC ABNORMALITIES

Of note, the ICC subdivides the previous category of B-ALL/LBL with *BCR::ABL1* into lymphoid only involvement and multilineage involvement. The previous entities B-ALL/LBL with hypodiploidy and B-ALL/LBL, *BCR::ABL1*-like are also further subdivided in the ICC. An additional nine new categories of B-ALL/LBL are defined, including seven entities with characteristic gene rearrangements and two new categories with specific single gene mutations.

B-ALL/LBL WITH t(9;22)(q34.1;q11.2)/*BCR::ABL1* WITH LYMPHOID ONLY INVOLVEMENT

Definition

B-lymphoblastic leukemia/lymphoma (B-ALL/LBL) with t(9;22)(q34.1;q11.2)/*BCR::ABL1* with lymphoid only involvement (*BCR::ABL1*+ ALL-L) is a neoplasm of lymphoblasts committed to the B-cell lineage in which the blasts harbor a translocation between *BCR* on chromosome 22 and the *ABL1* oncogene on chromosome 9. This translocation is only present in blasts and is not seen in cells of other lineages.

Synonyms

PH+ ALL (not recommended).

Epidemiology

Taken together, ALL/LBLs that harbor *BCR::ABL1* are more common in adults than children, accounting for <5% of pediatric cases, with the incidence increasing with age to comprise about 25% of adult B-ALL/LBL.

Although there are as yet limited data on the relative frequency of this subtype, *BCR::ABL1*+ ALL-L appears more common than *BCR::ABL1*+ ALL with multilineage involvement (*BCR::ABL1*+ ALL-M, see the following section).[1,2]

General clinical features

The presentation of *BCR::ABL1*+ ALL-L is similar to that of other types of de novo B-ALL/LBL.

Morphology

There are no unique morphologic features that distinguish this entity from other types of ALL.

Immunophenotype

Blasts are usually positive for CD19 (sometimes dim), CD10 (bright), TdT, and CD38 (dim). There is frequent expression of the myeloid-associated antigens CD13 and CD33 on the blasts, and CD66c expression is also typically seen. CD25 expression has been reported to be highly associated with *BCR::ABL1*+ B-ALL/LBL.[3] Immunophenotypic signatures have been described in pediatric patients with *BCR::ABL1*+ B-ALL/LBL by clustering analysis, including overexpression of CD33, CD34, CD45, CD52, HLA-DR, and TdT.[4] Acute leukemias with *BCR::ABL1* may also present with a B/myeloid mixed phenotype acute leukemia (MPAL) immunophenotype, in which case the neoplasm should be classified as B/myeloid MPAL with *BCR::ABL1* (see Chapter 39: Acute Leukemias of Ambiguous Lineage).

Genetics

The target cell for the transformation event in *BCR::ABL1*+ ALL-L is considered to be a lymphoid-committed hematopoietic progenitor. The t(9;22)(q34.1;q11.2)

TABLE 40.1 B-lymphoblastic leukemia/lymphoma (B-ALL)

B-ALL with recurrent genetic abnormalities
B-ALL with t(9;22)(q34.1;q11.2)/*BCR::ABL1*
with lymphoid only involvement
with multilineage involvement
B-ALL with t(v;11q23.3)/*KMT2A* rearranged
B-ALL with t(12;21)(p13.2;q22.1)/*ETV6::RUNX1*
B-ALL, hyperdiploid
B-ALL, low hypodiploid
B-ALL, near haploid
B-ALL with t(5;14)(p31.1;q32.3)/*IL3::IGH*
B-ALL with t(1;19)(q23.3;p13.3)/*TCF3::PBX1*
B-ALL, *BCR::ABL1*-like, *ABL1* class rearranged
B-ALL, *BCR::ABL1*-like, JAK-STAT activated
B-ALL, *BCR::ABL1*-like, NOS
B-ALL with iAMP21
B-ALL with *DUX4* rearrangement
B-ALL with *ZNF384* rearrangement
B-ALL with *MEF2D* rearrangement
B-ALL with *MYC* rearrangement
B-ALL with *NUTM1* rearrangement
B-ALL with *UBTF::ATXN7L3/PAN3, CDX2* (CDX2/UBTF)
B-ALL with *HLF* rearrangement
B-ALL with mutated PAX5 P80R
B-ALL with mutated IKZF1 N159Y
B-ALL, Not Otherwise Specified

results from the fusion of *BCR* at 22q11.2 and the cytoplasmic tyrosine kinase gene *ABL1* at 9q34.1, with production of a BCR::ABL1 fusion protein. Of note, variant/complex rearrangements may also be seen that also result in the fusion of *BCR* to *ABL1*, but do not generate the canonical Philadelphia (Ph) chromosome. The diagnosis can be rendered via FISH, as the fusion is seen exclusively in blasts (Figure 40.3). This is in contrast to *BCR::ABL1*+ ALL-M and chronic myeloid leukemia in lymphoid blast crisis (CML-LBP), in which the fusion protein is also seen in cell types other than blasts. Various BCR::ABL1 fusion protein isoforms have been identified, although p190 and p210 are the most common, with no definite clinical differences attributed to the length of the gene product. Although p190 is more strongly associated with B-ALL/LBL, the size of the fusion protein or transcript cannot be used to distinguish between CML-LBP and B-ALL/LBL, as both p190 and p210 can be seen in *BCR::ABL1*+ ALL. Other genetic abnormalities can be seen in *BCR::ABL1*+ ALL, including frequent *IKZF1* deletions.[5] In rare cases, concomitant abnormalities occur that might otherwise cause a case to be placed in one of the other categories such as B-ALL/LBL, hyperdiploid; however, it is generally believed that *BCR::ABL1* is the driving abnormality and will govern the clinical behavior of the neoplasm. Thus, in cases of *de novo* B-ALL that contain *BCR::ABL1*, classification as *BCR::ABL1*+ ALL-L is generally most appropriate. Rarely, however, *BCR::ABL1* fusion occurs in a subclone of an ALL with another driver mutation that is present in significantly higher frequency. It is unclear whether these cases behave like classic Ph+ ALL cases or whether ABL1 tyrosine kinase inhibitors (TKIs) are needed.

Prognosis and clinical comment

Overall, B-ALL/LBL with *BCR::ABL1* has historically been associated with a poor prognosis in both children and adults; however, therapy with TKIs has significantly improved outcomes in patients who lack a concomitant *IKZF1* alteration.[6] The achievement of minimal residual disease (MRD) negativity following treatment with chemotherapy/immunotherapy and TKIs may spare children the need for transplantation.[6]

Prognosis in children with *BCR::ABL1*+ ALL-L is affected by age, white blood cell (WBC) count, and response to therapy as assessed by MRD testing.[2]

B-ALL/LBL WITH t(9;22)(q34.1;q11.2)/*BCR::ABL1* WITH MULTILINEAGE INVOLVEMENT

Definition

B-ALL/LBL with t(9;22)(q34.1;q11.2) and multilineage involvement (*BCR::ABL1*+ ALL-M) is a neoplasm in which not only the B-lymphoblasts but also other cell types, including myeloid cells and mature lymphocytes, harbor a translocation between *BCR* on chromosome 22 and the *ABL1* oncogene on chromosome 9.[7]

Synonyms

CML-like Ph+ ALL; *BCR::ABL1*+ ALL-M (not recommended).

Epidemiology

This entity is reported in both children and adults. In children, *BCR::ABL1*+ ALL-M cases appear to comprise about 25% of all B-ALL/LBL associated with *BCR::ABL1*, although data are limited.[7] A similar percentage was seen in one small series of adult B-ALL/LBL cases.[1]

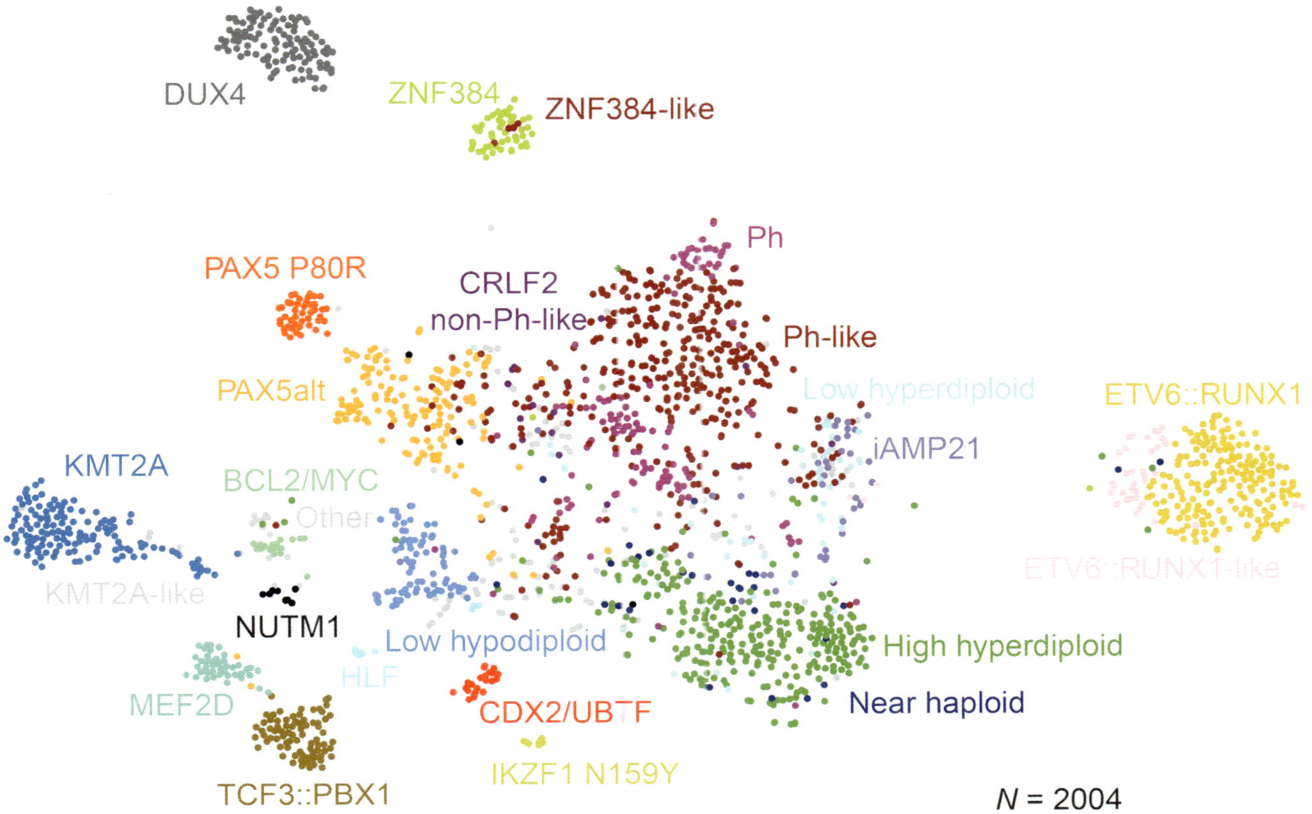

FIGURE 40.1 Gene expression clustering of B-ALL/LBL cases. Two-dimensional clustering using t-distributed stochastic neighbor embedding of whole transcriptome sequencing data from 2004 leukemia samples collected at diagnosis from children or adults with ALL. Cases are color coded by subtype. This approach, and much of the data, were first reported by Gu et al.[67] (Figure courtesy of Dr. Shunsuke Kimura, St. Jude Children's Research Hospital.)

General clinical features

The clinical presentation of *BCR::ABL1*+ ALL-M is similar to that of *BCR::ABL1*+ ALL-L, although in children the WBC count tends to be lower in *BCR::ABL1*+ ALL-M than in *BCR::ABL1*+ ALL-L.[7] Patients with *BCR::ABL1*+ ALL-M do not have an antecedent history of CML. The diagnosis may be suspected when the percentage of blasts in the specimen as quantified by morphology and/or flow cytometry is significantly lower than disease burden as quantified by FISH or reverse transcript (RT) PCR studies for the *BCR::ABL1* transcript. This pattern is seen because the latter studies will detect the fusion not only in the blasts but also in the other cell types.[1] Although this may be difficult to appreciate at presentation when blasts predominate, this discordance is often demonstrated in retrospect in the setting of minimal residual disease.[2] The distinction between *BCR::ABL1*+ ALL-M and CML-LBP can be difficult without a history of prior CML; however, *BCR::ABL1*+ ALL-M is not known to be associated with significant splenomegaly. Relapse may be medullary, extramedullary, or combined.[7]

Morphology

There are no unique morphologic features that distinguish this entity from other types of ALL. Additional study is needed, but basophilia has not been reported as a feature of this entity.

Immunophenotype

The immunophenotype of the blasts in *BCR::ABL1*+ ALL-M is similar to that seen in *BCR::ABL1*+ ALL-L (see the previous section).

Genetics

The target cell for the transformation event in *BCR::ABL1*+ ALL-M is believed to be a multipotent progenitor. Both p190 and p210 are reported in *BCR::ABL1*+ ALL-M. The frequency of secondary genomic alterations in *BCR::ABL1*+ ALL-M is variable, but this entity is often associated with *IKZF1* deletions.[8]

Prognosis and clinical comment

Data that compare outcomes of *BCR::ABL1*+ ALL-M patients to those with *BCR::ABL1*+ ALL-L are limited.

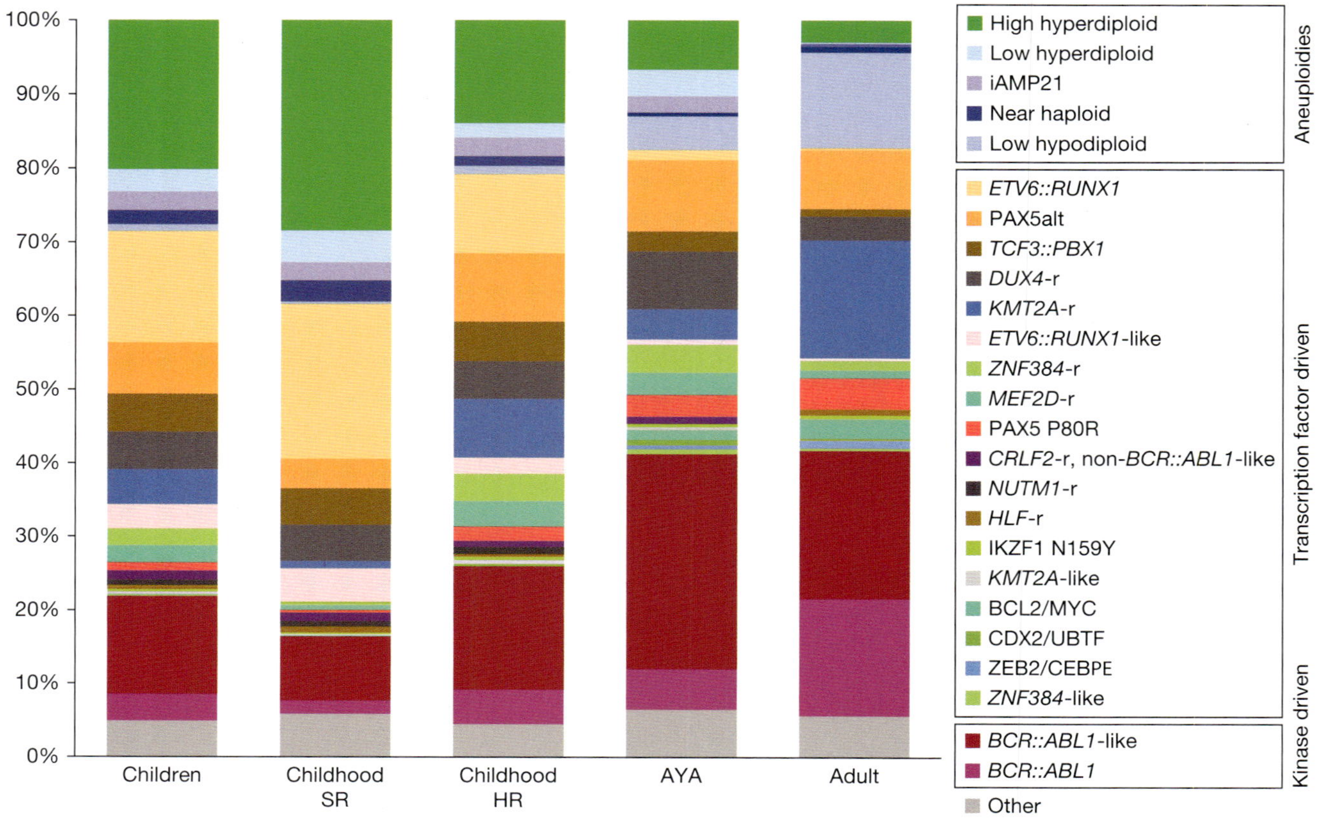

FIGURE 40.2 Age distribution among the various subtypes of B-ALL/LBL. The frequency of each B-ALL/LBL subtype is shown in children (1191 cases, birth-15 y), standard-risk children (childhood standard-risk, 515 cases), high-risk children (childhood high-risk, 676 cases), adolescents and young adults (AYA, 419 cases, 16-39 y), and adults (378 cases, 40+ years). Standard risk and high risk are defined according to the National Cancer Institute criteria. The colors denoting the various subtypes in the GEX clustering figure (Figure 40.1) correlate with the colors in the histograms. (Figure courtesy of Dr. Ilaria Iacobucci, St. Jude Children's Research Hospital.)

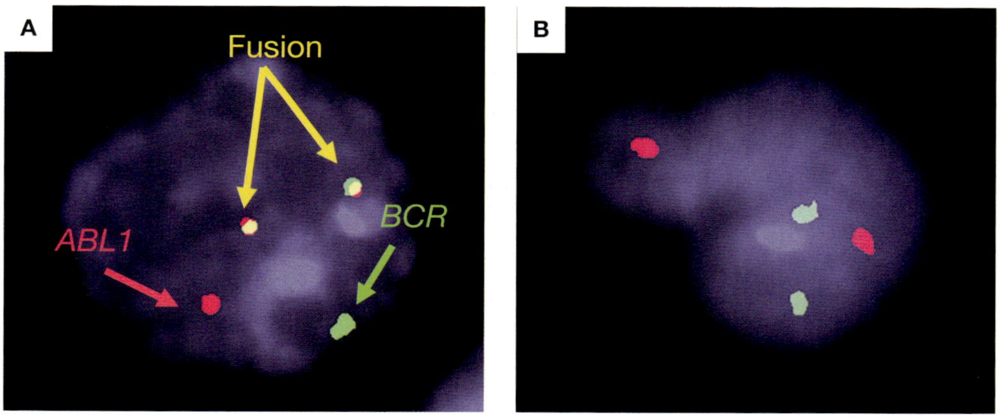

FIGURE 40.3 B-ALL with t(9;22)(q34.1;q11.2)/*BCR::ABL1* with lymphoid only involvement. **A:** Lymphoblasts were hybridized with the *BCR::ABL1* dual fusion probes, directed against *BCR* (22q11.2; green) and *ABL1* (9q34.1; red). The blasts show evidence of the rearrangement (yellow) with residual normal copies of *BCR* and *ABL1*. **B:** Rare residual neutrophils were identified and similarly hybridized, and show two copies of each gene with no fusion. By contrast, neutrophils from a case of B-ALL with *BCR::ABL1* ALL with multilineage involvement (not shown) would show evidence of *BCR::ABL1* fusion. (Images courtesy of Umut Aypar, PhD, FACMG, Memorial Sloan Kettering Cancer Center.)

Pediatric patients with *BCR::ABL1*+ ALL-M appear to have a similar survival as those with *BCR::ABL1*+ ALL-L.[2] In adults, patients with *BCR::ABL1*+ ALL-M appear to have a worse prognosis than patients with *BCR::ABL1*+ ALL-L.[1] Hyperleukocytosis is not known to be an adverse prognostic factor, and, in contrast to *BCR::ABL1*+ ALL-L, MRD status does not appear to affect prognosis in children.[2] As with *BCR::ABL1*+ ALL-M, the incorporation of TKIs into treatment protocols may spare patients transplant.

B-ALL/LBL WITH t(v;11q23.3)/*KMT2A*-REARRANGED

Definition

B-ALL/LBL with t(v;11q23.3) is a neoplasm of lymphoblasts committed to the B-cell lineage in which the blasts harbor a translocation between *KMT2A* (previously called *MLL*) at band 11q23.3 and any of a large number of fusion partners. Leukemias that have deletions of 11q23.3 without *KMT2A* rearrangement are not included in this group.

Synonyms

B-ALL/LBL with t(v;11q23); *MLL*-rearranged (not recommended).

Epidemiology

This entity is the most common leukemia in infants younger than 1 year of age, comprising 60% to 70% of all infant ALL. It is less common in older children, and then becomes increasingly common with age into adulthood. Although the specific etiology of B-ALL/LBL with *KMT2A* translocations is unknown, this rearrangement may occur in *utero*, and *KMT2A* translocations have been identified in neonatal blood spots of patients who subsequently developed leukemia.[9]

General clinical features

Patients with this leukemia typically present with very high WBC counts, often >100 × 10^9/L. There is also a high frequency of CNS involvement at diagnosis in infants, and a somewhat higher incidence in noninfants.[10] Although organ involvement may be seen, entirely lymphomatous presentations are not typical for this entity.

Morphology

There are no unique morphologic features that distinguish this entity from other types of ALL. In some cases of acute leukemia with *KMT2A* rearrangement, morphologically distinct populations of lymphoblasts and monoblasts may be seen. If immunophenotyping studies confirm separate populations of blasts or divergent B/myeloid differentiation, then the neoplasm should be classified as B/myeloid MPAL rather than B-ALL/LBL, *KMT2A*-rearranged.

Immunophenotype

This entity is characterized by lineage ambiguity; by definition it presents as B-ALL/LBL but may undergo lineage shifts over the course of the disease. Cases with t(4;11) typically have a CD19$^+$, CD10$^-$, and CD24$^-$ pro-B immunophenotype. The expression of NG2 is highly predictive for *KMT2A* rearrangement, as is the combination of CD10$^-$ and CD15$^+$ B-lymphoblasts. CD22 can be dim, absent, or partially expressed in cases with *KMT2A* gene rearrangement, and CD34 may be negative[11] (Figure 40.4).

Genetics

The *KMT2A* gene on chromosome 11q23.3 is known to have more than 100 fusion partners.[12] The most common partner gene is *AFF1* (AF4) on chromosome 4q21 (Figure 40.5), and other common fusions include *MLLT1* (ENL) on chromosome 19p13.3 (Figure 40.6), and *MLLT3* (AF9) on chromosome 9p21.3. These gene fusions are not specific for B-ALL, as *KMT2A::MLLT1* is also identified in T-ALL, and *KMT2A::MLLT3* is also seen in association with acute myeloid leukemia. Translocations involving *KMT2A* can be detected by standard karyotyping studies or by FISH with a break-apart probe directed against this gene. Targeted PCR studies may be used to identify the most common translocation partners; however, anchored multiplex PCR, whole transcriptome sequencing, or whole genome sequencing is needed to identify the full array of *KMT2A* fusion partners. Unlike most subtypes of B-ALL/LBL, B-ALL/LBL with *KMT2A* rearrangement in infants has very few associated additional mutations, and when mutations occur they typically involve Ras pathways.

Prognosis and Clinical Comment

Infants with *KMT2A* rearrangements, especially those less than 6 months of age, have a very poor prognosis. Adult patients with *KMT2A* rearrangements, regardless

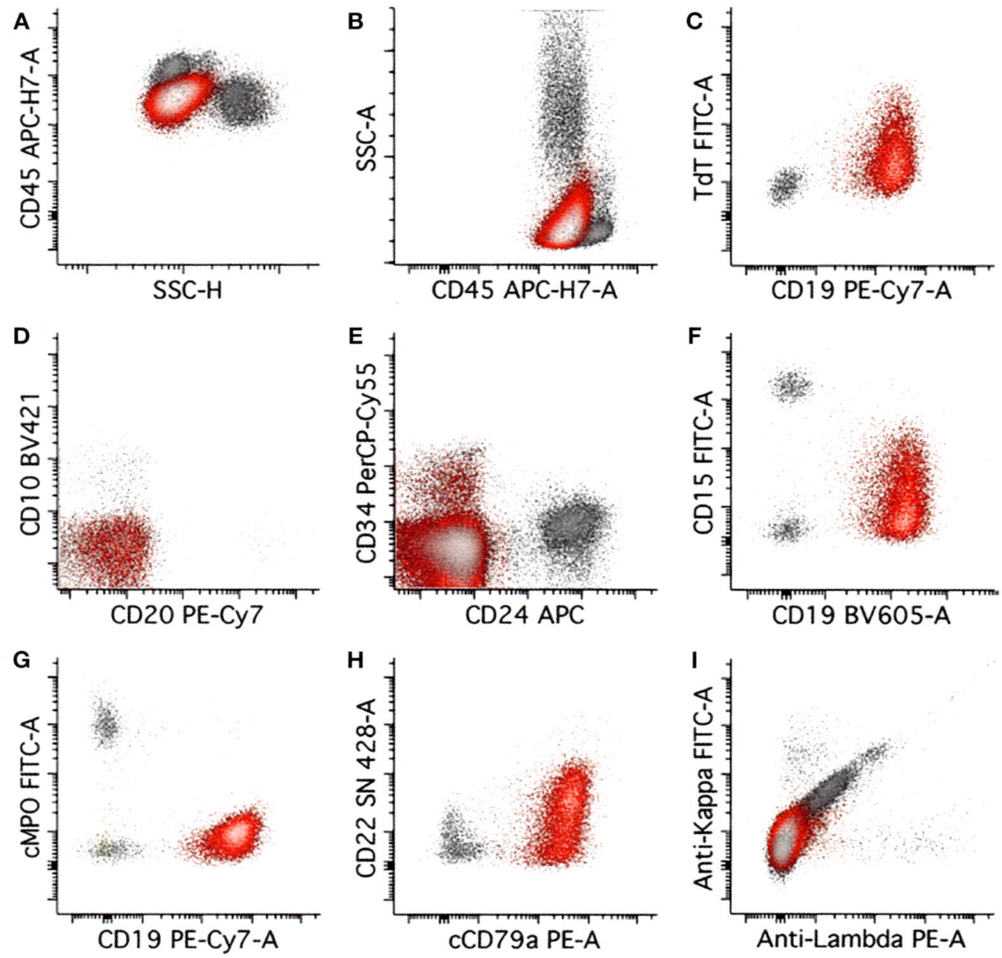

FIGURE 40.4 Flow cytometric analysis of B-ALL, *KMT2A*-rearranged. There is a distinct population of blasts (red) with dim CD45 and low right angle scatter (**A** and **B**); expressing CD19 and dim TdT (**C**), but lacking CD10 and CD20 (**D**), and with partial (minor subset) expression of CD34 (**E**). The blasts lack expression of CD24 (**E**), with partial expression of CD15 (**F**), and absent myeloperoxidase (**G**). The blasts also express cytoplasmic CD79a with partial dim CD22 (**H**), but lack expression of surface light chains (**I**).

of the partner, also have poor outcomes. In children other than infants, leukemias with the relatively common *KMT2A::AFF1* translocation have a poor prognosis, although the outcome for children with other *KMT2A* translocation partners is better.[10]

B-ALL/LBL WITH t(12;21)(p13.2;q22.1)/*ETV6::RUNX1*

Definition

B-ALL/LBL with t(12;21)(p13.2;q22.1) is a neoplasm of lymphoblasts committed to the B-cell lineage in which the blasts harbor a translocation between *ETV6* (previously called *TEL*) on chromosome 12 and *RUNX1* (previously called *AML1*) on chromosome 21.

Synonyms

B acute lymphoblastic leukemia/lymphoma with t(12;21)(p13.2;q22.1); *TEL/AML1* (not recommended).

Epidemiology

This leukemia is rarely seen in infants; however, it accounts for about 25% of cases of B-ALL/LBL in children. The incidence decreases with age, and it is rare in adulthood.

General Clinical Features

There are no unique clinical features that distinguish this entity from other types of ALL.

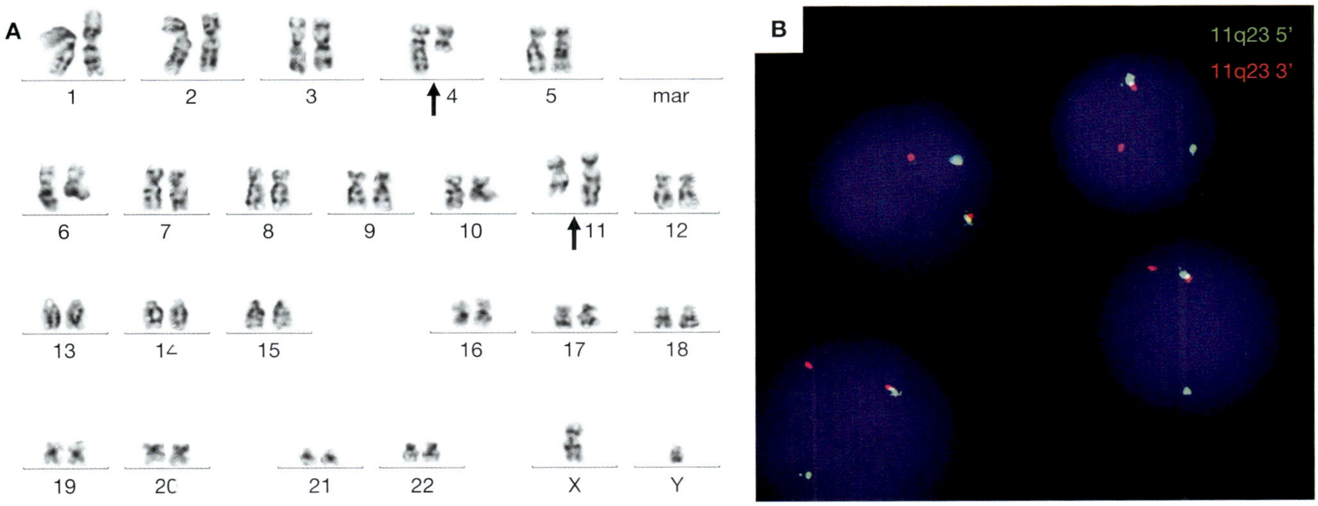

FIGURE 40.5 Cytogenetic characterization of B-ALL with t(4;11)(q21;q23)/*KMT2A::MLLT2(AFF1)*. **A:** G-banded karyotype showing translocation of genetic material from 4q to 11q. **B:** Fluorescence in situ hybridization (FISH) studies using a *KMT2A* (11q23) break-apart probe (5′ green, 3′ red) showing 4 blasts. All cells show one normal copy of *KMT2A*, with juxtaposition of 3′ and 5′ probes (yellow), as well as one copy of *KMT2A* disrupted by the translocation, with separation of the 5′ green and 3′ red probes. (Images courtesy of Umut Aypar, PhD, FACMG, Memorial Sloan Kettering Cancer Center.)

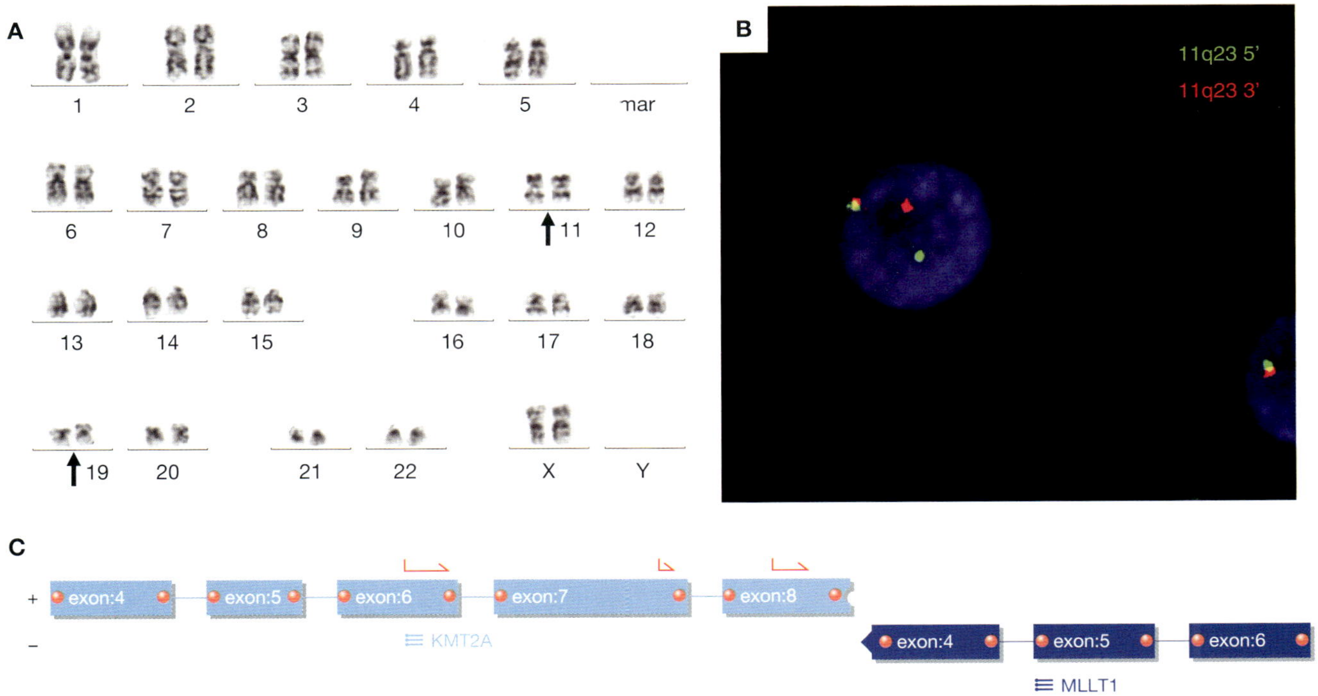

FIGURE 40.6 Cytogenetic characterization of a case of B-ALL with t(11;19)(q23;p13.3)/*KMT2A::MLLT1(ENL)*. **A:** G-banded karyotype showing translocation of genetic material from 11q to 19p. **B:** FISH using a *KMT2A* (11q23) break-apart probe, demonstrating that one copy of *KMT2A* is disrupted by the translocation, with separation of the 5′ green and 3′ red probes. One normal copy of *KMT2A* is also present (yellow). **C:** *KMT2A* (exon 8):*MLLT1* (exon 4) translocation, confirmed by anchored multiplex PCR. (Images courtesy of Umut Aypar, PhD, FACMG, Memorial Sloan Kettering Cancer Center.)

Morphology

There are no unique morphologic features that distinguish this entity from other types of ALL.

Immunophenotype

Blasts typically have a CD19^{+}, CD10^{+}, TdT+ phenotype, and are usually CD34 positive. The blasts also show expression of CD27, as well as a characteristic near or complete absence of CD9, CD20, CD44, and CD66c. Myeloid-associated antigens, such as CD13, are often expressed. This immunophenotype is relatively specific, but is also seen in the provisional entity B-ALL/LBL, *ETV6::RUNX1*-like.

Genetics

The *ETV6::RUNX1* translocation is thought to be an early lesion in leukemogenesis. The translocation is necessary but not sufficient for the development of disease, with the ETV6::RUNX1 fusion protein disrupting the function of the transcription factor *RUNX1*. Additional genetic alterations are common, particularly focal deletions mediated by aberrant recombination-activating gene activity, including deletion of the non-rearranged copy of *ETV6*, but none is specific. This entity has a characteristic GEX signature that is shared by the provisional entity B-ALL/LBL, *ETV6::RUNX1*-like (see Figure 40.1).

Prognosis and Clinical Comment

This entity has a very favorable prognosis, particularly in patients without adverse risk factors. Children with adverse prognostic factors do not have as favorable a prognosis, but tend to have better outcomes than B-ALL patients with the same adverse factors but different genetic lesions. Relapses often occur later than in other types of B-ALL. It has been suggested that these late relapses derive from persistent preleukemic clones that harbor the *ETV6::RUNX1* translocation without the additional genetic events required for the development of acute leukemia.

B-ALL/LBL, HYPERDIPLOID

Definition

B-ALL/LBL, hyperdiploid is a neoplasm of lymphoblasts committed to the B-cell lineage in which the blasts contain greater than 50 chromosomes, but usually fewer than 66 chromosomes.

Synonyms

Hyperdiploid acute lymphoblastic leukemia; high hyperdiploid acute lymphoblastic leukemia.

Epidemiology

This leukemia is not seen in infants but is common in children, accounting for about 30% of cases of B-ALL/LBL in this age group.[13] It decreases in frequency among older children, and is uncommon in adults, accounting for approximately 7% to 8% of cases.

General Clinical Features

There are no unique clinical features that distinguish this entity from other types of ALL.

Morphology

There are no unique morphologic features that distinguish this entity from other types of ALL.

Immunophenotype

Blasts are positive for CD19 and CD10, and express other markers typical of B-ALL/LBL. Most cases are CD34 positive, and CD45 is often decreased or absent. Altered (often higher) expression levels have been reported for several other antigens, including CD9, CD58, CD86, and CD123,[14] and CD66c positivity has also been reported.[15]

Genetics

Hyperdiploid B-ALL/LBL contains an increase in the number of chromosomes, usually without translocations or other structural abnormalities. Extra copies of chromosomes are non-random, and most commonly include chromosomes X, 4, 10, 14, 18, and 21.[13] Extra copies of chromosomes 1, 2, and 3 are the least often seen. Hyperdiploid B-ALL/LBL can be detected by karyotype, FISH, or flow cytometric DNA index. The identification of common trisomies by FISH, such as chromosomes 4 and 10 (double trisomy), is widely used as a surrogate marker for this entity, but only detects approximately two-thirds of hyperdiploid B-ALL/LBL cases. Some cases that appear to be hyperdiploid by conventional karyotyping may in fact be hypodiploid B-ALL/LBL that has undergone endoreduplication. In cases with endoreduplication, the aneuploidy is characterized mainly by tetrasomy rather than trisomy; this pattern is referred to as masked hypodiploidy (Figure 40.7), and these cases should not be classified as hyperdiploid B-ALL/

LBL.[16] Flow cytometric evaluation of the DNA index will often show an imperfect correlation between the DNA index and aneuploidy; for example, cases that have multiple gains of small chromosomes but fewer gains of large chromosomes often do not have a DNA index of >1.16. Hyperdiploidy may also be observed in a subset of cases with *BCR::ABL1*; as noted previously, these cases are best classified as B-ALL with *BCR::ABL1*. Rearrangement of *CRLF2* may also be observed, usually as a secondary event.[17]

Prognosis and Clinical Comment

Overall, this leukemia has a very favorable prognosis. Cure is achieved in >90% of children overall, and is even more common in children with a favorable risk profile. The specific chromosomes that appear as trisomies may be more important to prognosis than the total number of chromosomes, with simultaneous trisomies of chromosomes 4 and 10 associated with the best prognosis in some studies.[18] Factors such as advanced patient age and high WBC count may adversely affect the prognosis, but these patients may still have a favorable prognosis relative to other subtypes of B-ALL/LBL. Too few adult cases have been studied to determine the prognosis in this population.

B-ALL/LBL, LOW HYPODIPLOID

Definition

B-ALL/LBL, low hypodiploid is a neoplasm of lymphoblasts committed to the B-cell lineage in which the blasts harbor 32 to 39 chromosomes.

Synonyms

None.

Epidemiology

This entity is more common in adults than in children. There is an association with germline *TP53* mutations and Li Fraumeni syndrome, particularly in children.[19]

General Clinical Features

There are no unique clinical features that distinguish this entity from other types of ALL.

Morphology

There are no unique morphologic features that distinguish this entity from other types of ALL.

Immunophenotype

Blasts are typically CD19$^+$ and CD10$^+$, but there are no unique immunophenotypic features that distinguish this entity from other types of ALL.

Genetics

This leukemia definitionally exhibits multiple chromosomal losses. The most common targets of aneuploidy are chromosomes 2, 3, 4, 7, 9, 12, 13, 15, 16, 17 and 20. Chromosome 21 is never lost. The diagnosis can, however, be missed on standard karyotyping because of endoreduplication, which results in masked hypodiploidy (discussed previously in B-ALL/LBL, hyperdiploid) (see Figure 40.7). Structural abnormalities may be seen in the remaining chromosomes, although there are no specific structural abnormalities that are characteristically associated with this entity. The vast majority of low hypodiploid ALL cases have a *TP53* mutation, and this is present in the germline (Li Fraumeni syndrome) in about half of these cases in children. This subtype is also often associated with alterations in *IKZF2* and *RB1*, as well as activation of Ras-signaling and phosphoinositide 3-kinase-signaling pathways.[20]

Prognosis and Clinical Comment

B-ALL/LBL, low hypodiploid has a poor prognosis, especially in adults.

B-ALL/LBL, NEAR HAPLOID

Definition

B-ALL/LBL, near haploid is a neoplasm of lymphoblasts committed to the B-cell lineage in which the blasts harbor 24 to 31 chromosomes.

Synonyms

None.

Epidemiology

B-ALL/LBL, near haploid is most common in children.

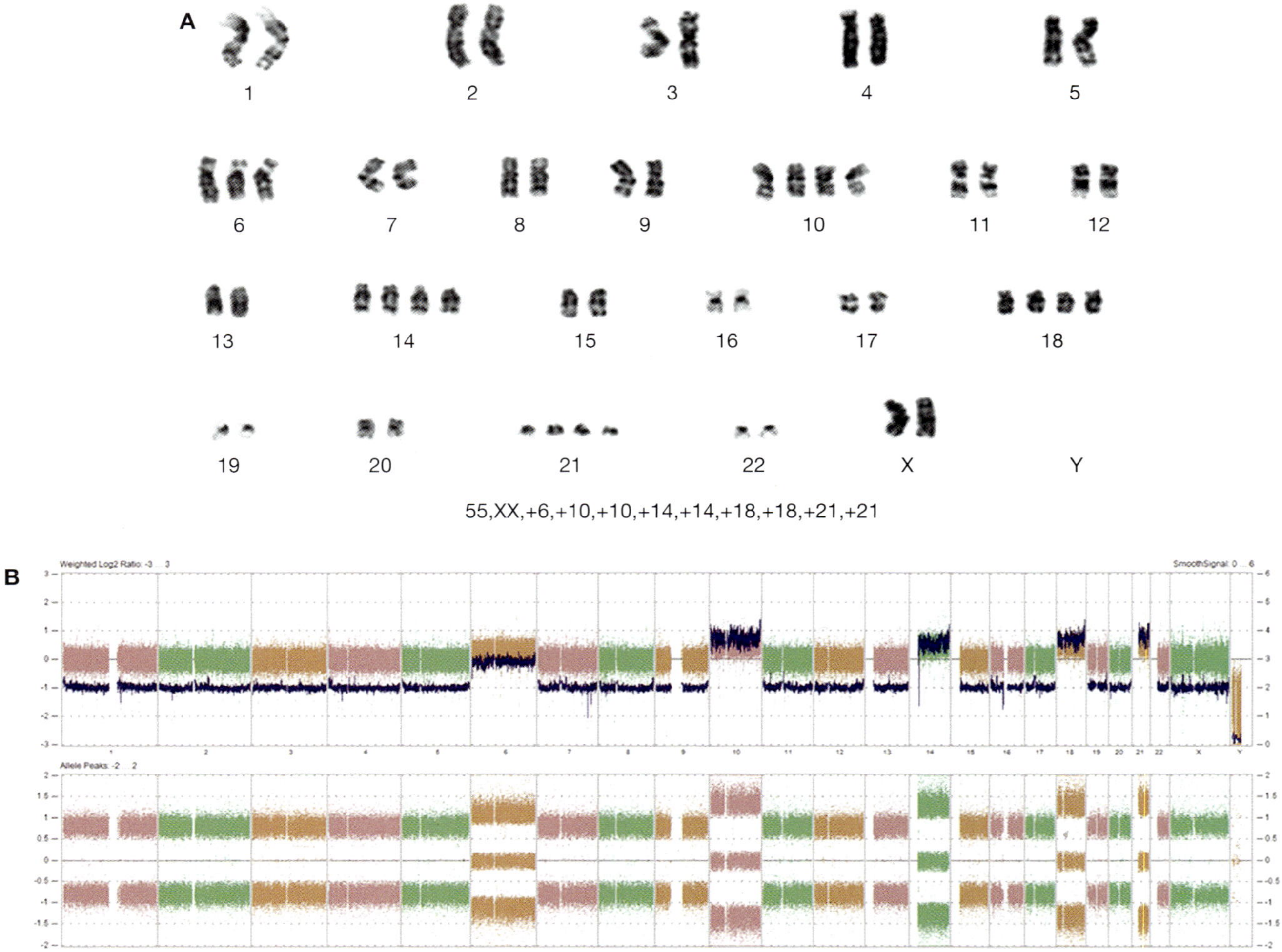

FIGURE 40.7 Karyotype and microarray analysis of a case of B-ALL, low hypodiploid with masked hypodiploidy. **A:** The karyotype shows an endoreduplicated clone containing 55 chromosomes. This clone exhibits tetrasomy of diploid chromosomes: 10, 14, 18 and 21; and disomy of aneuploid (monosomic) chromosomes: 1, 2, 3, 4, 5, 7, 8, 9, 11, 12, 13, 15, 16, 17, 19, 20 and 22. In this case, one copy of chromosome 6 was lost, resulting in trisomy. **B:** Microarray study confirming endoreduplication. The loss of chromosomes 1, 2, 3, 4, 5, 7, 8, 9, 11, 12, 13, 15, 16, 17, 19, 20 and 22 is represented by the decreased amplitude in copy number probe intensities as compared to reference DNA (log_2 ratio tracks; top panel). The allele tracks (bottom panel) show 2 alleles on chromosomes 6, 10, 14, 18 and 21, compatible with disomy. Only 1 allele is seen on other chromosomes, compatible with aneuploidy/monosomy. (Images courtesy of Umut Aypar, PhD, FACMG, Memorial Sloan Kettering Cancer Center.)

General Clinical Features

There are no unique clinical features that distinguish this entity from other types of ALL.

Morphology

There are no unique morphologic features that distinguish this entity from other types of ALL.

Immunophenotype

Blasts are typically $CD19^+$ and $CD10^+$, but there are no unique immunophenotypic features that distinguish this entity from other types of ALL.

Genetics

By definition, all cases exhibit severe aneuploidy.[20] The most common losses are chromosomes 1 to 7, 9, 11 to 13, 15 to 17, 19, 20 and 22. Notably, hypodiploid B-ALL/LBL with 23 chromosomes is never observed. Recurrent chromosomal rearrangements are uncommon. As with low hypodiploid B-ALL/LBL, masked hypodiploidy can be seen in near haploid B-ALL/LBL. This entity often has Ras pathway (particularly loss of function alterations of *NF1*) or receptor tyrosine kinase mutations, as well as mutations of *CREBBP* and *IKZF3*. The mutational spectrum and GEX profile of near haploid ALL is similar to high hyperdiploid ALL, suggesting commonalities in developmental origins.

Prognosis and Clinical Comment

This leukemia has a poor prognosis.

B-ALL/LBL WITH t(5;14)(q31.1;q32.1)/*IGH::IL3*

Definition

B-ALL/LBL with t(5;14)(q31.1;q32.1) is a neoplasm of lymphoblasts committed to the B-cell lineage in which the blasts harbor a translocation between *IL3* on chromosome 5 and *IGH* on chromosome 14. This genetic lesion is associated with eosinophilia, which may be striking, and diagnosis can be made on the basis of immunophenotypic and genetic findings even if the bone marrow blast count is low.

Synonyms

None.

Epidemiology

This subtype is very rare (<1% of cases of B-ALL/LBL) and has been reported in both children and adults.

General Clinical Features

The presenting clinical characteristics may be similar to those seen in patients with other ALLs, or patients may present with either symptomatic or asymptomatic eosinophilia. The complications of the pronounced eosinophilia are reported to include thromboembolic events, cardiac dysfunction, neurologic symptoms, and erythematous urticarial-like skin involvement.[21] Blasts may be very rare in the peripheral blood and sometimes in the marrow, and this diagnosis should be considered when even small numbers of B-cell precursors are identified in the blood or bone marrow of a patient with eosinophilia.

Morphology

This entity is characterized by eosinophilia in the blood and/or bone marrow. The eosinophils often show morphologic atypia but are not part of the leukemic clone. Lymphoblasts may be relatively rare, and do not show specific morphologic features (Figure 40.8).

Immunophenotype

The blasts have a typical CD19$^+$ and CD10$^+$ phenotype.

Genetics

The eosinophilia is driven by a functional rearrangement between the *IL3* gene on chromosome 5 and *IGH* on chromosome 14, resulting in constitutive overexpression of IL3. Other functional consequences of the rearrangement are not well understood. This abnormality can be detected by conventional karyotyping. It may, however, be difficult to detect because of the paucity of blasts relative to eosinophils, and FISH or molecular methods may be required for diagnosis.

Prognosis and Clinical Comment

Apart from the potential consequences of eosinophilia, the prognosis is not thought to be different from that of other types of ALL; however, there are too few cases to be certain. Blast percentage at diagnosis is not known to affect prognosis.

B-ALL/LBL WITH t(1;19)(q23;p13.3)/*TCF3::PBX1*

Definition

B-ALL/LBL with t(1;19)(q23;p13.3) is a neoplasm of lymphoblasts committed to the B-cell lineage in which the blasts harbor a translocation between the transcription factors *TCF3* (previously known as *E2A*) on chromosome 19 and *PBX1* on chromosome 1.

Synonyms

B acute lymphoblastic leukemia/lymphoma with t(1;19)(q23;p13.3); *E2A/PBX1* (not recommended).

Epidemiology

This leukemia accounts for about 6% of cases of B-ALL/LBL in children and is less common in adults. There is an increased prevalence in patients of African ancestry.[22]

General Clinical Features

There are no unique clinical features that distinguish this entity from other types of ALL.

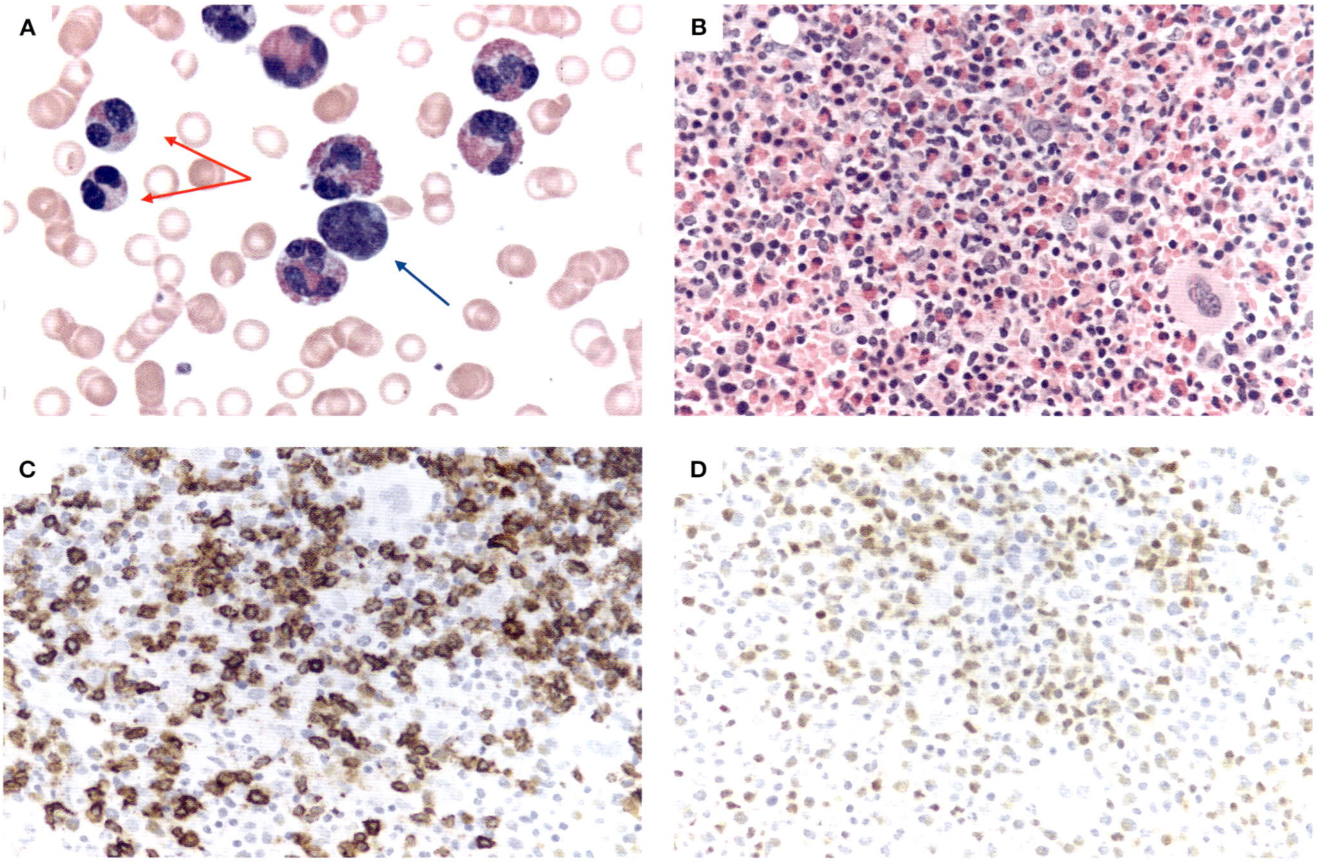

FIGURE 40.8 Morphology of B-ALL with t(5; 14) (*IL3::IGH*). **A:** Wright-Giemsa stained peripheral blood smear showing numerous eosinophils with some morphologic atypia (red arrows) along with rare blasts (blue arrow). **B:** Bone marrow H&E section showing numerous eosinophils with rare immature mononuclear cells that are morphologically consistent with blasts. **C:** Immunohistochemical stain for CD34 highlights B-lymphoblasts. **D:** Immunohistochemical stain for PAX5 highlights B-lymphoblasts.

Morphology

There are no unique morphologic features that distinguish this entity from other types of ALL.

Immunophenotype

Blasts typically have a pre-B phenotype, with expression of CD19 and CD10, and cytoplasmic mu heavy chain, but with very limited or absent expression of CD34. These leukemias characteristically show strong expression of CD9, and aberrant expression of myeloid markers is rare or absent. Although not common, surface light chain expression may occasionally be seen in this entity.[23]

Genetics

The *TCF3::PBX1* translocation produces a fusion protein that acts as a transcriptional activator, and also likely interferes with the normal function of both TCF3 and PBX1. The functional fusion gene is present on chromosome 19. Additional abnormalities of chromosome 1 may be seen, including loss of the derivative chromosome one in some cases. The demonstration of a *TCF3* rearrangement is not, by itself, diagnostic for this leukemia because rare cases of B-ALL/LBL with the alternative *TCF3* translocation t(17;19) are distinct, and are associated with a dismal prognosis (see B-ALL/LBL with *HLF*-rearrangement).[24] In addition, other subtypes of B-ALL/LBL, most commonly hyperdiploid B-ALL/LBL, may have a karyotypically identical t(1;19) that involves neither *TCF3* nor *PBX1*.[25]

Prognosis and Clinical Comment

This leukemia was historically associated with a poor prognosis, but the prognosis has improved with modern intensive therapy. When relapses occur, they tend to occur earlier than relapses in other B-ALL/LBL subtypes. There may be an increased relative risk of CNS relapse in these patients.

B-ALL/LBL, *BCR::ABL1*-LIKE, *ABL1*-CLASS REARRANGED

Definition

B-ALL/LBL, *BCR::ABL1*-like, *ABL1*-class rearranged is a neoplasm of lymphoblasts committed to the B-cell lineage that lack the *BCR::ABL1* translocation but have rearrangements of *ABL1* class genes and show a pattern of GEX very similar to that seen in *BCR::ABL1*+ B-ALL/LBL.

Synonyms

None.

Epidemiology

Overall, B-ALL/LBL, *BCR::ABL1*-like comprises 10% to 25% of patients with B-ALL/LBL, and the incidence increases with age.

The *ABL1*-class rearranged subtype comprises about 10% of *BCR::ABL1*-like B-ALL/LBL, and is slightly more common in children and adolescents than adults.[26,27]

General Clinical Features

The presenting clinical features are generally similar to those seen in patients with other ALLs, although patients tend to have a high WBC count at presentation.

Morphology

There are no unique morphologic features that distinguish this entity from other types of ALL.

Immunophenotype

There are no unique immunophenotypic features that distinguish this entity from other types of ALL.

Genetics

The *ABL1* class rearrangements include fusions between *ABL1*, *ABL2*, *CSF1R*, or *PDGFRA/B* and various partner genes, and can be detected by FISH or transcriptome sequencing. Although *PDGFRA/B*-rearranged neoplasms are typically included in the entity "myeloid/lymphoid neoplasms with *PDGFRA/B* rearrangement," those presenting as B-ALL/LBL (eg, *EBF1::PDGFRB*) are best classified as *BCR::ABL1*-like ALL, *ABL1*-class rearranged.

Prognosis and Clinical Comment

These cases, particularly those with *PDGFRB* fusions, are associated with poor early response and poor outcomes when treated with conventional chemotherapy. Cases with *EBF1::PDGFRB* may be particularly high risk.[28] The identification of this subtype is clinically important because these neoplasms may respond to TKIs that target ABL1.

B-ALL/LBL, *BCR::ABL1*-LIKE, JAK-STAT ACTIVATED

Definition

B-ALL/LBL, *BCR::ABL1*-like, JAK-STAT activated is a neoplasm of lymphoblasts committed to the B-cell lineage that show a pattern of GEX very similar to that seen in ALL with *BCR::ABL1*, but lacks *BCR::ABL1*. This subtype carries diverse mutations that result in the activation of JAK-STAT pathway signaling.

Synonyms

None.

Epidemiology

The JAK-STAT activated subtype is the most common subtype of *BCR::ABL1*-like B-ALL/LBL, comprising about two-thirds of *BCR::ABL1*-like cases in children and adults.[26,27] *GATA3* germline variants are associated with both Hispanic ancestry and an increased risk of developing B-ALL/LBL with *CRLF2* rearrangements.[29]

General Clinical Features

The presenting clinical features are generally similar to those seen in patients with other ALLs. Patients may have a high WBC count at presentation.

Morphology

There are no unique morphologic features that distinguish this entity from other types of ALL.

Immunophenotype

The lymphoblasts in this subtype show overexpression of CRLF2 on flow cytometry in cases with *CRLF2* rearrangement (Figure 40.9). CRLF2 overexpression is not,

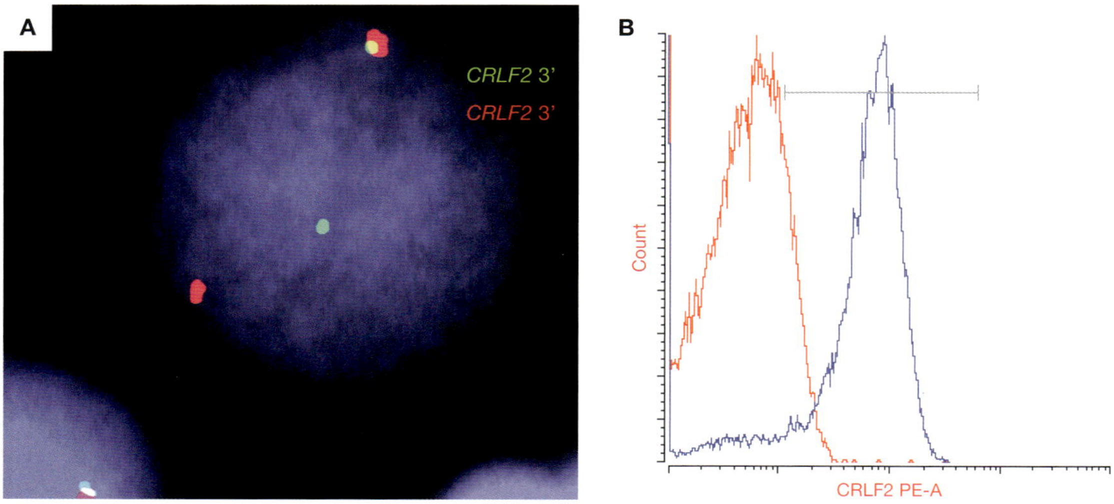

FIGURE 40.9 B-ALL with *CRLF2* rearrangement. **A:** Fluorescence in situ hybridization with a *CRLF2* break-apart probe (Xp22.33/Yp11.32) showing individual red and green signals indicating a *CRLF2* translocation, in addition to the normal copy of *CRLF2* (yellow). **B:** Flow cytometric analysis demonstrating upregulation of CRLF2 (blue curve) on blasts (gated on $CD19^+$, $CD10^+$ and dim CD45). A fluorescence minus one negative control omitting CRLF2 is shown in red. (**A:** Image courtesy of Umut Aypar, PhD, FACMG, Memorial Sloan Kettering Cancer Center.)

however, specific for this entity because translocations involving *CRLF2* have also been described in cases of B-ALL/LBL with iAMP21, among others.[30]

Genetics

The most common mutations in this subtype are *CRLF2* rearrangements with *IGH* or *P2RY8*, both of which result in CRLF2 overexpression (see Figure 40.9). *CRLF2* rearrangements may also be seen, usually as a secondary genetic alteration, in other subtypes such as B-ALL/LBL with *ETV6::RUNX1*, *DUX4*-rearrangement, and intrachromosomal amplification of chromosome 21 (iAMP21). In patients with a *CRLF2* rearrangement and genetic findings compatible with iAMP21, the iAMP21 classification should take precedence. Of note, patients with B-ALL and Down syndrome have a high frequency of *CRLF2*-rearrangements; however, these cases may require GEX profiling for definitive subclassification.[17] This occurs because B-ALL with *CRLF2*-rearrangements in patients with Down syndrome may lack the additional genomic alterations (eg, alteration of *IKZF1*) that contribute to the characteristic *BCR::ABL1*-like GEX profile. Less-common JAK-STAT activating alterations include *JAK2* fusions, truncating and activating rearrangements of *EPOR*, and *IL7R* or CRLF2 F232C mutations. Mutations in *JAK1*, *JAK2*, or *JAK3* are identified in approximately half of *CRLF2*-rearranged cases, and Ras pathway genes (*KRAS, NF1, NRAS,* and *PTPN11*) are also commonly mutated in *CRLF2*-rearranged cases.

Prognosis and Clinical Comment

This entity is generally considered to have a poor prognosis, but there may be some variability with age and specific genetic lesions. JAK inhibitors are being formally evaluated in trials, although there is variability in activity according to underlying alterations.

B-ALL/LBL, *BCR::ABL1*-LIKE, NOT OTHERWISE SPECIFIED

Definition

B-lymphoblastic leukemia/lymphoma, *BCR::ABL1*-like, not otherwise specified (B-ALL/LBL, *BCR::ABL1*-like, NOS) is a neoplasm of lymphoblasts committed to the B-cell lineage that show a pattern of GEX similar to that seen in *BCR::ABL1*+ B-ALL/LBL; however, this entity lacks not only the *BCR::ABL1* translocation, but also *ABL1*-class rearrangements and JAK-STAT activating mutations. The genetic alterations seen in this subtype are heterogeneous.

Synonyms

None.

Epidemiology

The NOS subtype comprises about 10% to 20% of *BCR::ABL1*-like cases in both children and adults.[26,27]

General Clinical Features

The presenting clinical features are thought to be similar to those seen in patients with other ALLs.

Morphology

There are no unique morphologic features that distinguish this entity from other types of ALL.

Immunophenotype

There are no unique immunophenotypic features that distinguish this entity from other types of ALL.

Genetics

This subtype encompasses heterogeneous alterations of other kinases and cytokine receptors, many of which are responsive to TKIs in preclinical models. The genetic alterations include kinase rearrangements, such as *FLT3*, *FGFR1*, *LYN*, *NTRK3*, *PTK2B* and *TYK2*, as well as mutations in Ras signaling pathway proteins, including *BRAF*, *CBL*, *KRAS*, *NF1*, *NRAS* and *PTPN11*.

Prognosis and Clinical Comment

Responsiveness of these cases to TKIs is variable and depends on the specific mutation and suitability of the inhibitor. Patients with fusions involving *NTKR3* may show responses to *TRK* inhibitors.[31]

B-ALL/LBL WITH INTRACHROMOSOMAL AMPLIFICATION OF CHROMOSOME 21 (iAMP21)

Definition

B-ALL/LBL with iAMP21 is a neoplasm of lymphoblasts committed to the B-cell lineage that is characterized by the amplification of a specific 7.8 Mb common region of chromosome 21 with ≥5 copies of this region (or ≥3 extra copies on a single abnormal chromosome 21).

Synonyms

None.

Epidemiology

This subtype accounts for about 2% of B-ALL/LBLcases, and is most often identified in children. The incidence in adults has not yet been established. Individuals with the rare constitutional Robertsonian translocation rob(15;21)(q10;q10) have an approximately 3000-fold increased risk of developing this leukemia.[32] The etiology in cases associated with the Robertsonian translocation appears related to chromothripsis, which likely plays a role in sporadic cases as well.

General Clinical Features

The median age of children with this leukemia is higher than that of other types of pediatric ALL, and it is associated with a low WBC count.

Morphology

There are no unique morphologic features that distinguish this entity from other types of ALL.

Immunophenotype

There are no unique immunophenotypic features that distinguish this entity from other types of ALL.

Genetics

These cases involve amplification of a specific region of chromosome 21 that encompasses 71 genes, commonly with flanking regions of genomic deletion.[33] In the majority of cases, the amplified region includes *RUNX1*, although *RUNX1* is not invariably present in the critical amplified region. Thus, although most cases of this leukemia can be recognized by FISH analysis using the probes for identification of the *ETV6::RUNX1* translocation, these probes will not identify cases where *RUNX1* is not contained in the region of amplification, or cases with variant rearrangements of portions of chromosome 21. The amplification of the critical area is the only structural chromosomal abnormality in about 20% of cases, but many other chromosomal abnormalities may be present, the most common of which are gains of the X chromosome and abnormalities of chromosome 7. This entity is associated with deletions, mutations, and/or loss-of-heterozygosity of *ETV6*, *RB1*, and *SH1B3*. Rearrangements of *CRLF2* are also observed in a minority of cases, most often as a secondary event. In some cases, these concomitant abnormalities might otherwise cause a case with iAMP21 to be placed in one of the other categories, as is the case with *CRLF2* translocations; however, given the unique nature of the iAMP21 alteration, it is generally believed that the iAMP21 classification should take precedence.

Prognosis and Clinical Comment

This entity previously had an unfavorable prognosis, although treatment with higher-intensity treatment regimens improves outcomes.[30]

B-ALL/LBL WITH *DUX4*-REARRANGEMENT

Definition

B-ALL/LBL with double homeobox 4 (*DUX4*)-rearrangement is a neoplasm of lymphoblasts committed to the B-cell lineage in which the blasts harbor rearrangement of *DUX4*.

Synonyms

None.

Epidemiology

This entity comprises 5% to 10% of B-ALL/LBL cases and is most common in adolescents and young adults.

General Clinical Features

There are no unique clinical features that distinguish this entity from other types of ALL.

Morphology

There are no unique morphologic features that distinguish this entity from other types of ALL.

Immunophenotype

The blasts in this entity are characterized by co-expression of CD2 and CD371.[34] With induction therapy, B lymphoblasts harboring rearrangements of *DUX4* may undergo immunophenotypic changes with acquisition of a myelomonocytic immunophenotype. Limited data suggest that this shift in immunophenotype does not have prognostic significance.[35]

Genetics

The most common rearrangement partners of *DUX4* are *IGH* enhancers, resulting in overexpression of a 3′ truncated isoform of DUX4. The *IGH::DUX4* translocation may be difficult to detect by transcriptome sequencing or FISH because of the repetitive nature of both the *DUX4* and *IGH* loci; however, the rearrangement results in overexpression of *DUX4* RNA and often the DUX4 protein, both of which may be helpful in identifying this entity. B-ALL/LBL with *DUX4* rearrangement is also associated with *ERG* and *IKZF1* deletions, as well as *CDKN2A* mutations.[36,37]

Prognosis and Clinical Comment

This entity is associated with an excellent prognosis in both children and adults even in the setting of otherwise poor risk features, including *IKZF1* deletion and elevated levels of MRD early in therapy.

B-ALL/LBL WITH *ZNF384*-REARRANGEMENT

Definition

B-ALL/LBL with zinc finger 384 (*ZNF384*)-rearrangements is a neoplasm of lymphoblasts committed to the B-cell lineage in which the blasts harbor rearrangement of *ZNF384*. B-ALL/LBL with *ZNF362* rearrangements was included in this category in the initial report of the ICC, but additional data suggest that these latter cases may be best considered in the B-ALL/LBL, *ZNF384*-rearranged-like provisional category.

Synonyms

None.

Epidemiology

This entity accounts for 5% to 10% of B-ALL/LBL cases and is relatively common in children and young adults.

General Clinical Features

There are no unique clinical features that distinguish this entity from other types of ALL.

Morphology

There are no unique morphologic features that distinguish this entity from other types of ALL.

Immunophenotype

The lymphoblasts of B-ALL/LBL with *ZNF384*-rearrangements often show dim or absent expression of CD10.[38] Myeloid antigen expression is typical. This entity is also characterized by lineage ambiguity, and cases with an identical rearrangement may present as B/myeloid MPAL. Lineage shifts may be seen over the course of disease or with therapy.[39] The GEX profiles and secondary genetic alterations of *ZNF384*-rearranged B/myeloid MPAL and B-ALL/LBL are similar.[40]

Genetics

ZNF384 has numerous fusion partners, although *CREBBP*, *EP300*, *TAF15*, and *TCF3* are most common.[41] This neoplasm is also associated with FLT3 overexpression because of epigenetic deregulation, but not FLT3 mutations, and may respond to FLT3 inhibition.[42] Ras pathway mutations and alterations in *ETV6* can also be seen in this entity.

Prognosis and Clinical Comment

The prognosis of this leukemia is variable and depends on the fusion partner: *EP300* fusions have the best prognosis, whereas *TCF3* fusions have the worst prognosis.

B-ALL/LBL WITH *MEF2D*-REARRANGEMENT

Definition

B-ALL/LBL with myocyte enhancer factor 2D (*MEF2D*)-rearrangement is a neoplasm of lymphoblasts committed to the B-cell lineage in which the blasts harbor rearrangement of the gene coding for the transcription factor MEF2D.

Synonyms

None.

Epidemiology

The entity accounts for 3% to 5% of B-ALL/LBL cases and is most commonly seen in children and young adults.

General Clinical Features

There are no unique clinical features that distinguish this entity from other types of ALL.

Morphology

The lymphoblasts in this entity may show morphologic features similar to those of Burkitt lymphoma.[43]

Immunophenotype

This subtype characteristically shows expression of cytoplasmic mu chain, with high levels of CD38 expression and low expression of CD10.[44,45]

Genetics

MEF2D can rearrange with multiple fusion partners, most often *BCL9* or, less frequently, *HNRNPUL1*.[46] These rearrangements result in enhanced and/or deregulated function of MEF2D, with over-expression of HDAC9. Diagnosis requires *MEF2D* break-apart probes or transcriptome sequencing. Coincident *CDKN2A* and Ras pathway mutations may be seen.

Prognosis and Clinical Comment

This subtype is associated with an unfavorable prognosis.[46,47] Because of the overexpression of HDAC9, HDAC inhibitors may have therapeutic potential in this entity.[46]

B-ALL/LBL WITH *MYC*-REARRANGEMENT

Definition

B-ALL/LBL with *MYC*-rearrangement is a neoplasm of lymphoblasts committed to the B-cell lineage in which the blasts harbor a *MYC*-rearrangement with immunoglobulin heavy or light chain genes. This entity does not include mature B-cell neoplasms that acquire features of immaturity on progression or transformation.

Synonyms

None.

Epidemiology

MYC translocations are reported in about 4% of adult B-ALL/LBL, and only rarely in pediatric B-ALL/LBL.

General Clinical Features

The clinical presentation of B-ALL/LBL with *MYC*-rearrangement is typically associated with bone marrow replacement, but mass lesions may be seen. Mature B-cell lymphomas can sometimes show immunophenotypic features of immaturity on progression or transformation, including TdT expression, and a diagnosis of B-ALL/LBL with *MYC*-rearrangement should be avoided in patients with such a history.[48]

Morphology

The lymphoblasts in this entity may show morphologic features similar to those of Burkitt lymphoma.[49,50]

Immunophenotype

The blasts in B-ALL/LBL with *MYC*-rearrangement typically but not invariably show expression of one or more markers of immaturity, specifically CD34 and/or TdT. CD45 and CD20 expression is weak or absent, and the lymphoblasts usually lack surface light chain expression. CD34 expression, in particular, favors a diagnosis of B-ALL/LBL.[51]

Genetics

The most frequent rearrangement partner for *MYC* in this entity is *IGH*, but rearrangements with *IGL* and *IGK* are rarely reported.[52] The clinical significance of possible non-immunoglobulin fusion partners is unclear, and currently non-immunoglobulin fusions are not included in the classification. B-ALL/LBLs with *MYC*-rearrangement are genetically distinct from mature B-cell lymphomas with a *MYC*-rearrangement. Prior work suggests that the target cell for the transformation event in B-ALL/LBL with *MYC*-rearrangement is a B-cell precursor undergoing variable-diversity-joining recombination, whereas the target cell for *MYC*-rearrangement in mature B-cell lymphomas is a germinal center B cell.[52] Accordingly, B-ALL/LBL with *MYC*-rearrangement is characterized by unmutated immunoglobulin heavy-chain variable region gene, whereas mature large B-cell lymphomas with *MYC*-rearrangements show evidence of somatic hypermutation. For this reason, somatic hypermutation analysis may be the most reliable means of recognizing this entity in clinically ambiguous cases. Mutational profiling of B-ALL/LBL with *MYC*-rearrangements may also be helpful in differentiating B-ALL/LBL from a progressing/transforming mature B-cell lymphoma, as B-ALL/LBL lacks mutations that are commonly seen in mature B-cell lymphomas, such as *CCND3*, *ID3*, *MYC*, and *SMARCA4*. In addition, B-ALL/LBL often contains Ras pathway mutations that are rare in transformed mature B-cell lymphomas.[48] Other genetic alterations that may be present in B-ALL/LBL with *MYC*-rearrangement include *TP53* mutations and gains of 1q. B-ALL/LBL with *MYC*-rearrangement and concomitant *BCL2* and/or *BCL6* rearrangements have also been described. Data about such cases are limited, and it is unclear whether they should be grouped together B-ALL/LBL with *MYC*-rearrangement; however, these cases have been observed to have a similar GEX profile, suggesting a common entity.[53]

Prognosis and Clinical Comment

This entity is associated with a very poor prognosis.

B-ALL/LBL WITH *NUTM1*-REARRANGEMENT

Definition

B-ALL/LBL with *NUTM1*-rearrangement is a neoplasm of lymphoblasts committed to the B-cell lineage in which the blasts harbor rearrangement of NUT midline carcinoma family member 1 (*NUTM1*).

Synonyms

None.

Epidemiology

This is a rare subtype, accounting for less than 2% of B-ALL/LBL. It is predominantly reported in infants and is rare in adults.

General Clinical Features

There are no known specific clinical features that distinguish this entity from other types of ALL.

Morphology

There are no known unique morphologic features that distinguish this entity from other types of ALL.

Immunophenotype

The blasts typically show dim to negative expression of CD10; this entity should be suspected in infants with CD10-negative B-ALL that lacks a *KMT2A* rearrangement. Myeloid antigen expression, including CD13, CD33, and CD15, has been described in this entity. The neoplastic cells show characteristic overexpression of NUT, which can be detected on immunohistochemical studies.[54]

Genetics

NUTM1 has numerous fusion partners including *ACIN1*, *BRD9*, *CUX1*, *IKZF1*, and *ZNF618*, and can be diagnosed via FISH studies using a *NUTM1* break-apart probe.[55]

Prognosis and Clinical Comment

This entity has a relatively favorable prognosis.[56]

B-ALL/LBL WITH *UBTF::ATXN7L3/PAN3,CDX2* (*CDX2/UBTF*)

Definition

B-ALL/LBL with *UBTF::ATXN7L3/PAN3,CDX2* (B-ALL/LBLwith CDX2/UBTF) is a neoplasm of lymphoblasts committed to the B-cell lineage in which the blasts harbor two alterations in all cases, namely a fusion oncoprotein-encoding rearrangement *UBTF::ATXN7L3* and a deletion upstream of *FLT3*.

Synonyms

None.

Epidemiology

This leukemia is rare, accounting for less than 1% of B-ALL/LBL cases, and tends to affect female adolescents and young adults.[57]

General Clinical Features

There are no known unique clinical features that distinguish this entity from other types of ALL.

Morphology

There are no known unique morphologic features that distinguish this entity from other types of ALL.

Immunophenotype

The lymphoblasts of this entity often show dim or absent expression of CD10.[57]

Genetics

This entity has two alterations: an interstitial deletion of chromosome 17 resulting in *UBTF::ATXN7L3* fusion, which can be detected by PCR; and a deletion upstream of *FLT3* that results in retargeting of the *PAN3* enhancer to *CDX2*, leading to its deregulation.[58,59] Both are obligate alterations that define this subtype, and are considered to be early disease-initiating events. These alterations may be detected by focused RT-PCR and/or genomic PCR assays. Co-occurring genetic alterations include *PAX5-ZCCHC7* deletions, and *PAX5* overexpression is seen in a subset of cases.

Prognosis and Clinical Comment

This entity has a poor prognosis.

B-ALL/LBL WITH *HLF*-REARRANGEMENT

Definition

B-ALL/LBL with *HLF* rearrangement is defined as a neoplasm of lymphoblasts committed to the B-cell lineage in which the blasts harbor a rearrangement between *HLF* and the gene coding for either transcription factor 3 or transcription factor 4 (*TCF3::HLF* and *TCF4::HLF*, respectively).

Synonyms

None.

Epidemiology

This entity is exceptionally rare, accounting for less than 1% of B-ALL/LBL cases, and is probably only found in children.

General Clinical Features

The incidence of disseminated intravascular coagulation and/or hypercalcemia is much higher in this leukemia than in other B-ALLs.[60,61]

Morphology

There are no known unique morphologic features that distinguish this from other types of ALL.

Immunophenotype

There are no known unique immunophenotypic features that distinguish this entity from other types of ALL.

Genetics

A limited series of *TCF3::HLF* cases showed overexpression of Aurora A kinase in all cases, which may represent a therapeutic target.[62]

Prognosis and Clinical Comment

B-ALL/LBL with either of these rearrangements has a very poor prognosis, although anti-CD19 therapy and transplant may improve outcomes.[63]

B-ALL/LBL WITH PAX5 P80R

Definition

B-ALL/LBL with PAX5 P80R is a neoplasm of lymphoblasts committed to the B-cell lineage in which the blasts harbor a PAX5 P80R missense variant with loss of the second wild-type *PAX5* allele.

Synonyms

None.

Epidemiology

This entity comprises 2% to 5% of B-ALL/LBL cases and is more common in adults.

General Clinical Features

There are no unique clinical features that distinguish this entity from other types of ALL.

Morphology

There are no unique morphologic features that distinguish this entity from other types of ALL.

Immunophenotype

There are no unique immunophenotypic features that distinguish this entity from other types of ALL. On induction therapy, B lymphoblasts harboring PAX5 P80R may undergo immunophenotypic changes with acquisition of a myelomonocytic immunophenotype. Limited data suggest that this shift in immunophenotype does not have prognostic significance, although further investigation is needed.[35]

Genetics

In general, *PAX5* mutations and deletions are common in many B-ALL/LBL subtypes, and *PAX5* translocations are also reported B-ALL/LBL.[64,65] However, the presence of this specific PAX5 P80R missense variant with concomitant disruption of the wild-type allele (via deletion, inactivating sequence mutation, or copy neutral loss of heterozygosity) is associated with a distinct GEX profile.[66] Rare cases have alternative hemizygous mutations of PAX5 also located in the DNA-binding paired domain, and exhibit the same GEX profile. This leukemia tends to have other cooperating lesions, including abnormalities in *CDKN2A*, *IL7R*, Ras pathways, JAK-STAT signaling pathways, and other kinase pathways, which may suggest additional therapeutic opportunities in these patients.

Prognosis and Clinical Comment

This leukemia has a relatively good prognosis in adults.

B-ALL/LBL WITH IKZF1 N159Y

Definition

B-ALL/LBL with IKZF1 N159Y is a neoplasm of lymphoblasts committed to the B-cell lineage in which the blasts harbor a heterozygous N159Y mutation in the DNA-binding protein Ikaros (IKZF1).

Synonyms

None.

Epidemiology

This entity is rare, and accounts for less than 1% of B-ALL/LBL cases. It is more common in adults.[67]

General Clinical Features

There are no unique clinical features that distinguish this entity from other types of ALL.

Morphology

There are no known unique morphologic features that distinguish this entity from other types of ALL.

Immunophenotype

There are no known unique immunophenotypic features that distinguish this entity from other types of ALL.

Genetics

Although various alterations in *IKZF1* are common in B-ALL/LBL, cases with the heterozygous IKZF1 N159Y mutation exhibit a distinct GEX profile.[67,68] Cases commonly have a tandem duplication of exon 5 of *IKZF1*, which harbors the N159Y mutation. The mutation is associated with abnormal cellular localization of IKZF1 and enhanced cell-cell adhesion. Co-occurring genetic abnormalities include gain of chromosome 21.

Prognosis and Clinical Comment

This leukemia has an intermediate prognosis.

B-ALL/LBL, NOS

Definition

B-ALL/LBL, NOS is a neoplasm of lymphoblasts committed to the B-cell lineage that do not have a cytogenetic abnormality, molecular alteration, or GEX profile that allows for classification as a specific entity.

Epidemiology, General Clinical Features, Immunophenotype, Genetics, Prognosis, and Clinical Comment

The features are generally those described for B-ALL/LBL in the introduction.

B-ALL/LBL: PROVISIONAL ENTITIES

The provisional entities (Table 40.2) include small clusters of cases that have essentially identical GEX profiles as one of the entities with a recurrent genetic abnormality but lack the specific subtype-defining abnormality. For other provisional subtypes, specific drivers are not well-defined or are highly variable. Comprehensive identification and classification of these cases require GEX studies.

TABLE 40.2 Provisional entities: B-lymphoblastic leukemia/lymphoma (B-ALL)

B-ALL, *ETV6::RUNX1*-like
B-ALL, *PAX5*-altered (PAX5Alt)
B-ALL, with coexisting H1038R mutations in *ZEB2* and *IGH::CEBPE*
B-ALL, *KMT2A* rearranged-like
B-ALL, *ZNF384* rearranged-like

B-ALL/LBL, *ETV6::RUNX1*-Like

Definition

B-ALL/LBL, *ETV6::RUNX1*-like is a neoplasm of lymphoblasts committed to the B-cell lineage that shares the same GEX profile and immunophenotype as B-ALL/LBL with t(12;21)(p13.2;q22.1)/*ETV6::RUNX1*, but lacks the defining translocation.

Synonyms

None.

Epidemiology

This provisional entity accounts for less than 5% of B-ALL/LBL cases. It is most common in children.[69]

General clinical features

There are no unique clinical features that distinguish this from other types of ALL.

Morphology

There are no unique morphologic features that distinguish this from other types of ALL.

Immunophenotype

The blasts have the same CD27 positive, CD44 dim/negative immunophenotype as B-ALL/LBL with t(12;21)(p13.2; q22.1)/*ETV6::RUNX1*.[70]

Genetics

These cases show fusions or copy number alterations in ETS family genes including *ETV6*, *FUS*, and *IKZF1*. Some cases harbor germline loss-of-function *ETV6* mutations.[36]

Prognosis and clinical comment

The prognosis is worse than B-ALL/LBL with t(12;21)(p13.2;q22.1)/*ETV6::RUNX1*.

B-ALL/LBL, *PAX5*-Altered

Definition

B-ALL/LBL, *PAX5*-altered is a neoplasm of lymphoblasts committed to the B-cell lineage that harbor a variety of different alterations in *PAX5*; however, all these cases exhibit a similar GEX profile.[67] A case should only be included in this provisional category if it does not fit into another category of B-ALL/LBL with recurrent genetic abnormalities.

Synonyms

None.

Epidemiology

This provisional entity comprises approximately 10% of B-ALL/LBL cases and is seen in both children and adults.

General clinical features

There are no unique clinical features that distinguish this from other types of ALL.

Morphology

There are no unique morphologic features that distinguish this from other types of ALL.

Immunophenotype

There are no unique immunophenotypic features that distinguish this from other types of ALL.

Genetics

The various mutations include point mutations (especially compound heterozygosity at R38 and R140), rearrangements/nonkinase fusions (most commonly *ETV6* and *NOL4L*), and focal intragenic amplification. *CDKN2A* co-mutations are common.[71]

Prognosis and clinical comment

The prognosis of this provisional entity appears to be intermediate to poor.[47,67]

B-ALL/LBL, WITH COEXISTING ZEB2 H1038R MUTATION AND *IGH::CEBPE*

Definition

B-ALL/LBL, with coexisting H1038R mutations in *ZEB2* and *IGH::CEBPE* is a neoplasm of lymphoblasts committed to the B-cell lineage that harbor a concomitant *ZEB2* H1038R mutation and *IGH::CEBPE* rearrangement.

Synonyms

None.

Epidemiology

This provisional entity is rare, accounting for less than 1% of B-ALL/LBL cases.[72]

General clinical features

There are no known unique clinical features that distinguish this from other types of ALL.

Morphology

There are no known unique morphologic features that distinguish this from other types of ALL.

Immunophenotype

There are no known unique immunophenotypic features that distinguish this from other types of ALL.

Genetics

These cases have a distinct GEX profile. The genetic basis of this subtype is not fully elucidated, as not all cases have *ZEB2* and/or *CEBPE* alterations, and ZEB2 H1038R mutations are observed in other entities. This entity is associated with *NRAS* mutations in about 50% of cases, as well as *LMO1* upregulation and downregulation of *BMP2* and *SMAD1*.[68]

Prognosis and clinical comment

This provisional entity appears to have a poor prognosis.[72]

B-ALL/LBL, *KMT2A*-Rearranged-Like

Definition

B-ALL/LBL, *KMT2A*-rearranged-like is a neoplasm of lymphoblasts committed to the B-cell lineage that share the same GEX profile and immunophenotype as *KMT2A*-rearranged B-ALL/LBL, but lack the defining *KMT2A* rearrangement.

Synonyms

None.

Epidemiology

This provisional entity is rare, and comprises less than 1% of B-ALL/LBL cases.[8,73]

General clinical features

There are no unique clinical features that distinguish this from other types of ALL.

Morphology

There are no unique morphologic features that distinguish this from other types of ALL.

Immunophenotype

Lymphoblasts may show dim or absent expression of CD10, similar to that seen in *KMT2A*-rearranged B-ALL/LBL.

Genetics

This provisional entity may also be associated with *HOXA* fusions.

Prognosis and clinical comment

Insufficient data are currently available regarding outcomes.

B-ALL/LBL, *ZNF384*-Rearranged-Like

Definition

B-ALL/LBL, *ZNF384*-rearranged-like is a neoplasm of lymphoblasts committed to the B-cell lineage that have a GEX profile similar to B-ALL/LBL with *ZNF384*-rearrangement but lack the defining rearrangement.

Synonyms

None.

Epidemiology

This provisional entity is rare, accounting for less than 1% of B-ALL/LBL cases.

General clinical features

There are no known unique clinical features that distinguish this from other types of ALL.

Morphology

There are no known unique morphologic features that distinguish this from other types of ALL.

Immunophenotype

There are no known unique immunophenotypic features that distinguish this from other types of ALL.

Genetics

Many, but not all, cases have translocations involving *ZNF362*.[74]

Prognosis and clinical comment

Insufficient data are currently available regarding outcomes.

References

1. Chen Z, Hu S, Wang SA, et al. Chronic myeloid leukemia presenting in lymphoblastic crisis, a differential diagnosis with Philadelphia-positive B-lymphoblastic leukemia. *Leuk Lymphoma*. 2020;61(12):2831-2838. doi: 10.1080/10428194.2020.1795160
2. Zuna J, Hovorkova L, Krotka J, et al. Minimal residual disease in BCR::ABL1-positive acute lymphoblastic leukemia—different significance in typical ALL and in CML-like disease. *Leukemia*. 2022;36(12):2793-2801. doi: 10.1038/s41375-022-01668-0
3. Chen P, Chu A, Zia H, et al. CD25 expression in B lymphoblastic leukemia/lymphoma predicts t(9;22)(q34;q11)/Philadelphia chromosome translocation (Ph) and is associated with residual disease in Ph-negative patients. *Am J Clin Pathol*. 2016;146(5):632-638. doi:10.1093/ajcp/aqw178
4. Buldini B, Zangrando A, Michielotto B, et al. Identification of immunophenotypic signatures by clustering analysis in pediatric patients with Philadelphia chromosome-positive acute lymphoblastic leukemia. *Am J Hematol*. 2010;85(2):138-141. doi:10.1002/ajh.21595
5. Martinelli G, Iacobucci I, Storlazzi CT, et al. IKZF1 (Ikaros) deletions in BCR-ABL1-positive acute lymphoblastic leukemia are associated with short disease-free survival and high rate of cumulative incidence of relapse: a GIMEMA AL WP report. *J Clin Oncol*. 2009;27(31):5202-5207. doi:10.1200/JCO.2008.21.6408
6. Slayton WB, Schultz KR, Kairalla JA, et al. Dasatinib plus intensive chemotherapy in children, adolescents, and young adults with Philadelphia chromosome-positive acute lymphoblastic leukemia: results of children's oncology group trial AALL0622. *J Clin Oncol*. 2018;36(22):2306-2314. doi:10.1200/JCO.2017.76.7228
7. Hovorkova L, Zaliova M, Venn NC, et al. Monitoring of childhood ALL using BCR-ABL1 genomic breakpoints identifies a subgroup with CML-like biology. *Blood*. 2017;129(20):2771-2781. doi:10.1182/blood-2016-11-749978
8. Brady SW, Roberts KG, Gu Z, et al. The genomic landscape of pediatric acute lymphoblastic leukemia. *Nat Genet*. 2022;54(9):1376-1389. doi:10.1038/s41588-022-01159-z
9. Gale KB, Ford AM, Repp R, et al. Backtracking leukemia to birth: identification of clonotypic gene fusion sequences in neonatal blood spots. *Proc Natl Acad Sci U S A*. 1997;94(25):13950-13954. doi:10.1073/pnas.94.25.13950
10. Attarbaschi A, Möricke A, Harrison CJ, et al. Outcomes of childhood noninfant acute lymphoblastic leukemia with 11q23/KMT2A rearrangements in a modern therapy era: a retrospective international study. *J Clin Oncol*. 2023;41(7):1404-1422. doi:10.1200/JCO.22.01297

11. Gao C, Liu SG, Yue ZX, et al. Clinical-biological characteristics and treatment outcomes of pediatric pro-B ALL patients enrolled in BCH-2003 and CCLG-2008 protocol: a study of 121 Chinese children. *Cancer Cell Int*. 2019;19:293. doi:10.1186/s12935-019-1013-9
12. Meyer C, Larghero P, Almeida Lopes B, et al. The KMT2A recombinome of acute leukemias in 2023. *Leukemia*. 2023;37(5):988-1005. doi:10.1038/s41375-023-01877-1
13. Paulsson K, Lilljebjörn H, Biloglav A, et al. The genomic landscape of high hyperdiploid childhood acute lymphoblastic leukemia. *Nat Genet*. 2015;47(6):672-676. doi:10.1038/ng.3301
14. Pierzyna-Świtała M, Sędek Ł, Kulis J, et al. Multicolor flow cytometry immunophenotyping and characterization of aneuploidy in pediatric B-cell precursor acute lymphoblastic leukemia. *Cent Eur J Immunol*. 2021;46(3):365-374. doi:10.5114/ceji.2021.109794
15. Hrusák O, Porwit-MacDonald A. Antigen expression patterns reflecting genotype of acute leukemias. *Leukemia*. 2002;16(7):1233-1258. doi:10.1038/sj.leu.2402504
16. Carroll AJ, Shago M, Mikhail FM, et al. Masked hypodiploidy: hypodiploid acute lymphoblastic leukemia (ALL) mimicking hyperdiploid ALL in children—a report from the Children's Oncology Group. *Cancer Genet*. 2019;238:62-68. doi:10.1016/j.cancergen.2019.07.009
17. Russell LJ, Jones L, Enshaei A, et al. Characterisation of the genomic landscape of CRLF2-rearranged acute lymphoblastic leukemia. *Genes Chromosomes Cancer*. 2017;56(5):363-372. doi:10.1002/gcc.22439
18. Harris MB, Shuster JJ, Carroll A, et al. Trisomy of leukemic cell chromosomes 4 and 10 identifies children with B-progenitor cell acute lymphoblastic leukemia with a very low risk of treatment failure: a Pediatric Oncology Group study. *Blood*. 1992;79(12):3316-3324.
19. Comeaux EQ, Mullighan CG. TP53 mutations in hypodiploid acute lymphoblastic leukemia. *Cold Spring Harb Perspect Med*. 2017;7(3):a026286. doi:10.1101/cshperspect.a026286
20. Holmfeldt L, Wei L, Diaz-Flores E, et al. The genomic landscape of hypodiploid acute lymphoblastic leukemia. *Nat Genet*. 2013;45(3):242-252. doi:10.1038/ng.2532
21. Fournier B, Balducci E, Duployez N, et al. B-ALL with t(5;14)(q31;q32); IGH-IL3 rearrangement and eosinophilia: a comprehensive analysis of a peculiar IGH-rearranged B-ALL. *Front Oncol*. 2019;9:1374. doi:10.3389/fonc.2019.01374
22. Pui C-H, Sandlund JT, Pei D, et al. Results of therapy for acute lymphoblastic leukemia in black and white children. *JAMA*. 2003;290(15):2001-2007. doi:10.1001/jama.290.15.2001
23. Kansal R, Deeb G, Barcos M, et al. Precursor B lymphoblastic leukemia with surface light chain immunoglobulin restriction: a report of 15 patients. *Am J Clin Pathol*. 2004;121(4):512-525. doi:10.1309/WTXC-Q5NR-ACVX-TYBY
24. Panagopoulos I, Micci F, Thorsen J, et al. A novel TCF3-HLF fusion transcript in acute lymphoblastic leukemia with a t(17;19)(q22;p13). *Cancer Genet*. 2012;205(12):669-672. doi:10.1016/j.cancergen.2012.10.004
25. Paulsson K, Harrison CJ, Andersen MK, et al. Distinct patterns of gained chromosomes in high hyperdiploid acute lymphoblastic leukemia with t(1;19)(q23;p13), t(9;22)(q34;q22) or MLL rearrangements. *Leukemia*. 2013;27(4):974-977. doi:10.1038/leu.2012.263
26. Roberts KG, Mullighan CG. Genomics in acute lymphoblastic leukaemia: insights and treatment implications. *Nat Rev Clin Oncol*. 2015;12(6):344-357. doi:10.1038/nrclinonc.2015.38
27. Tasian SK, Loh ML, Hunger SP. Philadelphia chromosome-like acute lymphoblastic leukemia. *Blood*. 2017;130(19):2064-2072. doi:10.1182/blood-2017-06-743252
28. Schwab C, Ryan SL, Chilton L, et al. EBF1-PDGFRB fusion in pediatric B-cell precursor acute lymphoblastic leukemia (BCP-ALL): genetic profile and clinical implications. *Blood*. 2016;127(18):2214-2218. doi:10.1182/blood-2015-09-670166
29. Madzio J, Pastorczak A, Sedek L, et al. GATA3 germline variant is associated with CRLF2 expression and predicts outcome in pediatric B-cell precursor acute lymphoblastic leukemia. *Genes Chromosomes Cancer*. 2019;58(9):619-626. doi:10.1002/gcc.22748
30. Harrison CJ, Moorman AV, Schwab C, et al. An international study of intrachromosomal amplification of chromosome 21 (iAMP21): cytogenetic characterization and outcome. *Leukemia*. 2014;28(5):1015-1021. doi:10.1038/leu.2013.317
31. Nardi V, Ku N, Frigault MJ, et al. Clinical response to larotrectinib in adult Philadelphia chromosome-like ALL with cryptic ETV6-NTRK3 rearrangement. *Blood Adv*. 2020;4(1):106-111. doi:10.1182/bloodadvances.2019000769
32. Li Y, Schwab C, Ryan S, et al. Constitutional and somatic rearrangement of chromosome 21 in acute lymphoblastic leukaemia. *Nature*. 2014;508(7494):98-102. doi:10.1038/nature13115
33. Gao Q, Ryan SL, Iacobucci I, et al. The genomic landscape of acute lymphoblastic leukemia with intrachromosomal amplification of chromosome 21. *Blood*. 2023;142(8):711-723. doi:10.1182/blood.2022019094
34. Schinnerl D, Mejstrikova E, Schumich A, et al. CD371 cell surface expression: a unique feature of DUX4-rearranged acute lymphoblastic leukemia. *Haematologica*. 2019;104(8):e352-e355. doi:10.3324/haematol.2018.214353
35. Novakova M, Zaliova M, Fiser K, et al. DUX4r, ZNF384r and PAX5-P80R mutated B-cell precursor acute lymphoblastic leukemia frequently undergo monocytic switch. *Haematologica*. 2021;106(8):2066-2075. doi:10.3324/haematol.2020.250423

36. Lilljebjörn H, Henningsson R, Hyrenius-Wittsten A, et al. Identification of ETV6-RUNX1-like and DUX4-rearranged subtypes in paediatric B-cell precursor acute lymphoblastic leukaemia. *Nat Commun*. 2016;7:11790. doi:10.1038/ncomms11790
37. Zaliova M, Potuckova E, Hovorkova L, et al. ERG deletions in childhood acute lymphoblastic leukemia with DUX4 rearrangements are mostly polyclonal, prognostically relevant and their detection rate strongly depends on screening method sensitivity. *Haematologica*. 2019;104(7):1407-1416. doi:10.3324/haematol.2018.204487
38. Janet NB, Kulkarni U, Arun AK, et al. Systematic application of fluorescence in situ hybridization and immunophenotype profile for the identification of ZNF384 gene rearrangements in B cell acute lymphoblastic leukemia. *Int J Lab Hematol*. 2021;43(4):658-663. doi:10.1111/ijlh.13580
39. Semchenkova A, Mikhailova E, Komkov A, et al. Lineage conversion in pediatric B-cell precursor acute leukemia under blinatumomab therapy. *Int J Mol Sci*. 2022;23(7):4019. doi:10.3390/ijms23074019
40. Alexander TB, Gu Z, Iacobucci I, et al. The genetic basis and cell of origin of mixed phenotype acute leukaemia. *Nature*. 2018;562(7727):373-379. doi:10.1038/s41586-018-0436-0
41. Hirabayashi S, Ohki K, Nakabayashi K, et al. ZNF384-related fusion genes define a subgroup of childhood B-cell precursor acute lymphoblastic leukemia with a characteristic immunotype. *Haematologica*. 2017;102(1):118-129. doi:10.3324/haematol.2016.151035
42. Zhao X, Wang P, Diedrich JD, et al. Epigenetic activation of the FLT3 gene by ZNF384 fusion confers a therapeutic susceptibility in acute lymphoblastic leukemia. *Nat Commun*. 2022;13(1):5401. doi:10.1038/s41467-022-33143-w
43. Sun J, Yu W, Zhang X. MEF2D-rearranged acute lymphoblastic leukemia resembles Burkitt lymphoma/leukemia. *Ann Hematol*. 2020;99(1):185-188. doi:10.1007/s00277-019-03857-x
44. Ohki K, Kiyokawa N, Saito Y, et al. Clinical and molecular characteristics of MEF2D fusion-positive B-cell precursor acute lymphoblastic leukemia in childhood, including a novel translocation resulting in MEF2D-HNRNPH1 gene fusion. *Haematologica*. 2019;104(1):128-137. doi:10.3324/haematol.2017.186320
45. Ohki K, Takahashi H, Fukushima T, et al. Impact of immunophenotypic characteristics on genetic subgrouping in childhood acute lymphoblastic leukemia: Tokyo Children's Cancer Study Group (TCCSG) study L04-16. *Genes Chromosomes Cancer*. 2020;59(10):551-561. doi:10.1002/gcc.22858
46. Gu Z, Churchman M, Roberts K, et al. Genomic analyses identify recurrent MEF2D fusions in acute lymphoblastic leukaemia. *Nat Commun*. 2016;7:13331. doi:10.1038/ncomms13331
47. Paietta E, Roberts KG, Wang V, et al. Molecular classification improves risk assessment in adult BCR-ABL1-negative B-ALL. *Blood*. 2021;138(11):948-958. doi:10.1182/blood.2020010144
48. Bhavsar S, Liu Y-C, Gibson SE, Moore EM, Swerdlow SH. Mutational landscape of TdT+ large B-cell lymphomas supports their distinction from B-lymphoblastic neoplasms: a multiparameter study of a rare and aggressive entity. *Am J Surg Pathol*. 2022;46(1):71-82. doi:10.1097/PAS.0000000000001750
49. Navid F, Mosijczuk AD, Head DR, et al. Acute lymphoblastic leukemia with the (8;14)(q24;q32) translocation and FAB L3 morphology associated with a B-precursor immunophenotype: the Pediatric Oncology Group experience. *Leukemia*. 1999;13(1):135-141. doi:10.1038/sj.leu.2401244
50. Li Y, Gupta G, Molofsky A, et al. B lymphoblastic leukemia/lymphoma with Burkitt-like morphology and IGH/MYC rearrangement: report of 3 cases in adult patients. *Am J Surg Pathol*. 2018;42(2):269-276. doi:10.1097/PAS.0000000000000982
51. Duffield AS, Dogan A, Amador C, et al. Progression of follicular lymphoma and related entities: report from the 2021 SH/EAHP Workshop. *Am J Clin Pathol*. 2023;159(6):572-597. doi:10.1093/ajcp/aqad042
52. Wagener R, López C, Kleinheinz K, et al. IG-MYC + neoplasms with precursor B-cell phenotype are molecularly distinct from Burkitt lymphomas. *Blood*. 2018;132(21):2280-2285. doi:10.1182/blood-2018-03-842088
53. Kelemen K, Holden J, Johnson LJ, Davion S, Robetorye RS. Immunophenotypic and cytogenetic findings of B-lymphoblastic leukemia/lymphoma associated with combined IGH/BCL2 and MYC rearrangement. *Cytometry B Clin Cytom*. 2017;92(4):310-314. doi:0.1002/cyto.b.21334
54. Pincez T, Landry J-R, Roussy M, et al. Cryptic recurrent ACIN1-NUTM1 fusions in non-KMT2A-rearranged infant acute lymphoblastic leukemia. *Genes Chromosomes Cancer*. 2020;59(2):125-130. doi:10.1002/gcc.22808
55. Hormann FM, Hoogkamer AQ, Beverloo HB, et al. NUTM1 is a recurrent fusion gene partner in B-cell precursor acute lymphoblastic leukemia associated with increased expression of genes on chromosome band 10p12.31-12.2. *Haematologica*. 2019;104(10):e455-e459. doi:10.3324/haematol.2018.206961
56. Boer JM, Valsecchi MG, Hormann FM, et al. Favorable outcome of NUTM1-rearranged infant and pediatric B cell precursor acute lymphoblastic leukemia in a collaborative international study. *Leukemia*. 2021;35(10):2978-2982. doi:10.1038/s41375-021-01333-y
57. Kimura S, Montefiori L, Iacobucci I, et al. Enhancer retargeting of CDX2 and UBTF::ATXN7L3 define a subtype of high-risk B-progenitor acute lymphoblastic leukemia. *Blood*. 2022;139(24):3519-3531. doi:10.1182/blood.2022015444

58. Passet M, Kim R, Gachet S, et al. Concurrent CDX2 cis-deregulation and UBTF::ATXN7L3 fusion define a novel high-risk subtype of B-cell ALL. *Blood.* 2022;139(24):3505-3518. doi:10.1182/blood.2021014723

59. Yasuda T, Sanada M, Kawazu M, et al. Two novel high-risk adult B-cell acute lymphoblastic leukemia subtypes with high expression of CDX2 and IDH1/2 mutations. *Blood.* 2022;139(12):1850-1862. doi: 10.1182/blood.2021011921

60. Hunger SP, Brown R, Cleary ML. DNA-binding and transcriptional regulatory properties of hepatic leukemia factor (HLF) and the t(17;19) acute lymphoblastic leukemia chimera E2A-HLF. *Mol Cell Biol.* 1994;14(9):5986-5996. doi:10.1128/mcb.14.9.5986-5996.1994

61. Inukai T, Hirose K, Inaba T, et al. Hypercalcemia in childhood acute lymphoblastic leukemia: frequent implication of parathyroid hormone-related peptide and E2A-HLF from translocation 17;19. *Leukemia.* 2007;21(2):288-296. doi:10.1038/sj.leu.2404496

62. Leonard J, Wolf JS, Degnin M, et al. Aurora A kinase as a target for therapy in TCF3-HLF rearranged acute lymphoblastic leukemia. *Haematologica.* 2021;106(11):2990-2994. doi:10.3324/haematol.2021.278692

63. Mouttet B, Vinti L, Ancliff P, et al. Durable remissions in TCF3-HLF positive acute lymphoblastic leukemia with blinatumomab and stem cell transplantation. *Haematologica.* 2019;104(6):e244-e247. doi:10.3324/haematol.2018.210104

64. Nebral K, Denk D, Attarbaschi A, et al. Incidence and diversity of PAX5 fusion genes in childhood acute lymphoblastic leukemia. *Leukemia.* 2009;23(1):134-143. doi:10.1038/leu.2008.306

65. Mullighan CG, Goorha S, Radtke I, et al. Genome-wide analysis of genetic alterations in acute lymphoblastic leukaemia. *Nature.* 2007;446(7137):758-764. doi:10.1038/nature05690

66. Passet M, Boissel N, Sigaux F, et al. PAX5 P80R mutation identifies a novel subtype of B-cell precursor acute lymphoblastic leukemia with favorable outcome. *Blood.* 2019;133(3):280-284. doi:10.1182/blood-2018-10-882142

67. Gu Z, Churchman ML, Roberts KG, et al. PAX5-driven subtypes of B-progenitor acute lymphoblastic leukemia. *Nat Genet.* 2019;51(2):296-307. doi:10.1038/s41588-018-0315-5

68. Li JF, Dai YT, Lilljebjörn H, et al. Transcriptional landscape of B cell precursor acute lymphoblastic leukemia based on an international study of 1,223 cases. *Proc Natl Acad Sci U S A.* 2018;115(50):E11711-E11720. doi:10.1073/pnas.1814397115

69. Zaliova M, Stuchly J, Winkowska L, et al. Genomic landscape of pediatric B-other acute lymphoblastic leukemia in a consecutive European cohort. *Haematologica.* 2019;104(7):1396-1406. doi:10.3324/haematol.2018.204974

70. Zaliova M, Kotrova M, Bresolin S, et al. ETV6/RUNX1-like acute lymphoblastic leukemia: a novel B-cell precursor leukemia subtype associated with the CD27/CD44 immunophenotype. *Genes Chromosomes Cancer.* 2017;56(8):608-616. doi:10.1002/gcc.22464

71. Bastian L, Schroeder MP, Eckert C, et al. PAX5 biallelic genomic alterations define a novel subgroup of B-cell precursor acute lymphoblastic leukemia. *Leukemia.* 2019;33(8):1895-1909. doi:10.1038/s41375-019-0430-z

72. Zaliova M, Potuckova E, Lukes J, et al. Frequency and prognostic impact of ZEB2 H1038 and Q1072 mutations in childhood B-other acute lymphoblastic leukemia. *Haematologica.* 2021;106(3):886-890. doi:10.3324/haematol.2020.249094

73. Fazio G, Bresolin S, Silvestri D, et al. PAX5 fusion genes are frequent in poor risk childhood acute lymphoblastic leukaemia and can be targeted with BIBF1120. *EBioMedicine.* 2022;83:104224. doi:10.1016/j.ebiom.2022.104224

74. Zaliova M, Winkowska L, Stuchly J, et al. A novel class of ZNF384 aberrations in acute leukemia. *Blood Adv.* 2021;5(21):4393-4397. doi:10.1182/bloodadvances.2021005318

Chapter 41

T-Lymphoblastic Leukemias/Lymphomas

Amy Duffield, Michael J. Borowitz, Sindhu Cherian, Mark D. Ewalt, Elias Jabbour, Charles G. Mullighan, Leonie Saft, and David T. Teachey

T-lymphoblastic leukemia/lymphoma (T-ALL/LBL) is subclassified into three entities: early T-cell precursor lymphoblastic leukemia/lymphoma (ETP ALL), *BCL11B*-activated; ETP ALL, Not Otherwise Specified (NOS); and T-ALL/LBL, NOS. Eight provisional entities are also described. (Table 41.1).

EARLY T-CELL PRECURSOR LYMPHOBLASTIC LEUKEMIA/ LYMPHOMA, *BCL11B*-ACTIVATED

Definition

ETP ALL, *BCL11B*-activated is a neoplasm composed of hematopoietic cells defined by an immunophenotype with limited evidence of T cell differentiation in the setting of a concurrent *BCL11B* activating genetic alteration(s). A subset of T/myeloid mixed phenotype acute leukemias and acute myeloid leukemias (AML) also harbor identical genomic and biologic features, and are distinguished only by immunophenotype.[1,2]

Synonyms

ETP ALL, *BCL11B*-rearranged.

Epidemiology

This is an uncommon neoplasm that occurs in both children and adults. It accounts for about one-third of cases of ETP ALL, and overall comprises <5% of cases of T-ALL.

General Clinical Features

The presentation of ETP, *BCL11B*-activated ALL is similar to those of other forms of *de novo* T-ALL. Although there are no distinguishing clinical features, in general ETP ALL is more likely to present with a lower white blood cell (WBC) count at diagnosis than other subtypes of T-ALL.[3]

Morphology

This entity does not have specific morphologic features.

Immunophenotype

By definition, ETP ALL expresses CD7, lacks CD8 and CD1a, and is positive for one or more of the myeloid/stem cell markers: CD11b, CD13, CD33, CD34, CD65, CD117, and/or HLA-DR (Figure 41.1). Blasts also express cytoplasmic CD3, which may be relatively dim. Rare cases can show dim or partial surface CD3 expression. The blasts may also express CD2 and/or CD4. By definition, in ETP ALL <75% of the blast population shows expression of CD5; however, the immunophenotype of *BCL11B*-activated ALL is notable for lack of CD5 expression.[4] Myeloperoxidase is, by definition, negative in ETP ALL.

Genetics

Gene expression (GEX) profiling studies of ETP ALL demonstrate a pattern similar to normal early thymocyte precursors, which is different from the pattern of GEX seen in cases of T-ALL with a more mature immunophenotype.[5] Many of the overexpressed genes are more typically associated with myeloid or stem cell profiles, and the mutational profile is also more similar to that of myeloid leukemias than other T-cell leukemias.[5-9] In 80% of cases, ETP ALL with *BCL11B* activation is associated with interchromosomal rearrangements to genomic regions that house superenhancers active in hematopoietic stem and progenitor cells (Figure 41.2). The remaining cases have focal amplifications that generate a neoenhancer distal to *BCL11B*.[2] Both alterations produce leukemias with similar GEX profiles, so this group has been termed "*BCL11B*-activated" to clarify that this subtype includes not only *BCL11B* rearrangements but also other *BCL11B*-activating genetic alterations. This entity excludes *BCL11B* rearrangements that do not result in activation of *BCL11B*, particularly *BCL11B::TLX3*, which is enriched in the provisional subtype of T-ALL, *TLX3*-rearranged.

TABLE 41.1 T-lymphoblastic leukemia/lymphoma (T-ALL)

Early T-precursor lymphoblastic leukemia/lymphoma, *BCL11B*-activated
Early T-precursor lymphoblastic leukemia/lymphoma, Not Otherwise Specified
T-Lymphoblastic Leukemia/Lymphoma, Not Otherwise Specified
Provisional Entities:
T-Lymphoblastic Leukemia/Lymphoma, *TAL1*/2-rearranged
T-Lymphoblastic Leukemia/Lymphoma, *TLX1*-rearranged
T-Lymphoblastic Leukemia/Lymphoma, *TLX3*-rearranged
T-Lymphoblastic Leukemia/Lymphoma, *HOXA* dysregulated
T-Lymphoblastic Leukemia/Lymphoma, *LMO1*/2-rearranged
T-Lymphoblastic Leukemia/Lymphoma, *NKX2*-rearranged
T-Lymphoblastic Leukemia/Lymphoma, *SPI1*-rearranged
T-Lymphoblastic Leukemia/Lymphoma, bHLH, Other

Identical *BCL11B*-activating alterations are present not only in ETP ALL, but also in other cases of acute leukemia that share a common GEX profile. These leukemias exhibit variable expression of cytoplasmic CD3 and myeloperoxidase, resulting in classification as ETP ALL, or T/myeloid mixed phenotype acute leukemias (approximately one-third of cases), or, less commonly, AML or acute undifferentiated leukemia (<5% of cases).[1,2,10,11] Thus, it may be best to consider *BCL11B*-activated leukemia a molecularly defined subset of acute leukemia irrespective of diagnostic immunophenotype. Other common genetic lesions seen in this subtype include *FLT3*-ITD mutations and *WT1* alterations, and the presence of a *FLT3* mutation in ETP ALL is suggestive of a *BCL11B*-activated leukemia.[2,12]

Prognosis and Clinical Comment

There are no published differences in prognosis or treatment response comparing *BCL11B*-activated ETP ALL and ETP ALL, NOS; a general comparison of ETP ALL with other types of T-ALL is discussed below.

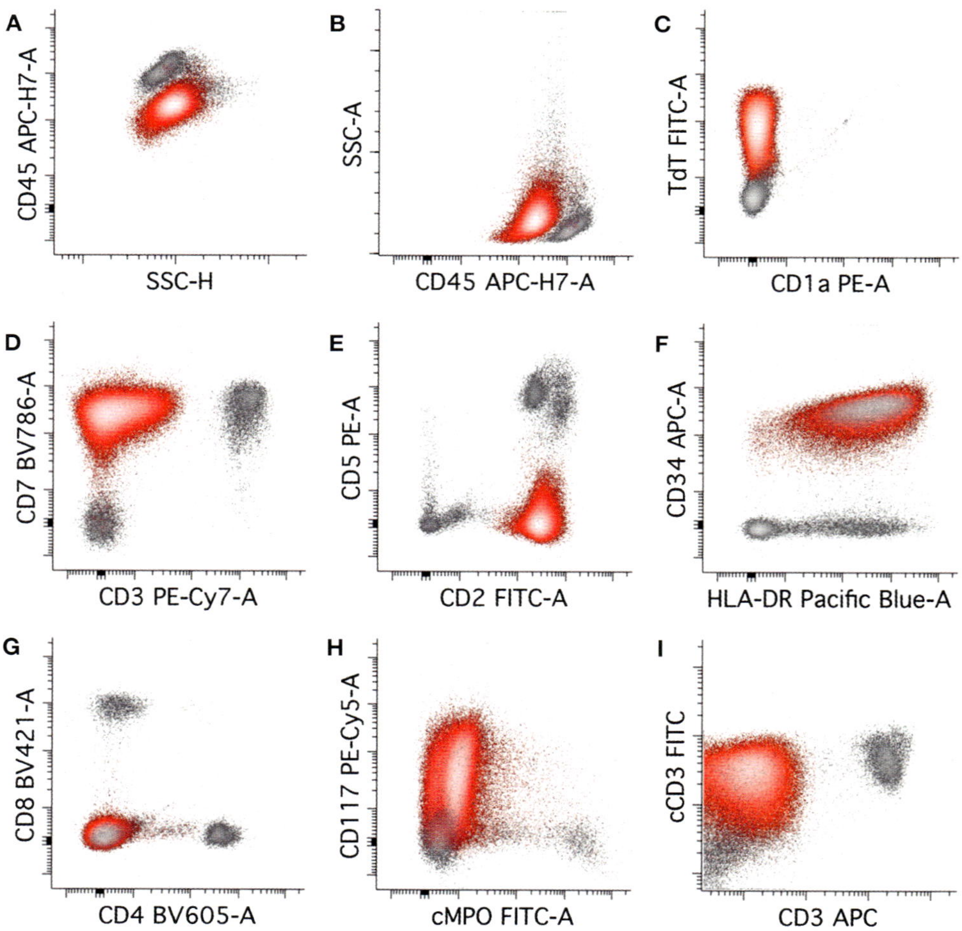

FIGURE 41.1 Flow cytometric analysis of a representative early T-cell precursor lymphoblastic leukemia. There is a distinct population of blasts (red) with dim CD45 and low right angle scatter (**A** and **B**). The blasts express TdT but are negative for CD1a **(C)**, are positive for strong CD7 with dim to absent surface membrane CD3 **(D)**, express CD2 but lack expression of CD5 **(E)**, are positive for CD34 and HLA-DR **(F)**, lack CD4 and CD8 **(G)**, show partial expression of CD117 with absent myeloperoxidase **(H)**, and express cytoplasmic CD3 **(I)**.

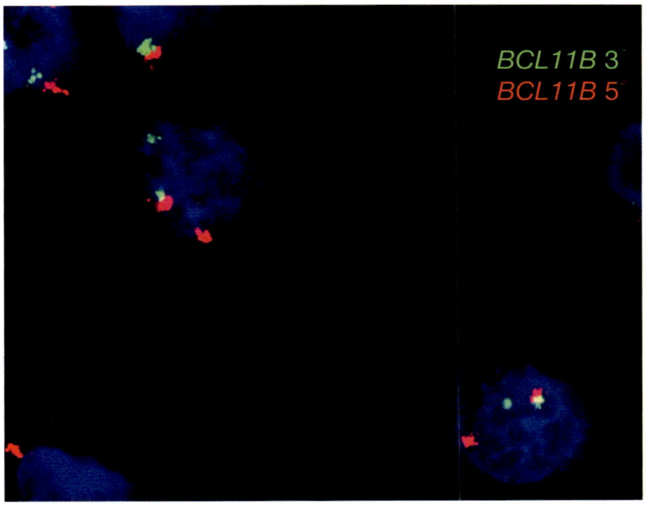

FIGURE 41.2 ETP ALL, *BCL11B*-activated. Fluorescence in situ hybridization (FISH) studies using a *BCL11B* (14q32.2) break apart probe (3′ green, 5′ orange). Both cells show one normal copy of *BCL11B*, with juxtaposition of 3′ and 5′ probes, as well as one copy of *KMT2A* disrupted by the translocation, with separation of the 3′ green and 5′ orange probes. (Image courtesy of Umut Aypar, PhD, FACMG, Memorial Sloan Kettering Cancer Center.)

EARLY T-CELL PRECURSOR LYMPHOBLASTIC LEUKEMIA/LYMPHOMA, NOS

Definition

ETP lymphoblastic leukemia (ETP ALL) is a neoplasm composed of hematopoietic cells defined by an immunophenotype with limited evidence of T cell differentiation. By definition this subtype lacks activating mutations of *BCL11B*.

Synonyms

None.

Epidemiology

This is an uncommon neoplasm found in both children and adults, accounting for approximately 5% to 10% of cases of T-ALL in childhood, and for <5% of cases of adult T-ALL.[13]

General Clinical Features

The presentation of ETP ALL, NOS is similar to other forms of *de novo* T-ALL, including ETP ALL, *BCL11B*-activated, and so-called "near-ETP" ALL (see Immunophenotype). The WBC count at diagnosis is generally lower in ETP ALL than in T-ALL, NOS or near-ETP ALL.

Morphology

This entity does not have specific morphologic features.

Immunophenotype

The immunophenotypic features of ETP ALL, NOS are the same as those seen in ETP ALL with *BCL11B*-activated (described previously, see Figure 41.1), although ETP ALL, NOS may show expression of CD5 on <75% of blasts. A subset of T-ALL cases that would otherwise meet phenotypic criteria for ETP ALL but with expression of CD5 on ≥75% of the blasts has been referred to as near-ETP ALL. Near-ETP ALL shows minor differences in clinical presentation and response to therapy, and has different genetic lesions than ETP ALL; it is not formally included in the classification because the drivers are not fully understood.[14,15]

Genetics

ETP ALL, NOS lacks activating mutations of *BCL11B*, but there are multiple other driver mutations. Common genetic lesions that are reported at high frequencies include gene mutations commonly associated with myeloid neoplasms, including alterations in *DNMT3A*, *FLT3*, *IDH1*, *IDH2*, and the *RAS* family of genes. Several mutations that are more characteristically associated with phenotypically more mature forms of T-ALL, such as mutations in *NOTCH1/FBXW7* and *CDKN1/2*, are reported at low frequencies in ETP ALL.[9] ETP ALL remains defined by immunophenotypic criteria, but recent large-scale genomic sequencing of childhood T-ALL indicated that the majority of ETP ALL cases are part of a larger group of both ETP and non-ETP cases that are characterized by the deregulation or mutation of genes encoding regulators of early hematopoietic development, including *ETV6*, *HOX* genes, *RUNX1*, and *ZFP36L2*.[16]

Prognosis and Clinical Comment

In general, minimal residual disease in ETP ALL tends to be higher at the end of induction therapy than in other patients with T-ALL.[17] Although the kinetics of response to therapy appears to be relatively slow in ETP ALL, in children the prognosis is similar to other T-ALLs,[18] although adults with ETP ALL may have a poorer prognosis.[3] Children and young adults with ETP ALL are more likely to relapse later in therapy or after completing treatment. Preclinical studies suggest that ETP ALL is more likely to be corticosteroid resistant as compared with non-ETP ALL, potentially explaining the higher frequency of minimal residual disease at the end of induction.[19]

T-LYMPHOBLASTIC LEUKEMIA/LYMPHOMA, NOS

Definition

T-ALL/LBL, NOS is a neoplasm composed of lymphoblasts committed to the T-cell lineage that lacks defining immunophenotypic findings or genetic lesions that permit for classification as a specific entity.

Synonyms

None.

Epidemiology, General Clinical Features, Immunophenotype, Genetics, Prognosis, and Clinical Comment

The features are generally as described for T-ALL in the Introduction.

T-ACUTE LYMPHOBLASTIC LEUKEMIA/LYMPHOBLASTIC LYMPHOMA: PROVISIONAL ENTITIES

There are eight new provisional entities of T-ALL/LBL that are classified based on aberrant activation of different families of transcription factors (see Table 41.1). To date, none of these has any known unique morphologic or clinical features. Many of the genetic abnormalities are rearrangements that can be detected using karyotyping, FISH probes, or PCR; however, aberrant transcription factor activation can be the result of various molecular abnormalities, including intragenic alterations. Thus, comprehensive genomic analysis may be necessary to classify all cases. Both the true frequency of these entities and characteristic features (other than defining genetic abnormalities) are often unclear due to the relative paucity of broad data collection across populations and uneven definitions of the entities within the literature. The classification of T-ALL/LBL, including the number of subtypes, their driver alterations, and associations with outcome, is rapidly changing as more cases undergo comprehensive genomic analysis.[16]

T-Lymphoblastic Leukemia/Lymphoma, *TAL1/2*-Rearranged

Definition

T-ALL/LBL, *TAL1/2*-rearranged is a neoplasm composed of lymphoblasts committed to the T-cell lineage in which the blasts harbor rearrangement of the genes T-cell acute lymphocytic leukemia protein 1 (*TAL1*) or T-cell acute lymphocytic leukemia protein 2 (*TAL2*).

Synonyms

None.

Epidemiology

This is a relatively common subtype, representing approximately 25% of cases.[20]

Immunophenotype

This entity often has a late cortical thymocyte ($CD4^+$ or $CD8^+$) immunophenotype.

Genetics

Rearrangements of *TAL1* are more common than rearrangements of *TAL2*. This subtype has variable fusion partners, most commonly *STIL* or *TRA/TRD*. *TRB* is a common fusion partner with *TAL2*. Other common genetic lesions deregulating *TAL1* include an interstitial deletion between *STIL* and *TAL1* at 1p32; and sequence variants within or flanking *TAL1* that generate a superenhancer. Common concomitant genomic alterations including deletions of *CDKN2A/CDKN2B*, sequence mutations of *NOTCH1/FBXW7* that activate NOTCH1 signaling, and deletions/mutations that inactivate *PTEN*. These alterations are also common in other non-ETP T-ALL subtypes. Mutations of *USP7* are enriched in *TAL1/2*-rearranged cases.[15,21,22]

Prognosis and Clinical Comment

The prognosis of this entity is heterogeneous.

T-Lymphoblastic Leukemia/Lymphoma, *TLX1*-Rearranged

Definition

T-ALL/LBL, *TLX1*-rearranged is a neoplasm composed of lymphoblasts committed to the T-cell lineage in which the blasts harbor rearrangement of T-cell leukemia homeobox 1 (*TLX1*).

Synonyms

None.

Epidemiology

The entity accounts for approximately 5% of T-ALL/LBL children, and increases with age to nearly 30% in adults.[20]

Immunophenotype

This entity often has a CD4/CD8 double positive and CD1a+ immunophenotype.[23]

Genetics

The most common rearrangement partner is *TCR*. Other common genetic lesions include alterations in *CDKN1B, BCL11B, DNM2, PHF6,* and *RB1*.[15,22] This entity can be separated from T-ALL/LBL, *TLX3*-rearranged (see below) by GEX profiling, or by identification of the driver alterations by FISH or genomic analyses.

Prognosis and clinical comment

The prognosis of this entity tends to be favorable in children and young adults, but is worse in adults.

T-Lymphoblastic Leukemia/Lymphoma, *TLX3*-Rearranged

Definition

T-ALL/LBL, *TLX3*-rearranged is a neoplasm composed of lymphoblasts committed to the T-cell lineage in which the blasts harbor rearrangement of T-cell leukemia homeobox 3 (*TLX3*).

Synonyms

None.

Epidemiology

The entity accounts for 15% to 25% of T-ALL/LBL in children, and <5% in adults.

Immunophenotype

This entity typically has a CD4/CD8 double positive and CD1a+ phenotype immunophenotype, although cases with a more immature immunophenotype are also described.[23]

Genetics

The most common rearrangement partners are *BCL11B, CDK6,* and *TCR*. The subset of cases with *BCL11B::TLX3* has a distinct pathogenesis, with hijacking of *BCL11B* enhancers resulting in *TLX3* deregulation[24]; this entity has a non-ETP immunophenotype, allowing it to be differentiated from ETP ALL, *BCL11B*-activated. Other common genetic lesions include alterations in *CDKN2A, FBXW7/NOTCH1,* and *PTEN*.[15,21,22] T-ALL/LBL, *TLX3*-rearranged, can be distinguished from T-ALL/LBL, *TLX1*-rearranged as discussed in the previous section.

Prognosis and clinical comment

The prognosis of this entity tends to be favorable.

T-Lymphoblastic Leukemia/Lymphoma, *HOXA* Dysregulated

Definition

T-ALL/LBL, homeobox gene cluster (*HOXA*) dysregulated is a neoplasm composed of lymphoblasts committed to the T-cell lineage in which the blasts harbor abnormalities that result in the dysregulation of the major homeobox gene cluster (*HOXA*).

Synonyms

None.

Epidemiology

The entity accounts for 15% to 25% of T-ALL/LBL childhood cases.

Immunophenotype

These cases tend to have an immature immunophenotype.

Genetics

This entity is often characterized by gene fusions, the most common of which are: *HOXA::TRB/TRG, KMT2A, PICALM::MLLT10,* and *SET::NUP214*.[15,21]

Prognosis and clinical comment

The prognosis of this entity is variable and may be dependent on the fusion partner.

T-Lymphoblastic Leukemia/Lymphoma, *LMO1/2*-Rearranged

Definition

T-ALL/LBL, *LMO1/2*-rearranged is a neoplasm composed of lymphoblasts committed to the T-cell lineage in which the blasts harbor rearrangement of either LIM domain only 1 (*LMO1*) or LIM domain only 2 (*LMO2*).

Synonyms

None.

Epidemiology

T-ALL/LBL, *LMO1*-rearranged accounts for <5% of T-ALL/LBL, and *LMO2*-rearranged cases account for approximately 10% of T-ALL/LBL.

Immunophenotype

This entity generally has an immature (CD4-CD8-) phenotype, although there are exceptions. This subtype is associated with very high expression of LMO proteins; however, this finding is not specific for this entity because high expression of LMO proteins is broadly seen across many different subtypes of T-ALL/LBL.[20]

Genetics

The most common rearrangement partner is *TCR*. Other common genetic lesions include alterations in *CDKN2A*, *FBXW7*/*NOTCH1*, *LEF1*, and *PTEN*.[15,21]

Prognosis and clinical comment

The prognosis of this entity is variable and may be dependent on the fusion partner.

T-Lymphoblastic Leukemia/Lymphoma, *NKX2*-Rearranged

Definition

T-ALL/LBL, *NKX2*-rearranged is a neoplasm composed of lymphoblasts committed to the T-cell lineage in which the blasts harbor rearrangements of NK2 homeobox gene cluster (*NKX2*).

Synonyms

None.

Epidemiology

This is an uncommon subtype in children, accounting for approximately 5% of T-ALL/LBL. It is rarely reported in adults.

Immunophenotype

This entity typically has a CD4/CD8 double positive and CD1a+ phenotype immunophenotype, and often shows deletion of *LEF1*.[23]

Genetics

The most common rearrangements are between *NKX2.1*/*NKX2.2*/*NKX2.5* and *BCL11B*, *CDK6*, or *TCR*. Other common genetic lesions include alterations in *CDKN2A*, *LEF1*, *NOTCH1*, *PHF6*, and *RPL10*.[21,22]

Prognosis and clinical comment

The prognosis of this rare entity is not well characterized.

T-Lymphoblastic Leukemia/Lymphoma, *SPI1*-Rearranged

Definition

T-ALL/LBL, *SPI1*-rearranged is a neoplasm composed of lymphoblasts committed to the T-cell lineage in which the blasts harbor rearrangements of Spi-1 proto-oncogene (*SPI1*).

Synonyms

None.

Epidemiology

This is a rare subtype, accounting for less than 2% of T-ALL/LBL. It is predominantly reported in children.

Immunophenotype

At least one case was reported to have a CD4-/CD8- immunophenotype.[25] The blasts in this entity characteristically express HLA-DR.

Genetics

The most common rearrangement partners are *BCL11B*, *STMN1*, and *TCF7*. Other common genetic lesions include alterations in *KRAS* and *NRAS*.[26]

Prognosis and clinical comment

This rare entity appears to have a very poor prognosis. It may relapse as a histiocytic/dendritic cell neoplasm, with preservation of the *SPI1* rearrangement and a common cell of origin.[16]

T-Lymphoblastic Leukemia/Lymphoma, BHLH, Other

Definition

T-ALL/LBL, basic helix-loop-helix (bHLH), Other is a neoplasm composed of lymphoblasts committed to the T-cell lineage in which the blasts harbor alterations that result in deregulation of bHLH transcription factors other than *TAL1*.

Synonyms

None.

Epidemiology

This is a rare subtype, accounting for less than 2% of T-ALL/LBL. It is predominantly reported in children.

Immunophenotype

This entity is reported to have a mature immunophenotype, and is associated with LMO overexpression.[27,28]

Genetics

bHLH transcription factors include lymphoblastic leukemia–associated hematopoiesis regulator 1 (*LYL1*) and oligodendrocyte transcription factor 2 (*OLIG2*); common rearrangements described in this entity are *TRB::LYL1* and *TCR::OLIG2/BHLHB1*.[27,28] Rearrangements involving the bHLH transcription factors *TAL1* or *TAL2* are included in the *TAL1/2* group rather than bHLH, Other.

Prognosis and clinical comment

The prognosis of this rare entity is not well characterized.

References

1. Di Giacomo D, La Starza R, Gorello P, et al. 14q32 rearrangements deregulating BCL11B mark a distinct subgroup of T-lymphoid and myeloid immature acute leukemia. *Blood*. 2021;138(9):773-784. doi:10.1182/blood.2020010510
2. Montefiori LE, Bendig S, Gu Z, et al. Enhancer hijacking drives oncogenic BCL11B expression in lineage-ambiguous stem cell leukemia. *Cancer Discov*. 2021;11:2846-2867. doi:10.1158/2159-8290.CD-21-0145
3. Jain N, Lamb AV, O'Brien S, et al. Early T-cell precursor acute lymphoblastic leukemia/lymphoma (ETP-ALL/LBL) in adolescents and adults: a high-risk subtype. *Blood*. 2016;127(15):1863-1869. doi:10.1182/blood-2015-08-661702
4. Fang H, Wang W, El Hussein S, et al. B-cell lymphoma/leukaemia 11B (BCL11B) expression status helps distinguish early T-cell precursor acute lymphoblastic leukaemia/lymphoma (ETP-ALL/LBL) from other subtypes of T-cell ALL/LBL. *Br J Haematol*. 2021;194(6):1034-1038. doi:10.1111/bjh.17681
5. Coustan-Smith E, Mullighan CG, Onciu M, et al. Early T-cell precursor leukaemia: a subtype of very high-risk acute lymphoblastic leukaemia. *Lancet Oncol*. 2009;10(2):147-156. doi:10.1016/S1470-2045(08)70314-0
6. Zhang J, Ding L, Holmfeldt L, et al. The genetic basis of early T-cell precursor acute lymphoblastic leukaemia. *Nature*. 2012;481(7380):157-163. doi:10.1038/nature10725
7. Neumann M, Heesch S, Schlee C, et al. Whole-exome sequencing in adult ETP-ALL reveals a high rate of DNMT3A mutations. *Blood*. 2013;121(23):4749-4752. doi:10.1182/blood-2012-11-465138
8. Neumann M, Coskun E, Fransecky L, et al. FLT3 mutations in early T-cell precursor ALL characterize a stem cell like leukemia and imply the clinical use of tyrosine kinase inhibitors. *PLoS One*. 2013;8(1):e53190. doi:10.1371/journal.pone.0053190
9. Van Vlierberghe P, Ambesi-Impiombato A, Perez-Garcia A, et al. ETV6 mutations in early immature human T cell leukemias. *J Exp Med*. 2011;208(13):2571-2579. doi:10.1084/jem.20112239
10. Wang W, Beird H, Kroll CJ, et al. T(6;14)(q25;q32) involves BCL11B and is highly associated with mixed-phenotype acute leukemia, T/myeloid. *Leukemia*. 2020;34(9):2509-2512. doi:10.1038/s41375-020-0761-9
11. Abbas S, Sanders MA, Zeilemaker A, et al. Integrated genome-wide genotyping and gene expression profiling reveals BCL11B as a putative oncogene in acute myeloid leukemia with 14q32 aberrations. *Haematologica*. 2014;99(5):848-857. doi:10.3324/haematol.2013.095604
12. Wang Q, Cai W, Wang Q, et al. Integrative genomic and transcriptomic profiling reveals distinct molecular subsets in adult mixed phenotype acute leukemia. *Am J Hematol*. 2023;98(1):66-78. doi:10.1002/ajh.26758
13. Xu X, Paxton CN, Hayashi RJ, et al. Genomic and clinical characterization of early T-cell precursor lymphoblastic lymphoma. *Blood Adv*. 2021;5(14):2890-2900. doi:10.1182/bloodadvances.2021004334
14. Morita K, Jain N, Kantarjian H, et al. Outcome of T-cell acute lymphoblastic leukemia/lymphoma: focus on near-ETP phenotype and differential impact of nelarabine. *Am J Hematol*. 2021;96(5):589-598. doi:10.1002/ajh.26144
15. Liu Y, Easton J, Shao Y, et al. The genomic landscape of pediatric and young adult T-lineage acute lymphoblastic leukemia. *Nat Genet*. 2017;49(8):1211-1218. doi:10.1038/ng.3909
16. Pölönen P, Di Giacomo D, Seffernick AE, et al. The genomic basis of childhood T-lineage acute lymphoblastic leukaemia. *Nature*. 2024;632(8027):1082-1091. doi: 10.1038/s41586-024-07807-0.
17. Teachey DT, Pui CH. Comparative features and outcomes between paediatric T-cell and B-cell acute lymphoblastic leukaemia. *Lancet Oncol*. 2019;20(3):e142-e154. doi:10.1016/S1470-2045(19)30031-2
18. Wood BL, Devidas M, Summers RJ, et al. Prognostic significance of ETP phenotype and minimal residual disease in T-ALL: a Children's Oncology Group study. *Blood*. 2023;142(24):2069-2078. doi:10.1182/blood.2023020678
19. Delgado-Martin C, Meyer LK, Huang BJ, et al. JAK/STAT pathway inhibition overcomes IL7-induced glucocorticoid resistance in a subset of human T-cell acute lymphoblastic leukemias. *Leukemia*. 2017;31(12):2568-2576. doi:10.1038/leu.2017.136
20. Girardi T, Vicente C, Cools J, De Keersmaecker K. The genetics and molecular biology of T-ALL. *Blood*. 2017;129(9):1113-1123. doi:10.1182/blood-2016-10-706465

21. Chang YH, Yu CH, Jou ST, et al. Targeted sequencing to identify genetic alterations and prognostic markers in pediatric T-cell acute lymphoblastic leukemia. *Sci Rep.* 2021;11(1):769. doi:10.1038/s41598-020-80613-6

22. Chen B, Jiang L, Zhong M-L, et al. Identification of fusion genes and characterization of transcriptome features in T-cell acute lymphoblastic leukemia. *Proc Natl Acad Sci U S A.* 2018;115(2):373-378. doi:10.1073/pnas.1717125115

23. Bardelli V, Arniani S, Pierini V, et al. T-cell acute lymphoblastic leukemia: biomarkers and their clinical usefulness. *Genes.* 2021;12(8):1118. doi:10.3390/genes12081118

24. Smits WK, Vermeulen C, Hagelaar R, et al. Elevated enhancer-oncogene contacts and higher oncogene expression levels by recurrent CTCF inactivating mutations in acute T cell leukemia. *Cell Rep.* 2023;42(4):112373. doi:10.1016/j.celrep.2023.112373

25. Van Thillo Q, De Bie J, Seneviratne JA, et al. Oncogenic cooperation between TCF7-SPI1 and NRAS(G12D) requires β-catenin activity to drive T-cell acute lymphoblastic leukemia. *Nat Commun.* 2021;12(1):4164. doi:10.1038/s41467-021-24442-9

26. Seki M, Kimura S, Isobe T, et al. Recurrent SPI1 (PU.1) fusions in high-risk pediatric T cell acute lymphoblastic leukemia. *Nat Genet.* 2017;49(8):1274-1281. doi:10.1038/ng.3900

27. Homminga I, Vuerhard MJ, Langerak AW, Buijs-Gladdines J, Pieters R, Meijerink JPP. Characterization of a pediatric T-cell acute lymphoblastic leukemia patient with simultaneous LYL1 and LMO2 rearrangements. *Haematologica.* 2012;97(2):258-261. doi:10.3324/haematol.2011.051722

28. Panagopoulos I, Gorunova L, Johannsdottir IMR, et al. Chromosome translocation t(14;21)(q11;q22) activates both OLIG1 and OLIG2 in pediatric T-cell lymphoblastic malignancies and may signify adverse prognosis. *Cancer Genomics Proteomics.* 2020;17(1):41-48. doi:10.21873/cgp.20166

Chapter 42
NK-Cell Acute Lymphoblastic Leukemia

Olga K. Weinberg, and Michael J. Borowitz

Definition

NK-cell acute lymphoblastic leukemia (NK-LL) is a rare acute leukemia composed of NK blasts that lack expression of lineage-specific markers of T cells, B cells, myeloid cells, or plasmacytoid dendritic cells. As absence of specific markers makes it difficult to clearly establish the origin of these malignancies, this is considered as a provisional entity. Early markers expressed by CD34-positive hematopoietic cells associated with propensity to differentiate into NK cells include CD7, CD10, CD45RA, and CD127.[1-3] The stages of NK cell maturation have been defined both in vitro and in vivo, and expression of CD94 and loss of CD117 mark an important step in this process.[4]

A diagnosis of NK-LL is considered in leukemic cases expressing CD56, typically uniform, along with immature markers and markers associated with both T cells and NK cells including CD2 and CD7 but lacking B-cell and myeloid markers. The phenotype of NK-LL can overlap with other CD56-positive hematopoietic neoplasms, which makes it difficult to define it precisely. Blastic plasmacytoid dendritic cell neoplasm (BPDCN) was previously known as NK cell leukemia/lymphoma before its biology and origin were understood to be a CD56$^+$ neoplasm that is derived from the precursors of plasmacytoid dendritic cells. NK-LL can be confused with T-cell lymphoblastic leukemia/lymphoma, where CD56 expression has been reported in a small subset of cases that appear to have distinct clinicopathologic findings, including association with higher rate of early T-cell precursor (ETP) subtype, and worse prognosis.[5,6] CD56 expression is also seen in a subset of acute myeloid leukemia (AML) cases[7] and some investigators have used "myeloid/NK acute leukemia" to suggest NK-cell origin, but these cases have been shown to have an immunophenotypic overlap with AML with minimal differentiation.[8] Acute undifferentiated leukemia (AUL) is a rare acute leukemia that lacks evidence of differentiation along any lineage and frequently shows coexpression of CD56 and T-cell markers, similar to NK-LL.[9]

Synonyms

Precursor NK-cell lymphoblastic leukemia/lymphoma.
NK lymphoblastic leukemia (not recommended).

Epidemiology

The overall incidence of NK-LL is unknown. The rarity of well-documented cases and the overlap with other CD56-positive hematopoietic neoplasms noted earlier make it difficult to establish the epidemiologic features of this provisional entity.

General Clinical Features

Only limited clinical information is available about patients with NK-LL and is based on isolated case reports and a single series.[10-12] In a series of six cases, patients with NK-LL at diagnosis had a median age of 13 years (range 4-72 years) and a white blood cell count, hemoglobin, platelet count, and bone marrow cellularity and blast percentage similar to that of patients with CD56-positive T-ALL.[12] As compared with patients with CD56$^+$ AUL, patients with NK-LL were significantly younger and presented with higher white blood cell counts and platelet count but with no difference in hemoglobin, circulating blasts, or bone marrow cellularity.[12]

Morphology

NK-LL blasts generally show scant, agranular cytoplasm and prominent nucleoli on aspirate smears (Figure 42.1A). Similar to other subtypes of ALL, bone marrow evaluation shows hypercellular marrow with predominance of blasts (Figure 42.1B). Dysplasia is rare, although a single reported NK-LL case showed granulocytic dysplasia.[11]

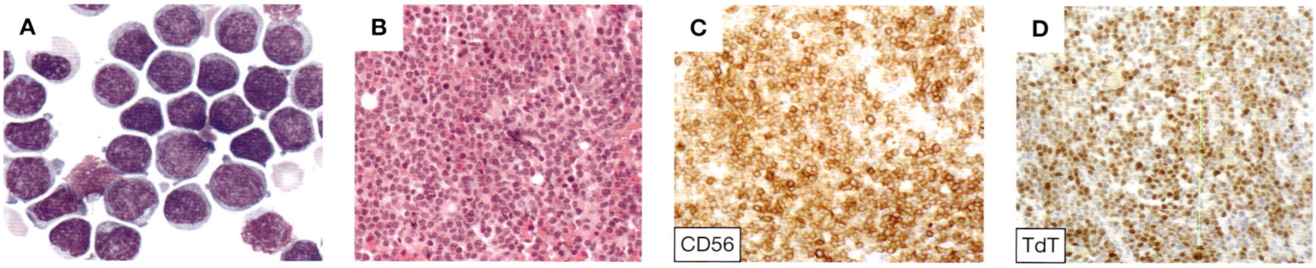

FIGURE 42.1 **A:** NK-LL blasts show scant, agranular cytoplasm and prominent nucleoli on aspirate smears. **B:** The biopsy is hypercellular with marked predominance of blasts. **C:** Blasts are diffusely positive for CD56 and also express TdT **(D)**.

Immunophenotype

Blasts in NK-LL typically express CD56, CD34, and CD7 but can be distinguished from BPDCN based on absence of CD4 and CD123 (Figure 42.1C and D). TdT may or may not be expressed. CD94 and CD16 are also positive, although these have not been reliably tested in all cases, and neither of these is absolutely NK specific. Because a subset of NK-LL cases can express cCD3,[12] distinction from T-ALL, and in particular from early T-precursor ALL, can be difficult, especially because CD56 expression has been reported in a small subset of cases ETP-ALL associated with worse prognosis.[5,6] CD56 expression is also seen not uncommonly in AML cases,[7] although it is often only dimly or partly expressed. Cases with myeloid markers and CD56 that were suggested to be "myeloid/NK acute leukemia" are now just considered AML.[8] Cases expressing CD56, CD34, and CD7 without TdT, cCD3, or myeloid markers can resemble AUL. This phenotypic overlap with other leukemias further emphasizes the reason that NK-LL remains a provisional entity at this time.

Genetics

T-cell receptor genes are in germline configuration, which can be useful to distinguish these from T-ALL, even though some cases of ETP-ALL will also lack TCR rearrangements.[13] Only limited data are available on karyotypic abnormalities in this entity, although complex karyotypes have been reported. Similarly, there are few studies of pathogenic mutations found in patients with NK-LL; the most common in one series were in *NOTCH1*, *ETV6*, and *JAK3* genes[12]; these abnormalities are also seen in ETP-ALL, although the latter sometimes have *FLT3* mutations, which to date have not been described in NK-LL.[14]

Prognosis and Clinical Comment

Because recognition of this entity is difficult it is difficult to describe prognosis or comment on therapy. Most patients with NK-LL received ALL-type therapy, and stem cell bone marrow transplant appears to be commonly employed. In a small series with six patients with median overall follow-up time of 36 months,[11] relapses were common but most patients were alive at last follow-up; to the extent overall outcome was favorable, this may be related to the relatively young age at presentation in this series.

References

1. Grzywacz B, Kataria N, Kataria N, Blazar BR, Miller JS, Verneris MR. Natural killer-cell differentiation by myeloid progenitors. *Blood*. 2011;117(13):3548-3558.
2. Carotta S, Pang SH, Nutt SL, Belz GT. Identification of the earliest NK-cell precursor in the mouse BM. *Blood*. 2011;117(20):5449-5452.
3. Renoux VM, Zriwil A, Peitzsch C, et al. Identification of a human natural killer cell lineage-restricted progenitor in fetal and adult tissues. *Immunity*. 2015;43(2):394-407.
4. Grzywacz B, Kataria N, Sikora M, et al. Coordinated acquisition of inhibitory and activating receptors and functional properties by developing human natural killer cells. *Blood*. 2006;108(12):3824-3833.
5. Jain N, Lamb AV, O'Brien S, et al. Early T-cell precursor acute lymphoblastic leukemia/lymphoma (ETP-ALL/LBL) in adolescents and adults: a high-risk subtype. *Blood*. 2016;127(15):1863-1869.
6. Dalmazzo LF, Jácomo RH, Marinato AF, et al. The presence of CD56/CD16 in T-cell acute lymphoblastic leukaemia correlates with the expression of cytotoxic molecules and is associated with worse response to treatment. *Br J Haematol*. 2009;144(2):223-229.
7. Alegretti AP, Bittar CM, Bittencourt R, et al. The expression of CD56 antigen is associated with poor prognosis in

patients with acute myeloid leukemia. *Rev Bras Hematol Hemoter*. 2011;33(3):202-206.

8. Suzuki R, Nakamura S, Suzumiya J, et al. Blastic natural killer cell lymphoma/leukemia (CD56-positive blastic tumor): prognostication and categorization according to anatomic sites of involvement. *Cancer*. 2005;104(5):1022-1031.
9. Weinberg OK, Hasserjian RP, Baraban E, et al. Clinical, immunophenotypic, and genomic findings of acute undifferentiated leukemia and comparison to acute myeloid leukemia with minimal differentiation: a study from the bone marrow pathology group. *Mod Pathol*. 2019;32(9):1373-1385.
10. Jain S, Kumar R, Purohit A, Pati HP. Precursor NK cell lymphoblastic leukemia/lymphoma-report of a case with literature review. *Indian J Hematol Blood Transfus*. 2014;30(suppl 1):283-285.
11. Sedick Q, Alotaibi S, Alshieban S, Naheet KB, Elyamany G. Natural killer cell lymphoblastic leukaemia/lymphoma: case report and review of the recent literature. *Case Rep Oncol*. 2017;10(2):588-595.
12. Weinberg OK, Chisholm KM, Ok CY, et al. Clinical, immunophenotypic and genomic findings of NK lymphoblastic leukemia: a study from the Bone Marrow Pathology Group. *Mod Pathol*. 2021;34(7):1358-1366.
13. Gutierrez A, Dahlberg SE, Neuberg DS, et al. Absence of biallelic TCRgamma deletion predicts early treatment failure in pediatric T-cell acute lymphoblastic leukemia. *J Clin Oncol*. 2010;28(24):3816-3823.
14. Booth CAG, Barkas N, Neo WH, et al. Ezh2 and Runx1 mutations collaborate to initiate lympho-myeloid leukemia in early thymic progenitors. *Cancer Cell*. 2018;33(2):274-291.e8.

INTERNATIONAL CONSENSUS CLASSIFICATION OF MATURE LYMPHOID AND HISTIOCYTIC/DENDRITIC CELL NEOPLASMS

Introduction to the International Consensus Classification of Mature Lymphoid Neoplasms

James R. Cook, Laurence de Leval, John R. Goodlad, and Rebecca L. King

Lymphomas are a heterogeneous group of neoplasms derived from mature B, T, or natural killer (NK) cells. They represent clonal expansions of lymphocytes harboring genetic abnormalities that result in altered expression of genes involved in growth control, usually resulting in autonomous and increased proliferation and/or reduced cell death. The fundamentals of modern lymphoma classification date from publication of the Revised European and American Lymphoma classification in 1994.[1] In this, and subsequent classifications, specific entities are recognized on the basis of shared morphological, immunophenotypic, genetic, and clinical features, ensuring relevant disease categories and diagnostic consistency. In addition, in many lymphoid neoplasms the constituent cells recapitulate normal stages of B-cell or T-cell development, albeit displaying some phenotypic and/or genotypic aberrancy, and to an extent can be classified according to their corresponding normal counterpart. However, for some entities, no normal counterpart exists, or has yet to be identified, meaning the putative physiological equivalent cannot be used as the sole determinant for classification.

Separation into benign and malignant categories, as is the norm in other forms of neoplasia (eg, neoplasms of epithelial origin), is not applicable to lymphoma classification. Instead, different entities are often regarded as displaying aggressive or indolent clinical behavior, although precise criteria for such separation is lacking. In addition, some newly defined entities, as well as some that were previously considered lymphoma, exhibit a benign, non-life-threatening clinical course despite showing morphologic, phenotypic, and genetic abnormalities similar to those seen in other lymphoid neoplasms. The term "lymphoproliferative disorder" is increasingly appended to this group of diseases in order to highlight their remarkably indolent evolution and separate them from overt lymphomas that have a propensity, albeit rare is some instances, to behave in a more aggressive manner.

According to the Cancer Surveillance Branch of the International Agency for Research on Cancer, in 2020 there were an estimated 544,352 new cases of lymphoma, 83,087 of Hodgkin lymphoma, and 176,404 of multiple myeloma worldwide in 2020.[2,3] The incidence of lymphoma, particularly B-cell lymphomas, increased significantly around the turn of the century but has since plateaued.[4] The increase may have been in part due to better detection, but other factors, such as human immunodeficiency virus (HIV)/acquired immunodeficiency syndrome and an increasing number of solid organ transplant recipients, likely also contributed. Regional variations in the incidence of lymphoma are also seen. For example, non-Hodgkin lymphoma is the 13th most common cancer worldwide but seventh most frequently encountered in the United States.[5,6] Regions with the highest incidence of Hodgkin and non-Hodgkin lymphoma include Australia and New Zealand, North America, and Northern and Western Europe, while the incidence is lower in middle and central Africa, Central America, and Eastern and Southeastern Asia (Figure 1).[6]

Globally, mature B-cell neoplasms account for approximately 90% of lymphoid neoplasms,[7,8] with diffuse large B-cell lymphoma (DLBCL) and follicular lymphoma representing the most frequently encountered entities. However, the relative frequency of different lymphoid neoplasms varies according to geographic location. For example, follicular lymphoma is the second most frequent lymphoma in the United States and Western Europe but is uncommon in South America, Eastern Europe, Africa, and Asia. Conversely, Burkitt lymphoma is endemic in equatorial Africa, where it is the most common type of childhood malignancy, but is rarely encountered in the United States and Western Europe. Lymphomas of T- and NK-cell origin generally constitute only a small proportion of lymphoma cases (~10% of all non-Hodgkin lymphomas worldwide in one epidemiological study), but certain entities have a significantly higher relative incidence in certain geographic locations and racial populations, including Asia, the Caribbean basin, and Native Americans from Central and South America and Mexico.[9-11]

Variations in geographic and subtype incidence are at least in part due to the multifactorial etiology and pathogenesis of various lymphoid neoplasms, which involves a complex interplay between genetic factors, environmental exposure, and the host immune system. Nonmodifiable risk factors associated with the development of non-Hodgkin lymphoma include age, gender, race/ethnicity, family history, autoimmune disease, and immune suppression. The incidence of lymphoma increases with age and is higher in males than in females. In the United States, whites and non-Hispanics are at greatest risk of developing non-Hodgkin lymphoma while Asian Pacific Islanders,

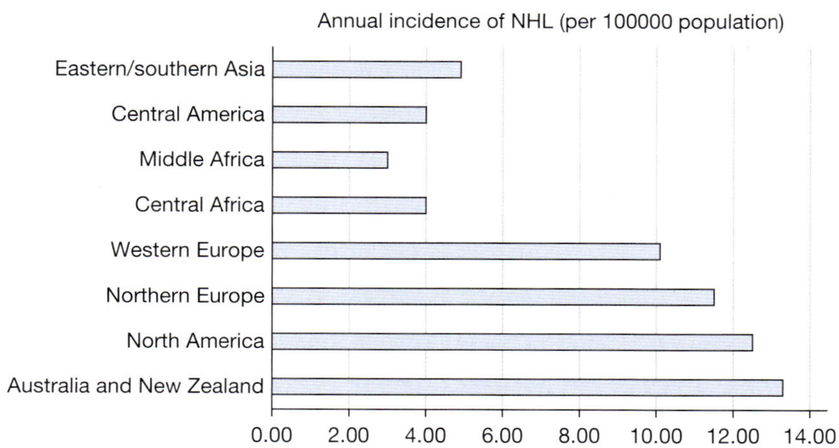

FIGURE 1 Annual incidence of non-Hodgkin lymphoma (NHL) by geographic location. (Data from Bispo JAB, Pinheiro PS, Kobetz EK. Epidemiology and etiology of leukemia and lymphoma. *Cold Spring Harb Perspect Med.* 2020;10(6):a034819. doi:10.1101/cshperspect.a034819.)

Native Americans, and black populations have the lowest risk.[10] The exception to this general rule is mycosis fungoides, which shows a higher incidence in African Americans.[10] First-degree relatives of patients with lymphoma are at greater risk of developing lymphoma than the general population as are those with autoimmune disease and individuals who are immunosuppressed as a consequence of HIV infection, following organ transplantation or due to other forms of iatrogenic immune suppression. In addition, radiation exposure, exposure to certain occupational chemicals, and a variety of infectious agents represent modifiable risk factors that have been implicated in the pathogenesis of lymphoma. Infectious agents linked with the development of lymphoma include Epstein-Barr virus (EBV), HIV, human T-lymphotropic virus 1, human herpesvirus 8, hepatitis C, and *Helicobacter pylori*.[6,10]

Overview of the Normal Immune Response

The immune response has been traditionally divided into two components—the innate immune system and the adaptive immune system. The innate immune system includes macrophages, monocytes, mast cells, NK cells, NK-like T cells, and other innate lymphoid cells, which utilize a variety of pattern recognition receptors that bind products found in many types of microbes in a non–major histocompatibility complex (MHC)-restricted fashion.[12] The innate immune system provides an initial response against pathogens and appears to be especially important at mucosal barriers. The adaptive immune system, in contrast, consists of B cells and T cells, which express immune receptors that recognize foreign antigens with high specificity in the context of MHC molecules. The adaptive response provides a secondary, more specific immune response with the capacity to develop immunologic memory that protects against future exposures to the same antigens.

B-Cell Development and Subsets

B lymphocytes are immune effector cells that play a central role in the adaptive immune system, which is responsible for humoral immunity. B cells recognize and interact with antigen in order to produce specific antibodies essential for host defense against infection, virus neutralization, opsonization of pathogens to facilitate phagocytosis, and antibody-dependent cellular cytotoxicity.

Interaction with antigen takes place via the B-cell receptor (BCR) comprising a transmembrane immunoglobulin (IG) molecule complexed with two transmembrane polypeptides, Igα (CD79a) and Igβ (CD79b), that are linked to immunoreceptor tyrosine-based activation motifs, which carry the activation signal across the cell membrane (Figure 2). IG molecules comprise two identical light chains and two identical heavy chains linked together by disulfide bonds. Constant and variable regions are present in both the light and heavy chains, the variable regions providing for antigen specificity and binding. Each B cell is limited to production of its own uniquely configured IG molecule. The diversity of IGs required to deal with possible encounter with huge numbers of antigens is generated by the process of IG gene rearrangement that takes place during B-cell development in the bone marrow (BM). Further evolution of the antibody response resulting in expanded clones of antigen-specific IG-producing cells (plasma cells) and memory cells for generating secondary responses takes place in secondary lymphoid organs via proliferation, somatic hypermutation, selection, and class switch recombination (CSR).[13]

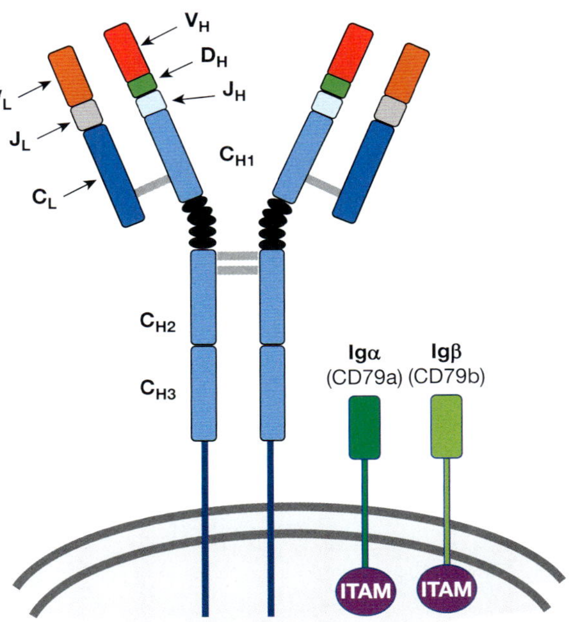

FIGURE 2 B-cell receptor complex. The B-cell receptor complex is made up by a membrane-bound immunoglobulin molecule complexed with two transmembrane polypeptides, Igα (CD79a) and Igβ (CD79b), each of which incorporates an immunoreceptor tyrosine-based activation motif (ITAM) and which carries the activation signal across the cell membrane. Immunoglobulin molecules comprise two identical light chains and two identical heavy chains, linked together by disulfide bonds. Heavy chains consist of constant (C_H), joining (J_H), diversity (D_H), and variable (V_H) regions. Light chains have constant (C_L), joining (J_L), and variable (V_L) regions but lack a diversity region. The light and heavy chain variable regions combine to provide antigen-binding sites.

In utero, B cells are generated in the fetal liver but subsequently are produced by differentiation of hematopoietic stem cells (HSCs) in the BM. HSCs have self-renewing capacity and sequentially give rise to multipotent, oligopotent, then fully committed progenitors, the last differentiating into mature blood cells.[14] Multipotent progenitors retain full lineage potential but with limited self-renewing capacity. Self-renewing capacity diminishes further and lineage potential becomes increasingly restricted during further stages of development.[14] An oligopotent common myeloid/lymphoid progenitor that can give rise to B cells, T cells, NK cells, granulocytes, and macrophages represents the earliest commitment to B-cell development. Further differentiation and development along B-lineage lines follows the pathway of pro-B-cell to pre-B-cell to fully mature B cell.[15] Transcription factors regulate each stage of differentiation and function in networks to define cell lineage, activating genes specific for the desired line of differentiation and silencing those specific for other lineages.[15,16] Transcription factors important in driving early B-cell differentiation are PU.1, IKAROS, PAX5, EBF2, and E2A, with PAX5 playing a central role in maintaining cellular identity throughout the life of a B cell.[16-20]

IG heavy chain genes are composed of multiple variable (V), diversity (D), joining (J), and constant (C) segments.[13] Light chain genes are similar but lack D regions. IG gene rearrangement is a hierarchical process that has potential to generate enormous diversity via the random selection and assembly of V, D, and J gene segments. Further diversity is introduced via imprecise joining mechanisms. IG rearrangement begins with joining of D and J segments ($D_H \rightarrow J_H$) at the very early pro-B-cell stage of maturation, under the control of recombination activating genes 1 and 2 (RAG-1 and RAG-2). $V_H \rightarrow DJ_H$ joining follows in the late pro-B-cell stage. During this process, terminal deoxynucleotidyl transferase (TdT) acts to insert N-nucleotides into the V(D)J segments, generating further variation into the antigen-binding site of the final BCR molecule. Following successful VDJ_H recombination, the constant region is produced along with the Igα/Igβ heterodimer and surrogate light chains (a heterodimer composed of germline encoded invariant proteins VpreB and λ5) (Figure 3). Transient expression of the resulting pre-BCR complex on the cell surface is associated with the pre-B-cell stage of maturation and triggers cell division and light chain gene rearrangement.[21] Following successful rearrangement of all variable regions, the BCR

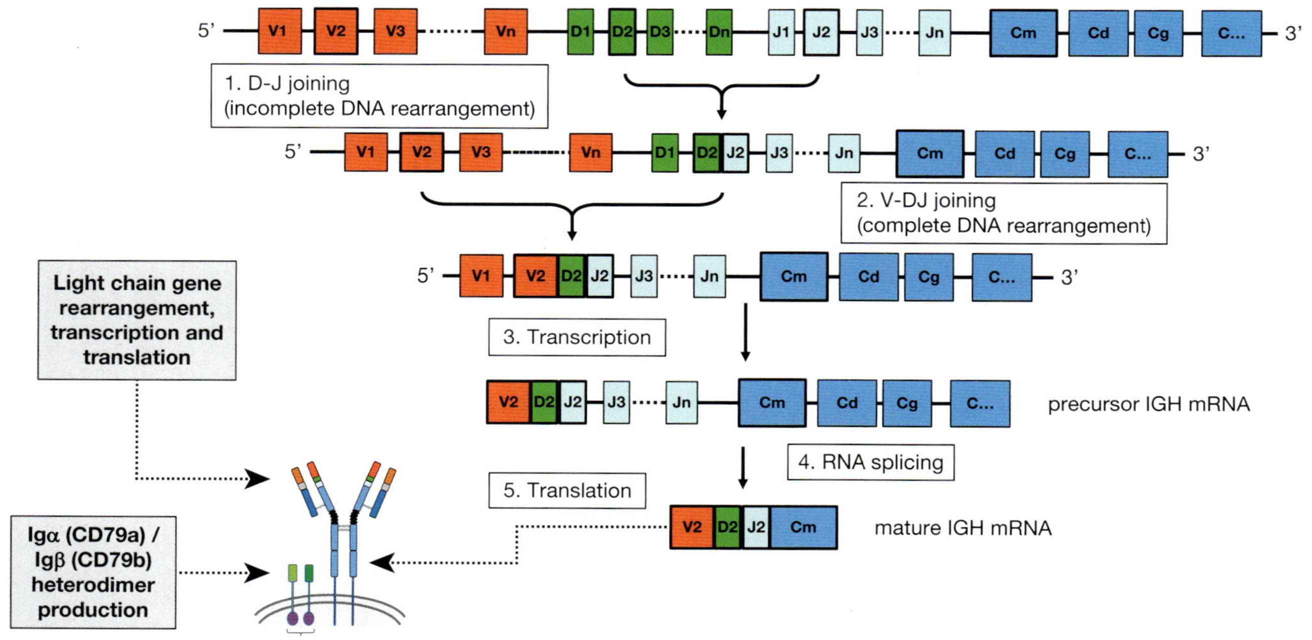

FIGURE 3 Immunoglobulin heavy chain gene rearrangement. Schematic representation of immunoglobulin heavy chain gene rearrangement. Immunoglobulin gene rearrangement generates enormous diversity by random selection and assembly of IG heavy chain (H), variable (V_H), diversity (D_H), and joining (J_H) gene segments. It is a hierarchical process beginning with joining of heavy chain D and J segments ($D_H \rightarrow J_H$). This takes place at the very early pro-B-cell stage of maturation (incomplete rearrangement). $V_H \rightarrow DJ_H$ joining follows in the late pro-B-cell stage (complete rearrangement). The rearranged VDJ_H segment is transcribed along with the constant region and intervening joining regions. This precursor immunoglobulin heavy chain gene mRNA is spliced to remove the redundant joining and heavy chain regions, leaving mature immunoglobulin heavy chain mRNA comprising the rearranged VDJ segment and the immunoglobulin M constant region (Cm). Light chain rearrangement follows along with production of Igα (CD79a) and Igβ (CD79b) heterodimers, the resulting products being assembled as a B-cell receptor complex on the cell surface.

is expressed on the cell surface as IgM, at which point the cell is recognizable as an immature B cell.

Before leaving the BM, immature B cells undergo a final selection process that serves to eliminate B cells with the ability to recognize self-antigen. Exposure to and reaction with self-antigen in the BM microenvironment results in clonal deletion, induction of anergy, or receptor editing where the light chain genes undergo repeated rounds of rearrangement to produce less self-specific antibody. Cells that do not recognize self-antigen are selected for survival, produce IgD molecules with the same variable domains as the IgM BCR via alternative splicing of the IGH locus, and enter the circulation as transitional IgM+ IgD+ B cells. Maturation is completed in the spleen during which time there is further elimination of self-reacting B cells as type 1 transitional B cells mature to type 2.

Fully mature, naïve B cells are short-lived in the absence of antigenic stimulation, but those that survive in the periphery are generally divided into three subtypes: B-1 cells, marginal zone cells, and follicular cells.[22,23] B-1 cells are long-lived with self-renewing capacity and are thought to be mainly of fetal liver origin, although some may be produced in the BM in later life.[22,23] They account for <10% of the total B-cell population in the spleen but are relatively abundant in the peritoneal and pleural cavities. Many express CD5 cf their cell surface.[22,23] B-1 and naïve marginal zone cells interact with T-independent antigens. T-independent (TI) antigens are nonproteins that express repeated molecular structures. Type 1 TI antigens (TI-1) are lipopolysaccharides and bacterial DNA, and type 2 TI antigens (TI-2) are large polysaccharide molecules comprising a nonimmunogenic backbone exhibiting recurring immunogenic epitopes with a periodicity that allows them to cross-link multiple BCRs. They act as B-cell mitogens at high concentration, engaging Toll-like receptors as well as BCRs, and only induce specific antibody at low concentration. TI antigen responses provide a rapid but low-affinity and short-lived IgM response, primarily to bacteria.[23]

Thymus-dependent (TD) antigens possess some epitopes recognizable by T cells and some by B cells. TD antigen presentation occurs in the context of MHC class II molecules and results in a humoral immune response characterized by specific antibody of high affinity, isotype switching, affinity maturation, and memory. Central to this response is the germinal center (GC) reaction. TD antigens activate naïve B cells in follicles and CD4-positive T cells in T zones. Cognate interactions at the border of the follicle follow, and the selected B cells begin to proliferate. A subset migrates to the medullary cords of the lymph node and differentiates into plasmablasts that secrete relatively low-affinity antibodies or develop directly into unswitched memory cells without traversing the GC reaction. The remainder (GC precursor B cells) and the activated T cells migrate to the center of the follicle. The T cells differentiate into T follicular helper (TFH) cells while the B cells rapidly divide and populate the follicular dendritic cell (FDC) network, pushing resident IgM+, IgD+ B cells to the periphery where they become a mantle to the developing GC. By day 7 after antigen exposure, the GC is fully developed with established light and dark zones, the former populated by a predominance of centrocytes together with FDC and macrophages and the latter containing a majority of centroblasts. High levels of antigen in the form of immune complexes are held on the surface of FDC in the GC light zone.[24] GC dark zones are rich in centroblasts that express CD10 and BCL6 as well as other markers of GC differentiation such as LMO2, GCET1, and HGAL. They switch off BCL2 expression and have only low levels of surface IG. Centroblasts proliferate rapidly in the dark zone undergoing somatic hypermutation (SHM). SHM involves the introduction and deletion of nucleotide bases during DNA replication resulting in changes in translated amino acid sequence with the potential to alter configuration of the eventually transcribed protein. It is a marker for a cell that has traversed the GC reaction. IGV regions are primarily affected, but other genes, such as *BCL2* and *BCL6*, can also be mutated in this way. Following division, centroblasts transit to the light zone, assuming morphological characteristics of centrocytes. Here, GC B cells harboring affinity-increasing mutations of their antigen-binding sites out-compete mutants with lower-affinity antigen receptors. Consequently, they are able to attach, internalize, and present a greater amount of antigen to TFH cells, thereby receiving the strongest signals to survive, reenter the dark zone, and undergo further rounds of division, SHM, and selection. GC B cells unable to compete successfully and lacking a BCL2 prosurvival signal undergo death by apoptosis. IG CSR, in which the IgM constant region is replaced by IgG, IgA, or IgE, also takes place during the repeated cycles of division and selection, resulting in expanded clones of high-affinity class-switched GC B cell coming to dominate the GC population. Both SHM and CSR are mediated by activation-induced cytidine deaminase. Ultimately, GCB cells receive signals that direct them to become long-lived plasma cells or memory cells and leave the GC. Long-lived plasma cells migrate to, and reside in, the BM while memory B cells circulate in peripheral blood (PB) and in part populate marginal zones in lymph nodes, the spleen, and mucosa-associated lymphoid tissue. Plasma cells leaving the GC lack surface IG and CD20 but express CD19, CD38, CD79a,

CD138, and IRF4. Memory cells express pan-B-cell antigens and CD27. They retain the ability to home to tissues in which they have undergone antigenic stimulation and upon reencounter with antigen rapidly differentiate into long-lived plasma cells or reenter GCs to undergo further rounds of division, SHM, and selection.[24] B-cell development and maturation is summarized in Figure 4.

Molecular control of the germinal center reaction (GCR) is highly complex, and a full discussion is beyond the scope of this section.[24,25] However, some facets are worthy of mention as deregulation of these mechanisms is implicated in the genesis of a variety of lymphomas. MYC, expressed by cells in the GC light zone, along with REL, is required for maintaining the GCR. BCL6 is the master regulator of the GCR and is central in establishing the GC dark zone expression profile that allows for SHM. In conjunction with BACH2, BCL6 also serves to repress genes involved in post–GC differentiation. Abrogation of the dark zone profile is facilitated by IRF4 expression, which is also required for CSR and, along with BLIMP1, plasma cell differentiation. Inhibition of terminal differentiation and maintenance of the dark zone phenotype is also subject to epigenetic regulation. The core catalytic component of polycomb recessive complex 2, enhancer of zeste homologue 2 (EZH2), silences the plasma cell regulators *IRF4* and *PRDM1,* which encodes BLIMP1.

Normal T-Cell Subsets and NK Cells

T cells are derived from a BM precursor and undergo a highly regulated maturation process in the thymus. Early T-cell precursors, which retain the ability to differentiate into B cells and myeloid cells, become committed to the T-cell lineage in the initial stages of intrathymic development. Thymocytes are initially

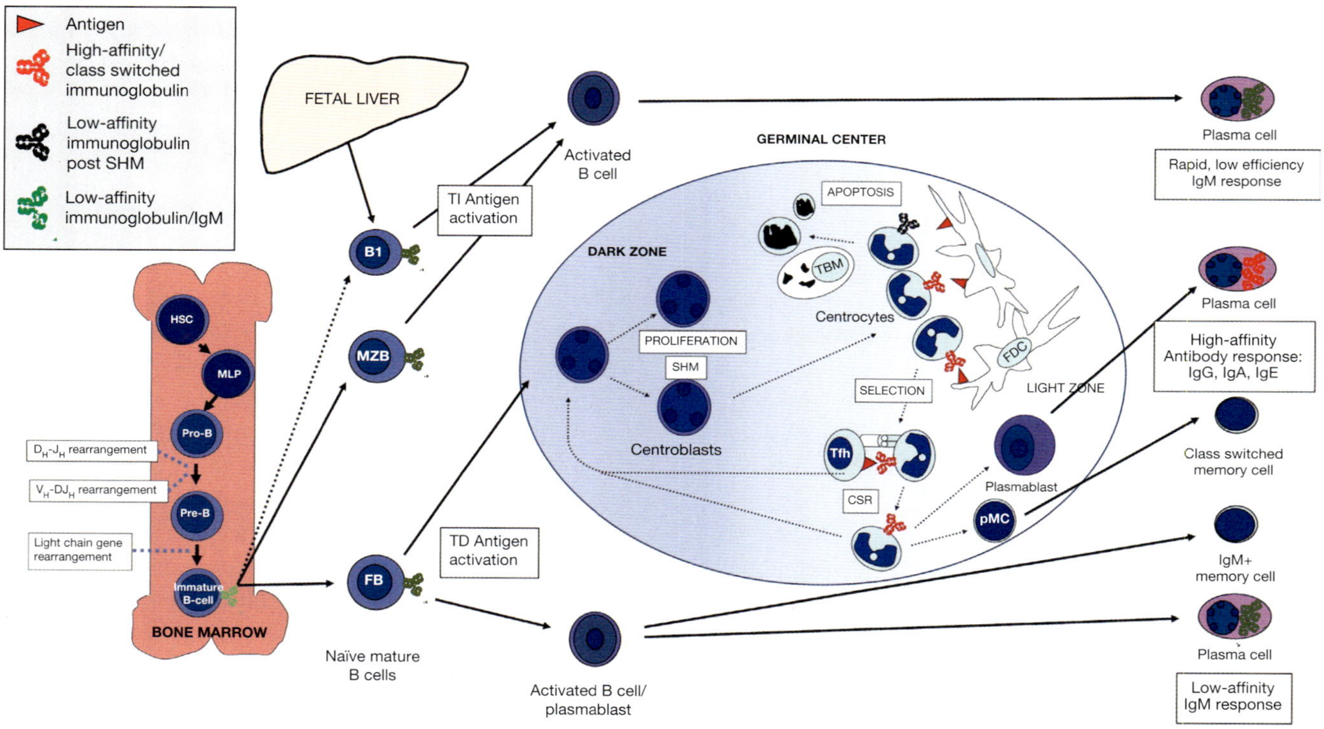

FIGURE 4 B-cell ontogeny and differentiation pathways. In the bone marrow, hematopoietic stem cells give rise to myeloid/lymphoid progenitors, which can differentiate into pro-B, pre-B, and immature B cells. Immunoglobulin heavy and light chain gene rearrangement occurs during this sequential maturation, resulting in assembly and expression of the B-cell receptor containing immunoglobulin of IgM type. Immature B cells undergo final selection in, and shortly after leaving, the bone marrow, ultimately becoming mature but antigen-naïve B cells in peripheral blood and lymphoid organs. Three types of naïve B cells are recognized. B-1 cells (largely produced by fetal liver) and marginal zone cells interact with T-independent antigens to produce a rapid, low-affinity, and short-lived IgM response, mainly to bacteria. Naïve follicular B cells are activated by T-dependent antigens and directly develop into IgM-positive plasma cells and memory cells or enter into a germinal center reaction. Repeated rounds of cell division take place within the germinal center, accompanied by somatic hypermutation, selection of high-affinity clones, and ultimately class switch recombination. Surviving cells exit the germinal center to become long-lived, class-switched memory cells or plasma cells that can secrete high-affinity antibodies of IgG, IgA, or IgE type. CSR, class switch recombination; FB, follicular B cell; FDC, follicular dendritic cell; HSC, hematopoietic stem cell; MLP, myeloid/lymphoid progenitor; MZB, marginal zone B-cell; pMC, precursor memory cell; SHM, somatic hypermutation; TBM, tingible body macrophage; TD, thymus dependent.

double-negative precursors, lacking both CD4 and CD8. At this stage, there is rearrangement of the T-cell receptor (TCR) loci, using mechanisms similar to those described earlier for IG gene rearrangements. The TCR beta chain locus contains approximately 50 V, 2 D, and 12 J segments while the alpha chain locus contains 45 V and 50 J segments. In contrast, the gamma and delta loci have many fewer segments, with only 7 V segments in total. Rearrangement of the TRG and TRD loci occur first, with cells producing functional rearrangements of these genes becoming γδ T cells (described further later in the discussion). T cells without functional TRG rearrangements may proceed to rearrange the TRA and TRB loci, becoming αβ T cells. αβ T cells in the thymus progress to a double-positive stage ($CD4^+CD8^+$) and undergo positive and negative selection based on the affinity of TCR binding to class I or class II major histocompatibility complexes. Finally, the thymocytes progress to mature single positive ($CD4^+$ or $CD8^+$) cells.

$CD4^+$ T cells become activated upon engagement of peptide/class II MHC complexes together with costimulatory receptors and various cytokines. Several distinct functional subsets of $CD4^+$ T cells have been described (Table 1), and the relationship of various T-cell neoplasms to these normal T-cell subsets is an active area of investigation. The most thoroughly characterized $CD4^+$ subsets are Th1, Th2, and TFH cells. Differentiation to the Th1 subset occurs upon TCR stimulation and signaling via IFN-γ and IL-12, leading to expression of the transcription factor T-bet (encoded by the *TBX21* gene). Th1 cells play an important role in responses to bacteria and viruses through production of IFN-γ. Differentiation toward the Th2 phenotype occurs via TCR signaling together with IL-2 and IL-4 stimulation. Th2 cells are characterized by expression of the GATA3 transcription factor, which suppresses the Th1 development program and leads to expression of Th2-derived cytokines including autocrine IL-4 signaling. Th2 cells are important mediators of allergy, asthma, and responses against helminth infection. Gene expression profiling studies have shown that peripheral T-cell lymphoma, not otherwise specified, can be divided into TBX21 versus GATA3 subsets, resembling normal Th1 versus Th2 subsets, and that this distinction may have biologic and clinical significance.[26] TFH cells are a unique subset of $CD4^+$ T cells that reside within the GCs and provide help to B cells during the GC reaction.[27] TFH cells coexpress CD4, CD10, CD57, PD1, BCL6, ICOS, and CXCL13. Neoplasms of TFH cells tend to retain their characteristic association of follicular dendritic cells and often show an exuberant background of reactive B cells. In the International Consensus Classification, these tumors are now grouped together under the umbrella term of "follicular helper T-cell (TFH-cell) lymphoma" and are further divided into the angioimmunoblastic type, follicular type, and not otherwise specified type.

Other $CD4^+$ subsets have also been characterized in recent years. Th9 cells are produced by TCR stimulation in the setting of IL-4 and TGF-β and coexpress GATA3, IRF4, and PU.1 transcription factors. Th17 cells are derived via TCR stimulation together with signaling via TGF-β, IL-6, IL-21, and IL-23. Expression of the transcription factor RORγt induces expression of IL-17, IL-21, and IL-10. While the specific functions of Th9 and Th17 subsets have not yet been fully characterized, they appear to play a role in defense against extracellular infectious agents.

Finally, regulatory T cells (Treg) play a specialized role in suppressing immune responses leading to development of immune tolerance. Tregs are distinguished by coexpression of the transcription factor FOXP3 and of the IL-2 receptor, CD25. The neoplastic cells of adult T-cell leukemia/lymphoma appear to correspond to Treg cells with characteristic expression of both FOXP3 and CD25.[28,29]

$CD8^+$ cytotoxic T cells function in responses against intracellular pathogens and tumor cells, with binding of TCR to peptide/class I MHC complexes together with costimulatory complexes. $CD8^+$ cells secrete the proinflammatory cytokines IFN-γ and TGF-β and release cytotoxic molecules including granzyme B and perforin, which lyse the target cell. Several distinct lymphomas of $CD8^+$ cytotoxic T cells are currently recognized,

TABLE 1 Characteristics of T-cell subsets

	Th1	Th2	Th9	TH17	TFH	Treg
Induced via	IFN-γ, IL-12	IL-2, IL-4	IL4, TGF-β	IL-6, TGF-β, IL-21, IL-23	IL-6, IL-21	TCR/CD28, IL-2, TGF-β
Transcription factors	T-bet (TBX21)	GATA3	IRF4, PU.1	RORγt	BCL6	FOXP3
Cytokines produced	IFN-γ	IL-4, IL-5, IL-13	IL-9, IL-10, IL-21	IL-17, IL-21, IL-10, IL-23, IL-22	IL-4, IL-21	IL-10, TGF-β, IL-35

such as T-cell large granular lymphocytic leukemia and subcutaneous panniculitis-like T-cell lymphoma.

γδ T cells have a limited repertoire of TCR rearrangements due to the smaller number of gene segments present in gamma and delta loci compared with the alpha and beta loci. γδ T cells have been described as bridging the innate and adaptive immune systems.[30] They recognize antigen in an MHC-independent fashion, and specific γδ TCR families provide responses against components of pathogens in part of the innate immune response. At the same time, γδ TCRs undergo recombination with junctional diversity and are capable of developing a memory phenotype, similar to other T cells and B cells of the adaptive immune system. γδ T cells are typically positive for CD2, CD3, and CD7 and negative for CD5. Commonly γδ T cells lack both CD4 and CD8, although a subset may show dim expression of CD8. γδ T-cell activation may produce a variety of effects including release of proinflammatory cytokines such INF-γ and IL-17, or antibody-dependent cellular cytotoxicity with release of granzyme and perforin. γδ T cells represent a minority of T cells overall, but they are particularly enriched at mucosal sites including skin, the gastrointestinal tract, and airways, as well as in the spleen. Like their nonneoplastic counterparts, lymphomas of γδ T cells also tend to have a predominantly extranodal presentation.[31]

NK cells are part of the innate immune system, responding to intracellular infections and tumor cells. An important feature is the lack of TCR gene rearrangements. NK cells express CD2 and CD7 but are negative for surface CD3, CD5, and TCRs. It is important to note that the CD3 epsilon chain, recognized by many clinically used anti-CD3 antibodies, is expressed in the cytoplasm of NK cells and thus CD3 staining by immunohistochemistry (IHC) with some antibodies may be seen in both NK cells and T cells. CD16, CD56, CD57, and the killer inhibitory receptors are characteristically expressed, although these are not restricted to NK cells and may also be seen on some T-cell subsets (termed "NK-like T cells").[32]

Principles of Classification—the Multiparameter Approach

Classification of lymphoid neoplasms requires a multiparametric approach incorporating both pathologic and clinical data for the highest level of diagnostic precision. The contemporary diagnostic pathologist must be prepared to incorporate morphologic review of well-fixed, hematoxylin and eosin–stained sections, as well as immunophenotyping by IHC and/or flow cytometry, and both cytogenetic and molecular genetic data. Applying this multiparametric approach in an efficient and cost-effective manner requires broad knowledge of both benign/reactive lymphoproliferations and the complete spectrum of lymphoid neoplasms. While not expected to be experts in clinical management, pathologists diagnosing lymphoma must have some knowledge of both typical clinical behavior and a general impression of critical clinical decision points faced by hematologist-oncologists. One example of this is regarding the diagnosis of high-grade B-cell lymphoma with *MYC* and *BCL2* rearrangements. Although many of these cases morphologically resemble DLBCL, there is ample evidence that this disease has unique and unifying aggressive biology. Many centers will treat these patients more aggressively than those with standard DLBCL, and so careful attention to detail in reporting of these cases is essential to ensure appropriate therapeutic options for patients.

Disease classification in some instances is heavily impacted by the site of disease, for example, in both primary cutaneous B- and T-cell neoplasms, which often have markedly different clinical behavior from their nodal counterparts. Another example of the importance of disease site is mediastinal gray zone lymphoma (MGZL), which represents evolution from prior classifications in which "B-cell lymphoma, unclassifiable, with features intermediate between DLBCL and classic Hodgkin lymphoma" could be diagnosed at nonmediastinal sites. Recent studies have shown that these extramediastinal cases do not share the same genetic features of MGZL, thus helping to refine our understanding and classification of this disease.

Tissue Sampling Considerations

The pathologist's ability to render an accurate and complete diagnosis is heavily reliant on the quality of the tissue specimen. Fine-needle aspiration alone, even with flow cytometric immunophenotyping, is discouraged, as assessment of tissue architecture is an essential element in diagnosis and classification of lymphoma, especially in the primary diagnostic setting.[33] Core needle biopsy (CNB) has been increasingly utilized across the world for lymph node and extranodal tissue sampling. While diagnostic material can often be obtained by CNB, the pathologist should use caution in this setting.[34-38] If CNB is to be used, multiple cores are recommended and the limitations of this type of specimen must be recognized and acknowledged.[38-41] Certain diagnoses, such as T-cell/histiocyte-rich large B-cell lymphoma, cannot be diagnosed on CNB, as it is not possible to adequately exclude differential diagnostic considerations in such a limited specimen. Other diagnoses, such as classic Hodgkin lymphoma, may be challenging to diagnose on CNB due to paucity of tumor cells.[34] Additionally, diagnoses that rely heavily on identification of architectural patterns such as nodal TFH lymphomas (including angioimmunoblastic T-cell lymphoma) can be exceptionally challenging on CNB.[34] While extensive immunophenotyping and molecular studies can aid in diagnosis in the setting of limited tissue, there is no substitute for comprehensive morphologic evaluation. Finally, adequacy issues with CNB specimens are likely going to become an increasing problem as the need for molecular and cytogenetic testing on lymphoma specimens increases.

Immunophenotyping in Lymphoma Diagnosis

Immunophenotyping remains a cornerstone of determining lineage and classifying lymphoid malignancies. Both IHC and flow cytometry are useful modalities in immunophenotyping of specimens suspected of involvement by a lymphoid neoplasm. Both can be used to help establish clonality and thus distinguish reactive from neoplastic lymphoid populations using basic principles that are beyond the scope of this text. Each chapter in this section outlines the expected phenotype of the respective disease, highlighting both pertinent positive and negative markers. It is important to remember that although many entities have a characteristic immunophenotype, such as CD5 and cyclin D1 expression in the B cells of mantle cell lymphoma, virtually no phenotypic findings are specific for any one neoplasm and all findings must be taken into context. For lymphomas involving PB, such as chronic lymphocytic leukemia/small lymphocytic lymphoma, flow cytometry provides a useful tool that in some cases may obviate the need for BM biopsy. In most cases, however, integration of phenotyping data with morphologic, and sometimes genetic, findings is paramount.

Flow cytometry is a useful tool for characterizing cell populations and can be applied on both liquid (PB/BM) and fresh tissue (lymph node, spleen) specimens. Since cells are queried singly during flow cytometric analysis, simultaneous evaluation of multiple surface or cytoplasmic markers is possible on a given cell. Especially in the setting of assays designed for minimal residual disease detection, this modality vastly surpasses what the human eye can accomplish via IHC alone. Flow cytometry is useful for establishing clonality in B-cell neoplasms via kappa and lambda restriction, and more recently in T-cell populations via expression of TRBC1 and TRBC2.[42] Identification of antigen aberrancy, such as loss of CD7 in T cells or expression of CD5 on B cells, is another example of the power of flow cytometry to easily identify populations that may be diagnostically pertinent. While flow cytometry is very sensitive for detecting small populations of cells, caution must be used as small "aberrant" populations or "clones" can be seen in the setting of reactive processes and thus correlation with other modalities remains critical. Other limitations of flow cytometry include the need for fresh tissue, the inability to directly correlate the cells being phenotyped with their morphologic equivalent, and the potential for sampling bias due to a variety of factors.

IHC remains the predominant method for immunophenotyping of lymphoma specimens. As correlation of phenotype with architecture is critical, visualizing the staining patterns of different cell populations by IHC on sequential sections remains a key tool of the hematopathologist. A major benefit is the ability to perform IHC on formalin-fixed paraffin-embedded (FFPE) tissue. While multiplex staining, including the use of digital imaging software, is now in widespread use via a variety of platforms in the research setting, this is not commonly used for diagnostic purposes. While some labs do have specialized flow cytometry panels for diseases with a paucity of tumor cells in a reactive background, such as classic Hodgkin lymphoma, in most practices IHC remains the best way to identify the sometimes-elusive Reed-Sternberg cells. Commonly used markers in lymphoma phenotyping such as BCL2, BCL6, MUM1, cyclinD1, and SOX11 are also not routinely available by flow cytometry but are well established for IHC in clinical practice. Chromogenic in situ hybridization on FFPE sections is also widely available and is typically applied for detection of EBV-encoded RNA, as well as in some labs for other uncommon viruses as well as kappa and lambda mRNA.

Molecular Cytogenetic Studies

Molecular and cytogenetic data play an increasingly important role in the diagnosis and classification of non-Hodgkin lymphomas.[43-45] Many different types of molecular abnormalities (single nucleotide variants, copy number changes, translocations, etc.) may be of diagnostic, prognostic, or therapeutic significance in different forms of lymphoma, and various types of molecular assays are required to efficiently identify different abnormalities (Table 2). While most cases of lymphoma do not require molecular studies for diagnostic purposes, such testing can be of great utility in selected settings and pathologists should be sufficiently familiar

TABLE 2 Genomic abnormalities detected by various methodologies

		Single nucleotide variants/InDels	Copy number aberrations	Structural variants	IG/TCR clonality	Cell of origin
Targeted	Fluorescence in situ hybridization		✓	✓		
	Single gene analyses	✓			✓	
	Next-generation sequencing panels	✓	✓	✓	✓	
Digital/Arrays	Genomic arrays		✓			
	Methylation arrays		✓			✓
	Gene expression					✓
Genome-wide	Metaphase Cytogenetics		✓	✓		
	Whole transcriptome sequencing			✓	✓	✓
	Whole exome sequencing	✓	✓	✓	✓	
	Whole genome sequencing	✓	✓	✓	✓	

Modified from de Leval L, Alizadeh AA, Bergsagel PLet al. Genomic profiling for clinical decision making in lymphoid neoplasms. *Blood.* 2022;140(21):2193-2227. doi:10.1182/blood.2022015854.

with molecular testing to select appropriate tests to be performed and to integrate molecular results with other ancillary findings in order to arrive at a final diagnosis.

One of the most commonly employed molecular techniques in lymphoma diagnostics is testing for clonal rearrangements of B-cell or T-cell receptors. Clonality testing is most commonly performed via polymerase chain reaction (PCR) assays with capillary electrophoresis, and the EuroClonality consortium has developed standardized primer sets and guidelines for interpretation.[46] A growing number of labs are transitioning clonality assays to next-generation sequencing (NGS) platforms. Compared with PCR-based assays, NGS-based methods provide additional information including the precise sequence of the clonal rearrangement detected. Such detailed sequence information may be helpful for comparing clones in different samples, identifying possible stereotyped rearrangements that may be clinically relevant, or (for B-cell rearrangements) documenting somatic hypermutation status. NGS-based clonality assays, however, currently tend to be more time consuming and expensive than traditional PCR-based approaches and are also less thoroughly standardized across institutions.

Identification of chromosomal translocations may be very helpful in classifying a variety of B-cell and T-cell lymphomas. Most lymphoma-associated translocations can be detected by metaphase karyotyping, but this is not often performed in routine practice because sufficient fresh tissue may not be available, especially given current trends toward widespread use of needle biopsies. Fluorescence in situ hybridization (FISH) testing therefore represents the most commonly used method to identify various recurrent translocations.[43,44] For example, *IGH::BCL2* translocations are characteristic of most cases of conventional follicular lymphoma, while rearrangements of *TCL1A* or *MTCP1* are found in most cases of T-cell prolymphocytic leukemia. Numerous probes are commercially available including break-apart probes (which identify a rearrangement of the gene of interest but do not identify the partner gene) and dual fusion probes (which specifically identify rearrangements involving both genes studied). RNA-based NGS testing can identify fusion genes such as the *NPM1::ALK* rearrangement associated with ALK-positive anaplastic large cell lymphoma, but such methods are generally not able to reliably detect translocations resulting in enhancer swaps, such as *IGH::MYC* rearrangements in Burkitt lymphoma.[43,47] Newer methods, such as optical genome mapping, may be capable of efficiently detecting translocations involving B-cell or T-cell receptors, but these assays are limited by a requirement for high-quality DNA that cannot be obtained from FFPE samples.

Chromosomal microarrays offer the potential to detect copy number changes too small to be detected by metaphase karyotyping or FISH studies. Using single nucleotide polymorphism arrays, areas of copy neutral loss of heterozygosity (also known as uniparental disomy or UPD) may also be identified. These assays are the method of choice in certain selected circumstances, such as identifying the characteristic pattern of chromosome 11q abnormalities seen in cases of large B-cell lymphoma with 11q abnormality (previously known as Burkitt-like lymphoma with 11q abnormality).[48] These techniques also allow for a genome-wide assessment of copy number changes that is not feasible by FISH methods.

Finally, targeted NGS panels for various lymphoma-associated single nucleotide variants and insertion/deletion mutations (indels) are increasingly important in routine diagnostic testing. NGS testing in isolation is rarely diagnostic of a specific entity, but patterns of mutational data can provide further diagnostic assistance when integrated with traditional morphology and phenotypic studies.[43] For example, in a difficult-to-classify small B-cell neoplasm with a differential diagnosis that includes follicular lymphoma versus marginal zone lymphoma, demonstration of mutations in *CREBP, EZH2, TNFRSF14,* or *STAT6* would favor classification as follicular lymphoma while mutations in *KLF2, NOTCH2,* or *PTPRD* would favor a diagnosis of marginal zone lymphoma. Mutational profiles characteristic of specific disease entities are discussed in detail in the following chapters. More advanced techniques, such as whole genome sequencing, may allow for even more detailed genetic characterization in the near future, but such methods generally remain a research tool at the current time.

Conclusion

The modern classification of lymphoma utilizes a multiparameter approach to define discrete clinicopathologic entities based in part on resemblance to normal lymphocyte subsets. This system is intended to provide specific diagnostic information to allow for individual patient treatment and management, and also to facilitate further research into specific disease entities in an effort to further enhance diagnosis, prognostic assessment, and therapy. As with all classifications, this system is a snapshot of a moment in time, and lymphoma classification will continue to evolve with advances in our understanding of these diverse neoplasms.

References

1. Harris NL, Jaffe ES, Stein H, et al. A revised European-American classification of lymphoid neoplasms: a proposal from the International Lymphoma Study Group. *Blood.* 1994;84(5):1361-1392. doi:10.1016/S0968-6053(00)80051-4
2. Ferlay J, Colombet M, Soerjomataram I, et al. Cancer statistics for the year 2020: an overview. *Int J Cancer.* 2021. doi:10.1002/ijc.33588
3. Wild C, Weiderpass E, Stewart B, eds. World Cancer Report: Cancer Research for Cancer Prevention. International Agency for Research on Cancer; 2020.
4. Global Burden of Disease Cancer Collaboration; Fitzmaurice C, Allen C, et al. Global, regional, and national cancer incidence, mortality, years of life lost, years lived with disability, and disability-adjusted life-years for 32 Cancer Groups, 1990 to 2015: a systematic analysis for the global burden of disease study. *JAMA Oncol.* 2017;3(4):524-548. doi:10.1001/jamaoncol.2016.5688
5. Sung H, Ferlay J, Siegel RL, et al. Global Cancer Statistics 2020: GLOBOCAN Estimates of Incidence and Mortality Worldwide for 36 Cancers in 185 countries. *CA Cancer J Clin.* 2021;71(3):209-249. doi:10.3322/caac.21660
6. Bispo JAB, Pinheiro PS, Kobetz EK. Epidemiology and Etiology of Leukemia and Lymphoma. *Cold Spring Harb Perspect Med.* 2020;10(6):a034819. doi:10.1101/cshperspect.a034819
7. A clinical evaluation of the International Lymphoma Study Group classification of non-Hodgkin's lymphoma. The Non-Hodgkin's Lymphoma Classification Project. *Blood.* 1997;89(11):3909-3918.
8. Armitage JO, Weisenburger DD. New approach to classifying non-Hodgkin's lymphomas: clinical features of the major histologic subtypes. Non-Hodgkin's lymphoma classification project. *J Clin Oncol.* 1998;16(8):2780-2795. doi:10.1200/JCO.1998.16.8.2780
9. Vose J, Armitage J, Weisenburger D; International T-Cell Lymphoma Project. International peripheral T-cell and natural killer/T-cell lymphoma study: pathology findings and clinical outcomes. *J Clin Oncol.* 2008;26(25):4124-30. doi:10.1200/JCO.2008.16.4558
10. Thandra KC, Barsouk A, Saginala K, Padala SA, Barsouk A, Rawla P. Epidemiology of Non-Hodgkin's Lymphoma. *Med Sci (Basel).* 2021;9(1):5. doi:10.3390/medsci9010005
11. de Leval L, Jaffe ES. Lymphoma classification. *Cancer J.* 2020;26(3):176-185. doi:10.1097/PPO.0000000000000451
12. Li D, Wu M. Pattern recognition receptors in health and diseases. *Signal Transduct Target Ther.* 2021;6(1):291. doi:10.1038/s41392-021-00687-0
13. Schroeder HW Jr, Cavacini L. Structure and function of immunoglobulins. *J Allergy Clin Immunol.* 2010;125(2 suppl 2):S41-S52. doi:10.1016/j.jaci.2009.09.046
14. Antoniani C, Romano O, Miccio A. Concise review: epigenetic regulation of hematopoiesis—biological insights and therapeutic applications. *Stem Cells Transl Med.* 2017;6(12):2106-2114. doi:10.1002/sctm.17-0192
15. Regalo G, Leutz A. Hacking cell differentiation: transcriptional rerouting in reprogramming, lineage infidelity and metaplasia. *EMBO Mol Med.* 2013;5(8):1154-1164. doi:10.1002/emmm.201302834
16. Cory S. Masterminding B cells. *J Immunol.* 2015;195(3):763-5. doi:10.4049/jimmunol.1501277
17. Zhuang Y, Soriano P, Weintraub H. The helix-loop-helix gene E2A is required for B cell formation. *Cell.* 1994;79(5):875-84. doi:10.1016/0092-8674(94)90076-0
18. Bain G, Maandag EC, Izon DJ, et al. E2A proteins are required for proper B cell development and initiation of immunoglobulin gene rearrangements. *Cell.* 1994;79(5):885-92. doi:10.1016/0092-8674(94)90077-9
19. Adams B, Dorfler P, Aguzzi A, et al. Pax-5 encodes the transcription factor BSAP and is expressed in B lymphocytes, the developing CNS, and adult testis. *Genes Dev.* 1992;6(9):1589-1607. doi:10.1101/gad.6.9.1589

20. Lin H, Grosschedl R. Failure of B-cell differentiation in mice lacking the transcription factor EBF. *Nature.* 1995;376(6537):263-267. doi:10.1038/376263a0
21. Zhang M, Srivastava G, Lu L. The pre-B cell receptor and its function during B cell development. *Cell Mol Immunol.* 2004;1(2):89-94.
22. Dorner T, Radbruch A, Burmester GR. B-cell-directed therapies for autoimmune disease. *Nat Rev Rheumatol.* 2009;5(8):433-441. doi:10.1038/nrrheum.2009.141
23. Allman D, Pillai S. Peripheral B cell subsets. *Curr Opin Immunol.* 2008;20(2):149-157. doi:10.1016/j.coi.2008.03.014
24. De Silva NS, Klein U. Dynamics of B cells in germinal centres. *Nat Rev Immunol.* 2015;15(3):137-148. doi:10.1038/nri3804
25. Song S, Matthias PD. The transcriptional regulation of germinal center formation. *Front Immunol.* 2018;9:2026. doi:10.3389/fimmu.2018.02026
26. Iqbal J, Wright G, Wang C, et al. Gene expression signatures delineate biological and prognostic subgroups in peripheral T-cell lymphoma. *Blood.* 2014;123(19):2915-2923. doi:10.1182/blood-2013-11-536359
27. Song W, Craft J. T follicular helper cell heterogeneity. *Annu Rev Immunol.* 2024;42(1):127-152. doi:10.1146/annurev-immunol-090222-102834
28. Karube K, Ohshima K, Tsuchiya T, et al. Expression of FoxP3, a key molecule in CD4CD25 regulatory T cells, in adult T-cell leukaemia/lymphoma cells. *Br J Haematol.* Jul 2004;126(1):81-84. doi:10.1111/j.1365-2141.2004.04999.x
29. Roncador G, Garcia JF, Garcia JF, et al. FOXP3, a selective marker for a subset of adult T-cell leukaemia/lymphoma. *Leukemia.* 2005;19(12):2247-2253. doi:10.1038/sj.leu.2403965
30. Hu Y, Hu Q, Li Y, et al. γδ T cells: origin and fate, subsets, diseases and immunotherapy. *Signal Transduct Target Ther.* 2023;8(1):434. doi:10.1038/s41392-023-01653-8
31. Swerdlow SH, Jaffe ES, Brousset P, et al. Cytotoxic T-cell and NK-cell lymphomas: current questions and controversies. *Am J Surg Pathol.* 2014;38(10):e60-e71. doi:10.1097/PAS.0000000000000295
32. Godfrey DI, Uldrich AP, McCluskey J, Rossjohn J, Moody DB. The burgeoning family of unconventional T cells. *Nat Immunol.* 2015;16(11):1114-1123. doi:10.1038/ni.3298
33. Frederiksen JK, Sharma M, Casulo C, Burack WR. Systematic review of the effectiveness of fine-needle aspiration and/or core needle biopsy for subclassifying lymphoma. *Arch Pathol Lab Med.* 2015;139(2):245-51. doi:10.5858/arpa.2013-0674-RA
34. Gonçalves M d C, de Oliveira C, Sandes AF, et al. Core needle biopsy in lymphoma diagnosis: the diagnostic performance and the role of the multidisciplinary approach in the optimization of results. *Am J Surg Pathol.* 2023;47(1):111-123. doi:10.1097/PAS.0000000000001991
35. Cohen OC, Brodermann MH, Dervin A, et al. Lymph node core biopsies reliably permit diagnosis of lymphoproliferative diseases. Real-World Experience from 554 sequential core biopsies from a single centre. *Eur J Haematol.* 2021;106(2):267-272. doi:10.1111/ejh.13545
36. Nguyen BM, Halprin C, Olimpiadi Y, Traum P, Yeh JJ, Dauphine C. Core needle biopsy is a safe and accurate initial diagnostic procedure for suspected lymphoma. *Am J Surg.* 2014;208(6):1003-1008. discussion 1007-1008. doi:10.1016/j.amjsurg.2014.09.001
37. Hu Q, Naushad H, Xie Q, Al-Howaidi I, Wang M, Fu K. Needle-core biopsy in the pathologic diagnosis of malignant lymphoma showing high reproducibility among pathologists. *Am J Clin Pathol.* 2013;140(2):238-247. doi:10.1309/AJCP9ZAGKVJ8PDAX
38. Syrykh C, Chaouat C, Poullot E, et al. Lymph node excisions provide more precise lymphoma diagnoses than core biopsies: a French lymphopath network survey. *Blood.* 2022;140(24):2573-2583. doi:10.1182/blood.2022015520
39. Johl A, Lengfelder E, Hiddemann W, Klapper W; German Low-grade Lymphoma Study Group GLSG. Core needle biopsies and surgical excision biopsies in the diagnosis of lymphoma-experience at the Lymph Node Registry Kiel. *Ann Hematol.* 2016;95(8):1281-1286. doi:10.1007/s00277-016-2704-0
40. Farmer PL, Bailey DJ, Burns BF, Day A, LeBrun DP. The reliability of lymphoma diagnosis in small tissue samples is heavily influenced by lymphoma subtype. *Am J Clin Pathol.* 2007;128(3):474-80. doi:10.1309/J7Y74D9DXEAJ9YUY
41. Ranheim EA. Pearls and pitfalls in the diagnostic workup of small lymph node biopsies. *Mod Pathol.* 2019;32(suppl 1):38-43. doi:10.1038/s41379-018-0151-2
42. Berg H, Otteson GE, Corley H, et al. Flow cytometric evaluation of TRBC1 expression in tissue specimens and body fluids is a novel and specific method for assessment of T-cell clonality and diagnosis of T-cell neoplasms. *Cytometry B Clin Cytom.* 2021;100(3):361-369. doi:10.1002/cyto.b.21881
43. de Leval L, Alizadeh AA, Bergsagel PL, et al. Genomic profiling for clinical decision making in lymphoid neoplasms. *Blood.* 2022;140(21):2193-2227. doi:10.1182/blood.2022015854
44. Grau M, Lopez C, Martin-Subero JI, Bea S. Cytogenomics of B-cell non-Hodgkin lymphomas: The "old" meets the "new". *Best Pract Res Clin Haematol.* 2023;36(4):101513. doi:10.1016/j.beha.2023.101513
45. Savage KJ, De Leval L. Introduction to the peripheral T-cell lymphoma review series: advances in molecular characterization, classification refinement and treatment optimization. *Haematologica.* 2023;108(12):3204-3210. doi:10.3324/haematol.2023.282719
46. Langerak AW, Groenen PJTATA, Brüggemann M, et al. EuroClonality/BIOMED-2 guidelines for interpretation and reporting of Ig/TCR clonality testing in suspected lymphoproliferations. *Leukemia.* 2012;26(10):2159-2171. doi:10.1038/leu.2012.246
47. Wang X, Johnson V, Johnson L, Cook JR. RNA-Based next generation sequencing complements but does not replace fluorescence in situ hybridization studies for the classification of aggressive B-Cell lymphomas. *Cancer Genet.* 2021;252-253:43-47. doi:10.1016/j.cancergen.2020.12.004
48. Quintanilla-Martinez L, Laurent C, Soma L, et al. Emerging entities: high-grade/large B-cell lymphoma with 11q aberration, large B-cell lymphoma with IRF4 rearrangement, and new molecular subgroups in large B-cell lymphomas. A report of the 2022 EA4HP/SH lymphoma workshop. *Virchows Arch.* 2023;483(3):281-298. doi:10.1007/s00428-023-03590-x

SECTION 11

Mature B-Cell Neoplasms

Chapter 43

Chronic Lymphocytic Leukemia/Small Lymphocytic Lymphoma and Monoclonal B-Cell Lymphocytosis

Birgitta Sander, Silvia Bea, John G. Gribben, Eric D. Hsi, Estella Matutes, and Andrew D. Zelenetz

Definitions

Chronic lymphocytic leukemia/small lymphocytic lymphoma

Chronic lymphocytic leukemia (CLL) and small lymphocytic lymphoma (SLL) are considered to be a single disease entity with different clinical presentation. The diagnosis of CLL requires ≥ $5*10^{(9)}$ CLL cells/L in the blood. Patients with less degree of lymphocytosis but with nodal, splenic, or other extranodal involvement are diagnosed with SLL. Patients with cytopenia caused by a typical marrow infiltrate may be also be diagnosed as CLL per International Workshop on CLL (iwCLL) guidelines.

Monoclonal B-cell lymphocytosis

Monoclonal B-cell lymphocytosis (MBL) is defined by the presence of a small clonal proliferation of B lymphocytes ($<5*10^{(9)}$/L) in the blood. MBL patients are asymptomatic without lymphadenopathy >1.5 cm, organomegaly or other signs of a lymphoproliferative disorder. MBL clones are defined as CLL-type MBL and non-CLL type MBL and are detected by flow cytometry of peripheral blood in approximately 3% to 5% of individuals >40 years of age. CLL-type MBL has the same phenotype as CLL with expression of CD5 and CD23 and is further divided into low-count MBL ($<0.5*10^{(9)}$ clonal B cells/L) and high count MBL (≥0.5 but $<5*10^{(9)}$ cells/L). The risk of low-count MBL to progress to CLL is negligible in spite of persistence over time, while the progression risk for high-count MBL is 1%/year. Non-CLL-type MBL has a phenotype that differs from CLL (bright CD20, $CD5^+$, variable CD23 or $CD5^-$, $CD23^+$), and some cases may represent marginal zone B-cell proliferations. The B-cell receptor (BCR) immunoglobulin gene usage is more similar to CLL in high-count MBL than in low-count MBL. Longitudinal studies of MBL evolving to CLL suggest gradual accumulations of recurrent, CLL-associated, gene mutations.[1]

Tissue-based MBL (tMBL) can be considered when a monoclonal B-cell population is detected by flow cytometry in lymph nodes or other tissues, usually biopsied for other reasons than suspicion of lymphoma.[2-4] In some, but not all, of these cases the clonal B cells can be visualized by immunohistochemistry. On clinical evaluation some patients may also have MBL in peripheral blood.[4] Lymph node size of <1.5 cm, preserved lymph node architecture, and absence of proliferation centers have been suggested to be features favoring tMBL rather than partial lymph node involvement by CLL/SLL.[3,4]

Synonyms

Chronic lymphoid leukemia (not recommended).

Epidemiology

CLL is the most common low-grade B-cell leukemia in the Western world with an incidence of 3 to 5/100,000 individuals/year and a median age at diagnosis of 70 years.[5] There is a slight male predominance (M:F = 1.7:1).

General Clinical Features

Most patients (70%) are asymptomatic and are incidentally diagnosed on blood findings while the remaining cases have symptoms related to lymphadenopathy, hepatosplenomegaly, or, in a minority of cases, weight loss, night sweats, or fatigue. Cytopenia at diagnosis can be due to bone marrow involvement or autoimmune mechanisms.[5] Less commonly, paraproteinemia or recurrent infections are present at time of diagnosis.[5]

Morphology

Peripheral blood smears show lymphocytosis composed of small lymphocytes with scant cytoplasm and condensed chromatin (Figure 43.1A). The cells may

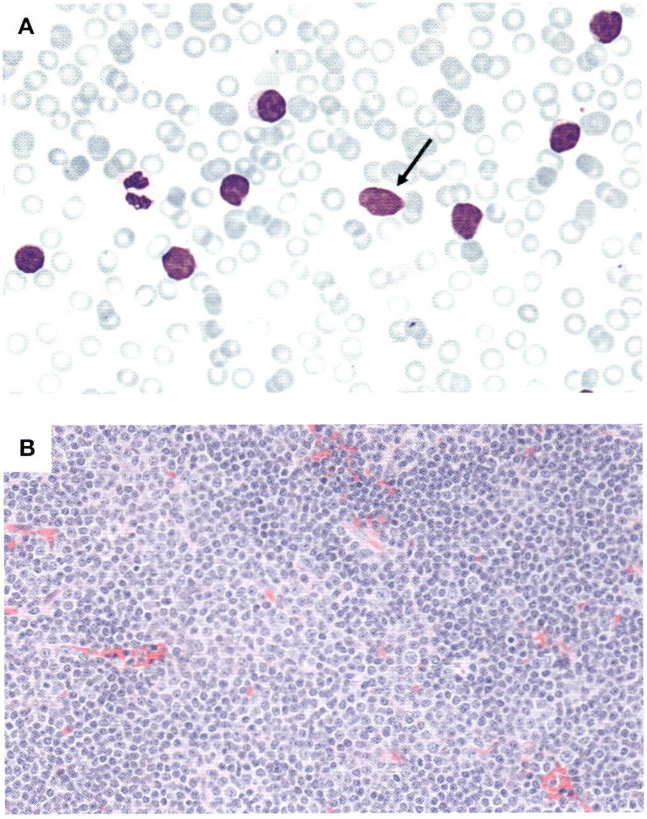

FIGURE 43.1 **A:** The blood smear shows small lymphocytes with sparse cytoplasm and occasional smudge cells (arrow). **B:** The lymph node shows a diffuse proliferation of small lymphocytes and a paler area containing a proliferation center.

be fragile and break due to pressure, leaving remnants without a clear cytoplasmic border, so-called smudge cells. Prolymphocytes are of intermediate size (1.5 times the size of a normal lymphocyte) and have open chromatin and a central nucleolus. Prolymphocytes are usually <15% of lymphocytes, and >10% prolymphocytes has been associated with worse prognosis.[6] If prolymphocytes are >55%, a diagnosis of prolymphocytic progression of CLL or a de novo B-cell prolymphocytic leukemia should be considered.[7]

In tissue, CLL/SLL is characterized by a diffuse proliferation of small round lymphocytes with scattered prolymphocytes and paraimmunoblasts that partially or totally efface the lymph node architecture (Figure 43.1B). Proliferation centers consist of pale nodules of prolymphocytes and paraimmunoblasts with cells that have a higher proliferation than the surrounding small lymphocytes. Cases with large or confluent proliferation centers that fill a 20× microscopic field or that show a Ki67 index >40% per proliferation center have been termed accelerated CLL/SLL (aCLL).[8] These cases are associated with an unfavorable genetic profile[9] and aggressive clinical behavior.[8] Richter transformation (RT) is defined as the development of a high-grade lymphoma in a patient with concurrent or previously diagnosed CLL/SLL.[10] The estimated incidence of RT is 0.5% to 1%/year, and the most common transformation is to diffuse large B-cell lymphoma (DLBCL-RT), followed by Hodgkin-like (HL-RT), and, more rarely, plasmablastic lymphoma. In DLBCL-RT sheets of large, transformed cells (nuclear size equal or larger than macrophage nuclei or >2 times larger than a normal lymphocyte) and a diffuse growth pattern are present (Figure 43.2A). There are two types of HL-RT, type 1 with isolated Hodgkin-Reed-Sternberg (HRS) cells in a background of CLL/SLL cells and type 2 with HRS cells in a mixed inflammatory background similar to classic Hodgkin lymphoma (Figure 43.2B).[7] The 2022 International Consensus Classification[2] emphasizes the need to distinguish aCLL from RT and from the phenomenon of "pseudo-RT," which can occur in patients treated with BTK inhibitors (BTKis) that temporarily are off-treatment.[11] In these patients cessation of BTK inhibition leads to lymph node enlargement with an histology similar to that of DLBCL; however, after reintroduction of ibrutinib the clinical manifestations resolve and the morphology reverts to CLL/SLL.[7,11]

Immunophenotype

Flow cytometry can usually distinguish CLL/SLL from other small cell lymphomas (Figure 43.3). Typically, the cells are positive for CD19, CD5, CD23, CD43, and CD200; weakly positive for CD20, CD79b, and monotypic immunoglobulin light chains; and negative for CD10. Immunohistochemistry shows expression of CD19, CD20, CD79a, CD5, CD23, and LEF1, while cyclin D1, SOX11, and CD10 are negative. Cells in proliferation centers may be weakly cyclin D1 positive but without t(11;14)(q13;q32) and are always SOX11 negative. Proliferation centers in CLL/SLL are often positive for LEF1, which may be diagnostically helpful since LEF1 is negative in mantle cell lymphoma and in marginal zone lymphoma.[12] DLBCL-RT can have a non-germinal center (GC) or GC phenotype (69% and 31%, respectively), and cells are usually highly proliferative (Ki67 median 80%, range 10%-100%).[13] In HL-RT the HRS cells express CD30, CD15, and PAX5 and may be EBV positive[14] (Figure 43.2B-G).

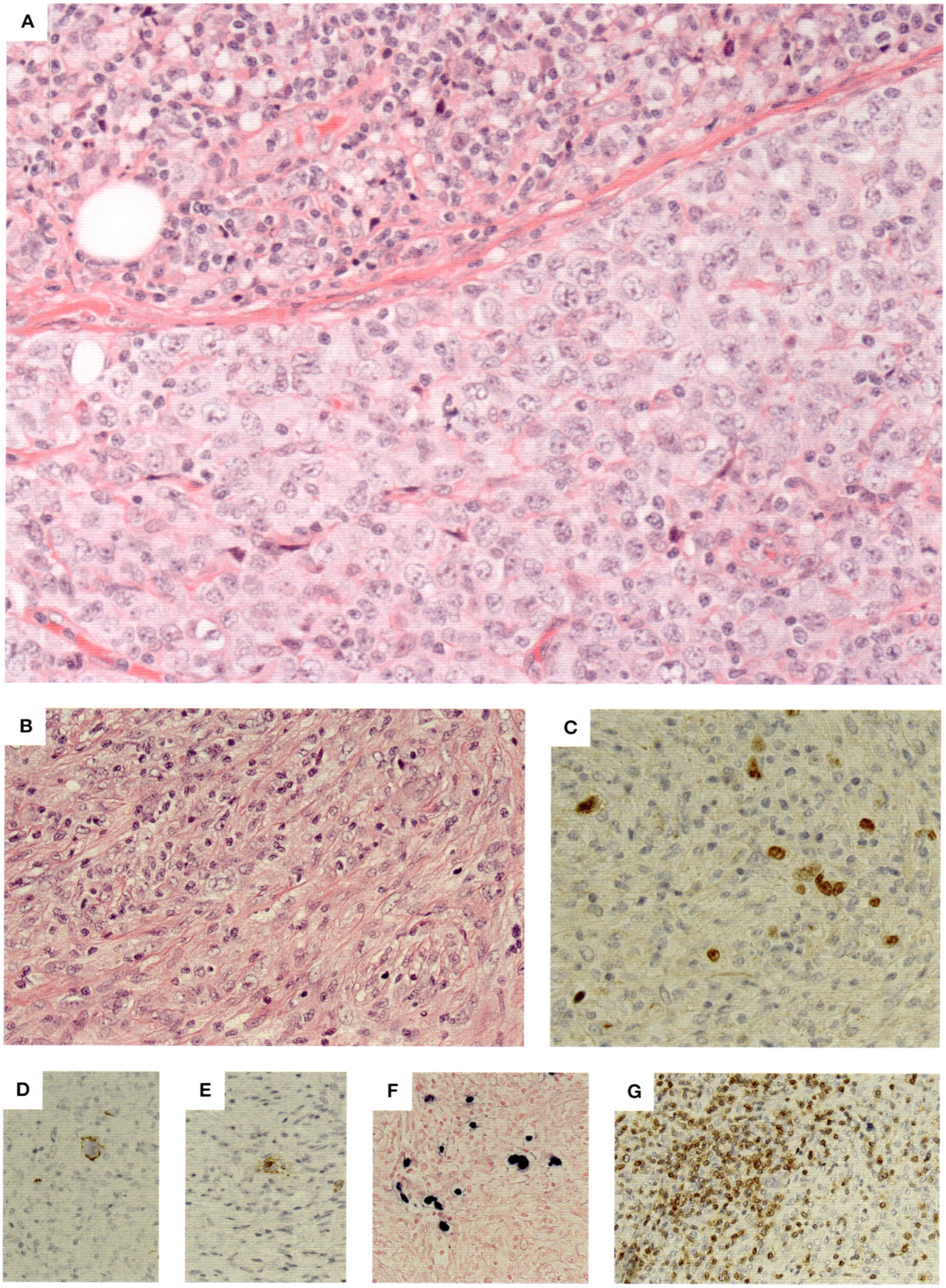

FIGURE 43.2 Examples of Richter transformation. **A:** Diffuse large B-cell lymphoma Richter transformation in the lower part of the figure. **B:** Hodgkin-like transformation with increased fibrosis and scattered large atypical cells that are positive for PAX5 **(C)**, CD30 **(D)**, CD15 **(E)**, and EBER **(F)**. The atypical cells are negative for CD20 and for CD3 (double staining for CD20 in red and CD3 in brown) **(G)**.

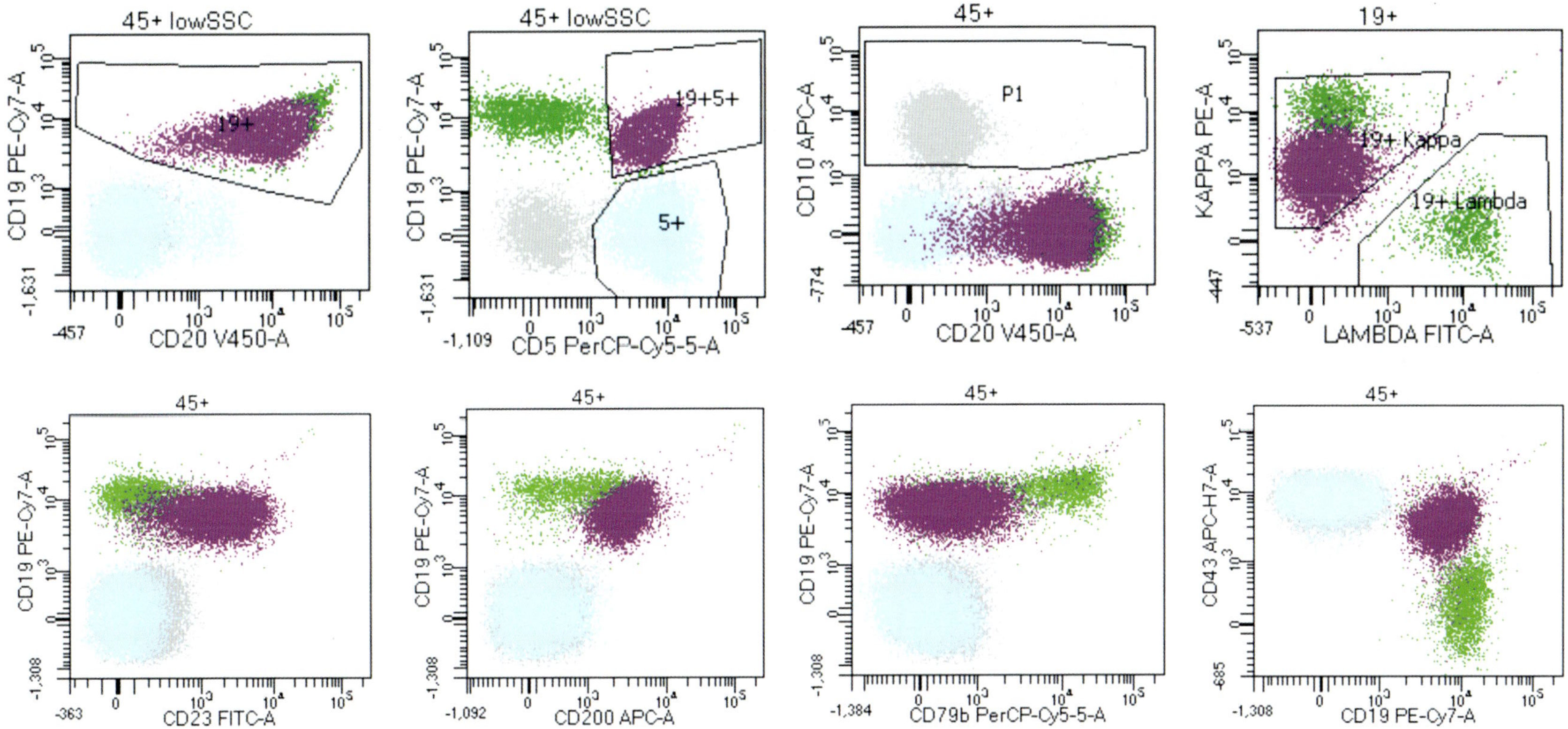

FIGURE 43.3 Flow cytometry of blood shows a chronic lymphocytic leukemia (CLL) population (in purple) in a background of polyclonal B cells (in green). The CLL population is positive for CD19, dim positive for CD20, positive for CD5, negative for CD10, and weakly positive for kappa. Further analysis shows positivity for CD23, CD200, and CD43 while CD79b is negative (lower panels).

Genetics

CLL/SLL is characterized by an accumulation of small, CD5-positive, clonal B lymphocytes with impaired apoptosis and increased proliferation due to abnormal activation of the BCR signaling pathway. CLL is usually preceded by high-count MBL, and it has been suggested that the persistent stimulation by foreign antigens or autoantigens leads to polyclonal expansion of premalignant cells. Some of these cells may acquire chromosomal aberrations and recurrent gene mutations that lead to clonal precursor populations and finally overt CLL (Figure 43.4). Further enrichment of mutated subclones occur during disease development, and clonal selection can also follow treatment leading to enrichment of clones carrying *TP53* abnormalities (after chemotherapy), Bruton tyrosine kinase (*BTK*) mutations (after ibrutinib), and *BCL2* mutations (after venetoclax).

The first described and most commonly defined cytogenetic abnormalities in previously untreated CLL, usually detected by fluorescence in situ hybridization, are deletion (del) 13q (55%-65%), del(11q) (5%-20%), trisomy 12 (10%-20%), and del(17p) (3%-8%) (Table 43.1). Chromosome banding analyses or genomic microarrays[18] can be used to determine the genomic complexity as cases with a highly complex karyotype (≥5 abnormalities) have adverse prognosis[18,19] while cases with a complex karyotype (≥3 abnormalities) follow an aggressive disease course only if they include *TP53* abnormalities.[19] Other alterations in CLL include del(6q) and del(8p) as well as 2p and 8q gains. Translocations of IGH genes are infrequent and include *BCL2, BCL3, BCL11A,* and *ZFP36L1* as partner genes. Genetically, high-count MBL may harbor the same aberrations seen in CLL, such as del(13q), trisomy 12, and del(17p) and *TP53* mutations.[1,20]

The somatic hypermutation status of the immunoglobulin heavy chain variable region gene (IGHV) plays an important role in the pathophysiology of CLL/SLL. In general, 50% of patients with CLL/SLL have an unmutated BCR IGHV gene (≥98% similarity with the germline sequence) (U-CLL) and these patients typically have a shorter time from diagnosis to progressive disease and more adverse outcome than patients with a mutated IGHV (<98% similarity with germline) (M-CLL). It is hypothesized that M-CLL is derived from germinal center–experienced memory cells while U-CLL are either naïve B cells or germinal center–independent memory cells. Further immunogenetic studies have shown similarities in the amino acids of the BCR immunoglobulin among cases so-called stereotypes, and 29 major stereotypes have been defined based on the sequence of the IGH V, D, and J genes.[21] These stereotypes are present in 40% of CLL/SLL cases and suggest antigen selection in CLL/SLL pathogenesis. Importantly, the stereotype subsets identify patients with similar clinical course and outcome. Subset #8 cases have unmutated IGHV, class switching to IgG, enrichment for trisomy 12, and *NOTCH1* mutations

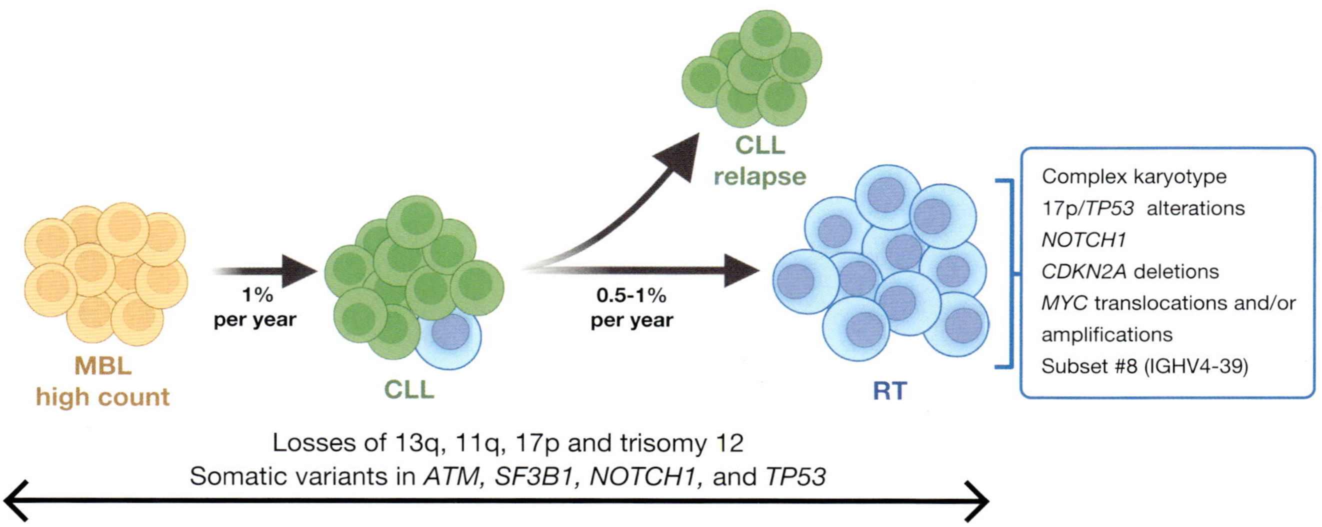

FIGURE 43.4 Evolution of high-count monoclonal B-cell lymphocytosis (MBL) to chronic lymphocytic leukemia (CLL) and Richter transformation (RT). High-count MBL may harbor the same genetic aberrations seen in CLL such as del(13q), trisomy 12, and del(17p) and *TP53* mutations. The risk of progression to CLL is 1%/year. RT cases show complex karyotypes, increased incidence of del(17p) and *TP53* mutations, *NOTCH1* mutations, *CDKN2A/B* deletions, *MYC* translocations or amplifications, as well as subset #8 (IGHV4-39). The risk of transformation is 0.5%-1%/year.

TABLE 43.1 Frequent copy number alterations and mutations in CLL according to IGHV mutational status

Alteration/gene	M-CLL (%)	U-CLL (%)
del(13q)	55-65	39-48
Trisomy 12	9-15	19-22
del(11q)	4	15-28
del(17p)	2-3	10-15
del(6q)	3-7	6-8
del(8p)	0-1	5
gain(2p)	0-2	10-12
gain(8q)	2	4-6
SF3B1	6-12	14-24
ATM	6	18
NOTCH1	2-4	16-18
TP53	4-5	10-15
CHD2	8	3
XPO1	1	8-10
POT1	1-3	6-9
BIRC3	2	3-4
EGR2	1	4-6
MYD88	4-6	0-1
NFKBIE	0-1	1-6
IGLV3-21^{R110}	6	5

The numbers are a summary of different studies.[15-17] Regions and genes with at least 4% mutations have been considered.
CLL, chronic lymphocytic leukemia; del, deletion; IGHV, immunoglobulin heavy chain variable region gene; M-CLL, CLL with mutated IGHV; U-CLL, CLL with unmutated IGHV.
Nadeu F, Royo R, Clot G, et al. IGLV3-21R110 identifies an aggressive biological subtype of chronic lymphocytic leukemia with intermediate epigenetics. *Blood.* 2021;137(21):2935-2946; Knisbacher BA, Lin Z, Hahn CK, et al. Molecular map of chronic lymphocytic leukemia and its impact on outcome. *Nat Genet.* 2022;54(11):1664-1674; and Mansouri L, Thorvaldsdottir B, Sutton LA, et al. Different prognostic impact of recurrent gene mutations in chronic lymphocytic leukemia depending on IGHV gene somatic hypermutation status: a study by ERIC in HARMONY. *Leukemia.* 2023;37(2):339-347.

and have a higher risk for RT. Subset #2 cases are enriched for mutations in the *SF3B1* gene and *ATM* aberrations and have a poor outcome, in spite of being IGHV-mutated.[21] Interestingly, subset #2 BCR immunoglobulins are encoded by the IGHV3-21/IGLV3-21 genes with distinctive, restricted VH and VL CDR3 sequences. A particular mutation in the lambda light chain variable region, IGLV3-21^{R110}, has been detected not only in stereotype #2 cases but also in other CLL cases lacking this BCR configuration. The IGLV3-21^{R110} mutation induces autonomous BCR signaling and confers poor prognosis independent of IGHV mutation status.[15]

Analysis of gene mutations in CLL reveals putative driver genes (Table 43.1). Some of these drivers are relatively more frequent while the majority of drivers are mutated in <2% of patients.[16] The most common driver mutations are *SF3B1* (mutated in 17.5% of cases), *NOTCH1* (12.3%), *ATM* (11.2%), IGLV3-21^{R110} (5.5%), and *TP53* (9.1%). Increased number of putative driver gene mutations are found in U-CLL compared with M-CLL, and the putative driver gene mutations also differ according to IGHV mutation status.[16,17] Subclonal *TP53* alterations with low variant allele frequency (<10%) may be associated with clinically adverse outcome.[22]

Approximately 80% of cases of DLBCL-RT are clonally related to the underlying CLL/SLL as shown by IGH rearrangement studies while clonally unrelated cases represent de novo DLBCL. The latter have similar overall survival as de novo DLBCL while clonally related DLBCL-RT has a median overall survival of less than 1 year.[10] Genomic studies of RT show alterations in genes that regulate tumor suppression, cell cycle, and proliferation pathways including *TP53, CDKN2A/B, NOTCH1,* and *MYC* in a high number of cases[10,23,24] (Figure 43.4). Overall, RT accumulates alterations in genes involved in NF-κB and NOTCH pathways. Studies of sequential samples from patients have shown that small subclones carrying genetic alterations characteristic of the RT are already present in CLL at diagnosis, up to 19 years before the transformation.[24] The HRS cells of HL-RT are clonally related to the CLL in some cases, but not all. Clonal relatedness does not appear to influence survival in the limited available data.[14]

Prognosis and Clinical Comment

Most patients with CLL/SLL remain relatively asymptomatic at the time of presentation, and the disease remains incurable. The goals of therapy are therefore to improve quality of life and to prolong survival. Most patients with CLL do not require initiation of treatment at diagnosis, and newly diagnosed patients and patients on follow-up who remain without signs of bone marrow failure should be monitored and not treated until there are signs of disease progression. This "watch and wait approach" is supported by a number of clinical trials that showed no survival benefit for an early start of treatment and has been confirmed with current standard chemoimmunotherapy (fludarabine, cyclophosphamide, plus rituximab FCR)[25] and with ibrutinib.[26] International workshop for CLL (iWCLL) guidelines[27] have been established. Treatment indications are progressive bone marrow failure (anemia and/or thrombocytopenia), progressive or symptomatic lymphadenopathy or splenomegaly, progressive lymphocytosis with an increase of >50% over a 2-month period, lymphocyte doubling time of less than 6 months, or disease-related symptoms such as weight loss, fever, night sweats, or fatigue. Treatment may also be indicated in patients with CLL with autoimmune anemia and/or thrombocytopenia that poorly responds to corticosteroids.

The treatment approach for treatment-naïve and relapsed/refractory disease has changed enormously over the last few years.[28] Chemoimmunotherapy was previously the treatment of choice but has largely been now supplanted with novel agents targeting either the BCR pathway using the BTKis ibrutinib, acalabrutinib, or zanubrutinib or the BCL2 pathway using venetoclax (usually used in combination with anti-CD20 mAbs).[28] BTKi therapy is given as continuous therapy until drug intolerance or resistance occurs, whereas venetoclax, when given in combination with the anti-CD20 monoclonal antibody obinutuzumab, has an advantage of being given as a 1-year fixed duration therapy and this can therefore be an attractive option for many patients. A number of prognostic models have been developed, and these continue to be refined as new data on predictive factors for each of the approved agents in CLL are verified. However, it is still premature to use these models in clinical decisions outside the setting of clinical trials. IGHV mutational status and high-risk cytogenetics can be used to assist in determining the treatment approach. Fixed-duration approaches with venetoclax are very attractive in patients with mutated IGHV disease, whereas patients with deletion and/or mutation of *TP53* appear to have better outcome with continuous therapy approaches. Patients who progress after fixed-duration venetoclax can be re-treated with the same approach if they have had long treatment-free intervals or can be treated by switching to BTKi therapy. The major mechanisms of resistance to BTKi therapy involve mutations in the BCR-binding site or in the downstream BCR signaling pathway, and these patients can then respond to venetoclax alone or in combination with anti-CD20 mAbs. Since ibrutinib, acalabrutinib, or zanubrutinib all bind to the same site on BTK there is no value in changing to another covalent BTK-binding agent. Novel BTKis that do not bind covalently to this binding site are in clinical development and have demonstrated high response rates in patients resistant to ibrutinib, acalabrutinib, or zanubrutinib.

The approval of novel BTKi and BCL2i agents has had an impact on the role of allo–stem cell transplantation, and the number of transplants being performed continues to decrease markedly in both Europe and the United States.[29]

Chimeric antigen receptor (CAR) T cells have also been explored as potentially curative approaches in CLL/SLL and RT, but despite promising results in phase II studies,[30] there are still no approved CAR-T cell products in this disease setting. Addition of ibrutinib at the time of collection of T cells and after infusion improves CAR-T function in this disease setting.

References

1. Semenzato G, Ghobrial IM, Ghia P. Monoclonal B-cell lymphocytosis, monoclonal gammopathy of undetermined significance, and T-cell clones of uncertain significance: are these premalignant conditions sharing a common identity? *Lancet Haematol.* 2023;10(7):e549-e556.
2. Campo E, Jaffe ES, Cook JR, et al. The International Consensus classification of mature lymphoid neoplasms: a report from the clinical advisory committee. *Blood.* 2022;140(11):1229-1253.
3. Gibson SE, Swerdlow SH, Ferry JA, et al. Reassessment of small lymphocytic lymphoma in the era of monoclonal B-cell lymphocytosis. *Haematologica.* 2011;96(8):1144-1152.

4. Habermehl GK, Durkin L, Hsi ED. A tissue counterpart to monoclonal B-cell lymphocytosis. *Arch Pathol Lab Med*. 2021;145(12):1544-1551.
5. Shadman M. Diagnosis and treatment of chronic lymphocytic leukemia: a review. *JAMA*. 2023;329(11):918-932.
6. Oscier D, Else M, Matutes E, Morilla R, Strefford JC, Catovsky D. The morphology of CLL revisited: the clinical significance of prolymphocytes and correlations with prognostic/molecular markers in the LRF CLL4 trial. *Br J Haematol*. 2016;174(5):767-775.
7. Sander B, Campo E, Hsi ED. Chronic lymphocytic leukaemia/small lymphocytic lymphoma and mantle cell lymphoma: from early lesions to transformation. *Virchows Arch*. 2023;482(1):131-145.
8. Gine E, Martinez A, Villamor N, et al. Expanded and highly active proliferation centers identify a histological subtype of chronic lymphocytic leukemia ("accelerated" chronic lymphocytic leukemia) with aggressive clinical behavior. *Haematologica*. 2010;95(9):1526-1533.
9. Lapierre L, Syrykh C, Largeaud L, et al. "Accelerated phase" chronic lymphocytic leukemia: still an intermediate risk disease in the era of targeted therapies. *Hematol Oncol*. 2022;40(4):805-808.
10. Condoluci A, Rossi D. Biology and treatment of Richter transformation. *Front Oncol*. 2022;12:829983.
11. Barnea Slonim L, Ma S, Behdad A, Chen Q. Pseudo-Richter transformation of chronic lymphocytic leukaemia/small lymphocytic lymphoma following ibrutinib interruption: a diagnostic pitfall. *Br J Haematol*. 2020;191(1):e22-e25.
12. Patel N, Durkin L, Bodo J, Hsi ED. Immunohistochemical expression of lymphoid enhancer binding factor 1 in CD5-positive marginal zone, lymphoplasmacytic, and follicular lymphomas. *Am J Clin Pathol*. 2020;153(5):646-655.
13. Wang Y, Ding W. Richter transformation of chronic lymphocytic leukemia in the era of novel agents. *Clin Adv Hematol Oncol*. 2020;18(6):348-357.
14. Xiao W, Chen WW, Sorbara L, et al. Hodgkin lymphoma variant of Richter transformation: morphology, Epstein-Barr virus status, clonality, and survival analysis-with comparison to Hodgkin-like lesion. *Hum Pathol*. 2016;55:108-116.
15. Nadeu F, Royo R, Clot G, et al. IGLV3-21R110 identifies an aggressive biological subtype of chronic lymphocytic leukemia with intermediate epigenetics. *Blood*. 2021;137(21):2935-2946.
16. Knisbacher BA, Lin Z, Hahn CK, et al. Molecular map of chronic lymphocytic leukemia and its impact on outcome. *Nat Genet*. 2022;54(11):1664-1674.
17. Mansouri L, Thorvaldsdottir B, Sutton LA, et al. Different prognostic impact of recurrent gene mutations in chronic lymphocytic leukemia depending on IGHV gene somatic hypermutation status: a study by ERIC in HARMONY. *Leukemia*. 2023;37(2):339-347.
18. Ramos-Campoy S, Puiggros A, Bea S, et al. Chromosome banding analysis and genomic microarrays are both useful but not equivalent methods for genomic complexity risk stratification in chronic lymphocytic leukemia patients. *Haematologica*. 2022;107(3):593-603.
19. Baliakas P, Jeromin S, Iskas M, et al. Cytogenetic complexity in chronic lymphocytic leukemia: definitions, associations, and clinical impact. *Blood*. 2019;133(11):1205-1216.
20. Griffin R, Wiedmeier-Nutor JE, Parikh SA, et al. Differential prognosis of single and multiple TP53 abnormalities in high-count MBL and untreated CLL. *Blood Adv*. 2023;7(13):3169-3179.
21. Agathangelidis A, Chatzidimitriou A, Chatzikonstantinou T, et al. Immunoglobulin gene sequence analysis in chronic lymphocytic leukemia: the 2022 update of the recommendations by ERIC, the European Research Initiative on CLL. *Leukemia*. 2022;36(8):1961-1968.
22. Rossi D, Khiabanian H, Spina V, et al. Clinical impact of small TP53 mutated subclones in chronic lymphocytic leukemia. *Blood*. 2014;123(14):2139-2147.
23. Chakraborty S, Martines C, Porro F, et al. B-cell receptor signaling and genetic lesions in TP53 and CDKN2A/CDKN2B cooperate in Richter transformation. *Blood*. 2021;138(12):1053-1066.
24. Nadeu F, Royo R, Massoni-Badosa R, et al. Detection of early seeding of Richter transformation in chronic lymphocytic leukemia. *Nat Med*. 2022;28(8):1662-1671.
25. Herling CD, Cymbalista F, Gross-Ophoff-Muller C, et al. Early treatment with FCR versus watch and wait in patients with stage Binet A high-risk chronic lymphocytic leukemia (CLL): a randomized phase 3 trial. *Leukemia*. 2020;34(8):2038-2050.
26. Langerbeins P, Zhang C, Robrecht S, et al. The CLL12 trial: ibrutinib vs placebo in treatment-naive, early-stage chronic lymphocytic leukemia. *Blood*. 2022;139(2):177-187.
27. Hallek M, Cheson BD, Catovsky D, et al. iwCLL guidelines for diagnosis, indications for treatment, response assessment, and supportive management of CLL. *Blood*. 2018;131(25):2745-2760.
28. Hallek M. First line therapy of CLL. *Hematol Oncol*. 2023;41(suppl 1):129-135.
29. Tournilhac O, van Gelder M, Eikema DJ, et al. The European landscape on allogeneic haematopoeietic cell transplantation in chronic lymphocytic leukaemia between 2009 and 2019: a perspective from the chronic malignancies working party of the EBMT. *Bone Marrow Transplant*. 2023;58(6):621-624.
30. Siddiqi T, Maloney DG, Kenderian SS, et al. Lisocabtagene maraleucel in chronic lymphocytic leukaemia and small lymphocytic lymphoma (TRANSCEND CLL 004): a multicentre, open-label, single-arm, phase 1-2 study. *Lancet*. 2023;402(10402):641-654.

Chapter 44
B-Cell Prolymphocytic Leukemia

Birgitta Sander, Elias Campo, Martin Dreyling, and Estella Matutes

Definition

B-cell prolymphocytic leukemia (B-PLL) is a neoplasm involving peripheral blood, bone marrow, and usually the spleen with prolymphocytes that represent >55% of lymphoid cells in the peripheral blood. This diagnosis should be rendered only after rigorous exclusion of other B-cell lymphomas such as mantle cell lymphoma (MCL), splenic marginal zone lymphoma, or progression from chronic lymphocytic leukemia (CLL).[1,2]

Epidemiology

B-PLL is a rare leukemia and constitutes <1% of lymphoid leukemias. Patients are elderly (median age 72 years) with a male to female ratio of 1.4.

General Clinical Features

There is peripheral blood lymphocytosis and involvement of the bone marrow. Approximately 60% of patients have splenomegaly while lymphadenopathy is less frequent.[3,4] Symptomatic patients (56% of cases) more frequently have cytopenias and tumoral disease.[4]

Morphology

In peripheral blood smears, prolymphocytes are medium-sized lymphoid cells (larger than CLL cells) with a moderate amount of basophilic cytoplasm. The nucleus is round and contains a distinct nucleolus (Figure 44.1).

Immunophenotype

The cells of B-PLL express CD19, CD20, CD22, CD79a, and FMC7, with intense surface IgM/IgD. CD5 has been reported to be expressed in 56% and CD23 in 30% of cases, respectively.[3] CD200 is variable, and hairy cell markers (CD25, CD103, CD123) as well as markers for MCL (Cyclin D1 and SOX11) are negative.

Genetics

Complex karyotype (CK) (≥3 numerical or structural chromosomal abnormalities) is found in 73% of cases and a highly CK (≥5 numerical or structural chromosomal abnormalities) in 45%. More than 50% of cases have a *MYC* translocation to the IGH, IGL, or IGK locus, and 15% of cases have extra copies of the *MYC* gene. Other frequent alterations are del(17p), del(13q), del(8p), and trisomy of chromosomes 3, 12, and 18. IGHV may be mutated in 80% of the cases with common use of IGHV3, particularly IGHV3-23, or IGHV4.[3] *TP53* has been identified as the most frequent mutated gene, followed by *MYD88, BCOR, MYC,* and *SF3B1*.[3] Rearrangements of *CCND1, CCND2,* and *CCNDD3* are typical of mantle cell lymphoma and are negative in B-PLL.

Prognosis and Clinical Comment

Based on the presence of *MYC* aberrations (translocations or copy number gain) and/or del(17p), three prognostic groups have been suggested with better overall survival (OS) in patients without *MYC* aberrations, intermediate risk in patients with *MYC* aberrations and no del(17p), and lowest OS in patients with both *MYC* aberrations and del(17p).[3] Response to standard treatment (eg, R-FC in *TP53* wild type) or targeted therapy (ibrutinib, venetoclax, alemtuzumab in *TP53*-mutated cases) is usually only short term, and transplantation strategies may be considered for relapsed disease in suitable patients.

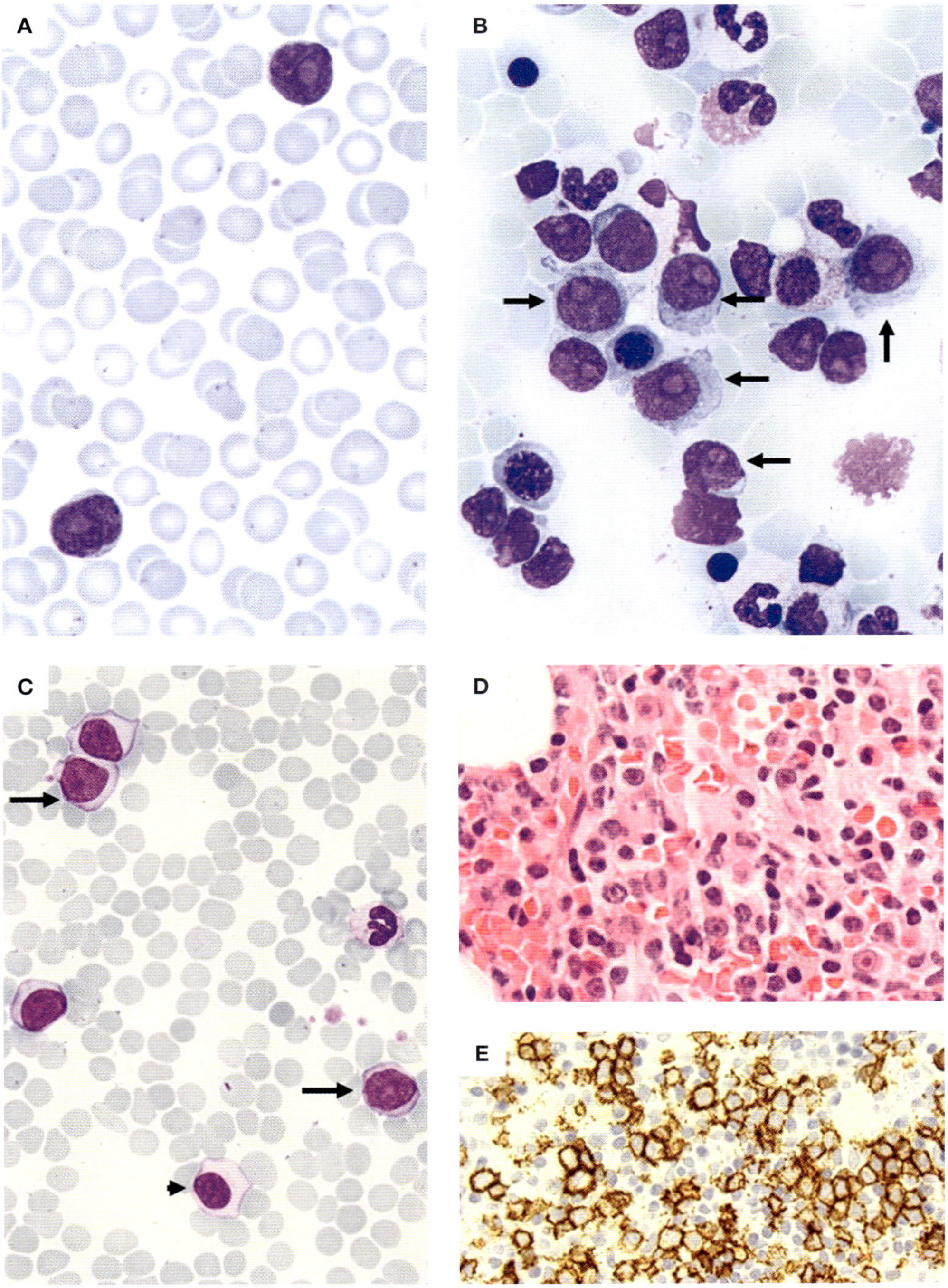

FIGURE 44.1 **A:** Peripheral blood smear with two prolymphocytes. **B:** Bone marrow smear with numerous prolymphocytes (arrows). **C:** Blood smear from a patient with marked lymphocytosis and splenomegaly. Visualized are several prolymphocytes (arrows) and a normal lymphocyte (arrowhead). **D:** Bone marrow from the same patient. Groups of intermediate-sized lymphocytes with prominent nucleoli. **E:** CD20 immunohistochemistry. This case had a very complex karyotype with del(17)(p22) and a *TP53* mutation. Fluorescence in situ hybridization was negative for del(13)(q24), del(11)(q22.3), and trisomy 12 as well as t(11;14)(q13;q32) and *MYC* split.

References

1. Campo E, Jaffe ES, Cook JR, et al. The International consensus classification of mature lymphoid neoplasms: a report from the Clinical Advisory Committee. *Blood.* 2022;140(11):1229-1253.
2. Sander B, Campo E, Hsi ED. Chronic lymphocytic leukaemia/small lymphocytic lymphoma and mantle cell lymphoma: from early lesions to transformation. *Virchows Arch.* 2023;482(1):131-145.
3. Chapiro E, Pramil E, Diop M, et al. Genetic characterization of B-cell prolymphocytic leukemia: a prognostic model involving MYC and TP53. *Blood.* 2019;134(21):1821-1831.
4. Algrin C, Perol L, Chapiro E, et al. Retrospective analysis of a cohort of 41 de novo B-cell prolymphocytic leukemia patients: impact of genetics and targeted therapies (a FILO study). *Haematologica.* 2023;108(6):1691-1696.

Chapter 45
Splenic Marginal Zone Lymphoma

Alexandar Tzankov, Stefan Dirnhofer, and Emanuele Zucca

Definition

Splenic marginal zone lymphoma (SMZL) is a mature small B-cell lymphoma involving the spleen and frequently the bone marrow with a nodular infiltration pattern that replaces preexisting splenic structures of the white pulp by surrounding and supplanting germinal centers and expanding the follicle mantles and marginal zones. It often shows a characteristic micronodular and sinus-associated infiltration pattern of the splenic red pulp and of the bone marrow as well as villous lymphocytes in the peripheral blood.[1]

Synonyms

Splenic lymphoma with villous lymphocytes (not recommended).

Epidemiology

SMZL accounts for approximately 1% of all lymphomas but it is probably underestimated, as historically some insufficiently worked-up cases have been misclassified as, eg, (CD5-negative) chronic lymphocytic leukemia (CLL)/small lymphocytic lymphoma, or referred to as small B-cell lymphoma, without a specific phenotype/not otherwise specified. The age-standardized incidence rate for SMZL is 1.8 per 1.000.000 person-years, which is on the rise partly due to advancements in diagnostic techniques that enable more accurate categorization of patients, and also due to a general increase in the exposure to and prevalence of risk factors such as infections, autoimmune disorders, and other conditions of immune dysregulation. The male-to-female ratio is approximately 1:1, although some studies report a slight female predominance. The median age of the affected individuals is 67 years (age range: 20-96). The general association of B-cell lymphomas with chronic hepatitis C virus (HCV) infection seems to be particularly pronounced in SMZL, and recent data also suggest a possible association with hepatitis B virus.[1-5]

General Clinical Features

SMZL patients present with splenomegaly, often with peripheral blood absolute lymphocytosis that may include villous lymphocytes. Occasionally, an immune-mediated thrombocytopenia can be observed. Cytopenias related to hypersplenism and/or bone marrow infiltration are evident in higher tumor-burden instances. Bone marrow infiltration is regularly detected, while lymph node involvement occurs rarely and is initially limited to the hilar splenic lymph nodes. One-third of patients display a monoclonal protein without hyperviscosity or hypergammaglobulinemia.

Morphology

Splenectomy is rarely performed as a diagnostic procedure. However, when it is performed, a gross examination of the spleen would typically reveal a significant enlargement, usually exceeding 18 cm. This enlargement is accompanied by a noticeable expansion of the white pulp (Figure 45.1).

Microscopically, the preexisting structures of the splenic white pulp appear replaced by small round lymphocytes with slightly more abundant cytoplasm

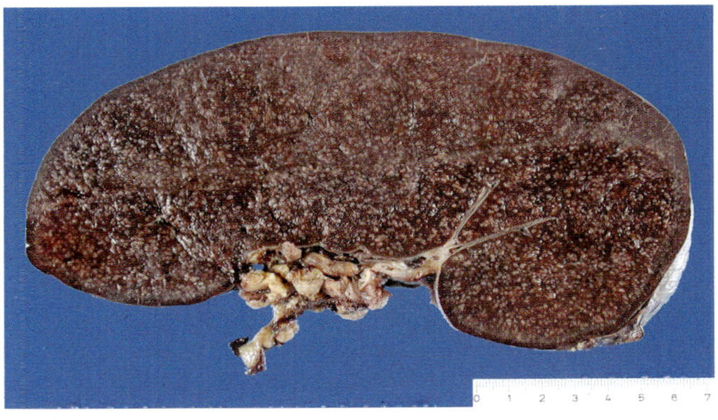

FIGURE 45.1 Splenic marginal zone lymphoma. Enlarged spleen (20 cm) with marked expansion of the white pulp.

than seen in CLL, which surround and supplant the germinal centers and expand the follicle mantles and the marginal zones. At the periphery of the nodules and resembling normal marginal zone cells, the neoplastic lymphocytes often appear medium sized with abundant cytoplasm (Figure 45.2A and B). The red pulp is always infiltrated in a micronodular and often intrasinusoidal pattern (Figure 45.3). Occasionally, more pronounced monocytoid or plasmacytoid differentiation can be observed.

The hilar splenic lymph nodes show dilated and often tumor-infiltrated sinuses, and a nodular, marginal zone-pattern infiltration of germinal centers.

The bone marrow, which is the most commonly biopsied organ in SMZL, may show nodular, at times peritrabecular, interstitial and a very characteristic intrasinusoidal infiltration that may become less pronounced as the disease progresses (Figure 45.4).

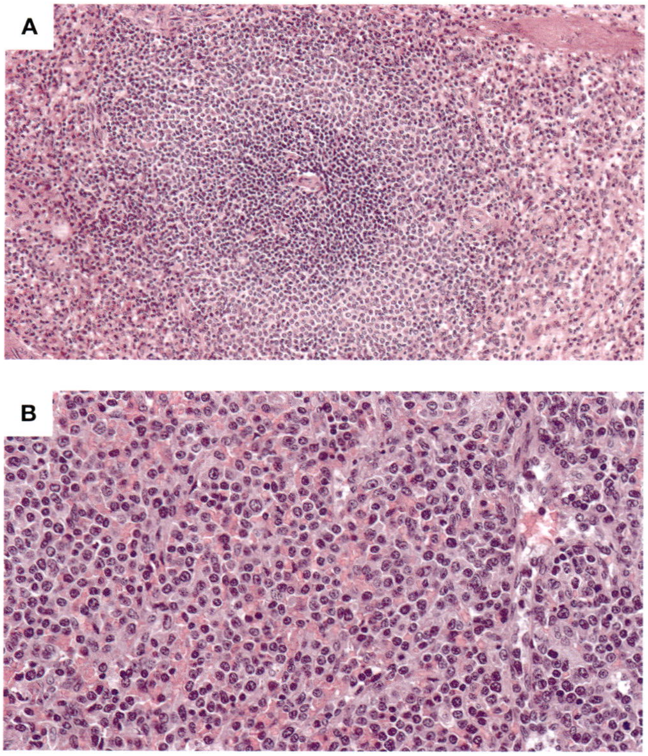

FIGURE 45.2 Splenic marginal zone lymphoma. **A:** Infiltration of the white pulp with a central small lymphocytic core of cells with condensed chromatin replacing a germinal center with effacement of the follicle mantle and merging with a peripheral zone of medium-sized lymphocytes with dispersed chromatin and more abundant and paler cytoplasm that resemble marginal zone cells. **B:** Higher-magnification view of marginal zone–resembling cells with occasional plasmacytoid and monocytoid appearance and isolated paraimmunoblastoid cells.

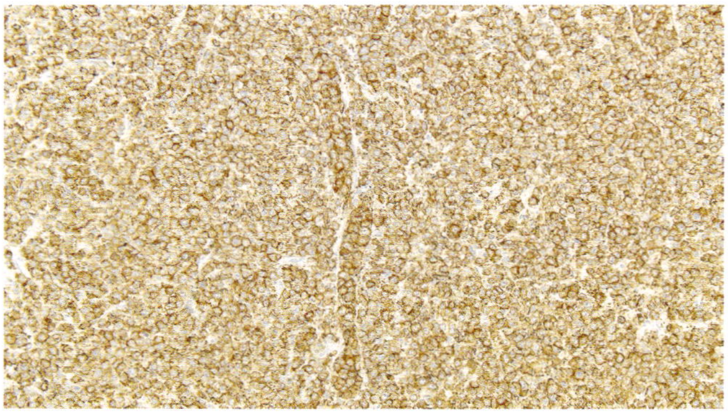

FIGURE 45.3 Splenic marginal zone lymphoma. Moderate but diffuse expression of CD20 with a characteristic paler to negative-appearing broader cytoplasm of the neoplastic lymphocytes and a perceptible intrasinusoidal pattern.

SMZL in the peripheral blood can present with various characteristics. These include the presence of short polar villi (Figure 45.5), a plasmacytoid appearance, or an unremarkable small lymphocytic morphology.

SMZL cannot be diagnosed on the basis of the pattern and extent of bone marrow or peripheral blood involvement alone. However, the presence of a clonal B-cell population in these locations with a phenotype consistent with SMZL (see **Immunophenotype**), supported by clinical and/or imaging evidence of splenic involvement, enables establishing the diagnosis even in the absence of splenectomy. Applying ancillary techniques, SMZL can be distinguished from most of the other mature small B-cell lymphomas, but definitive distinction from splenic diffuse red pulp small B-cell lymphoma (SDRPL), which is considerably rarer than SMZL, is not possible without evaluation of the splenic histology.[6]

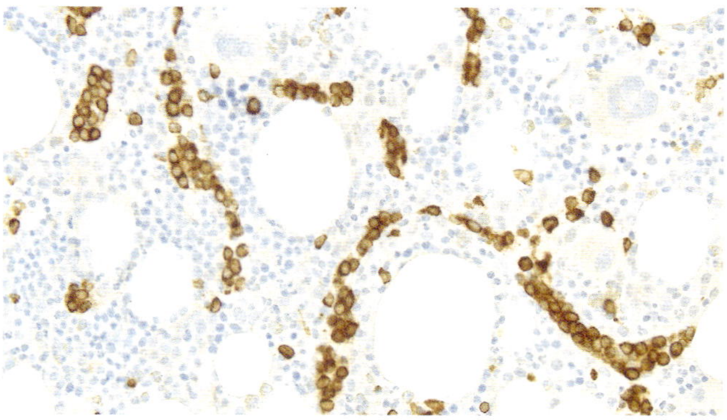

FIGURE 45.4 Splenic marginal zone lymphoma. Characteristic intrasinusoidal infiltration of the bone marrow.

Immunophenotype

Almost all SMZL cases express CD20 (Figure 45.3), CD79a, PAX5, and tartrate-resistant acid phosphatase (TRAP) and are dim IgM positive and bright CD180 positive, the latter being potentially helpful in discriminating from other mature small B-cell lymphomas with a nonspecific (CD5 negative, CD10 negative) phenotype. Approximately half of the cases (range 30%-70%) display positivity for IgD, CD11c, dim CD21, immune receptor translocation-associated protein 1 (IRTA1), myeloid nuclear differentiation antigen (MNDA), multiple myeloma oncogene 1 (MUM1), T-box expressed in T cells (T-Bet), and T-cell leukemia/lymphoma protein 1 (TCL1a). A fraction, 15% to 45%, of SMZL is positive for CD72 (DBA.44). A minor proportion (≤5%) shows positivity for BRAF V600E, CD5 (especially cases with more pronounced lymphocytosis), CD23, CD25, CD43, CD103, or cyclin D1 (weak and variable staining; highly likely in *BRAF*-mutated cases). SMZL does not express annexin A1, CD10, CD123, CD200, and lymphoid enhancer-binding factor 1 (LEF1).[7-9]

Discerning SMZL from other mature small B-cell lymphomas presenting with splenomegaly, especially on nonsplenic specimens such as bone marrow biopsies, on which the great majority is currently being diagnosed, may be challenging. Expression of germinal center markers, such as BCL6, CD10, GCET1, HGAL, LMO2, and MEF2B, especially in the context of dim CD19 and/or *BCL2* rearrangement supports a diagnosis of follicular lymphoma rather than SMZL. Demonstration of *CCND1* rearrangement in the context of positivity for CD5 and/or SOX11 establishes the diagnosis of mantle cell lymphoma. CLL usually shows a characteristic phenotype with coexpression of CD5, CD20, CD23, CD43, CD200, and LEF1. Hairy cell leukemia displays a characteristic phenotype with expression of annexin A1, BRAF V600E, CD25, CD103, CD123, and often cyclin D1. Expression of CD72 (DBA.44) and cyclin D3 in the context of negativity for CD11c may favor a SDRPL. Expression of CD72 (DBA.44) and CD103, and/or the presence of *MAP2K1* mutations, may help establishing the diagnosis of hairy cell leukemia variant in instances with interstitial bone marrow involvement; CD11c is not discriminant in this context.[1,6,10-12]

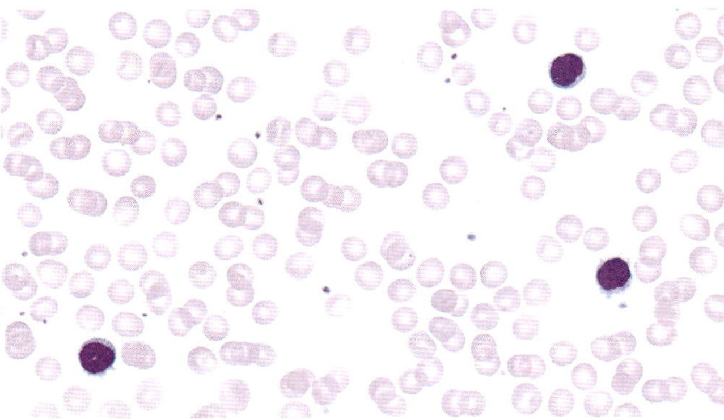

FIGURE 45.5 Splenic marginal zone lymphoma. Characteristic villous lymphocytosis in the peripheral blood. (Smear provided by Dr. Patrick Baettig.)

Genetics

SMZL displays three characteristic chromosomal aberrations, namely, del(7q)(32.1-32.2), in up to 40% of cases (Figure 45.6), and t(2;7)(p12;q21) with *CDK6::IGK* fusion or t(7;22)(q22;q22) with *CDK6::IGL* fusion in single cases.[1] In addition, rather nonspecific gains of chromosomes 3, 12, and 18 have been observed. Deletions of 17p13 (*TP53*) affect approximately 10% of patients.

Several recurrent mutations have been detected in SMZL. In descending order, the 10 most commonly mutated genes are *KLF2* and *NOTCH2* (in 30% each, cooccurring in 50% of the mutated cases), *TNFAIP3* and *KMT2D* (in 20% each), *TP53* and *NOTCH1* (in 15%), and *TRAF3, SPEN, CARD11,* and *CREBBP* (in roughly 10% each).[13] Except for *KLF2* mutations, which are regularly found in both SMZL and nodal MZL, and the higher occurrence of *TP53* mutations in SMZL, the mutational patterns in SMZL overlap with those of other MZL subtypes. Consequently, relying solely on single gene profiling is not sufficient for establishing a diagnosis of SMZL. However, this may not be the case for

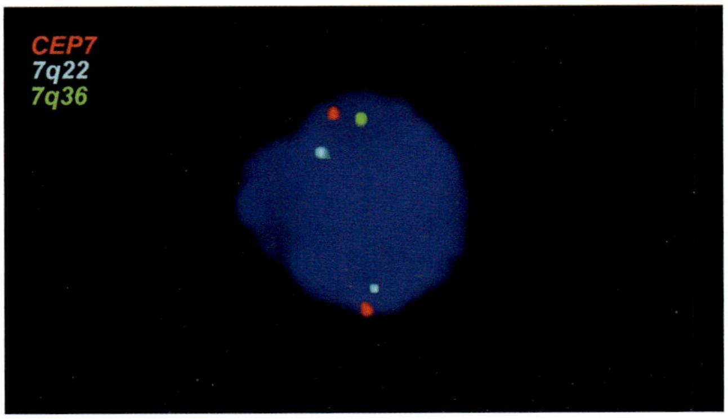

FIGURE 45.6 Splenic marginal zone lymphoma. Deletion of 7q32 demonstrated by fluorescence in situ hybridization using a tricolor probe against the centromere 7 (red), the 7q22 region (aqua), and 7q36 (green). Note that the examined lymphoma cell contains two red and blue signals, but only one green signal, indicating a respective deletion. 7q36 is codeleted along del (7q32).

approximately 15% of cases that are *KLF* and *NOTCH2* comutated, especially when they also exhibit a del(7q); in such instances, the genetic profile strongly suggests a diagnosis of SMZL. *MYD88* is rarely mutated, and its mutations usually map outside the L265 hotspot.

Mathematic modeling[13] suggests that SMZL comprises two main genetic clusters characterized either by mutations affecting **N**F-κB, **N**OTCH, and ***K**LF2* (called NNK) or by mutations of *TP53* and/or genes encoding for other **D**NA-damage response proteins, **M**APK-encoding compounds, and genes encoding modules of the **T**LR-signaling cascade (called DMT). The NNK cluster accounts for 60% of cases and is characterized by enrichment for del(7q) and IGHV1-2*4 usage. The DMT cluster accounts for 30% and is characterized by mutations in genes that are affected in different B-cell lymphomas.

Prognosis and Clinical Comment

Several clinical prognostic factors for SMZL have been proposed, including leukocytosis, lymphocytosis, anemia, thrombocytopenia, monoclonal component, β2-microglobulin, performance status, involvement of nonhematopoietic sites, age, and bone marrow infiltration pattern. The most commonly used prognostic score is calculated from lactate dehydrogenase and hemoglobin levels, platelet count, and the presence of extrahilar lymphadenopathy.[14] Molecular studies on SMZL are revealing promising prognostic biomarkers (such as *NOTCH2* and *KLF2* mutations, *TP53* abnormalities, and an immunosuppressive tumor microenvironment) that may enhance risk stratification.[13] Whether the suggested more tailored efficacies of drugs that target the B-cell receptor-dependent NF-κB activation (eg, BTK inhibitors) in NNK-SMZL and of drugs that activate the apoptotic machinery when the DNA damage response pathway is disrupted (eg, BCL2 inhibitors) in DMT-SMZL hold true remains to be determined.

While splenectomy has been progressively replaced by rituximab (with or without chemotherapy) as the preferred initial therapy,[15] compared with other so-called indolent B-cell lymphomas, the life expectancy of patients with SMZL has not improved in the last decade. The 5-year overall survival of roughly 80% remains inferior to the age-matched general population.[2,3,13] Patients with SMZL are at increased risk for infectious and cardiovascular complications,[3] and transformation (SMZL-T), mostly to diffuse large B-cell lymphoma,[16] but occasionally to classic Hodgkin lymphoma.[17] SMZL-T displays higher genomic complexity, higher incidence of *TNFAIP3* and *TP53* alterations, and 9p21.3 (*CDKN2A/B*) losses and 6p gains, and usually arises by divergent evolution from a common altered precursor cell.[16]

A large population-based analysis for the period 1999 to 2016[3] suggested no significant differences in overall survival or SMZL-specific survival based on the treatment strategy employed, including observation, splenectomy, chemotherapy, or combination of splenectomy and chemotherapy. However, this study did not take into account the effects of rituximab, which has shown significant activity in SMZL,[15,18] nor did it consider the impact of other factors that may have influenced the clinical choice of therapy. Nevertheless, in this US-based study, older age, Hispanic ethnicity, SMZL-T, and B-symptoms were linked to a worse prognosis. Although age <60 years and female sex were significantly associated with splenectomy, splenectomy had no effect on overall or SMZL-specific survival compared with active surveillance.

In SMZL, rituximab monotherapy leads to an overall response rate of approximately 90%, the majority being long-lasting and nearly half being complete responses.[15] The BRISMA trial showed that bendamustine and rituximab should be considered when a chemotherapy combination with rituximab is deemed necessary for high-risk patients with symptomatic progressive disease.[18]

The efficacies of HCV eradication[19] and front-line checkpoint blockade in SMZL[20] have also been reported. These treatment approaches are rational due to the association of SMZL with chronic viral hepatitis[4,5] and the presence of an immunosuppressive/checkpoint inhibiting microenvironment in selected cases,[13] indicating that targeting the underlying viral infection and modulating the immune response can be beneficial in managing selected SMZL.

References

1. Piris MA, Pittaluga S, Isaacson PG, et al. Splenic marginal zone lymphoma. In: Swerdlow SH, Campo E, Harris NL, et al, eds. WHO Classification of Tumours of Haematopoietic and Lymphoid Tissues. 4th rev ed. IARC Press; 2017:223-225.
2. Cerhan JR, Habermann TM. Epidemiology of marginal zone lymphoma. *Ann Lymphoma*. 2021;5:1.
3. Florindez JA, Alderuccio JP, Reis IM, Lossos IS. Splenic marginal zone lymphoma: a US population-based survival analysis (1999-2016). *Cancer*. 2020;126(21):4706-4716.

4. Yi S, Yan Y, Xiong W, et al. Distinct clinical characteristics draw a new prognostic model for splenic marginal zone lymphoma in HBV high prevalent region. *Oncotarget*. 2017;8(58):98757-98770.
5. Zucca E, Bertoni F, Vannata B, Cavalli F. Emerging role of infectious etiologies in the pathogenesis of marginal zone B-cell lymphomas. *Clin Cancer Res*. 2014;20:5207-5216.
6. Yilmaz E, Chhina A, Nava VE, Aggarwal A. A review on splenic diffuse red pulp small B-cell lymphoma. *Curr Oncol*. 2021;28(6):5148-5154.
7. Turakhia S, Lanigan C, Hamadeh F, Swerdlow SH, Tubbs RR, Cook JR. Immunohistochemistry for BRAF V600E in the differential diagnosis of hairy cell leukemia vs other splenic B-cell lymphomas. *Am J Clin Pathol*. 2015;144(1):87-93.
8. Wang Z, Cook JR. IRTA1 and MNDA expression in marginal zone lymphoma: utility in differential diagnosis and implications for classification. *Am J Clin Pathol*. 2019;151(3):337-343.
9. Miguet L, Lennon S, Baseggio L, et al. Cell-surface expression of the TLR homolog CD180 in circulating cells from splenic and nodal marginal zone lymphomas. *Leukemia*. 2013;27(8):1748-1750.
10. Bikos V, Darzentas N, Hadzidimitriou A, et al. Over 30% of patients with splenic marginal zone lymphoma express the same immunoglobulin heavy variable gene: ontogenetic implications. *Leukemia*. 2012;26(7):1638-1646.
11. Pillonel V, Juskevicius D, Ng CKY, et al. High-throughput sequencing of nodal marginal zone lymphomas identifies recurrent BRAF mutations. *Leukemia*. 2018;32(11):2412-2426.
12. Vela V, Juskevicius D, Dirnhofer S, Menter T, Tzankov A. Mutational landscape of marginal zone B-cell lymphomas of various origin: organotypic alterations and diagnostic potential for assignment of organ origin. *Virchows Arch*. 2022;480(2):403-413.
13. Bonfiglio F, Bruscaggin A, Guidetti F, et al. Genetic and phenotypic attributes of splenic marginal zone lymphoma. *Blood*. 2022;139(5):732-747.
14. Montalbán C, Abraira V, Arcaini L, et al. Risk stratification for Splenic Marginal Zone Lymphoma based on haemoglobin concentration, platelet count, high lactate dehydrogenase level and extrahilar lymphadenopathy: development and validation on 593 cases. *Br J Haematol*. 2012;159(2):164-171.
15. Kalpadakis C, Pangalis GA, Sachanas S, et al. Rituximab monotherapy in splenic marginal zone lymphoma: prolonged responses and potential benefit from maintenance. *Blood*. 2018;132(6):666-670.
16. Grau M, López C, Navarro A, et al. Unraveling the genetics of transformed splenic marginal zone lymphoma. *Blood Adv*. 2023;7(14):3695-3709.
17. Menter T, Dirnhofer S, Tzankov A. Transformation of a splenic marginal zone lymphoma into classic Hodgkin lymphoma. *J Clin Pathol*. 2019;72(5):391-392.
18. Iannitto E, Bellei M, Amorim S, et al. Efficacy of bendamustine and rituximab in splenic marginal zone lymphoma: results from the phase II BRISMA/IELSG36 study. *Br J Haematol*. 2018;183(5):755-765.
19. Hermine O, Lefrère F, Bronowicki JP, et al. Regression of splenic lymphoma with villous lymphocytes after treatment of hepatitis C virus infection. *N Engl J Med*. 2002;347(2):89-94.
20. Miller PG, Sperling AS, Gibson CJ, et al. A deep molecular response of splenic marginal zone lymphoma to front-line checkpoint blockade. *Haematologica*. 2021;106(2):651-654.

Chapter 46
Hairy Cell Leukemia

Miguel A. Piris, Brunangelo Falini, and Catherine Thieblemont

Definition

Hairy cell leukemia (HCL) is an indolent small B-cell neoplasm, commonly associated with *BRAF* V600E mutation, characterized by bone marrow, spleen, and peripheral blood involvement by small B cells with hairy projections.

Synonyms

None.

Epidemiology

HCL is a rare disease accounting for 2% of all leukemias, with an incidence of 0.28 to 0.3 cases/100,000 people/year in Europe and the United States.[1,2] HCL is less frequent in Asians, Africans, and Arabs than in individuals of European descent.

Multiple studies show a clear male predominance (M:F ratio: 4:1). The median age at diagnosis is 59 years.

General Clinical Features

Patients usually present with pancytopenia and a low percentage of peripheral blood circulating leukemic cells. About 15% of cases present with leukocytosis. Monocytopenia is frequent. Splenomegaly occurs in about 85% of patients and may be marked. General symptoms are related to the degree of bone marrow infiltration and splenomegaly.

Peripheral lymphadenopathy is exceptional at diagnosis. Retroperitoneal or mesenteric lymph node infiltration is occasionally observed, especially in long-standing progressive disease.

Morphology

Hairy cells in the peripheral blood have a characteristic cytology, consisting of medium-sized cells with oval or cleaved nucleus and homogeneous chromatin. Nucleoli are absent. The characteristic hairy cytoplasmic projections are mainly observable in peripheral blood smears (Figure 46.1).

In bone marrow biopsies, the prominent clear cytoplasm of the neoplastic cells makes a pattern that has been described as "fried egg" or "honeycomb" (Figure 46.1). The primary growth pattern is interstitial with some aggregates but with partial preservation of fat and other hematopoietic elements. In other cases, the bone marrow may show massive infiltration with replacement of all other components. Some cases are hypocellular with a low degree of infiltration that may be overlooked unless immunohistochemistry (IHC) staining for CD20 and other B-cell markers is performed (Figure 46.2). After progression, fibrosis may mask the cytology. Mitotic figures are very rare.

The spleen shows expansion of the red pulp by neoplastic cells occupying the sinuses and typically contains red blood cell lakes where neoplastic cells surround collections of erythrocytes. Liver and abdominal lymph nodes show a characteristic sinusoidal infiltration.

Immunophenotype

The neoplastic cells express all B-cell markers, including CD19, CD20, CD22, PAX5, and CD79a. There is also expression of marginal zone markers such T-Bet and MNDA (Figure 46.3). HCL cells show a very characteristic phenotypic profile, including the expression of Cyclin D1, Annexin A1, CD103, CD25, CD123, FMC7, and CD200. Cyclin D1 expression, a useful marker for HCL cells (Figure 46.3), is independent of the presence of the t(11;14)(q13;q32), which is never found in this condition. The most specific marker for HCL cells is Annexin A1, not observed in any other lymphoproliferative disorder, and also expressed by myeloid cells. Immunohistochemical staining for the *BRAF* V600E mutant protein using the mutant-specific VE1 antibody clone is helpful to identify HCL.[3]

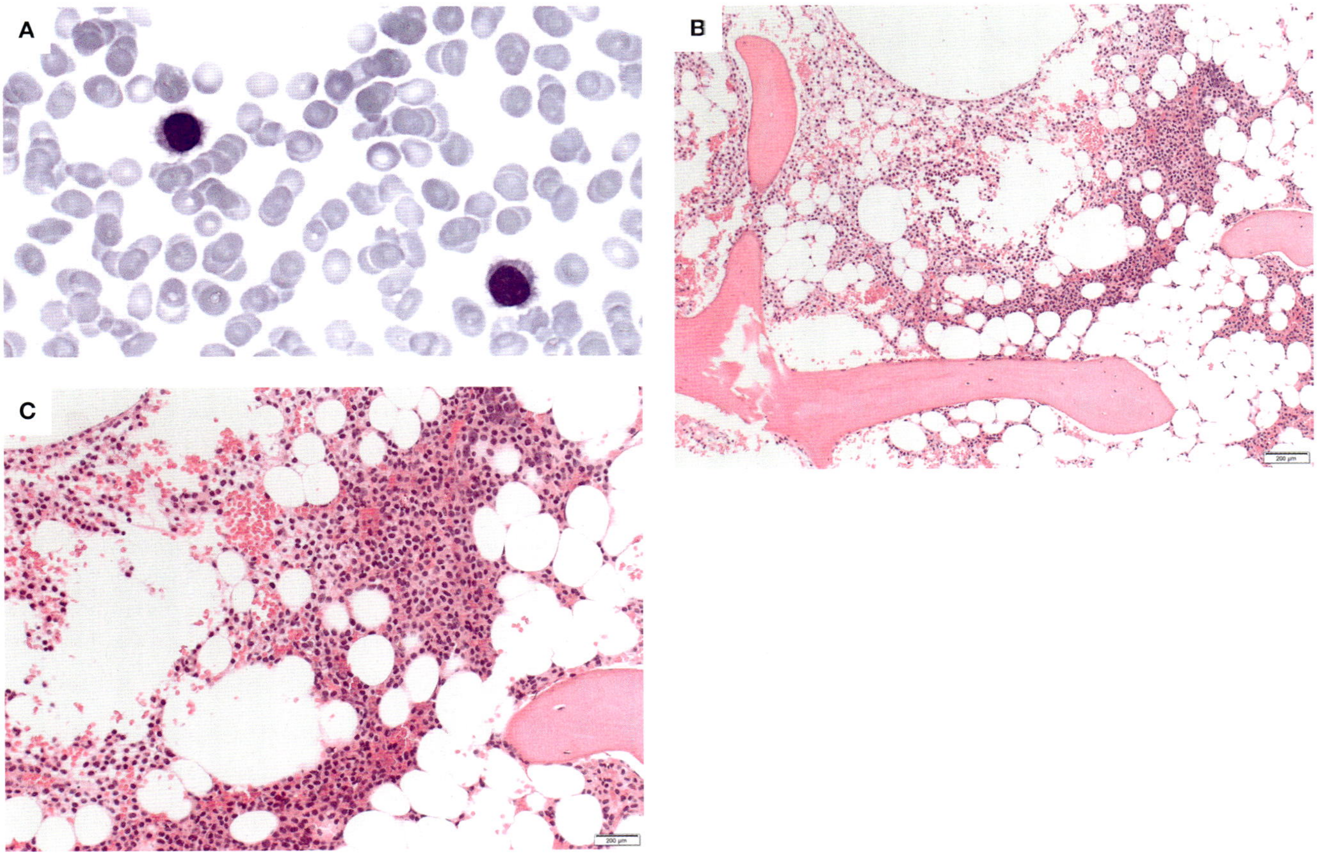

FIGURE 46.1 **A:** Hairy cell leukemia cells in peripheral blood. Medium-sized cells with typical hairy projections. **B:** Bone marrow infiltration. Interstitial pattern with mild fibrosis and partial preservation of fat. **C:** Bone marrow histology, medium power. Medium-sized cells with clear cytoplasm, partial preservation of other hematopoietic components. (**A:** Courtesy Dr E Matutes, Hospital Clinic, Barcelona.)

Genetics

The underlying genetic cause for a large majority (>90%) of HCL cases is the *BRAF* V600E kinase-activating mutation, which is somatically present through the entire disease spectrum and clinical course.[4] This driver mutation aberrantly activates the RAF-MEK-ERK signaling pathway, shaping some of the key HCL biologic features of HCL, including its distinct expression signature, hairy morphology, and apoptosis inhibition.[5] Accompanying mutations of the *KLF2* transcription factor or the *CDKN1B* (p27) cell cycle inhibitor are recurrent in 16% of patients with HCL and likely cooperate with *BRAF* V600E in HCL pathogenesis.[5-7]

Prognosis and Clinical Comment

HCL is an indolent neoplasm, with a median overall survival of 27 years and a median relapse-free survival of 11 years. Patients with HCL require long-term follow-up because of their relatively increased risk of second malignancies.[8]

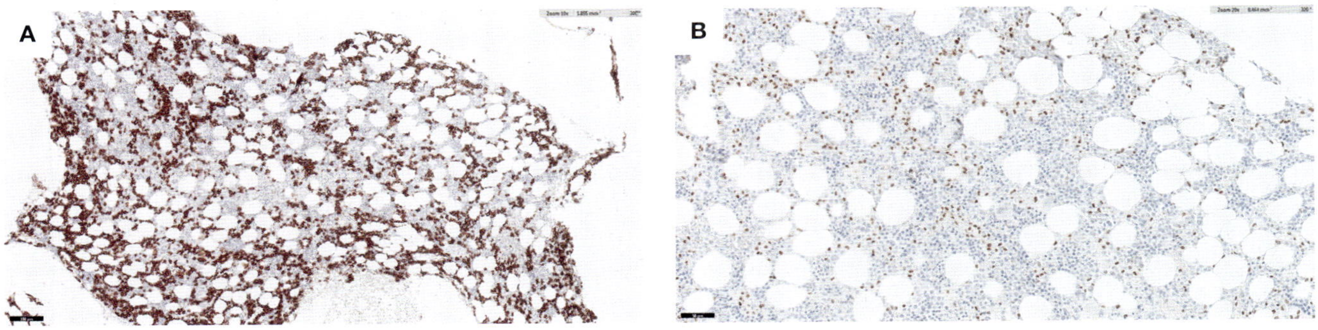

FIGURE 46.2 Bone marrow with subtle infiltration. **A** and **B:** CD20 (**A**) and PAX5 (**B**) staining outline the interstitial pattern.

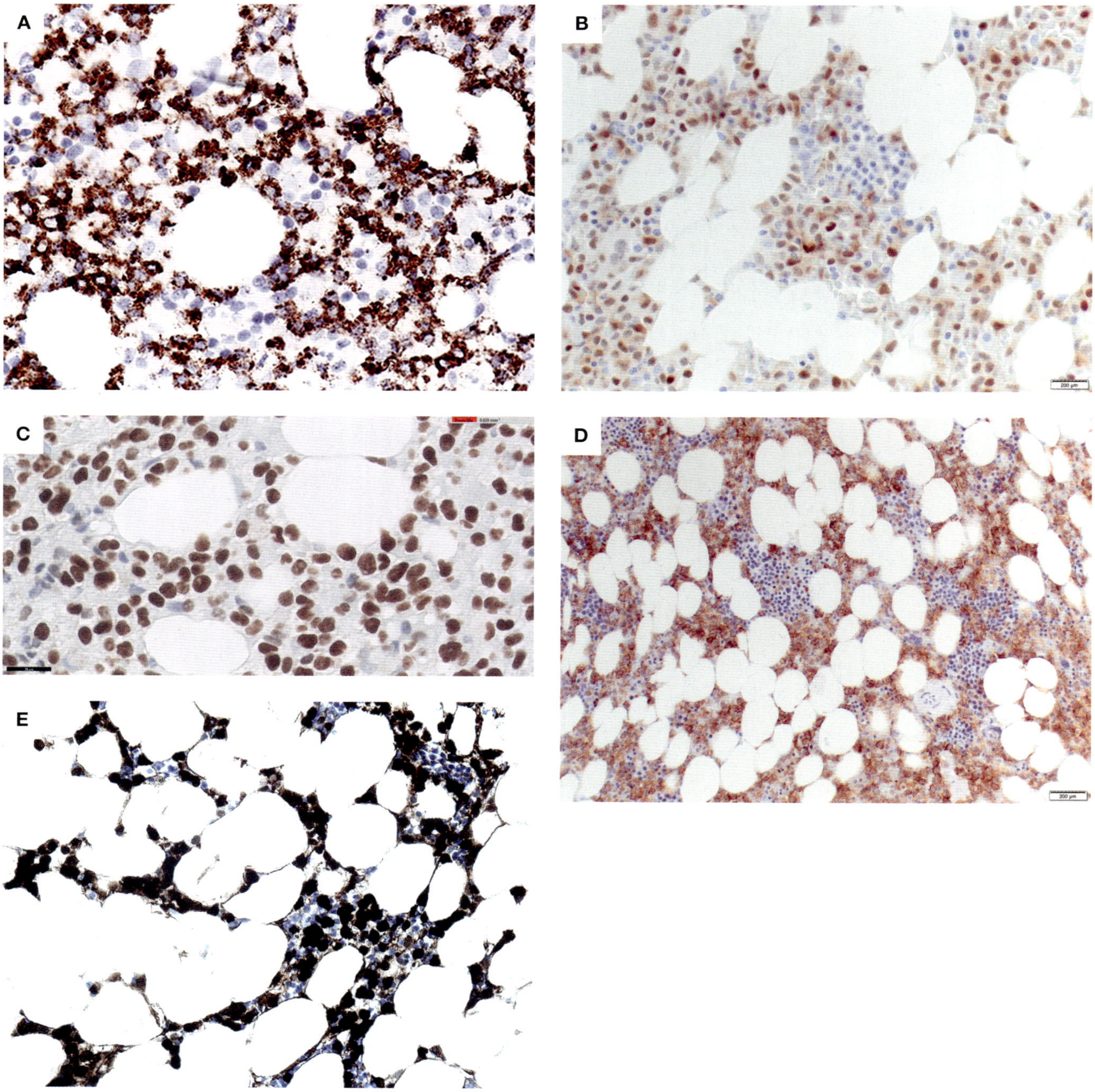

FIGURE 46.3 Bone marrow. **A:** pERK nuclear and cytoplasmic staining. **B:** CyclinD1 nuclear immunostaining is a useful marker for hairy cell leukemia (HCL) cells. **C:** MNDA staining. HCL cells show expression of marginal zone markers such as MNDA and T-bet. **D:** CD11c positivity is detectable either by flow cytometry or immunohistochemistry. **E:** Annexin A1 staining. Positive HCL cells with a background of positive myeloid cells and negative red blood cells.

HCL is highly responsive to the purine analogues cladribine and pentostatin (PNAs). A poorer response to these agents is observed in patients with more marked leukocytosis, bulky splenomegaly, an unmutated immunoglobulin variable heavy chain (IgVH) gene profile, use of IGH VH4-34, or *TP53* mutations.[9]

For patients with refractory or relapsed HCL, chemotherapy-free, nonmyelotoxic regimen of vemurafenib plus rituximab is associated with a durable complete response in most patients.[10-13] Cases resistant to this regimen may respond to venetoclax.[14]

References

1. Teras LR, DeSantis CE, Cerhan JR, Morton LM, Jemal A, Flowers CR. 2016 US lymphoid malignancy statistics by World Health Organization subtypes. *CA Cancer J Clin.* 2016;66(6):443-459.
2. Gatta G, Capocaccia R, Botta L, et al. Burden and centralised treatment in Europe of rare tumours: results of RARECAREnet—a population-based study. *Lancet Oncol.* 2017;18(8):1022-1039.
3. Turakhia S, Lanigan C, Hamadeh F, Swerdlow SH, Tubbs RR, Cook JR. Immunohistochemistry for BRAF V600E in the differential diagnosis of hairy cell leukemia vs other splenic B-cell lymphomas. *Am J Clin Pathol.* 2015;144(1):87-93.
4. Tiacci E, Trifonov V, Schiavoni G, et al. BRAF mutations in hairy cell leukemia. *N Engl J Med.* 2011;364(24):2305-2315.
5. Tiacci E, Pettirossi V, Schiavoni G, Falini B. Genomics of hairy cell leukemia. *J Clin Oncol.* 2017;35(9):1002-1010.
6. Piva R, Deaglio S, Famà R, et al. The Krüppel-like factor 2 transcription factor gene is recurrently mutated in splenic marginal zone lymphoma. *Leukemia.* 2015;29(2):503-507.
7. Maitre E, Tomowiak C, Lebecque B, et al. Deciphering genetic alterations of hairy cell leukemia and hairy cell leukemia-like disorders in 98 patients. *Cancers.* 2022;14(8):1904.
8. Paillassa J, Cornet E, Noel S, et al. Analysis of a cohort of 279 patients with hairy-cell leukemia (HCL): 10 years of follow-up. *Blood Cancer J.* 2020;10(5):62.
9. Cornet E, Delmer A, Feugier P, et al. Recommendations of the SFH (French Society of Haematology) for the diagnosis, treatment and follow-up of hairy cell leukaemia. *Ann Hematol.* 2014;93(12):1977-1983.
10. Falini B, Martelli MP, Tiacci E. BRAF V600E mutation in hairy cell leukemia: from bench to bedside. *Blood.* 2016;128(15):1918-1927.
11. Pettirossi V, Santi A, Imperi E, et al. BRAF inhibitors reverse the unique molecular signature and phenotype of hairy cell leukemia and exert potent antileukemic activity. *Blood.* 2015;125(8):1207-1216.
12. Tiacci E, De Carolis L, Simonetti E, et al. Vemurafenib plus rituximab in refractory or relapsed hairy-cell leukemia. *N Engl J Med.* 2021;384(19):1810-1823.
13. Falini B, De Carolis L, Tiacci E. How I treat refractory/relapsed hairy cell leukemia with BRAF inhibitors. *Blood.* 2022;139(15):2294-2305.
14. Tiacci E, De Carolis L, Santi A, et al. Venetoclax in relapsed or refractory hairy-cell leukemia. *N Engl J Med.* 2023;388(10):952-954.

Chapter 47

Splenic B-Cell Lymphoma/Leukemia, Unclassifiable

Miguel A. Piris, Brunangelo Falini, and Catherine Thieblemont

Introduction

Several forms of incompletely characterized splenic-based small B-cell neoplasms have been described that do not meet criteria for any of the clearly defined entities in the International Consensus Classification. Two types of rare neoplasms, splenic diffuse red pulp small B-cell lymphoma (SDRPL) and hairy cell leukemia variant (HCLv), are recognized as provisional entities. The precise relationship of SDRPL and HCLv to each other and to splenic marginal zone lymphoma remains controversial, and establishing these diagnoses may sometimes require evaluation of peripheral blood (PB), bone marrow (BM), and splenic histology together. Other cases of unusual splenic-based small B-cell neoplasms that do not meet criteria for these provisional entities should be diagnosed as splenic B-cell lymphoma/leukemia, unclassifiable.

SPLENIC DIFFUSE RED PULP SMALL B-CELL LYMPHOMA

Definition

SDRPL is a small B-cell lymphoma involving the spleen, BM, and PB. A peculiar diffuse infiltration of the splenic red pulp by small B cells is associated in these cases with PB infiltration by small lymphocytes with surface projections.

Synonyms

Splenic marginal zone lymphoma with diffuse red pulp involvement (not recommended).

Splenic red pulp lymphoma with numerous basophilic villous lymphocytes (not recommended).

Epidemiology

SDRPL is a rare neoplasm where precise data on incidence rates are not yet available, but it corresponds to approximately 10% of the splenic lymphoma specimens and 0.5% of all chronic lymphoid malignancies with PB involvement.[1-3] The median ages in the larger published series were 65.5 and 77 years (range 40-91 years), with a clear male predominance (male:female ratio of 1.64-2.4).

General Clinical Features

Clinical manifestations are mainly due to splenomegaly. This is a leukemic condition, where the spleen, BM, and PB are regularly infiltrated. Lymph node infiltration at initial diagnosis has not been described. Paraproteinemia is observed in a low proportion of cases, always at a low level.[2,3] A preexistent phase of monoclonal B-cell lymphocytosis with non-chronic lymphocytic leukemia phenotype has been described in some cases.[4,5]

Morphology

Neoplastic cells in the PB smears are small to medium in size with round or oval nuclei, without conspicuous nucleoli (Figure 47.1). Typically, the cytoplasm of neoplastic cells exhibit distinct villous projections unevenly distributed around the cells, frequently with a polar distribution.[3]

BM biopsy shows some degree of neoplastic infiltration in all cases, albeit with a variable amount of residual hematopoiesis (Figure 47.2). The most distinctive feature is the intrasinusoidal infiltration pattern. Additionally, there may be interstitial aggregates, without forming lymphoid follicles, without follicular dendritic cells, in contrast with SMZL.

Diffuse splenic infiltration is the main feature of this neoplasm (Figure 47.3). Both splenectomy specimens and splenic needle core biopsies show a diffuse pattern of infiltration that seems to originate in the red pulp, progressively replacing the lymphoid follicles of white pulp. Massive intrasinusoidal infiltration is a useful finding, and red blood cell lakes lined by neoplastic lymphocytes can be found, similar to those in hairy cell leukemia. The neoplastic B cells in tissue sections

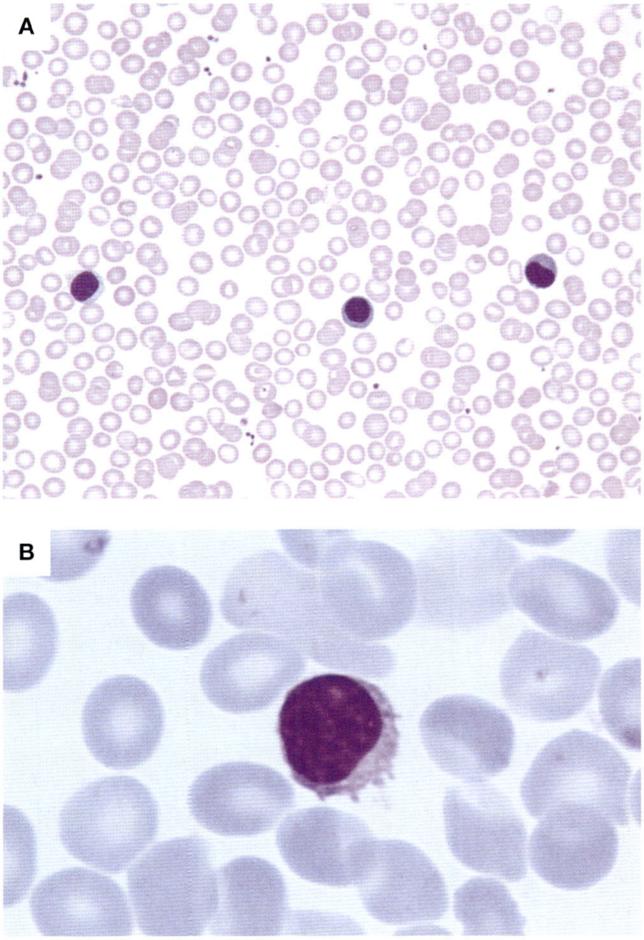

FIGURE 47.1 Splenic diffuse red pulp small B-cell lymphoma. Peripheral blood cytology (**A** and **B**). Medium-sized cells with villous projections with a polar distribution.

have a relatively round hyperchromatic nucleus with clumped chromatin, without discernible nucleolus, and a slightly basophilic cytoplasm, which gives them a plasmacytoid appearance.

Immunophenotype

SDRPL is positive for B-cell markers (CD20, CD19, CD79a), marginal zone markers (MNDA, T-Bet), DBA44, and IgG or IgM/IgD, but negative for SOX11, CD5, CD23, CD43, cyclin D1, CD21, CD10, CD25, CD38, and Annexin A1 [1,2,6,7]. Cyclin D3 is expressed in 70% of cases [8] and in the appropriate context is a valuable diagnostic marker.[9] Expression of CD123 and CD103 has been reported in very few cases. The proliferation index (Ki67) is usually low. P53 seems to be more frequently expressed than in SMZL. By flow cytometry (FCM), an increased expression of CD180 has been proposed as a useful feature in the recognition of SDRPL.[10] CD11c, as detected by FCM or immunohistochemistry, is frequently positive.[11]

Genetics

Losses of 7q31, a quite characteristic finding in SMZL, is only rarely found in SDRPL. In contrast, these cases show a variable number of chromosomal changes and recurrent losses.[12]

Most cases express B-cell receptor immunoglobulin with somatically hypermutated *IGHV* genes. The *IGHV* gene repertoire is biased, with a predominance of the *IGHV3-23* and *IGHV4-34* genes [3,13,14]. Use of IGVH1-2, as seen in SMZL, is an unusual finding.

Recurrent mutations and copy number variations have been found in a series of genes including *NOTCH1, NOTCH2, TP53, MAP2K1, CCND3, BCOR, ARIDIA-A1,* and *SYK.*[1,8,13–17]

No molecular assay is diagnostic of SDRPL, but the presence of *CCND3* or *BCOR* mutation seem to be more frequent in this disorder. Neoplastic cells lack the *BRAF* V600E mutation, and *MYD88* L265P and *NOTCH2* mutations are very rare.[1]

Prognosis and Clinical Comment

The available information is limited. A shorter progression-free survival has been noted in cases associated with mutations in *NOTCH1, TP53,* or *MAP2K1* genes in a recent study.[12] Transformation to diffuse large B-cell lymphoma is rarely observed.[18,19]

HAIRY CELL LEUKEMIA VARIANT

Definition

HCLv is a designation that has been used for B-cell chronic lymphoproliferative disorders that display some, but not all, features of hairy cell leukemia (HCL) and lack the *BRAF* V600E mutation. These cases exhibit features that are unusual in HCL such as leukocytosis, monocytosis, and PB cytology that is intermediate between prolymphocytes and classic HCL cells. HCLv is now known to be biologically unrelated to HCL, lacking the distinctive molecular or clinical features of HCL. This is a disorder that requires a redefinition based on additional studies including common clinical, phenotypical, morphological, and molecular features. A striking overlap with splenic red pulp lymphoma is being progressively recognized.[20]

Synonyms

Splenic B-cell lymphoma/leukemia with prominent nucleoli (not recommended).

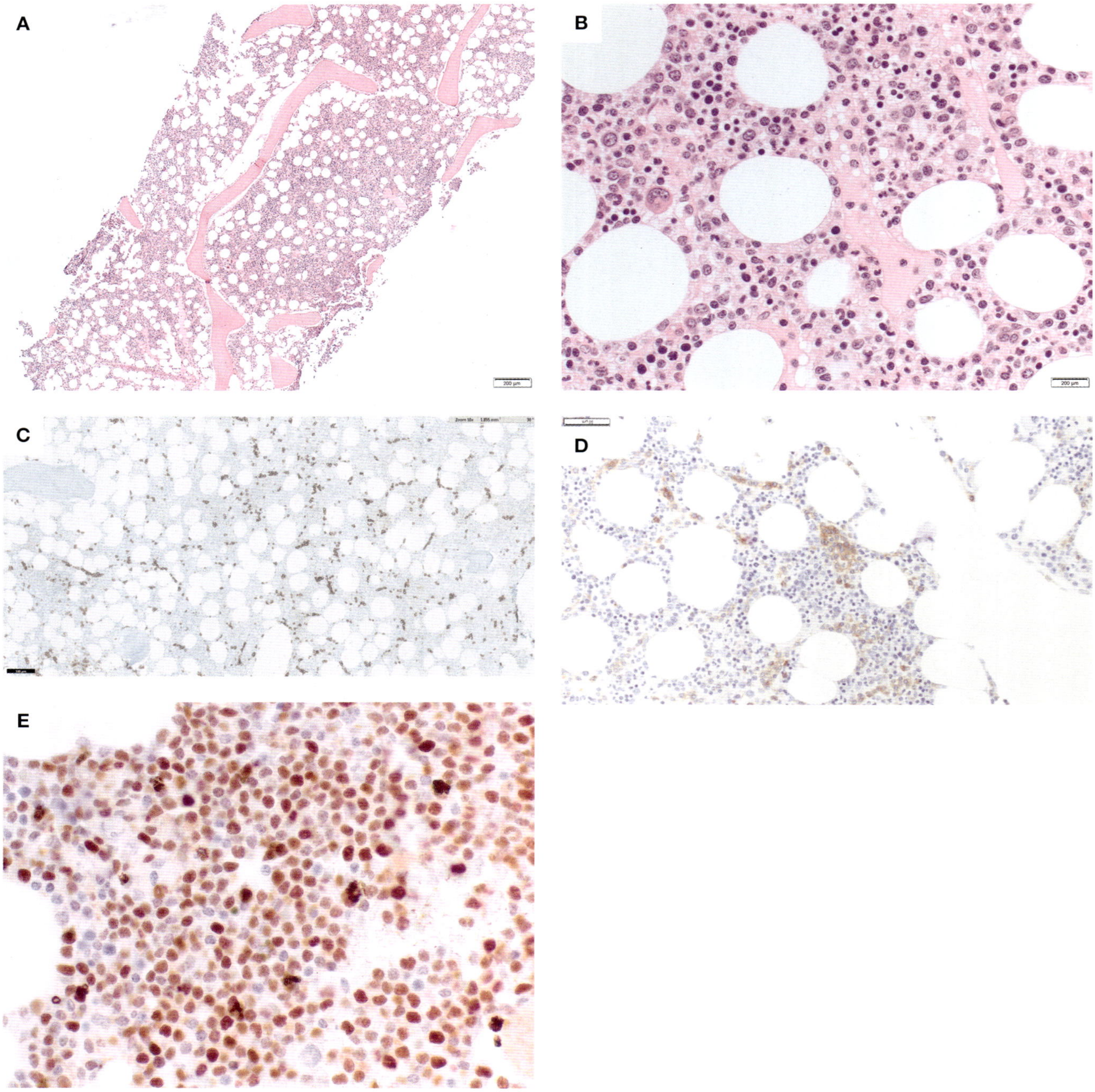

FIGURE 47.2 Bone marrow infiltration by splenic diffuse red pulp small B-cell lymphoma. Interstitial and intrasinusoidal pattern (**A** and **B**); more evident after CD20 staining (**C**). Neoplastic cells express CD11c (**D**) and frequently CyclinD3 (**E**).

Epidemiology

HCLv is a rare B-cell disorder that accounts for approximately 10% of HCL cases. It affects elderly or middle-aged patients with a male predominance.[21]

General Clinical Features

The main features are splenomegaly, PB lymphocytosis, and absence of monocytopenia.[21] Signs and symptoms may be due to either splenomegaly or cytopenias.

Morphology

The neoplastic cells in the PB exhibit cytologic features that are a hybrid of B-cell prolymphocytic leukemia and classic HCL (Figure 47.4A). A combination of prominent central nucleoli and cytoplasmic hairy projections is the most typical feature.

BM histology shows mostly an interstitial and/or sinusoidal pattern without lymphoid nodules (Figure 47.4B-E). Fibrosis is usually absent.[22]

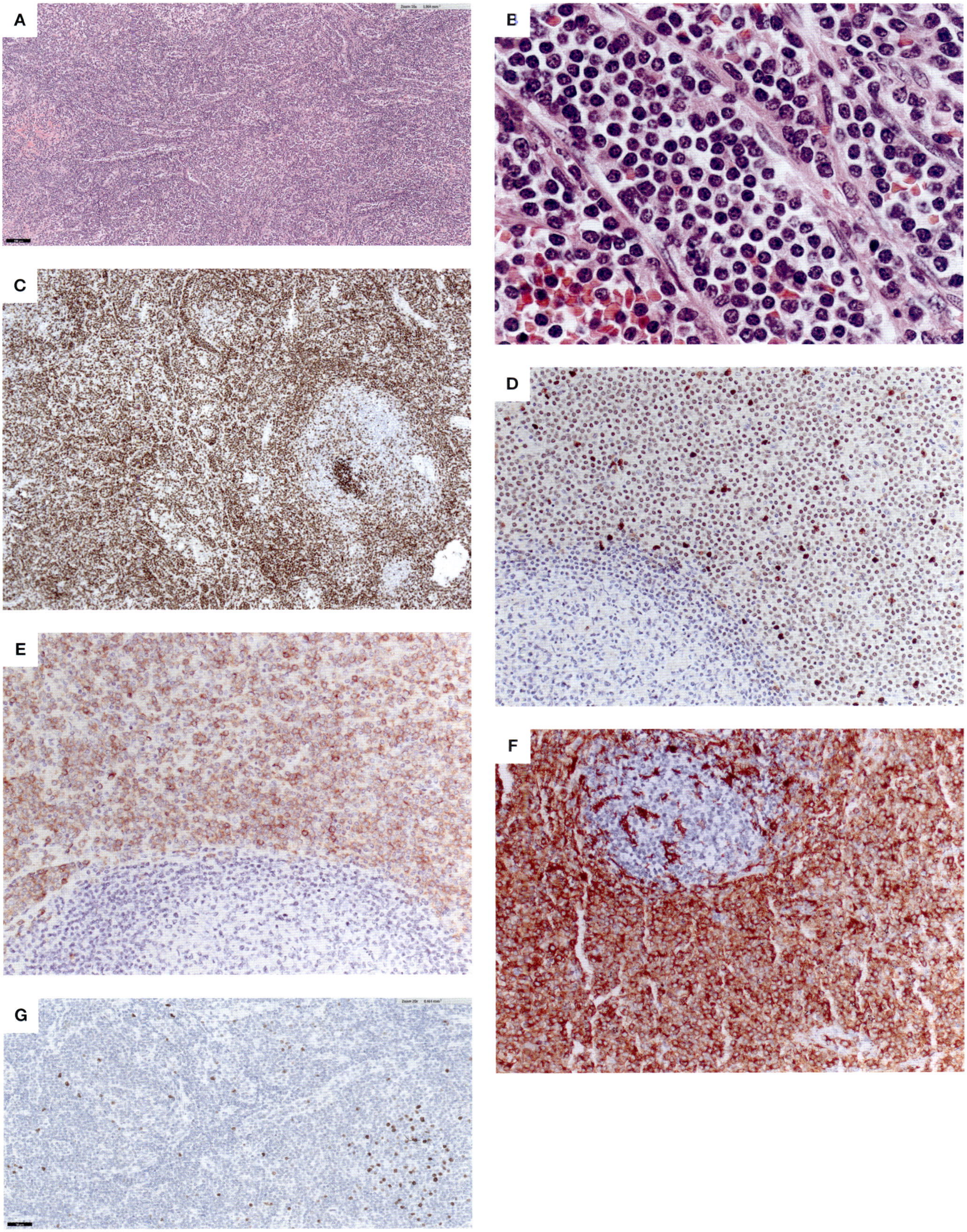

FIGURE 47.3 Spleen infiltration by splenic diffuse red pulp small B-cell lymphoma has a characteristic pattern, with red pulp expansion **(A)**, intrasinusoidal infiltration **(B)** by small monomorphous lymphocytes and residual lymphoid follicles. Neoplastic cells express B-cell markers such as PAX5 **(C)** and marginal zone markers, such as MNDA **(D)**, DBA44 **(E)**, and CD11c **(F)**. Low Ki67 **(G)**, contrast with the higher proliferation present in a partially replaced germinal center.

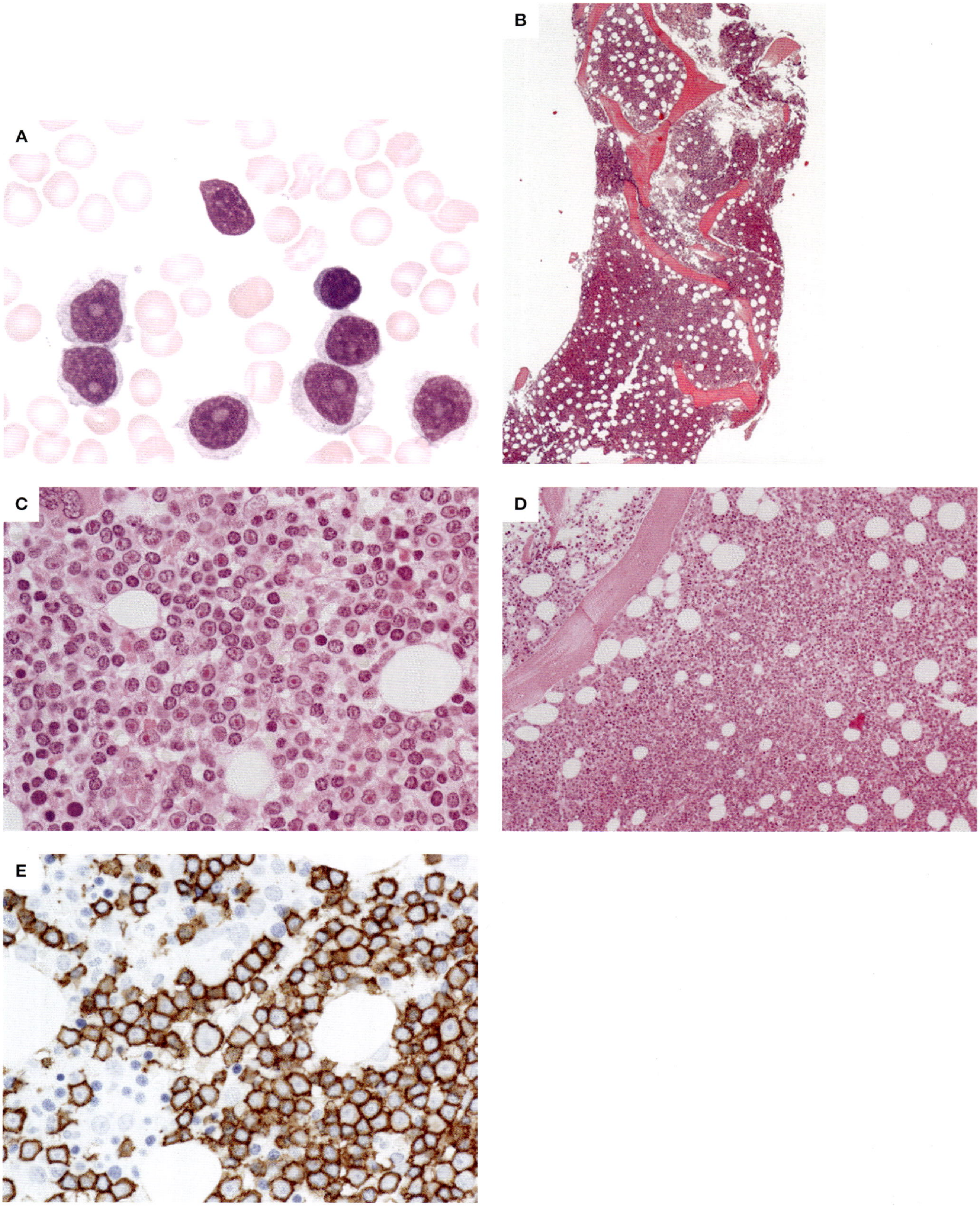

FIGURE 47.4 Peripheral blood characteristic cytology of hairy cell leukemia variant, showing large cells with prominent nucleolus and hairy cytoplasmatic projections (**A**). Bone marrow infiltration (**B-D**) with a diffuse and interstitial pattern. High-power view illustrates the large cells with large nucleolus. Neoplastic cells are CD20-positive (**E**).

Spleen histology shows an expansion of the red pulp, with partial or total disappearance of the white pulp. The neoplastic cells infiltrate the sinusoids and may form red blood cell lakes, like in classic HCL.

Immunophenotype

The immunophenotype is that of a clonal B cell with expression of both CD11c and CD103. However, unlike classical HCL, the tumor cells are negative for CD25, CD123, and CD200.[23] In contrast with classic HCL, HCLv cells are also negative for Annexin A1 and Cyclin D1.

Genetics

Mutational studies of HCLv have not identified *BRAF* V600E mutations but have shown frequent mutations in *MAP2K1* (48% of cases), a potential therapeutic target for MEK inhibitors.[24-26] Approximately 38% of patients with HCLv have an abnormal p53 gene either as a result of deletion or mutation.

HCLv frequently uses IGHV4-34 in the unmutated conformation (40% of all HCLv). This group typically has higher blood cell count at diagnosis, shorter overall survival, and poor response to single-agent cladribine.[27,28]

Prognosis and Clinical Comment

The course is chronic but more aggressive than in classic HCL, with median survival of 7 to 9 years. The five-year survival probability is 57%.[29] There remains no clear optimal treatment for HCLv. Durable remissions of HCLv have been observed with the combination of cladribine plus rituximab.[30] Ibrutinib has been shown to induce objective responses, resulting in prolonged disease control.[31,32] Patients with HCLv should be possibly entered into clinical trials.[33] A potential role for MEK inhibitors has been proposed for *MAP2K1*-mutated HCLv cases.[34,35]

References

1. Traverse-Glehen A, Verney A, Gazzo S, et al. Splenic diffuse red pulp lymphoma has a distinct pattern of somatic mutations amongst B-cell malignancies. *Leuk Lymphoma*. 2017;58(3):666-675.
2. Kanellis G, Mollejo M, Montes-Moreno S, et al. Splenic diffuse red pulp small B-cell lymphoma: revision of a series of cases reveals characteristic clinico-pathological features. *Haematologica*. 2010;95(7):1122-1129.
3. Traverse-Glehen A, Baseggio L, Bauchu EC, et al. Splenic red pulp lymphoma with numerous basophilic villous lymphocytes: a distinct clinicopathologic and molecular entity? *Blood*. 2008;111(4):2253-2260.
4. Xochelli A, Kalpadakis C, Gardiner A, et al. Clonal B-cell lymphocytosis exhibiting immunophenotypic features consistent with a marginal-zone origin: is this a distinct entity? *Blood*. 2014;123(8):1199-1206.
5. Heraud I, Mauduit C, Golfier C, Grange B, Baseggio L. Monoclonal B-cell lymphocytosis with a non-CLL immunophenotype—review of 34 cases. *Ann Biol Clin*. 2023;81(2):162-167. doi:10.1684/abc.2023.1803
6. Traverse-Glehen A, Baseggio L, Salles G, Coiffier B, Felman P, Berger F. Splenic diffuse red pulp small-B cell lymphoma: toward the emergence of a new lymphoma entity. *Discov Med*. 2012;13(71):253-265.
7. Papadaki T, Stamatopoulos K, Belessi C, et al. Splenic marginal-zone lymphoma: one or more entities? A histologic, immunohistochemical, and molecular study of 42 cases. *Am J Surg Pathol*. 2007;31(3):438-446.
8. Curiel-Olmo S, Mondéjar R, Almaraz C, et al. Splenic diffuse red pulp small B-cell lymphoma displays increased expression of cyclin D3 and recurrent CCND3 mutations. *Blood*. 2017;129(8):1042-1045.
9. Ozkaya N, Jaffe ES. Splenic diffuse red pulp small B-cell lymphoma with cyclin D3 expression cyclin D3 expression. *Blood*. 2022;140(7):793. doi:10.1182/blood.2022016694
10. Favre R, Manzoni D, Traverse-Glehen A, et al. Usefulness of CD200 in the differential diagnosis of SDRPL, SMZL, and HCL. *Int J Lab Hematol*. 2018;40(4):e59-e62.
11. Baseggio L, Traverse-Glehen A, Callet-Bauchu E, et al. Relevance of a scoring system including CD11c expression in the identification of splenic diffuse red pulp small B-cell lymphoma (SRPL). *Hematol Oncol*. 2011;29(1):47-51.
12. Martinez D, Navarro A, Martinez-Trillos A, et al. NOTCH1, TP53, and MAP2K1 mutations in splenic diffuse red pulp small B-cell lymphoma are associated with progressive disease. *Am J Surg Pathol*. 2016;40(2):192-201.
13. Bikos V, Darzentas N, Hadzidimitriou A, et al. Over 30% of patients with splenic marginal zone lymphoma express the same immunoglobulin heavy variable gene: ontogenetic implications. *Leukemia*. 2012;26(7):1638-1646.
14. Jallades L, Baseggio L, Sujobert P, et al. Exome sequencing identifies recurrent BCOR alterations and the absence of KLF2, TNFAIP3 and MYD88 mutations in splenic diffuse red pulp small B-cell lymphoma. *Haematologica*. 2017;102(10):1758-1766.
15. Salido M, Baró C, Oscier D, et al. Cytogenetic aberrations and their prognostic value in a series of 330 splenic marginal zone B-cell lymphomas: a multicenter study of the Splenic B-Cell Lymphoma Group. *Blood*. 2010;116(9):1479-1488.

16. Traverse-Glehen A, Bachy E, Baseggio L, et al. Immunoarchitectural patterns in splenic marginal zone lymphoma: correlations with chromosomal aberrations, IGHV mutations, and survival. A study of 76 cases. *Histopathology*. 2013;62(6):876-893.
17. Oscier D, Stamatopoulos K, Mirandari A, Strefford J. The genomics of hairy cell leukaemia and splenic diffuse red pulp lymphoma cell leukaemia and splenic diffuse red pulp lymphoma. *Cancers*. 2022;14(3):697. doi:10.3390/cancers14030697
18. Christensen LM, Severinsen MT, Katoch P, et al. An aggressive course of transformed splenic diffuse red pulp small B-cell lymphoma with novel somatic loss-of-function mutation in RB1. *J Hematol*. 2023;12(3):118-122.
19. Lopedote P, Nawaiseh AA, Malek A, et al. Early progression and transformation of a splenic diffuse red pulp small B-cell lymphoma with NOTCH1, ARID2, CREBBP, and TNFRSF14 gene mutations. *Leuk Res Rep*. 2023;20:100384.
20. Traverse-Glehen A, Baseggio L, Callet-Bauchu E, et al. Hairy cell leukaemia-variant and splenic red pulp lymphoma: a single entity? *Br J Haematol*. 2010;150(1):113-116.
21. Matutes E, Wotherspoon A, Catovsky D. The variant form of hairy-cell leukaemia. *Best Pract Res Clin Haematol*. 2003;16(1):41-56.
22. Cessna MH, Hartung L, Tripp S, Perkins SL, Bahler DW. Hairy cell leukemia variant: fact or fiction. *Am J Clin Pathol*. 2005;123(1):132-138.
23. Matutes E, Martínez-Trillos A, Campo E. Hairy cell leukaemia-variant: disease features and treatment. *Best Pract Res Clin Haematol*. 2015;28(4):253-263.
24. Waterfall JJ, Arons E, Walker RL, et al. High prevalence of MAP2K1 mutations in variant and IGHV4-34-expressing hairy-cell leukemias. *Nat Genet*. 2014;46(1):8-10.
25. Maitre E, Tomowiak C, Lebecque B, et al. Deciphering genetic alterations of hairy cell leukemia and hairy cell leukemia-like disorders in 98 patients. *Cancers*. 2022;14(8):1904.
26. Xi L, Arons E, Navarro W, et al. Both variant and IGHV4-34-expressing hairy cell leukemia lack the BRAF V600E mutation. *Blood*. 2012;119(14):3330-3332.
27. Arons E, Kreitman RJ. Molecular variant of hairy cell leukemia with poor prognosis. *Leuk Lymphoma*. 2011;52(suppl 2):99-102.
28. Hockley SL, Giannouli S, Morilla A, et al. Insight into the molecular pathogenesis of hairy cell leukaemia, hairy cell leukaemia variant and splenic marginal zone lymphoma, provided by the analysis of their IGH rearrangements and somatic hypermutation patterns. *Br J Haematol*. 2010;148(4):666-669.
29. Hockley SL, Else M, Morilla A, et al. The prognostic impact of clinical and molecular features in hairy cell leukaemia variant and splenic marginal zone lymphoma. *Br J Haematol*. 2012;158(3):347-354.
30. Chihara D, Arons E, Stetler-Stevenson M, et al. Long term follow-up of a phase II study of cladribine with concurrent rituximab with hairy cell leukemia variant. *Blood Adv*. 2021;5(23):4807-4816.
31. Paillassa J, Safa F, Troussard X. Updates in hairy cell leukemia (HCL) and variant-type HCL (HCL-V): rationale for targeted treatments with a focus on ibrutinib. *Ther Adv Hematol*. 2022;13:20406207221090886.
32. Rogers KA, Andritsos LA, Wei L, et al. Phase 2 study of ibrutinib in classic and variant hairy cell leukemia. *Blood*. 2021;137(25):3473-3483.
33. Parry-Jones N, Joshi A, Forconi F, Dearden C; BSH Guidelines Committee. Guideline for diagnosis and management of hairy cell leukaemia (HCL) and hairy cell variant (HCL-V). *Br J Haematol*. 2020;191(5):730-737.
34. Andritsos LA, Grieselhuber NR, Anghelina M, et al. Trametinib for the treatment of IGHV4-34, MAP2K1-mutant variant hairy cell leukemia. *Leuk Lymphoma*. 2018;59(4):1008-1011.
35. Grever M, Andritsos L, Anghelina M, et al. Hairy cell leukemia variant and WHO classification correspondence Re: 5th edition WHO classification haematolymphoid tumors: lymphoid neoplasms. *Leukemia*. 2024;38(7):1642-1644.

Chapter 48
Lymphoplasmacytic Lymphoma

James R. Cook, Pei Lin, and Steven Treon

Definition

Lymphoplasmacytic lymphoma (LPL) is a neoplasm of small B cells, plasmacytoid cells, and plasma cells that usually involves the bone marrow and sometimes lymph node and spleen and is associated with a *MYD88* L265P mutation in >95% of cases. Waldenstrom macroglobulinemia (WM) is defined as an IgM paraprotein due to bone marrow involvement by LPL; many, but not all, patients with LPL meet criteria for WM.

Synonyms

None.

Epidemiology

LPL presents at a median age in the seventh decade and is approximately twice as common in white populations than in other ethnic groups.[1,2] There is a male predominance (male:female ratio approximately 2:1). IgM monoclonal gammopathy of undetermined significance (MGUS) is considered a precursor lesion with an approximately 200-fold risk of developing LPL/WM.[1,3] A familial predisposition has been reported in approximately 20% of cases, and an increased risk has been described in association with autoimmune disorders.

General Clinical Features

Approximately 30% of patients are asymptomatic and identified incidentally upon serum protein electrophoresis studies. In symptomatic cases, patients may present with weakness, fatigue, or anemia. Most cases are associated with a monoclonal IgM paraprotein, but a minority of cases may show an IgG or IgA monoclonal protein or may be nonsecretory. Hyperviscosity, identified in 10% to 30% of patients, is associated with higher levels of IgM protein, especially above 60 g/L.[4] Other symptoms attributable to the monoclonal IgM protein may include cryoglobulinemia (found in approximately 20% of patients), peripheral neuropathy due to anti-myelin sheath antigen reactivity, or amyloid deposition. IgM reactivity against clotting factors, fibrin, or platelets may produce coagulopathy and/or thrombocytopenia. Primary cold agglutinin disease is now considered to represent a distinct lymphoproliferative disorder.

Morphology

Bone marrow and peripheral blood

The neoplastic cells display a characteristic spectrum of morphology ranging from small mature lymphocytes with clumped chromatin and scant cytoplasm to lymphoplasmacytoid forms and well-differentiated plasma cells. This cytologic spectrum may be best

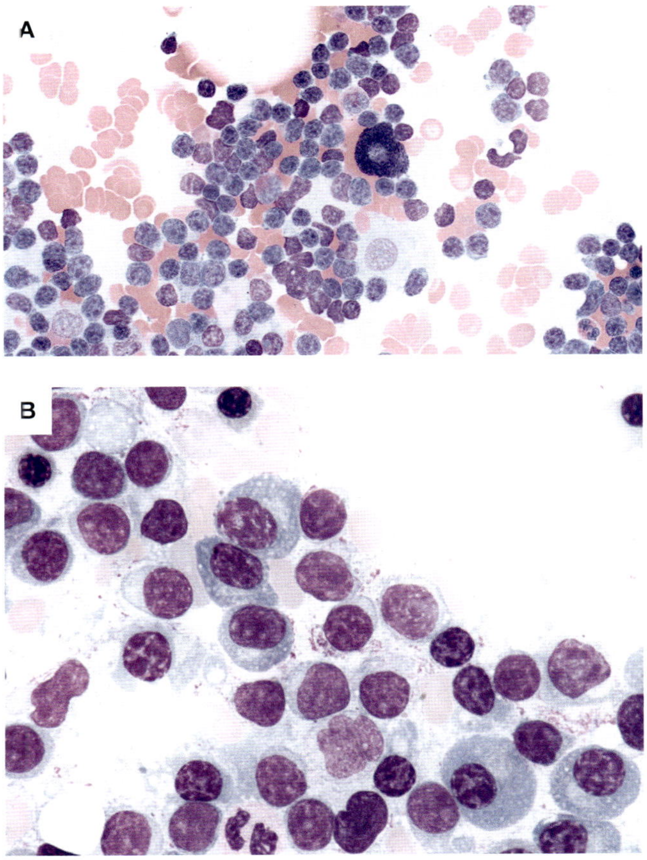

FIGURE 48.1 Lymphoplasmacytic lymphoma. **A:** Bone marrow aspirate smear with numerous small mature lymphocytes and an admixed mast cell. **B:** The lymphocytes exhibit a spectrum of morphology from small mature forms with scant cytoplasm to plasmacytoid forms with eccentric nuclei and occasional well-differentiated plasma cells.

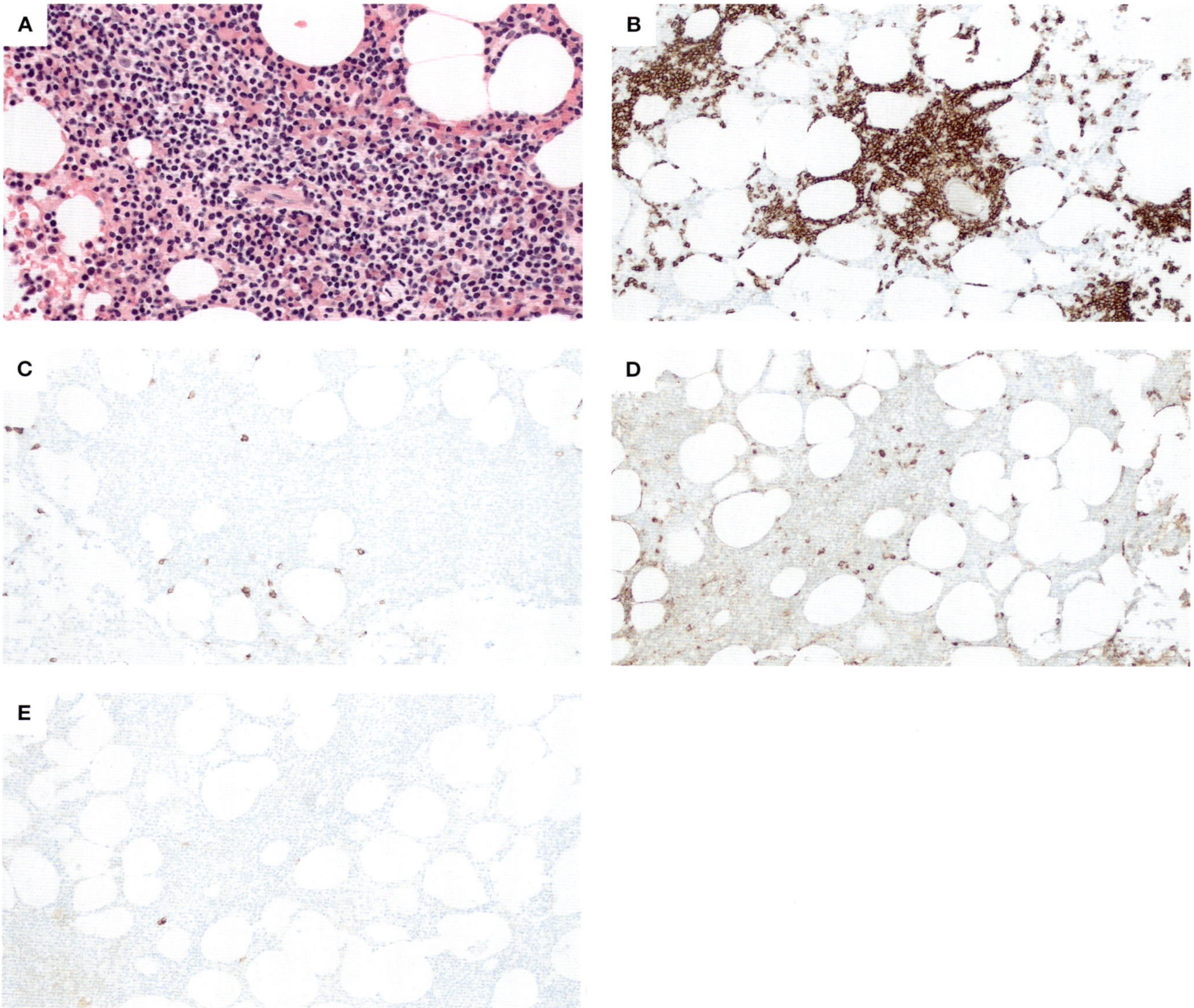

FIGURE 48.2 Lymphoplasmacytic lymphoma. **A:** Bone marrow trephine biopsy with an interstitial lymphoplasmacytic aggregate. **B:** The aggregate contains predominantly small B cells (CD20 stain). **C:** Few plasma cells are admixed (CD138 stain). **D:** The plasmacytic cells are monotypic for kappa light chains. **E:** Only rare background lambda-positive plasma cells are present.

appreciated on aspirate smears (Figure 48.1). Increased mast cells are common within the lymphoplasmacytic aggregates. In bone marrow biopsies, LPL typically exhibits an interstitial or diffuse growth pattern (Figure 48.2). In some cases a paratrabecullar pattern may be identified. A distinctly intrasinusoidal growth pattern should prompt consideration of a diagnosis of splenic marginal zone lymphoma rather than LPL.[2,5,6]

In the 2016 World Health Organization classification, establishing a diagnosis of LPL required finding a lymphoplasmacytic infiltrate in ≥10% of a trephine core biopsy.[7] However, this requirement conflicted with the longstanding criteria of the International Workshop on Waldenstrom's Macroglobulinemia, which recognized LPL/WM with <10% bone marrow infiltration.[8] The International Consensus Classification clinical advisory committee concluded that a diagnosis of LPL may be rendered in cases with abnormal lymphoplasmacytic aggregates in the setting of clonal B cells and clonal plasma cells, even with <10% of a core biopsy cellularity.[9] In challenging cases where it remains unclear whether aggregates are reactive rather than neoplastic, a diagnosis of IgM MGUS may be more appropriate.

Peripheral blood involvement is common in LPL. While absolute lymphocyte counts are typically lower than in chronic lymphocytic leukemia, approximately half show monoclonal B cells by flow cytometry and an even higher proportion show evidence of clonality by molecular methods.[10] The neoplastic cells in the peripheral blood show a spectrum of features similar to that seen in the bone marrow, ranging from small mature forms with scant cytoplasm to lymphoplasmacytoid or plasmacytic forms.

Lymph nodes and other extramedullary tissues

The most classic pattern of lymph node involvement by LPL, which is usually associated with WM, displays preserved architecture with patent sinuses and scattered residual germinal centers (Figure 48.3).[6,11-14] The paracortical and medullary areas contain a relatively monotonous infiltrate of small mature lymphocytes admixed with fewer plasmacytoid forms and mature plasma cells. Dutcher bodies may be present. Hemosiderin deposits and increased mast cells are also frequently identified. Occasional large cells may be present but are generally inconspicuous. Amyloid deposition, nonamyloid immunoglobulin deposits, or crystal-storing histiocytes may be seen in some cases. Other LPL cases show a more varied histologic appearance with architectural effacement, extension into extracapsular soft tissues, prominent epithelioid histiocytes, a more extensive plasmacytic component, or increased numbers of scattered large cells (Figure 48.4).

The histologic findings at other sites have been incompletely described. In the spleen, a diffuse or nodular lymphocytic infiltrate may be seen in the red pulp, sometimes with involvement of the white pulp nodules.[2,6] The diagnosis of LPL at other extramedullary sites should be made only with extreme caution in the absence of a known diagnosis of LPL in bone marrow or lymph nodes. Central nervous system (CNS) involvement (Bing-Neel syndrome; BNS) may be diagnosed by demonstration of LPL infiltration of CNS parenchyma or meningeal biopsies or with involvement of cerebrospinal fluid. Molecular testing for mutated *MYD88* (see later discussion) may also be helpful in the diagnosis of BNS.

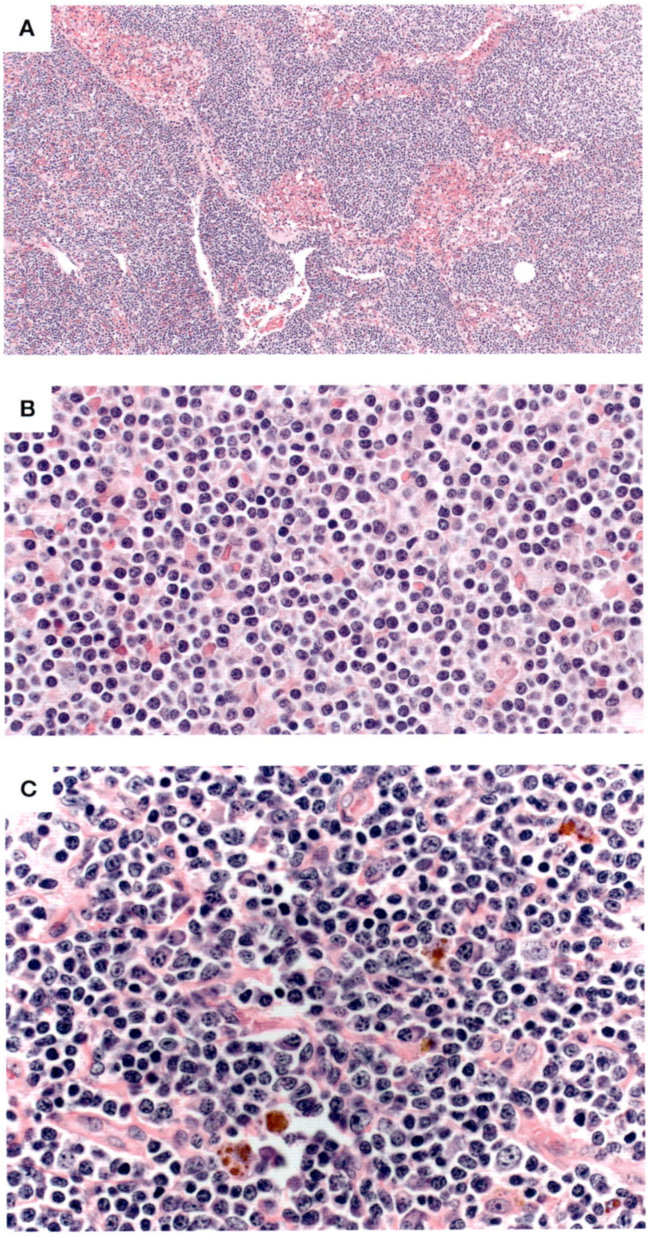

FIGURE 48.3 Lymphoplasmacytic lymphoma (LPL). **A:** Classic pattern of lymph node involvement by LPL with widely patent sinuses and a monomorphic small lymphocytic infiltrate. **B:** The infiltrate is composed predominantly of small lymphocytes with mature chromatin and scant cytoplasm and occasional plasmacytoid forms with more abundant cytoplasm. **C:** This nodal LPL shows conspicuous hemosiderin deposition within an infiltrate of small lymphocytes and plasmacytoid forms.

Immunophenotype

The neoplastic B cells are positive for CD19, CD20, CD22, CD79a, and CD45. CD25 and CD38 are often present. The B cells show surface immunoglobulin light chain restriction, and most cases express IgM heavy chains. The B cells are typically negative for CD5, CD10, and CD23, although rare cases may express any of these markers.[2,6,15] By immunohistochemistry, LPL is negative for LEF1 and Cyclin D1. Expression of IRTA1 and CD180 appears to be rare and favors a diagnosis of marginal zone lymphoma over LPL.

Plasma cells in LPL are positive for CD19 and negative for CD56 or CD117, in contrast to multiple

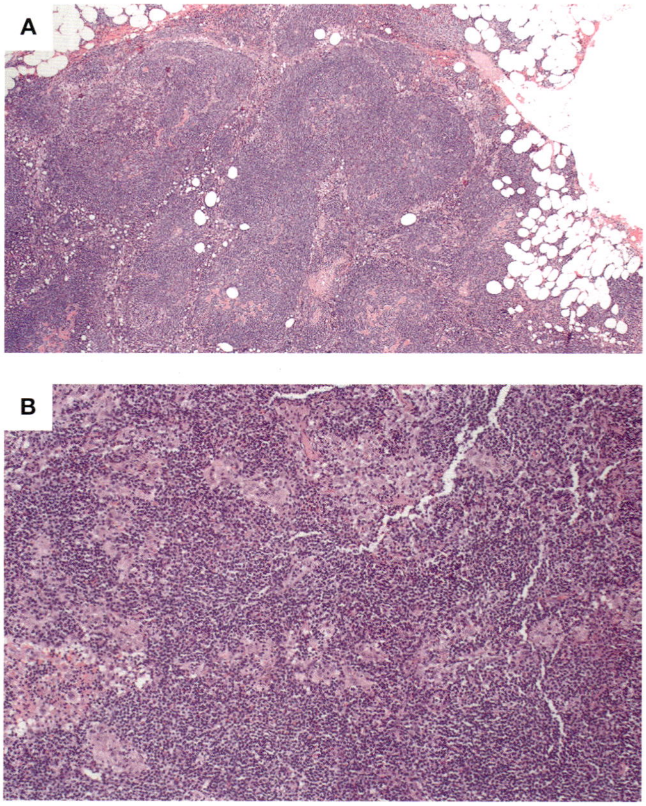

FIGURE 48.4 Lymphoplasmacytic lymphoma (LPL). **A:** Nodal LPL with a vaguely nodular pattern, patent sinuses, and extension of the neoplastic infiltrate into perinodal soft tissues. **B:** LPL with architectural effacement and prominent epithelioid histiocytes.

myeloma or other plasma cell neoplasms. CD38 and CD138 are generally positive, and plasma cells exhibit light chain restriction. In some cases, the clonal plasma cells may be masked by background polytypic plasma cells, but the inability to document clonal plasma cells by either flow cytometry or immunohistochemistry should raise the possibility of alternate diagnoses. The diagnosis of IgM myeloma should be considered in patients with very high IgM levels and plasma cell predominant bone marrow disease, and evaluation for *MYD88* mutation, t(11;14) *IGH::CCND1*, and Cyclin D1 protein expression should be performed.[16]

Genetics

LPL exhibits monoclonal immunoglobulin heavy chain (IGH) and light chain rearrangements detectable by polymerase chain reaction (PCR). The IGH variable regions show somatic hypermutation without ongoing mutations.[17] There is evidence of biased IGHV segment usage.

The *MYD88* L265P mutation is found in >95% of cases utilizing sensitive methods, with a lower incidence reported in non-IgM cases.[2,6,15-17] The mutated *MYD88* gene triggers phosphorylation of IRAK-1/IRAK-4 as well as BTK leading to activation of downstream prosurvival signaling pathways including NF-KB and ERK1/2 (Figure 48.5).[18] Cases of LPL lacking *MYD88* L265P may show other mutations in *MYD88* or other mutations in the downstream NF-KB pathway.[2,15,16] *MYD88* mutations are not specific for LPL, being identified in diffuse large B-cell lymphoma, not otherwise specified (DLBCL, NOS) of activated B-cell type, primary cutaneous DLBCL of leg type, primary CNS or testicular DLBCL, and a small percentage of other small B-cell neoplasms including marginal zone lymphomas.

Somatic *CXCR4* mutations are identified in approximately 30% to 40% of cases. More than 40 different missense and nonsense *CXCR4* mutations have been described, most commonly truncating mutations at codon S338, similar to the germline mutations seen in warts, hypogammaglobulinemia, immunodeficiency, and myelokathexis syndrome.[2,16,17] Next-generation sequencing (NGS) may miss two-thirds of patients who carry *CXCR4* mutations, particularly those with lower bone marrow (BM) disease burden (<40%).[19] Newer NGS platforms utilizing molecular barcoding with deeper sequencing may improve detection. Recent consensus recommendations recommend allele-specific PCR to evaluate for the most common *CXCR4* nonsense variant S338X.[20]

Routine testing for *MYD88* and *CXCR4* is strongly encouraged at initial diagnosis.[15,17] *TP53* alterations should also be evaluated, which are more common in previously treated patients with WM.[20] Other recurrent mutations include *CD79B*, *KMT2D*, and *ARID1A*.

The most common recurrent cytogenetic abnormality is deletion of chromosome 6q, reported in 30% to 60% of bone marrow–based cases.[2,6,9,15,16,21] Del(6q) is a nonspecific finding that may also be seen in other B-cell neoplasms and may be less common in nodal LPL.[22] Other recurrent cytogenetic abnormalities include +4, del(11q), del(17p), and +18.

Prognosis and Clinical Comment

The extent of bone marrow involvement by LPL does not necessarily correlate with the presence or absence of symptoms, the serum monoclonal protein concentration, or need for therapy. Treatment-naïve patients with LPL/WM with <10% bone marrow can present with symptomatic disease and require therapy as evidenced by their participation in numerous clinical trials.[8] Many of these patients have morbidity attributable to the monoclonal IgM protein including but not

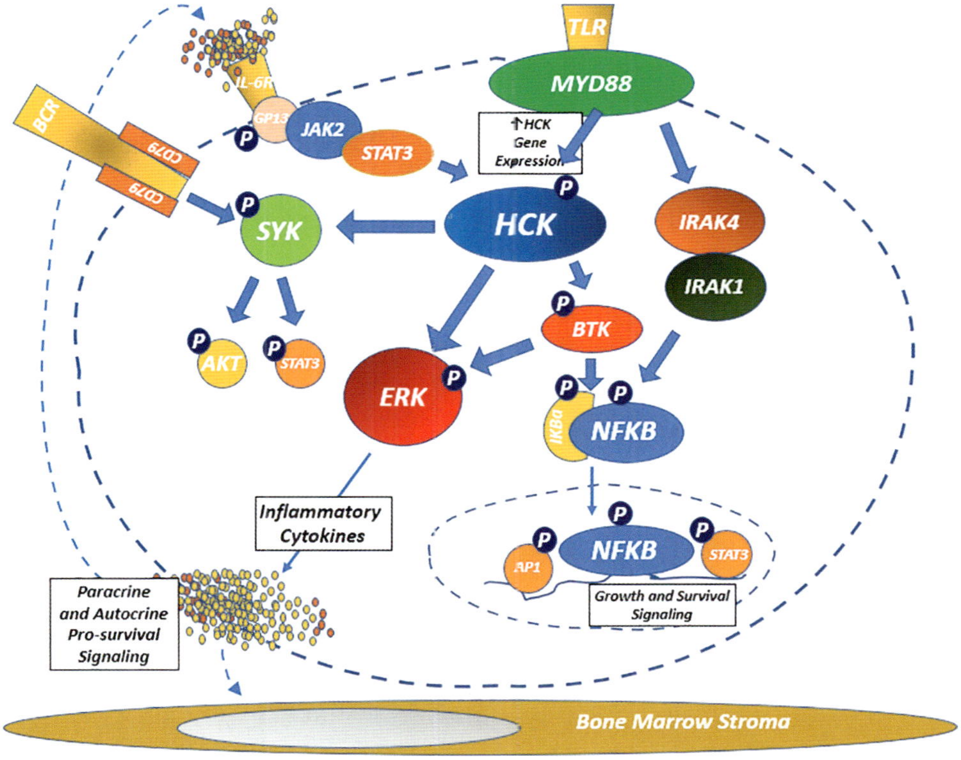

FIGURE 48.5 Lymphoplasmacytic lymphoma. Increased activation of the MYD88 signaling pathway in the presence of *MYD88* mutations leads to activation of the NF-KB and ERK pathways, promoting growth and survival.

limited to demyelinating peripheral neuropathy, cryoglobulinemia, cold agglutinemia, anti-phospholipid antibody syndrome, and hyperviscosity syndrome. Conversely, other patients may fulfill the diagnostic criteria for LPL/WM without symptoms related to their disease. These patients are termed as having "asymptomatic WM," also referred to as "smoldering WM." Asymptomatic patients do not meet criteria for initiation of treatment based on consensus criteria.[8]

The mutational profile in LPL impacts disease presentation, prognosis, treatment outcomes, and survival. Patients with *MYD88* wild-type WM have a high risk for disease transformation and/or shorter overall survival.[16] Patients with *MYD88* wild-type show poor response to the BTK inhibitor ibrutinib but appear more sensitive to zanubrutinib.[23] Outcomes with bendamustine-based therapy are also impacted by *MYD88* mutation status, with shorter progression-free survival noted for patients with *MYD88* wild-type WM.[24] Patients with nonsense *CXCR4* mutations such as S338X show higher BM disease burden, higher serum IgM levels and/or symptomatic hyperviscosity, shorter time to initial treatment, and/or shorter overall survival in WM. *CXCR4* mutations, particularly nonsense variants can also impact treatment outcomes with BTK inhibitors.[20,23,25] A longer time to major response attainment and fewer major responses, as well as shorter progression-free survival, have been reported in BTK inhibitor trials. Alterations in *TP53* ($TP53^{Alt}$) that include somatic mutations and 17p deletions occur in 5% to 10% of treatment-naïve patients with WM. A recent study showed that $TP53^{Alt}$ were markedly higher (up to 30%) among previously treated patients with WM, nearly all of whom received prior alkylator (85%) or nucleoside analogue (22%) therapy.[23,26] Patients with WM with $TP53^{Alt}$ show shorter overall survival and/or progression-free survival with BTK inhibitors.[23,27]

References

1. McMaster ML. The epidemiology of Waldenstrom macroglobulinemia. *Semin Hematol.* 2023;60(2):65-72. doi:10.1053/j.seminhematol.2023.03.008
2. Wang W, Lin P. Lymphoplasmacytic lymphoma and Waldenstrom macroglobulinaemia: clinicopathological features and differential diagnosis. *Pathology.* 2020;52(1):6-14. doi:10.1016/j.pathol.2019.09.009
3. Kyle RA, Rajkumar SV, Therneau TM, Larson DR, Plevak MF, Melton LJ III. Prognostic factors and predictors of outcome of immunoglobulin M monoclonal gammopathy of undetermined significance. *Clin Lymphoma.* 2005;5(4):257-260. doi:10.3816/clm.2005.n.011

4. Gustine JN, Meid K, Dubeau T, et al. Serum IgM level as predictor of symptomatic hyperviscosity in patients with Waldenstrom macroglobulinaemia. *Br J Haematol.* 2017;177(5):717-725. doi:10.1111/bjh.14743
5. Bassarova A, Trøen G, Spetalen S, Micci F, Tierens A, Delabie J. Lymphoplasmacytic lymphoma and marginal zone lymphoma in the bone marrow: paratrabecular involvement as an important distinguishing feature. *Am J Clin Pathol.* 2015;143(6):797-806. doi:10.1309/AJCP6ZODWV1CIDME
6. Lin P, Molina TJ, Cook JR, Swerdlow SH. Lymphoplasmacytic lymphoma and other non-marginal zone lymphomas with plasmacytic differentiation. *Am J Clin Pathol.* 2011;136(2):195-210. doi:10.1309/AJCP8FOIVTB6LBER
7. Swerdlow SH, Sohani AR, Pileri SA, Harris NL, Jaffe ES, Stein H. Lymphoplasmacytic lymphoma. In: Swerdlow SHCE, Harris NL, Jaffe ES, eds. WHO Classification of Tumours of Haematopoietic and Lymphoid Tissues. Revised 4th ed. IARC Press; 2017:232-235.
8. Treon SP, Tedeschi A, San-Miguel J, et al. Report of consensus Panel 4 from the 11th International Workshop on Waldenstrom's macroglobulinemia on diagnostic and response criteria. *Semin Hematol.* 2023;60(2):97-106. doi:10.1053/j.seminhematol.2023.03.009
9. Campo E, Jaffe ES, Cook JR, et al. The International consensus classification of mature lymphoid neoplasms: a report from the clinical advisory committee. *Blood.* 2022;140(11):1229-1253. doi:10.1182/blood.2022015851
10. Montesdeoca S, Garcia-Gisbert N, Calvo X, et al. Leukemic involvement is a common feature in Waldenstrom macroglobulinemia at diagnosis. *Cancers.* 2023;15(16):4152. doi:10.3390/cancers15164152
11. Hamadeh F, MacNamara SP, Aguilera NS, Swerdlow SH, Cook JR. MYD88 L265P mutation analysis helps define nodal lymphoplasmacytic lymphoma. *Mod Pathol.* 2015;28(4):564-574. doi:10.1038/modpathol.2014.120
12. Lin P, Bueso-Ramos C, Wilson CS, Mansoor A, Medeiros LJ. Waldenstrom macroglobulinemia involving extramedullary sites: morphologic and immunophenotypic findings in 44 patients. *Am J Surg Pathol.* 2003;27(8):1104-1113.
13. Cook JR, Aguilera NI, Reshmi-Skarja S, et al. Lack of PAX5 rearrangements in lymphoplasmacytic lymphomas: reassessing the reported association with t(9;14). *Hum Pathol.* 2004;35(4):447-454. doi:S004681770300618X [pii].
14. Andriko JAWA, Swerdlow SH, Aguilera NI, Abbondanzo SL. Is lymphoplasmacytic lymphoma/immunocytoma a distinct entity? A clinicopathologic study of 20 cases. *Am J Surg Pathol.* 2001;25(6):742-751.
15. Fend F, Dogan A, Cook JR. Plasma cell neoplasms and related entities-evolution in diagnosis and classification. *Virchows Arch.* 2023;482(1):163-177. doi:10.1007/s00428-022-03431-3
16. Treon SP, Gustine JN, Xu L, et al MYD88 wild-type Waldenstrom macroglobulinaemia: differential diagnosis, risk of histological transformation, and overall survival. *Br J Haematol.* 2018;180(3):374-380.
17. Wagner SD, Martinelli V, Luzzatto L. Similar patterns of V kappa gene usage but different degrees of somatic mutation in hairy cell leukemia, prolymphocytic leukemia, Waldenstrom's macroglobulinemia, and myeloma. *Blood.* 1994;83(12):3647-3653.
18. Yang G, Zhou Y, Liu X, et al. A mutation in MYD88 (L265P) supports the survival of lymphoplasmacytic cells by activation of Bruton tyrosine kinase in Waldenström macroglobulinemia. *Blood.* 2013;122(7):1222-1232.
19. Gustine JN, Xu L, Yang G, et al. Bone marrow involvement and subclonal diversity impairs detection of mutated CXCR4 by diagnostic next-generation sequencing in Waldenström macroglobulinaemia. *Br J Haematol.* 2021;194(4):730-733.
20. Garcia-Sanz R, Varettoni M, Jimenez C, et al. Report of consensus panel 3 from the 11th International workshop on Waldenstrom's macroglobulinemia: recommendations for molecular diagnosis in Waldenstrom's macroglobulinemia. *Semin Hematol.* 2023;60(2):90-96. doi:10.1053/j.seminhematol.2023.03.007
21. de Leval L, Alizadeh AA, Bergsagel PL, et al. Genomic profiling for clinical decision making in lymphoid neoplasms. *Blood.* 2022;140(21):2193-2227. doi:10.1182/blood.2022015854
22. Cook JR, Aguilera NI, Reshmi S, et al. Deletion 6q is not a characteristic marker of nodal lymphoplasmacytic lymphoma. *Cancer Genet Cytogenet.* 2005;162(1):85-88. S0165-4608(05)00220-7 [pii]. doi:10.1016/j.cancergencyto.2005.04.013
23. Dimopoulos MA, Opat S, D'Sa S, et al. Zanubrutinib versus ibrutinib in symptomatic Waldenstrom Macroglobulinemia: final analysis from the randomized phase III ASPEN study. *J Clin Oncol.* 2023;2023:JCO2202830. Published online doi:10.1200/JCO.22.02830
24. Laribi K, Poulain S, Willems L, et al. Bendamustine plus rituximab in newly-diagnosed Waldenström macroglobulinaemia patients. A study on behalf of the French Innovative Leukaemia Organization (FILO). *Br J Haematol.* 2019;186(1):146-149.
25. Treon SP, Cao Y, Xu L, Yang G, Liu X, Hunter ZR. Somatic mutations in MYD88 and CXCR4 are determinants of clinical presentation and overall survival in Waldenstrom macroglobulinemia. *Blood.* 2014;123(18):2791-2796.
26. Dimopoulos MA, Opat S, D'Sa S, et al. ASPEN biomarker analysis: response to BTK inhibitor treatment in patients with Waldenström Macroglobulinemia harboring CXCR4, TP53, and TERT mutations. *Proceedings of the 11th Internation Workshop on Waldenstrom's Macroglobulinemia*. 2020. Abstract WM041.
27. Poulain S, Roumier C, Bertrand E, et al. TP53 mutation and its prognostic significance in Waldenstrom's macroglobulinemia. *Clin Cancer Res.* 2017;23(20):6325-6335.

Chapter 49

IgM Monoclonal Gammopathy of Undetermined Significance

James R. Cook, Megan O. Nakashima, and Steven Treon

Definition

IgM monoclonal gammopathy of undetermined significance (IgM MGUS) is defined by a serum IgM monoclonal protein <30 g/L in the absence of features diagnostic of multiple myeloma, light chain amyloidosis, lymphoplasmacytic lymphoma, or other overt lymphoproliferative disorder (Table 49.1). IgM MGUS is further divided into two subtypes: IgM MGUS of plasma cell type, which represents a precursor of multiple myeloma or other plasma cell neoplasm, and IgM MGUS not otherwise specified (IgM MGUS, NOS), which may progress to lymphoplasmacytic lymphoma or other overt lymphoma (Table 49.2).

TABLE 49.1 Diagnostic criteria for IgM monoclonal gammopathy of undetermined significance

- Serum IgM monoclonal protein concentration <30 g/L
- Clonal bone marrow plasma cells <10%
- Criteria not met for lymphoplasmacytic lymphoma, other overt B-cell lymphoma, multiple myeloma, or other plasma cell neoplasm.

Modified from Rajkumar SV, Dimopoulos MA, Palumbo A, et al. International Myeloma Working Group updated criteria for the diagnosis of multiple myeloma. *Lancet Oncol.* 2014; 15(2):e538-e548.

TABLE 49.2 Criteria for plasma cell subtype of IgM monoclonal gammopathy of undetermined significance (IgM MGUS). Cases not meeting criteria for plasma cell subtype of IgM MGUS should be designated IgM MGUS, not otherwise specified

- Presence of t(11;14)(q13;q32) *IGH::CCND1* or other myeloma-associated *IGH* translocation.

or

- Clonal plasma cell population detected without clonal B-cell population and *MYD88* is wild-type.

Synonyms

None.

Epidemiology

Population-based studies indicate that IgM MGUS accounts for 15% to 18% of all MGUS and is present in 0.5% of people 50 years or older.[1,2] Median age at diagnosis is 74 years, and there is a mild male predominance (male:female 1.4:1).[3] While MGUS is overall more prevalent in people of African heritage, IgM is less common in this population (2%-10% of all MGUS).[4]

General Clinical Features

Patients with IgM MGUS lack the typical signs and symptoms of multiple myeloma or overt lymphoproliferative disorders. However, symptoms attributable to the monoclonal paraprotein, such as peripheral neuropathy or cryoglobulinemia, have been reported in 30% to 50% of patients with clinical IgM MGUS.[5-7] The terms "IgM-related disorder" or "Monoclonal gammopathy of clinical significance" have been used to describe this subset of patients.[8]

Morphology

Bone marrow biopsy may show mildly increased and scattered B cells or plasma cells, but plasma cells are <10% of cellularity and abnormal lymphoid aggregates diagnostic of lymphoplasmacytic lymphoma or other overt lymphoma are not identified.

Immunophenotype

In plasma cell–type IgM MGUS, clonal B-cell populations are absent. Plasma cells may show light chain restriction by immunohistochemistry and/or flow cytometry. Cases with an *IGH::CCND1* translocation may show strong nuclear Cyclin D1 in plasma cells by immunohistochemistry.

In IgM MGUS, NOS, clonal B-cell populations may be detected by flow cytometry, and in most cases the B cells are negative for CD5 and CD10.[5,9] Clonal CD5-positive B-cell populations, when detected, may represent concurrent clones unrelated to the IgM paraprotein.[5]

Genetics

The *MYD88* L265P mutation has been reported in 54% to 87% of cases,[5,10,11] and *CXCR4* mutations have been reported in 4% to 39%.[12-14] Specific karyotypic abnormalities have not been identified in IgM MGUS NOS. Cases of plasma cell–type IgM MGUS are *MYD88* wild type.

Prognosis and Clinical Comment

In a series by Kyle et al, the cumulative probability of progression to symptomatic lymphoplasmacytic lymphoma/Waldenstrom's macroglobulinemia (LPL/WM) in patients with IgM MGUS was 10% at 5 years, 18% at 10 years, and 24% at 15 years, or approximately 1.5% per year.[15] By comparison in the same series, the cumulative probability of progression for patients with asymptomatic (smoldering) LPL/WM to symptomatic LPL/WM was 6% at 1 year, 39% at 3 years, 59% at 5 years, and 65% at 10 years. The concentration of serum monoclonal protein at diagnosis and the initial serum albumin value were the only independent predictors of progression with multivariate analysis in patients with IgM MGUS. A minority of patients with IgM MGUS (<10%) may progress to immunoglobulin light chain amyloidosis, and progression to multiple myeloma is rare.[3]

References

1. Eisele L, Durig J, Huttmann A, et al. Prevalence and progression of monoclonal gammopathy of undetermined significance and light-chain MGUS in Germany. *Ann Hematol.* 2012;91(2):243-248. doi:10.1007/s00277-011-1293-1
2. Kyle RA, Therneau TM, Rajkumar SV, et al. Prevalence of monoclonal gammopathy of undetermined significance. *N Engl J Med.* 2006;354(13):1362-1369. doi:10.1056/NEJMoa054494
3. Kyle RA, Therneau TM, Rajkumar SV, et al. Long-term follow-up of IgM monoclonal gammopathy of undetermined significance. *Blood.* 2003;102(10):3759-3764. doi:10.1182/blood-2003-03-0801
4. Greenberg AJ, Vachon CM, Rajkumar SV. Disparities in the prevalence, pathogenesis and progression of monoclonal gammopathy of undetermined significance and multiple myeloma between blacks and whites. *Leukemia.* 2012;26(4):609-614. doi: 10.1038/leu.2011.368
5. Bruehl FK, Mannion P, Barbato E, Nakashima MO, Cook JR. IgM monoclonal gammopathy of undetermined significance: clinicopathologic features with and without IgM-related disorders. *Haematologica.* 2023;108(10):2764-2773. doi:10.3324/haematol.2022.282389
6. Nobile-Orazio E, Barbieri S, Baldini L, et al. Peripheral neuropathy in monoclonal gammopathy of undetermined significance: prevalence and immunopathogenetic studies. *Acta Neurol Scand.* 1992;85(6):383-390. doi:10.1111/j.1600-0404.1992.tb06033.x
7. Talamo G, Mir MA, Pandey MK, Sivik JK, Raheja D. IgM MGUS associated with anti-MAG neuropathy: a single institution experience. *Ann Hematol.* 2015;94(6):1011-1016. doi:10.1007/s00277-014-2294-7
8. Khwaja J, D'Sa S, Minnema MC, Kersten MJ, Wechalekar A, Vos JM. IgM monoclonal gammopathies of clinical significance: diagnosis and management. *Haematologica.* 2022;107(9):2037-2050. doi:10.3324/haematol.2022.280953
9. Paiva B, Montes MC, Garcia-Sanz R, et al. Multiparameter flow cytometry for the identification of the Waldenstrom's clone in IgM-MGUS and Waldenstrom's Macroglobulinemia: new criteria for differential diagnosis and risk stratification. *Leukemia.* 2014;28(1):166-173. doi:10.1038/leu.2013.124
10. Jiménez C, Sebastián E, Chillón MC, et al. MYD88 L265P is a marker highly characteristic of, but not restricted to, Waldenström's macroglobulinemia. *Leukemia.* 2013;27:1722-1728. doi:10.1038/leu.2013.62
11. Xu L, Hunter ZR, Yang G, et al. MYD88 L265P in Waldenström macroglobulinemia, immunoglobulin M monoclonal gammopathy, and other B-cell lymphoproliferative disorders using conventional and quantitative allele-specific polymerase chain reaction. *Blood.* 2013;121(11):2051-2058. doi:10.1182/blood-2012-09-454355
12. Moreno DF, Lopez-Guerra M, Paz S, et al. Prognostic impact of MYD88 and CXCR4 mutations assessed by droplet digital polymerase chain reaction in IgM monoclonal gammopathy of undetermined significance and smouldering Waldenstrom macroglobulinaemia. *Br J Haematol.* 2023;200(2):187-196. doi:10.1111/bjh.18502
13. Varettoni M, Zibellini S, Defrancesco I, et al. Pattern of somatic mutations in patients with Waldenstrom macroglobulinemia or IgM monoclonal gammopathy of undetermined significance. *Haematologica.* 2017;102(12):2077-2085. doi:10.3324/haematol.2017.172718
14. Xu L, Hunter ZR, Tsakmaklis N, et al. Clonal architecture of CXCR4 WHIM-like mutations in Waldenstrom macroglobulinaemia. *Br J Haematol.* 2016;172(5):735-744. doi:10.1111/bjh.13897
15. Kyle RA, Therneau TM, Dispenzieri A, et al. Immunoglobulin m monoclonal gammopathy of undetermined significance and smoldering Waldenström macroglobulinemia. *Clin Lymphoma Myeloma Leuk.* 2013;13(2):184-186.

Chapter 50
Primary Cold Agglutinin Disease

Jan Delabie, Christine Cserti-Gazdewich, Ahmet Dogan, and Anne Tierens

Definition

Primary cold agglutinin disease (pCAD) is a small B-cell lymphoproliferative disorder of the bone marrow that secretes a monoclonal antibody, typically binding to ABO(H) precursor substance i/I and causing autoimmune hemolytic anemia. It is to be distinguished from cold agglutinin *syndrome* secondary to other diseases such as infections, autoimmune diseases, or neoplasia, including other defined types of lymphoma.

Synonyms

Cold-agglutinin-associated lymphoproliferative disorder (not recommended).

Epidemiology

The incidence of pCAD is less than 2/million/y and is higher and more severe in colder climate zones and by season.[1] The latter is likely due to humoral effects of the lymphoproliferative disease being physically enhanced at colder temperatures.

General Clinical Features

pCAD is characterized by a monoclonal IgM antibody secreted by the B-cell lymphoproliferative disorder.[1] The secreted pentameric IgM antibody binds to red blood cells at cold temperatures, usually in acral parts of the body. Once bound, the antibody fixes complement leading to deposition of C3b on red cell membranes. C3b opsonization by C3b receptors on macrophages, mainly in the liver, leads to erythrophagocytosis. The latter causes anemia. Full complement activation is rare due to the dissociation of the antibody from the red blood cell once it recirculates to warmer central parts of the body. However, when full complement activation occurs, it may give rise to intravascular hemolysis. The most common presenting features are hemolytic anemia and acrocyanosis. Raynaud-like symptoms are seen in about 25% of patients, while gangrene or ulcerations are rare (1.5% patients). Cold agglutinins with a titer of more than 64 at 4 °C and a positive monospecific direct antiglobulin test for C3d are required for the diagnosis, together with absence of underlying clinical disease to account for the anemia.[2] About 70% of patients with serologic evidence of pCAD show detectable evidence of a small B-cell lymphoproliferative disorder in the bone marrow.

Morphology

The major importance of the proper diagnosis of pCAD is to avoid misdiagnosis of other small B-cell lymphoma types, which may rarely be associated with cold agglutinins and warrant specific therapy. The bone marrow trephine may show several intraparenchymatous nodular lymphoid infiltrates, usually not comprising more than 10% of nucleated cells in the marrow (Figure 50.1).[3] Paratrabecular or intrasinusoidal lymphoid infiltration is not seen. Occasionally, the aggregates may show a small germinal center. The lymphoid cells are small with round nuclei without prominent nucleolus and without Dutcher body inclusions. Lymphoplasmacytic cells and paraimmunoblasts are not seen. Plasma cells are not numerous. When present, plasma cells surround the infiltrates or are diffusely scattered throughout the marrow.

Immunophenotype

The lymphoid aggregates in the bone marrow consist of CD20+ small B cells, which are best characterized by flow cytometry. The B cells are $CD5^-$ or $CD5^+$, $CD10^-$, $CD11c^-$, $CD19^+$, $CD20^+$, $CD23^-$, $CD38^-$, $CD79b^+$, $CD200^+$, IgM^+, and in most instances IgK^+. BCL6 is not expressed, but BCL2 is. When present, small reactive germinal centers are $BCL6^+$, $BCL2^-$. Plasma cells surrounding the infiltrates are few but express IgM and show restricted immunoglobulin light chain expression. The clonal B cells express CD27 and display somatic hypermutation of immunoglobulin genes, features of IgM-expressing memory B cells.

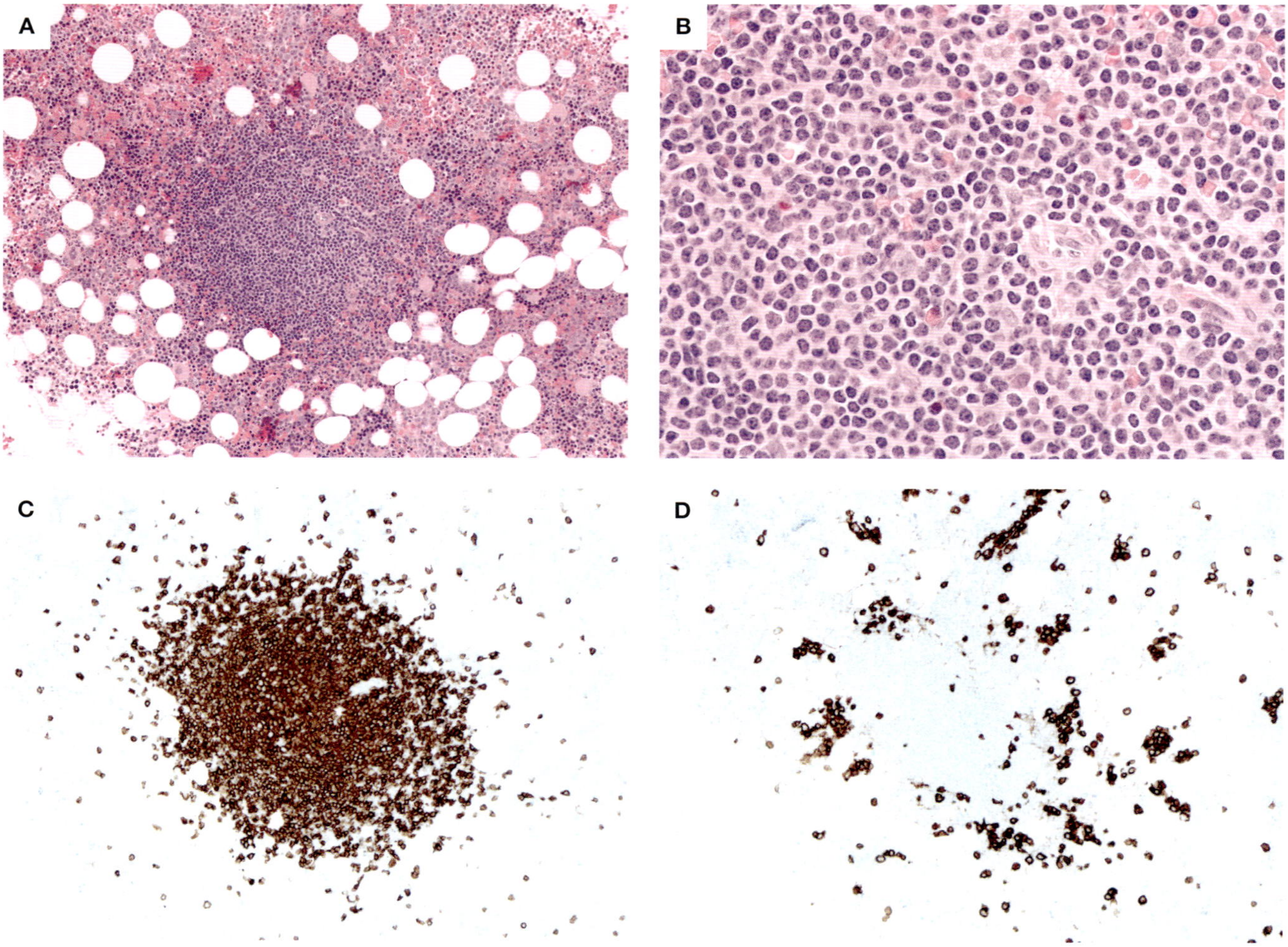

FIGURE 50.1 Hematoxylin and eosin–stained section of a bone marrow trephine biopsy showing an intraparenchymatous nodular aggregate of small lymphoid cells (**A:** 100×), with round nuclei without prominent nucleoli and with scant but visible cytoplasm (**B:** 400×). The cells express CD20 (**C:** 100×), and this B-cell aggregate is surrounded by CD138-expressing plasma cells (**D:** 100×).

Genetics

Trisomy 3, 12, and 18 are commonly present. Mutations of *KMT2D*, *CARD11*, and *CXCR4* are present in 50%, 30%, and 25% of cases, respectively. When present, *CARD11* and *CXCR4* mutations occur in addition to *KMT2D* mutation. *MYD88* L265P mutation is rare to absent.[3]

Prognosis and Clinical Comment

The 5-year overall survival is 83% and may not be significantly lower than expected for an age-matched population. Anemia and vascular symptoms determine disease severity. These symptoms are less related to the extent of the clonal B-cell proliferation or to the titer of the cold agglutinin antibody, and rather more related to the thermal amplitude of the antibody. The latter is defined as the highest temperature at which the antibody binds red blood cells. Transformation to large B-cell lymphoma is rare, with a 3.4% incidence at 8 years of follow-up.[1]

References

1. Berentsen S, Barcellini W, D'Sa S, et al. Cold agglutinin disease revisited: a multinational, observational study of 232 patients. *Blood*. 2020;136(4):480-488.
2. Jäger U, Barcellini W, Broome CM, et al. Diagnosis and treatment of autoimmune hemolytic anemia in adults: recommendations from the First International Consensus Meeting. *Blood Rev*. 2020;41:100648. doi:10.1016/j.blre.2019.100648
3. Guenther A, Tierens A, Malecka A, Delabie J. The histopathology of cold agglutinin disease-associated B-cell lymphoproliferative disease. *Am J Clin Pathol*. 2023;160(3):229-237.

Chapter 51
Heavy Chain Diseases

James R. Cook, David Dingli, and Elaine S. Jaffe

Introduction

The heavy chain diseases are a group of rare neoplasms defined by the presence of a serum or urine monoclonal protein composed of a truncated immunoglobulin heavy chain that often has deletions in the switch-CH1 region and therefore lacks the ability to bind light chains (Figure 51.1A). The truncated protein may be difficult to identify by serum protein electrophoresis alone and is best identified by immunofixation or immunoelectrophoresis studies or matrix-assisted laser desorption ionization–time of flight mass spectrometry, which show a monoclonal heavy chain without a corresponding light chain (Figure 51.1B).

Some cases of heavy chain disease show histologic similarities to other well-defined B-cell neoplasms. For example, some cases of gamma heavy chain disease (gHCD) are morphologically consistent with splenic marginal zone lymphoma, while mu heavy chain disease (mHCD) has been reported to resemble chronic lymphocytic leukemia and alpha heavy chain disease (aHCD) is considered a clinical variant of an extranodal marginal zone lymphoma of the intestines. The clinical features of the heavy chain diseases, however, are felt to be sufficiently distinctive to warrant recognition as separate diagnostic entities.

GAMMA HEAVY CHAIN DISEASE

Definition

Gamma heavy chain disease (gHCD) is a small B-cell neoplasm with plasmacytic differentiation that produces a truncated IgG heavy chain that is incapable of associating with immunoglobulin light chains. Once considered a variant of lymphoplasmacytic lymphoma (LPL), gHCD is now thought to be biologically unrelated to LPL.

Synonyms

Franklin disease.

Epidemiology

gHCD is rare, with approximately 200 cases reported in the literature. The median age at presentation is in the seventh decade, with a slight female predominance.[1-3]

General Clinical Features

Systemic symptoms are common, including weight loss, fatigue, and fever. Associated autoimmune disorders, which may precede the diagnosis of gHCD by many years, have been reported in 25% to 70% of patients. These most frequently include rheumatoid arthritis and systemic lupus erythematosus, although other disorders such as Sjögren syndrome, myasthenia gravis, and autoimmune hemolytic anemia or immune thrombocytopenia have also been described.

Most patients present with disseminated disease, including generalized adenopathy, splenomegaly, and less frequently hepatomegaly. Swelling of the soft palate and uvula is an uncommon manifestation. Bone marrow involvement has been reported in 30% to 60% of cases. Lytic bone disease is usually not present. Coexisting T-cell large granular lymphocyte proliferations have been reported in a subset of patients. In 10% to 20% of patients, an overt lymphoplasmacytic proliferation is not identified.

Morphology

The histologic findings in gHCD are variable. Most commonly, lymph nodes show diffuse effacement by a polymorphous infiltrate of small lymphocytes, plasmacytoid lymphocytes, plasma cells, histiocytes, and eosinophils (Figure 51.2). Variable numbers of scattered large cells may be present. A smaller number of cases are histologically typical of splenic marginal zone lymphoma or extranodal marginal zone lymphoma (Figure 51.3).

The peripheral blood may show an absolute lymphocytosis with small lymphocytes and/or plasmacytoid forms. In the bone marrow, some cases exhibit infiltration by distinct lymphoplasmacytic aggregates, while other cases may show only scattered abnormal plasmacytoid cells.

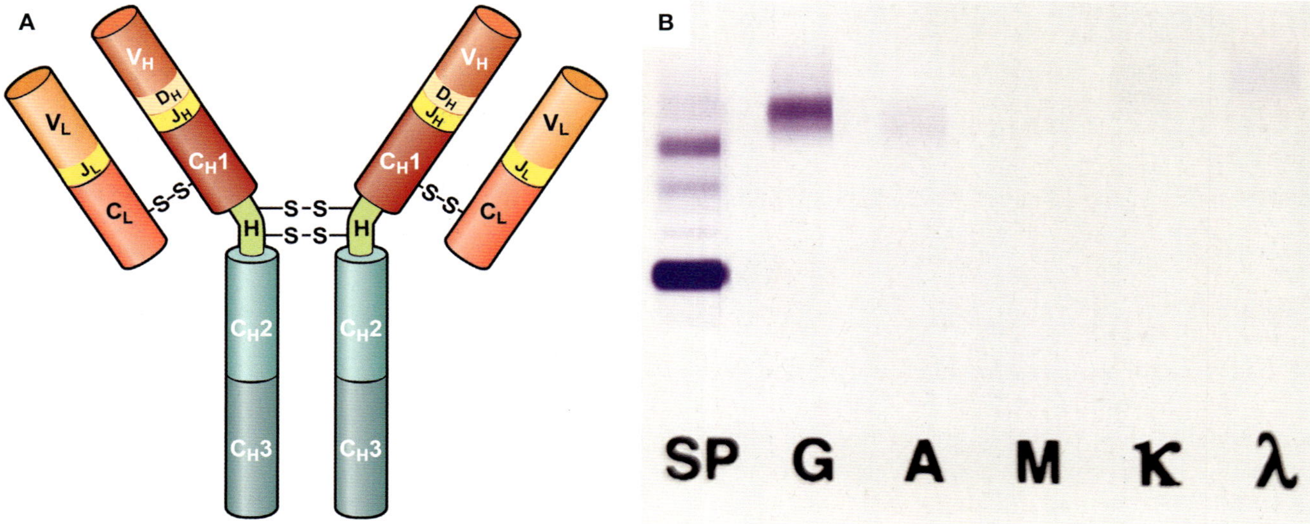

FIGURE 51.1 Heavy chain disease. **A:** Structure of the normal IgG protein. In gamma heavy chain disease, variably sized deletions occur in the CH1 domain leading to loss of the light chain–binding site. **B:** Immunofixation analysis showing a monoclonal band in the IgG lane without matching band in kappa or lambda lanes. (**A:** Reprinted by permission from Molina TJ, ed. *Hematopathology (Encyclopedia of Pathology)*. Springer Nature. 2020. https://doi.org/10.1007/978-3-319-95309-0

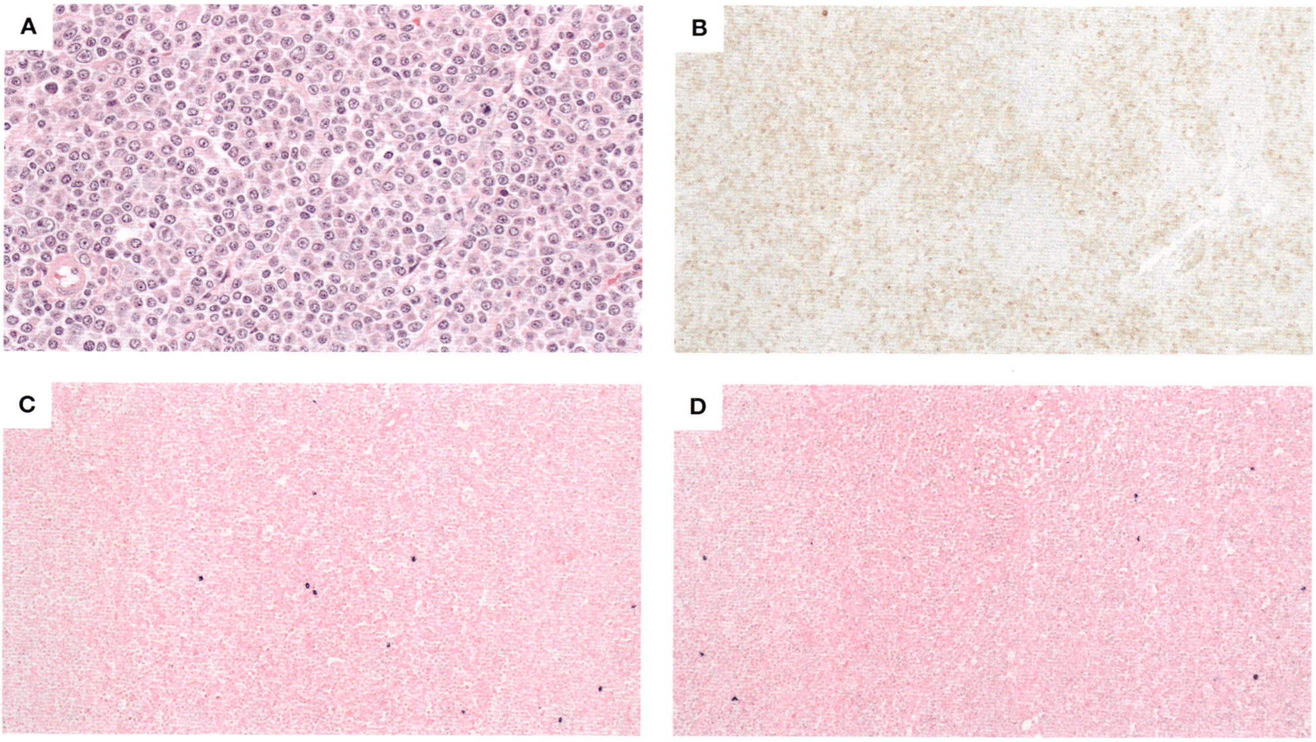

FIGURE 51.2 Gamma heavy chain disease. **A:** The lymph node is effaced by a diffuse proliferation of small lymphocytes, plasmacytoid forms, and occasional large cells. **B:** The neoplastic cells are positive for IgG heavy chain. By conventional in situ hybridization, the neoplastic cells are negative for both kappa (**C**) and lambda (**D**) light chains.

Immunophenotype

The neoplastic cells are positive for CD79a and IgG heavy chains, with variable CD20 and CD138 on the lymphoid and plasmacytic elements, respectively. The B cells are negative for CD5 and CD10. Immunoglobulin light chain proteins are generally not detectable by immunohistochemistry, although light chain RNA may be demonstrated by in situ hybridization in some cases.

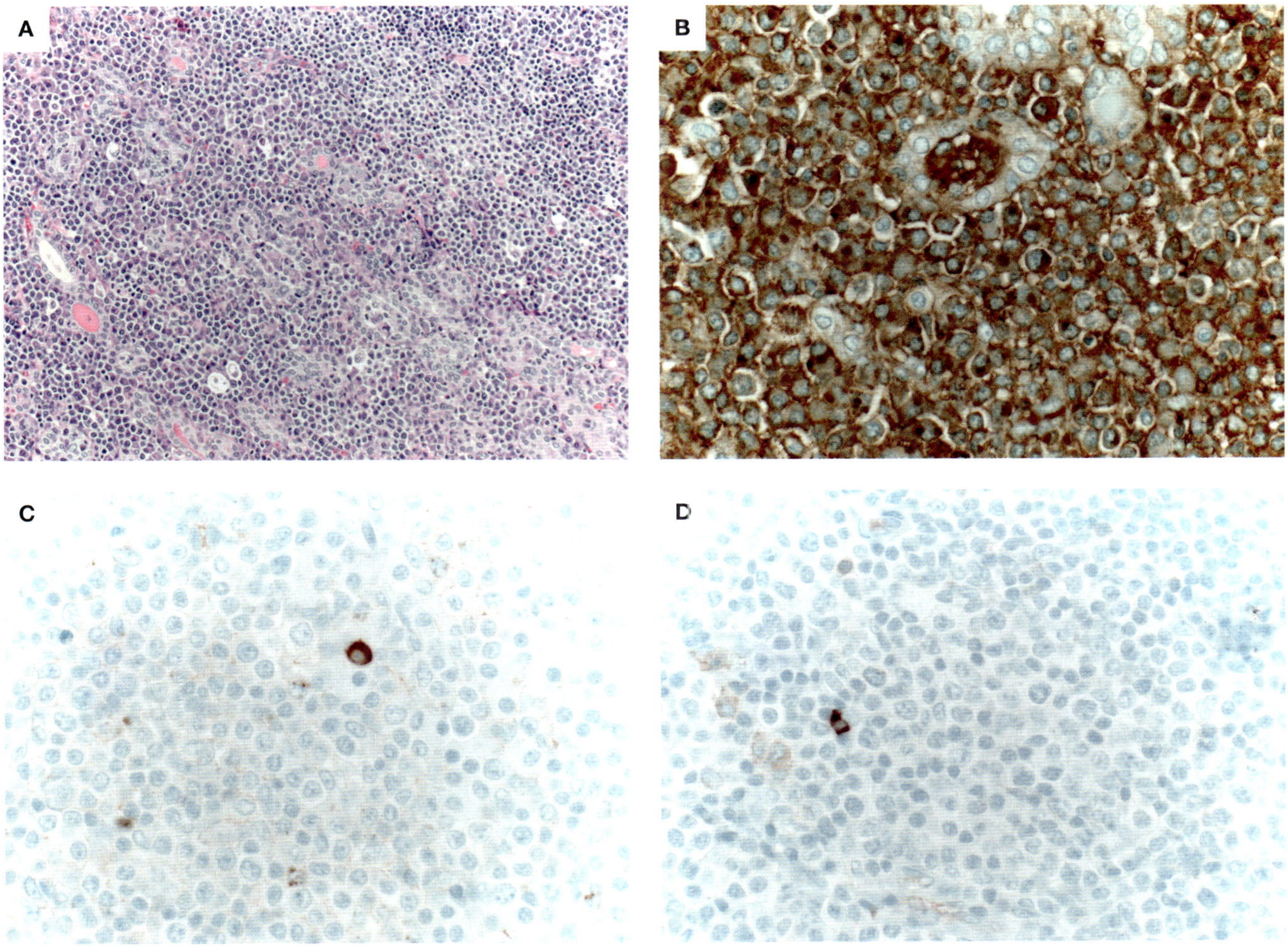

FIGURE 51.3 Gamma heavy chain disease. **A:** A thyroid mass contains an infiltrate of small lymphocytes and plasma cells including lymphoepithelial lesions resembling thyroid extranodal marginal zone (MALT) lymphoma. By immunohistochemistry, the neoplastic cells are positive for IgG heavy chains **(B)** and negative for both kappa **(C)** and lambda **(D)** light chains.

Genetics

The immunoglobulin gamma heavy chain gene shows variably sized deletions of the variable region and CH1 domains. No specific recurrent cytogenetic abnormality has been described. The *MYD88* L265P mutation, characteristic of lymphoplasmacytic lymphoma, is absent in gHCD. Polymerase chain reaction studies for immunoglobulin rearrangement are typically negative in clinical testing, likely secondary to genomic deletions.

Prognosis and Clinical Comment

The clinical course is variable from the indolent to rapidly progressive. Patients with symptomatic disease may be treated with a "CHOP"-like regimen (cyclophosphamide, doxorubicin, vincristine, and prednisone), and if the clonal cells express CD20, rituximab may be added. Anecdotal reports attest to the efficacy of myeloma regimens such as CyBorD (cyclophosphamide, bortezomib, and dexamethasone) if the cell population is predominantly plasmacytic. The prognosis varies from indolent disease (monoclonal gammopathy) to rapidly progressive akin to an aggressive lymphoma with a survival of several weeks. Median survival in one series was 7.4 years.[3]

MU HEAVY CHAIN DISEASE

Definition

Mu heavy chain disease (mHCD) is a small B-cell neoplasm that produces a truncated monoclonal IgM heavy chain that lacks associated light chains.

Synonyms

None.

Epidemiology

Mu heavy chain disease is extremely rare with 30 to 40 cases reported in the literature to date.[1,4,5] The median age of diagnosis is in the seventh decade, and roughly equal numbers of men and women have been described.

General Clinical Features

Mu heavy chain disease involves the bone marrow, often with enlargement of the liver and spleen. Peripheral blood absolute lymphocytosis occurs in a subset of patients. Lymph node involvement or extranodal disease is uncommon.[1,4,5] By definition, protein electrophoresis and immunofixation of the serum shows a monoclonal IgM heavy chain without associated light chains. Hypogammaglobulinemia is frequently present. Monotypic light chains (Bence-Jones proteins) are reported in the urine in approximately half of cases, and some patients have been reported to develop amyloidosis or light chain cast nephropathy.

Morphology

The bone marrow contains small lymphocytes with mature chromatin and scant cytoplasm, frequently described as resembling chronic lymphocytic leukemia/small lymphocytic lymphoma. Plasma cells frequently show vacuolated cytoplasm (Figure 51.4).

Immunophenotype

The B cells are reported to be negative for CD5 and CD10. Monotypic light chains, which are often still produced despite being unable to bind to the defective heavy chain, may be detected in a subset of cases.

Genetics

The immunoglobulin heavy chain locus is clonally rearranged, with variably sized deletions of the variable region and CH1 domain. Insertions of large amounts of DNA of unknown origin may occur. Recently, three cases have been reported to harbor *MYD88* L265P mutations,[6,7] raising a possible relationship with lymphoplasmacytic lymphoma in at least some cases.

Prognosis and Clinical Comment

Patients needing therapy often will receive combination therapy similar to other non-Hodgkin lymphomas including monoclonal antibodies that may target cell surface markers expressed by the clonal cells. Prognosis is variable: patients may survive for many years with indolent disease while others succumb to their illness in a few months.

ALPHA HEAVY CHAIN DISEASE

Definition

aHCD is a variant of extranodal marginal zone lymphoma that secretes abnormal IgA heavy chains that lack associated immunoglobulin light chains.

Synonyms

Mediterranean lymphoma; immunoproliferative small intestinal disease; Seligmann disease.

Epidemiology

aHCD historically is the most common of the heavy chain disorders, with more than 400 cases reported in the literature. Most cases occur in the Middle East and Mediterranean regions.[8-10] Patients typically present in the second or third decade of life, and there is a male predominance. There is an association with lower socioeconomic status and poor sanitation. Infection with *Campylobacter jejuni* or other gastrointestinal infections has been proposed to contribute to lymphomagenesis.[10-13] The incidence appears to have decreased in recent years, likely due to changes in socioeconomic conditions and reduced infections.

General Clinical Features

Most patients present with malabsorption, diarrhea, weight loss, and abdominal pain due to involvement of the duodenum and/or jejunum. Adenopathy or hepatosplenomegaly is uncommon. Rare cases have been reported to involve other sites including the respiratory tract or thyroid.

Morphology

The small bowel lamina propria displays an infiltrate of small lymphocytes and plasma cells (Figure 51.5). Marginal zone–type cells and lymphoepithelial lesions may be present, and villous atrophy is common.[10,14] Variable numbers of scattered large transformed cells may be present, but the presence of sheets of large transformed cells indicates progression to diffuse large B-cell lymphoma.

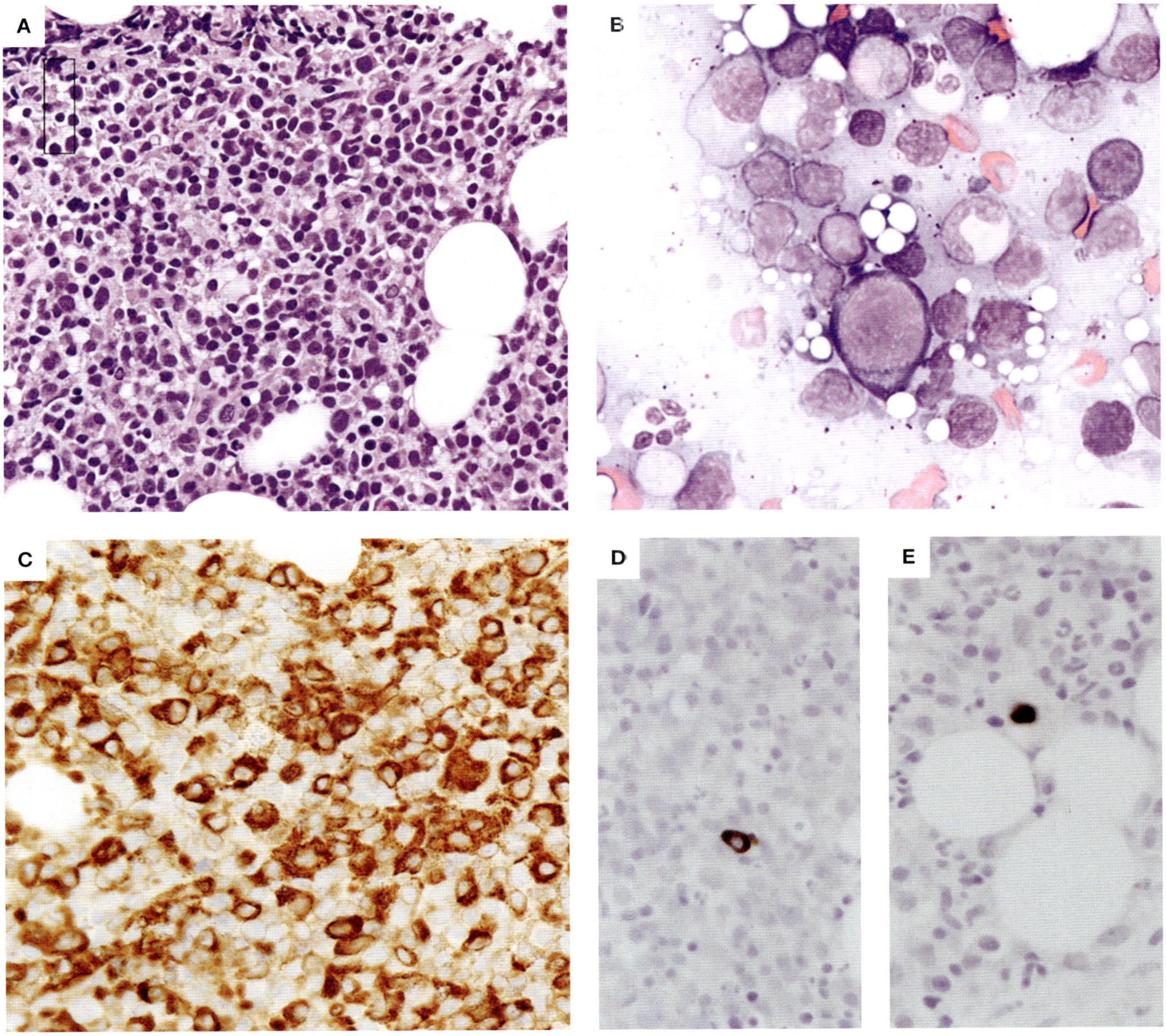

FIGURE 51.4 Mu heavy chain disease. **A:** Bone marrow biopsy with aggregates of small lymphocytes and plasma cells. **B:** In bone marrow aspirate smears, the plasmacytoid cells and lymphocytes contain cytoplasmic vacuoles. **C-E:** The neoplastic cells are positive for IgM **(C)** heavy chains and negative for kappa **(D)** and lambda **(E)** light chains.

Immunophenotype

The B cells are positive for CD20 and negative for CD5 and CD10.[10,14] Plasma cells are typically positive for IgA heavy chains and negative for immunoglobulin light chains.

Genetics

The immunoglobulin heavy and light chains are clonally rearranged. The IgA heavy chain shows variable sized deletions leading to loss of the variable region and the CH1 domain.[1,5] Recurrent cytogenetic abnormalities, including *MALT1* translocations, have not been described to date in aHCD.

Prognosis and Clinical Comment

Therapy with antimicrobial agents targeting concomitant intestinal infections is often used for early-stage disease, but if patients do not respond to antimicrobials, therapy directed at the underlying lymphoma should be given such as rituximab with cyclophosphamide, doxorubicin, vincristine, and prednisone. With this approach, up to 70% of patients may experience long-term survival.

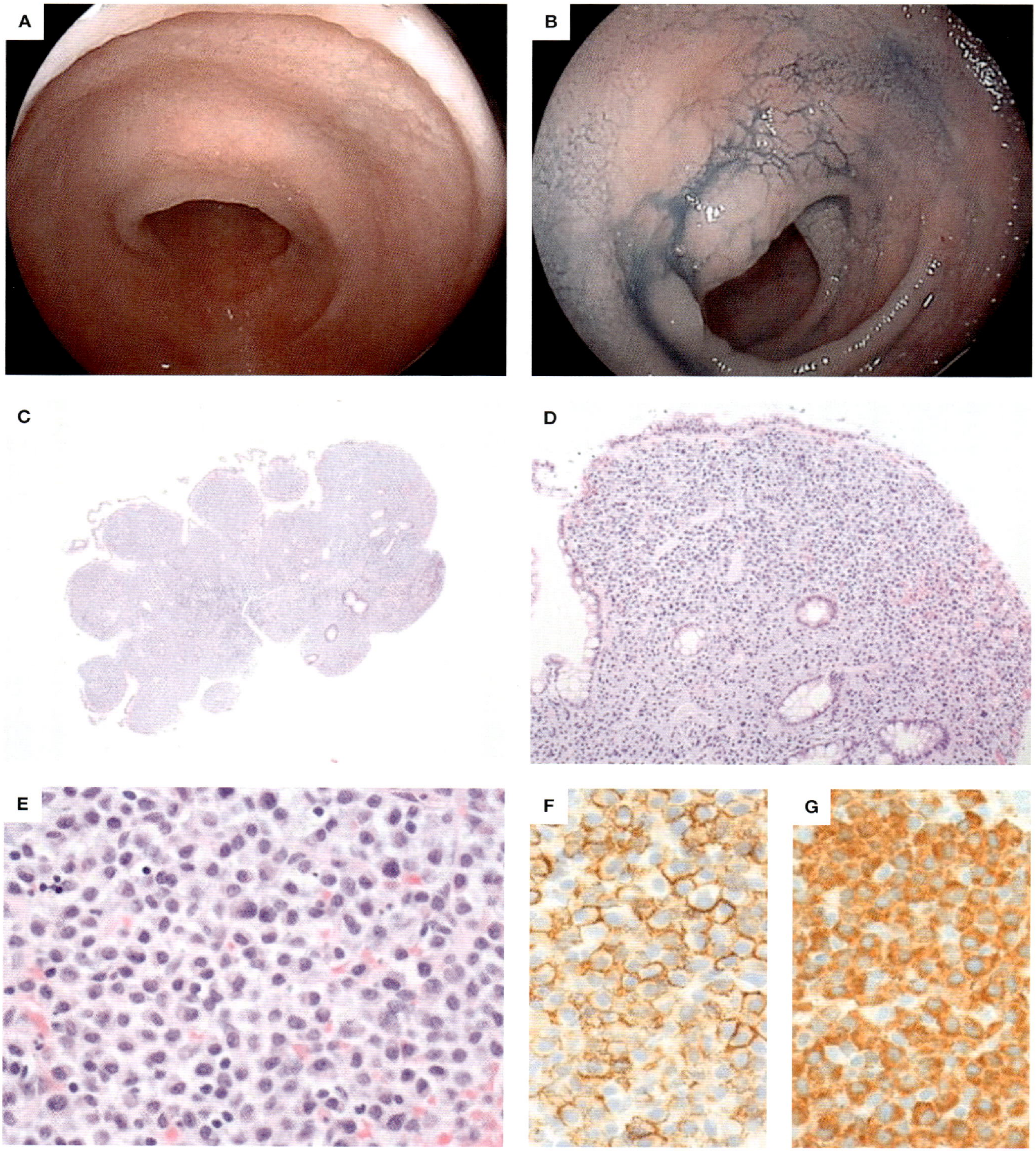

FIGURE 51.5 Alpha heavy chain disease. **A** and **B:** Double-balloon endoscopy showing villous edema in the ileum. **C-E:** Villi are blunted by a dense lymphoplasmacytic lymphoma. **F** and **G:** The tumor cells are positive for CD138 **(F)** and IgA **(G)** but lack light chains (not illustrated). (Reproduced from Ishikawa E, Nakamura M, Satou A, Shimada K, Nakamura S. Mucosa-Associated Lymphoid Tissue (MALT) lymphoma in the gastrointestinal tract in the modern era. *Cancers (Basel)*. 2022;14(2):446. doi:10.3390/cancers14020446.)

References

1. Bianchi G, Anderson KC, Harris NL, Sohani AR. The heavy chain diseases: clinical and pathologic features. *Oncology (Williston Park)*. 2014;28(1):45-53.
2. Bieliauskas S, Tubbs RR, Bacon CM, et al. Gamma heavy-chain disease: defining the spectrum of associated lymphoproliferative disorders through analysis of 13 cases. *Am J Surg Pathol*. 2012;36(4):534-543. doi:-DOI: 10.1097/PAS.0b013e318240590a
3. Wahner-Roedler DL, Witzig TE, Loehrer LL, Kyle RA. Gamma-heavy chain disease: review of 23 cases. *Medicine (Baltim)*. 2003;82(4):236-250. doi:10.1097/01.md.0000085058.63483.7f
4. Wahner-Roedler DL, Kyle RA. Mu-heavy chain disease: presentation as a benign monoclonal gammopathy. *Am J Hematol*. 1992;40(1):56-60. doi:10.1002/ajh.2830400112
5. Wahner-Roedler DL, Kyle RA. Heavy chain diseases. *Best Pract Res Clin Haematol*. 2005;18(4):729-746. S1521-6926(05)00030-7 [pii]. doi:10.1016/j.beha.2005.01.029
6. Vergneault H, Bengoufa D, Frazier-Mironer A, et al. Light chain proteinuria revealing mu-heavy chain disease: an atypical presentation of Waldenstrom macroglobulinemia in two cases. *Haematologica*. 2021;106(7):2034-2036. doi:10.3324/haematol.2020.277137
7. Baloda V, Wheeler SE, Murray DL, et al. Mu heavy chain disease with MYD88 L265P mutation: an unusual manifestation of lymphoplasmacytic lymphoma. *Diagn Pathol*. 2022;17(1):63. doi:10.1186/s13000-022-01244-1
8. Al Yamany R, Kharfan-Dabaja MA, Hamadani M, Alshaibani A, Aljurf M. The evolution of our understanding of Immunoproliferative Small Intestinal Disease (IPSID) over time. *Curr Oncol*. 2022;29(5):3759-3769. doi:10.3390/curroncol29050301
9. Al-Saleem T, Al-Mondhiry H. Immunoproliferative small intestinal disease (IPSID): a model for mature B-cell neoplasms. *Blood*. 2005;105(6):2274-2280. doi:10.1182/blood-2004-07-2755
10. Bianchi G, Sohani AR. Heavy chain disease of the small bowel. *Curr Gastroenterol Rep*. 2018;20(1):3. doi:10.1007/s11894-018-0608-y
11. Ewers EC, Sheffler RL, Wang J, Ngauy V. Immunoproliferative small intestinal disease associated with overwhelming polymicrobial gastrointestinal infection with transformation to diffuse large B-cell lymphoma. *Am J Trop Med Hyg*. 2016;94(5):1177-1181. doi:10.4269/ajtmh.15-0831
12. Lecuit M, Abachin E, Martin A, et al. Immunoproliferative small intestinal disease associated with Campylobacter jejuni. *N Engl J Med*. 2004;350(3):239-248. doi:10.1056/NEJMoa031887
13. Diss TC, Baginsky L, Ye H, et al. Campylobacter jejuni is a strong candidate for involvement in the development of immunoproliferative small intestinal disease. Meeting Abstract. *J Pathol*. 2004;204:8A-8A.
14. Isaacson PG, Dogan A, Price SK, Spencer J. Immunoproliferative small-intestinal disease. An immunohistochemical study. *Am J Surg Pathol*. 1989;13(12):1023-1033. doi:10.1097/00000478-198912000-00004

Chapter 52

Plasma Cell Neoplasms

Falko Fend, P. Leif Bergsagel, Dragan Jevremovic, Robert B. Lorsbach, Megan O. Nakashima, and Jesus F. San-Miguel

Introduction

The plasma cell neoplasms are a group of related entities characterized by a clone of plasma cells that frequently secrete a monoclonal immunoglobulin (IG) protein, also known as an M protein. This chapter includes non-IgM monoclonal gammopathy of undetermined significance (MGUS), multiple myeloma (MM), and plasmacytoma. The neoplastic plasma cells in these disorders share many morphologic and phenotypic features, but there are marked differences in clinical behavior. These entities are distinguished by a multiparameter approach that integrates clinical, laboratory, pathologic, and radiographic features. IgM MGUS, which most frequently progresses to lymphoma rather than MM, is discussed in a separate chapter, as are the monoclonal IG deposition diseases.

NON-IGM MONOCLONAL GAMMOPATHY OF UNDETERMINED SIGNIFICANCE

Definition

Non-IgM monoclonal gammopathy of undetermined significance (non-IgM MGUS) is a clonal premalignant proliferation of plasma cells—or rarely of lymphoplasmacytic cells—defined by a non-IgM monoclonal protein <30 g/L in the serum or a single light chain with an abnormal free light chain (FLC) ratio (<0.26 or >1.65) and urinary M protein <500 mg/24 h, with <10% clonal bone marrow (BM) plasma cells in the absence of features diagnostic of MM, IG light chain amyloidosis, lymphoplasmacytic lymphoma, or other overt lymphoproliferative disorders (Table 52.1).[2-5] Cases with renal or other clinical symptoms associated with clonal IG secretion, but not fulfilling the diagnostic criteria for MM, lymphoplasmacytic lymphoma, or amyloidosis, remain within this category, but the terms monoclonal gammopathy of renal or clinical significance (MGRS and MGCS, respectively) can be added as clinical descriptors.[6-8]

TABLE 52.1 Diagnostic criteria for non-IgM MGUS

For IgA and IgG MGUS:
- Serum M protein (non-IgM) <30 g/L - Clonal BM plasma cells <10% - Absence of myeloma-defining events (SLiM-CRAB criteria) or amyloidosis attributable to the plasma cell proliferative disorder
For light chain MGUS:
- Abnormal free light chain ratio (<0.26 or >1.65) - Increased level of the involved free light chain - No immunoglobulin heavy chain expression on immunofixation - Urinary M protein <500 mg/24 h - Clonal BM plasma cells <10% - Absence of SLiM-CRAB criteria or amyloidosis attributable to the plasma cell proliferative disorder

BM, bone marrow; MGUS, monoclonal gammopathy of undetermined significance. Modified from McKenna RW, Kyle RD, Kuehl WM, Harris NL, Coupland R, Fend F. Plasma cell neoplasms. In: Swerdlow SH, Campo E, Harris NL, Jaffe ES, Pileri S, Stein H, et al, eds. *WHO Classification of Tumours of Hematopoietic and Lymphoid Tissues*. IARC; 2017:241-253.

Synonyms

Monoclonal gammopathy (not recommended).

Epidemiology

Non-IgM MGUS is rare below 40 years of age but affects approximately 3% to 4% of individuals >50 years and >5% above 70 years. There is a slight male predominance, and non-IgM MGUS incidence is more than twice in individuals of African heritage.[9] An increased prevalence has been observed in families with lymphoid or plasma cell disorders.

General Clinical Features

Patients with non-IgM MGUS by definition lack the typical signs and symptoms of MM or overt lymphoproliferative disorders and are usually asymptomatic. In most patients, the M protein is detected in serum electrophoresis performed for the evaluation of another disorder. Approximately 60% are of IgG, 20% light chains only, 15% IgA, 1% each IgD and IgE, and 3% to 5% are biclonal.[2,4,9] Reduction of uninvolved Ig isotypes is found in 30% to 40% and monoclonal light chain in urine in nearly a third of cases.[3] Approximately 1.5% of patients with non-IgM MGUS have renal damage with various pathologies attributed to the monoclonal protein, but not fulfilling MM criteria, termed MGRS.[7,8] MGUS can also be associated with neurologic or skin systemic manifestations. Patients with BM plasma cells at MGUS levels, but fulfilling criteria for POEMS or TEMPI syndrome, are classified accordingly.

Morphology

BM biopsy and aspirate show normal to mildly increased, usually mature-appearing plasma cells, which account for <10% of cellularity and are usually regularly dispersed with occasional small clusters.[1] Cytoplasmic inclusions or nucleoli can occasionally be observed. Abnormal larger aggregates of plasma cells or lymphoplasmacytic cells diagnostic of MM or B-cell lymphoma are not identified.

Immunophenotype

Plasma cells can be quantified by stains for CD138 or MUM1 and may show light chain restriction by immunohistochemistry (IHC) and/or flow cytometry (FCM). Owing to the presence of normal polyclonal plasma cells, light chain restriction may not be identified in cases with a small clonal population. The presence of two populations of plasma cells, including reactive polytypic cells and abnormal ones with an aberrant immunophenotype, including loss of CD19, expression of CD56, or decreased CD38 expression is frequently detected by FCM and/or IHC.[10] Cases with an *IGH::CCND1* translocation (15%-25%) show strong nuclear cyclin D1 staining in clonal plasma cells.

Genetics

Non-IgM MGUS is derived from antigen-experienced, post–germinal center, class-switched plasma cells with somatic hypermutation of IG genes. The genetic profile of non-IgM MGUS is similar to that of MM, albeit with some differences in frequency of certain alterations. By fluorescence in situ hybridization (FISH) of enriched plasma cells, 74% of cases show abnormalities (presumably lower than the >95% in MM because of some cases with low numbers of clonal plasma cell [PC]), which are rarely detectable by conventional cytogenetics due to the low proliferation rate of the clonal population. Considering only samples in which at least one abnormality is detected by FISH, around 44% of cases show recurrent *IGH* translocations involving *CCND* family genes (32%), primarily t(11;14)(q23;q32) *IGH::CCND1*, *MAF* family genes (8%), t(4;14) (p16.3;q32) *IGH::NSD2*, (4%), multiple trisomies of chromosomes 3, 7, 9, 11, 15, 17 (27%), and something other than recurrent IgH translocations or trisomies (29%)[11-14] Deletions of chromosome 13q occur in 38%. As compared with MM, in MGUS the frequency of t(11;14) is higher, while t(4;14) and hyperdiploidy are lower, and in those with *CCND* or *MAF* translocation the frequency of del(13q) is lower.[15] Genetic alterations typical for overt and advanced MM are found at much lower frequencies in non-IgM MGUS, such as gains of chromosome 1q, activating mutations of *KRAS* and *NRAS*, del(17p), and *TP53* mutations.[16]

Prognosis and Clinical Comment

Most individuals with non-IgM MGUS show no progression to an overt malignancy for prolonged periods of time. The average rate of transformation to MM, or rarely amyloidosis or B-cell lymphoma, is around 1% per year, ranging from 0.3% per year for light chain MGUS to 1.5% for IgA MGUS. In addition to the isotype and the amount of the M protein, reduction in polyclonal Ig, a high percentage (>90%) of clonal plasma cells with aberrant immunophenotype by FCM, plasma cell aneuploidy, t(4;14), t(14;16), gain(1q), and del(13/13q) are associated with an increased progression risk of non-IgM MGUS.[2,10,17,18] Proposed risk models can stratify individuals with non-IgM MGUS into subgroups progressing to MM at rates ranging from approximately 0.3% to 12% per year.

Recent, albeit small scale, genome-wide studies have shown that non-IgM MGUS progressing to MM shows distinct genetic profiles compared with those with stable disease, which may provide a more refined risk stratification in the future.[1,19,20]

MULTIPLE MYELOMA

Definition

MM is a BM-based, multifocal neoplastic proliferation of monoclonal plasma cells associated with an M protein in serum or urine in most cases and evidence of organ damage related to the plasma cell neoplasm, termed CRAB criteria (hyperCalcemia, Renal dysfunction, Anemia, and Bone involvement).[5] In virtually all cases, MM is preceded by non-IgM MGUS.[21] Thus, MM originates in the BM in nearly all cases, and most patients show disseminated BM involvement. The clinical spectrum ranges from asymptomatic to highly aggressive disease. Owing to the stepwise evolution from its precursor lesion non-IgM MGUS, from which it needs to be distinguished, MM diagnosis is based on a combination of clinical, morphological, radiological, and laboratory features. Asymptomatic patients surpassing the limits for MGUS as described earlier are designated smoldering (asymptomatic) MM, unless they show biological markers of high disease activity with risk for rapid progression to symptomatic disease, including BM plasmacytosis >60%, serum free light chain ratio >100, and >1 focal lesion detected by magnetic resonance imaging (MRI) (so-called SLiM criteria).[5] The diagnostic criteria for symptomatic and smoldering MM are listed in Table 52.2.

TABLE 52.2 Diagnostic criteria for symptomatic and smoldering multiple myeloma

Plasma cell myeloma
≥10% clonal plasma cells or biopsy-proven plasmacytoma and ≥1 myeloma-defining event - Evidence of end-organ damage (CRAB) attributable to the plasma cell neoplasm • Hypercalcemia: 0.25 mmol/L above upper limit of normal or > 2.75 mmol/L • Renal insufficiency: creatinine clearance <40 mL/min or serum creatinine >177 µmol/L (>2 mg/dL) • Anemia: hemoglobin <20 g/L below lower limit of normal or <100 g/L • Bone lesions: one or more osteolytic lesions on skeletal radiography, computed tomography (CT), or positron emission tomography-CT - ≥1 biomarker of malignancy • ≥ 60% clonal bone marrow plasma cells • Involved:uninvolved serum free light chain ratio ≥100 (involved free light chain level must be ≥100 mg/L and urine monoclonal protein level at least 200 mg per 24 h on urine protein electrophoresis) • >1 focal lesion on magnetic resonance imaging (at least 5 mm in size)
Asymptomatic (smoldering) myeloma (both criteria must be met)
- Monoclonal serum protein >30 g/L ***or*** urinary M protein >500 mg/24 h **and/or** 10%-60% clonal bone marrow plasma cells - No myeloma-defining events or amyloidosis

Modified from McKenna RW, Kyle RD, Kuehl WM, Harris NL, Coupland R, Fend F. Plasma cell neoplasms. In: Swerdlow SH, Campo E, Harris NL, Jaffe ES, Pileri S, Stein H, et al, eds. *WHO Classification of Tumours of Hematopoietic and Lymphoid Tissues*. IARC; 2017:241-253 and Visram A, Rajkumar SV, Kapoor P, et al. Monoclonal proteinuria predicts progression risk in asymptomatic multiple myeloma with a free light chain ratio ≥100. *Leukemia*. 2022;36(5):1429-1431.

Synonyms

Plasma cell myeloma, medullary plasmacytoma, Kahler disease (not recommended).

Epidemiology

MM comprises about 1% to 1.5% of malignant tumors and 10% to 15% of hematopoietic and lymphoid neoplasms.[1,23] An estimated 35,800 cases will be diagnosed and more than 12,000 patients are expected to die from MM in the United States in 2024 (https://seer.cancer.gov/statfacts/html/mulmy.html). MM is slightly more common in men (1.1-1.2:1) and nearly twice as frequent in patients of African descent.[9] MM development is exceptional in children and rare in adults <30 years of age. The incidence increases progressively with age, with 90% of MM cases occurring in individuals >50 years, with a median age at diagnosis of 70 years. Individuals with a first-degree relative with MM have 2.1- to 3.7-fold risk for developing the disease.[24]

General Clinical Features

Symptomatic MM is characterized by the presence of end-organ damage and appropriate clinical symptoms in patients with a monoclonal plasma cell population in the BM and M protein in serum or urine. Bone destruction, replacement and suppression of normal hematopoiesis by the neoplastic plasma cell proliferation, immunoparesis, hypercalcemia, and kidney damage or hyperviscosity caused by deposition, and toxic levels of M protein are responsible for the majority of clinical symptoms in patients with symptomatic MM.

The most prevalent symptom, seen in more than half of the patients with newly diagnosed MM, is bone pain due to multiple osteolytic lesions or osteoporosis, mostly affecting the axial skeleton and the long bones.[25] Pathological fractures occur commonly and occasionally are the presenting symptom. Loss of height or kyphosis due to vertebral compression fractures can be seen in advanced disease. Other presenting findings can include infections, hemorrhagic diathesis due to thrombopenia, symptoms caused by renal failure or hypercalcemia, and, less commonly, neurologic manifestations due to spinal cord or radicular compression or peripheral neuropathy.[25,26] Involvement of other extramedullary sites is a common feature of advanced disease, and extramedullary myeloma infiltrates are to be distinguished from solitary extraosseous plasmacytoma (EOP). MM is frequently diagnosed in an asymptomatic individual following discovery of an M protein. Smoldering MM progresses to symptomatic MM at a rate of 10%/year in the first 5 years, with the frequency declining to 3%/year in the subsequent 5 years, underlining the clinical and biological heterogeneity of this intermediate disease stage.[27-29]

Imaging

A conventional radiographic survey will detect skeletal abnormalities in 70% to 80% of patients, whereas MRI and positron emission tomography/computed tomography (PET/CT) identify bone lesions in an even higher percentage of patients.[25,30,31] Osteolytic lesions (70%) and osteoporosis are the most common findings and most frequently involve the vertebral column, the long bones, pelvis, shoulder girdle, and ribs. Osteosclerotic lesions are very rare and are associated with osteosclerotic MM and POEMS syndrome. Owing to the adapted International Myeloma Working Group criteria for active MM, MRI or PET/CT need to be performed during initial staging.[5]

Laboratory features

Almost all patients show a monoclonal paraprotein in serum or urine, with IgG in >50%, IgA in 20%, and light chains only (Bence-Jones proteins) in 15% to 20%, with rare cases (<1%) showing IgD, IgE, or IgM or biclonal paraproteins.[1,5,25,27] Although total Ig is commonly increased due to the M protein, uninvolved polyclonal Ig (<50% of normal serum Ig) is decreased in most patients, termed immunoparesis.

Cytopenias are common, with anemia of usually moderate severity in about 50% of patients, leukopenia in approximately 20%, and thrombocytopenia in 5% at presentation.[25] Erythrocyte sedimentation rate is variably increased and correlates with the level of M protein. Renal failure, which may be a presenting symptom, is due to tubular damage by secreted light chains, especially the lambda isotype.[8] Other laboratory findings include hypercalcemia (20%), creatinine elevation (20%-30%), hyperuricemia (>30%), and hypoalbuminemia (~15%).[25,32]

Staging

Staging of symptomatic MM is performed according to the International Staging System (ISS),[32] which has been revised by including cytogenetic risk factors (R-ISS),[33] shown in Table 52.3. Since plasma cell percentages are of central importance for separation of smoldering from symptomatic MM, correct enumeration is crucial. Counts should be assessed both in the aspirate and the BM trephine, aided by immunostaining in the latter. In the case of discrepancies, the higher estimate should be used. Owing to possible dilution effects, counts based on FCM should not be used.[34]

Clinical variants

Nonsecretory MM

Approximately 1% of cases are nonsecretory, also lacking an abnormal FLC ratio.[5] Nevertheless, in most of these cases cytoplasmic IG can be demonstrated in the neoplastic plasma cells, pointing to defects in Ig secretion. In around 15% of nonsecretory cases, molecular alterations in IG genes result in lack of Ig translation.[35] Clinically and genetically, nonsecretory MM is similar to conventional MM, but with a lower incidence of renal insufficiency, hypercalcemia, and immunoparesis due to the absence of an M protein and a higher frequency of the t(11;14) translocation.[36,37]

Plasma cell leukemia

Plasma cell leukemia (PCL) is defined as clonal plasma cells constituting >5% of peripheral blood cells.[38] This new, lower threshold replaces the old PCL definition of >20% of total leukocytes or an absolute count $>2.0 \times 10^9$/L, since it has been shown that these

TABLE 52.3 Revised international staging system for multiple myeloma

Stage	Criteria	Median PFS	5-y PFS (%)
I	β2MG ≤ 3.5 mg/L Serum albumin ≥35 g/L Standard risk cytogenetics LDH ≤ upper normal limit	66 mo	55
II	Not stage I or III	42 mo	36
III	β2MG ≥5.5 mg/L and high-risk cytogenetics (del(17p) and/or t(4;14) and/or t(14;16)) or LDH > upper normal limit	29 mo	24

β2MG, β2-microglobulin LDH, lactic dehydrogenase; PFS, progression-free survival.

Modified according to Palumbo A, Avet-Loiseau H, Oliva S, et al. Revised international staging system for multiple myeloma: a report from International myeloma working group. *J Clin Oncol.* 2015;33(26):2863-2869.

patients have a similarly poor prognosis.[6,39] Primary PCL accounts for about 2% to 4% of newly diagnosed MM, but it may also occur as secondary leukemic transformation in end-stage disease.[40] Most patients show massive BM infiltration and frequent extramedullary infiltrates including hepatosplenomegaly and/or lymphadenopathy and body cavity effusions, whereas osteolytic lesions are less common. Patients with primary PCL are, on average, younger than those with conventional MM, and primary PCL shows a higher proportion of cases with only light chains or rare heavy chain isotypes. CD20 and cyclin D1 expression, associated with the t(11;14) translocation, is more frequent in PCL, whereas CD56 is usually negative.[41]

Plasma cell neoplasms with an associated paraneoplastic syndrome

POEMS syndrome (synonyms: Osteosclerotic myeloma, Crow-Fukase syndrome)

POEMS syndrome is a rare paraneoplastic disorder accounting for less than 1% of plasma cell neoplasms. It is characterized by a clonal plasma cell neoplasm, frequent osteosclerotic and fibrotic changes in the bone, and, in 11% to 30% of cases, lymph node changes of the multicentric plasma cell variant of Castleman disease. The acronym POEMS stands for Polyneuropathy, Organomegaly, Endocrinopathy, Monoclonal gammopathy, and Skin lesions. The diagnostic criteria are shown in Table 52.4. POEMS syndrome shows a wide spectrum of clinical features, including the ones included in the acronym, and others such as extravascular fluid overload with effusions, papilledema, and lung disease may occur. The markedly elevated levels of vascular endothelial growth factor correlate with disease activity.[43] Most patients (90%-95%) show an M protein with lambda light chains. The BM features of POEMS syndrome are distinct from those of MM. A lambda light chain–restricted plasma cell population can be identified in most, but not all, patients. Half of the cases show lymphoid aggregates, frequently rimmed by monotypic plasma cells. The majority of patients show hypercellular hematopoiesis with marked megakaryocyte proliferation.[44] Fibrosis and osteosclerosis is usually not observed, unless lesional tissue is biopsied.

TEMPI syndrome

TEMPI syndrome is a very rare paraneoplastic syndrome with a clonal plasma cell proliferation.[45] The acronym stands for Telangiectasias, elevated Erythropoietin levels, Erythrocytosis, Monoclonal gammopathy, Perinephric fluid accumulations and Intrapulmonary shunting. The predominant M protein is IgG kappa. BM shows marked reactive erythroid hyperplasia as a result of significantly elevated erythropoietin and a clonal plasma cell population, which usually is in the percentage range of MGUS, ie, less than 10%.[46]

TABLE 52.4 Diagnostic criteria for POEMS syndrome

	Symptoms and findings	Frequency
Mandatory criteria		
	(Demyelinating) polyneuropathy	100%
	Clonal plasma cell proliferation (mostly λ)	100%
Other major criteria (1 required)		
	Multicentric Castleman disease	11%-25%
	Sclerotic bone lesions	27%-97%
	VEGF elevation	common
Minor criteria		
	Organomegaly	45%-85%
	Endocrinopathy	67%-84%
	Extravascular volume overload	29%-87%
	Skin changes	68%-89%
	Papillary edema	29%-64%
	Thrombocytosis/polycythemia	54%-88%

The diagnosis of POEMS syndrome is confirmed when both of the mandatory major criteria, one of the three other major criteria, and one of the six minor criteria are present.

VEGF, vascular endothelial growth factor.

Modified according to Dispenzieri A. POEMS syndrome: 2021 Update on diagnosis, risk-stratification, and management. *Am J Hematol.* 2021;96(7):872-888.

Morphology

BM aspirate and biopsy are complementary for the diagnosis of MM. The number and distribution of neoplastic cells is extremely variable from case to case. Their cytomorphology shows a broad spectrum, ranging from mature plasma cells without cytologic atypia to plasmablastic and anaplastic cells (Figures 52.1 and 52.2A and B). Mature plasma cells show a typical eccentrically located clockface nucleus and basophilic cytoplasm with a lighter-stained perinuclear hof. The lymphoplasmacytic or small cell variant of MM is characterized by small lymphoid-appearing cells with a narrow rim of basophilic cytoplasm with a small hof; approximately 50% of cases with this morphology are associated with the t(11;14) translocation and cyclin D1 overexpression (Figure 52.3A and B). Immature forms show a reduced nuclear/cytoplasmic ratio with larger, sometimes irregular nuclei frequently with prominent nucleoli. Multinucleation, nuclear pseudoinclusions (Dutcher bodies), and nuclear lobulations can be observed. Immaturity, prominent nucleoli, and nuclear atypia are usually lacking in reactive plasmacytosis and therefore are good indicators of malignancy. Plasmablastic morphology is found in almost 10% of cases. Plasmablasts may either resemble immunoblasts with central, prominent eosinophilic nucleoli or occasionally show myeloblast-like features (Figure 52.1D-F). The plasmablastic subtype of MM shows a poor prognosis and an aggressive course. Anaplastic MM can be difficult to discern from aggressive lymphoma or nonhematopoietic neoplasms. IgA-secreting MM frequently exhibits large, mature plasma cells with broad, "flaming" cytoplasm

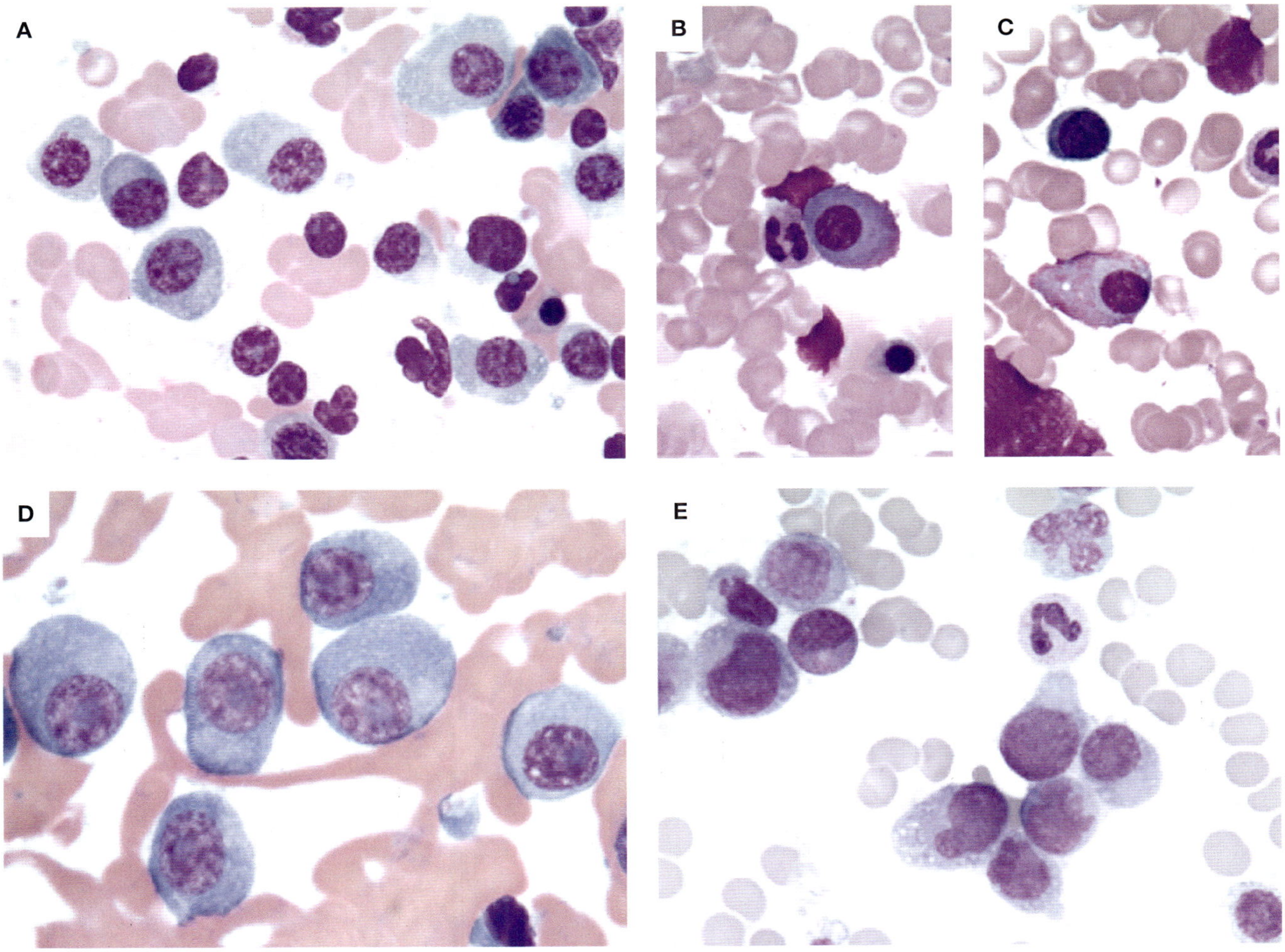

FIGURE 52.1 Multiple myeloma. Cytological features in the bone marrow aspirate. **A:** Mature plasma cells with condensed chromatin, mostly eccentrically located nucleus and variably broad, basophilic cytoplasm. **B** and **C:** So-called flame cells with vermilion-staining cytoplasm in IgA myeloma. **D:** Plasmablastic myeloma with large cells with enlarged nuclei with more open chromatin and prominent central nucleoli. **E:** Immature myeloma: Cells with increased nucleus to cytoplasm ratio, irregular nuclei with open chromatin and sometimes blastoid features.

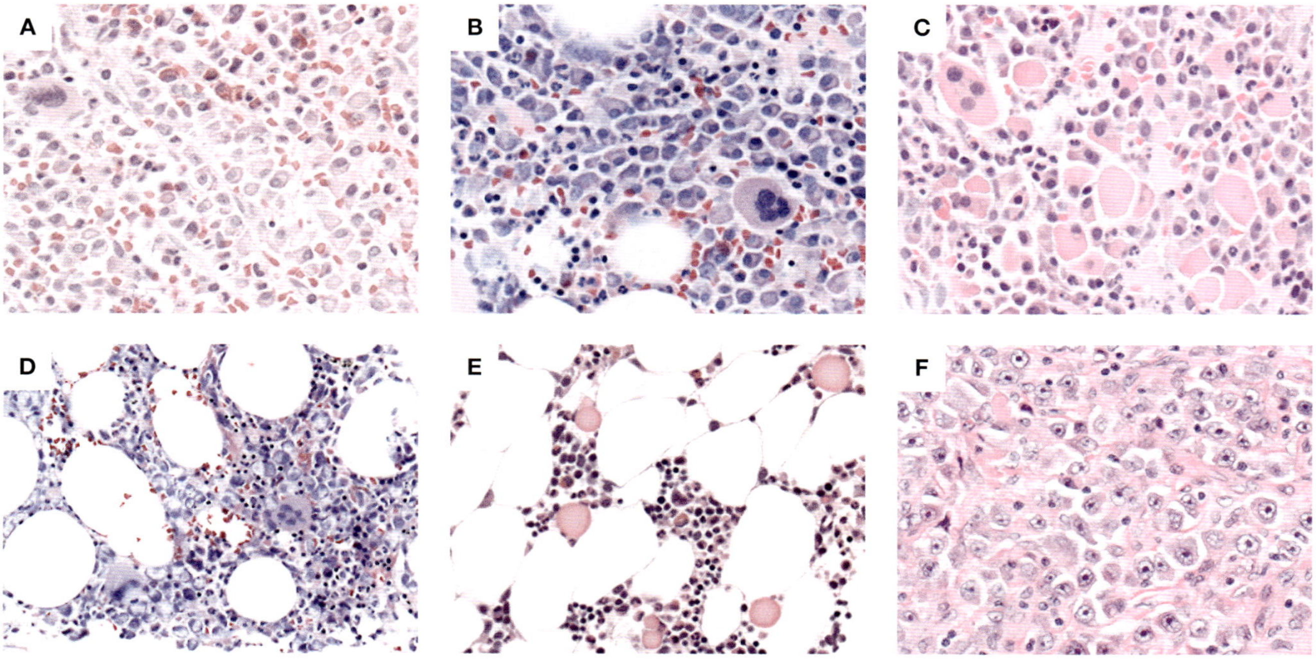

FIGURE 52.2 Multiple myeloma in the bone marrow biopsy. **A:** Conventional myeloma with mostly mature, excentrically located nuclei. **B:** Same case in Giemsa staining highlights the basophilic cytoplasm and perinuclear hof. **C:** Amorphous immunoglobulin inclusions in plasma cells. **D:** So-called signet ring cells in myeloma. **E:** Abundant Russell bodies in a case of myeloma. **F:** Extramedullary infiltrate of multiple myeloma with plasmablastic features with large, central nucleoli.

(Figure 52.1B and C). Disturbances in Ig secretion can cause cytoplasmic changes, including Mott cells, eosinophilic Russell bodies, pseudo-signet ring cells, and rarely pseudo-Gaucher cells with fibrillary deposits or crystalline inclusions[1,47] (Figures 52.2C-E and 52.4). Crystal storing histiocytosis with macrophages containing abundant granular or crystalline inclusions can accompany MM and may obscure the underlying plasma cell neoplasm.[48]

In the BM trephine, the distribution and arrangement of plasma cells are important for the distinction from reactive plasmacytosis. Plasma cell clusters in the fatty marrow and small nodular aggregates are highly suspicious for malignancy. Tumorous aggregates and sheet-like infiltrates with displacement of hematopoiesis are diagnostic of MM (Figure 52.2). Of note, the distribution of infiltrates may be very heterogenous, underlying the importance of an adequate specimen. Interstitial infiltrates, especially of small cell MM may be obscured by reactive hyperplasia of hematopoiesis, making IHC mandatory to assess the presence and extent of a plasma cell infiltrate. Irregularly contoured bone trabeculae and prominent osteoclastic activity are observed in active bone disease. Amyloidosis is observed in a subset of MM, either as vascular amyloid or more extensive interstitial deposits.

Immunophenotype

Overall, neoplastic plasma cells share the antigen profile of normal plasma cells with loss of most B-cell surface markers but usually exhibit some aberrant immunophenotypic features. The immunophenotype of MM is summarized in Table 52.5. Of note, the frequencies of expression of any given marker given in the literature may vary depending on the mode of detection (IHC vs FCM). In normal and most malignant plasma cells, upregulation of the master transcription factor IRF4/MUM1 results in downregulation of PAX5 and consecutive loss of expression of surface IG and several B-cell markers including CD20 and CD22, whereas plasma cell antigens are expressed. Loss of CD19, however, discriminates most malignant from benign plasma cells, which partially retain CD19 expression. The most commonly used plasma cell markers in the BM trephine are MUM1 and CD138 (Figure 52.5), and additional useful antigens are CD79a and CD38.[47,49] Epithelial membrane antigen (EMA, MUC1) is expressed in most normal and malignant plasma cells. Of note, none of these markers is specific for plasma cells and may be expressed by various other cell types. MM often shows no or only weak expression of CD45. CD56 (NCAM) is expressed by 70% to 80% of MM and is a good, although not entirely specific, marker of malignancy[50]

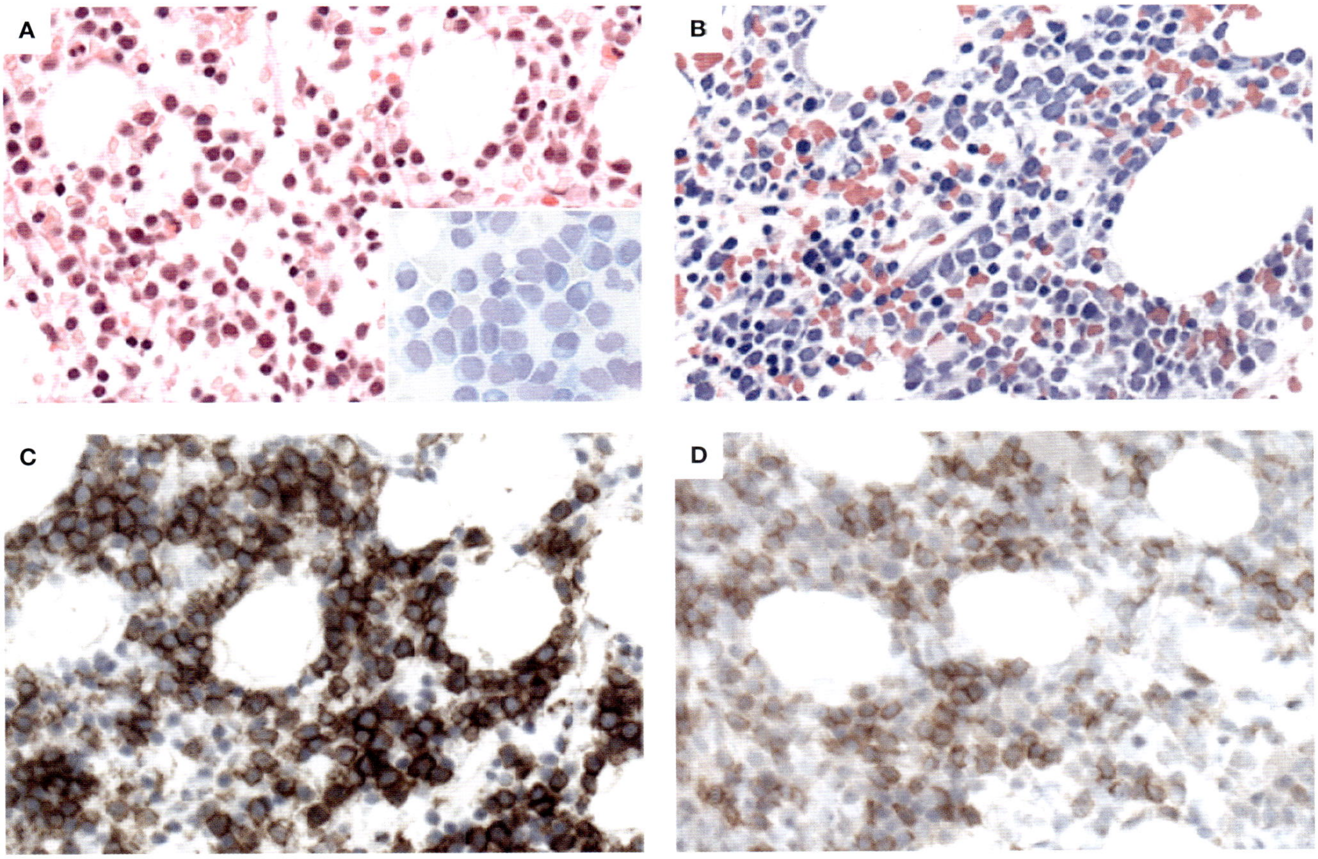

FIGURE 52.3 Multiple myeloma with small cell/lymphoplasmacytic morphology, IgD kappa paraprotein, multiple osteolytic lesions, and t(11;14) translocation. **A:** Conventional morphology shows a small cell infiltrate with scant cytoplasm, reminiscent of small B-cell lymphoma or lymphoplasmacytic lymphoma. The inset shows identical features in the cytology. **B:** Giemsa stain reveals narrow, eccentric cytoplasm of the plasma cells. **C:** Strong CD20 expression and **D:** heterogeneous CD56 expression. This case additionally partially expressed CD19 and CD22 and was strongly positive for CD138 and cyclin D1.

(Figure 52.3D). Of note, clonal plasma cells in lymphoplasmacytic lymphoma are always CD56 negative.[51] Other surface markers aberrantly expressed in a subset of MM are CD117, CD20, and CD10. CD20 is positive in about 20% of cases, with strong and homogeneous positivity in a subset[52] (Figure 52.3C). These cases are frequently associated with lymphoplasmacytic morphology and may rarely express other B-cell markers, such as PAX5 and/or CD22, but usually retain strong and homogeneous expression of CD138.[53] Cyclin D1, which is absent from normal B cells and plasma cells, is expressed in approximately 50% of MM, with strong and homogeneous nuclear expression in cases carrying the t(11;14) translocation[54] (Figure 52.5C). Upregulation of MYC protein to a variable degree is a hallmark of MM, unrelated to the presence or absence of *MYC* translocations, but is typically absent from MGUS.[55]

Stains for Ig light chains, complemented if necessary by staining for heavy chains, are essential to confirm a monotypic plasma cell population. Since IG expression may be low in neoplastic plasma cells, demonstration of light chain restriction can be difficult by IHC in some patients. Colorimetric/chromogenic in situ hybridization for Ig light chains is a robust alternative method.[56] IgM-positive MM, which does not undergo heavy chain class switch, is rare, making up less than 1% of cases. It shows conventional morphology and homogeneous expression of plasma cell markers, usually lacks CD56 and CD117 and is often positive for CD20 and cyclin D1, and shows a higher frequency of the t(11;14) translocation but lacks the *MYD88* L265P mutation.[57,58] Biclonal MM with production of different heavy chains or light chains is rare (<1%).[59]

By FCM, plasma cells are typically detected by gating on CD45 versus CD38 or CD138 (Figure 52.6). While plasma cells are frequently negative for surface IG light chains, monotypic expression of kappa or lambda can be detected in the cytoplasm. Aberrant surface marker expression can be detected in nearly all cases, especially lack of CD19 (95%). Other markers seen on normal

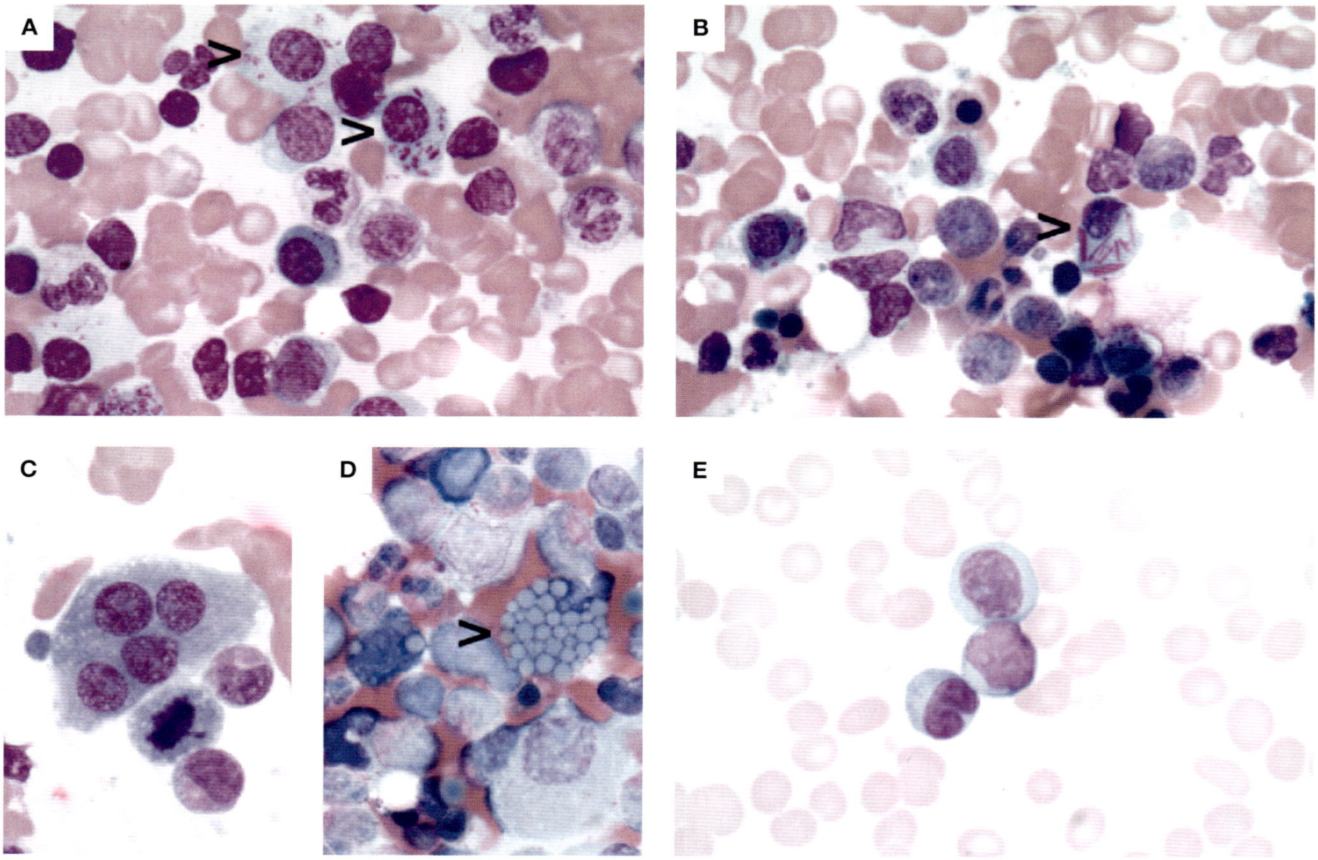

FIGURE 52.4 Multiple myeloma. Unusual cytological features. **A** and **B:** Plasma cells with diverse crystalline cytoplasmic inclusions (arrowheads). **C:** Multinucleated plasma cell. **D:** Mott cell with globular immunoglobulin inclusions (arrowhead). **E:** Plasma cell leukemia: Circulating plasma cells with blastoid features.

TABLE 52.5 Common immunophenotypic markers for multiple myeloma (MM)

Marker	Reactivity in normal cells	Frequency in MM
CD138 (syndecan)	PC, epithelia	>95%
MUM1/IRF4	PC, late/post-GC B cells	>95%
CD79a	PC, Pan-B cell	>95%
CD38	PC, T cells	>95%
CD19	B cells, normal PC	<5%
CD20	B cells, normal PC neg.	10%-20%
PAX5	B cells, normal PC neg.	Rare
CD45	Pan leukocyte marker, variable in normal PC	20%-30%, frequently weak
CD56 (NCAM)	NK cells, normal PC neg.	70%-80%
Cytoplasmic immunoglobulins		IgG > 50%; IgA 15%; Light chain only 20%; IgD, IgE, IgM < 1%
Cyclin D1	Proliferating nonlymphoid cells	40%-50%, associated with t(11;14) and trisomy 11
CD117	Mast cells, myeloblasts	20%-35%
EMA	Epithelial cells, normal PC	60%-90%

EMA, epithelial membrane antigen; PC, plasma cell.

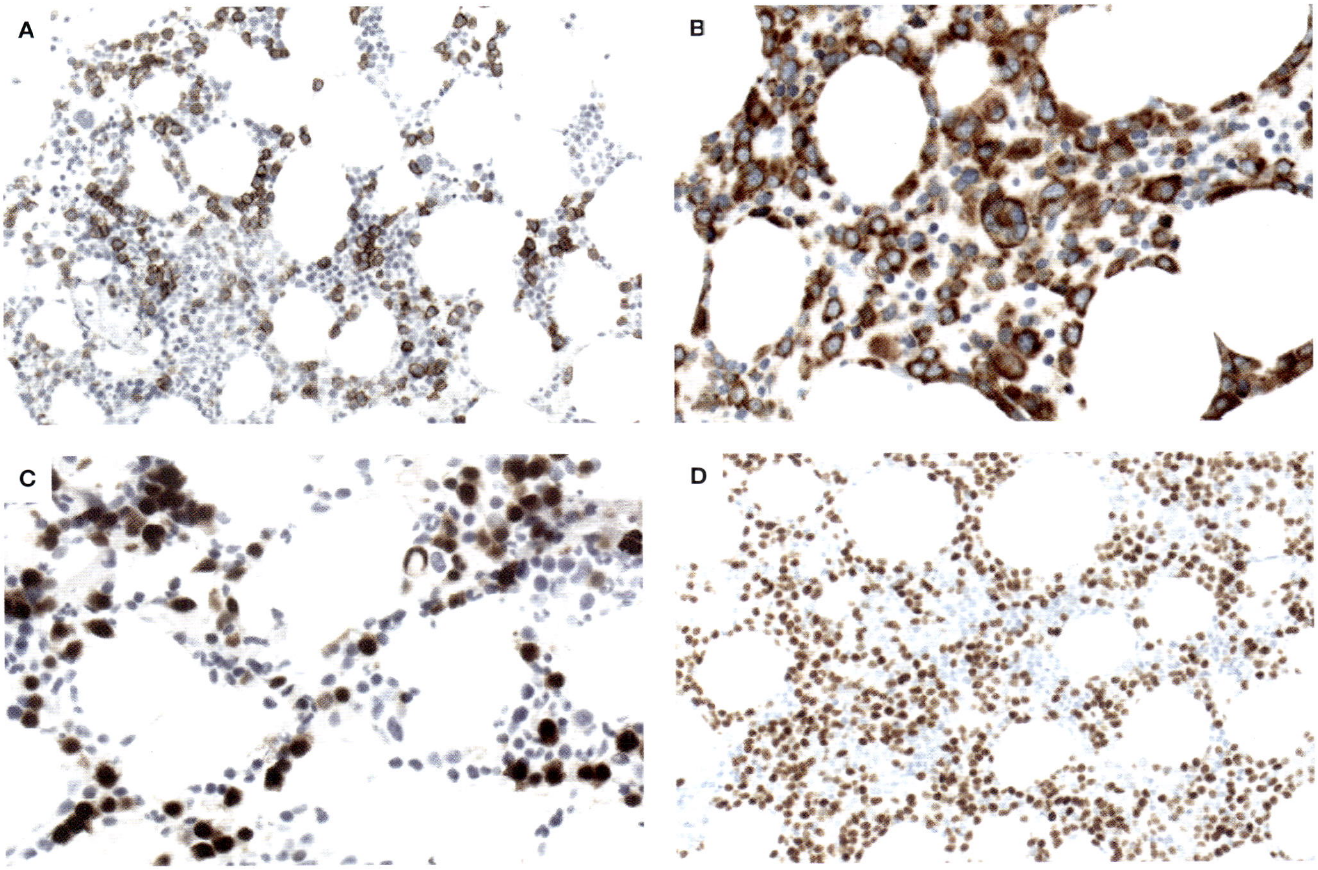

FIGURE 52.5 Immunohistochemistry of multiple myeloma in the bone marrow biopsy. **A:** CD138-positive plasma cells in an interstitial distribution. **B:** Strong kappa light chain expression in atypical plasma cells. **C:** Strong and homogeneous nuclear cyclin D1 expression in myeloma with t(11;14) translocation. **D:** Strong nuclear expression of MUM1 in myeloma with small cell morphology.

plasma cells may be decreased or aberrantly dim such as CD27 and CD81. Aberrant expression of markers not seen on normal plasma cells can also be detected, such as CD56 and CD200, which are present in a majority of cases (75%-80% and 60%-75%, respectively). Other markers of aberrancy include CD20, CD28, and CD117. FCM can also detect aberrancies in the intensity of plasma cell markers, including relatively dim CD38 and bright CD138, relative to normal plasma cells.[60]

Assessing a large panel of surface markers may aid in detecting malignant plasma cells in difficult cases such as biclonal disease or in the presence of a polytypic background. Most diagnostic panels include CD19, CD27, CD38, CD45, CD81, and cytoplasmic kappa and lambda. However, utilizing an extended panel of markers is helpful in patients who receive therapy targeted against plasma cell markers, such as anti-CD38 antibodies. In these patients CD38 cannot be reliably used to gate plasma cells, with potential alternatives including CD229 and VS38c.[61] Reliable alternative gating strategies are also important when using FCM to assess for minimal residual disease (MRD). The EuroFlow consortium proposes the combined surface plus intracellular staining of CD38 using a multiepitope (ie, polyclonal) antibody.[62] The next-generation FCM method proposed by the consortium for the assessment of MRD includes two eight-color combinations: CD138/CD27/CD38/CD56/CD45/CD117/CD81 and CD138/CD27/CD38/CD56/CD45/CyKappa/cyLambda.[62] FCM underestimates the percent of plasma cells present compared with CD138 IHC on the trephine or clot.[34]

Patterns of antigen expression detected by FCM may also have prognostic significance, with some markers being associated with worse prognosis, including positivity for CD19, CD28, and CD200 and negativity for CD45 and CD117. While there are some conflicting data, a retrospective analysis suggested aberrantly dim CD38, presence of CD81, and absence of CD117 was associated with worse prognosis in multivariate analysis.[63] The proportion of clonal plasma cells compared with background normal plasma cells appears to have prognostic significance both in MGUS and myeloma.[64,65]

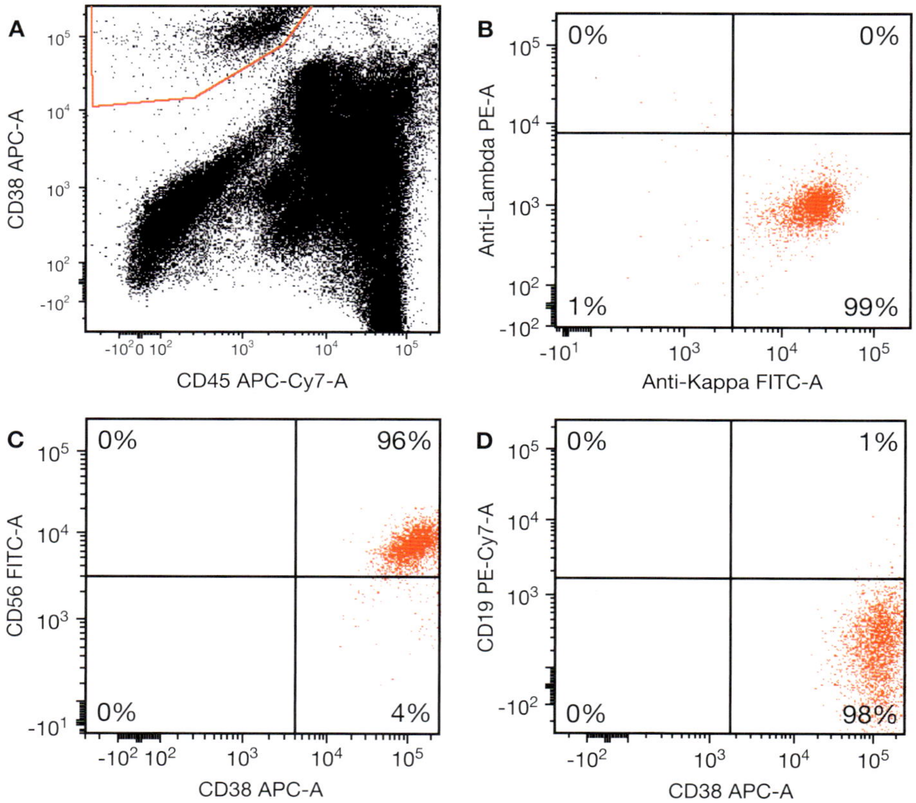

FIGURE 52.6 Flow cytometry histograms from myeloma in the bone marrow. **A:** Gating of plasma cells with CD38 and CD45. The plasma cells show **B:** cytoplasmic kappa light chain expression, **C:** CD38 and strong CD56 expression, and **D:** lack of CD19.

Genetics

In keeping with its post–germinal center derivation, MM shows clonally rearranged IG genes with a high load of somatic hypermutation, but without ongoing mutations.

MM is probably one of the genetically most diverse hematological neoplasms. This heterogeneity is associated with a broad spectrum of clinical aggressiveness and differences in therapy response, which has prompted the formal separation of MM into cytogenetic groups in the International Consensus Classification as shown in Table 52.6.[49,67] Both numerical and structural aberrations occur at high frequency and in part have important prognostic implications.[33,68]

Two major cytogenetic groups can be discerned in MM. Approximately 40% to 50% of cases are nonhyperdiploid and show translocations involving the immunoglobulin heavy chain (IGH) locus on 14q32, with rare translocations involving the light chain loci.[69-71] These cytogenetic features are already present in MGUS and thus represent primary alterations.[12,72] They persist throughout the disease course and are strongly correlated with clinical and phenotypic features, prognosis, therapy response, and the gene expression profile.[33,73-75] The IGH translocations in most, but not all, cases do not occur during primary VDJ IGH rearrangement, but rather during the heavy chain switch recombination, which takes place in the germinal center. In contrast to most small B-cell lymphomas, the translocations are promiscuous and involve a large variety of partner genes. The most common recurrent translocation partners can be divided into three groups: *CCND* family translocations, with the t(11;14)(q13;q32) *CCND1::IGH* being most common; *MAF* family translocations; and t(4;14)(p16;q32) *NSD2::IGH*.[67,73] A variety of rare partner genes have been described. Cases with t(11;14)(q13;q32), approximately 15% to 20% of all MM, can be recognized by their strong and homogeneous nuclear expression of cyclin D1 and exhibit some clinical and phenotypic peculiarities, including frequent response to the BCL2 inhibitor venetoclax.[54,76,77] This translocation is overrepresented in PCL and nonsecretory and IgM-positive MM.[36] About half of t(11;14)+ MM show lymphoplasmacytic morphology, often in combination with the expression of B-cell markers such as CD20.[76] The second major cytogenetic group encompasses

TABLE 52.6 Cytogenetic subclassification of multiple myeloma (MM)

Type of alteration/category	Involved genes	Frequency	Risk
Multiple myeloma, NOS	-	9%	Standard
MM with recurrent alterations			
- Hyperdiploid	—	45%	Standard
- Nonhyperdiploid	IGH translocations	40%-45%	
- *CCND* family		18%-22%	
- t(11;14)(q13;q32)	*CCND1*/cyclin D1	15%	Standard
- t(12;14)(p13;q32)	*CCND2*/cyclin D2	2%	
- t(6;14)(p21;q32)	*CCND3*/cyclin D3	<1%	
- *NSD2*/t(4;14)(p16;q32)	*NSD2*	13%-15%	High
- *MAF* family		6%-8%	
- t(14;16)(q32;q23)	*MAF*	5%	High
- t(14;20)(q32;q11)	*MAFB*	2%	
- t(8;14)(q24;q32)	*MAFA*	<1%	
Other frequent alterations			
- Monosomy 13 or del(13q)		45%-50%	Standard for MM, high for SMM
add(1q)	*MCL1/CKS1B*	40%	High
del(1p)	*CDKN2C*	7%-40%	High (?)
del(17p)	*TP53*	7%-10%	High

IGH, immunoglobulin heavy chain; NOS, not otherwise specified; SMM, smoldering multiple myeloma.
Modified from Bergsagel PL, Kuehl WM. Critical roles for immunoglobulin translocations and cyclin D dysregulation in multiple myeloma. *Immunol Rev.* 2003;194:96-104.

approximately 45% of cases and is characterized by hyperdiploidy with gains of 3 or more odd-numbered chromosomes including 3, 5, 7, 9, 11, 15, 19, and 21. In the future, this group may be further subdivided according to presence of trisomy 11 and *CCND1*/cyclin D1 expression.[54,78] About 9% of MM cases cannot be assigned to the above-mentioned groups and are termed MM, not otherwise specified. The frequencies of the recurrent primary genetic abnormalities and their prognostic features are listed in Table 52.5 and illustrated in Figure 52.7. The role of mutational profiling in MM remains to be determined in future studies, but mutational analysis of *TP53* is recommended for relapsed MM.[79,80] The current standard

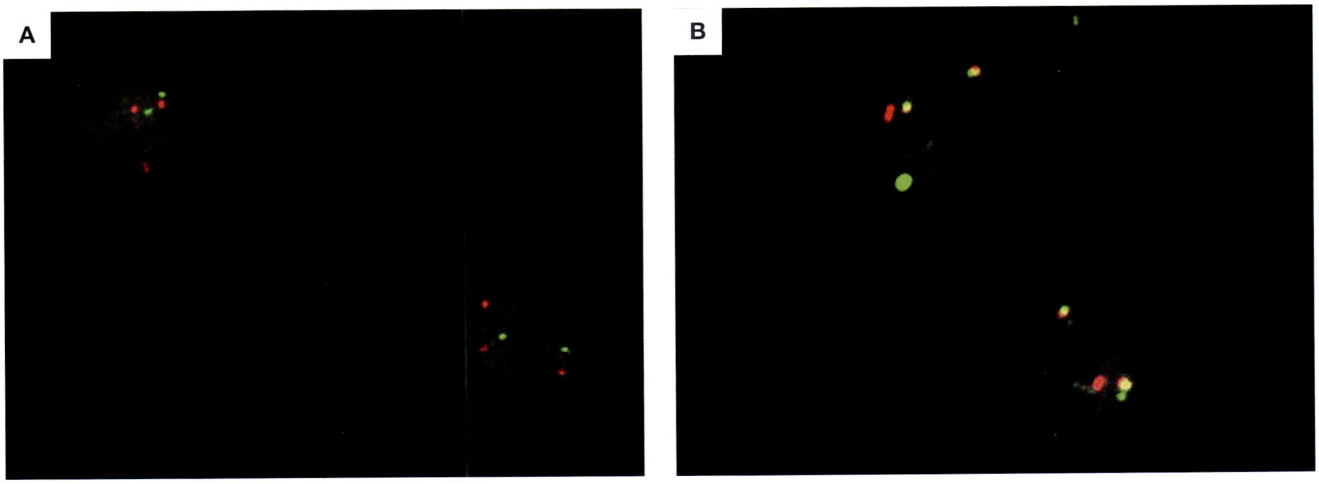

FIGURE 52.7 Fluorescence in situ hybridization in myeloma. **A:** Two cells with gain of 1q (red, three signals) and normal 1p (green, two signals). **B:** Two plasma cells with t(14;16) with yellow fusion signals.

for genetic subclassification is FISH, and minimal and comprehensive FISH panels have been published.[73] In the future, high-throughput techniques may gain importance, since they allow a more comprehensive assessment of genetic alterations including cryptic translocations, copy number changes and mutations, as well as gene expression profile.[66,75,81,82]

Prognosis and Clinical Comment

MM is a unique cancer paradigm for investigating the mechanisms involved in the transition from a premalignant condition (MGUS) into a malignant disease (MM). In the pathogenesis of myeloma, the dialogue between plasma cells and their microenvironment is as important as the genotypic characteristics of the tumor clone, and it is likely that myeloma will soon no longer be considered as a single entity.[83,84] The outcome of patients with MM is highly heterogeneous, and the identification of those features influencing survival and response to therapy is mandatory in order to achieve the purpose of patients' treatment individualization. The most relevant prognostic factor in MM include (i) the genetic factors (described previously), (ii) the tumor load (clinical stage, elevated LDH, circulating PC, extramedullary disease), and (iii) factors related to the host (age, comorbidities, renal insufficiency, frailty). Nevertheless, the most important prognostic factor is the depth of response to therapy, and at present, MRD strategies, by next-generation sequencing or FCM, have become the most relevant tools to monitor treatment efficacy, with the goal to achieve and sustain MRD negativity.[85-87] The outcome of patients with MM has significantly improved in the last 2 decades, and in fact, the term "incurable" usually used to define MM has now been challenged with median survivals that exceed 10 years for many patients. This has been possible first through the introduction of high-dose therapy followed by autologous stem cell transplant, subsequently due to the use of proteasome inhibitors (bortezomib, carfilzomib) and immunomodulatory agents (thalidomide, lenalidomide, and pomalidomide) and more recently with the development of immunotherapeutic strategies based on anti-CD38 monoclonal antibodies, bispecific antibodies, and CAR-T cells.[88-91] Moreover, the introduction of new diagnostic criteria of early MM and the possibility of early intervention at the stage of smoldering MM opens up new therapeutic avenues with the ultimate aim of achieving a cure for this disease.[68,92]

PLASMACYTOMA

Definition

Plasmacytoma is a localized tumor composed of clonal plasma cells that are cytologically and immunophenotypically similar to those of MM. MM-defining clinical, laboratory, or radiologic findings (SLiM-CRAB criteria) are absent. Two major types of plasmacytoma are recognized: solitary plasmacytoma of bone (SBP) and EOP.[49]

Solitary Plasmacytoma of Bone

Definition

SBP is defined as a localized, destructive tumor of bone consisting of clonal, neoplastic PCs that share cytologic, immunophenotypic, and genetic similarities with MM. Clinical and laboratory features of MM are absent. Although overt disseminated BM involvement is lacking in all cases, SBP is subclassified according to the absence or presence of minimal BM involvement (<10% clonal PCs).

Synonyms

Plasmacytoma of bone; osseous plasmacytoma; solitary plasmacytoma; plasma cell tumor; solitary myeloma (nor recommended).

Epidemiology

SBP comprises 3% to 5% of PC neoplasms and accounts for 70% of all plasmacytomas.[3] SBP develops more commonly in males (M:F of 2:1) with a median age at diagnosis of 50 to 55 years.

General clinical features

A single painful bone lesion or pathologic fracture is the most common presenting feature of SBP. Bones of the axial skeleton are affected most frequently, in particular the skull, vertebrae, ribs, scapula, and femur.[93] Involvement of distal long bones of the extremities is rare. Vertebral involvement may cause compression of the spinal cord or nerve root.

Morphology

The morphologic features of SBP are similar to those of MM. Extension of the neoplastic PCs into adjacent soft tissue may be present in some cases. A staging BM aspirate and biopsy should be obtained in all cases of SBP to evaluate for disseminated BM involvement and subclassification of SBP according to the absence of minimal BM involvement (no clonal PCs detected) or presence of minimal BM involvement (clonal PCs present at <10%).

Immunophenotype

The immunophenotypic features of SBP are similar to those of MM (Table 52.5).

Genetics

The genetics of SBP are similar to those of MM (Table 52.6). Myeloma FISH should be performed on either the plasmacytoma or enriched BM PCs, if present, to assess for high-risk cytogenetic abnormalities.[94]

Prognosis and clinical comment

Approximately 50% of patients progress to MM within 10 years of initial diagnosis. The likelihood of disease progression is significantly influenced by the presence of minimal BM involvement as assessed by conventional flow cytometric MRD with 10^{-4} sensitivity. MM develops in approximately 70% and 10%, respectively, of patients with SBP with and without minimal BM involvement.[95,96] The presence of high-risk cytogenetic abnormalities, including del(17p), gain 1q, t(4;14), t(14;16), and t(14;20), is predictive of a significantly shorter interval for progression to MM.[94] Skeletal surveys, which were historically used to stage patients with SBP, are insufficiently sensitive to detect additional small lytic lesions, the presence of which would be diagnostic of MM. Therefore, more sensitive imaging modalities, eg, MRI or PET/CT should be performed as part of the diagnostic workup. SBP is exquisitely sensitive to radiotherapy, which is the mainstay of treatment in most patients.[93] The therapeutic value of chemotherapy in SBP is not well defined. Baseline and posttherapy serum protein studies (serum protein electrophoresis, immunofixation electrophoresis, and serum free light chain [SFLC]) should be performed. An abnormal SFLC ratio at diagnosis or persistence of a serum M protein following radiotherapy is associated with an increased risk for progression to MM.[93]

Extraosseous Plasmacytoma

Definition

EOP is a localized PC neoplasm arising, by definition, in a nonosseous site. EOP must be distinguished from extramedullary MM and from lymphomas with prominent plasmacytic differentiation, such as extranodal marginal zone (MALT) lymphoma and lymphoplasmacytic lymphoma.

Synonyms

Extramedullary plasmacytoma.

Epidemiology

EOP is rare and accounts for <2% of all PC neoplasms. EOP develops more commonly in males (M:F of 2:1-6:1) with a median age at diagnosis of 50 to 55 years.[97,98]

General clinical features

EOP presents as a solitary mass lesion. EOP may develop at a wide array of anatomic sites; however, 60% to 65% of lesions develop in the upper respiratory tract including the nasal cavity, sinuses, oropharynx, and larynx.[97] A serum M protein is present in about 20% of patients. SLiM-CRAB criteria are absent.

Morphology

EOP is morphologically similar to SBP and consists of a dense, sheetlike infiltrate of clonal PCs. The neoplastic PCs have mature morphology in most cases. Low-grade lymphomas with plasmacytic differentiation, such as extranodal MALT lymphoma and lymphoplasmacytic lymphoma, are the main considerations in the differential diagnosis and may be challenging to distinguish from EOP on solely a morphologic basis (Table 52.7). The presence of monocytoid cells or lymphoplasmacytic cells favors a diagnosis of lymphoma. Plasmablastic lymphoma is readily distinguished from EOP in most instances by virtue of the high-grade cytologic features of the neoplastic cells in the former (Table 52.7). EOP rarely occurs in children and younger adults; these lesions are primarily nodal, are composed of mature-appearing PCs, and express IgA.[99] Similar to SBP, a staging BM aspirate and biopsy should be obtained in all cases of EOP to exclude disseminated myelomatous BM involvement and for subclassification of EOP based on minimal (clonal PCs present at <10%) or absent BM involvement.

Immunophenotype

Similar to MM, the clonal PCs of EOP express CD38, CD138, and MUM1, and they show cytoplasmic light chain (LC) restriction assessed by either IHC or in situ hybridization (Table 52.5).[100] The proliferative activity of the clonal PCs is quite variable, with >80% Ki-67-positive cells in some cases. In contrast to MM, EOP lacks expression of CD56 in most cases.[98] CD20 is usually negative. EBV LMP and EBER are negative in most cases. Detection of an LC-restricted B-cell population by FCM favors a diagnosis of lymphoma.

Genetics

Scant data are available on the genetics of EOP. There is overlap of the genetic abnormalities present in EOP

TABLE 52.7 Distinguishing features of extramedullary plasmacytic/plasmablastic neoplasms

	LPL	EMZL	EOP	EMM	PBL
Morphology	Small lymphocytes, lymphoplasmacytic cells, and variable PC component	Small lymphocytes, centrocytoid and/or monocytoid cells, and variable PC component	Diffuse, sheetlike infiltrate of mature PCs in most cases	Diffuse, sheetlike infiltrate of PCs with variable cytology ranging from mature to plasmablastic or anaplastic	Diffuse proliferation of large cells with inclusion-like nucleoli; mature-appearing PCs usually absent
Immunophenotype	$CD19^+$, $CD20^+$, $CD5^{-/+}$, $CD23^{-/+}$ PCs negative for CD56, cyclin D1, and CD117 EBV-	$CD19^+$, $CD20^+$, $CD5^{-/+}$, $CD43^{-/+}$ PCs negative for CD56, cyclin D1, and CD117 EBV-	$CD138^+$, $CD38^+$, MUM1+, monotypic LC; $CD56^{-/+}$ Negative for CD19, CD20, PAX5, cyclin D1, MYC, or p53 overexpression EBV+ in <15% of cases	$CD138^+$, $CD38^+$, MUM1+, monotypic LC; $CD56^{+/-}$; variable positivity for CD20, PAX5, and cyclin D1; frequent MYC and/or p53 overexpression Negative for CD19 EBV-	$CD138^+$, $CD38^+$, MUM1+, monotypic LC; frequent MYC and/or p53 overexpression; high Ki-67 labeling Negative for CD19, CD20 EBV+ in 50%-75% of cases
Genetic findings	*MYD88* L265P in >90%; *CXCR4*^{mut} in 30%-40% MM-related lesions absent	EMZL-type translocations depending on location MM-related lesions absent	Primary MM-related lesions present, except for t(11;14) Secondary mutations undefined	Primary MM-related lesions present; secondary and high-risk alterations common, including 1q gains, del(17p), *MYC* translocations, and *TP53* mutations	*MYC* translocations in 50% of cases RAS-RAF, JAK-STAT, and NOTCH pathway mutations; MM-related lesions absent

EMM, extramedullary multiple myeloma; EMZL, extranodal marginal zone B-cell lymphoma; EOP, extraosseous plasmacytoma; LC, light chain; LPL, lymphoplasmacytic lymphoma; MM, multiple myeloma; PBL, plasmablastic lymphoma; PC, plasma cell.

Table modified from Fend F, Dogan A, Cook JR. Plasma cell neoplasms and related entities-evolution in diagnosis and classification. *Virchows Arch.* 2023;482(1):163-177.

and MM, including polysomy of odd-numbered chromosomes and translocations targeting the IGH locus at 14q32, although differences exist (Table 52.6). The t(11;14) *CCND1::IGH* appears to be significantly less frequent in EOP than in MM.[101]

Prognosis and clinical comment

Approximately 12% to 35% of EOPs progress to MM within 10 years of initial diagnosis. Similar to SBP, the likelihood of disease progression is significantly influenced by the presence of minimal BM involvement; MM develops in approximately 20% and 6%, respectively, of patients with EOP with and without minimal BM involvement.[95,96] In addition to BM examination, MRI or PET/CT imaging should be performed as part of the diagnostic workup of EOP. Depending on the anatomic site, complete surgical excision may be an effective therapy for EOP. For lesions involving the head and neck and other sites where excision is not feasible, radiotherapy is curative in most patients. Baseline and posttherapy serum protein studies should be performed. An abnormal SFLC ratio at diagnosis or persistence of a serum M protein following radiotherapy is associated with an increased risk for progression to MM.

References

1. McKenna RW, Kyle RD, Kuehl WM, Harris NL, Coupland R, Fend F. Plasma cell neoplasms. In: Swerdlow SH, Campo E, Harris NL, Jaffe ES, Pileri S, Stein H, et al, eds. WHO Classification of Tumours of Hematopoietic and Lymphoid Tissues. IARC; 2017:241-253.
2. Kyle RA, Larson DR, Therneau TM, et al. Long-term follow-up of monoclonal gammopathy of undetermined significance. *N Engl J Med.* 2018;378(3):241-249.
3. Kyle RA, Rajkumar SV. Monoclonal gammopathy of undetermined significance. *Br J Haematol.* 2006;134(6):573-589.
4. Kyle RA, Therneau TM, Rajkumar SV, et al. Prevalence of monoclonal gammopathy of undetermined significance. *N Engl J Med.* 2006;354(13):1362-1369.
5. Rajkumar SV, Dimopoulos MA, Palumbo A, et al. International Myeloma Working Group updated criteria for the diagnosis of multiple myeloma. *Lancet Oncol.* 2014;15(12):e538-e548.
6. Fermand JP, Bridoux F, Dispenzieri A, et al. Monoclonal gammopathy of clinical significance: a novel concept with therapeutic implications. *Blood.* 2018;132(14):1478-1485.
7. Leung N, Bridoux F, Batuman V, et al. The evaluation of monoclonal gammopathy of renal significance:

a consensus report of the International Kidney and Monoclonal Gammopathy Research Group. *Nat Rev Nephrol.* 2019;15(1):45-59.

8. Leung N, Bridoux F, Nasr SH. Monoclonal gammopathy of renal significance. *N Engl J Med.* 2021;384(20):1931-1941.
9. Landgren O, Gridley G, Turesson I, et al. Risk of monoclonal gammopathy of undetermined significance (MGUS) and subsequent multiple myeloma among African American and white veterans in the United States. *Blood.* 2006;107(3):904-906.
10. Pérez-Persona E, Mateo G, García-Sanz R, et al. Risk of progression in smouldering myeloma and monoclonal gammopathies of unknown significance: comparative analysis of the evolution of monoclonal component and multiparameter flow cytometry of bone marrow plasma cells. *Br J Haematol.* 2010;148(1):110-114.
11. Brousseau M, Leleu X, Gerard J, Intergroupe Francophone du Myélome, et al. Hyperdiploidy is a common finding in monoclonal gammopathy of undetermined significance and monosomy 13 is restricted to these hyperdiploid patients. *Clin Cancer Res.* 2007;13(20):6026-6031.
12. Kaufmann H, Ackermann J, Baldia C, et al. Both IGH translocations and chromosome 13q deletions are early events in monoclonal gammopathy of undetermined significance and do not evolve during transition to multiple myeloma. *Leukemia.* 2004;18(11):1879-1882.
13. Mikulasova A, Smetana J, Wayhelova M, et al. Genomewide profiling of copy-number alteration in monoclonal gammopathy of undetermined significance. *Eur J Haematol.* 2016;97(6):568-575.
14. Schmidt-Hieber M, Gutiérrez ML, Pérez-Andrés M, et al. Cytogenetic profiles in multiple myeloma and monoclonal gammopathy of undetermined significance: a study in highly purified aberrant plasma cells. *Haematologica.* 2013;98(2):279-287.
15. Chesi M, Stein CK, Garbitt VM, et al. Monosomic loss of MIR15A/MIR16-1 is a driver of multiple myeloma proliferation and disease progression. *Blood Cancer Discov.* 2020;1(1):68-81.
16. Mikulasova A, Wardell CP, Murison A, et al. The spectrum of somatic mutations in monoclonal gammopathy of undetermined significance indicates a less complex genomic landscape than that in multiple myeloma. *Haematologica.* 2017;102(9):1617-1625.
17. Kyle RA, Durie BG, Rajkumar SV; International Myeloma Working Group, et al. Monoclonal gammopathy of undetermined significance (MGUS) and smoldering (asymptomatic) multiple myeloma: IMWG consensus perspectives risk factors for progression and guidelines for monitoring and management. *Leukemia.* 2010;24(6):1121-1127.
18. van Nieuwenhuijzen N, Spaan I, Raymakers R, Peperzak V. From MGUS to multiple myeloma, a paradigm for clonal evolution of premalignant cells. *Cancer Res.* 2018;78(10):2449-2456.
19. Oben B, Froyen G, Maclachlan KH, et al. Whole-genome sequencing reveals progressive versus stable myeloma precursor conditions as two distinct entities. *Nat Commun.* 2021;12(1):1861.
20. Sun F, Cheng Y, Ying J, et al. A gene signature can predict risk of MGUS progressing to multiple myeloma. *J Hematol Oncol.* 2023;16(1):70.
21. Landgren O, Kyle RA, Pfeiffer RM, et al. Monoclonal gammopathy of undetermined significance (MGUS) consistently precedes multiple myeloma: a prospective study. *Blood.* 2009;113(22):5412-5417.
22. Visram A, Rajkumar SV, Kapoor P, et al. Monoclonal proteinuria predicts progression risk in asymptomatic multiple myeloma with a free light chain ratio ≥100. *Leukemia.* 2022;36(5):1429-1431.
23. Kyle RA, Therneau TM, Rajkumar SV, Larson DR, Plevak MF, Melton LJ III. Incidence of multiple myeloma in Olmsted county, Minnesota: trend over 6 decades. *Cancer.* 2004;101(11):2667-2674.
24. Greenberg AJ, Rajkumar SV, Vachon CM. Familial monoclonal gammopathy of undetermined significance and multiple myeloma: epidemiology, risk factors, and biological characteristics. *Blood.* 2012;119(23):5359-5366.
25. Kyle RA, Gertz MA, Witzig TE, et al. Review of 1027 patients with newly diagnosed multiple myeloma. *Mayo Clin Proc.* 2003;78(1):21-33.
26. International Myeloma Working Group. Criteria for the classification of monoclonal gammopathies, multiple myeloma and related disorders: a report of the International Myeloma Working Group. *Br J Haematol.* 2003;121(5):749-757.
27. Kyle RA, Remstein ED, Therneau TM, et al. Clinical course and prognosis of smoldering (asymptomatic) multiple myeloma. *N Engl J Med.* 2007;356(25):2582-2590.
28. Lakshman A, Rajkumar SV, Buadi FK, et al. Risk stratification of smoldering multiple myeloma incorporating revised IMWG diagnostic criteria. *Blood Cancer J.* 2018;8(6):59. doi:10.1038/s41408-018-0077-4
29. Mateos MV, Kumar S, Dimopoulos MA, et al. International Myeloma Working Group risk stratification model for smoldering multiple myeloma (SMM). *Blood Cancer J.* 2020;10(10):102. doi:10.1038/s41408-020-00366-3
30. Hillengass J, Moulopoulos LA, Delorme S, et al. Whole-body computed tomography versus conventional skeletal survey in patients with multiple myeloma: a study of the International Myeloma Working Group. *Blood Cancer J.* 2017;7(8):e599.
31. Regelink JC, Minnema MC, Terpos E, et al. Comparison of modern and conventional imaging techniques in establishing multiple myeloma-related bone disease: a systematic review. *Br J Haematol.* 2013;162(1):50-61.
32. Greipp PR, San Miguel J, Durie BG, et al. International staging system for multiple myeloma. *J Clin Oncol.* 2005;23(15):3412-3420.

33. Palumbo A, Avet-Loiseau H, Oliva S, et al. Revised international staging system for multiple myeloma: a report from International myeloma working group. *J Clin Oncol.* 2015;33(26):2863-2869.
34. Matsue K, Matsue Y, Kumata K, et al. Quantification of bone marrow plasma cell infiltration in multiple myeloma: usefulness of bone marrow aspirate clot with CD138 immunohistochemistry. *Hematol Oncol.* 2017;35(3):323-328.
35. Coriu D, Weaver K, Schell M, et al. A molecular basis for nonsecretory myeloma. *Blood.* 2004;104(3):829-831.
36. Avet-Loiseau H, Garand R, Lode L, Harousseau JL, Bataille R; Intergroupe Francophone du Myélome. Translocation t(11;14)(q13;q32) is the hallmark of IgM, IgE, and nonsecretory multiple myeloma variants. *Blood.* 2003;101(4):1570-1571.
37. Nandakumar B, Kumar SK, Dispenzieri A, et al. Cytogenetic features and clinical outcomes of patients with non-secretory multiple myeloma in the era of novel agent induction therapy. *Clin Lymphoma Myeloma Leuk.* 2020;20(1):53-56.
38. Fernandez de Larrea C, Kyle R, Rosinol L, et al. Primary plasma cell leukemia: consensus definition by the International Myeloma Working Group according to peripheral blood plasma cell percentage. *Blood Cancer J.* 2021;11(12):192.
39. Jelinek T, Bezdekova R, Zihala D, et al. More than 2% of circulating tumor plasma cells defines plasma cell leukemia-like multiple myeloma. *J Clin Oncol.* 2023;41(7):1383-1392.
40. Avet-Loiseau H, Daviet A, Brigaudeau C, et al. Cytogenetic, interphase, and multicolor fluorescence in situ hybridization analyses in primary plasma cell leukemia: a study of 40 patients at diagnosis, on behalf of the Intergroupe Francophone du Myelome and the Groupe Francais de Cytogenetique Hematologique. *Blood.* 2001;97(3):822-825.
41. Pellat-Deceunynck C, Barille S, Jego G, et al. The absence of CD56 (NCAM) on malignant plasma cells is a hallmark of plasma cell leukemia and of a special subset of multiple myeloma. *Leukemia.* 1998;12(12):1977-1982.
42. Dispenzieri A. POEMS syndrome: 2021 Update on diagnosis, risk-stratification, and management. *Am J Hematol.* 2021;96(7):872-888.
43. Dispenzieri A. POEMS syndrome: update on diagnosis, risk-stratification, and management. *Am J Hematol.* 2023;98(12):1934-1950.
44. Dao LN, Hanson CA, Dispenzieri A, Morice WG, Kurtin PJ, Hoyer JD. Bone marrow histopathology in POEMS syndrome: a distinctive combination of plasma cell, lymphoid, and myeloid findings in 87 patients. *Blood.* 2011;117(24):6438-6444.
45. Bazari H, Attar EC, Dahl DM, Uppot RN, Colvin RB. Case records of the Massachusetts General Hospital. Case 23-2010. A 49-year-old man with erythrocytosis, perinephric fluid collections, and renal failure. *N Engl J Med.* 2010;363(5):463-475.
46. Rosado FG, Oliveira JL, Sohani AR, et al. Bone marrow findings of the newly described TEMPI syndrome: when erythrocytosis and plasma cell dyscrasia coexist. *Mod Pathol.* 2015;28(3):367-372.
47. Grogan TM. Plasma cell myeloma marrow diagnosis including morphologic and phenotypic features. *Semin Diagn Pathol.* 2003;20(3):211-225.
48. Fang H, Chiu A, Reichard KK. Crystal-storing histiocytosis in bone marrow: a clinicopathologic study of eight cases and review of the literature. *Am J Clin Pathol.* 2018;149(2):148-163.
49. Fend F, Dogan A, Cook JR. Plasma cell neoplasms and related entities-evolution in diagnosis and classification. *Virchows Arch.* 2023;482(1):163-177.
50. Ely SA, Knowles DM. Expression of CD56/neural cell adhesion molecule correlates with the presence of lytic bone lesions in multiple myeloma and distinguishes myeloma from monoclonal gammopathy of undetermined significance and lymphomas with plasmacytoid differentiation. *Am J Pathol.* 2002;160(4):1293-1299.
51. San Miguel JF, Vidriales MB, Ocio E, et al. Immunophenotypic analysis of Waldenstrom's macroglobulinemia. *Semin Oncol.* 2003;30(2):187-195.
52. Robillard N, Avet-Loiseau H, Garand R, et al. CD20 is associated with a small mature plasma cell morphology and t(11;14) in multiple myeloma. *Blood.* 2003;102(3):1070-1071.
53. Lin P, Mahdavy M, Zhan F, Zhang HZ, Katz RL, Shaughnessy JD. Expression of PAX5 in CD20-positive multiple myeloma assessed by immunohistochemistry and oligonucleotide microarray. *Mod Pathol.* 2004;17(10):1217-1222.
54. Specht K, Haralambieva E, Bink K, et al. Different mechanisms of cyclin D1 overexpression in multiple myeloma revealed by fluorescence in situ hybridization and quantitative analysis of mRNA levels. *Blood.* 2004;104(4):1120-1126.
55. Chng WJ, Huang GF, Chung TH, et al. Clinical and biological implications of MYC activation: a common difference between MGUS and newly diagnosed multiple myeloma. *Leukemia.* 2011;25(6):1026-1035.
56. Beck RC, Tubbs RR, Hussein M, Pettay J, Hsi ED. Automated colorimetric in situ hybridization (CISH) detection of immunoglobulin (Ig) light chain mRNA expression in plasma cell (PC) dyscrasias and non-Hodgkin lymphoma. *Diagn Mol Pathol.* 2003;12(1):14-20.
57. Castillo JJ, Jurczyszyn A, Brozova L, et al. IgM myeloma: a multicenter retrospective study of 134 patients. *Am J Hematol.* 2017;92(8):746-751.
58. Lu H, Durkin L, Zhao X, Nakashima MO. IgM plasma cell myeloma. *Am J Clin Pathol.* 2022;157(1):47-53.
59. Campbell JP, Heaney JLJ, Pandya S, et al. Active multiple myeloma suppresses and typically eliminates coexisting MGUS. *Br J Cancer.* 2017;117(6):835-839.

60. Tembhare PR, Yuan CM, Venzon D, et al. Flow cytometric differentiation of abnormal and normal plasma cells in the bone marrow in patients with multiple myeloma and its precursor diseases. *Leuk Res*. 2014;38(3) 371-376.
61. Wang HW, Lin P. Flow cytometric immunophenotypic analysis in the diagnosis and prognostication of plasma cell neoplasms. *Cytometry B Clin Cytom*. 2019;96(5):338-350.
62. Flores-Montero J, Sanoja-Flores L, Paiva B, et al. Next Generation Flow for highly sensitive and standardized detection of minimal residual disease in multiple myeloma. *Leukemia*. 2017;31(10):2094-2103.
63. Arana P, Paiva B, Cedena MT, et al. Prognostic value of antigen expression in multiple myeloma: a PETHEMA/GEM study on 1265 patients enrolled in four consecutive clinical trials. *Leukemia*. 2018;32(4):971-978.
64. Perez-Persona E, Vidriales MB, Mateo G, et al. New criteria to identify risk of progression in monoclonal gammopathy of uncertain significance and smoldering multiple myeloma based on multiparameter flow cytometry analysis of bone marrow plasma cells. *Blood*. 2007;110(7):2586-2592.
65. Rodriguez-Otero P, Mateos MV, Martinez-Lopez J, et al. Predicting long-term disease control in transplant-ineligible patients with multiple myeloma: impact of an MGUS-like signature. *Blood Cancer J*. 2019;9(4):36.
66. Bergsagel PL, Kuehl WM. Critical roles for immunoglobulin translocations and cyclin D dysregulation in multiple myeloma. *Immunol Rev*. 2003;194:96-104.
67. Campo E, Jaffe ES, Cook JR, et al. The International consensus classification of mature lymphoid neoplasms: a report from the clinical Advisory Committee. *Blood*. 2022;140(11):1229-1253.
68. Mateos M, Martinez-Lopez J, Rodriguez-Otero P. Curative strategy (GEM-CESAR) for high-risk smoldering myeloma (SMM): carfilzomib, lenalidomide and dexamethasone (KRd) as induction followed by HDT-ASCT, consolidation with Krd and maintenance with Rd. *Blood*. 2019;134:781.
69. Bergsagel PL, Kuehl WM. Molecular pathogenesis and a consequent classification of multiple myeloma. *J Clin Oncol*. 2005;23(26):6333-6338.
70. Fonseca R, Barlogie B, Bataille R, et al. Genetics and cytogenetics of multiple myeloma: a workshop report. *Cancer Res*. 2004;64(4):1546-1558.
71. Fonseca R, Bergsagel PL, Drach J; International Myeloma Working Group, et al. International Myeloma Working Group molecular classification of multiple myeloma: spotlight review. *Leukemia*. 2009;23(12):2210-2221.
72. Drach J, Angerler J, Schuster J, et al. Interphase fluorescence in situ hybridization identifies chromosomal abnormalities in plasma cells from patients with monoclonal gammopathy of undetermined significance. *Blood*. 1995;86(10):3915-3921.
73. de Leval L, Alizadeh AA, Bergsagel PL, et al. Genomic profiling for clinical decision making in lymphoid neoplasms. *Blood*. 2022;140(21):2193-2227.
74. Schinke C, Hoering A, Wang H, et al. The prognostic value of the depth of response in multiple myeloma depends on the time of assessment, risk status and molecular subtype. *Haematologica*. 2017;102(8):e313-e316.
75. Zhan F, Huang Y, Colla S, et al. The molecular classification of multiple myeloma. *Blood*. 2006;108(6):2020-2028.
76. Bal S, Kumar SK, Fonseca R, et al. Multiple myeloma with t(11;14): unique biology and evolving landscape. *Am J Cancer Res*. 2022;12(7):2950-2965.
77. Gupta VA, Barwick BG, Matulis SM, et al. Venetoclax sensitivity in multiple myeloma is associated with B-cell gene expression. *Blood*. 2021;137(26):3604-3615.
78. Bergsagel PL, Kuehl WM, Zhan F, Sawyer J, Barlogie B, Shaughnessy , J Jr. Cyclin D dysregulation: an early and unifying pathogenic event in multiple myeloma. *Blood*. 2005;106(1):296-303..
79. Manier S, Salem KZ, Park J, Landau DA, Getz G, Ghobrial IM. Genomic complexity of multiple myeloma and its clinical implications. *Nat Rev Clin Oncol*. 2017;14(2):100-113.
80. Pawlyn C, Morgan GJ. Evolutionary biology of high-risk multiple myeloma. *Nat Rev Cancer*. 2017;17(9):543-556.
81. Bustoros M, Sklavenitis-Pistofidis R, Park J, et al. Genomic profiling of smoldering multiple myeloma identifies patients at a high risk of disease progression. *J Clin Oncol*. 2020;38(21):2380-2389. doi:10.1200/JCO.20.00437
82. Walker BA, Mavrommatis K, Wardell CP, et al. Identification of novel mutational drivers reveals oncogene dependencies in multiple myeloma. *Blood*. 2018;132(6):587-597.
83. Nakamura K, Smyth MJ, Martinet L. Cancer immunoediting and immune dysregulation in multiple myeloma. *Blood*. 2020;136(24):2731-2740.
84. Soekojo CY, Chng WJ. The evolution of immune dysfunction in multiple myeloma. *Eur J Haematol*. 2022;109(5):415-424.
85. Jimenez-Ubieto A, Paiva B, Puig N; GEM Grupo Español de Mieloma/PETHEMA Programa Español de Tratamientos en Hematología Cooperative Study Group, et al. Validation of the International Myeloma Working Group standard response criteria in the PETHEMA/GEM2012MENOS65 study: are these times of change? *Blood*. 2021;138(19):1901-1905.
86. Lahuerta JJ, Paiva B, Vidriales MB, GEM Grupo Español de Mieloma/PETHEMA Programa para el Estudio de la Terapéutica en Hemopatías Malignas Cooperative Study Group, et al. Depth of response in multiple myeloma: a pooled analysis of three PETHEMA/GEM clinical trials. *J Clin Oncol*. 2017;35(25):2900-2910.

87. Paiva B, Puig N, Cedena MT, GEM Grupo Español de Mieloma/PETHEMA Programa Para el Estudio de la Terapéutica en Hemopatías Malignas Cooperative Study Group, et al. Measurable residual disease by next-generation flow cytometry in multiple myeloma. *J Clin Oncol.* 2020;38(8):784-792.
88. Facon T, Kumar SK, Plesner T, et al. Daratumumab, lenalidomide, and dexamethasone versus lenalidomide and dexamethasone alone in newly diagnosed multiple myeloma (MAIA): overall survival results from a randomised, open-label, phase 3 trial. *Lancet Oncol.* 2021;22(11):1582-1596.
89. Holstein SA, Grant SJ, Wildes TM. Chimeric antigen receptor T-cell and bispecific antibody therapy in multiple myeloma: moving into the future. *J Clin Oncol.* 2023;41(27):4416-4429.
90. Ludwig H, Terpos E, van de Donk N, et al. Prevention and management of adverse events during treatment with bispecific antibodies and CAR T cells in multiple myeloma: a consensus report of the European Myeloma Network. *Lancet Oncol.* 2023;24(6):e255-e269.
91. Rodriguez-Otero P, Paiva B, San-Miguel JF. Roadmap to cure multiple myeloma. *Cancer Treat Rev.* 2021;100:102284.
92. Lahuerta JJ, Paiva B, Jimenez-Ubieto A, et al. Early detection of treatment failure and early rescue intervention in multiple myeloma: time for new approaches. *Blood Adv.* 2021;5(5):1340-1343.
93. Caers J, Paiva B, Zamagni E, et al. Diagnosis, treatment, and response assessment in solitary plasmacytoma: updated recommendations from a European Expert Panel. *J Hematol Oncol.* 2018;11(1):10.
94. Yadav U, Kumar SK, Baughn LB, et al. Impact of cytogenetic abnormalities on the risk of disease progression in solitary bone plasmacytomas. *Blood.* 2023;142(22):1871-1878.
95. Hill QA, Rawstron AC, de Tute RM, Owen RG. Outcome prediction in plasmacytoma of bone: a risk model utilizing bone marrow flow cytometry and light-chain analysis. *Blood.* 2014;124(8):1296-1299.
96. Paiva B, Chandia M, Vidriales MB, et al. Multiparameter flow cytometry for staging of solitary bone plasmacytoma: new criteria for risk of progression to myeloma. *Blood.* 2014;124(8):1300-1303.
97. Holler A, Cicha I, Eckstein M, et al. Extramedullary plasmacytoma: tumor occurrence and therapeutic concepts-A follow-up. *Cancer Med.* 2022;11(24):4743-4755.
98. Kremer M, Ott G, Nathrath M, et al. Primary extramedullary plasmacytoma and multiple myeloma: phenotypic differences revealed by immunohistochemical analysis. *J Pathol.* 2005;205(1):92-101.
99. Shao H, Xi L, Raffeld M, et al. Nodal and extranodal plasmacytomas expressing immunoglobulin a: an indolent lymphoproliferative disorder with a low risk of clinical progression. *Am J Surg Pathol.* 2010;34(10):1425-1435.
100. Boll M, Parkins E, O'Connor SJ, Rawstron AC, Owen RG. Extramedullary plasmacytoma are characterized by a "myeloma-like" immunophenotype and genotype and occult bone marrow involvement. *Br J Haematol.* 2010;151(5):525-527.
101. Bink K, Haralambieva E, Kremer M, et al. Primary extramedullary plasmacytoma: similarities with and differences from multiple myeloma revealed by interphase cytogenetics. *Haematologica.* 2008;93(4):623-626.

Chapter 53

Monoclonal Immunoglobulin Deposition Diseases

Ellen D. McPhail, Angela Dispenzieri, and Falko Fend

Introduction

Systemic AL (immunoglobulin light chain) amyloidosis, localized AL amyloidosis, and light and heavy chain deposition disease (LHCDD) are closely related entities in which clonal plasma cells or, less commonly, clonal B cells produce abnormal immunoglobulins that form extracellular deposits, resulting in tissue damage and/or impaired organ function. In both systemic and localized AL amyloidosis the abnormal deposits are amyloid, manifesting as insoluble extracellular fibrillar deposits with cross beta sheet conformation that bind Congo red with typical birefringence. In LHCDD, however, the ultrastructure is not organized as such; there are no beta-pleated sheets and no Congo red binding. Systemic AL amyloidosis often involves vital organs such as heart and kidney and typically has an aggressive clinical course, while localized AL amyloidosis involves a single extramedullary organ system such as urinary bladder or lung and usually has an excellent prognosis. LHCDD may be multisystem or localized.

SYSTEMIC IMMUNOGLOBULIN LIGHT CHAIN AMYLOIDOSIS

Definition

Systemic AL amyloidosis is characterized by production of amyloidogenic light chains by clonal bone marrow plasma cells that form extracellular fibrillar aggregates in multiple anatomic sites, resulting in end-organ damage.

Synonyms

Light chain amyloidosis, primary amyloidosis (obsolete term) (not recommended).

Epidemiology

Systemic AL amyloidosis is a rare disease, with an estimated annual incidence worldwide of approximately 10 cases per 1 million population.[1] The incidence has remained stable over time, but the prevalence has increased to 51 cases per million population, likely due to increased awareness, earlier diagnosis, and extended patient survival. Mean age at diagnosis is 63 years, and there is a slight male predominance (M:F = 1.3:1).

General Clinical Features

Systemic AL amyloidosis involves multiple organs, but presenting symptoms are often nonspecific and include fatigue, weight loss, and edema. Heart and kidney are frequently affected, commonly manifesting as heart failure with preserved ejection fraction and nephrotic syndrome, respectively. Liver, peripheral and autonomic nervous system, gastrointestinal tract, and many other sites may also be involved. Systemic AL amyloidosis is typically caused by a clonal bone marrow plasma cell neoplasm that produces abnormal immunoglobulin fragments that subsequently misfold and form AL amyloid fibrils. Rarely, B-cell lymphomas that secrete clonal immunoglobulins, such as lymphoplasmacytic lymphoma or marginal zone lymphoma, can cause systemic AL amyloidosis.

Morphology

Amyloid of any type appears as amorphous eosinophilic extracellular material on hematoxylin and eosin–stained sections. Systemic AL amyloidosis often surrounds adipocytes in fat pad biopsies. In bone marrow, it typically involves blood vessels, stroma, and periosteal soft tissue.[2] The median clonal plasma cell percentage is around 10%, and about three-quarters of cases are lambda light chain restricted; the remainder

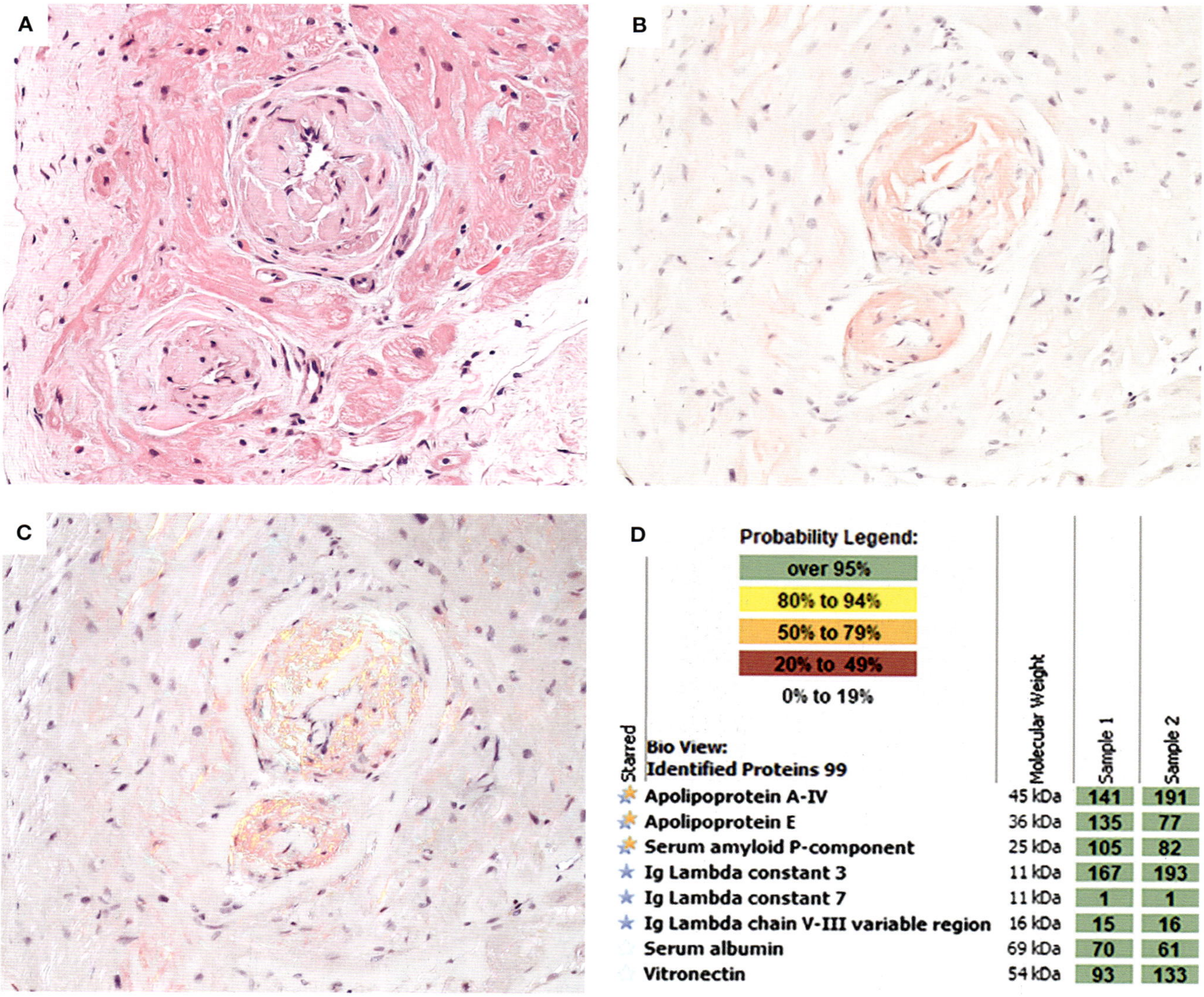

FIGURE 53.1 A 69-year-old woman with new-onset heart failure with preserved ejection fraction. **A:** Amorphous, pale pink amyloid deposits in a vascular and interstitial distribution (hematoxylin and eosin). **B:** Congophilic amyloid deposits (Congo red stain). **C:** The amyloid deposits show green birefringence under polarized light (Congo red stain). **D:** Scaffold display of AL-lambda amyloid proteome by liquid chromatography and tandem mass spectrometry amyloid typing. The dual yellow/blue stars indicate the amyloid signature proteins (apolipoprotein E, serum amyloid P, and apolipoprotein A4), and the blue stars indicate the amyloidogenic lambda proteins. Numbers in the green boxes specify the total number of tandem mass spectrometry spectra matching a protein in a sample, which is a semiquantitate measure of its abundance.

are kappa restricted. AL amyloid deposits are often interstitial, vascular, and/or endocardial in heart (Figure 53.1); glomerular, vascular, and/or interstitial in kidney; and sinusoidal in liver. However, amyloid type cannot be reliably determined by histopathologic pattern.

Congo red, which binds to amyloid and produces typical birefringence under polarized light, is commonly used to confirm the presence of amyloid. For optimal results, strict adherence to Congo red stain protocols is recommended. Amyloid may also be identified using other special stains, such as sulfated Alcian blue and thioflavin T. By transmission electron microscopy, amyloid fibrils are straight, randomly oriented, and 9 to 11 nm in diameter.

Amyloid typing

There are currently 42 canonical amyloid types.[3] Mass spectrometry–based proteomics, which identifies all amyloid types with very high sensitivity and specificity in a single assay performed on paraffin-embedded tissue or wet fat aspirate specimens, is now considered the gold-standard method for amyloid typing.[4,5] Correct typing is crucial as prognosis and treatment regimens vary dramatically according to amyloid type. The presence of monoclonal gammopathy of undetermined significance (MGUS) does not guarantee systemic AL-type amyloidosis, as MGUS is present in up to 40% of patients with ATTR (transthyretin)-type cardiac amyloidosis, which is the most common cardiac amyloid type.[6] In a survey of biopsy specimens, the constellation of bone marrow amyloid, cardiac amyloidosis, and a monoclonal protein proved to be ATTR-type amyloidosis in over 10% of cases.[2]

Genetics

The t(11;14)(q13;q32) translocation is present in approximately 40% to 50% of patients with systemic AL amyloidosis.[7] This translocation is associated with lower response rates to bortezomib but very high response rates to venetoclax. Other adverse prognostic indicators include gain of 1q with deletion of 14q, deletion of 1p, and hyperdiploidy.[8,9]

Prognosis and Clinical Comment

Clinical outcome in systemic AL amyloidosis is largely dictated by extent of cardiac involvement. Biomarkers of cardiac injury, such as serum troponin T and N-terminal pro–brain natriuretic peptide (NT-proBNP), are excellent predictors of survival. Amyloidogenic light chains are also toxic to involved organs, so both larger plasma cell clones and elevated free light chains are associated with inferior survival. The aim of treatment is to eliminate production of amyloidogenic light chains by suppressing the plasma cell clone. Treatment is usually chemotherapy based and typically includes the anti-CD38 antibody daratumumab and bortezomib. High-dose chemotherapy followed by stem cell transplant may be an option for eligible patients. However, the nonspecific nature of the presenting symptoms often results in a delay in diagnosis, which may limit the patient's ability to tolerate therapy. Median overall survival (OS) is 4.0 years but varies dramatically depending on stage (stage I: median OS = 12 years; stage IIIB: median OS = 0.4 years).[10]

LOCALIZED IMMUNOGLOBULIN LIGHT CHAIN AMYLOIDOSIS

Definition

Localized AL amyloidosis is characterized by localized production of amyloidogenic light and/or heavy chains, often in association with a localized, minor clonal plasmacytic or lymphoplasmacytic infiltrate.

Synonyms

None.

Epidemiology

Localized AL amyloidosis is a rare disease that represents approximately 10% of all AL amyloidoses.

General Clinical Features

Localized AL amyloidosis arises in a single extramedullary organ system such as urinary tract, upper respiratory tract, lung, breast, or skin. The amyloid usually forms a single tumor-like lesion, although there may be multiple masses/nodules within a single organ system. An association with connective tissue disorders such as Sjögren syndrome has been reported, most commonly among patients with nodular pulmonary amyloidosis.[11] However, the presence of AL amyloidosis in these organ systems does not guarantee localized disease, as systemic AL amyloidosis may also involve diverse extramedullary sites.

Morphology

Local production of amyloidogenic light and/or heavy chains results in formation of a tumor-like mass ("amyloidoma") (Figure 53.2), sometimes with associated foreign body giant cells. An underlying, minor monoclonal lymphoplasmacytic infiltrate may be identified by immunophenotyping or clonality analysis, although these infiltrates may be difficult to see as they are partially obliterated by the amyloid fibrils. The amyloid typically dominates the picture, and cases with manifest mucosa-associated lymphoid tissue (MALT) lymphoma or plasmacytoma should be classified as such. Monoclonal plasma cells and monoclonal B cells are absent in the bone marrow.

Genetics

Clonal immunoglobulin gene rearrangements are often present.

Prognosis and Clinical Comments

Localized AL amyloidosis is typically treated with excision, observation, or radiotherapy. Outcome is excellent and does not differ from that of the general population.[11]

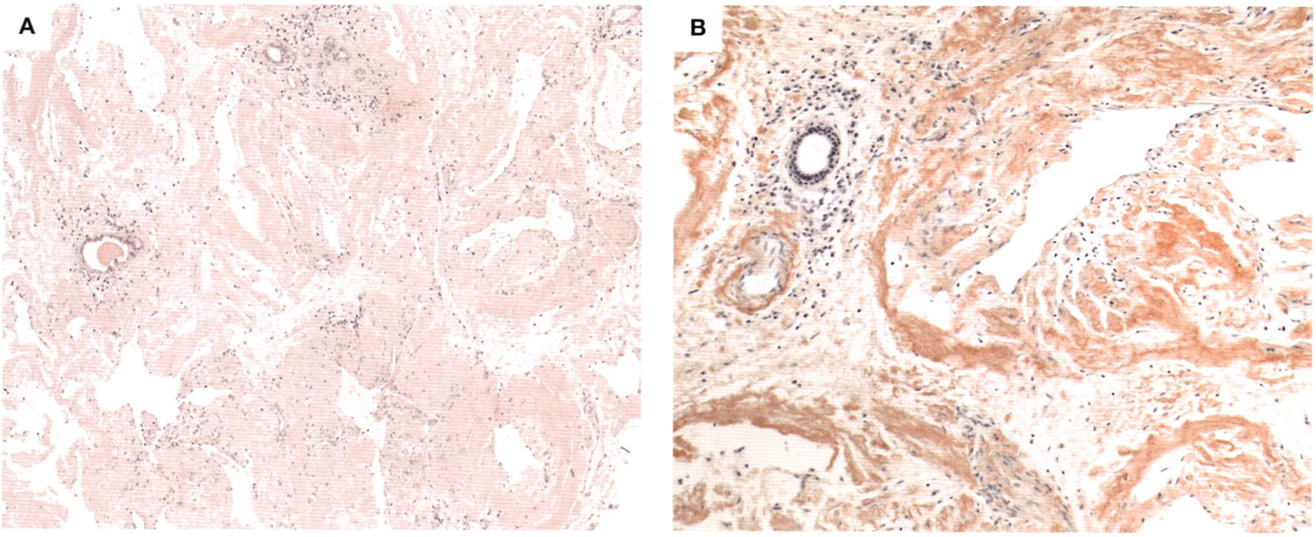

FIGURE 53.2 Nasal mass in a 46-year-old woman without evidence of systemic amyloidosis or plasma cell disorder. **A:** Extensive deposition of amorphous eosinophilic material in the nasal mucosa accompanied by rare plasma cells and lymphocytes. Hematoxylin and eosin staining, 50×. **B:** Strong Congo red positivity, confirming the amyloid nature of the deposits. 100×.

LIGHT CHAIN AND HEAVY CHAIN DEPOSITION DISEASE

Definition

Multisystem LHCDD is a rare disease characterized by deposits of abnormal nonamyloidogenic light and/or heavy chain immunoglobulins that are secreted by a plasma cell neoplasm or low-grade B-cell lymphoma. There is also a localized form of LHCDD.

Synonyms

Light chain deposition disease; heavy chain deposition disease; Randall-type monoclonal immunoglobulin deposition disease; monoclonal immunoglobulin deposition disease.

Epidemiology

No formal epidemiological studies exist, but these conditions are even more rare than AL amyloidosis.

General Clinical Features

Multisystem LHCDD presents in middle age with a male predominance and typically involves kidney. Heart, liver, and peripheral nerves are less commonly involved. An associated plasma cell neoplasm is almost invariably present in the bone marrow. The clinical features of localized LHCDD vary depending on the anatomic site, and there is often an associated low-grade B-cell lymphoma such as MALT lymphoma.

Morphology

In multisystem LHCDD, light or heavy chain–restricted, linear immunoglobulin deposits can be demonstrated in the kidney along glomerular, tubular, and vascular wall basement membranes on immunofluorescence (Figure 53.3). Finely granular "powdery" electron-dense deposits are present on electron microscopy. In localized LHCDD, amorphous eosinophilic extracellular Congo red–negative deposits, which may be tumor-like, are present, typically involving sites such as lung and gastrointestinal tract. The proteinaceous deposits show light chain and/or heavy chain restriction by immunohistochemistry or mass spectrometry–based proteomics, and associated monoclonal small B cells and/or monoclonal plasma cells can usually be identified.

Genetics

The t(11;14)(q13;q32) translocation is present in approximately 50% of patients with multisystem LHCDD.[12]

Prognosis and Clinical Comments

Treatment of multisystem LHCDD is tailored to control the plasma cell neoplasm to preserve kidney function and improve survival.[12] Patients with multisystem

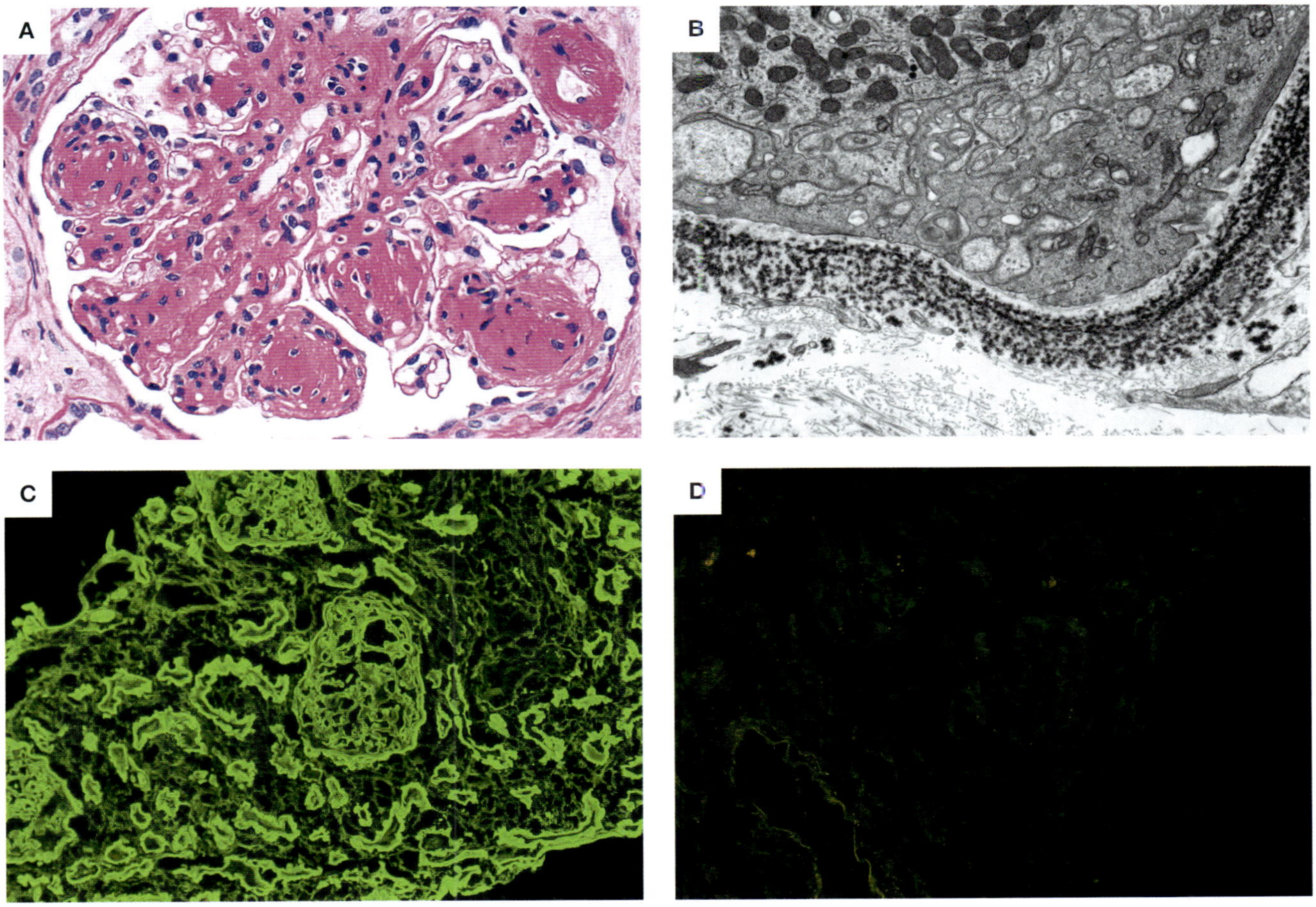

FIGURE 53.3 **A:** A glomerulus exhibits global nodular sclerosis with mild mesangial hypercellularity. There is segmental duplication of the glomerular basement membrane with associated cellular interposition. Nodular sclerosing glomerulopathy reminiscent of diabetic glomerulosclerosis is seen in two-thirds of cases of light chain deposition disease (PAS, X400). **B:** An electron microscopy figure showing abundant finely granular "powdery" electron-dense deposits along the outer aspect of a distal tubule basement membrane (X15,4000). **C:** On immunofluorescence, there is diffuse linear staining of the glomerular and tubular basement membranes and mesangial staining for kappa light chain (X100). **D:** In contrast, staining for lambda light chain is negative (X100). PAS, periodic acid-schiff. (**D:** Image courtesy of Dr. Samih Nasr, MD.)

LHCDD are treated similarly to multiple myeloma as long as there is not cardiac involvement, and similarly to AL amyloidosis if cardiac involvement is present.

References

1. Kumar N, Zhang NJ, Cherepanov D, Romanus D, Hughes M, Faller DV. Global epidemiology of amyloid light-chain amyloidosis. *Orphanet J Rare Dis*. 2022;17(1):278. doi:10.1186/s13023-022-02414-6
2. Chiu A, Dasari S, Kurtin PJ, et al. Bone marrow amyloid: a comprehensive analysis of 1,469 samples, including amyloid type, clinical features, and morphologic distribution. *Amyloid*. 2022;29(3):156-164. doi:10.1080/13506129.2022.2031963
3. Buxbaum JN, Dispenzieri A, Eisenberg DS, et al. Amyloid nomenclature 2022: update, novel proteins, and recommendations by the International Society of Amyloidosis (ISA) Nomenclature Committee. *Amyloid*. 2022;29(4):213-219. doi:10.1080/13506129.2022.2147636
4. Hill MM, Dasari S, Mollee P, et al. The clinical impact of proteomics in amyloid typing. *Mayo Clin Proc*. 2021;96(5):1122-1127. doi:10.1016/j.mayocp.2020.12.002
5. Dasari S, Theis JD, Vrana JA, et al. Amyloid typing by mass spectrometry in clinical practice: a comprehensive review of 16,175 samples. *Mayo Clin Proc*. 2020;95(9):1852-1864. doi:10.1016/j.mayocp.2020.06.029
6. Phull P, Sanchorawala V, Connors LH, et al. Monoclonal gammopathy of undetermined significance in systemic transthyretin amyloidosis (ATTR). *Amyloid*. 2018;25(1):62-67. doi:10.1080/13506129.2018.1436048
7. Dumas B, Yameen H, Sarosiek S, Sloan JM, Sanchorawala V. Presence of t(11;14) in AL amyloidosis as a marker of response when treated with a bortezomib-based regimen. *Amyloid*. 2020;27(4):244-249. doi:10.1080/13506129.2020.1778461

8. Muchtar E, Dispenzieri A, Kumar SK, et al. Interphase fluorescence in situ hybridization in untreated AL amyloidosis has an independent prognostic impact by abnormality type and treatment category. *Leukemia.* 2017;31(7):1562-1569. doi:10.1038/leu.2016.369
9. Granzow M, Hegenbart U, Hinderhofer K, et al. Novel recurrent chromosomal aberrations detected in clonal plasma cells of light chain amyloidosis patients show potential adverse prognostic effect: first results from a genome-wide copy number array analysis. *Haematologica.* 2017;102(7):1281-1290. doi:10.3324/haematol.2016.160721
10. Abdallah N, Dispenzieri A, Muchtar E, et al. Prognostic restaging after treatment initiation in patients with AL amyloidosis. *Blood Adv.* 2021;5(4):1029-1036. doi:10.1182/bloodadvances.2020003782
11. Kourelis TV, Kyle RA, Dingli D, et al. Presentation and outcomes of localized immunoglobulin light chain amyloidosis: the mayo clinic experience. *Mayo Clin Proc.* 2017;92(6):908-917. doi:10.1016/j.mayocp.2017.02.016
12. Kourelis TV, Nasr SH, Dispenzieri A, et al. Outcomes of patients with renal monoclonal immunoglobulin deposition disease. *Am J Hematol.* 2016;91(11):1123-1128. doi:10.1002/ajh.24528

Chapter 54

Extranodal Marginal Zone Lymphoma of Mucosa-Associated Lymphoid Tissue (MALT Lymphoma)

Sarah E. Gibson, Ahmet Dogan, and Gilles Salles

Definition

Extranodal marginal zone lymphoma of mucosa-associated lymphoid tissue (MALT lymphoma) is an indolent B-cell lymphoma that may arise at a variety of extranodal sites and is often associated with an underlying chronic inflammatory disorder. The lymphoma is composed of heterogeneous B cells that include marginal zone (centrocyte-like) cells, monocytoid cells, small lymphocytes, and scattered immunoblasts and centroblast-like cells and is an architectural mimic of Peyer patches. Plasma cell differentiation is present in a proportion of cases. Although MALT lymphomas at different anatomic sites have overlapping morphological features, there are also site-specific etiologic, genetic, and clinical differences. In the 2022 International Consensus Classification, primary cutaneous cases are designated separately as primary cutaneous marginal zone lymphoproliferative disorder (see Chapter 55).

Synonyms

None.

Epidemiology

MALT lymphomas comprise 5% to 8% of all B-cell lymphomas, with an incidence rate of 0.3 to 1.6 per 100,000 person-years.[1-5] While the incidence of nongastric MALT lymphomas has increased over time, a decline in gastric cases has been observed, likely reflecting widespread antibiotic therapy for *Helicobacter pylori* and early treatment of patients with peptic disease symptoms.[1,5-7] The lymphoma typically occurs in adults (median age in the seventh decade of life) and is rare in children. Although the overall incidence is similar in males and females, there are site-specific differences, such as a female predominance reported with salivary gland, thyroid, and breast MALT lymphomas and a male predominance with primary cutaneous marginal zone lymphoproliferative disorder.[1,7] There is also geographical variability, with a higher frequency reported in developed regions (8.8%) compared with developing regions (5.2%).[4] Alpha heavy chain disease (also known as immunoproliferative small intestinal disease [IPSID]) is a special subtype of MALT lymphoma that most commonly occurs in the Middle East, Africa, and other tropical and subtropical locations and is linked to factors associated with low socioeconomic status (see Chapter 51).[5]

MALT lymphoma is described in almost all extranodal tissues (Table 54.1) but paradoxically is rarely seen in sites with native MALT (eg, tonsil or terminal ileum).[8] The stomach remains the most common site (30% of cases), followed by cases arising in the ocular adnexa/orbit (12%), skin (10%), lung (9%), other gastrointestinal sites (8%), salivary glands (7%), breast (3%), and thyroid gland (2%).[1] In many cases, there is a history of a chronic inflammatory disorder resulting in acquired MALT. The preceding inflammation may result from chronic infection, autoimmune disease, or other unknown stimuli.[8]

The most well-established association between infection and MALT lymphoma is that of *H. pylori* infection and gastric MALT lymphoma. *H. pylori* has been shown to promote the development of gastric MALT lymphomas via the activation of T cells and/or direct oncogenic effects on B cells.[5,8] *H. pylori* eradication with antibiotics results in regression of the gastric MALT lymphoma in up to 75% of *H. pylori*-positive cases.[1,5,7] However, the proportion of gastric MALT lymphomas that are positive for *H. pylori* at diagnosis has decreased from >90% of cases in the 1990s to 17% to 32% of cases in the current era.[6,9] Other infectious organisms have been implicated in the development of MALT lymphomas, including *Chlamydia psittaci* (ocular

TABLE 54.1 Anatomic site distribution of MALT lymphomas and associated conditions

Site of disease	Proportion of cases[a]	Associated conditions
Gastrointestinal tract		
Stomach	30%	*Helicobacter pylori*
Colon/rectum	5%	
Small intestine	3%	*Campylobacter jejuni?*
Ocular adnexa/orbit	12%	*Chlamydia psittaci*, hepatitis C virus?, Sjögren syndrome
Skin	10%	*Borrelia burgdorferi*, hepatitis C virus?
Lung	9%	*Achromobacter xylosoxidans?*
Salivary glands	7%	Sjögren syndrome, hepatitis C virus?
Breast	3%	
Thyroid gland	2%	Hashimoto thyroiditis
Oral cavity/oropharynx	2%	
Soft tissue	2%	
Genitourinary tract (kidney, bladder, prostate gland)	1%	
Nasopharynx	1%	
Other sites	13%	

MALT, mucosa-associated lymphoid tissue.
[a]United States, SEER-18, 2001 to 2017.
Cerhan JR, Habermann TM. Epidemiology of marginal zone lymphoma. Ann Lymphoma. 2021;5:1.

adnexa), *Borrelia burgdorferi* (skin), *Campylobacter jejuni* (IPSID), *Achromobacter xylosoxidans* (lung), and hepatitis C virus (ocular adnexa, salivary gland, skin/subcutaneous).[1,5,7] The strength of these associations is quite variable, relating, at least in part, to geographical diversity, as well as limited data sets for some proposed infectious agents.

Other MALT lymphomas arise from acquired MALT resulting from B cell–mediated autoimmune diseases, such as Sjögren syndrome or Hashimoto thyroiditis.[1,7] Individuals with Sjögren syndrome have a 14- to 19-fold risk of developing lymphoma compared with the general population and up to a 1000-fold risk of parotid gland MALT lymphoma.[1,10] Similarly, patients with Hashimoto thyroiditis have a 3-fold risk of lymphoma compared with the general population and up to a 67-fold risk of primary thyroid lymphoma.[1,11] Rare MALT lymphomas arise in patients with immune deficiency/dysregulation, including a subset of cases associated with Epstein-Barr virus.[12]

General Clinical Features

The majority of patients with MALT lymphoma present with localized disease (stage I-II), but involvement of two or more extranodal sites may occur at initial presentation as well as during the disease course.[2,5,7] Bone marrow involvement is present in only a minority of patients (2%-15% of cases in more recent series).[7,13,14] Involvement of multiple extranodal sites and bone marrow is more common in nongastric MALT lymphomas.[2,5,7] Generalized lymphadenopathy is infrequent (<10% of cases).[2] As MALT lymphomas may involve virtually any organ or tissue, presenting signs and symptoms are quite variable (Figure 54.1). Most individuals will have a good performance status and will not display systemic B symptoms or laboratory abnormalities that may be seen in other B-cell lymphomas (eg, elevation of lactate dehydrogenase [LDH] or β2-microglobulin).[2,7] A serum monoclonal gammopathy may be detectable in up to one-third of patients, most frequently of IgM type, and often associated with plasmacytic differentiation.[15]

Morphology

The morphologic features of MALT lymphoma are similar across anatomic sites. The marginal zone B cells are small to medium in size, resemble centrocytes with slightly irregular nuclei, and have moderately dispersed chromatin and inconspicuous nucleoli but have more abundant pale cytoplasm (Figure 54.2). Some cells contain even more abundant pale cytoplasm imparting a monocytoid appearance, which is more prominent at certain locations, such as the salivary gland and thymus. In other cases, the marginal zone B cells resemble

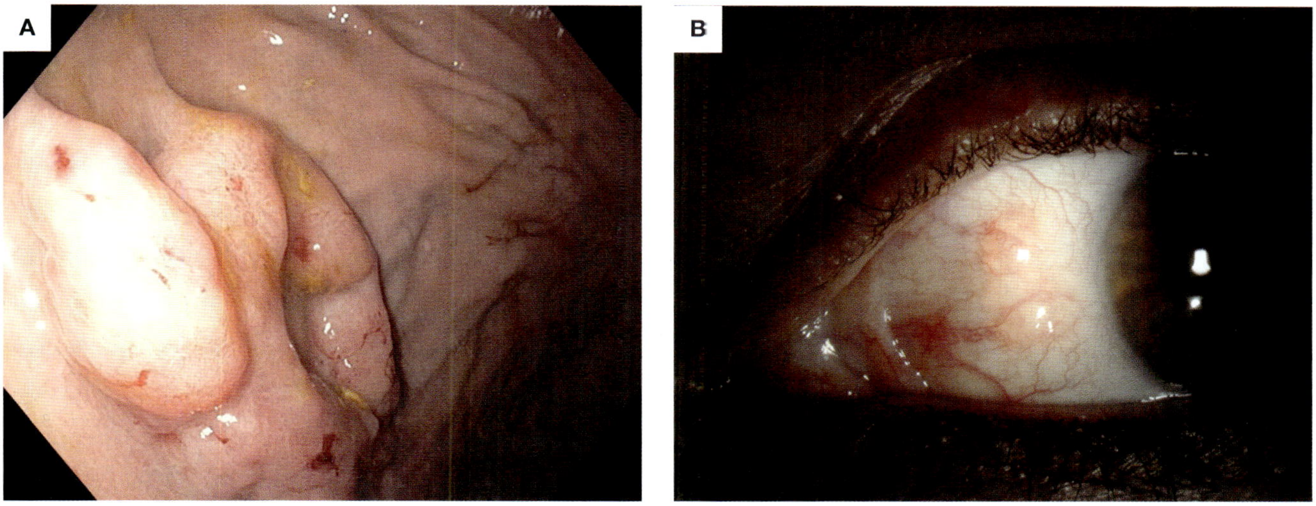

FIGURE 54.1 Extranodal marginal zone lymphoma of mucosa-associated lymphoid tissue (MALT lymphoma). **A:** Esophagogastroduodenoscopy image of a MALT lymphoma involving the gastric body. **B:** MALT lymphoma involving the conjunctiva.

small lymphocytes. Scattered transformed lymphoid cells, with centroblast-like or immunoblast-like cytology, are usually present. Plasmacytic differentiation is present in up to one-third of gastric MALT lymphomas and may occasionally mimic an extramedullary plasmacytoma. Localized immunoglobulin light chain–associated amyloid deposition or crystal-storing histiocytosis may be seen in some cases.

Architecturally, the neoplastic B cells surround the periphery of reactive follicles in a marginal zone distribution external to the mantles and spread out to form confluent areas between germinal centers (GCs) (Figure 54.3). The infiltrate eventually replaces the follicle, disrupting and expanding follicular dendritic cell (FDC) meshworks and often leaving small remnants of nonneoplastic GCs. In some MALT lymphomas, the neoplastic cells extensively colonize reactive GCs and may mimic follicular lymphoma (FL) (Figure 54.4). Lymphoepithelial lesions (aggregates of ≥3 marginal zone cells with distortion or destruction of the epithelium) are variable across anatomic sites but are present in almost all gastric or parotid MALT lymphomas and are less frequent in the colon or conjunctiva (Figures 54.5 and 54.6).[14] MALT lymphoma involving regional lymph nodes occupies marginal zone areas and may show an interfollicular expansion or perisinusoidal growth pattern. Plasmacytic differentiation and follicular colonization may also be present.

There is currently no consensus for grading MALT lymphomas based on the number of transformed centroblast-like or immunoblast-like cells present. However, when solid, sheet-like proliferations of large cells are present, the tumor should be diagnosed as a diffuse large B-cell lymphoma (DLBCL), with the presence of an accompanying MALT lymphoma noted. The term "high-grade MALT lymphoma" is not recognized, and the diagnosis of MALT lymphoma should not be applied to a DLBCL arising at a MALT site.

Immunophenotype

The neoplastic cells are positive for pan-B-cell antigens (CD19, CD20, CD22, CD79a, PAX5) and are generally negative for CD5, CD10, CD23, LEF1, cyclin D1, and SOX11. Infrequent CD5- or CD10-positive cases are described. CD43 is expressed in up to 50% of cases.[2,14] Disrupted and expanded meshworks of FDCs, related to colonized follicles, can be highlighted with stains for CD21, CD23, and/or CD35. Similarly, remnants of nonneoplastic GCs may be highlighted by positive staining for BCL6 and/or CD10 and negative staining for BCL2 (Figure 54.4). Most MALT lymphomas express IgM heavy chains, but not IgD; occasional cases are class switched expressing either IgG or IgA.[2,7] Demonstration of immunoglobulin light chain restriction in B cells with flow cytometry or sensitive immunohistochemistry/in situ hybridization techniques is helpful in the differential diagnosis with a reactive hyperplasia. Immunoglobulin heavy chain and light chain assessment is also useful in cases with plasmacytic differentiation. MNDA may be a helpful marker to distinguish MALT lymphoma from FL, as it is expressed by 61% to 95% of MALT lymphomas and only rare FLs.[14] Similarly, IRTA1 is reported to be positive in 52% to 93% of MALT lymphomas and only rare in nonmarginal zone lymphomas.[14]

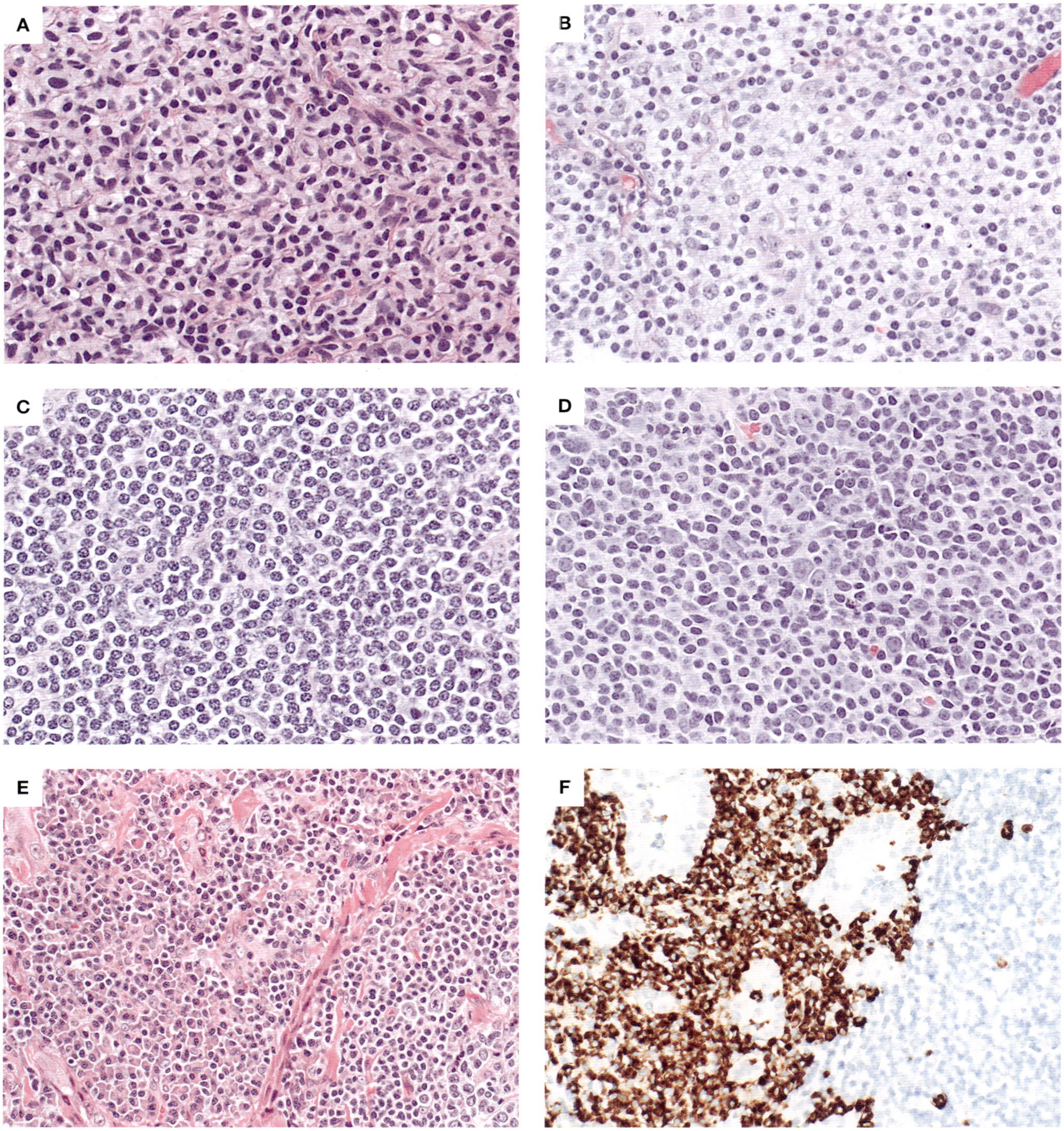

FIGURE 54.2 Morphologic spectrum of extranodal marginal zone lymphoma of mucosa-associated lymphoid tissue (MALT lymphoma). **A:** Marginal zone B cells with centrocyte-like nuclei but more abundant pale cytoplasm. **B:** The abundant pale cytoplasm of these lymphoma cells results in a monocytoid appearance. **C:** MALT lymphoma cells resembling small lymphocytes, with few scattered large, transformed cells. **D:** This MALT lymphoma contains heterogeneous marginal zone B cells and scattered transformed cells. **E:** Plasmacytic differentiation may be prominent in some MALT lymphomas. **F:** Plasma cells show kappa light chain restriction in this example.

Genetics

Immunoglobulin heavy and light chain genes are rearranged and show evidence of somatic hypermutation in most cases. There is biased usage of specific IGH variable gene families at different anatomic sites, supporting the concept of a common antigen-induced clonal expansion during lymphomagenesis.[8,14] Balanced chromosomal

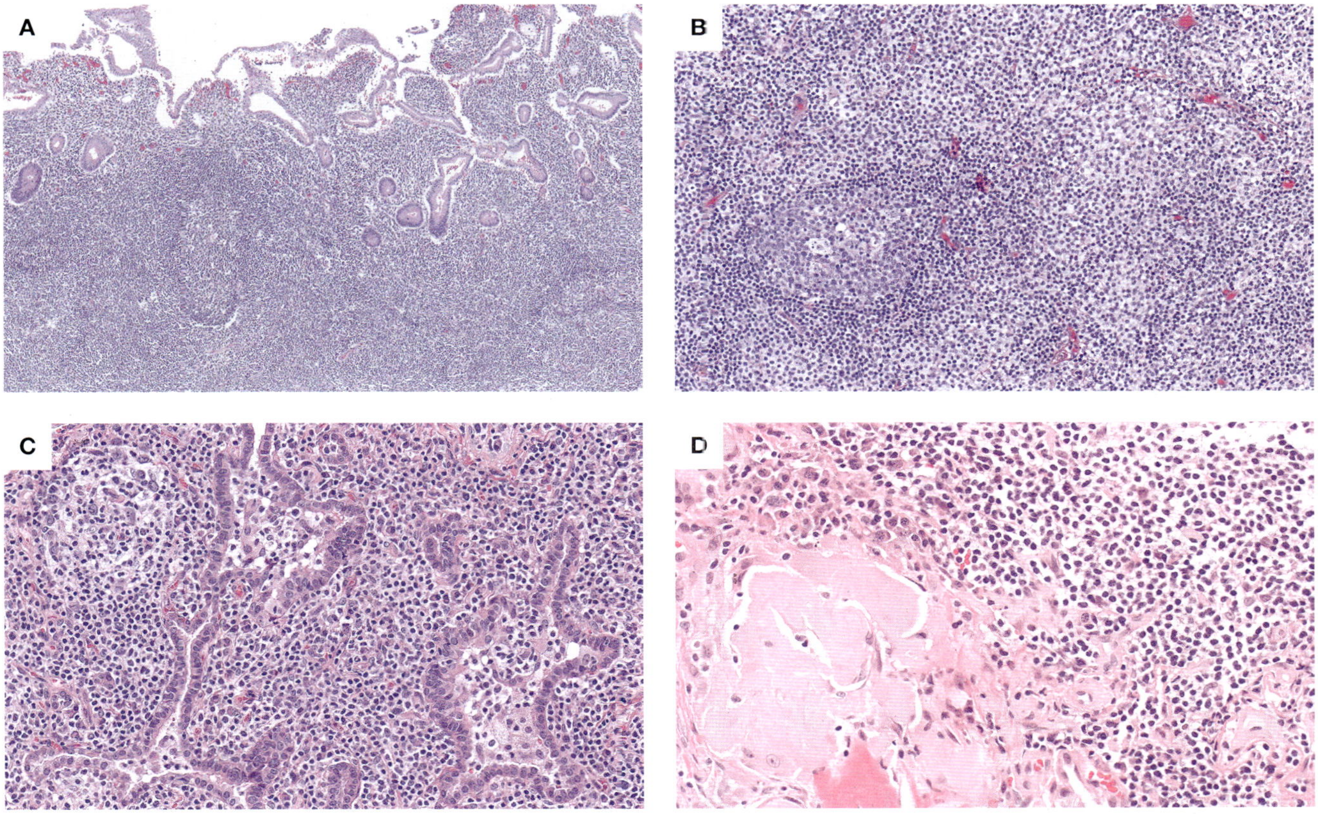

FIGURE 54.3 Extranodal marginal zone lymphoma of mucosa-associated lymphoid tissue (MALT lymphoma). **A:** Neoplastic cells surround reactive follicles and infiltrate the lamina propria in this small intestinal MALT lymphoma. **B:** The tumor cells surrounding a reactive follicle have a monocytoid appearance in this MALT lymphoma involving the bladder. **C:** Pulmonary MALT lymphoma demonstrating marginal zone B cells that infiltrate a reactive germinal center (top left) and form lymphoepithelial lesions in the adjacent bronchiolar epithelium. **D:** Localized amyloid (AL lambda) deposition is associated with this pulmonary MALT lymphoma.

translocations specifically associated with MALT lymphomas include t(11;18)(q21;q21);*BIRC3*::*MALT1*, t(14;18)(q32;q21);*IGH*::*MALT1*, t(1;14)(p22;q32);*BCL10*::*IGH*, t(3;14)(p14;q32);*FOXP1*::*IGH*, and t(X;14)(p11;q32);*GPR34*::*IGH* (Figure 54.7). These chromosomal alterations lead to dysregulation of the NFKB pathway, with frequencies that vary by the primary site of disease.[7,14,16-20] Identification of these translocations may be useful diagnostically, as they are only rarely present in other small B-cell lymphomas. Fluorescence in situ hybridization or next-generation sequencing (NGS) to detect the t(11;18)(q21;q21);*BIRC3*::*MALT1* fusion may guide treatment in patients with gastric MALT lymphomas, as cases harboring this alteration are resistant to antibiotic therapy.[2,14] Trisomies of chromosomes 3 and 18 are recurrent in MALT lymphomas and also occur in primary nodal and splenic marginal zone lymphomas. A large number of recurrently mutated genes have been identified by NGS (eg, *TNFAIP3*, *TBL1XR1*, *KMT2C*, *KMT2D*, *CREBBP*, *TET2*, *LRP1B*, *TNFRSF14*, *NOTCH1*, *NOTCH2*, *GPR34*, *SPEN*, and *PRDM1*).[16,21] Many of these alterations result in activation of the NFKB or NOTCH pathways or impact chromatin modifier-encoding genes.[21] Mutation frequency varies across anatomic sites, again indicating site-specific differences in lymphomagenesis.[14,16,21] The *MYD88* L265P mutation is found in <10% of MALT lymphomas, and *CXCR4* mutations are only rarely reported.[8,14]

Prognosis and Clinical Comment

MALT lymphomas have an indolent clinical course regardless of stage and are slow to disseminate, with 5- and 10-year overall survival rates reaching 90% and 80%, respectively.[2,7] A small proportion of patients with adverse features (age ≥70 years, advanced stage, and elevated serum LDH) have a less favorable outcome; such features are incorporated into the MALT lymphoma International Prognostic Index.[22,23] Relapses are common, can occur in the same primary site (50%-60% of cases) or involve nodal or other extranodal sites, and may occur decades after treatment.[2,7] A higher rate of recurrence is noted in nongastric versus gastric cases.[2,5] The treatment of MALT

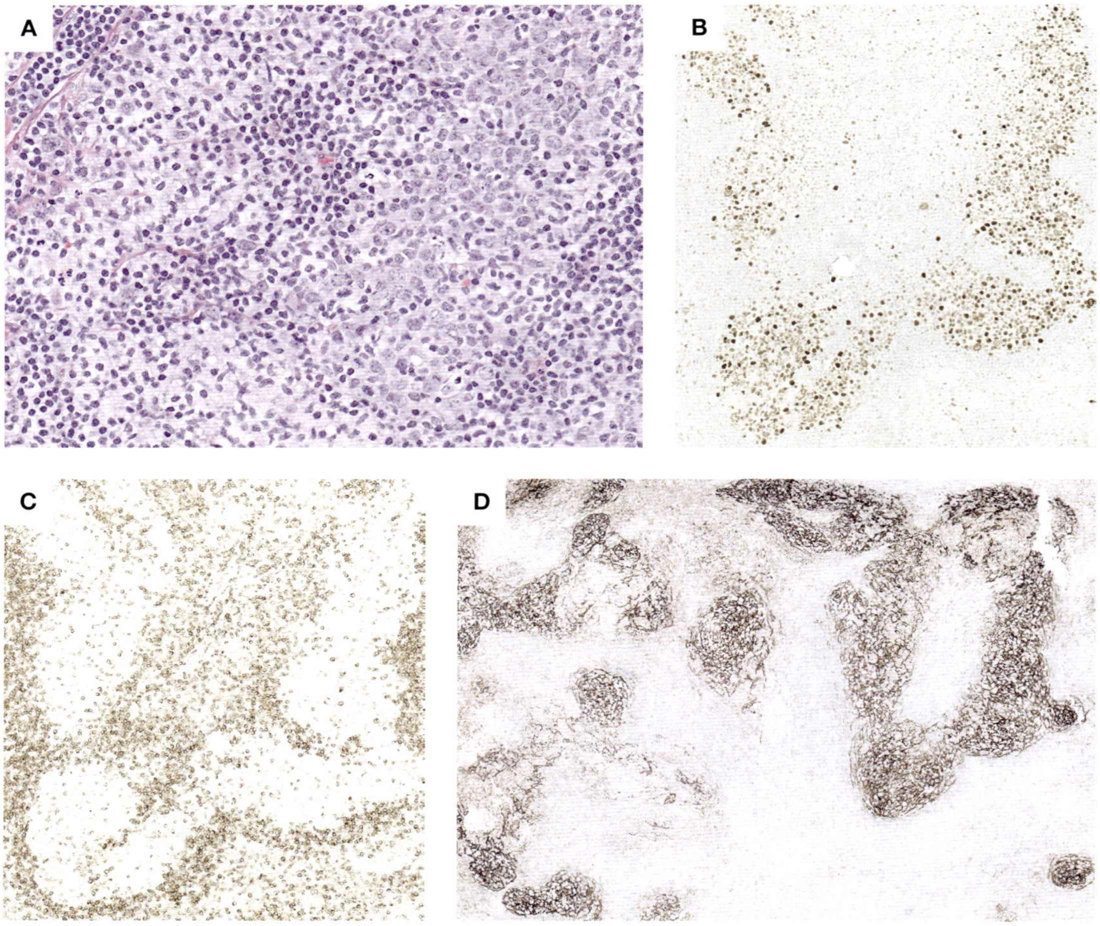

FIGURE 54.4 Extranodal marginal zone lymphoma of mucosa-associated lymphoid tissue (MALT lymphoma) demonstrating follicular colonization. **A:** This MALT lymphoma arising in the bladder shows neoplastic cells infiltrating a reactive germinal center. **B:** The remaining reactive germinal center cells are positive for BCL6. **C:** BCL2 negativity also highlights the germinal center remnants. **D:** Expanded and distorted follicular dendritic cell meshworks are highlighted with a CD21 stain.

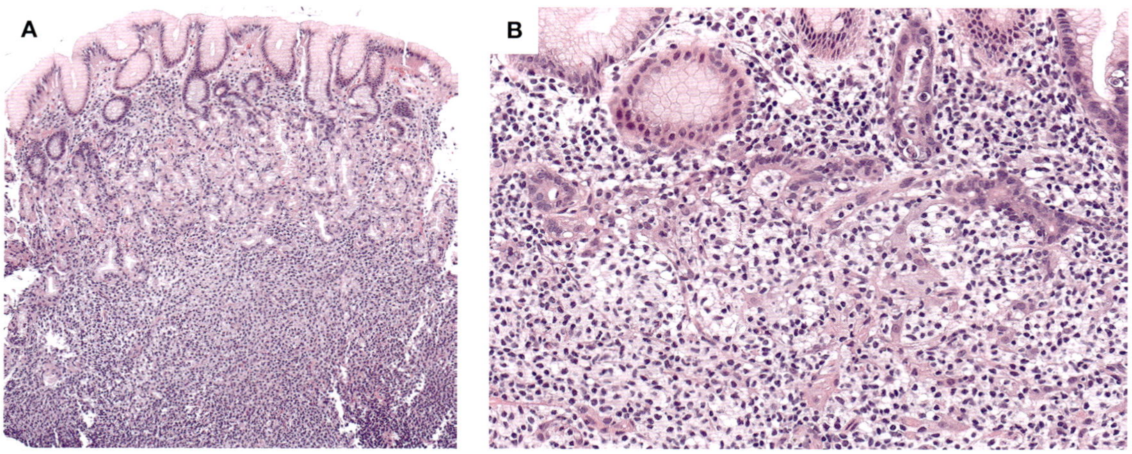

FIGURE 54.5 Gastric extranodal marginal zone lymphoma of mucosa-associated lymphoid tissue (MALT lymphoma). **A:** Marginal zone B cells infiltrate the lamina propria. **B:** Prominent lymphoepithelial lesions are present.

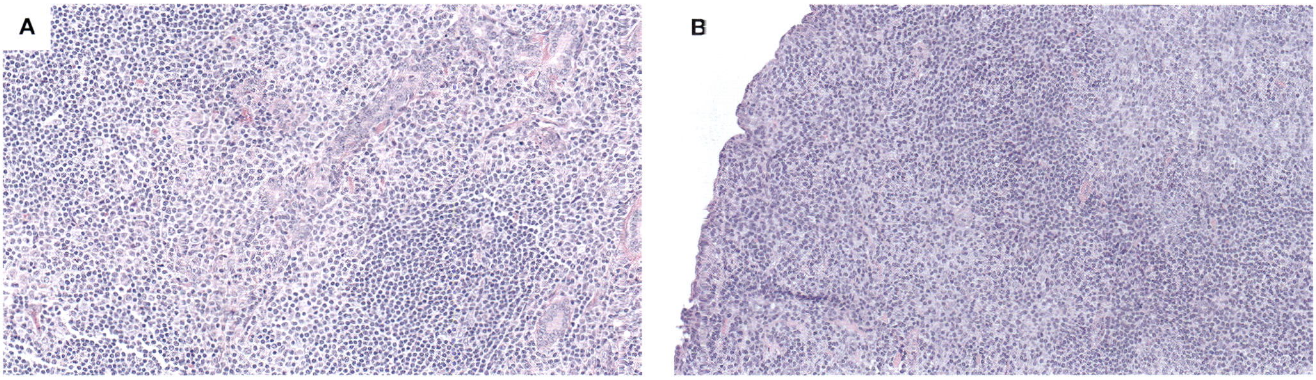

FIGURE 54.6 Extranodal marginal zone lymphoma of mucosa-associated lymphoid tissue (MALT lymphoma). **A:** Neoplastic lymphoid cells with pale cytoplasm are present in and around the lymphoepithelial lesions of this salivary gland MALT lymphoma. **B:** Conjunctival MALT lymphoma showing marginal zone B cells, some of which have a monocytoid appearance, which surround a reactive follicle (top right) and infiltrate the overlying epithelium.

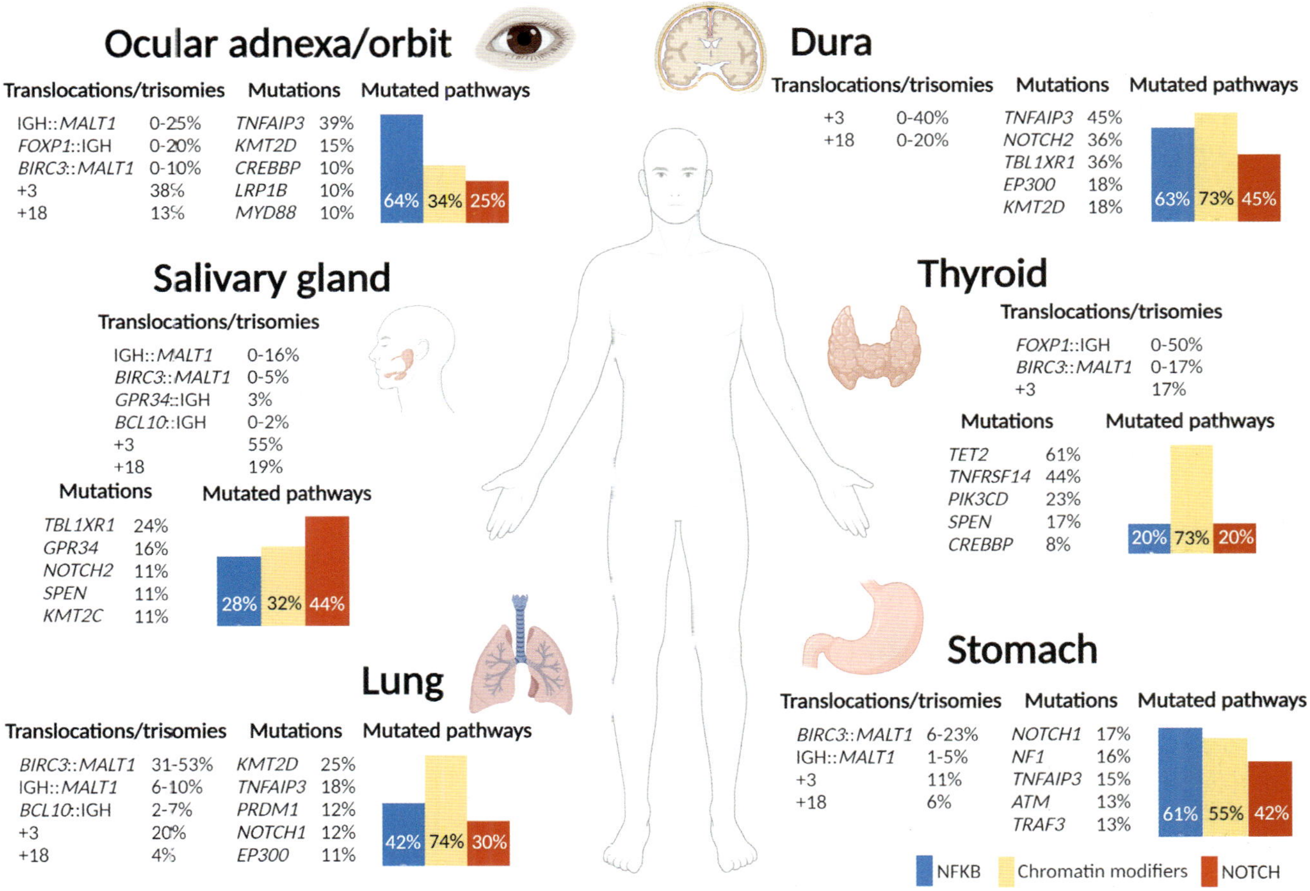

FIGURE 54.7 Frequency of genetic abnormalities in extranodal marginal zone lymphoma of mucosa-associated lymphoid tissue (MALT lymphoma) based on anatomic site. (Data summarized from Laurent C, Cook JR, Yoshino T, et al. Follicular lymphoma and marginal zone lymphoma: how many diseases? *Virchows Arch.* 2023;482:149-162; Moody S, Thompson JS, Chuang SS, et al. Novel GPR34 and CCR6 mutation and distinct genetic profiles in MALT lymphomas of different sites. *Haematologica.* 2018;103:1329-1336; Nomani L, Cotta CV, Hsi ED, et al. Extranodal marginal zone lymphoma of the central nervous system includes parenchymal-based cases with characteristic features. *Am J Clin Pathol.* 2020;154:124-132; Remstein ED, Dogan A, Einerson RR, et al. The incidence and anatomic site specificity of chromosomal translocations in primary extranodal marginal zone B-cell lymphoma of mucosa-associated lymphoid tissue (MALT lymphoma) in North America. *Am J Surg Pathol.* 2006;30:1546-1553; Streubel B, Simonitsch-Klupp I, Mullauer L, et al. Variable frequencies of MALT lymphoma-associated genetic aberrations in MALT lymphomas of different sites. *Leukemia.* 2004;18:1722-1726; Tu PH, Giannini C, Judkins AR, et al. Clinicopathologic and genetic profile of intracranial marginal zone lymphoma: a primary low-grade CNS lymphoma that mimics meningioma. *J Clin Oncol.* 2005;23:5718-5727; and Vela V, Juskevicius D, Dirnhofer S, et al. Mutational landscape of marginal zone B-cell lymphomas of various origin: organotypic alterations and diagnostic potential for assignment of organ origin. *Virchows Arch.* 2022;480:403-413. Created with BioRender.com.)

lymphoma differs based on the site of origin and extent of disease and varies from a watch-and-wait approach to surgery, antibiotic or antiviral therapy, radiotherapy, and single-agent or multiagent immunochemotherapy.[2,7] Antibiotic therapy may be the only initial treatment required for patients with *H. pylori*-associated gastric MALT lymphomas; however, cases with t(11;18)(q21;q21);*BIRC3*::*MALT1* are resistant to *H. pylori* eradication.[2,7] Antibiotics have also been used successfully in the treatment of selected other MALT lymphomas that are associated with infectious agents (eg, ocular adnexa and skin). MALT lymphomas are sensitive to radiation therapy, which may be curative in patients with localized disease. Various single-agent or multiagent immunochemotherapy approaches used for other indolent lymphomas are also generally effective in the treatment of MALT lymphomas.[2,7] Early progression within 24 months after initiation of therapy is associated with an inferior outcome.[23] Transformation to DLBCL may uncommonly occur (<10% of cases).[2,5]

References

1. Cerhan JR, Habermann TM. Epidemiology of marginal zone lymphoma. *Ann Lymphoma.* 2021;5:1.
2. Kalpadakis C, Pangalis GA, Vassilakopoulos TP, et al. Clinical aspects of MALT lymphomas. *Curr Hematol Malig Rep.* 2014;9(3):262-272.
3. Monga N, Nastoupil L, Garside J, et al. Burden of illness of follicular lymphoma and marginal zone lymphoma. *Ann Hematol.* 2019;98(1):175-183.
4. Perry AM, Diebold J, Nathwani BN, et al. Non-Hodgkin lymphoma in the developing world: review of 4539 cases from the International non-Hodgkin lymphoma classification project. *Haematologica.* 2016;101(10):1244-1250.
5. Zucca E, Bertoni F. The spectrum of MALT lymphoma at different sites: biological and therapeutic relevance. *Blood.* 2016;127(17):2082-2092.
6. Luminari S, Cesaretti M, Marcheselli L, et al. Decreasing incidence of gastric MALT lymphomas in the era of anti-Helicobacter pylori interventions: results from a population-based study on extranodal marginal zone lymphomas. *Ann Oncol.* 2010;21(4):855-859.
7. Raderer M, Kiesewetter B, Ferreri AJ. Clinicopathologic characteristics and treatment of marginal zone lymphoma of mucosa-associated lymphoid tissue (MALT lymphoma). *CA Cancer J Clin.* 2016;66(2):153-171.
8. Du MQ. MALT lymphoma: a paradigm of NF-κB dysregulation. *Semin Cancer Biol.* 2016;39:49-60.
9. Sena Teixeira Mendes L, D Attygalle A, C Wotherspoon A. *Helicobacter pylori* infection in gastric extranodal marginal zone lymphoma of mucosa-associated lymphoid tissue (MALT) lymphoma: a re-evaluation. *Gut.* 2014;63(9):1526-1527.
10. Liang Y, Yang Z, Qin B, Zhong R. Primary Sjogren's syndrome and malignancy risk: a systematic review and meta-analysis. *Ann Rheum Dis.* 2014;73(6):1151-1156.
11. Kato I, Tajima K, Suchi T, et al. Chronic thyroiditis as a risk factor of B-cell lymphoma in the thyroid gland. *Jpn J Cancer Res.* 1985;76(11):1085-1090.
12. Rea B, Liu YC, Maguire A, et al. Genomic landscape of Epstein-Barr virus-positive extranodal marginal zone lymphomas of mucosa-associated lymphoid tissue. *Mod Pathol.* 2022;35(7):938-945.
13. Alderuccio JP, Reis IM, Koff JL, et al. Predictive value of staging PET/CT to detect bone marrow involvement and early outcomes in marginal zone lymphoma. *Blood.* 2023;141(15):1888-1893.
14. Laurent C, Cook JR, Yoshino T, Quintanilla-Martinez L, Jaffe ES. Follicular lymphoma and marginal zone lymphoma: how many diseases? *Virchows Arch.* 2023;482(1):149-162.
15. Epperla N, Zhao Q, Karmali R, et al. Impact of detectable monoclonal protein at diagnosis on outcomes in marginal zone lymphoma: a multicenter cohort study. *Blood Adv.* 2023;7(17):5038-5046.
16. Moody S, Thompson JS, Chuang SS, et al. Novel GPR34 and CCR6 mutation and distinct genetic profiles in MALT lymphomas of different sites. *Haematologica.* 2018;103(8):1329-1336.
17. Nomani L, Cotta CV, Hsi ED, Ferry JA, Cook JR. Extranodal marginal zone lymphoma of the central nervous system includes parenchymal-based cases with characteristic features. *Am J Clin Pathol.* 2020;154(1):124-132.
18. Remstein ED, Dogan A, Einerson RR, et al. The incidence and anatomic site specificity of chromosomal translocations in primary extranodal marginal zone B-cell lymphoma of mucosa-associated lymphoid tissue (MALT lymphoma) in North America. *Am J Surg Pathol.* 2006;30(12):1546-1553.
19. Streubel B, Simonitsch-Klupp I, Mullauer L, et al. Variable frequencies of MALT lymphoma-associated genetic aberrations in MALT lymphomas of different sites. *Leukemia.* 2004;18(10):1722-1726.
20. Tu PH, Giannini C, Judkins AR, et al. Clinicopathologic and genetic profile of intracranial marginal zone lymphoma: a primary low-grade CNS lymphoma that mimics meningioma. *J Clin Oncol.* 2005;23(24):5718-5727.
21. Vela V, Juskevicius D, Dirnhofer S, Menter T, Tzankov A. Mutational landscape of marginal zone B-cell lymphomas of various origin: organotypic alterations and diagnostic potential for assignment of organ origin. *Virchows Arch.* 2022;480(2):403-413.
22. Thieblemont C, Cascione L, Conconi A, et al. A MALT lymphoma prognostic index. *Blood.* 2017;130(12):1409-1417.
23. Tracy SI, Larson MC, Feldman AL, et al. The utility of prognostic indices, early events, and histological subtypes on predicting outcomes in non-follicular indolent B-cell lymphomas. *Am J Hematol.* 2019;94(6):658-666.

Chapter 55

Primary Cutaneous Marginal Zone Lymphoproliferative Disorder

John R. Goodlad, Sarah E. Gibson, Steven T. Rosen, and Alberto Zamò

Definition

Primary cutaneous marginal zone lymphoproliferative disorder (PCMZLPD) is an indolent neoplasm, confined to the skin at presentation and composed of varying proportions of small lymphocytes and plasma cells. In contrast to the World Health Organization revised fourth edition, which did not differentiate between extranodal marginal zone lymphoma of mucosa-associated lymphoid tissue arising primarily in the skin and those occurring at other sites, this is now considered a distinct entity. Moreover, the term lymphoproliferative disorder rather than lymphoma is applied to reflect the remarkably benign behavior exhibited by nearly all cases. Two subtypes are recognized, a class-switched variant comprising the majority of cases (76%-86%) and a non-class-switched form.[1-3]

Synonyms

Primary cutaneous immunocytoma (not recommended). Primary cutaneous marginal zone lymphoma (not recommended).

Epidemiology

PCMZLPD accounts for around a quarter of all primary cutaneous B-cell lymphomas.[4] Most cases arise in adults with a median age of around 50 years, but a broad age range, including rare pediatric cases, is described.[4,5] Most, if not all cases, likely arise on a background of chronic inflammation. There is a variable relationship with *Borrelia burgdorferi*. An association between prior infection with *B. burgdorferi* and PCMZLPD has been demonstrated in certain geographic locations in Europe where infection is endemic, such as the Scottish Highlands and Austria, but is not evident in other locations, including parts of North America and Asia.[6-9] A relationship with hepatitis C virus and PCMZLPD has been described in Northern Italy, a region with a high prevalence of infection.[10]

General Clinical Features

Patients typically present with erythematous papules, plaques, or nodules. These are solitary or present in clusters in approximately half of patients and are multifocal in the remainder. The trunk and upper extremities are most frequently involved.

Morphology

The neoplastic cells in PCMZLPD may have the appearance of small lymphocytes, often with slightly cleaved nuclei, monocytoid cells, lymphoplasmacytic cells, or plasma cells. The proportion of these cell types and prominence of associated reactive lymphoid tissue is variable. A large majority of cases, mostly corresponding to the class-switched variant, manifest as nodular dermal infiltrates that sometimes involve subcutaneous fat (Figure 55.1). Lymphoid follicles, most with reactive germinal centers, are usually present. These are surrounded by a majority of small lymphocytes, most of which are reactive T cells, with variably sized aggregates of plasma cells placed around the deep and lateral peripheries of the infiltrate as well as in subepidermal locations (Figure 55.1). The latter may be the only easily identifiable component of the PCMZLPD. Scattered immunoblasts, histiocytes, and eosinophils may be seen among the small T cells. Less often, a more diffuse infiltrate is present. This pattern is more frequently associated with IgM expression and involvement of subcutaneous fat (Figure 55.2). The infiltrate in such cases comprises sheets of small B cells or monocytoid cells that overrun and obscure reactive follicles admixed with lesser numbers of small T cells[11] (Figure 55.2). A variable degree of plasmacytic differentiation may be seen.

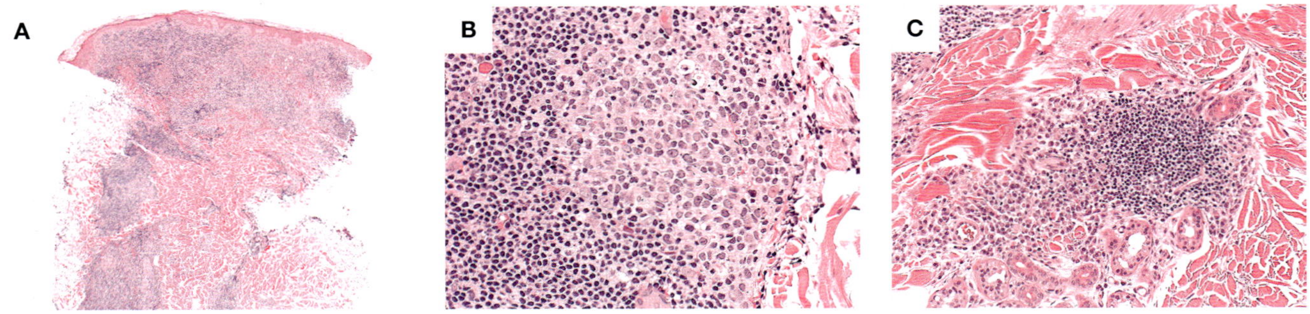

FIGURE 55.1 Primary cutaneous marginal zone lymphoproliferative disorder (PCMZLPD), class-switched variant. **A:** Class-switched PCMZLPD often presents as relatively sparse nodular, perivascular, and periadnexal infiltrates. **B:** Reactive lymphoid follicles are often present, with surrounding small lymphocytes (T cells). **C:** Aggregates of plasma cells are found at the peripheries of the infiltrate and may represent the majority of identifiable neoplastic cells.

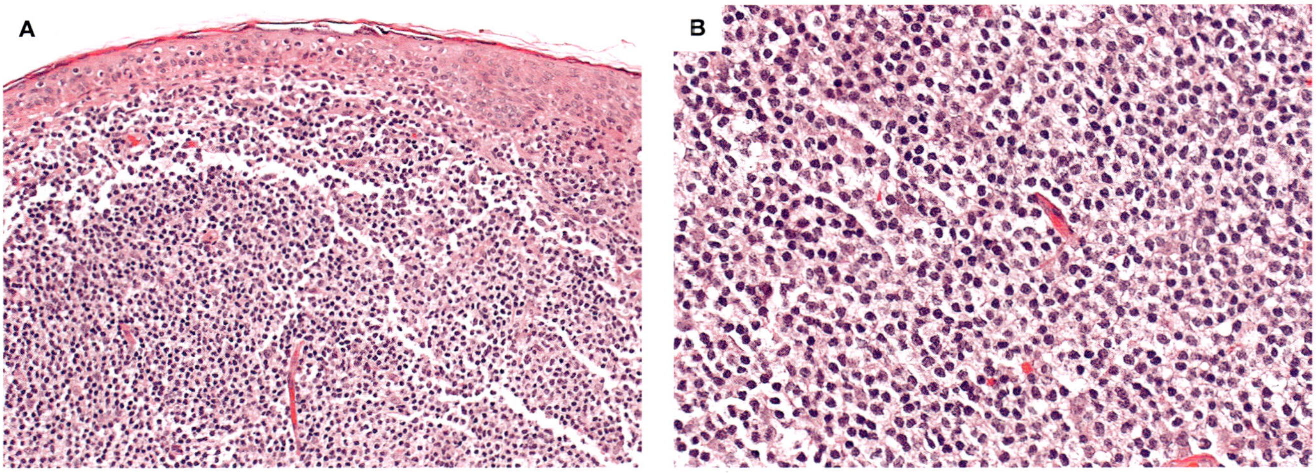

FIGURE 55.2 Primary cutaneous marginal zone lymphoproliferative disorder (PCMZLPD), IgM-positive variant. **A:** IgM-positive PCMZLPD typically presents as a solid/diffuse infiltrate of lymphoid cells. **B:** This variant of PCMZLPD consists predominantly of B cells, in this case displaying monocytoid morphology.

Immunophenotype

The neoplastic B cells have an indeterminate phenotype, expressing CD20 and other B-cell markers together with BCL2 but lacking CD5, CD10, CD23, BCL6, and cyclin D1.[12] Cells showing plasmacytic differentiation usually lack CD20 and other B-cell antigens such as PAX5 but react with antibodies to CD79A, CD138, and/or IRF4/MUM1. In most instances light chain restriction can be demonstrated in the plasma cells by immunohistochemistry (Figure 55.3). In cases with prominent plasmacytic differentiation and a significant background of reactive lymphoid tissue the plasma cells most frequently express IgG, but occasionally IgA and rarely IgE.[1] The IgG is often of IgG4 subtype (up to 40% of class-switched cases).[3] Conversely, cases in which sheets of marginal zone or monocytoid B cells predominate more usually express IgM and, in contrast with class-switched cases, are more frequently positive for IRTA1 and CXCR3[1,2,13] (Figure 55.4).

Genetics

Unlike other types of extranodal marginal zone lymphoma, mutations of the *FAS* gene are frequent, being found in 63% of PCMZLPD, including some of IgM type. Mutations of *SLAMF1, SPEN,* and *NCOR2* have also been documented in 24%, 18%, and 13% of cases, respectively.[14] Rearrangements of *MALT1* and *FOXP1* have been identified in a minority of cases, but fluorescence in situ hybridization analysis does not form part of the typical diagnostic workup.

Prognosis and Clinical Comment

Treatment is usually locally directed in the form of radiotherapy and/or surgical excision. For multifocal lesions, the preference is for observation or intralesional steroids when there are cosmetic considerations. Complete remission is the norm, but relapse is relatively frequent (approximately 50% of cases). Despite

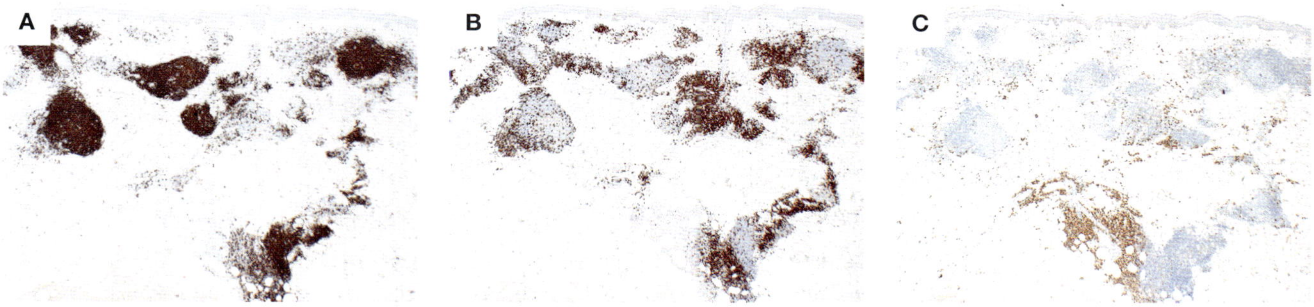

FIGURE 55.3 Primary cutaneous marginal zone lymphoproliferative disorder, class-switched variant. **A:** Antibodies to CD20 highlight nonneoplastic B-cell follicles. **B:** The small lymphocytes surrounding the follicles are CD3-positive, reactive T cells. **C:** Aggregates of IRF4/MUM1-positive plasma cells, representing the neoplastic component, are seen at the peripheries of the infiltrate.

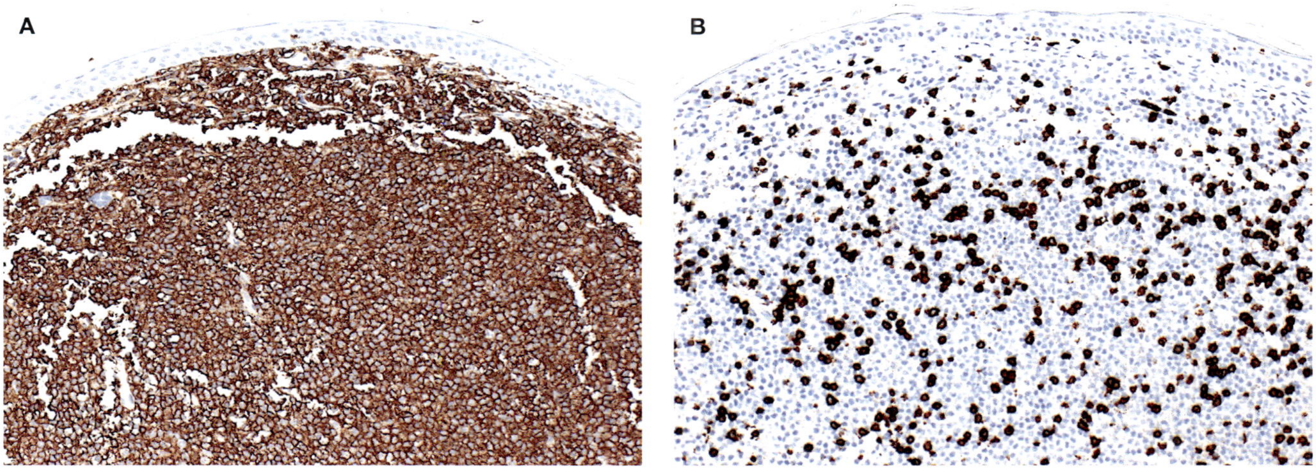

FIGURE 55.4 Primary cutaneous marginal zone lymphoproliferative disorder (PCMZLPD), IgM-positive variant. **A:** CD20-positive neoplastic B cells constitute the majority of the infiltrate. **B:** Reactive CD3-positive T cells are also present but are less prominent than in class-switched PCMZLPD.

the high incidence of relapse, extracutaneous spread is rare (<5%) and the long-term prognosis is excellent, with 5-year disease-specific survivals greater than 98% quoted.[4] Because of this remarkably indolent behavior and distinctive mutational profile, MALT-type lymphoma arising primarily in the skin has been recognized as a specific entity and redesignated as a lymphoproliferative disorder.

References

1. Edinger JT, Kant JA, Swerdlow SH. Cutaneous marginal zone lymphomas have distinctive features and include 2 subsets. *Am J Surg Pathol.* 2010;34(12):1830-1841.
2. van Maldegem F, van Dijk R, Wormhoudt TA, et al. The majority of cutaneous marginal zone B-cell lymphomas expresses class-switched immunoglobulins and develops in a T-helper type 2 inflammatory environment. *Blood.* 2008;112(8):3355-3361.
3. Brenner I, Roth S, Puppe B, Wobser M, Rosenwald A, Geissinger E. Primary cutaneous marginal zone lymphomas with plasmacytic differentiation show frequent IgG4 expression. *Mod Pathol.* 2013;26(12):1568-1576.
4. Senff NJ, Hoefnagel JJ, Jansen PM, et al. Reclassification of 300 primary cutaneous B-Cell lymphomas according to the new WHO-EORTC classification for cutaneous lymphomas: comparison with previous classifications and identification of prognostic markers. *J Clin Oncol.* 2007;25(12):1581-1587.
5. Fink-Puches R, Chott A, Ardigó M, et al. The spectrum of cutaneous lymphomas in patients less than 20 years of age. *Pediatr Dermatol.* 2004;21(5):525-533.
6. Wood GS, Kamath NV, Guitart J, et al. Absence of Borrelia burgdorferi DNA in cutaneous B-cell lymphomas from the United States. *J Cutan Pathol.* 2001;28(10):502-507.
7. Cerroni L, Zöchling N, Pütz B, Kerl H. Infection by Borrelia burgdorferi and cutaneous B-cell lymphoma. *J Cutan Pathol.* 1997;24(8):457-461.
8. Goodlad JR, Davidson MM, Hollowood K, et al. Primary cutaneous B-cell lymphoma and Borrelia burgdorferi infection in patients from the Highlands of Scotland. *Am J Surg Pathol.* 2000;24(9):1279-1285.

9. Li C, Inagaki H, Kuo TT, Hu S, Okabe M, Eimoto T. Primary cutaneous marginal zone B-cell lymphoma: a molecular and clinicopathologic study of 24 asian cases. *Am J Surg Pathol.* 2003;27(8):1061-1069.
10. Arcaini L, Burcheri S, Rossi A, et al. Prevalence of HCV infection in nongastric marginal zone B-cell lymphoma of MALT. *Ann Oncol.* 2007;18(2):346-350.
11. Goodlad JR, Cerroni L, Swerdlow SH. Recent advances in cutaneous lymphoma-implications for current and future classifications. *Virchows Arch.* 2023;482(1):281-298.
12. de Leval L, Harris NL, Longtine J, Ferry JA, Duncan LM. Cutaneous b-cell lymphomas of follicular and marginal zone types: use of Bcl-6, CD10, Bcl-2, and CD21 in differential diagnosis and classification. *Am J Surg Pathol.* 2001;25(6):732-741.
13. Carlsen ED, Bhavsar S, Cook JR, Swerdlow SH. IRTA1 positivity helps identify a MALT-lymphoma-like subset of primary cutaneous marginal zone lymphomas, largely but not exclusively defined by IgM expression. *J Cutan Pathol.* 2022;49(1):55-60.
14. Maurus K, Appenzeller S, Roth S, et al. Panel sequencing shows recurrent genetic FAS alterations in primary cutaneous marginal zone lymphoma. *J Invest Dermatol.* 2018;138(7):1573-1581.

Chapter 56
Nodal Marginal Zone Lymphoma

Ahmet Dogan, Adam Bagg, and Emanuele Zucca

Definition

Nodal marginal zone lymphoma (NMZL) is an indolent B-cell lymphoma composed of small- to intermediate-sized cells that often phenotypically mimic physiological marginal zone B cells. Although dissemination to extranodal sites such as the bone marrow can be seen, by definition, clinical and/or histological demonstration of lymph node involvement is required for the diagnosis.

Synonyms

None.

Epidemiology

NMZL is a rare disorder accounting less than 2% of all lymphomas with an age-adjusted incidence rate (IR) of 6 per 1,000,000 people. The disease typically presents at sixth or seventh decade of life with the incidence increasing sharply with age. Overall IR for NMZL appears to be highest in non-Hispanic whites, followed by Hispanics of all races, and then non-Hispanic Blacks and Asian/Pacific Islanders.[1] NMZL shows equal distribution between the sexes. Although genetic predisposition, autoimmunity, and infections such as hepatitis C virus (HCV) have been implicated in the pathogenesis of other marginal zone lymphoma (MZL),[1] only an association with prior HCV infections has been suggested for NMZL.[2]

General Clinical Features

The most common presentation is with painless localized or systemic lymphadenopathy. Evidence for systemic disease such as anemia and elevated LDH can be seen in approximately 20% of cases.[3,4] Approximately 60% of patients present with stage 3 to 4 disease and bone marrow involvement can be seen up to 40%. A low-level serum M-spike, often IgM type, can be detected in around 30% of cases.[5]

Morphology

Histology shows effacement of the lymph node architecture by an infiltrate of small- or intermediate-sized lymphoid cells often arranged in a nodular architecture (Figure 56.1). Cytologically, the neoplastic B cells in prototypical cases are intermediate in size, with clear cytoplasm (the so-called monocytoid appearance), and small oval nuclei showing minimal indentations and indistinct nucleoli (Figure 56.1). Scattered larger cells with immunoblastic or centroblastic morphology are often present. Plasma cell differentiation can be identified in one-third of cases. NMZL frequently retains follicular architecture, and in prototypical cases, the neoplastic B cells surround reactive germinal centers mimicking physiological marginal zones of organized lymphoid tissues. However, in many other cases, the infiltrate may have different architectural patterns including a more nodular pattern reminiscent of follicular lymphoma, a more paracortical pattern resembling lymphoplasmacytic lymphoma, or occasionally a diffuse pattern. When bone marrow involvement is documented, the infiltrate is typically nodular, sometimes interstitial, but intrasinusoidal pattern characteristic of splenic marginal zone lymphoma (SMZL) is not seen.

NMZL may contain substantial numbers of large cells, in some cases accounting for up to 20% of all cells, that are intermixed within the smaller cells[6] (Figure 56.1G). There are limited studies examining the risk of transformation in NMZL. Although NMZL appears to have a more aggressive clinical behavior than other MZL, the transformation risk appears to be low as compared with other indolent B-cell lymphomas, with one study suggesting a 3% transformation rate[7] and another reporting a cumulative incidence of 15% at 10 years.[3] There are no well-established, evidence-based criteria to delineate NMZL with increased large cells from transformation to a diffuse large B-cell lymphoma (DLBCL), but the presence of sheets of large cells is recommended as a minimum requirement for diagnosis of transformation to a DLBCL.

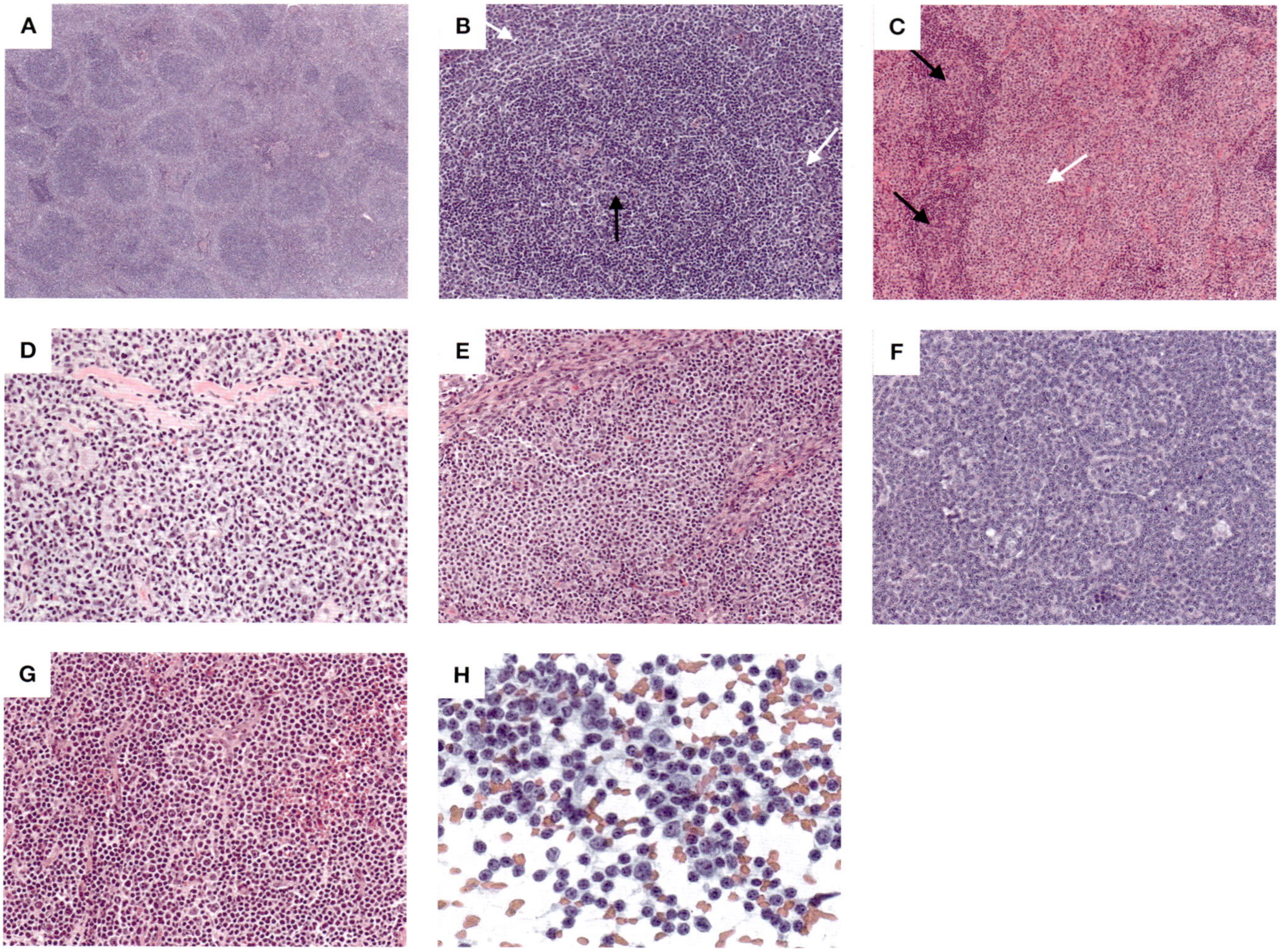

FIGURE 56.1 Histological features of nodal marginal zone lymphoma (NMZL). **A:** Low-power view of the lymph node involved by NMZL showing nodular architecture with attenuated follicle centers surrounded by mantle zone B cells and expanded marginal zone occupied by neoplastic B cells. **B** and **C:** Medium-power view of NMZL, black arrows indicate reactive follicle centers and white arrows highlight neoplastic marginal zones. **D-F:** High-power view of neoplastic B cells in three different cases of NMZL highlighting cytological heterogeneity. **G:** High-power view of NMZL with increased large cells. **H:** Cytological appearances of NMZL in a fine needle aspiration smear.

Immunophenotype

Given that morphological features of NMZL overlap with other indolent B-cell lymphomas, immunophenotyping is essential for diagnosis. The phenotype of NMZL is similar to the physiological marginal zone B cells of organized lymphoid tissues. The neoplastic B cells express mature B-cell markers such as CD19, CD20, CD79a, and PAX5 and lack expression of germinal center B-cell markers CD10 and BCL6, and in most cases, no or only partial expression of CD5 or CD23 is seen (Figure 56.2). BCL6 and to a lesser extent CD10 may highlight residual physiologic germinal centers surrounded by the neoplastic NMZL cells (Figure 56.3D). The residual germinal centers are distinguished by lack of BCL2 expression, whereas NMZL cells often show weak/variable BCL2 expression. Even if no morphologically identifiable residual germinal centers are present, the presence of disrupted follicular dendritic cells can be demonstrated by CD23 and CD21, indicating the presence of underlying follicular infrastructure in virtually all cases. In line with this, increased number of follicular helper T cells can be detected with CD10 or PD1 stains (Figure 56.3). The proliferation fraction in NMZL as detected by Ki-67 stain is quite variable, between 10% and 50%, and often parallels the numbers of neoplastic large cells observed in hematoxylin and eosin sections. Ki-67 stain frequently highlights residual germinal centers with high proliferation fractions up to 80% to 90% (Figure 56.2H).

Like physiological marginal zone B cells, the NMZL cells express IgM and sometimes also IgD. Up to 25%

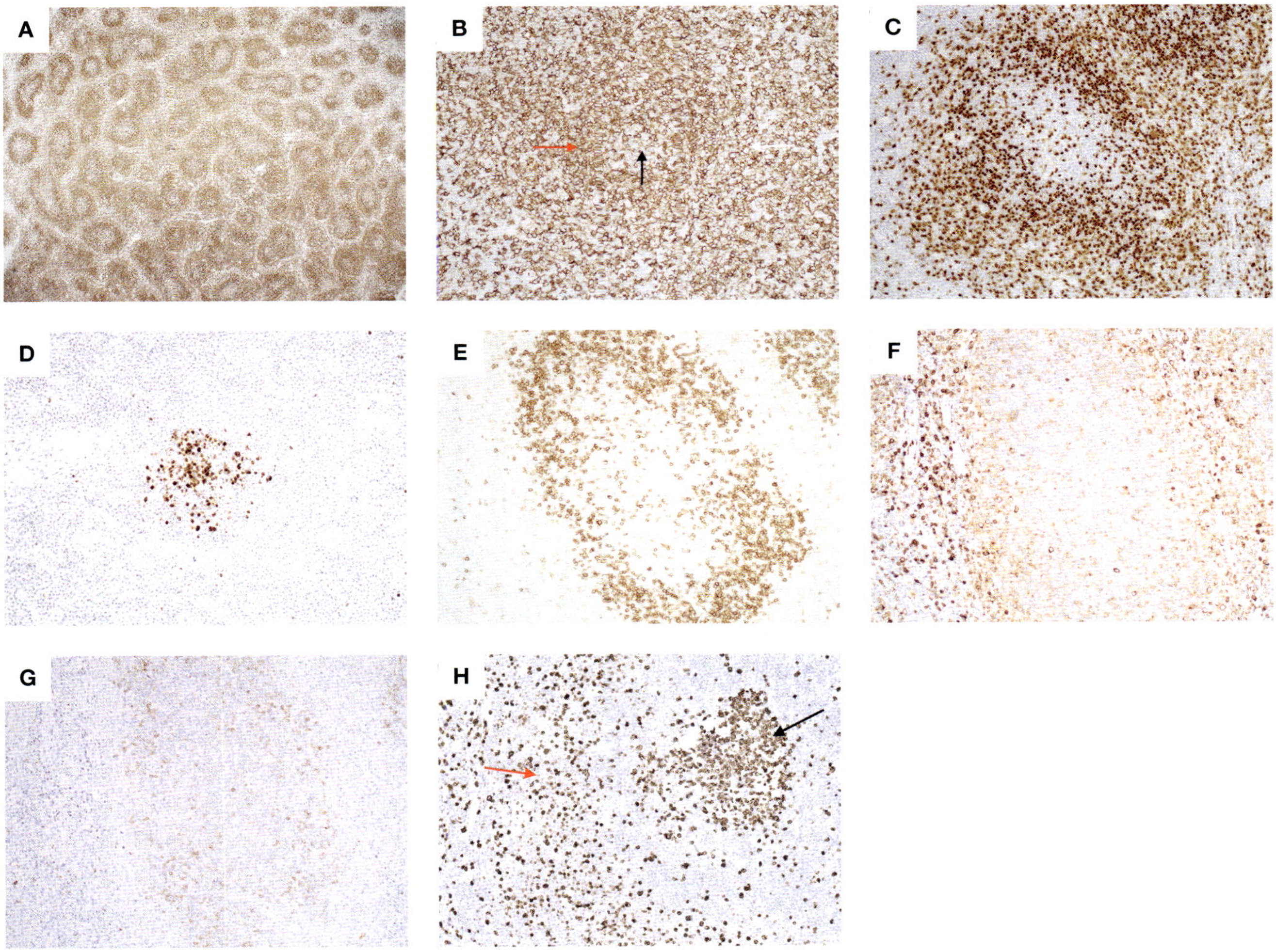

FIGURE 56.2 Immunohistochemical features of nodal marginal zone lymphoma (NMZL). **A:** Low-power view of CD79a highlighting residual depleted follicle centers, surrounding benign mantle zones, and expanded neoplastic marginal zones. **B:** CD20 highlights residual reactive follicle center cells (black arrow), the mantle zones (red arrow), and the neoplastic marginal zone (white arrow). **C:** The neoplastic cells express dimmer PAX5 distinguishing them from benign B cells. **D:** Residual reactive follicle centers express BCL6 but the NMZL cells are negative. **E:** IgD highlights reactive mantle zone, but the NMZL cells are negative. **F:** The NMZL cells are kappa light chain restricted and show partial plasma cell differentiation. **G:** The NMZL cells are negative for lambda light chains. **H:** Ki-67 stain shows the so-called targetoid pattern with high expression in residual reactive follicles (black arrow) and moderate expression in the neoplastic marginal zone (red arrow), whereas there is low expression in the mantle zone separating the reactive follicles form the neoplastic marginal zone.

of cases express CD43 aberrantly, a feature that may be helpful in distinguishing NMZL from benign mimics. Markers such as LEF1 characteristic of small lymphocytic lymphoma/chronic lymphocytic leukemia or cyclin D1 and SOX11 characteristic of mantle cell lymphomas are not expressed by NMZL.

By flow cytometry, bright CD19, CD20, CD22, and immunoglobulin light chain expression is characteristic, and variable CD38 expression is seen, but CD5 or CD10 is not usually expressed (Figure 56.4).

As noted, the immunophenotype of NMZL is nonspecific and the diagnosis rests on exclusion of other indolent B-cell neoplasms. Although not widely accepted in clinical practice, two markers may be fairly specific for MZL, including NMZL, which may help in the differential diagnosis.[8] Immunoglobulin super family receptor translocation associated 1 (IRTA1) has been reported to be expressed by MZL but not by other low-grade B-cell lymphomas including follicular lymphoma, small lymphocytic lymphoma/chronic lymphocytic leukemia, and lymphoplasmacytic lymphoma.[9] Another marker that has been investigated is myeloid cell nuclear differentiation antigen (MNDA), a nuclear protein expressed by myeloid cells and a subset of B cells. MNDA is expressed by most cases of MZL including NMZL but also by other B-cell lymphomas

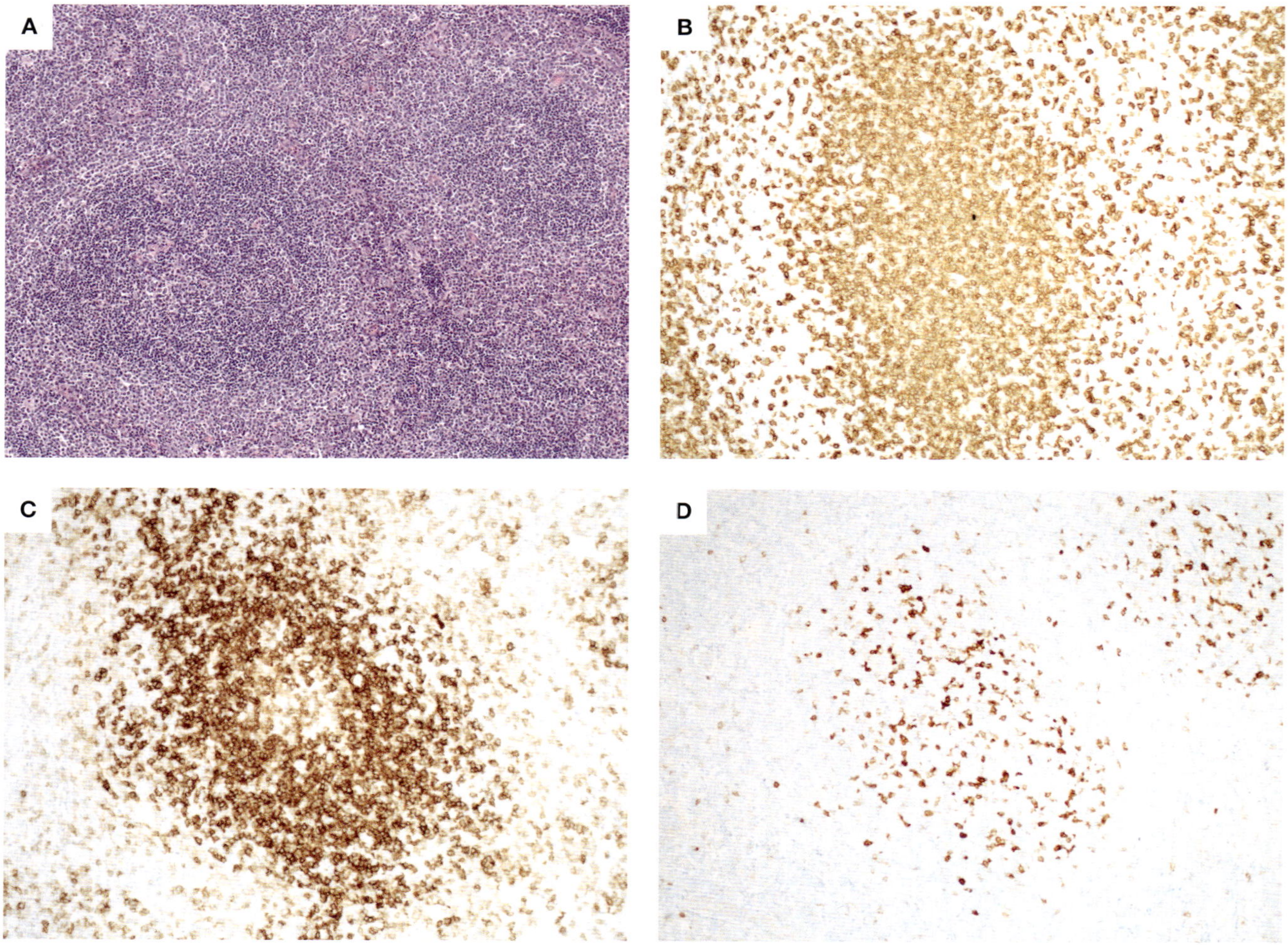

FIGURE 56.3 Enrichment of follicular helper T cells in nodal marginal zone lymphoma (NMZL). **A:** Medium power of a case of NMZL with follicle centers enriched in small lymphoid cells distinct from mantle zone B cells. **B:** Immunohistochemistry for CD3 shows that most of these cells are T cells. **C** and **D:** The T cells express bright PD1 (**C**) and partial CD10 (**D**).

with the exception of follicular lymphoma and may provide help in differential diagnosis of NMZL from follicular lymphoma in some cases.[10]

Genetics

Only limited studies have been published about the genetic features of NMZL. Though not specific, common numerical abnormalities at the chromosome level include trisomies of chromosome 3 and 18 and less frequently chromosome 12.[11,12] Structural alterations such as chromosomal translocations characteristic of other B-cell lymphomas including those involving *BCL2*, *BCL6*, *MYC*, or *MALT1* and IGH translocations have been only rarely reported in NMZL.

High-throughput sequencing studies have led to the exploration of the mutational profile of NMZL.[12,13] Although there are some differences between published studies, the main biological pathways altered by the mutations include chromatin remodeling genes such as *KMT2D, CREBBP, TET2,* and *EZH2* seen in 70%, NF-kB pathway regulating genes such as *CARD11, BCL10, TNFAIP3, TNFRSF14,* and *KLF2* seen in 50%, and NOTCH pathway genes such as *NOTCH2* and *SPEN* seen in 40% of cases. Other mutations of interest include missense *BRAF* mutations in 16% of the NMZL cases reported in one study[13] and mutations of *PTPRD* in 15% of NMZL cases reported by another study.[12] PTPRD is a receptor-type protein tyrosine phosphatase regulating cell growth, with mutations leading to the loss of its phosphatase activity and deregulation of the cell cycle transcriptional program.

Mutations characteristics of lymphoplasmacytic lymphoma such as *MYD88* and *CXCR4* have been reported only in 5% of NMZL cases. The overall mutational profile of NMZL overlaps with other indolent

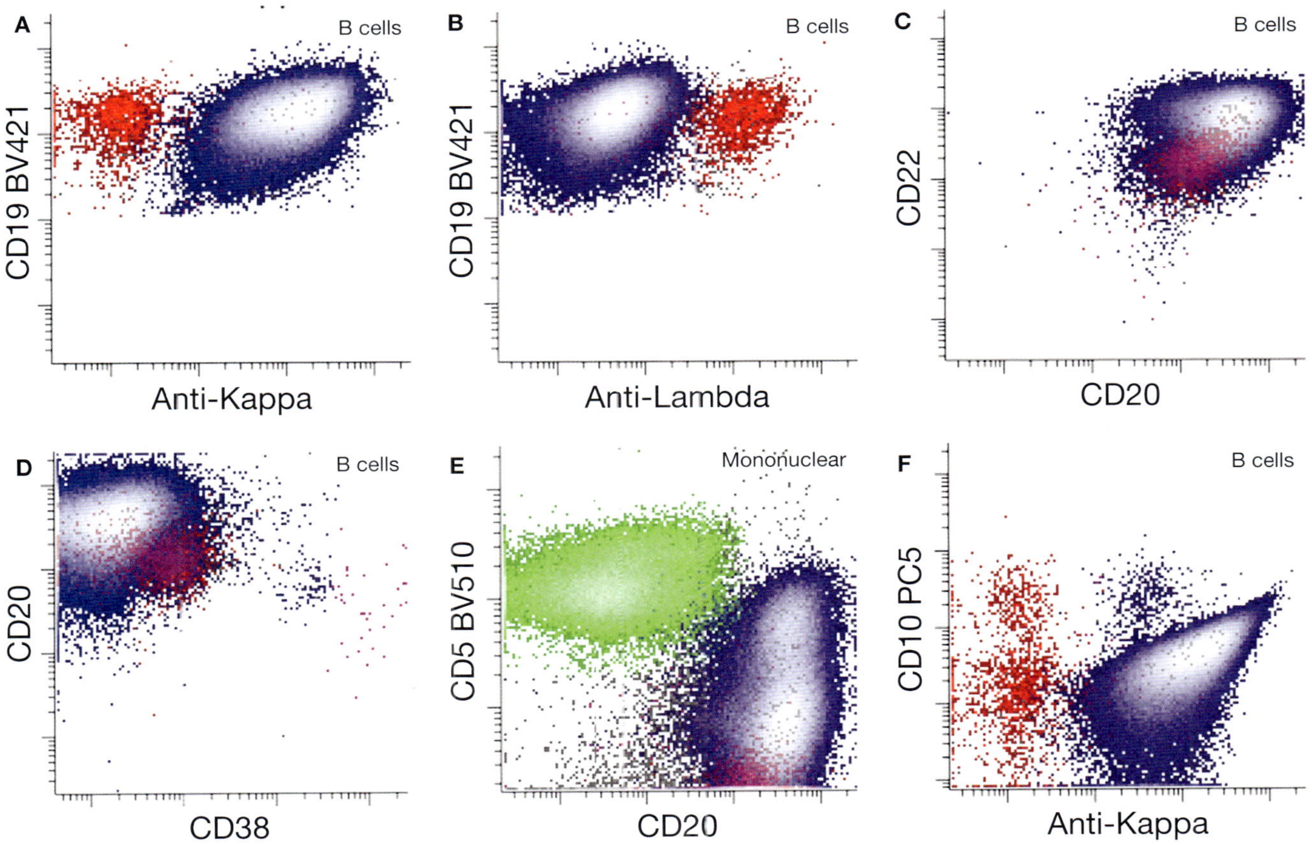

FIGURE 56.4 Flow cytometric immunophenotyping in nodal marginal zone lymphoma (NMZL). **A** and **B:** The neoplastic NMZL B cells express CD19 and kappa light chains (blue population) but not lambda light chains (red population). **C:** The NMZL B cells express bright CD20 and CD19 (blue population) compared to benign B cells (red population). **D:** They are negative for CD38. **E:** They show partial CD5 expression (blue population) but at a lower level compared to T cells (green population). **F:** The NMZL B cells do not express CD10. However, note the presence of residual CD10-positive, polytypic, reactive follicle center B cell populations. This is a characteristic finding in NMZL.

lymphomas including follicular lymphoma, SMZL, and extranodal MZL except for *PTPRD* mutations, which appear to be enriched in NMZL. The diagnostic utility of comprehensive mutational profiling remains unclear in the context of NMZL. The absence of *MYD88* mutations in the appropriate clinical, histologic, and immunophenotypic context would favor a diagnosis of NMZL over lymphoplasmacytic lymphoma.

The genetic basis of large cell transformation in NMZL has not been well established. However, recent studies have identified a subset of de novo DLBCLs showing mutational profiles similar to that seen in NMZL including mutations affecting *NOTCH2, SPEN, TNFAIP3, BCL10*, and *KLF2*, in addition to frequent *BCL6* alterations.[14] It has been suggested that such tumors may represent transformation of underlying occult MZL.

Prognosis and Clinical Comment

There are no specific prognostic indices to predict clinical outcome for NMZL. However, progression of disease at 24 months and event-free survival at 12 months have been shown to predict overall survival in some cohorts.[15] The baseline Follicular Lymphoma International Prognostic Index, which was validated for follicular lymphoma, has been shown to have limited value in risk stratifying NMZL.[3]

NMZL is an indolent disorder with prolonged survival over 90% at 5 years in retrospective studies.[3] Like most indolent B-cell lymphomas, NMZL is not curable with current therapeutic modalities. Therefore, initial management can be quite conservative with observation in asymptomatic, low tumor burden patients, which accounts up 40% of cases or with localized radiotherapy for limited stage presentation.[3] Eventually most patients will require systemic therapy due to a variety of clinical factors including bulky disease, systemic symptoms, and development of paraneoplastic syndromes such as autoimmune hemolytic anemia and immune-mediated renal disease. Choice of systemic therapy includes single-agent anti-CD20 antibody therapy or chemoimmunotherapy.[4] Causes of death in NMZL include large cell transformation, infections, and also other malignancies and cardiovascular disease.[3]

References

1. Cerhan JR, Habermann TM. Epidemiology of marginal zone lymphoma. *Ann Lymphoma*. 2021;5:1. doi:10.21037/aol-20-28
2. Arcaini L, Paulli M, Boveri E, et al. Splenic and nodal marginal zone lymphomas are indolent disorders at high hepatitis C virus seroprevalence with distinct presenting features but similar morphologic and phenotypic profiles. *Cancer*. 2004;100(1):107-115. doi:10.1002/cncr.11893
3. Stuver RN, Drill E, Qualls D, et al. Retrospective characterization of nodal marginal zone lymphoma. *Blood Adv*. 2023;7(17):4838-4847. doi:10.1182/bloodadvances.2022009587
4. Rossi D, Bertoni F, Zucca E. Marginal-zone lymphomas. *N Engl J Med*. 2022;386(6):568-581.
5. Berger F, Traverse-Glehen A, Felman P, et al. Clinicopathologic features of Waldenstrom's macroglobulinemia and marginal zone lymphoma: are they distinct or the same entity? *Clin Lymphoma*. 2005;5(4):220-224. doi:10.3816/clm.2005.n.003
6. Traverse-Glehen A, Bertoni F, Thieblemont C, et al. Nodal marginal zone B-cell lymphoma: a diagnostic and therapeutic dilemma. *Oncol (Williston Park, NY)*. 2012;26(1):92-104. 92-9, 103-4.
7. Conconi A, Franceschetti S, Hohenstaufen KA, et al. Histologic transformation in marginal zone lymphomas †. *Ann Oncol*. 2015;26(11):2329-2335. doi:10.1093/annonc/mdv368
8. Wang Z, Cook JR. IRTA1 and MNDA expression in marginal zone lymphoma utility in differential diagnosis and implications for classification. *Am J Clin Pathol*. 2019;151(3):337-343.
9. Falini B, Agostinelli C, Bigerna B, et al. IRTA1 is selectively expressed in nodal and extranodal marginal zone lymphomas. *Histopathology*. 2012;61(5):930-941.
10. Kanellis G, Roncador G, Arribas A, et al. Identification of MNDA as a new marker for nodal marginal zone lymphoma. *Leukemia*. 2009;23(10):1847-1857.
11. Braggio E, Dogan A, Keats JJ, et al. Genomic analysis of marginal zone and lymphoplasmacytic lymphomas identified common and disease-specific abnormalities. *Mod Pathol*. 2012;25(5):651-660.
12. Spina V, Khiabanian H, Messina M, et al. The genetics of nodal marginal zone lymphoma. *Blood*. 2016;128(10):1362-1373.
13. Pillonel V, Juskevicius D, Ng CKY, et al. High-throughput sequencing of nodal marginal zone lymphomas identifies recurrent BRAF mutations. *Leukemia*. 2018;32(11):2412-2426.
14. Wright GW, Huang DW, Phelan JD, et al. A probabilistic classification tool for genetic subtypes of diffuse large B cell lymphoma with therapeutic implications. *Cancer Cell*. 2020;37(4):551-568 e14.
15. Luminari S, Merli M, Rattotti S, et al. Early progression as a predictor of survival in marginal zone lymphomas: an analysis from the FIL-NF10 study. *Blood*. 2019;134(10):798-801.

Chapter 57
Follicular Lymphoma

Camille Laurent, Steve M. Ansell, Leticia Quintanilla-Martinez, and Gilles Salles

Definition

Follicular lymphoma (FL) is characterized by a clonal proliferation of mature B cells with phenotype and genotype of germinal center (GC) B cells composed of varying proportions of centrocytes and centroblasts, which usually has at least a partial follicular pattern. FL harbors the t(14;18) *IGH::BCL2* translocation leading to the overexpression of BCL2 in up to 90% of cases. Diffuse areas of any size, composed of predominantly centroblasts, are evidence of progression to diffuse large B-cell lymphoma (DLBCL). Two early lesions closely related to conventional FL are recognized as variants, namely, in situ follicular neoplasia (ISFN) and duodenal-type follicular lymphoma (DTFL). Additionally, alternative forms of FL without *BCL2* rearrangements (*BCL2*-R) are recognized as distinct entities, including the new provisional entity of *BCL2*-R-negative CD23^{+} follicle center lymphoma (*BCL2*R-, CD23^{+} FCL), pediatric-type follicular lymphoma (PTFL), testicular follicular lymphoma (TFL), primary cutaneous follicle center lymphoma (PCFL), and large B-cell lymphoma with *IRF4* rearrangement (LBCL-*IRF4*),[1] and are classified separately from conventional FL.[2]

Synonyms

None.

Epidemiology

FL is the second most common lymphoma worldwide (after DLBCL) accounting for 20% of all non-Hodgkin lymphomas.[3] Conventional FL predominantly affects adults with a median age of 60 years with most studies reporting no gender predilection and occurs very rarely in patients <18 years.[3] It is more frequent in developed countries (25.5%) compared with developing countries (15.3%). In the United States, FL constitutes almost 40% of non-Hodgkin lymphoma and shows the highest incidence rate at 3.5 per 100,000. Furthermore, FL is most frequent in white populations followed by African and Asian/Pacific populations.[3,4] The risk of FL increases in patients with a family history of non-Hodgkin lymphoma, obesity, and Sjögren syndrome. Among environmental factors, pesticide exposure in agriculture (malathion and dichlorodiphenyltrichoroethane), living in industrial areas, smoking especially in females, professional spray painters, and hepatitis C virus infection increase the risk of FL.[3]

General Clinical Features

Sites of involvement

Most patients with FL have widespread disease at diagnosis (stage III or IV) including peripheral and central (abdominal, retroperitoneal, and mediastinal) lymphadenopathy. The bone marrow is involved in more than 40% to 50% of cases.[5] The majority of patients probably have circulating neoplastic cells, and a small proportion are frankly leukemic. Despite widespread disease, patients are usually asymptomatic and B symptoms such as fever and weight loss are uncommon. A nonnodal presentation is less frequent and might involve the spleen, tonsils, skin, testis, or gastrointestinal tract. Notably, primary FL arising in the small intestine (particularly duodenum) is considered an early, localized FL lesion referred to as DTFL (see following discussion). Extranodal involvement of FL can have the same morphological and genetic characteristics as nodal FL. Alternative FL forms, especially those lacking *BCL2*-R such as *BCL2*R- CD23^{+} FCL, PCFL, PTFL, TFL, and LBCL-*IRF4*, should be distinguished from conventional FL and will be discussed in Chapters 58-62, respectively.

Clinical evaluation and staging

FL diagnosis is best made on an excisional lymph node biopsy, which provides the best opportunity to assess FL grade and growth pattern and also excludes possible areas of DLBCL transformation. The staging procedures for FL include physical examination, blood investigations (complete blood count, renal function and liver function tests, lactate dehydrogenase, and β2-microglobulin), whole body computed tomography (CT) scan, and fluorodeoxyglucose positron emission tomography (FDG-PET). FDG-PET is more sensitive than CT scan (especially at detecting extranodal FL or for up-staging early-stage patients to advanced-stage disease),[6-8] and therefore, it is now the gold-standard imaging investigation at initial staging.[9] It might also help guide the biopsy site in lesions with high glucose uptake (high standard uptake value) to rule out potential histologic transformation. The extent of the disease is then classified according to the Lugano classification. Assessment of bone marrow (BM) involvement with a BM biopsy is not necessary for staging but is recommended if the results modify patient management.

Morphology

Cytology

FL is composed of a mixture of centrocytes and centroblasts, which typically exhibit a follicular growth pattern (Figure 57.1). In most cases, centrocytes appear relatively small and more monomorphic than those in normal follicles and the few centroblasts stand out sharply from the monotonous background of centrocytes. The nuclei of centrocytes are usually less than twice the size of small lymphocytes but may be as large as nuclei of histiocytes or centroblasts. The nuclei of

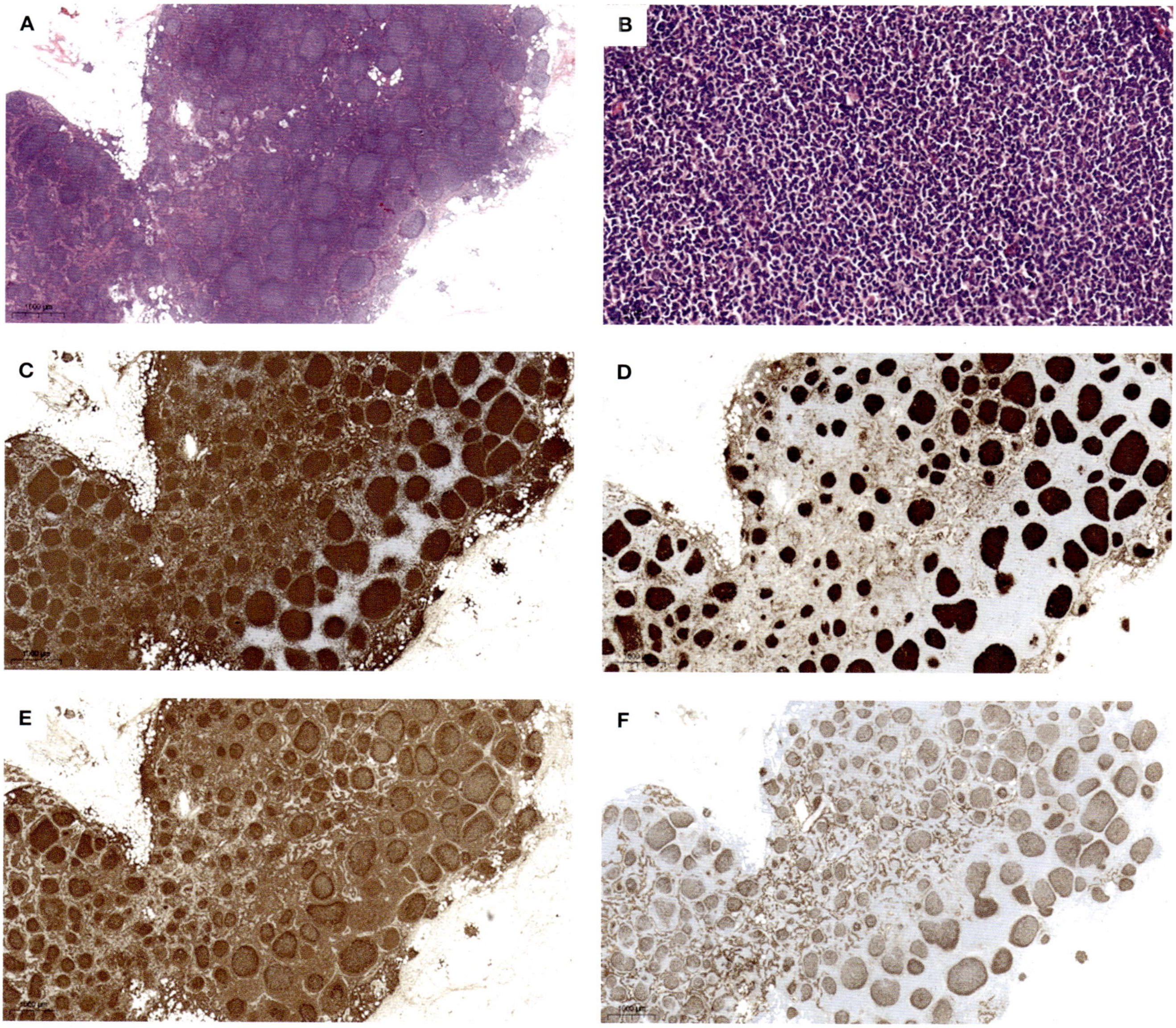

FIGURE 57.1 Lymph node with follicular lymphoma grade 1 to 2. **A:** The normal architecture of the lymph node is effaced by a neoplasia with follicular growth pattern. The neoplastic follicles are relatively uniform and closely packed without mantle zone. Focally there is extension into the extranodal adipose tissue. **B:** Most follicles are composed of centrocytes. **C-E:** Neoplastic cells strongly express CD20 (**C**), CD10 (**D**), and BCL2 (**E**). **F:** Tumor follicles are sustained by expanded CD21+ follicular dendritic cell meshworks.

centrocytes often are irregular or angulated with pale and evenly dispersed chromatin giving the nucleus a gray-blue appearance. They are surrounded by scant pale cytoplasm that is usually not visible on the hematoxylin and eosin (H&E)- or Giemsa-stained sections. Large centrocytes with dispersed chromatin and inconspicuous nucleoli may predominate. The nuclei of centroblasts are usually three to four times the size of small lymphocytes, similar to or larger than the nuclei of histiocytes. The nuclei are round or oval but may be irregular, indented, or even split. The nucleus is vesicular with a clear center and some peripheral chromatin condensation. One to three basophilic nucleoli are often attached to the nuclear membrane. The proportion of centroblasts may vary among follicles. Mitotic activity is usually low, and a starry-sky pattern with tingible body macrophages is rare. Rare cases of FL are composed of blastoid-appearing cells, with dispersed chromatin resembling lymphoblasts. This morphology is associated with a more aggressive clinical course.

Cytological variant of conventional FL

Cytological variants of FL are well recognized. In about 10% of conventional FL, marginal zone differentiation or monocytoid appearing B cells are observed in the periphery of the follicles.[10] Plasmacytic differentiation, although uncommon, might be observed (Figure 57.2).[10] The plasma cells are believed to be part of the neoplastic population, carry the t(14;18) translocation, and are distributed predominantly in the interfollicular area. The morphology of the plasma cells ranges from small mature cells to somewhat atypical forms. Rarely, the neoplastic cells may have a signet ring cell appearance with clear cytoplasmic vacuoles and others may contain Dutcher bodies. Other rare cases may contain intrafollicular amorphous deposits that stain strongly for CD10 and CD20.[11] FL cases with hyaline-vascular Castleman-like feature have been also reported.[12] Finally, few FL cases can contain some intrafollicular giant or multinucleated cells resembling Hodgkin-Reed-Sternberg cells.

Grading

FL follicles are composed of various proportions of centrocytes and centroblasts. FL grading is determined by the number of centroblasts (CBs) per high-power field (HPF) (10-20 HPF in randomly selected follicles 40×): grade 1 ≤ 5CB/HPF, grade 2 = 5 to 15 CB/HPF, and grade 3 or high grade ≥ 15 CB/HPF. Grade 3 is subdivided into grades 3A and 3B (Figures 57.3 and 57.4);

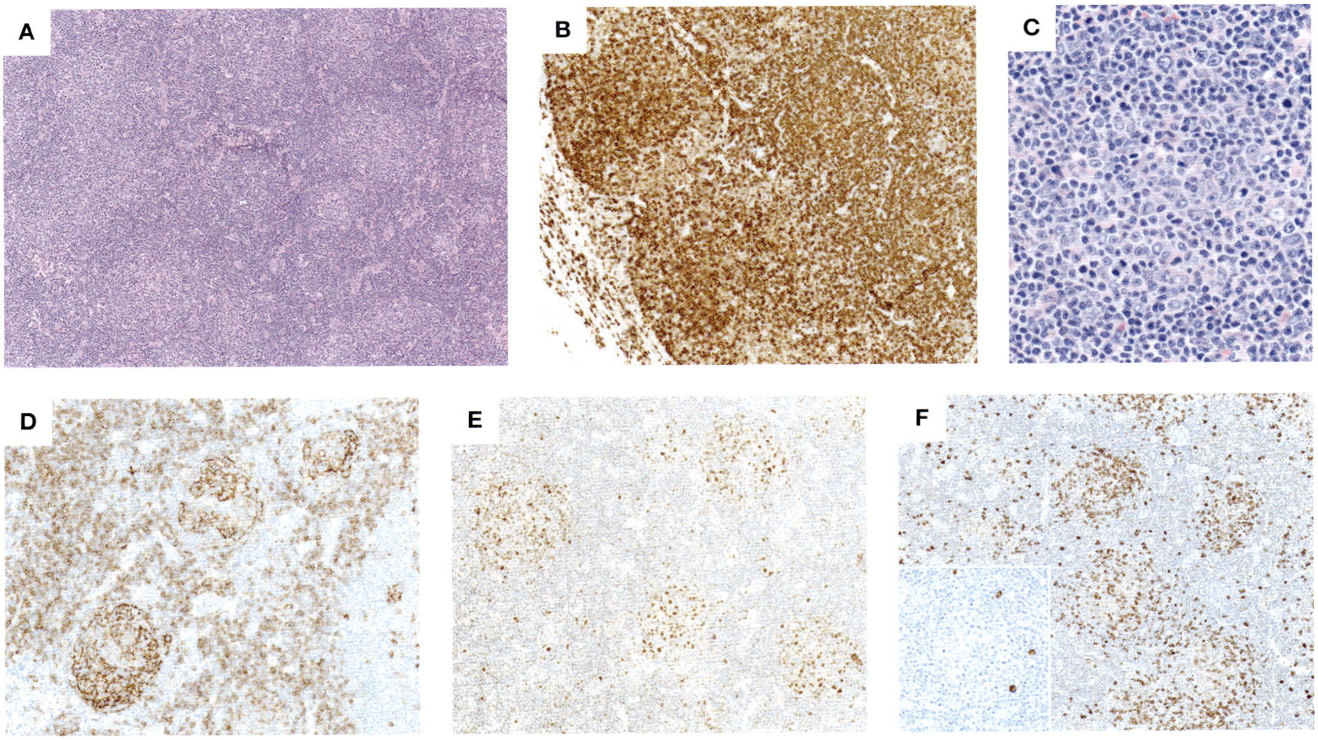

FIGURE 57.2 Follicular lymphoma (FL) with plasma cell differentiation. **A:** The lymph node architecture is effaced by a follicular neoplasm. **B:** Neoplastic cells are BCL2 positive. **C:** Giemsa stain shows neoplastic cells with plasmacytic differentiation. The cells have small nucleoli and scant basophilic cytoplasm. **D:** CD23 shows follicular dendritic cell meshwork and a variable expression on FL cells in interfollicular area. **E:** Neoplastic cells are BCL6 positive. **F:** The neoplastic cells are kappa positive **(F)** and lambda negative (inset).

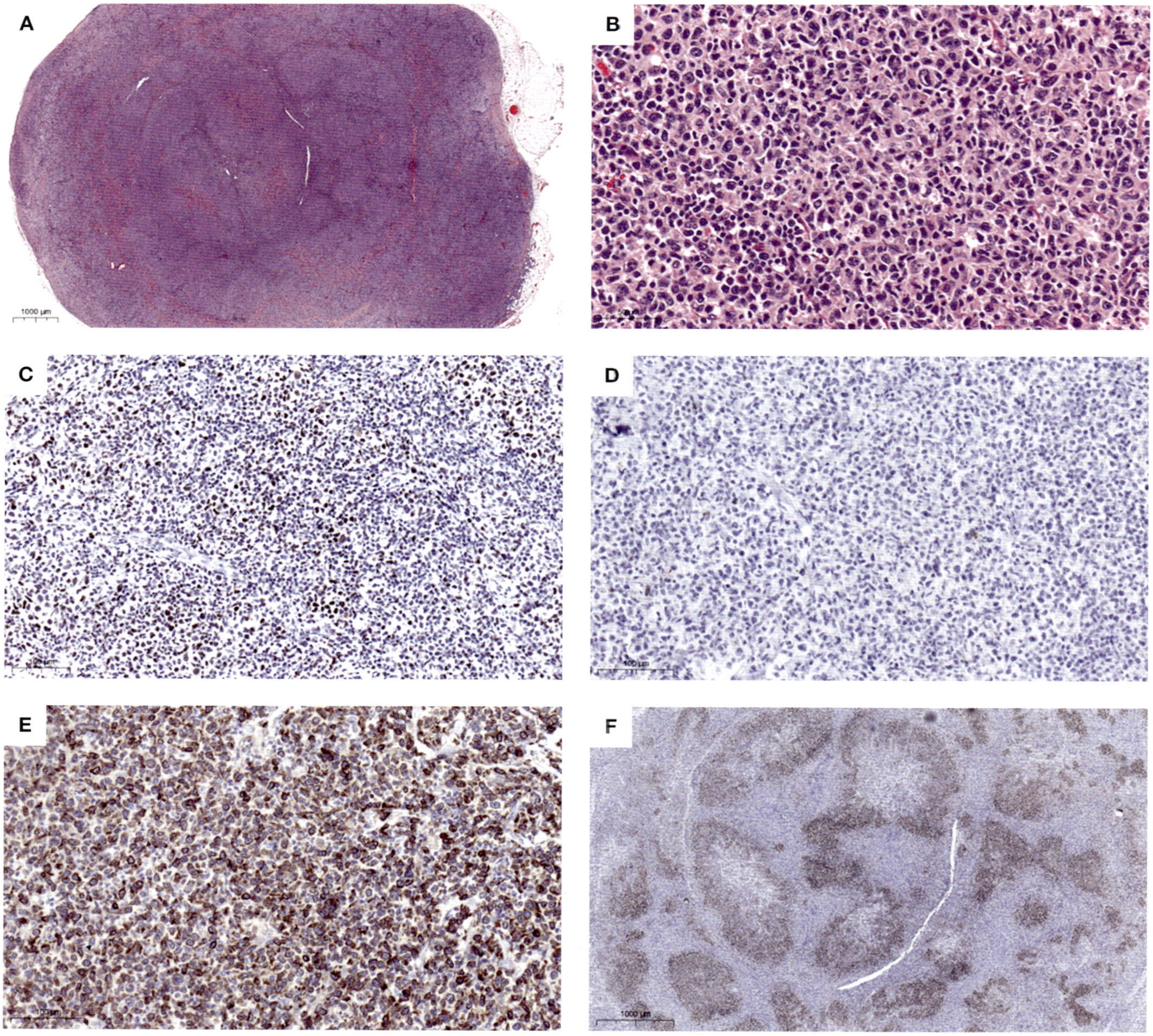

FIGURE 57.3 Lymph node with follicular lymphoma grade 3A. **A:** The lymph node architecture is completely effaced by a follicular proliferation. **B:** The neoplastic follicles are composed of centrocytes and numerous centroblasts (>15 CB/HPF). **C** and **D:** Neoplastic cells are BCL6 positive **(C)** and CD10 negative **(D)**. **E:** Neoplastic cells strongly express BCL2. **F:** CD21 staining shows follicular dendritic cell meshworks.

the latter is assigned to FL cases in which neoplastic follicles are essentially composed of sheets of centroblasts and are usually treated as DLBCL.[5] Moreover, because grades 1 and 2 comprise a morphologic continuum and are both clinically indolent, the designation grade 1 to 2 (low-grade FL) introduced in the 2008 World Health Organization classification[5] is still recommended (Figure 57.1). However, FL grading based on strict counting methods of centroblasts and centrocytes lacks reproducibility in some cases,[13] and its clinical impact, especially between grade 1 to 2 and 3A, appears to be less significant in the era of rituximab.[14,15] Some grade 3 FL cases, composed of neoplastic cells that are not classic centroblasts but rather small-sized blasts or large cleaved cells, are still considered as grade 3.[1] In these difficult cases, the demonstration of *BCL2*-R and CD10 expression that both favor grade 3A is useful and recommended. Finally, despite the biological relationship between grade 1 to 2 and 3A, and the difficulties in FL grading,[1] histologic grading is still maintained, in part to allow for investigation of response of new agents and pursue clinical investigation.[1,2] Notably, new

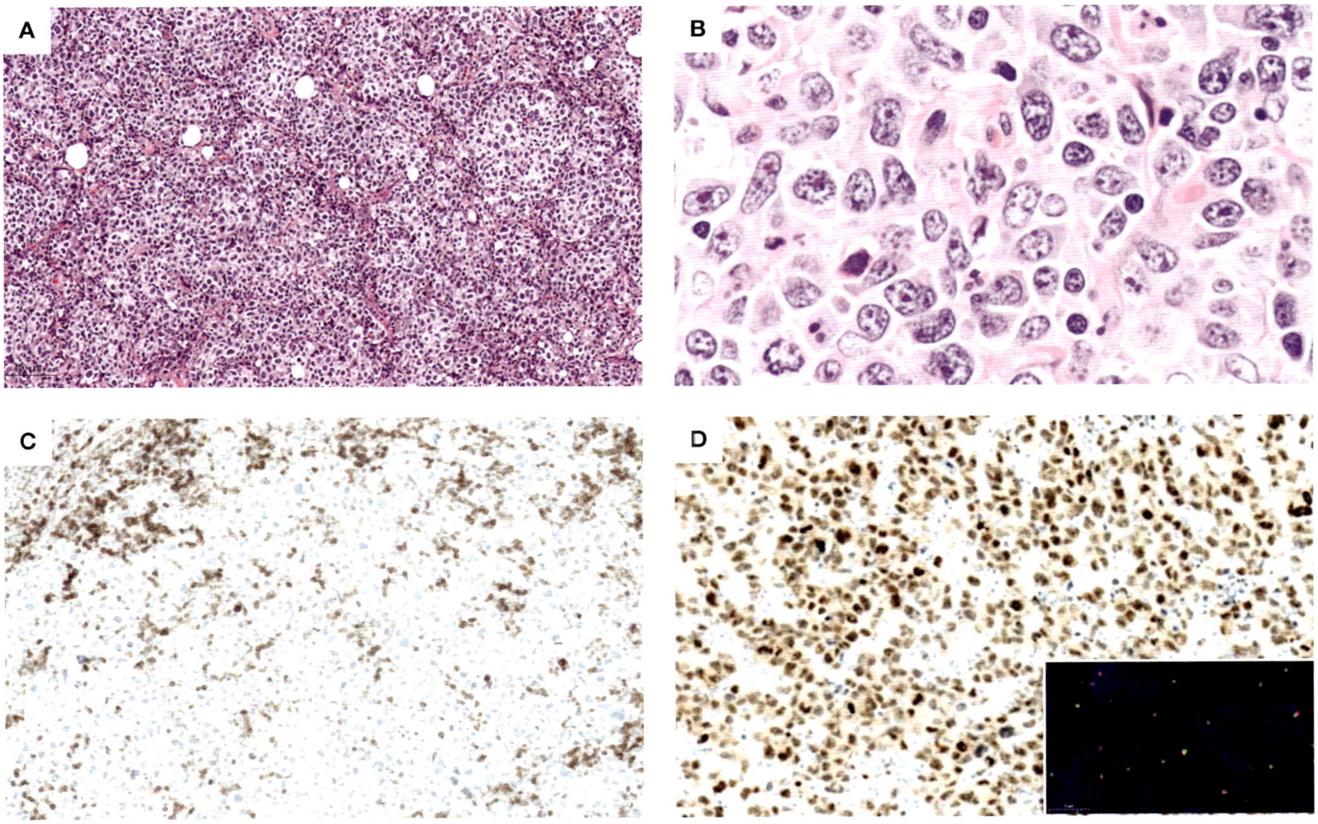

FIGURE 57.4 Lymph node with follicular lymphoma grade 3B. **A:** The lymph node architecture is effaced by a follicular neoplasia with back-to-back follicles and absent mantle zone. **B:** Higher magnification demonstrates that the neoplastic follicles are composed of sheets of centroblasts with no evidence of centrocytes. **C:** The neoplastic cells are negative for BCL2. **D:** IRF4/MUM1 is strong and homogeneously expressed in the tumor cells (inset: fluorescence in situ hybridization using *IRF4* break apart probes is negative).

genetic studies have shown that the separation between FL grade 1/2 and 3A matters and has clinical impact.[16]

Pattern

FL is characterized by an effacement of normal lymph node architecture by closely packed neoplastic follicles sustained by a follicular dendritic cell (FDC) network. However, sometimes more and less extended diffuse areas can be observed. Diagnostic reports traditionally identify the growth pattern, with designations of mainly follicular pattern (at least 75%), FL with follicular and diffuse pattern (25%-75%), predominantly diffuse (<25%), and totally diffuse (no follicles). Diffuse FL diagnosis should be made with caution after excluding other lymphomas, especially DLBCL in case of predominant large B-cell proliferation (Figure 57.5). Moreover, the new provisional entity *BCL2*R- CD23$^+$ FCL (see Chapter 58) often has a diffuse growth pattern and should be distinguished from conventional FL.[1,2] Neoplastic follicles may vary in size from a primary follicle to much larger than reactive follicles. They usually are round and monotonous with loss of follicle polarization, absence of body macrophages, and attenuated mantle zones. Sometimes follicles may be irregular and serpiginous, mimicking florid reactive hyperplastic follicles. Mantle zones are attenuated or absent.

Tumor microenvironment

In addition to FDC, neoplastic follicles contain numerous CD4$^+$ follicular helper T cells (T_{FH}), some classic regulatory T cells (T_{REG}), and follicular regulatory T cells (T_{FR}).[17] The interfollicular region usually shows a reduced normal T-cell zone with variable amounts of T_{REG}, CD8$^+$ T cells frequently exhibiting an exhausted phenotype and some cytotoxic T cells that are usually observed at the follicle border.[18,19] There are few plasma cells. Macrophages and stroma cells also contribute to FL's tumor microenvironment (TME) and are usually present in the interfollicular region.[20] FL may contain numerous blood vessels with high endothelial venules often infiltrated by neoplastic centrocytes. Subcapsular and medullary sinuses are typically obliterated but may be partially preserved in some cases. Sclerosis is common and may present surrounding the follicle, in diffuse areas (especially when FL is in mesenteric and retroperitoneal regions) or less often in the follicle. Extrascapular extension is common and leads to the formation of fibrous bands in the extranodal tissue.

Immunophenotype

FL cells express the pan B-lymphocyte antigens (CD19, CD20, CD22, CD79a, PAX-5) and express IgM with or without IgD. Similar to normal GC cells, FL cells also express CD10 and BCL6, usually stronger in the neoplastic follicles than in interfollicular areas. However, a subset of FL, especially grade 3B, can be negative for CD10 and/or BCL6. In this context, other GC markers including GCET1, HGAL (GCET2), LMO2, and/or MEF2B should be performed to rule out other B-cell lymphomas diagnoses. They are negative for CD5 and CD43.

FL cells typically overexpress BCL2 as a result of the genetic hallmark of FL, t(14;18) *IGH::BCL2* translocation. Similar to CD10 staining, the frequency of BCL2 expression is higher in grade 1 to 2 (85%-90%) than in grade 3 (50%-70%) FL. However, some FL cases do not express BCL2 protein due to the absence of *BCL2*-R.[21] In addition, some FL cases harboring t(14;18) may be falsely negative when stained with an anti-BCL2 antibody, due to mutations in the *BCL2* gene that alter the epitopes recognized by some monoclonal antibodies. In these "pseudonegative" cases, other anti-BCL2 antibodies (clones E17 or SP66) and/or fluorescence in situ hybridization for *BCL2*-R should be tested.[22]

IRF4/MUM1 is typically not expressed except in some cases of high-grade FL, especially grade 3B (see later discussion). In the case of FL grade 3 expressing MUM1/IRF4, the International Consensus Classification (ICC) recommends evaluating *IRF4* alterations, especially in younger patients, to rule out the diagnosis of LBCL *IRF4*-R (discussed in Chapter 62).[1,2] A nodular pattern is assessed by the presence of CD21, CD23, and/or CD35 positivity in the FDC meshwork but absent in cases with diffuse areas. Some FL neoplastic cells can also express CD21 or CD23. Most, but not all, grade 1-2 FL have a low Ki-67 proliferation index (<20%), but due to heterogeneity of distribution, it is still difficult to assess and alone, its clinical significance remains uncertain. Finally, Ki67 is not required for grading.

Genetics

Antigen receptor genes

The immunoglobulin (IG) heavy chain and light chain genes are clonally rearranged, and IG variable gene regions show extensive and ongoing somatic mutations. Similar to normal GC B cells, FL cells express activation-induced cytidine deaminase (AID) in >25% of FL, an essential requirement for somatic hypermutations (SHMs) and isotype switch.[23] About 40% to 50% of FL have undergone isotype switching and express IgG, and surprisingly, most IgM^+ FLs show class-switch recombination (CSR) on the translocated allele and IGHC deletions on the expressed IGH allele.[24] Retention of IgM expression in FL cells could be advantageous for (pre)malignant cells, as it appears that IgM^+ memory B cells have a greater propensity to reenter GC than class-switched memory B cells.

Although linear clonal evolution has been described, most FL cases follow a subclonal evolution from a common precursor cell, leading to multiple subclones

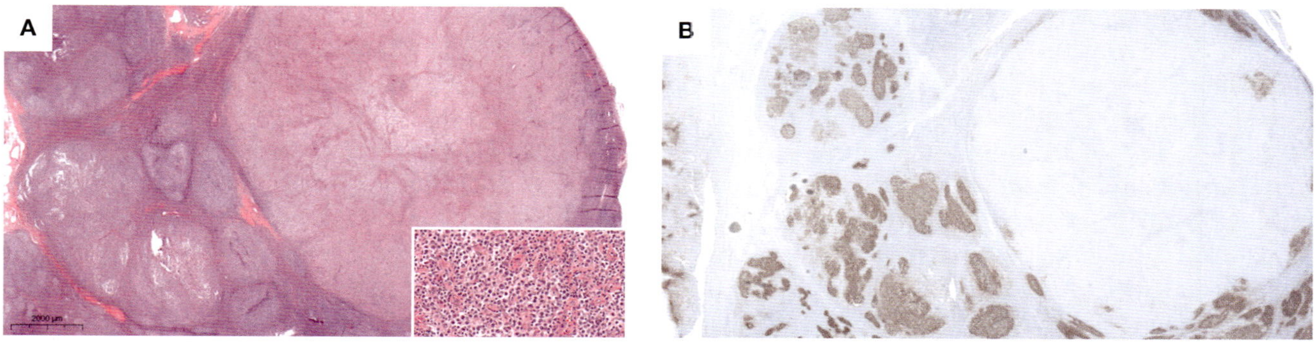

FIGURE 57.5 Lymph node infiltrated by follicular lymphoma (FL) with a component of diffuse large B-cell lymphoma (DLBCL). **A:** This lymph node shows two different areas. On the left side there is infiltration by neoplastic follicles without mantle zones. The infiltrate is composed of admixed centrocytes and centroblasts corresponding to FL grade1-2. The second area on the right side shows a diffuse area composed of sheets of large cells consistent with DLBCL (inset: high magnification showing diffuse proliferation of large centrocytes and centroblasts). **B:** CD21 staining shows follicular dendritic cell meshworks in the follicular areas but not in the DLBCL.

already identified in the early stages of FL (early FL lesions, see later discussion) that provide the substrate for FL progression and transformation.[25]

In addition, FL cells have a high incidence of N-glycosylation sites (Asn-X-Ser/Thr) introduced by SHM, mostly in the IG variable gene regions[26] that induce FL interactions with TME via surface structures (C-type lectins, dendritic cell–specific ICAM-grabbing nonintegrin, and mannose receptors) and that promote FL survival.

Cytogenetic abnormalities

FL with *BCL2* rearrangement

The translocation t(14;18)(q32;q21), or on rare occasions its variants t(2;18)(p12;q21) or t(18;22)(q21;q11), is the hallmark of conventional FL occurring in 85% to 90% of cases and leading to the overexpression of the antiapoptotic protein BCL2. *BCL2*-R is more often observed in low-grade than in high-grade FL. The t(14;18) can also be detected at very low levels (~1-100 cells per million B cells) in the peripheral blood (PB) of >70% healthy adults (referred as "FL-like cells"). The frequency of FL-like cells in PB increases with age and risk exposure (pesticides).[27] Although higher levels of circulating FL-like cells are associated with an increased risk of developing an overt FL, the vast majority of those healthy individuals will never develop FL,[28] indicating that the translocation alone is not sufficient for the development of FL and additional genetic alterations are needed for full transformation. In fact, the acquisition of t(14;18) allows FL-like cells to iteratively reenter GC and engage in multiple cycles of SHM and CSR, thereby increasing the risk of accumulation of genomic instability.

FL without *BCL2* rearrangement (*BCL2*-R negative)

BCL2-R-negative FL represents 10% to 15% of FL cases and constitutes a heterogeneous group of FL.[21,29,30] Based on clinical presentation, *BCL2*-R-negative FL can be divided into three groups: (1) nodal presentation, (2) extranodal presentation including the PCFL, and (3) those affecting predominantly children and young adults such as PTFL, TFL, and LBCL *IRF4*-R. Of note, PCFL, PTFL, TFL, and LBCL *IRF4*-R are considered as distinct entities separate from conventional FL in the ICC 2022[1,2] (see Chapters 59-62). Regarding nodal *BCL2*-R-negative FLs, genetic studies comparing *BCL2*-R negative and *BCL2*-R positive FLs have pointed out subtle differences in the developmental stages of the neoplastic B cells, the usage of divergent oncogenic pathways, and the composition of the microenvironment.[31] Likewise, genetic alterations frequently observed in *BCL2*-R+ FL have been reported in nodal *BCL2*-R-negative cases but at different frequencies, showing an enrichment of *STAT6* (57%) mutations followed by *CREBBP* (49%), *TNFRSF14* (39%), and *KMT2D* mutations[21] as well as some variations in chromosomal alterations such as the most frequent *BCL6*-R and 1p36 deletion.

Based on their molecular profiles, three groups of nodal *BCL2*-R-negative FLs are identified: (1) *BCL2*R-, CD23+ FCL, discussed in Chapter 58; (2) nodal *BCL2*-R-negative FL with *BCL6*-R (excluding FL3B, see later discussion); and (3) nodal *BCL2*-R-negative and *BCL6*-R-negative FLs. Nodal *BCL2*-R-negative FL with *BCL6*-R, grade 1-3A represents ~20% of *BCL2*-R-negative FLs. Patients with FL *BCL6*-R present with a more advanced clinical stage.[30] *BCL6*-R involving 3q27 with a variety of partners leads to anomalous upregulation and prevents the cell from progressing past the GC stage, thus facilitating neoplastic transformation. FL with *BCL6*-R grade 1 to 2 and 3A has a follicular pattern, usually conserves a GC phenotype, and shares similar genetic alterations with conventional FL *BCL2*-R+. However, it shows a more complex genetic profile and fewer *CREBBP* and *STAT6* mutations than other nodal *BCL2*-R-negative FLs.[21,30] Nodal *BCL2*-R-negative and *BCL6*-R-negative FL grades 1 to 2 and 3A are characterized by few genetic alterations, noninguinal presentation with follicular growth pattern, and lack of both *STAT6* mutations and CD23 expression.[29] The differential diagnosis of nodal marginal zone lymphoma (MZL) can be challenging. However, these cases express at least one GC marker and lack typical mutations of nodal MZL.

Other genetic alterations

Copy-number alterations are found in most FLs and include chromosomal gains of 18, X, 1q, 2p, and 7, and less commonly gains of 17q, 6p, 8q, 12q as well as deletions of 6q and 1p and less frequently deletions of 10q and 9p.[5,32] Genomic alterations in *TP53* or *CDKN2A* and *MYC* translocations are rare and have been reported to be associated with high-grade features and/or increased risk of transformation. However, the prognostic value of de novo *BCL2*-R positive FL with *MYC*-R is still controversial. Based on the limited data available, de novo *BCL2*-R/*MYC*-R positive FL with should not be considered as high grade B-cell lymphoma with *MYC* and *BCL2* rearrangements.[2]

Recurrent mutations in epigenetic regulators and chromatin remodeling genes are the most frequent mutations in conventional FL.[33] Among them, mutations in chromatin-remodeling genes such as

KMT2D/MLL2, *CREBBP*, and *EP300* represent common drivers of conventional FL. *KMT2D/MLL2* is the most frequently observed in 90% of cases followed by *CREBBP* in 33% to 75% of cases. Additional epigenetic dysregulation comprises gain-of-function mutations of *EZH2* (25%), a histone methyltransferase catalyzing trimethylation of lysine on histone H3 (H3K24me3). Other less frequent epigenetic modifier mutations are seen in *ARID1A*, *MEF2B*, and *KMT2C* genes. *BCL2* mutations are common due to AID activity. *TNFRSF14* mutations or 1p36 deletion (including *TNFRSF14* gene) can be observed in FL, irrespective of t(14;18). *STAT6*, *CARD11*, *FOXO1*, *NOCTH1/2*, and *TNFAIP3* mutations are less frequently seen in FL with *BCL2*-R. However, as mentioned previously, these frequencies of genetic alterations differ in nodal *BCL2*-R-negative FL, showing enrichment of *STAT6* mutations followed by *CREBBP*, *TNFRSF14*, and *KMT2D* mutated genes. Besides clonal evolution over time, studies have also demonstrated significant spatial heterogeneity in mutation and genomic profiles in different disease sites in a given patient.[34,35] This hampers the development of prognostic biomarkers based on tumor genetic architecture.

Follicular Lymphoma Grade 3B

FL grade 3B, accounting for ~5 to 10% of all FL cases,[36] is defined by the presence of solid sheets of centroblasts (>15 CB/HPF) with at least a partial follicular pattern (Figure 57.4). Coexistence with DLBCL is frequent. FL3B should also be distinguished from FL3A. As mentioned earlier, ICC recommends evaluating the status of *BCL2*-R and CD10 expression in FL grade 3 (absence of *BCL2*-R and the CD10 expression favor the diagnosis of FL3B).[1,2] *BCL2*-R is less frequently observed (9%-50%) in FL3B, whereas *BCL6*-R is reported in up to 40% and *MYC*-R in 20% of cases. The tumor cells are often negative for CD10 (40%-100%) and BCL6 (0%-50%) and have a lower expression of BCL2 and increased p53 expression.[21,37] Moreover, IRF4/MUM1 has been variably reported (42%-100%). In addition, $CD10^-$ $MUM1/IRF4^+$ FL grade 3 lacking *BCL2*-R and *BCL6*-R may be associated with poorer prognosis.[36] As mentioned earlier, FL 3B should be tested for *IRF4* alterations to exclude LBCL *IRF4*-R diagnosis (see Chapter 62). Additional cytogenetic abnormalities such as gain of chromosome 7 or 3 and 6q deletion have been reported.[38] As in conventional FL, epigenetic mutations including *KMT2D/2C* and *CREBBP* are the most frequent in pure FL3B.[39] *TP53* and *MYD88* mutations may also be observed.[39] Two gene expression profiling studies concluded that FL3B has a distinct signature closer to that of FL3A and different from DLBCL and FL grades 1 to 2,[40,41] supporting the contention that FL3B belongs to the group of FL rather DLBCL. However, further studies are needed to clarify this issue.

Prognosis and Clinical Outcome

FL is usually a disseminated but indolent disease with a median overall survival (OS) of patients between 15 and 20 years. Its prognosis is related to disease extent at diagnosis and other disease and patient characteristics. The Follicular Lymphoma International Prognostic Index (FLIPI) distinguishes three groups of patients (approximately one-third each) with significant differences in OS.[42,43] The FLIPI uses five independent adverse predictors: age >60 years, hemoglobin <12 g/dL, elevated serum lactate dehydrogenase, Ann Arbor stage III/IV (disseminated disease in the Lugano system), and >4 involved nodal areas. The presence of 0 to 1, 2, 3-5 of these factors defines low-risk, intermediate-risk, and high-risk disease, respectively. Other clinical prognostic indices, such as FLIPI-2 and PRIMA-PI, are not commonly used in daily practice.[44,45] Except for grade 3B, histological grade has no significant impact on outcome in patients treated with rituximab, cyclophosphamide, doxorubicin, vincristine and prednisone (R-CHOP) regimens.[1,2] For patients requiring treatment, the use of combined immunochemotherapy results in a 10-year OS of around 80%. Despite recent therapeutic progress and improved OS, progression occurs over time in most patients. Early progression within 24 months of treatment initiation (POD24), occurring in 15% to 20% of FL, has a poor prognosis, with a variable but significant proportion of those patients experiencing histological transformation.

Recently, the m7-FLIPI (integrating FLIPI with seven common gene mutations) and some gene expression signatures related to dark zone CBs have been identified as prognostic indices but remain investigational.[33,46-48] The composition and spatial distribution of the FL microenvironment have shown a prognostic impact of distinct subpopulations (Treg, T_{FH}, cytotoxic T cells, and stromal cells) in numerous studies, but there is still a lack of consensus regarding biomarkers.[49-51]

Histologic transformation of FL to high-grade lymphoma, occurring at a risk of 1% to 3% per year,[52,53] might affect 5% to 12% of patients with FL within 5 years of follow-up.[52] The most common histology is DLBCL (mainly GCB rather than ABC subtype, 80% vs. 20%)

and more rarely Burkitt lymphoma, lymphoblastic lymphoma, or Hodgkin disease.[52,54] High FLIPI score and resistance to first-line therapy have been reported as risk factors for transformation.[5] In addition, genetic factors including deletions and gains (del 1q, del 6q, +2, +3q, +5), loss of *B2M*, and alteration of *CDKN2A*/B, *MYC*, and *TP53*[55,56] have been associated with the risk of transformation, but early detection of molecular alterations predicting transformation has not been so far successful.

EARLY LESIONS OF FOLLICULAR LYMPHOMA

In Situ Follicular Neoplasia

Definition

ISFN is an FL variant characterized by a monoclonal proliferation of B cells carrying t(14;18) translocation and partially or totally colonizing the GC of some follicles in lymphoid tissue. ISFN is biologically similar to the presence of t(14;18) found in PB of healthy individuals, referred as FL-like B cells.[5]

Synonyms

None.

Epidemiology

ISFN is an incidental finding reported in 2% to 3% of unselected reactive lymph nodes from middle-aged or older individuals. However, some ISFN can occur syn- or metachronously with confirmed FL, as well as with other B-cell lymphomas.

General Clinical Features

For patients with incidentally diagnosed ISFN and no other evidence of FL on clinical evaluation, the risk of subsequent FL is very low (5%). The number of follicles involved by ISFN cannot predict the subsequent risk of developing FL. High levels of FL-like B cells in PB are associated with an increased risk of subsequent FL.

Morphology

ISFN is generally not apparent in routine H&E-stained sections. The lymph node has a preserved nodal architecture and contains reactive follicles with well-defined GC and intact mantle zones (Figure 57.6). The affected follicles are similar in size and shape to uninvolved follicles. ISFN is distinct from partial involvement by FL, in which only selected follicles within an lymph node may be involved. Moreover, ISFN can only be observed with subsequent immunohistochemistry, whereas partial involvement by FL can be suspected on H&E-stained sections with at least focal areas of architectural effacement. Partial involvement by FL is associated with lower-stage disease that can histologically progress to full FL in 53% of the cases versus 5% of ISFN.[57]

Immunophenotype

BCL2 is strongly expressed by the tumor B cells (mostly cleaved centrocytes-like cells) confined to the GC. BCL2 staining in tumor cells shows a higher intensity than in adjacent T cells or mantle zones. BCL2+ tumor cells also show strong expression of CD10 and BCL6 (Figure 57.6).

Genetics

ISFN cells carry the t(14;18) *IGH::BCL2* and share genetic alterations similar to systemic FL but at lower frequencies,[58,59] suggesting that ISFN is a very early step in FL lymphomagenesis. Mutations in *CREBBP*, *KMT2D*, *TNFRSF14*, and *EZH2*; deletions in 1p36; and acquisition of N-glycosylation sites have been reported in ISFN.[58,59] Recently, the *CREBBP* mutation has been shown to be the most commonly observed precursor lesion and may distinguish patients developing FL from healthy adults with or without detected *BCL2*-R.[60] In cases where ISFN and overt FL are seen in the same patient, there are additional genetic alterations in the FL not detected in ISFN. Recently, branched clonal evolution, rather than a linear one between early FL lesions and systemic FL, has been reported, suggesting that ISFN and FL evolve from a common progenitor.[61]

Duodenal-Type Follicular Lymphoma

Definition

DTFL is another FL variant defined by distinctive clinical and biological features.[5] The lesions are predominantly found in the second portion of the duodenum, presenting as multiple polyps, often as an incidental finding on endoscopy performed for other reasons. Most patients have localized disease (stage IE or IIE). Cases without the typical features of DTFL should be investigated for evidence of conventional FL involvement at other sites. It also must be differentiated from primary intestinal FL,

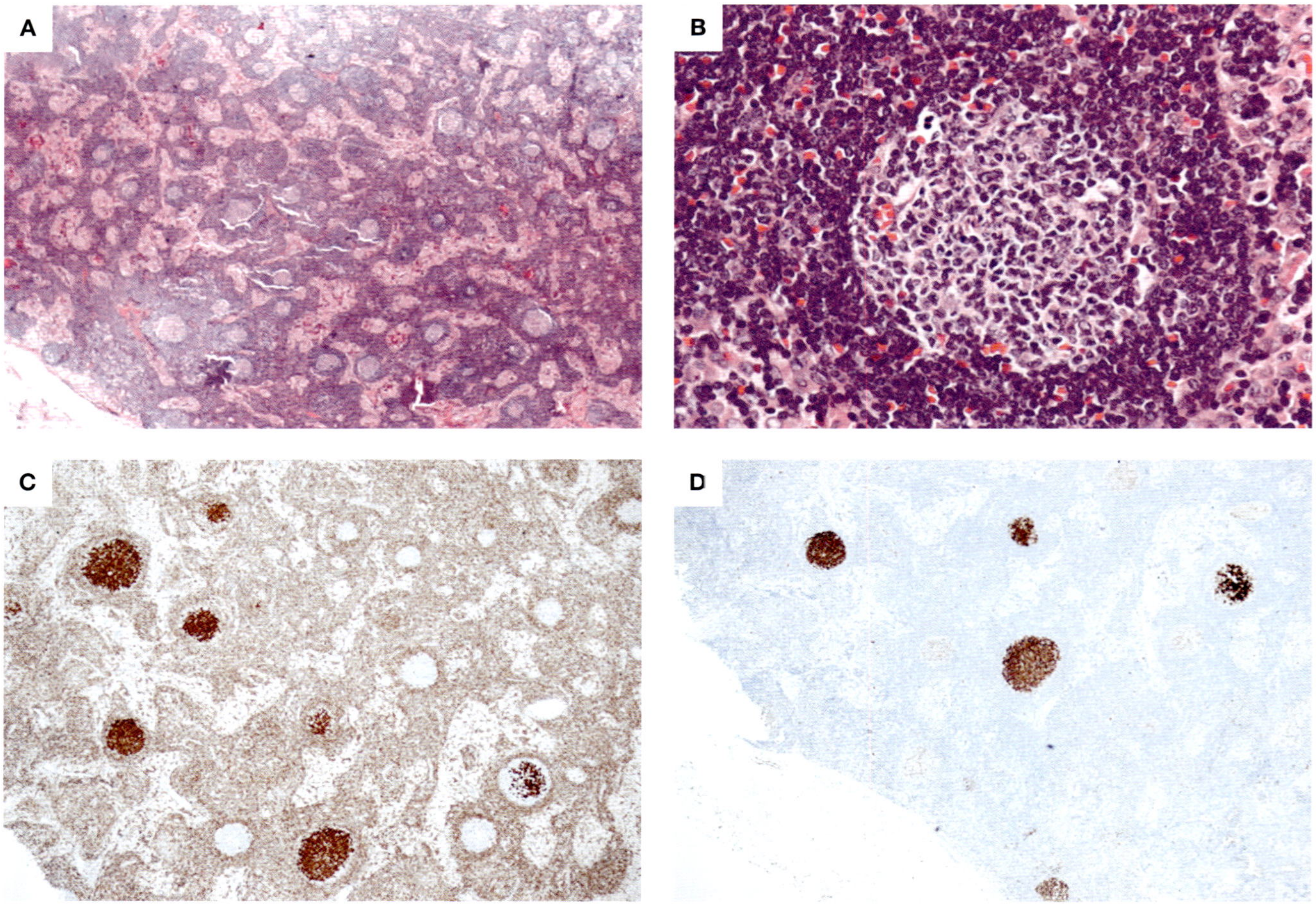

FIGURE 57.6 In situ follicular neoplasia. **A:** Lymph node biopsy shows preserved nodal architecture with reactive follicles and open sinuses. **B:** The follicle is small with a well-defined germinal center surrounded by an intact mantle zone. It contains mainly centrocytes. **C:** BCL2 stain highlights the few follicles, which are BCL2 positive. Note that the expression of BCL2 in the follicles is stronger than in reactive B and T cells. **D:** Neoplastic cells show increased expression of CD10 when compared with the residual normal germinal centers.

which often shows transmural infiltration with systemic spread and variation in cytological grade.

Synonyms

None.

General Clinical Features

DTFL has an indolent clinical course, often without therapy. Local recurrences can occur. There is a low progression to nodal disease. Clinical evaluation and staging are essential to exclude systemic FL secondarily involving the bowel, which follows a more aggressive course.

Epidemiology

DTFL accounts for 4% of all primary gastrointestinal lymphomas. The small intestine, especially duodenum, is most often involved, although stomach and colorectum may be affected. Most patients are middle aged, with an equal male-to-female ratio in most series.

Morphology

DTFL is characterized by a neoplastic follicular proliferation localized to the mucosa/submucosa and composed of mostly centrocytes, corresponding to grades 1 to 2 in the grading system for nodal FL (Figure 57.7).

Immunophenotype

The DTFL immunophenotype is similar to that of nodal FL. The cells are positive for CD10, CD20, BCL6, and BCL2. There is also frequent expression of IgA and alpha4 beta7 integrin, which is a mucosal homing receptor. FDCs demonstrated by CD21 or CD23 expression are characteristically restricted to the periphery of the follicles.[62] The proliferation rate is generally low.

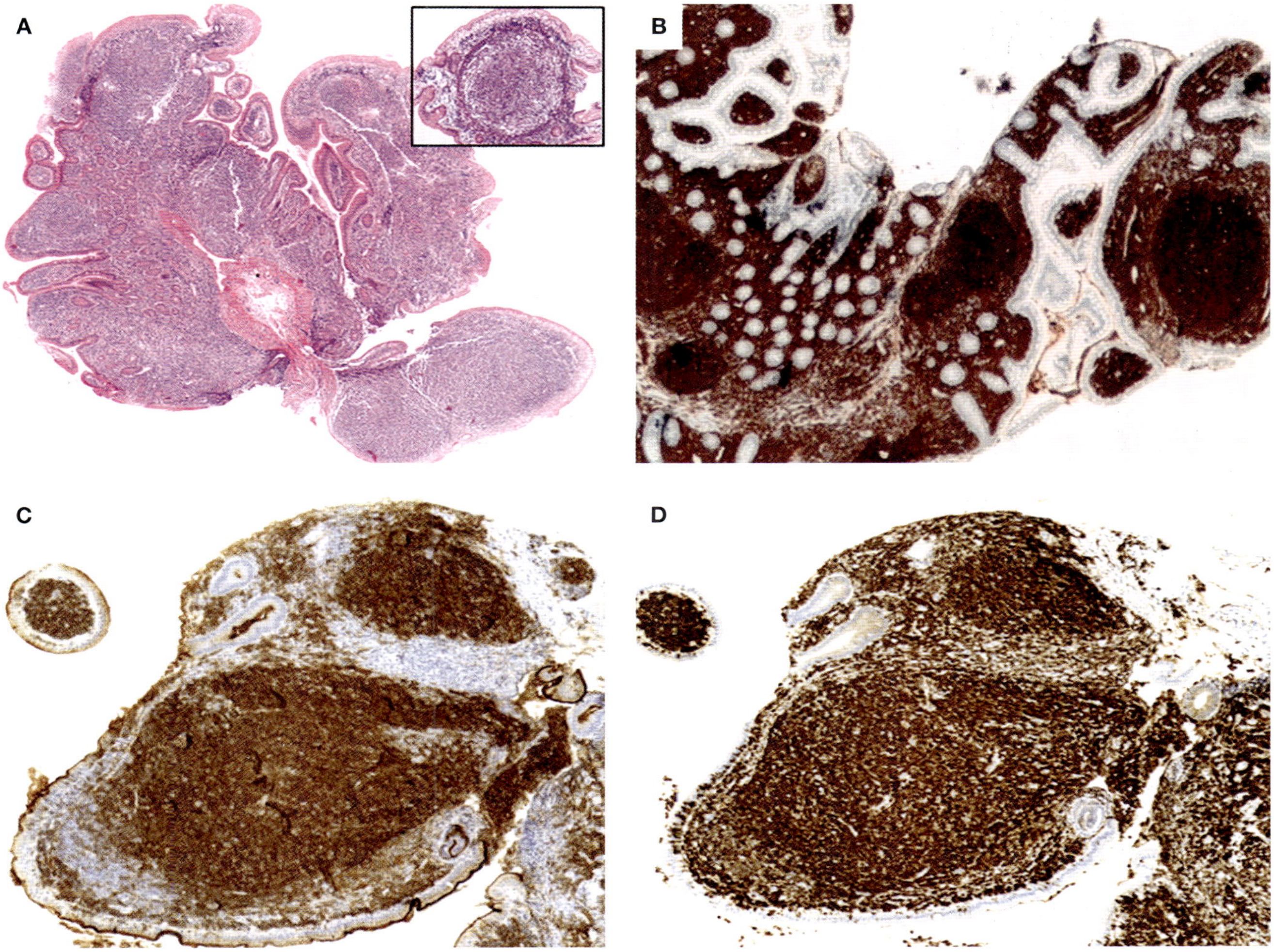

FIGURE 57.7 Duodenal-type follicular lymphoma. **A:** Duodenal polyp found incidentally in a patient undergoing screening endoscopy (inset: high magnification of atypical lymphoid follicle showing mostly centrocytes with lack of polarization). **B:** CD20 stain. **C:** Neoplastic cells express CD10. **D:** Neoplastic cells are BCL2 positive.

Genetics

Tumor cells carry the t(14;18) translocation and also mutations typically encountered in conventional FL such as *TNFRSF14* (or del 1p), *EZH2*, *KMT2D*, and *CREBBP*. The frequency of *KMT2D* mutations is lower than in conventional FL, as is its genetic complexity. DTFL is thought to derive from memory B cells and show evidence of SHM of the IGH gene. Restricted IGHV usage (VH4 and VH5) suggests similarities to mucosa-associated lymphoid tissue (MALT) lymphoma. Genomic expression profiling also suggest an overlap with MALT lymphoma, showing an enrichment for a chronic inflammation signature including overexpression of *MADCAM1* and *CCL20*, which recruits proinflammatory Th17^{+} cells.[63]

References

1. Campo E, Jaffe ES, Cook JR, et al. The international consensus classification of mature lymphoid neoplasms: a report from the Clinical Advisory Committee. *Blood.* 2022;140(11):1229-1253. doi:10.1182/blood.2022015851
2. Laurent C, Cook JR, Yoshino T, Quintanilla-Martinez L, Jaffe ES. Follicular lymphoma and marginal zone lymphoma: how many diseases? *Virchows Arch.* 2023;482(1):149-162. doi:10.1007/s00428-022-03432-2
3. Cerhan JR. Epidemiology of follicular lymphoma. *Hematol Oncol Clin North Am.* 2020;34(4):631-646. doi:10.1016/j.hoc.2020.02.001
4. Shirley MH, Sayeed S, Barnes I, Finlayson A, Ali R. Incidence of haematological malignancies by ethnic group in England, 2001-7. *Br J Haematol.* 2013;163(4):465-477. doi:10.1111/bjh.12562

5. Swerdlow S, Campo E, Harris NL, et al. World Health Organization (WHO) Classification of Tumours of Haematopoietic and Lymphoid Tissues. Revised 4th ed, Vol. 2. International Agency for Research on Cancer Press; 2017.
6. Luminari S, Biasoli I, Arcaini L, et al. The use of FDG-PET in the initial staging of 142 patients with follicular lymphoma: a retrospective study from the FOLL05 randomized trial of the Fondazione Italiana Linfomi. *Ann Oncol.* 2013;24(8):2108-2112. doi:10.1093/annonc/mdt137
7. Tychyj-Pinel C, Ricard F, Fulham M, et al. PET/CT assessment in follicular lymphoma using standardized criteria: central review in the PRIMA study. *Eur J Nucl Med Mol Imaging.* 2014;41(3):408-415. doi:10.1007/s00259-013-2441-8
8. Adams HJA, Nievelstein RAJ, Kwee TC. Systematic review on the additional value of 18F-Fluoro-2-Deoxy-D-Glucose positron emission tomography in staging follicular lymphoma. *J Comput Assist Tomogr.* 2017;41(1):98-103. doi:10.1097/RCT.0000000000000485
9. Trotman J, Fournier M, Lamy T, et al. Positron emission tomography-computed tomography (PET-CT) after induction therapy is highly predictive of patient outcome in follicular lymphoma: analysis of PET-CT in a subset of PRIMA trial participants. *J Clin Oncol.* 2011;29(23):3194-3200. doi:10.1200/JCO.2011.35.0736
10. Gradowski JF, Jaffe ES, Warnke RA, et al. Follicular lymphomas with plasmacytic differentiation include two subtypes. *Mod Pathol.* 2010;23(1):71-79. doi:10.1038/modpathol.2009.146
11. Harris J, Cherry D, Lazarchick J. Follicular lymphoma with PAS-positive amorphous material: report of two cases. *Ann Clin Lab Sci.* 2002;32(3):299-304.
12. Pina-Oviedo S, Miranda RN, Lin P, Manning JT, Medeiros LJ. Follicular lymphoma with hyaline-vascular Castleman-like features: analysis of 6 cases and review of the literature. *Hum Pathol.* 2017;68:136-146. doi:10.1016/j.humpath.2017.08.024
13. Laurent C, Adélaïde J, Guille A, et al. High-grade follicular lymphomas exhibit clinicopathologic, cytogenetic, and molecular diversity extending beyond grades 3A and 3B. *Am J Surg Pathol.* 2021;45(10):1324-1336. doi:10.1097/PAS.0000000000001726
14. Koch K, Hoster E, Ziepert M, et al. Clinical, pathological and genetic features of follicular lymphoma grade 3A: a joint analysis of the German low-grade and high-grade lymphoma study groups GLSG and DSHNHL. *Ann Oncol.* 2016;27(7):1323-1329. doi:10.1093/annonc/mdw185
15. Mustafa Ali M, Rybicki L, Nomani L, et al. Grade 3 follicular lymphoma: outcomes in the rituximab era. *Clin Lymphoma Myeloma Leuk.* 2017;17(12):797-803. doi:10.1016/j.clml.2017.07.002
16. Dreval K, Hilton LK, Cruz M, et al. Genetic subdivisions of follicular lymphoma defined by distinct coding and noncoding mutation patterns. *Blood.* 2023;142(6):561-573. doi:10.1182/blood.2022018719
17. Tarte K. Role of the microenvironment across histological subtypes of NHL. *Hematology Am Soc Hematol Educ Program.* 2017;2017(1):610-617. doi:10.1182/asheducation-2017.1.610
18. Laurent C, Müller S, Do C, et al. Distribution, function, and prognostic value of cytotoxic T lymphocytes in follicular lymphoma: a 3-D tissue-imaging study. *Blood.* 2011;118(20):5371-5379. doi:10.1182/blood-2011-04-345777
19. Gravelle P, Do C, Franchet C, et al. Impaired functional responses in follicular lymphoma CD8+TIM-3+ T lymphocytes following TCR engagement. *OncoImmunology.* 2016;5(10):e1224044. doi:10.1080/2162402X.2016.1224044
20. Amé-Thomas P, Tarte K. The yin and the yang of follicular lymphoma cell niches: role of microenvironment heterogeneity and plasticity. *Semin Cancer Biol.* 2014;24:23-32. doi:10.1016/j.semcancer.2013.08.001
21. Salaverria I, Weigert O, Quintanilla-Martinez L. The clinical and molecular taxonomy of t(14;18)-negative follicular lymphomas. *Blood Adv.* 2023;7(18):5258-5271. doi:10.1182/bloodadvances.2022009456
22. Adam P, Baumann R, Schmidt J, et al. The BCL2 E17 and SP66 antibodies discriminate 2 immunophenotypically and genetically distinct subgroups of conventionally BCL2-"negative" grade 1/2 follicular lymphomas. *Hum Pathol.* 2013;44(9):1817-1826. doi:10.1016/j.humpath.2013.02.004
23. Smit LA, Bende RJ, Aten J, Guikema JEJ, Aarts WM, van Noesel CJM. Expression of activation-induced cytidine deaminase is confined to B-cell non-Hodgkin's lymphomas of germinal-center phenotype. *Cancer Res.* 2003;63(14):3894-3898.
24. Scherer F, Navarrete MA, Bertinetti-Lapatki C, Boehm J, Schmitt-Graeff A, Veelken H. Isotype-switched follicular lymphoma displays dissociation between activation-induced cytidine deaminase expression and somatic hypermutation. *Leuk Lymphoma.* 2016;57(1):151-160. doi:10.3109/10428194.2015.1037758
25. Green MR, Alizadeh AA. Common progenitor cells in mature B-cell malignancies: implications for therapy. *Curr Opin Hematol.* 2014;21(4):333-340. doi:10.1097/MOH.0000000000000049
26. Zhu D, McCarthy H, Ottensmeier CH, Johnson P, Hamblin TJ, Stevenson FK. Acquisition of potential N-glycosylation sites in the immunoglobulin variable region by somatic mutation is a distinctive feature of follicular lymphoma. *Blood.* 2002;99(7):2562-2568. doi:10.1182/blood.v99.7.2562
27. Agopian J, Navarro JM, Gac AC, et al. Agricultural pesticide exposure and the molecular connection to lymphomagenesis. *J Exp Med.* 2009;206(7):1473-1483. doi:10.1084/jem.20082842

28. Roulland S, Kelly RS, Morgado E, et al. t(14;18) Translocation: a predictive blood biomarker for follicular lymphoma. *J Clin Oncol.* 2014;32(13):1347-1355. doi:10.1200/JCO.2013.52.8190
29. Nann D, Ramis-Zaldivar JE, Müller I, et al. Follicular lymphoma t(14;18)-negative is genetically a heterogeneous disease. *Blood Adv.* 2020;4(22):5652-5665. doi:10.1182/bloodadvances.2020002944
30. Los-de Vries GT, Stevens WBC, van Dijk E, et al. Genomic and microenvironmental landscape of stage I follicular lymphoma, compared with stage III/IV. *Blood Adv.* 2022;6(18):5482-5493. doi:10.1182/bloodadvances.2022008355
31. Leich E, Salaverria I, Bea S, et al. Follicular lymphomas with and without translocation t(14;18) differ in gene expression profiles and genetic alterations. *Blood.* 2009;114(4):826-834. doi:10.1182/blood-2009-01-198580
32. Qu X, Li H, Braziel RM, et al. Genomic alterations important for the prognosis in patients with follicular lymphoma treated in SWOG study S0016. *Blood.* 2019;133(1):81-93. doi:10.1182/blood-2018-07-865428
33. Pastore A, Jurinovic V, Kridel R, et al. Integration of gene mutations in risk prognostication for patients receiving first-line immunochemotherapy for follicular lymphoma: a retrospective analysis of a prospective clinical trial and validation in a population-based registry. *Lancet Oncol.* 2015;16(9):1111-1122. doi:10.1016/S1470-2045(15)00169-2
34. Araf S, Wang J, Korfi K, et al. Correction: genomic profiling reveals spatial intra-tumor heterogeneity in follicular lymphoma. *Leukemia.* 2019;33(6):1540. doi:10.1038/s41375-019-0425-9
35. Haebe S, Shree T, Sathe A, et al. Single-cell analysis can define distinct evolution of tumor sites in follicular lymphoma. *Blood.* 2021;137(21):2869-2880. doi:10.1182/blood.2020009855
36. Ott G, Katzenberger T, Lohr A, et al. Cytomorphologic, immunohistochemical, and cytogenetic profiles of follicular lymphoma: 2 types of follicular lymphoma grade 3. *Blood.* 2002;99(10):3806-3812. doi:10.1182/blood.v99.10.3806
37. Salaverria I, Siebert R. Follicular lymphoma grade 3B. *Best Pract Res Clin Haematol.* 2011;24(2):111-119. doi:10.1016/j.beha.2011.02.002
38. Bosga-Bouwer AG, van Imhoff GW, Boonstra R, et al. Follicular lymphoma grade 3B includes 3 cytogenetically defined subgroups with primary t(14;18), 3q27, or other translocations: t(14;18) and 3q27 are mutually exclusive. *Blood.* 2003;101(3):1149-1154. doi:10.1182/blood.V101.3.1149
39. Koch K, Richter J, Hanel C, Huttmann A, Duhrsen U, Klapper W. Follicular lymphoma grade 3B and diffuse large B-cell lymphoma present a histopathological and molecular continuum lacking features of progression/transformation. *Haematologica.* 2022;107(9):2144-2153. doi:10.3324/haematol.2021.279351
40. Piccaluga PP, Califano A, Klein U, et al. Gene expression analysis provides a potential rationale for revising the histological grading of follicular lymphomas. *Haematologica.* 2008;93(7):1033-1038. doi:10.3324/haematol.12754
41. Horn H, Kohler C, Witzig R, et al. Gene expression profiling reveals a close relationship between follicular lymphoma grade 3A and 3B, but distinct profiles of follicular lymphoma grade 1 and 2. *Haematologica.* 2018;103(7):1182-1190. doi:10.3324/haematol.2017.181024
42. Solal-Céligny P, Roy P, Colombat P, et al. Follicular lymphoma international prognostic index. *Blood.* 2004;104(5):1258-1265. doi:10.1182/blood-2003-12-4434
43. Batlevi CL, Sha F, Alperovich A, et al. Follicular lymphoma in the modern era: survival, treatment outcomes, and identification of high-risk subgroups. *Blood Cancer J.* 2020;10(7):74. doi:10.1038/s41408-020-00340-z
44. Freedman A, Jacobsen E. Follicular lymphoma: 2020 update on diagnosis and management. *Am J Hematol.* 2020;95(3):316-327. doi:10.1002/ajh.25696
45. Bachy E, Maurer MJ, Habermann TM, et al. A simplified scoring system in de novo follicular lymphoma treated initially with immunochemotherapy. *Blood.* 2018;132(1):49-58. doi:10.1182/blood-2017-11-816405
46. Huet S, Tesson B, Jais JP, et al. A gene-expression profiling score for prediction of outcome in patients with follicular lymphoma: a retrospective training and validation analysis in three international cohorts. *Lancet Oncol.* 2018;19(4):549-561. doi:10.1016/S1470-2045(18)30102-5
47. Bolen CR, Mattiello F, Herold M, et al. Treatment dependence of prognostic gene expression signatures in de novo follicular lymphoma. *Blood.* 2021;137(19):2704-2707. doi:10.1182/blood.2020008119
48. Tsukamoto T, Tokuda Y, Nakano M, Tashiro K, Kuroda J. Expression of activated B-cell gene signature is predictive of the outcome of follicular lymphoma. *Blood Adv.* 2022;6(6):1932-1936. doi:10.1182/bloodadvances.2021005876
49. Bolen CR, McCord R, Huet S, et al. Mutation load and an effector T-cell gene signature may distinguish immunologically distinct and clinically relevant lymphoma subsets. *Blood Adv.* 2017;1(22):1884-1890. doi:10.1182/bloodadvances.2016000786
50. Xerri L, Huet S, Venstrom JM, et al. Rituximab treatment circumvents the prognostic impact of tumor-infiltrating T-cells in follicular lymphoma patients. *Hum Pathol.* 2017;64:128-136. doi:10.1016/j.humpath.2017.03.023
51. Tobin JWD, Keane C, Gunawardana J, et al. Progression of disease within 24 Months in follicular lymphoma is associated with reduced intratumoral immune infiltration. *J Clin Oncol.* 2019;37(34):3300-3309. doi:10.1200/JCO.18.02365

52. Link BK, Maurer MJ, Nowakowski GS, et al. Rates and outcomes of follicular lymphoma transformation in the immunochemotherapy era: a report from the University of Iowa/MayoClinic Specialized Program of Research Excellence molecular epidemiology resource. *J Clin Oncol.* 2013;31(26):3272-3278. doi:10.1200/JCO.2012.48.3990

53. Federico M, Caballero Barrigón MD, Marcheselli L, et al. Rituximab and the risk of transformation of follicular lymphoma: a retrospective pooled analysis. *Lancet Haematol.* 2018;5(8):e359-e367. doi:10.1016/S2352-3026(18)30090-5

54. Kridel R, Mottok A, Farinha P, et al. Cell of origin of transformed follicular lymphoma. *Blood.* 2015;126(18):2118-2127. doi:10.1182/blood-2015-06-649905

55. Pasqualucci L, Khiabanian H, Fangazio M, et al. Genetics of follicular lymphoma transformation. *Cell Rep.* 2014;6(1):130-140. doi:10.1016/j.celrep.2013.12.027

56. Kridel R, Chan FC, Mottok A, et al. Histological transformation and progression in follicular lymphoma: a clonal evolution study. *PLoS Med.* 2016;13(12):e1002197. doi:10.1371/journal.pmed.1002197

57. Jegalian AG, Eberle FC, Pack SD, et al. Follicular lymphoma in situ: clinical implications and comparisons with partial involvement by follicular lymphoma. *Blood.* 2011;118(11):2976-2984. doi:10.1182/blood-2011-05-355255

58. Schmidt J, Ramis-Zaldivar JE, Bonzheim I, et al. CREBBP gene mutations are frequently detected in in situ follicular neoplasia. *Blood.* 2018;132(25):2687-2690. doi:10.1182/blood-2018-03-837039

59. Schmidt J, Salaverria I, Haake A, et al. Increasing genomic and epigenomic complexity in the clonal evolution from in situ to manifest t(14;18)-positive follicular lymphoma. *Leukemia.* 2014;28(5):1103-1112. doi:10.1038/leu.2013.307

60. Schroers-Martin JG, Soo J, Brisou G, et al. Tracing founder mutations in circulating and tissue-resident follicular lymphoma precursors. *Cancer Discov.* 2023;13(6):1310-1323. doi:10.1158/2159-8290.CD-23-0111

61. Vogelsberg A, Steinhilber J, Mankel B, et al. Genetic evolution of in situ follicular neoplasia to aggressive B-cell lymphoma of germinal center subtype. *Haematologica.* 2021;106(10):2673-2681. doi:10.3324/haematol.2020.254854

62. Takata K, Sato Y, Nakamura N, et al. Duodenal follicular lymphoma lacks AID but expresses BACH2 and has memory B-cell characteristics. *Mod Pathol.* 2013;26(1):22-31. doi:10.1038/modpathol.2012.127

63. Hellmuth JC, Louissaint A, Szczepanowski M, et al. Duodenal-type and nodal follicular lymphomas differ by their immune microenvironment rather than their mutation profiles. *Blood.* 2018;132(16):1695-1702. doi:10.1182/blood-2018-03-837252

Chapter 58

BCL2-Rearrangement Negative, CD23-Positive Follicle Center Lymphoma

Leticia Quintanilla-Martinez, Itziar Salaverria, and Oliver Weigert

Definition

BCL2-rearrangement-negative, CD23-positive follicle center lymphoma (*BCL2*-R-, CD23^{+} FCL) is an uncommon nodal follicular lymphoma that occurs primarily in adults with stage I/II disease. It is considered a provisional entity. The terminology of "follicle center lymphoma" is employed to emphasize the parallelism to primary cutaneous FCL, in which a predominantly diffuse growth pattern is observed despite the follicle center derivation of the tumor cells. By definition, *BCL2* translocations are absent and the neoplastic cells are CD23 positive. This entity is characterized by recurrent *STAT6* and/or *SOCS1* mutations. *BCL2*-R negative follicular lymphoma (FL) without CD23 expression should not be included in this category.

Synonyms

Predominantly diffuse follicular lymphoma.
BCL2-negative nodal follicular lymphoma (not recommended).

Epidemiology

BCL2-R-, CD23^{-} FCL accounts for approximately 8% to 10% of all nodal FLs grade 1-3A in adults and approximately 65% of the nodal *BCL2*-R-negative FL.[1,2] The disease has a female predominance (male-to-female ratio, 1:2).[2-6]

General Clinical Features

Patients present frequently with localized but often clinically impressive lymphadenopathy (median size 5 cm). Most patients present in Ann Arbor clinical stage I/II and no B symptoms.[2,4,7] Inguinal lymph nodes are the most common site of involvement (40%-83%), but other regions can also be involved such as axillary lymph nodes (9%-24%), head and neck (9%-15%), and other regions (1%-20%).[2,4]

Morphology

Most cases have a predominantly diffuse (Figure 58.1) or vaguely nodular growth pattern characterized by >75% diffuse growth with microfollicle formation, which represents abnormal follicles predominantly composed of centrocytes lacking follicular dendritic cell (FDC) meshworks as demonstrated with CD21/CD23 stains (Figure 58.2). Some cases have a follicular and diffuse growth pattern (25%-75% diffuse).[4-6] Residual lymphoid follicles with reactive-appearing germinal centers and preserved mantle zones are often observed either intermingled or in the periphery of the lymph node (Figure 58.1). Around 35% of the cases have a follicular pattern (ie, <25% diffuse), with closely packed follicles and attenuated or absent mantle zones indistinguishable from conventional t(14;18)-positive FL (Figure 58.3).[2] Other notable features include frequent sclerosis and interstitial fibrosis. Cases with inguinal presentation have higher frequency of diffuse growth pattern. The diagnosis of *BCL2*-R-, *CD23*$^{+}$ FCL should be made with caution in core needle biopsies.

Cytologically, most cases are composed of centrocyte-like cells characterized by small to medium-sized cells with angulated or cleaved nuclei, mature chromatin, and scant cytoplasm. Intermingled scattered large cells with oval nuclei, open chromatin, several nucleoli, and abundant basophilic cytoplasm characteristic of centroblasts are observed (Figure 58.2). Although the majority of the cases are classified as grade 1 to 2, some cases, mostly with pure follicular pattern might show grade 3A cytology.[2]

Immunophenotype

The lymphoma cells show a mature B-cell phenotype with positivity for B-cell markers (CD20, CD19, CD22, CD79a, PAX5) and express at least one germinal center marker (CD10, BCL6, LMO2, HGAL).[3] BCL2 is mostly negative, but some cases with weak expression are reported (Figure 58.3F).[4,6,9] FDC meshworks are absent

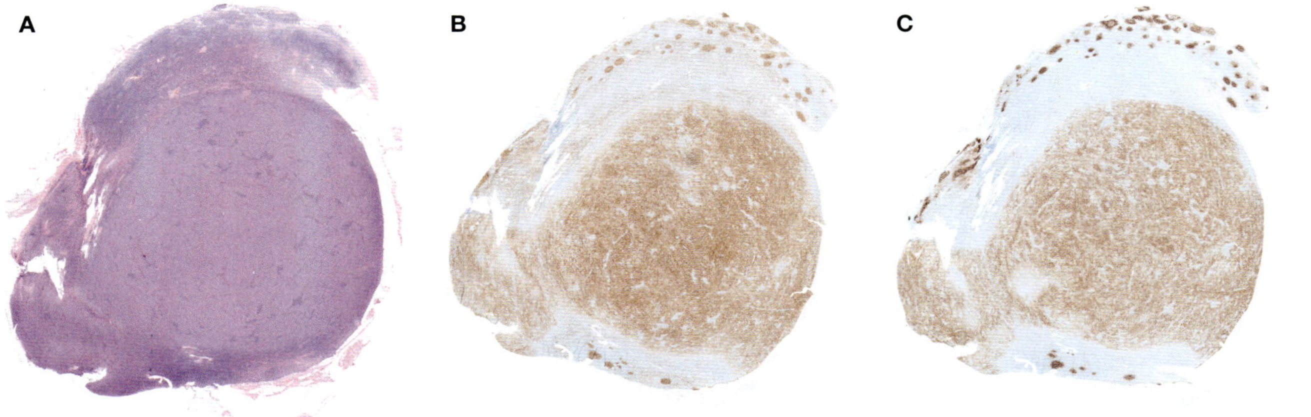

FIGURE 58.1 *BCL2*-R-, CD23⁺ follicle center lymphoma. Diffuse growth pattern. **A:** Hematoxylin and eosin stain of an inguinal lymph node with partial involvement of a diffuse lymphoid infiltrate that leaves a rim of normal lymph node in the periphery. The tumor is composed mainly of centrocyte-like cells. **B:** The tumor cells are strongly positive for CD10. Note that the residual normal germinal centers in the periphery of the lymph node are CD10 positive. **C:** The tumor cells are CD23 positive. In the residual normal germinal centers CD23 highlights the follicular dendritic cell meshworks. In this case *STAT6* and a *SOCS1* mutations were identified. (Modified from Salaverria I, Weigert O, Quintanilla-Martinez L. The clinical and molecular taxonomy of t(14;18)-negative follicular lymphomas. *Blood Adv*. 2023;7(18):5258-5271.)

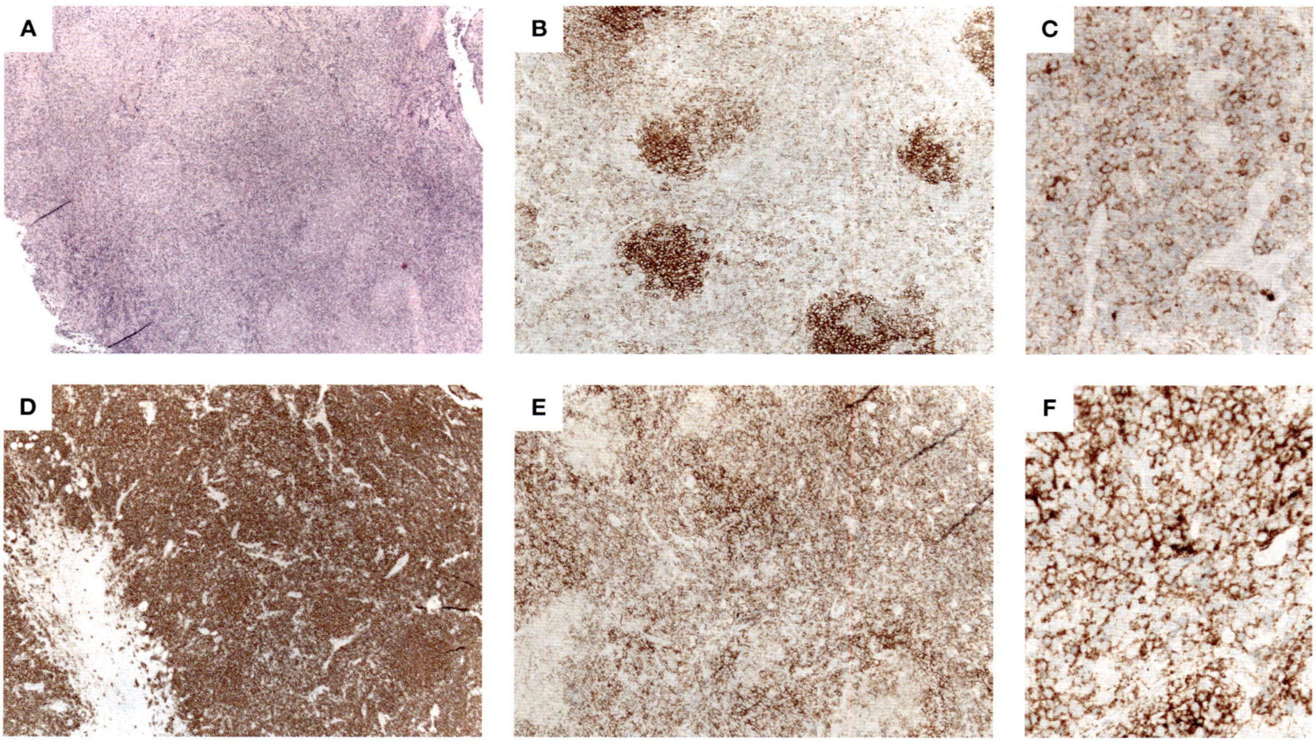

FIGURE 58.2 *BCL2*-R-, CD23+ follicle center lymphoma. Diffuse growth pattern with microfollicles. **A:** Hematoxylin and eosin stain of an inguinal lymph node showing infiltration by a vaguely nodular infiltrate. The follicles lack a mantle zone, and the interfollicular area is expanded. **B:** CD10 stain highlights the presence of the small follicles so-called microfollicles. Note that the interfollicular component is also positive for CD10. **C:** Higher magnification to demonstrate the CD10 positivity in the interfollicular component. **D:** CD20 stain demonstrates that both the follicular and the interfollicular components are CD20 positive. **E:** CD23 is positive in the interfollicular component but negative in the small follicles. Note that the follicles lack follicular dendritic cells. **F:** Higher magnification shows the CD23 positivity in the tumor cells. In this case several gene mutations were identified targeting *STAT6, TNFRSF14* (2x), *FOXO1, EP300,* and *HIST1H1B*.

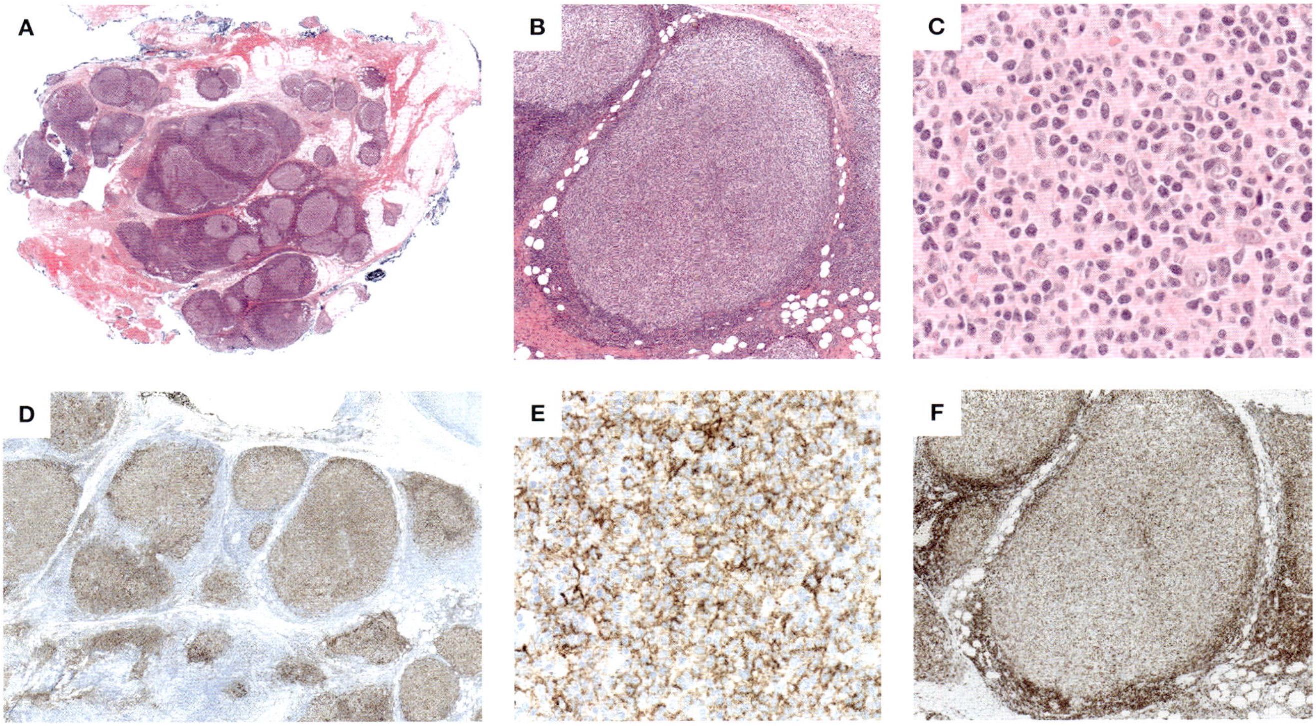

FIGURE 58.3 *BCL2*-R-, CD23+ follicle center lymphoma. Follicular growth pattern. **A:** Hematoxylin and eosin stain of a lesion demonstrating a follicular infiltrate in a lymph node that extended into the fat and soft tissue. The lymphoma is composed of follicles and lacks mantle zones. **B:** Higher magnification of one of the follicles shows lack of polarization with a monotonous cellular composition. **C:** Higher magnification view shows that the follicles are composed of small-sized centrocytes with irregular nuclei, without nucleoli, and with scant cytoplasm. Intermingled follicular dendritic cells and few centroblasts are present. **D:** CD23 stain reveals that the follicles are positive, whereas the interfollicular areas are negative. Note that in the periphery of the follicles some follicular dendritic cells are strongly positive. **E:** Higher magnification shows that the tumor cells are CD23 positive. **F:** In this case the tumor cells were weak BCL2 positive despite the absence of *BCL2* rearrangement. In contrast, the reactive T cells surrounding the follicles are strong BCL2 positive. In this case *STAT6* and a *CREBBP* mutations were identified.

in the diffuse areas and sparse or absent in the so-called microfollicles (Figure 58.2). In contrast, FDCs are readily demonstrated in the cases with follicular growth pattern. By definition the tumor cells express CD23 (Figures 58.1-58.3). The Ki-67 proliferation index ranges from 10% to 70% with a slight accentuation in the atypical follicles.[3,4,10]

Genetics

Immunoglobulin genes are clonally rearranged. The cases lack *BCL2* and *MYC* rearrangements; however, in rare cases *BCL6* rearrangements can be detected.[2] The characteristic genetic finding, although not exclusive to this entity, is the presence of activating *STAT6* gene mutations targeting the DNA-binding domain (Figure 58.4). *STAT6* mutations are found in 85% to 100% of the cases and co-occur with *CREBBP* missense mutations identified in the HAT-KAT domain, typical of FL, and/or *TNFRSF14* mutations.[2,6-9,11,12] *STAT6* mutations show a strong positive correlation with CD23 expression, which is therefore a good surrogate marker in routine diagnosis.[2] *STAT6* activating mutations enhance interleukin 4 (IL-4)/STAT6 target gene expression including *FCER2* (CD23), *CCL17,* and *CCL22.*[13] A minority of cases without *STAT6* mutations carry *SOCS1* mutations, which are upstream of STAT6 contributing to STAT6 activation and upregulation of CD23. *SOCS1* mutations may be identified alone or together with *STAT6* mutations. Mutations in *EZH2, KMT2D,* and another chromatin modifier genes, which are highly recurrent in conventional FL, are rare. Copy number (CN) profiles are similar between t(14;18)-positive and negative cases.[2] The most recurrently gained regions are 1q21-qter, 2p25-p15, 2q22-q36, 8q, 9q21-qter, 11p, 12p, and 12q. Recurrent regions of loss are observed at 1p36/*TNFRSF14* and 6q21/*TNFAIP3*. CN neutral loss of heterozygosity are mostly detected in 1p36/*TNFRSF14*, 16p13-p12/*CREBBP,* and 6p25-p21.[2] Of note, 1p36 losses, originally reported in 93% of cases

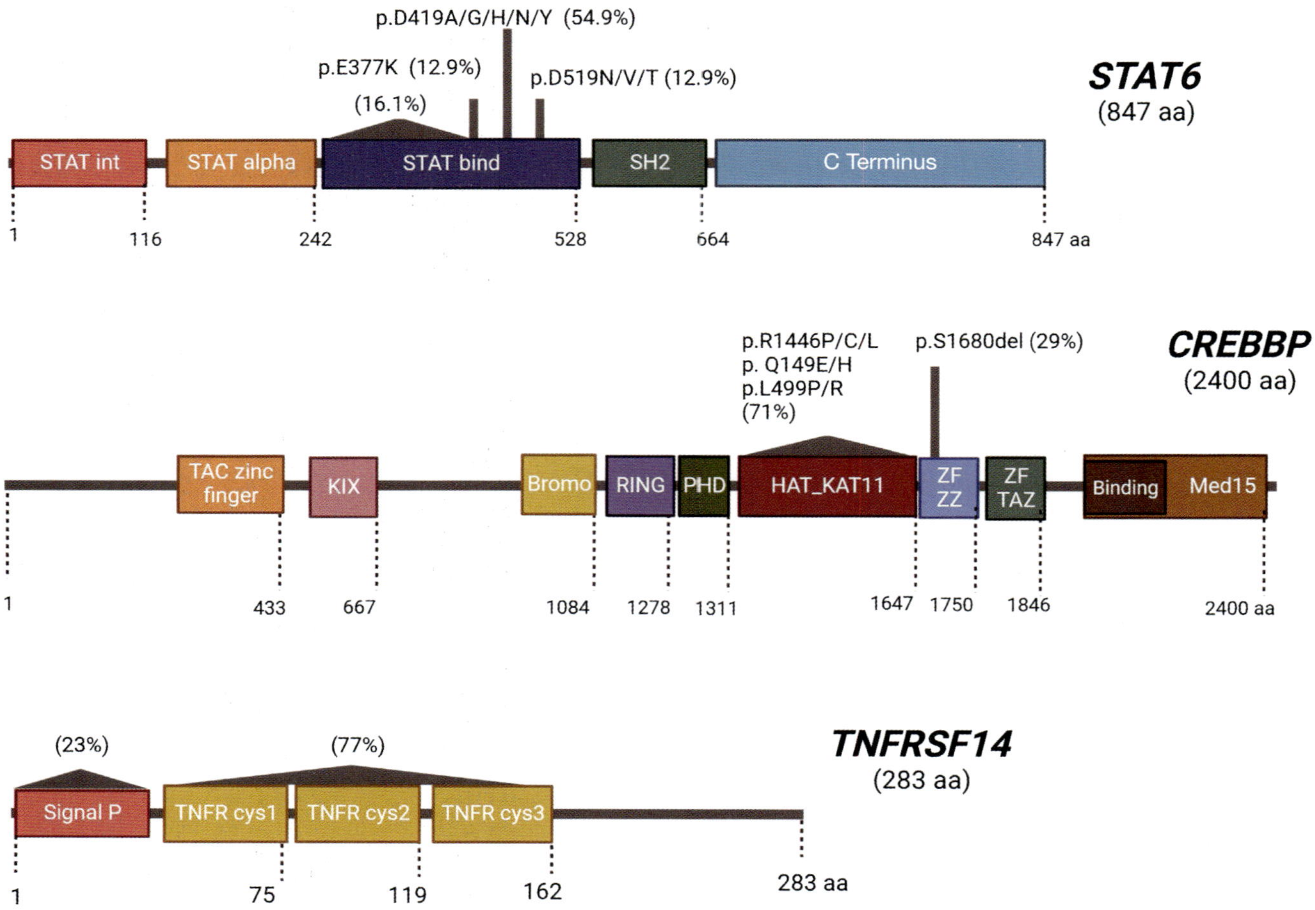

FIGURE 58.4 Mutational landscape of *BCL2*-R-, CD23+ follicle center lymphoma. A diagram of the relative positions of driver mutations is depicted for *STAT6, CREBBP,* and *TNFRSF14*. *STAT6* mutations target the DNA domain with three hot spots. Mutations in *CREBBP* are mainly identified in the HAT-KAT domain and a hot spot in p.S1680del. Mutations in *TNFRSF14* are identified mainly in the first three exons. (Data from Nann D, Ramis-Zaldivar JE, Muller I, et al. Follicular lymphoma t(14;18)-negative is genetically a heterogeneous disease. *Blood Adv*. 2020;4(22):5652-5665.)

and suggested to be the genetic hallmark of the disease, have been shown to occur in 20% to 30% of cases in subsequent studies.[2,4-6] Gene expression and microRNA profiles in t(14;18)-negative FL resemble a late germinal center B cell that has not yet exited the germinal center stage of differentiation.[1,14]

Prognosis and Clinical Comment

Since the majority of patients present with localized disease, the most commonly used treatment regimens are radiation-based therapies with very high rates of complete remission (>90%) and low rates of recurrence and/or progression reported after initial therapy. However, the available data are still limited and based on relatively small and retrospective studies that used different inclusion criteria.[2,4,5,10] Transformation to a high-grade lymphoma has not yet been documented.

References

1. Leich E, Salaverria I, Bea S, et al. Follicular lymphomas with and without translocation t(14;18) differ in gene expression profiles and genetic alterations. *Blood*. 2009;114(4):826-834.
2. Nann D, Ramis-Zaldivar JE, Muller I, et al. Follicular lymphoma t(14;18)-negative is genetically a heterogeneous disease. *Blood Adv*. 2020;4(22):5652-5665.
3. Adam P, Baumann R, Schmidt J, et al. The BCL2 E17 and SP66 antibodies discriminate 2 immunophenotypically and genetically distinct subgroups of conventionally BCL2-"negative" grade 1/2 follicular lymphomas. *Hum Pathol*. 2013;44(9):1817-1826.
4. Katzenberger T, Kalla J, Leich E, et al. A distinctive subtype of t(14;18)-negative nodal follicular non-Hodgkin lymphoma characterized by a predominantly diffuse growth pattern and deletions in the chromosomal region 1p36. *Blood*. 2009;113(5):1053-1061.

5. Siddiqi IN, Friedman J, Barry-Holson KQ, et al. Characterization of a variant of t(14;18) negative nodal diffuse follicular lymphoma with CD23 expression, 1p36/TNFRSF14 abnormalities, and STAT6 mutations. *Mod Pathol.* 2016;29(6):570-581.
6. Xian RR, Xie Y, Haley LM, et al. CREBBP and STAT6 co-mutation and 16p13 and 1p36 loss define the t(14;18)-negative diffuse variant of follicular lymphoma. *Blood Cancer J.* 2020;10(6):69.
7. Los-de Vries GT, Stevens WBC, van Dijk E, et al. Genomic and microenvironmental landscape of stage I follicular lymphoma, compared with stage III/IV. *Blood Adv.* 2022;6(18):5482-5493.
8. Salaverria I, Weigert O, Quintanilla-Martinez L. The clinical and molecular taxonomy of t(14;18)-negative follicular lymphomas. *Blood Adv.* 2023;7(18):5258-5271.
9. Zamo A, Pischimarov J, Horn H, Ott G, Rosenwald A, Leich E. The exomic landscape of t(14;18)-negative diffuse follicular lymphoma with 1p36 deletion. *Br J Haematol.* 2018;180(3):391-394.
10. Leich E, Hoster E, Wartenberg M, et al. Similar clinical features in follicular lymphomas with and without breaks in the BCL2 locus. *Leukemia.* 2016;30(4):854-860.
11. Yildiz M, Li H, Bernard D, et al. Activating STAT6 mutations in follicular lymphoma. *Blood.* 2015;125(4):668-679.
12. Crouch S, Painter D, Barrans SL, et al. Molecular subclusters of follicular lymphoma: a report from the United Kingdom's Haematological Malignancy Research Network. *Blood Adv.* 2022;6(21):5716-5731.
13. Mentz M, Keay W, Strobl CD, et al. PARP14 is a novel target in STAT6 mutant follicular lymphoma. *Leukemia.* 2022;36(9):2281-2292.
14. Leich E, Zamo A, Horn H, et al. MicroRNA profiles of t(14;18)-negative follicular lymphoma support a late germinal center B-cell phenotype. *Blood.* 2011;118(20):5550-5558.

Chapter 59

Primary Cutaneous Follicle Center Lymphoma

John R. Goodlad, and Steven T. Rosen

Definition

Primary cutaneous follicle center lymphoma (PCFCL) is a neoplasm of germinal center cells confined to the skin at presentation. In all cases, small and large cells resembling centrocytes constitute the predominant cell type. Centroblasts may also be present but should be in a minority. Unlike follicular lymphoma of the usual type, a follicular architecture is not a prerequisite for diagnosis: PCFCL may have a follicular, follicular and diffuse, or purely diffuse growth pattern. Nevertheless, lymphomas with a diffuse growth pattern composed entirely of immunoblast- or centroblast-like cells are excluded from this category, most of these fulfilling criteria for primary cutaneous diffuse large B-cell lymphoma, leg type, irrespective of site.

Synonyms

Primary cutaneous follicle center cell lymphoma.[1]
Reticulohistiocytoma of the dorsum (not recommended)
Crosti lymphoma (not recommended).

Epidemiology

PCFCL accounts for just less than 60% all primary cutaneous B-cell lymphomas in larger series.[2,3] Middle-aged adults are most commonly affected with a male:female ratio of approximately 1.5:1.[2,3]

General Clinical Features

Approximately 80% of patients present with localized lesions, most frequently on the head and neck, especially the scalp (Figure 59.1) and trunk. Presentation at other sites, including legs, is less commonly encountered. Up to 15% have multifocal lesions at the outset.[2,3] Individual lesions typically manifest as firm erythematous plaques, nodules, or tumors. Tumors may be surrounded by erythematous papules and/or figurate plaques. Disease should be restricted to cutaneous sites at presentation in order to qualify as PCFCL.

Morphology

The neoplastic cells in PCFCL comprise a majority of centrocytes with centroblasts few in number and always in the minority.[1] Centrocytes have angulate, twisted, or cleaved nuclei with inconspicuous nucleoli and scant cytoplasm. They may be small, intermediate, or large in size. Centroblasts have round or oval nuclei with vesicular chromatin, one to three nucleoli, and a narrow rim of cytoplasm.

The growth pattern may be follicular, follicular and diffuse, or entirely diffuse (Figure 59.2A and B). Low-power examination often reveals a variably dense, nodular perivascular and periadnexal infiltrate within the dermis, sometimes extending into subcutaneous fat but sparing the epidermis. Follicles are often present when this pattern of growth is seen (Figure 59.2A). They tend to be ill-defined with poorly formed or absent mantles, few if any tingible body macrophages, and no polarization, giving rise to a relatively monotonous appearance. Centrocytes predominate within follicles, but histological grading is not relevant in PCFCL.[4] Centrocytes also predominate in diffuse lesions where they tend to be of large size; variable numbers may possess multilobated nuclei[1] (Figure 59.2C). In rare cases, the centrocytes show a spindled morphology in part or whole[5] (Figure 59.3).

Immunophenotype

The neoplastic B cells express B-cell markers (CD20, CD79a, PAX5) and BCL6. Expression of CD10 is variable but most frequently seen when there is a prominent follicular growth pattern.[6] Other antigens associated with germinal center differentiation, such as stathmin, MEF2B, LMO2, and HGAL, are almost always expressed, even when CD10 is absent.[7-9]

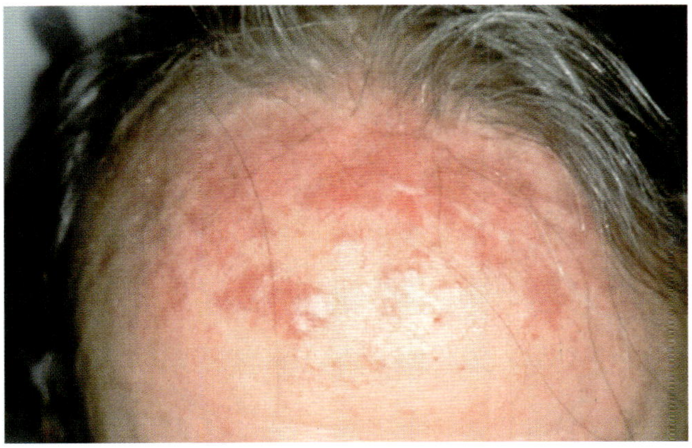

FIGURE 59.1 Classic clinical presentation of primary cutaneous follicle center lymphoma on the scalp.

A variable incidence of BCL2 expression has also been reported, ranging from 0 to >60%. In practice, while some cases are entirely negative, BCL2 is often expressed but weakly compared with the surrounding T cells and often only in a proportion of the neoplastic cells[6,8] (Figure 59.4A-C). Strong expression of BCL2 is rarely seen and usually only in cases with follicular architecture (Figure 59.4D). False-negative immunohistochemical staining for BCL2 protein due to BCL2 mutation does not appear to contribute to the low rate of detection, since mutation of BCL2 is virtually absent in PCFCL and since cases negative with the BCL2 124 clone are also negative with the E17 antibody.[7,8] Rare cases express CD23 and CD30 but staining for CD5, IRF4/MUM1, and Cyclin D1 is usually negative.

Genetics

The molecular landscape of PCFCL lymphoma shows some similarities and also distinct differences to that of nodal FL, reinforcing its recognition as a distinct but related entity. In PCFCL, immunoglobulin genes are clonally rearranged and somatically hypermutated. The reported incidence of *BCL2* rearrangements is variable, ranging from 0% to 41%, but likely it is present in around 10% of cases.[8,10,11] Occasional cases harbor *BCL6* rearrangements.[9,12] Deletions of 1p36/*TNFRSF14* are frequent in PCFCL and usually occur in the absence of *BCL2* rearrangement. Conversely, loss of 1p36 is also common in nodal follicular lymphoma but is typically concurrent with BCL2 rearrangement.[7-9] Mutations of *TNFRSF14* are encountered at similar frequency in PCFCL and *BCL2*-rearranged systemic FL (30%-40%). However, mutations in the chromatin modifiers, *CREBBP* (25%), *KMT2D* (21%), and *EZH2* (0%-6%), as well as *BCL2* (0%), are much less frequent in PCFCL, while *TNFAIP3* mutations (25%) are more common.[7,12] Despite a virtual absence of *EZH2* mutations involving common hotspots, the majority of PCFCL show high levels of *EZH2* expression.[10] The gene expression profile of PCFCL is similar to that of diffuse large B-cell lymphoma of germinal center type.[13,14] Amplification of *REL* is common, but in contrast to diffuse large B-cell lymphoma, leg type, deletions of *CDKN2A* and *CDKN2B* are rare.

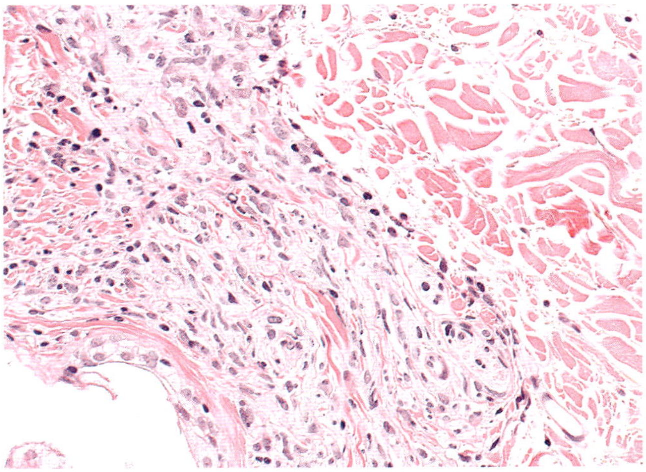

FIGURE 59.3 A case of primary cutaneous follicle center lymphoma exhibiting spindle cell morphology.

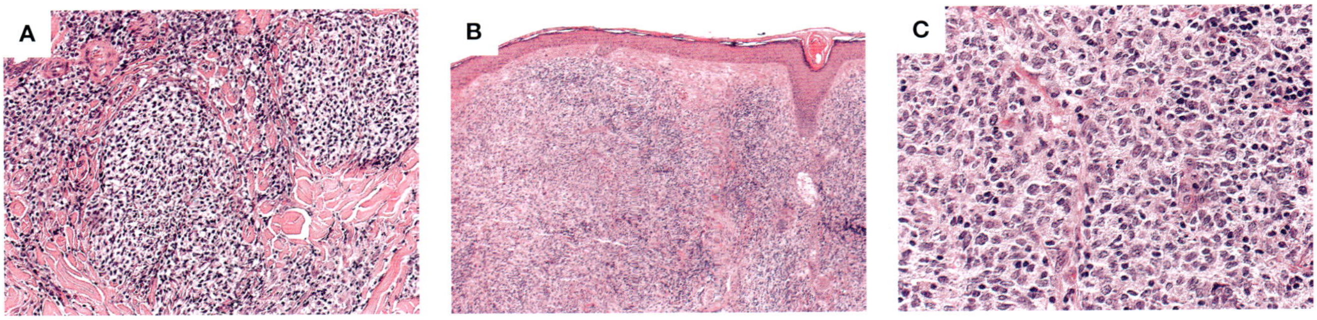

FIGURE 59.2 Primary cutaneous follicle center lymphoma shows varied with follicular, follicular and diffuse, or purely diffuse patterns recognized. **A:** Predominantly follicular. **B:** Predominantly diffuse **C:** All cases contain a predominance of centrocytes, even when the neoplastic lymphocytes are large and growing in diffuse sheets.

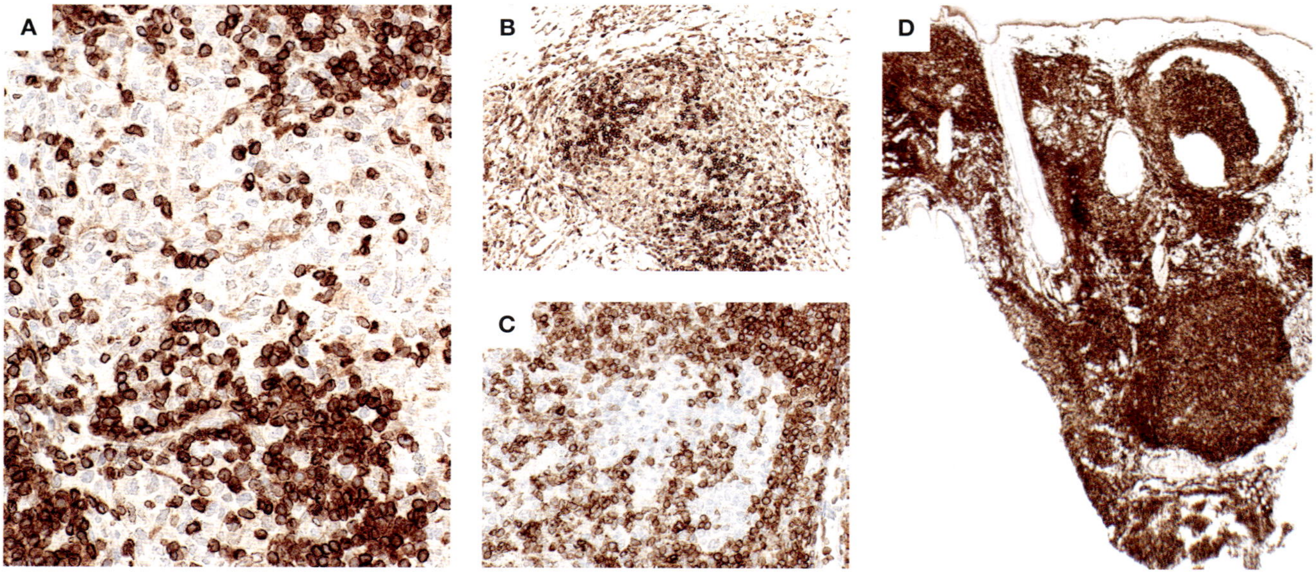

FIGURE 59.4 Patterns of BCL2 staining in primary cutaneous follicle center lymphoma. **A:** In the majority of cases there is a mixture of BCL2 negative and weakly positive cells. **B:** Some cases show weak uniform expression of BCL2 when compared with surrounding reactive T cells. **C:** BCL2 may be entirely negative. **D:** In rare cases there is overexpression of BCL2.

Prognosis and Clinical Comment

For solitary or localized lesions, the recommended treatment is radiotherapy and/or excision. Intralesional steroid injections can be considered for multiple scattered small nodules, with systemic therapies similar to those employed for nodal follicular lymphoma reserved for progressive, more advanced disease.[15] Complete remission is the norm after primary treatment, and although cutaneous relapse is not uncommon (~30%), extracutaneous spread is relatively rare (10%).[2,3] Outcome is usually very favorable with quoted 5-year overall and disease-specific survivals of 87% and 95% quoted.[2]

References

1. Willemze R, Kerl H, Sterry W, et al. EORTC classification for primary cutaneous lymphomas: a proposal from the cutaneous lymphoma study Group of the European Organization for Research and treatment of Cancer. *Blood*. 1997;90(1):354-371.
2. Senff NJ, Hoefnagel JJ, Jansen PM, et al. Reclassification of 300 primary cutaneous B-Cell lymphomas according to the new WHO-EORTC classification for cutaneous lymphomas: comparison with previous classifications and identification of prognostic markers. *J Clin Oncol*. 2007;25(12):1581-1587.
3. Zinzani PL, Quaglino P, Pimpinelli N, et al. Prognostic factors in primary cutaneous B-cell lymphoma: the Italian Study Group for cutaneous lymphomas. *J Clin Oncol*. 2006;24(9):1376-1382.
4. Cerroni L, Arzberger E, Pütz B, et al. Primary cutaneous follicle center cell lymphoma with follicular growth pattern. *Blood*. 2000;95(12):3922-3928.
5. Charli-Joseph Y, Cerroni L, LeBoit PE. Cutaneous spindle-cell B-cell lymphomas: most are neoplasms of follicular center cell origin. *Am J Surg Pathol*. 2015;39(6):737-743.
6. Goodlad JR, Krajewski AS, Batstone PJ, et al. Primary cutaneous follicular lymphoma: a clinicopathologic and molecular study of 16 cases in support of a distinct entity. *Am J Surg Pathol*. 2002;26(6):733-741.
7. Barasch NJK, Liu YC, Ho J, et al. The molecular landscape and other distinctive features of primary cutaneous follicle center lymphoma. *Hum Pathol*. 2020;106:93-105.
8. Szablewski V, Ingen-Housz-Oro S, Baia M, Delfau-Larue MH, Copie-Bergman C, Ortonne N. Primary cutaneous follicle center lymphomas expressing BCL2 protein frequently harbor BCL2 gene break and may present 1p36 deletion: a study of 20 cases. *Am J Surg Pathol*. 2016;40(1):127-136.
9. Verdanet E, Dereure O, René C, et al. Diagnostic value of STMN1, LMO2, HGAL, AID expression and 1p36 chromosomal abnormalities in primary cutaneous B cell lymphomas. *Histopathology*. 2017;71(4):648-660.
10. Gángó A, Bátai B, Varga M, et al. Concomitant 1p36 deletion and TNFRSF14 mutations in primary cutaneous follicle center lymphoma frequently expressing high levels of EZH2 protein. *Virchows Arch*. 2018;473(4):453-462.
11. Pham-Ledard A, Cowppli-Bony A, Doussau A, et al. Diagnostic and prognostic value of BCL2 rearrangement in 53 patients with follicular lymphoma presenting as primary skin lesions. *Am J Clin Pathol*. 2015;143(3):362-373.

12. Zhou XA, Yang J, Ringbloom KG, et al. Genomic landscape of cutaneous follicular lymphomas reveals 2 subgroups with clinically predictive molecular features. *Blood Adv*. 2021;5(3):649-661.
13. Hoefnagel JJ, Dijkman R, Basso K, et al. Distinct types of primary cutaneous large B-cell lymphoma identified by gene expression profiling. *Blood*. 2005;105(9):3671-3678.
14. Schrader AMR, de Groen RAL, Willemze R, et al. Cell-of-origin classification using the Hans and Lymph2Cx algorithms in primary cutaneous large B-cell lymphomas. *Virchows Arch*. 2022;480(3):667-675.
15. Willemze R, Hodak E, Zinzani PL, Specht L, Ladetto M. Primary cutaneous lymphomas: ESMO Clinical Practice Guidelines for diagnosis, treatment and follow-up. *Ann Oncol*. 2013;24(suppl 6):vi149-vi154.

Chapter 60
Pediatric-Type Follicular Lymphoma

Elaine S. Jaffe, Junhun Cho, Robert S. Ohgami, and Leticia Quintanilla-Martinez

Definition

Pediatric-type follicular lymphoma (PTFL) is an uncommon B-cell lymphoma that occurs almost exclusively in nodal sites. It presents primarily in children and young adults, with a marked male predominance.[1,2] This term should not be used for other lymphomas of follicle center derivation that may occur in the pediatric age group, such as testicular follicular lymphoma and large B-cell lymphomas with *IRF4* rearrangement (see Chapters 61 and 62).[3] The prognosis is excellent, and many patients are in continuous complete remission following only complete surgical excision of the affected lymph node. The usual genetic aberrations seen in other B-cell lymphomas of follicle center origin (*BCL2, BCL6*) are absent. Most cases show biallelic inactivation of *TNFRSF14* along with mutations affecting the *IRF8* and *MAP2K1* genes.[4,5]

Synonyms

PTFL with and without marginal zone differentiation.[6]

Epidemiology

Nearly all cases occur in children or young adults, with a median age of onset of 15 to 18 years.[2,5] Some cases present in older adults, but diagnosis beyond the age of 45 years is rare and should raise concern for follicular lymphoma (FL), grade 3A or 3B. The male:female ratio is approximately 10:1. No particular racial or ethnic predisposition has been recognized.

General Clinical Features

Most patients present with localized enlarged lymph nodes in the head and neck region, in the absence of systemic symptoms.[1,7] Rare cases with similar histological and genetic features may present in the conjunctiva.[8] Other extranodal sites of involvement have not been identified.

Morphology

The lymph node architecture is effaced by large expansile follicles, often with a serpiginous growth pattern.[9] Partial involvement can be seen with a rim of normal node surrounding the atypical follicles. At low power the follicles exhibit a starry sky pattern and have thin or absent mantle zones (Figure 60.1). The cellular composition is monotonous; the atypical cells are intermediate in size, often with a blastoid appearance, lacking prominent nucleoli.[2] Some cases may contain more typical centroblasts. Areas of diffuse large B-cell lymphoma exclude the diagnosis of pediatric-type FL. Grading is not utilized.

Some degree of marginal zone differentiation is very common, with a rim of paler cells surrounding the atypical follicles, although marked plasmacytic differentiation is uncommon.[1,2] In some cases, the interfollicular component is dominant, encroaching upon the remaining serpiginous follicles, with limited and attenuated mantle zones (Figure 60.2). The residual follicles resemble progressive transformation of germinal centers. In such cases the interfollicular component is polymorphous with cells of varied size with pale cytoplasm and focal plasmacytic differentiation. Admixed eosinophils may be present. Cases with this histological appearance have been diagnosed in the past as pediatric marginal zone lymphoma (PMZL).[10] However, genomic studies have shown common features between PMZL and PTFL, leading to the proposal to name the entity PTFL with and without marginal zone differentiation.[6]

Immunophenotype

The neoplastic cells are CD20$^+$ CD79a$^+$ PAX5$^+$ B cells with consistent expression of BCL6 and a high proliferation fraction as shown by Ki-67. The atypical follicles are positive for CD10 and usually do not express BCL2 but sometimes show faint BCL2 staining in a subset of neoplastic B cells.[1,2] Staining for IRF4/MUM1 is usually negative. Follicles are associated with CD21$^+$ and CD23$^+$ follicular dendritic cell meshworks. IgD

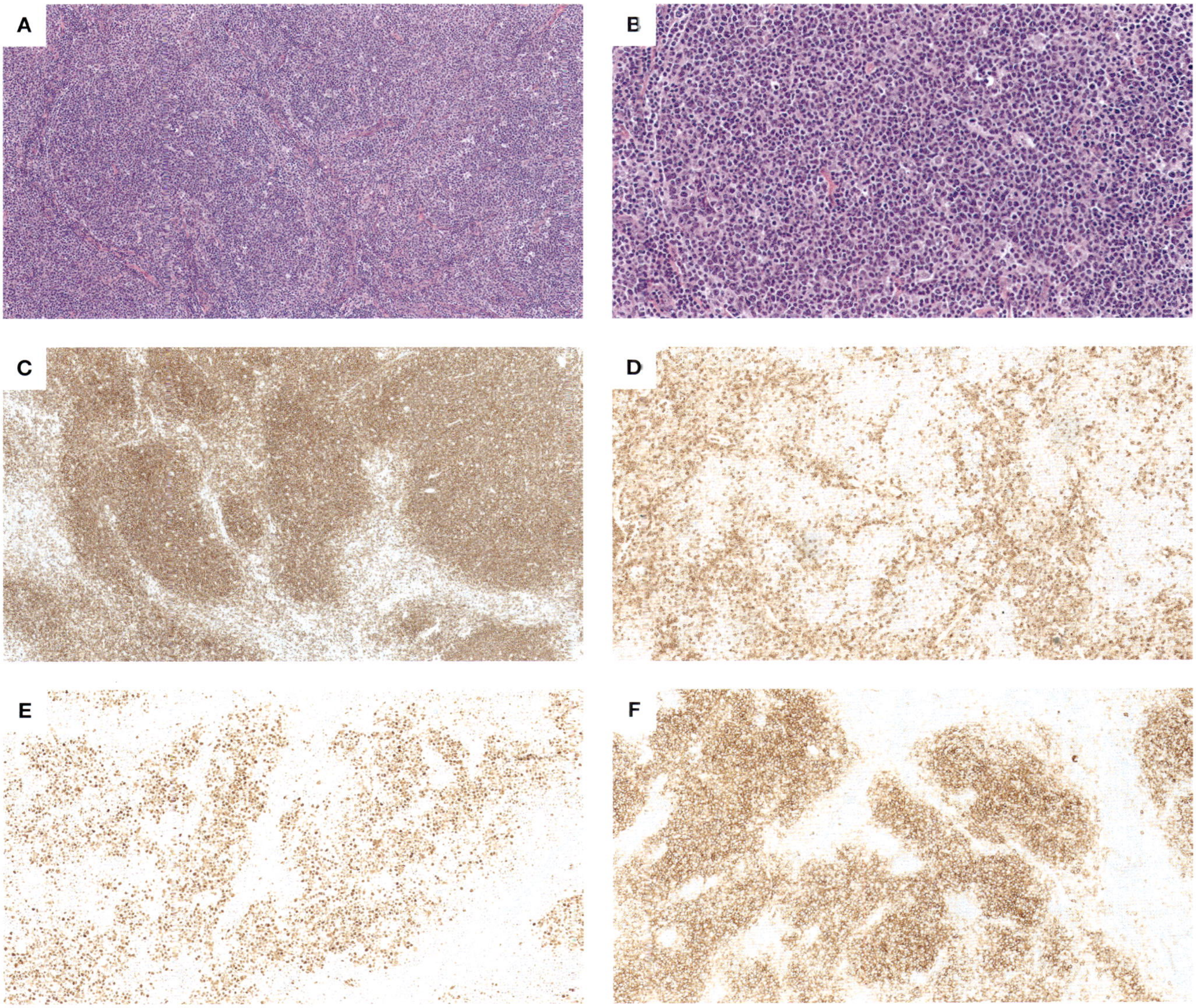

FIGURE 60.1 Pediatric-type follicular lymphoma, cervical lymph node. **A:** At low power large follicles have a starry sky pattern and have loss of a well-formed lymphoid cuff. A thin rim of pale cells surrounding the follicle is indicative of focal marginal zone differentiation. **B:** At high power the cells are medium in size with a monotonous cellular composition. **C:** The follicles are positive for CD20, with irregular shapes and sizes. Follicles are negative for BCL2 (**D**) but positive for BCL6 (**E**) and CD10. (**F**). Note irregular and sometimes serpentine configuration.

delineates the attenuated mantle cuffs surrounding the atypical follicles. In cases with marginal zone differentiation, this component is negative for BCL6 and CD10 but expresses B-cell markers including CD20 and CD79a.[6] Focal expression of MUM1/IRF4 may be seen in this population, but strong and uniform staining for MUM1 is absent. Cytoplasmic light chain restriction can be seen in the interfollicular cells.

Genetics

PTFL shows very low levels of genomic complexity. *BCL2*, *BCL6*, *IRF4,* and *MYC* gene rearrangements are not seen.[4] The most common alteration is mutation of *MAP2K1*, identified in 40% to 50% of the cases.[5,11] This alteration is associated with constitutive expression of phospho-ERK, which can be detected in a subset by immunohistochemistry in routine paraffin-embedded sections.[11] PTFL lacks mutations in epigenetic regulators such as *KMT2D, CREBBP*, or *EZH2*, which are hallmarks of FL with *BCL2* rearrangement. In common with other t(14;18)-negative FLs, PTFL shows biallelic inactivation of *TNFRSF14* via insertions/deletions, point mutations, and copy number neutral loss of heterozygosity at 1p36.[4,12] *IRF8* mutations in PTFL are identified in ~30% of cases, with hotspot mutations at p.K66R and p.Y23H. Mutations in *IRF8* often co-occur with *TNFRSF14* mutations, suggesting

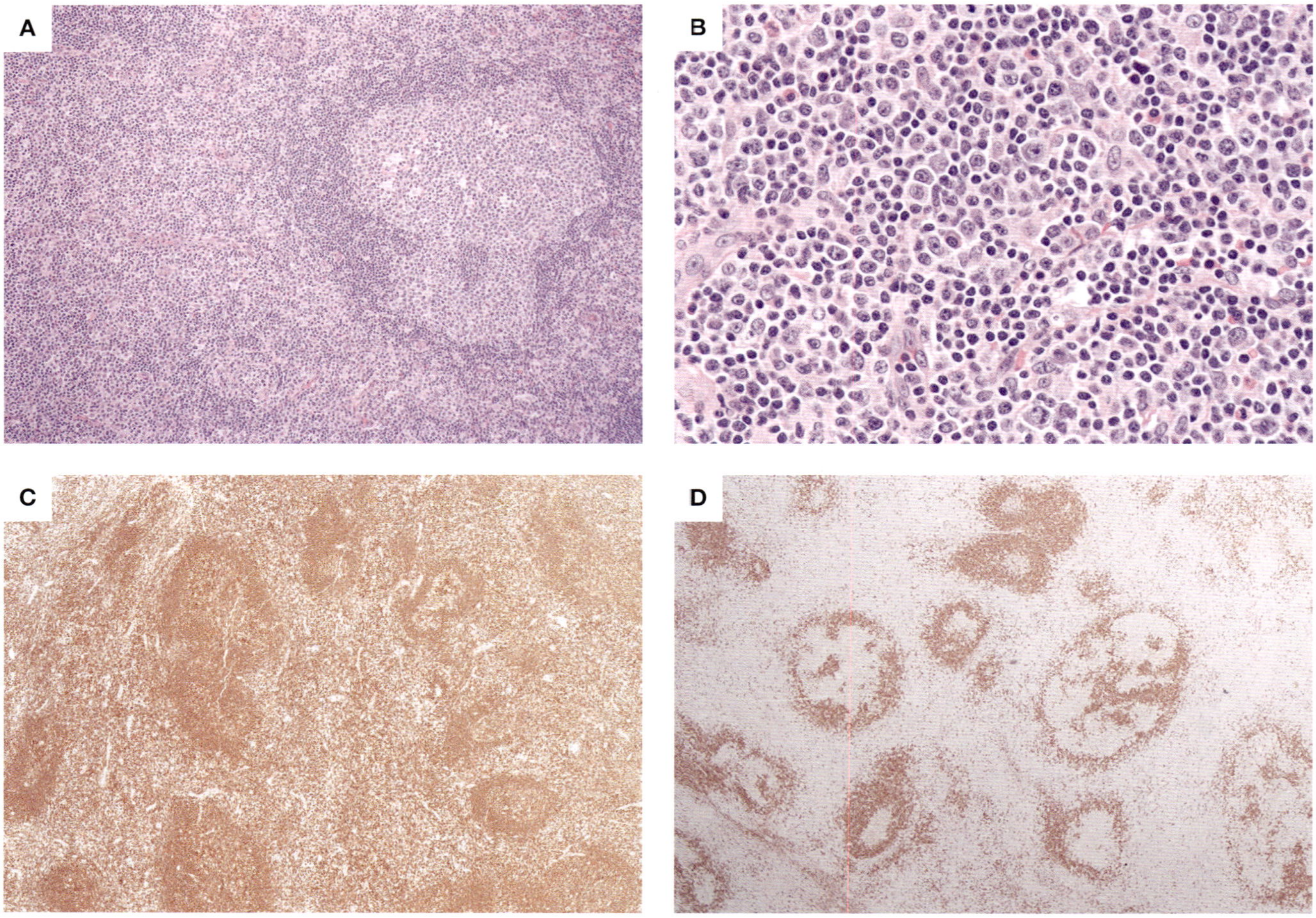

FIGURE 60.2 Pediatric-type follicular lymphoma with prominent marginal zone differentiation. **A:** Focal atypical follicles are present, but the process is largely interfollicular. **B:** The expanded interfollicular zone contains a polymorphous infiltrate, with some cells showing plasmacytoid features. **C:** CD20 stains the follicles and also shows increased B cells in the expanded marginal zone. **D:** IgD highlights the mantle cuffs, which show fragmentation resembling progressive transformation of germinal centers. Follicles were positive for CD10 and BCL6 but negative for BCL2 (not shown).

possible cooperation between these two genes.[3] The *IRF4* gene is not altered in PTFL, which is helpful in excluding the diagnosis of large B-cell lymphoma with *IRF4* rearrangement.

PTFL with marginal zone differentiation shares a similar genomic profile with more purely follicular cases, suggesting that they are part of a common entity.[6] DNA-methylation analysis also showed no major differences between PTFL and PMZL. Supporting this view, both variants have very similar clinical features in terms of median age, gender, and anatomic sites of presentation.

Prognosis and Clinical Comment

PTFL, with or without marginal zone differentiation, has an excellent prognosis. Most patients present with localized stage I disease without systemic symptoms. There is a high cure rate with simple surgical excision, although rare recurrences have been reported. Chemotherapy or radiation therapy are generally not indicated.

References

1. Louissaint, A Jr, Ackerman AM, Dias-Santagata D, et al. Pediatric-type nodal follicular lymphoma: an indolent clonal proliferation in children and adults with high proliferation index and no BCL2 rearrangement. *Blood.* 2012;120(12):2395-2404. blood-2012-05-429514 [pii]. doi:10.1182/blood-2012-05-429514
2. Liu Q, Salaverria I, Pittaluga S, et al. Follicular lymphomas in children and young adults: a comparison of the pediatric variant with usual follicular lymphoma. *Am J Surg Pathol.* 2013;37(3):333-343. doi:10.1097/PAS.0b013e31826b9b57

3. Salaverria I, Weigert O, Quintanilla-Martinez L. The clinical and molecular taxonomy of t(14;18)-negative follicular lymphomas. *Blood Adv*. 2023;7(18):5258-5271. doi:10.1182/bloodadvances.2022009456
4. Schmidt J, Gong S, Marafioti T, et al. Genome-wide analysis of pediatric-type follicular lymphoma reveals low genetic complexity and recurrent alterations of TNFRSF14 gene. *Blood*. 2016;128(8):1101-1111. doi:10.1182/blood-2016-03-703819
5. Louissaint A Jr, Schafernak KT, Geyer JT, et al. Pediatric-type nodal follicular lymphoma: a biologically distinct lymphoma with frequent MAPK pathway mutations. *Blood*. 2016;128(8):1093-1100. doi:10.1182/blood-2015-12-682591
6. Salmeron-Villalobos J, Egan C, Borgmann V, et al. A unifying hypothesis for PNMZL and PTFL: morphological variants with a common molecular profile. *Blood Adv*. 2022;6(16):4661-4674. doi:10.1182/bloodadvances.2022007322
7. Laurent C, Cook JR, Yoshino T, Quintanilla-Martinez L, Jaffe ES. Follicular lymphoma and marginal zone lymphoma: how many diseases? *Virchows Arch*. 2023;482(1):149-162. doi:10.1007/s00428-022-03432-2
8. Okudolo JO, Bagg A, Meghpara BB, Sieber MR, Eagle RC Jr, Milman T. Conjunctival pediatric-type follicular lymphoma. *Ophthalmic Plast Reconstr Surg*. 2020;36(2):e46-e49. doi:10.1097/iop.0000000000001556
9. Koo M, Ohgami RS. Pediatric-type follicular lymphoma and pediatric nodal marginal zone lymphoma: recent clinical, morphologic, immunophenotypic, and genetic insights. *Adv Anat Pathol*. 2017;24(3):128-135. doi:10.1097/pap.0000000000000144
10. Taddesse-Heath L, Pittaluga S, Sorbara L, Bussey M, Raffeld M, Jaffe ES. Marginal zone B-cell lymphoma in children and young adults. *Am J Surg Pathol*. 2003;27(4):522-531.
11. Schmidt J, Ramis-Zaldivar JE, Nadeu F, et al. Mutations of MAP2K1 are frequent in pediatric-type follicular lymphoma and result in ERK pathway activation. *Blood*. 2017;130(3):323-327. doi:10.1182/blood-2017-03-776278
12. Martin-Guerrero I, Salaverria I, Burkhardt B, et al. Recurrent loss of heterozygosity in 1p36 associated with TNFRSF14 mutations in IRF4 translocation negative pediatric follicular lymphomas. *Haematologica*. 2013;98(8):1237-1241. haematol.2012.073916 [pii]. doi:10.3324/haematol.2012.073916

Chapter 61
Testicular Follicular Lymphoma

Chris M. Bacon, and Ahmet Dogan

Definition

Testicular follicular lymphoma is a neoplasm of germinal center B cells with at least a partially follicular growth pattern arising within the testicular parenchyma and rarely the epididymis. These cases lack *BCL2* translocations and evidence of systemic disease.

Synonyms

None.

Epidemiology

Testicular follicular lymphoma is very rare, with fewer than 30 cases reported in detail to date. Most reported cases have occurred in boys with a median age of approximately 4 years, but a small number of cases occurring in adult men (27-69 years old) have also been described.[1-10] The etiology and risk factors of testicular follicular lymphoma are unknown. None of the reported patients have had known conditions predisposing to lymphoma development, and there is little evidence of preceding testicular pathology.

General Clinical Features

Patients with testicular follicular lymphoma present with painless diffuse enlargement of, or a palpable mass within, one testis, often identified during routine physical examination. Bilateral disease has not been reported. Some cases have been associated with hydrocele,[3,9] but systemic symptoms are absent. Macroscopic examination of the testis reveals areas of white/gray/tan, soft to firm, infiltration 15 to 80 mm in diameter. The rete testis, epididymis, and tunica albuginea are each often involved, but the spermatic cord generally is not. Except for a single adult patient with lymphadenopathy,[1] staging investigations showed no evidence of involvement of lymph nodes or other extratesticular sites in the patients reported in detail.[1-5,7-10]

Morphology

The testicular parenchyma is replaced by lymphoma with a follicular or follicular and diffuse growth pattern, which effaces or infiltrates between seminiferous tubules. The follicles are generally small and uniform in size and may be well defined, either back-to-back or widely spaced, or appear as vague nodularity on hematoxylin and eosin–stained sections (Figures 61.1 and 61.2). They lack polarization and tingible body macrophages and have attenuated or absent mantle zones. The neoplastic intrafollicular cells in most cases include numerous large centroblasts admixed with large or small centrocytes. The centroblasts typically have round or ovoid nuclei, vesicular chromatin, and one to three peripheral nucleoli, but in some cases centroblasts with large multilobulated nuclei are also present. Most cases thus correspond to grade 3A morphology, although occasional cases in adults may correspond to grade 1 to 2. Mitotic figures may be easily identified.

The interfollicular and diffuse areas contain varying proportions of neoplastic centrocytes and centroblasts along with small reactive lymphocytes and sometimes a few plasma cells. In up to half of the cases there are areas of diffuse neoplastic cell infiltration, which may focally contain more than 15 centroblasts per 0.159 mm^2 high-power field. Although such a finding raises the consideration of a diffuse large B-cell lymphoma, not otherwise specified, no well-documented cases of large cell transformation have been documented.[1,2,5,7-10] Therefore, unless there is compelling evidence of a diffuse large B-cell lymphoma (such as topologically distinct diffuse cohesive sheets of centroblasts), the mixture of centroblasts and centrocytes in diffuse areas should be best considered within the spectrum of follicular lymphoma. In some cases, there is either interstitial fibrosis or foci of more dense fibrosis, sometimes involving the tunica albuginea and/or associated with chronic inflammation. Necrosis is not a feature.

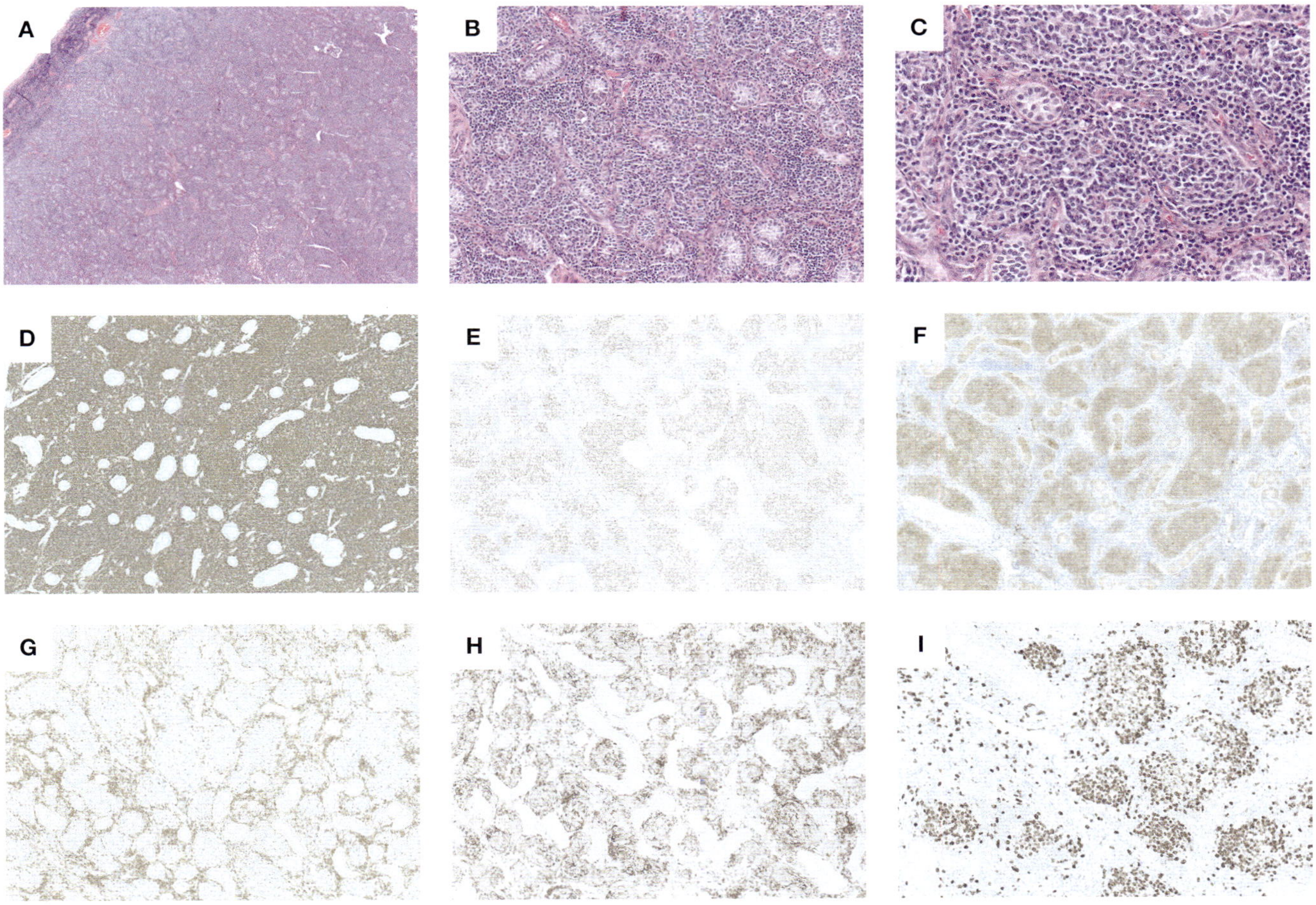

FIGURE 61.1 Histological and immunophenotypic features of a testicular follicular lymphoma in a 4-year-old child. Low-power view shows replacement of the testis parenchyma by dense lymphoid infiltrate with a subtle nodular pattern (**A**). In medium-power view, atypical lymphoid cells forming small nodules/follicles between the preserved seminiferous tubules is evident (**B**). In high-power view, the neoplastic follicles are composed of numerous centroblasts intermixed with centrocytes (**C**). Low-power view, CD20 immunostain highlights extensive infiltrate of neoplastic B cells (**D**). The neoplastic B cells express follicle center B-cell markers BCL6 (**E**) and CD10 (**F**) but appear negative for BCL2 (**G**). CD23 immunostain labels follicular dendritic cells underlying the follicles as well as a subset of the B cells (**H**). The neoplastic follicles show a high proliferation fraction with Ki67 immunostain (**I**). (Images courtesy of Dr Rebecca King, Mayo Clinic, Rochester, MN, USA.)

Immunophenotype

The neoplastic cells of testicular follicular lymphoma are germinal center B cells. Accordingly, they express pan B-cell antigens, such as CD20, CD79a, and Pax5, as well as the germinal center B-cell antigens BCL6 and, usually, CD10 (Figures 61.1 and 61.2). As in follicular lymphomas at other sites, the neoplastic B cells outwith the follicles may show relative downregulation of BCL6 and/or CD10. The intrafollicular lymphoma cells are negative for BCL2. The expression of other antigens is inconsistently documented in the literature: CD23 may be expressed by a proportion of the B cells; MUM1/IRF4 is negative or positive in only a minority of B cells. Specific markers of other lymphoma types, such as cyclin D1 and LEF1, should be negative. Staining for CD21 and CD23 identifies follicular dendritic cell meshworks and helps identify the follicular architecture in areas that are morphologically only vaguely nodular. The Ki67 proliferation fraction may be high in both follicles and diffuse areas. Reactive CD3-positive T cells are present, predominantly between follicles.

Genetics

Unlike the majority of follicular lymphomas, but in common with 10% to 15% of follicular lymphomas and with pediatric-type follicular lymphoma, testicular follicular lymphoma lacks the *IGH::BCL2* translocation or variants. Cases of follicular lymphoma arising in the testis or epididymis that do

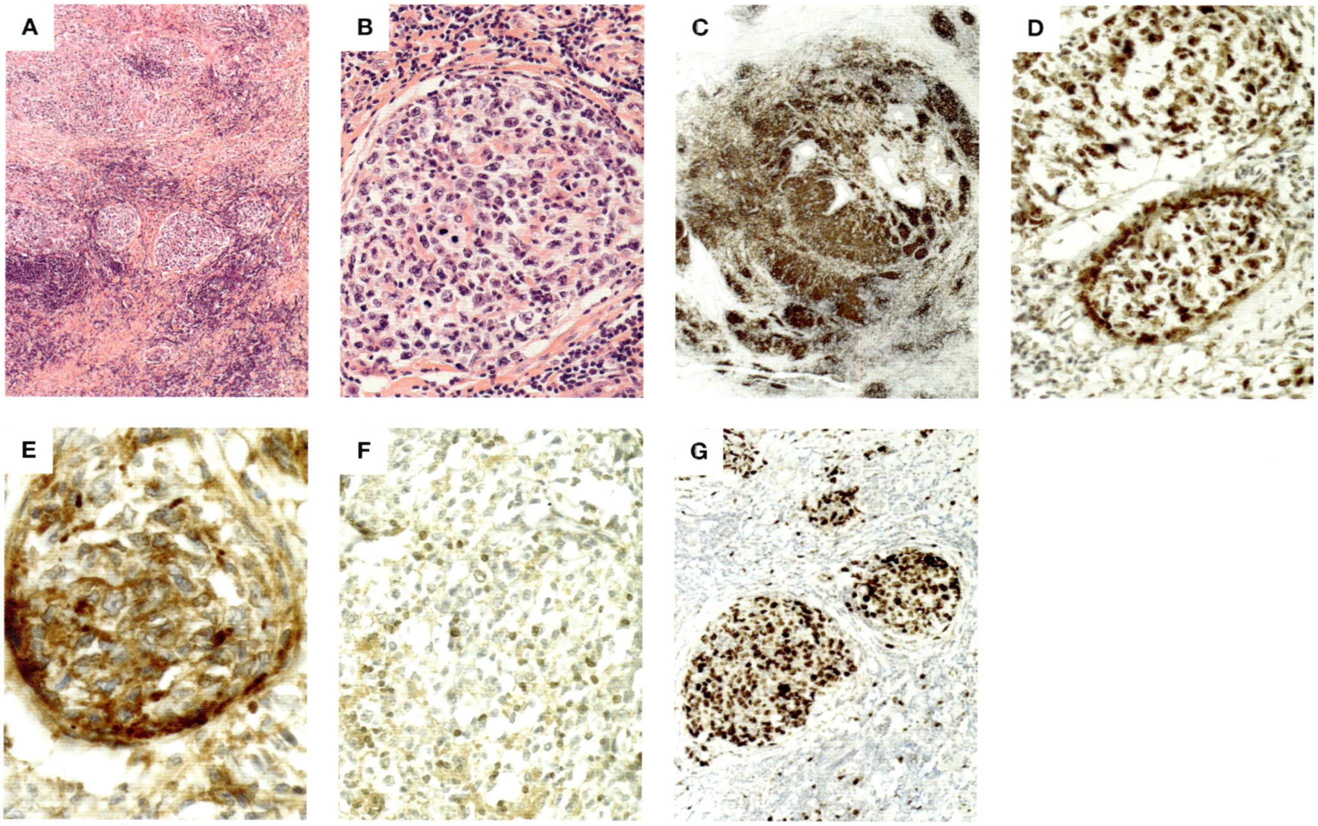

FIGURE 61.2 Histological and immunophenotypic features of a testicular follicular lymphoma in a young adult. Low-power view shows replacement of the testis parenchyma by a nodular dense lymphoid infiltrate with surrounding fibrosis and chronic inflammatory changes **(A)**. In high-power view, the neoplastic follicles are composed of numerous centroblasts intermixed with centrocytes **(B)**. Low-power view, CD20 immunostain highlights the infiltrate of neoplastic B cells with follicular pattern **(C)**. The neoplastic B cells express follicle center B-cell markers BCL6 **(D)** and CD10 **(E)** but appear negative for BCL2 **(F)**. The neoplastic follicles show a high proliferation fraction with Ki67 immunostain **(G)**.

carry a *IGH::BCL2* translocation or variant may be more appropriately diagnosed as follicular lymphoma of conventional type. A *BCL6* rearrangement was detected in one case by Southern blot analysis.[2] Limited information is available on the spectrum of somatic mutations seen in testicular follicular lymphoma.[6] Two cases subjected to whole exome sequencing carried missense variants in the epigenetic modifiers *EZH2* or *KMT2D*; one had a MAPK pathway variant and showed immunohistochemical evidence of pathway activation (phospho-ERK), and the other had an *IRF8* variant distinct from the K66R variant recurrent in pediatric-type follicular lymphoma. A mutation in *TNFRSF14* was identified in a third case. The molecular relationship between testicular follicular lymphoma and other follicular lymphoma subtypes thus remains a topic for further investigation.

Prognosis and Clinical Comment

The prognosis of testicular follicular lymphoma is good, regardless of age, with all children reported in detail, and all but one adult (who developed nodal follicular lymphoma 22 years later) disease free at last reported follow-up (6-96 months, median 36 months).[1-5,7-10] Most children have been treated with orchidectomy and short-duration, risk-adapted chemotherapy, but in others, and in some adults, longer or more intense regimens have been used. In some patients, orchidectomy alone has resulted in durable remissions.[1,3,4]

References

1. Bacon CM, Ye H, Diss TC, et al. Primary follicular lymphoma of the testis and epididymis in adults. *Am J Surg Pathol.* 2007;31(7):1050-1058.

2. Finn LS, Viswanatha DS, Belasco JB, et al. Primary follicular lymphoma of the testis in childhood. *Cancer.* 1999;85(7):1626-1635.
3. Heller KN, Teruya-Feldstein J, La Quaglia MP, Wexler LH. Primary follicular lymphoma of the testis: excellent outcome following surgical resection without adjuvant chemotherapy. *J Pediatr Hematol Oncol.* 2004;26(2):104-107.
4. Liu Q, Salaverria I, Pittaluga S, et al. Follicular lymphomas in children and young adults: a comparison of the pediatric variant with usual follicular lymphoma. *Am J Surg Pathol.* 2013;37(3):333-343.
5. Lones MA, Raphael M, McCarthy K, et al. Primary follicular lymphoma of the testis in children and adolescents. *J Pediatr Hematol Oncol.* 2012;34(1):68-71.
6. Lovisa F, Binatti A, Coppe A, et al. A high definition picture of key genes and pathways mutated in pediatric follicular lymphoma. *Haematologica.* 2019;104(9):e406-e409.
7. Lu D, Medeiros LJ, Eskenazi AE, Abruzzo LV. Primary follicular large cell lymphoma of the testis in a child. *Arch Pathol Lab Med.* 2001;125:551-554.
8. Moertel CL, Watterson J, McCormick SR, Simonton SC. Follicular large cell lymphoma of the testis in a child. *Cancer.* 1995;75(5):1182-1186.
9. Pakzad K, MacLennan GT, Elder JS, et al. Follicular large cell lymphoma localized to the testis in children. *J Urol.* 2002;168(1):225-228.
10. Pileri SA, Sabattini E, Rosito P, et al. Primary follicular lymphoma of the testis in childhood: an entity with peculiar clinical and molecular characteristics. *J Clin Pathol.* 2002;55(9):684-688.

Chapter 62

Large B-Cell Lymphoma With *IRF4* Rearrangement

Stefania Pittaluga, Jan Delabie, and Itziar Salaverria

Definition

Large B-cell lymphoma with *IRF4* rearrangement (LBCL-IRF4) is an uncommon subtype of lymphoma that typically has LBCL morphology with or without a diffuse component, shows moderate/high IRF4/MUM1 expression, and usually carries a detectable *IRF4* rearrangement.[1-3] It occurs primarily in children and young adults, with Waldeyer ring or head and neck lymph node involvement, although it can also occasionally occur in adults with features similar to those in children.[4,5] When occurring in the pediatric age group, it should not be considered as part of the pediatric-type follicular lymphomas, even if exclusively follicular. Also, the definition does not include aggressive B-cell lymphomas with *IRF4* rearrangements that are associated with *BCL2* or *MYC* rearrangements. LBCL-IRF4 was introduced as a provisional entity in the 2017 World Health Organization classification and has been now upgraded to a definite entity.[6]

Synonyms

None.

Epidemiology

LBCL-IRF4 is rare (0.05% of diffuse large B-cell lymphoma). The median age at presentation is 12 years with an equal gender distribution. It is significantly more frequent in children (≤18 years) than in adults (>18 years; 15% vs 2%) $P < .001$.

General Clinical Features

Most patients present with enlarged lymph nodes of the head and neck region. Waldeyer ring involvement is also a frequent site of disease; other reported sites of involvement include the gastrointestinal tract. Most patients present with localized disease (stage I-II).

Morphology

LBCL-IRF4 is often follicular and diffuse, but it may be purely follicular or diffuse in some cases. It is composed predominantly of medium-sized centroblast-like cells with clumped chromatin and basophilic nucleoli. Typically, there is a high proliferation rate and sometimes a starry sky pattern. When follicular, the neoplastic follicles are large, with a back-to-back growth pattern and absent or attenuated mantle cuffs (Figure 62.1). In contrast to pediatric-type follicular lymphomas, the follicles lack a serpiginous outline, progressive transformation of germinal centers- like changes, and a starry sky pattern.

Immunophenotype

The atypical cells have a mature B-cell phenotype and are positive for CD20, CD79a, and PAX5. IRF4/MUM1 is typically strongly expressed, with positivity as well for BCL6, while PRDM1/BLIMP1 is usually negative (Figure 62.2). CD10 and BCL2 expression is also observed in 66% of cases and CD5 in about half of the cases.[2] The proliferative rate is usually high without evidence of polarization in the neoplastic follicles. Cases with coexpression of the germinal center cell markers CD10 and BCL6 together with IRF4/MUM1 in the appropriate clinical context should be screened for *IRF4* rearrangements.

Genetics

Immunoglobulin gene analysis shows clonal rearrangements. A cytogenetically cryptic rearrangement of the *IRF4* gene, which can be detected by a break-apart probe (Figure 62.3),[1,3] with an IGH locus is detected in the majority of cases, whereas rearrangements with immunoglobulin (IG) light chain genes seem to be rare. A subset of LBCL-IRF4 carries *BCL6* locus breakpoints, while *MYC* and *BCL2* rearrangements are absent. LBCL-IRF4 displays a complex pattern of genetic changes. Losses of 17p, frequently in the

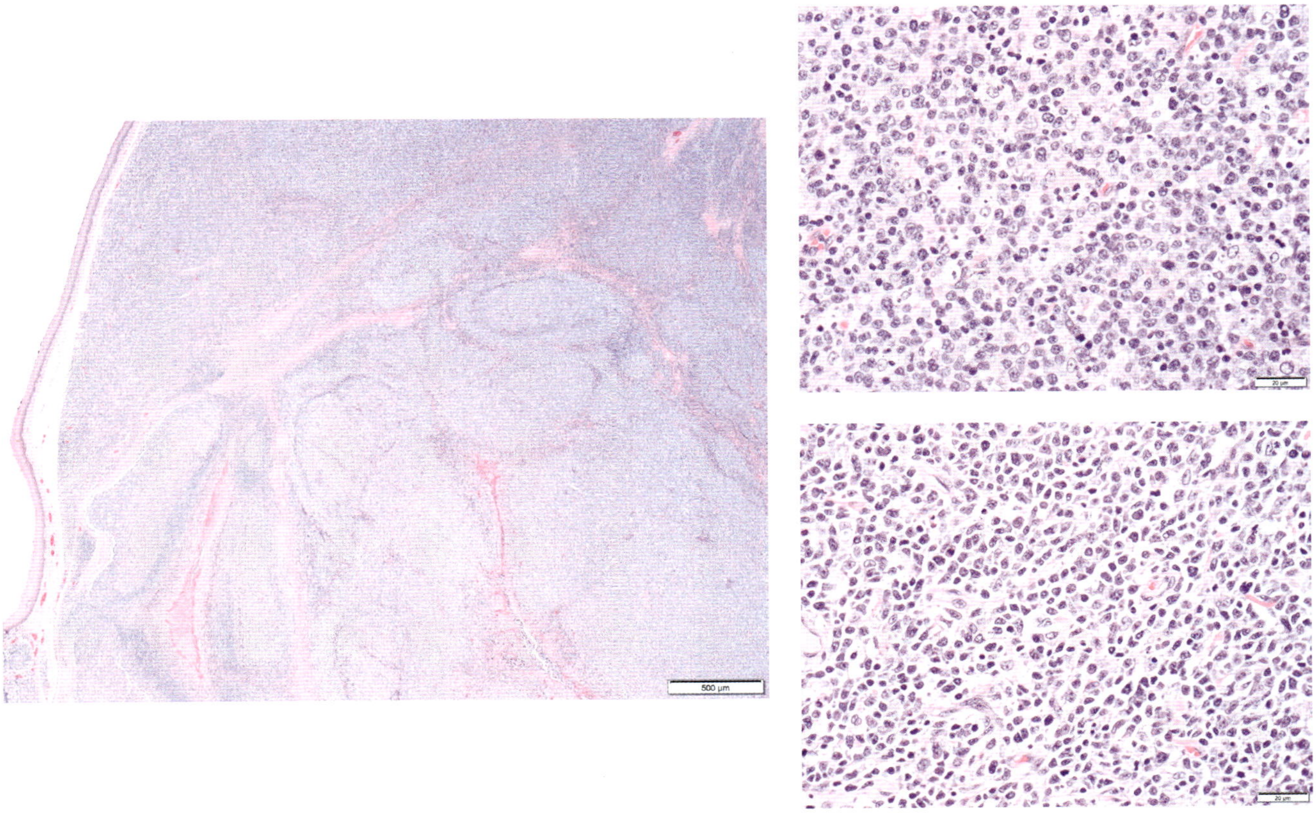

FIGURE 62.1 Large B-cell lymphoma with *IRF4* rearrangement. (Left) Low magnification of a tonsil with large abnormal follicles and diffuse areas. (Right) Higher magnification showing frequent apoptotic bodies cytologically distinct from typical centrocytes and centroblasts (top) and monotonous proliferation of medium-sized to large atypical cells that lack a starry sky pattern (bottom).

context of isochromosome 17, and 11q12-qter gains are characteristic of this entity.[3,7,8]

LBCL-IRF4 has mainly a germinal centre B-cell (GCB) of origin either by gene expression profiling or by immunohistochemistry despite the constitutive IRF4 overexpression; however, it has a unique signature by gene expression profiling pattern that is distinct from GCB and activated B-cell.[7]

Somatic mutations of *IRF4*, most likely by its juxtaposition to the IG gene, and *BCL6* are frequent, as are mutations of NF-kB pathway genes (*CARD11*, *CD79B*, and *MYD88*).[3,7] A single study reported that mutations affecting the NF-kB pathway seem to be exclusively observed in cases with a pure diffuse morphology, while *MAP2K1* mutations, characteristic of PTFL, were detected in two of nine cases with a follicular component.[7] More studies are needed to confirm this observation.

In cases with the same constellation of pathological and clinical features but absence of *IRF4* rearrangement by fluorescence in situ hybridization, the demonstration of an IGH rearrangement without *BCL2*, *BCL6*, and *MYC* breaks and/or identification of *IRF4* somatic mutations could support inclusion in this diagnostic category.[2,7,9]

Prognosis and Clinical Comment

Invariably patients have a favorable outcome after systemic treatment despite a diffuse growth pattern and a high cytologic grade. Age at presentation is a favorable predictor. This is in contrast with pediatric follicular lymphomas that tend to do well with local management.[1,3,7,10]

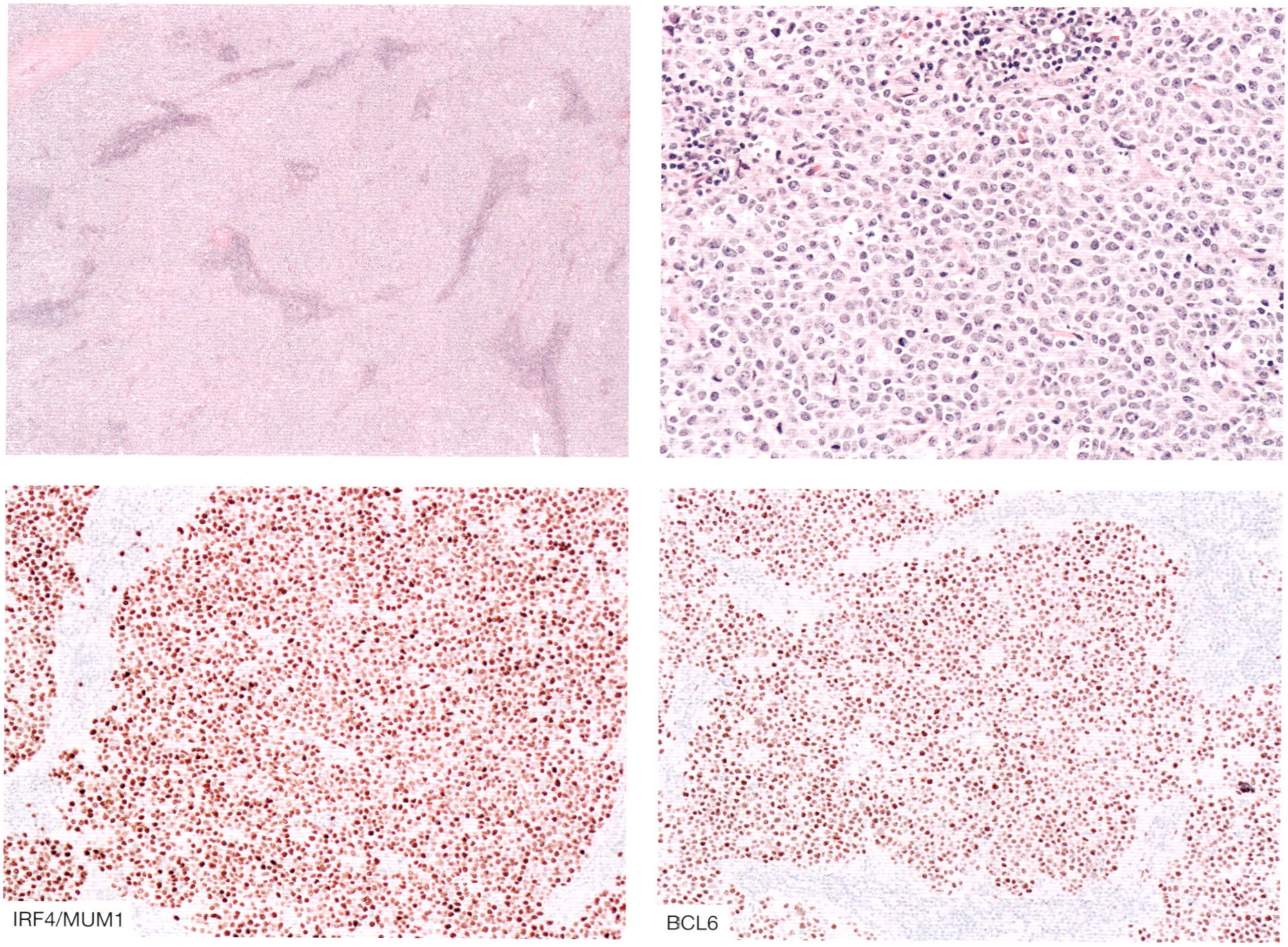

FIGURE 62.2 Large B-cell lymphoma with *IRF4* rearrangement. Hematoxylin and eosin–stained sections from a lymph node show expanded follicles with attenuated mantes (left) and higher magnification a monotonous proliferation of medium to large atypical cells. By immunohistochemical stains the neoplastic cells are uniformly positive for IRF4/MUM1 (bottom left) and BCL6 (bottom right).

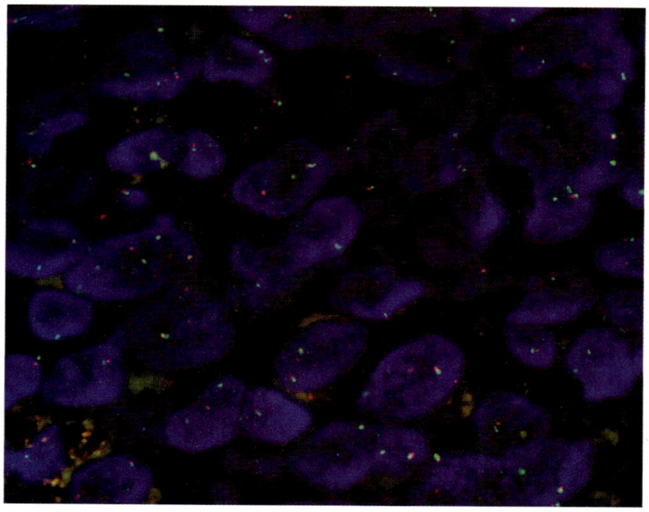

FIGURE 62.3 Large B-cell lymphoma with *IRF4* rearrangement. Fluorescence in situ hybridization for *IRF4* rearrangement using a break-apart probe demonstrated split signal (1 red and 1 green) indicative of the rearrangement and one intact copy (colocalized signal red/green).

References

1. Au-Yeung RKH, Arias Padilla L, Zimmermann M, et al. Experience with provisional WHO-entities large B-cell lymphoma with IRF4-rearrangement and Burkitt-like lymphoma with 11q aberration in paediatric patients of the NHL-BFM group. *Br J Haematol*. 2020;190(5):753-763. doi:10.1111/bjh.16578
2. Quintanilla-Martinez L, Laurent C, Soma L, et al. Emerging entities: high-grade/large B-cell lymphoma with 11q aberration, large B-cell lymphoma with IRF4 rearrangement, and new molecular subgroups in large B-cell lymphomas. A report of the 2022 EA4HP/SH lymphoma workshop. *Virchows Arch*. 2023;483(3):281-298. doi:10.1007/s00428-023-03590-x
3. Salaverria I, Philipp C, Oschlies I; et al. Translocations activating IRF4 identify a subtype of germinal center-derived B-cell lymphoma affecting predominantly children and young adults. *Blood*. 2011;118(1):139-147. doi:10.1182/blood-2011-01-330795

4. Frauenfeld L, Castrejon-de-Anta N, Ramis-Zaldivar JE, et al. Diffuse large B-cell lymphomas in adults with aberrant coexpression of CD10, BCL6, and MUM1 are enriched in IRF4 rearrangements. *Blood Adv.* 2022;6(7):2361-2372. doi:10.1182/bloodadvances.2021006034
5. Streich S, Frauenfeld L, Otto F, et al. Prevalence of IRF4 rearrangement in large B-cell lymphomas of the Waldeyer's ring in adults. *Virchows Arch.* 2023;482(3):551-560. doi:10.1007/s00428-023-03516-7
6. Pittaluga SH, N, Siebert R, Salaverria I. Large B-Cell Lymphoma with IRF4 Rearrangement. IARC; 2017.
7. Ramis-Zaldivar JE, Gonzalez-Farre B, Balague O, et al. Distinct molecular profile of IRF4-rearranged large B-cell lymphoma. *Blood.* 2020;135(4):274-286. doi:10.1182/blood.2019002699
8. Salaverria I, Martin-Guerrero I, Burkhardt B, et al. High resolution copy number analysis of IRF4 translocation-positive diffuse large B-cell and follicular lymphomas. *Genes Chromosomes Cancer.* 2013;52(2):150-155. doi:10.1002/gcc.22014
9. Liu Q, Salaverria I, Pittaluga S, et al. Follicular lymphomas in children and young adults: a comparison of the pediatric variant with usual follicular lymphoma. *Am J Surg Pathol.* 2013;37(3):333-343. doi:10.1097/PAS.0b013e31826b9b57
10. Chisholm KM, Mohlman J, Liew M, et al. IRF4 translocation status in pediatric follicular and diffuse large B-cell lymphoma patients enrolled in Children's Oncology Group trials. *Pediatr Blood Cancer.* 2019;66(8):e27770. doi:10.1002/pbc.27770

Chapter 63

Mantle Cell Lymphoma: Conventional and Leukemic Nonnodal Subtypes

Elias Campo, Martin Dreyling, Birgitta Sander, and Andrew D. Zelenetz

Definition

Mantle cell lymphoma (MCL) is a mature B-cell neoplasm that is generally composed of monomorphic small to medium-sized lymphoid cells with irregular nuclei, frequently expresses CD5, and carries *CCND1* rearrangements with immunoglobulin (IG) genes, leading to overexpression of cyclin D1. Some tumors with similar morphology and phenotype are cyclin D1 negative and have instead *CCND2* or *CCND3* translocations and overexpression.[1-3] Two molecular MCL subtypes are now recognized: conventional MCL (cMCL), which is the most common, and leukemic nonnodal MCL (nnMCL). These subtypes differ in their cell of origin, molecular profiles, and clinical behavior (Figure 63.1).[4] Both subtypes carry *CCND1* rearrangements, but cMCL derives from germinal center unexperienced cells, usually with unmutated or low-mutated IGHV and overexpression of the transcription factor SOX11. nnMCL derives from a cell that has passed through the germinal center, carries mutated IGHV, and is SOX11 negative. nnMCL usually has an indolent behavior for long periods.

Synonyms

None.

Epidemiology

MCL represents 2.5% to 10% of all non-Hodgkin lymphomas and occurs predominantly in older adult men (male-to-female ratio, 2.1-3.9:1; median age approximately 65 years; range, 23-96). The mean annual incidence is 0.71 per 100,000 (range, 0.42-1.01).[1]

General Clinical Features

Most patients present with stage IV disease, generalized lymphadenopathy, hepatosplenomegaly, and bone marrow involvement; bulky disease and B symptoms are less common.[1] Extranodal involvement is frequent and may occur in virtually any site but is usually associated with lymphadenopathy. Frequent locations are the Waldeyer ring and gastrointestinal tract. Gastrointestinal involvement may be isolated and can present as lymphomatoid polyposis.[5] Central nervous system involvement rarely occurs at diagnosis but may appear late in evolution.[6] Peripheral blood involvement is frequent and may be detected by flow cytometry in virtually all patients.[7] Some patients may present with a very aggressive leukemic form with blastoid morphology mimicking acute leukemia.[8] nnMCL usually presents in leukemic phase with no or minimal lymphadenopathy and may be asymptomatic for long periods followed by the development of splenomegaly without nodal dissemination. Some of these patients may eventually progress to an aggressive disease with or without nodal dissemination.

Morphology

MCL usually effaces the lymph node architecture with mantle zone, nodular, or diffuse patterns (Figure 63.2). In the mantle zone pattern the tumor cells expand the follicle mantle surrounding a reactive germinal center. Transitional areas between nodular and diffuse patterns are common. Residual germinal centers can be seen focally in tumors with a diffuse pattern. Four major cytological variants are recognized (Figure 63.3). Classic MCL is the most common and characterized by a monotonous proliferation of small to medium-sized lymphoid cells with scant cytoplasm, irregular nuclei, evenly distributed condensed chromatin, and inconspicuous nucleoli. The small cell variant is less frequent, predominantly seen in nnMCL, and composed of small lymphocytes with round nuclei mimicking chronic lymphocytic leukemia (CLL), but proliferation centers and prolymphocytes are absent. Blastoid and pleomorphic variants are associated with more aggressive behavior. Blastoid cells have round nuclei with finely dispersed chromatin mimicking lymphoblasts,

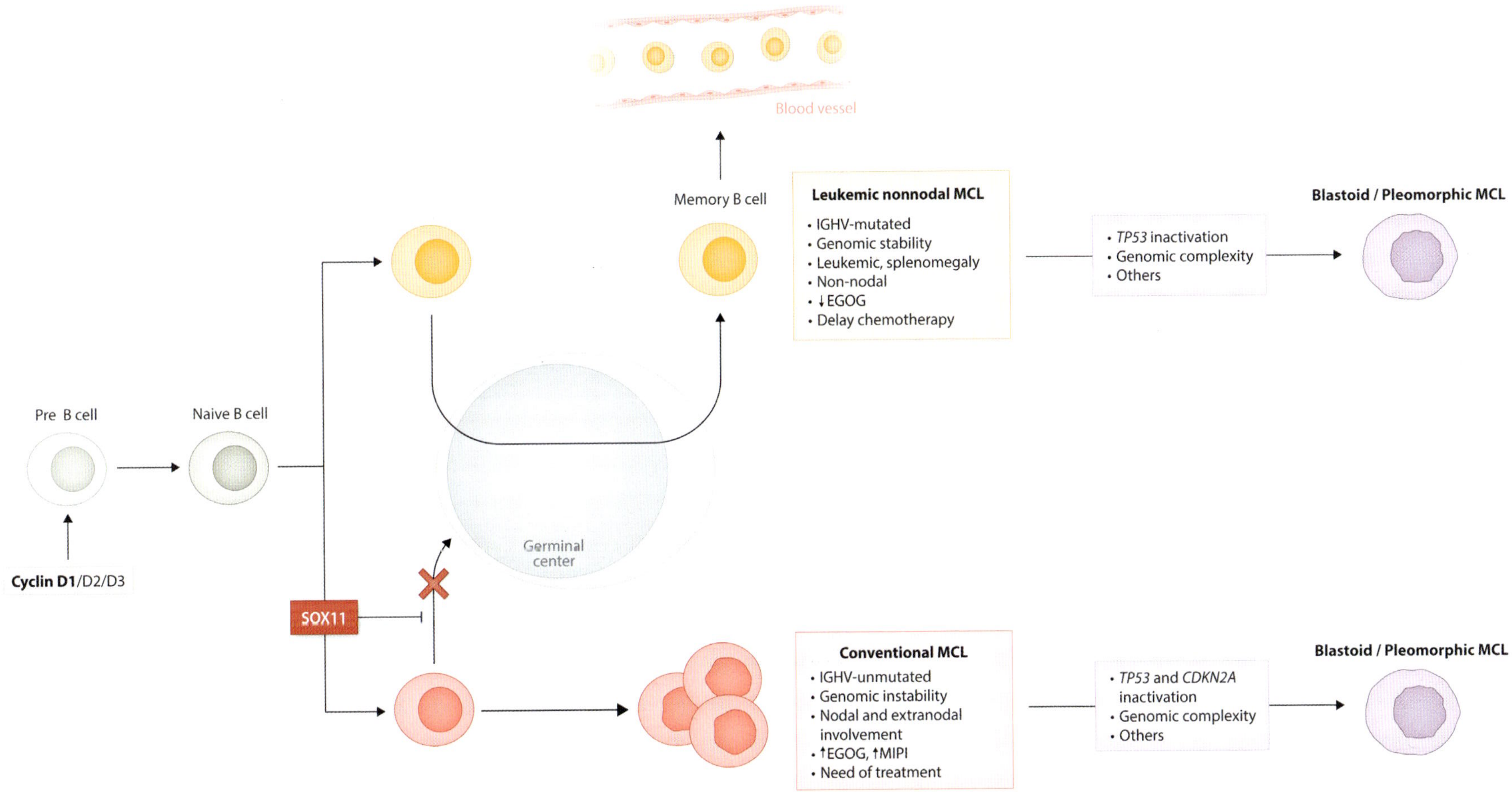

FIGURE 63.1 Mantle cell lymphoma (MCL) cell of origin and molecular subtypes. CCND1 and to less extent CCND2 or D3 rearrangements with Ig genes are acquired in pre-B cell in the bone marrow. The leukemic nonnodal MCL subtype derives from a cell that has transited the germinal center, whereas the conventional MCL derives from a cell that expresses SOX11 and has not experienced the germinal center microenvironment. Both molecular subtypes may transform to blastoid/pleomorphic variants of MCL in association with the acquisition of subsequent oncogenic events.

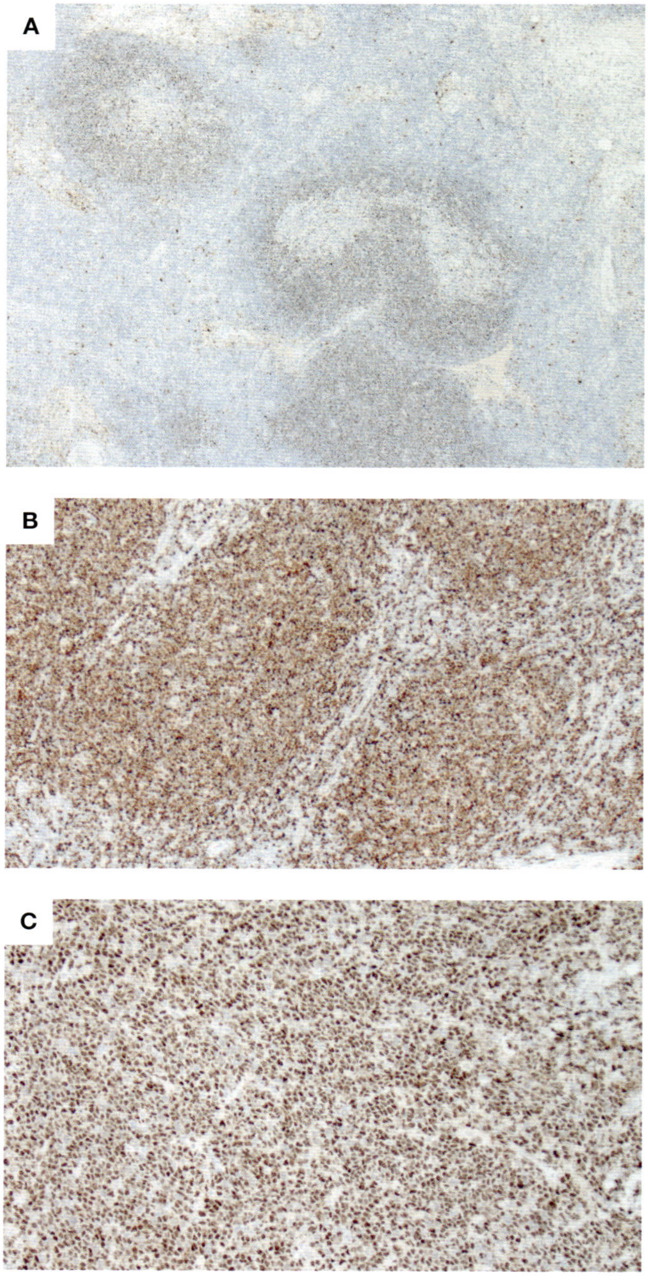

FIGURE 63.2 Lymph node architecture in mantle cell lymphoma as illustrated by cyclin D1 staining. **A:** Mantle zone pattern. **B:** Nodular pattern. **C:** Diffuse pattern.

whereas pleomorphic cells are larger with irregular nuclei, resembling diffuse large B-cell lymphoma, with occasional small or inconspicuous nucleoli. Although most blastoid/pleomorphic MCLs are detected at initial diagnosis, around 20% to 35% of classic/small cell variants may progress to these aggressive variants in subsequent relapses. Some MCLs have cells with abundant pale cytoplasm, mimicking monocytoid B cells. CD5 and cyclin D1 positivity are helpful to distinguish from marginal zone lymphomas or hairy cell leukemia.[1] Clonally related plasmacytoid differentiation has been observed in some nnMCLs.[9] Proliferation may be variable in classic MCL, usually low in the small cell variant and very high in blastoid/pleomorphic tumors. Scattered histiocytes with broad, pale cytoplasm, and fine capillaries with hyalinized walls are common. A "starry sky" pattern may be seen in blastoid/pleomorphic tumors.

Tumor cells in blood and bone marrow have similar features, but some leukemic tumors may have prominent nucleoli mimicking B prolymphocytic leukemia, but the nuclei in MCL are more irregular. Identification of *CCND1/D2/D3* rearrangement or overexpression in these cases is essential for the diagnosis of MCL. Bone marrow infiltrates may be nodular, interstitial, paratrabecular, or diffuse. An intrasinusoidal pattern may also be seen, mainly in nnMCL.

Splenic involvement expands the white pulp nodules, with variable involvement of the red pulp. A common manifestation of gastrointestinal disease is lymphomatoid polyposis, in which multiple lymphoid polyps are identified in the small and large bowels and may be associated with larger tumor masses. Although characteristic, this presentation is not specific for MCL. Gastrointestinal involvement without the macroscopic appearance of polyposis may also occur. Asymptomatic involvement of the gastrointestinal tract with microscopic infiltration of endoscopically normal mucosa is very common (above 80%).

MCL may be occasionally associated with a second lymphoid neoplasm particularly follicular lymphoma, CLL/small lymphocytic lymphoma, splenic and nodal marginal-zone lymphomas, plasma cell neoplasms, and Hodgkin lymphoma.[10]

Immunophenotype

MCL is a mature B-cell neoplasm expressing the B-cell markers CD19, CD20, CD21, PAX5, and CD79a with frequent coexpression of CD5 and CD43. Surface IGs are usually of moderate to strong intensity, with frequent coexpression of immunoglobulin M (IgM) and IgD with lambda more frequently expressed than kappa light chain. CD23 and CD200 are usually negative in cMCL but may be expressed by nnMCL, sometimes with negativity for CD5.[3] CD10 and BCL6 are usually negative, although occasional positive cases have been documented, particularly with blastoid/pleomorphic morphology, high Ki-67, complex cytogenetics, and poor prognosis.[3] LEF1 is negative but may be seen in occasional blastoid/pleomorphic variants. IRF4/MUM1 may be detected in a minor subset of cells,

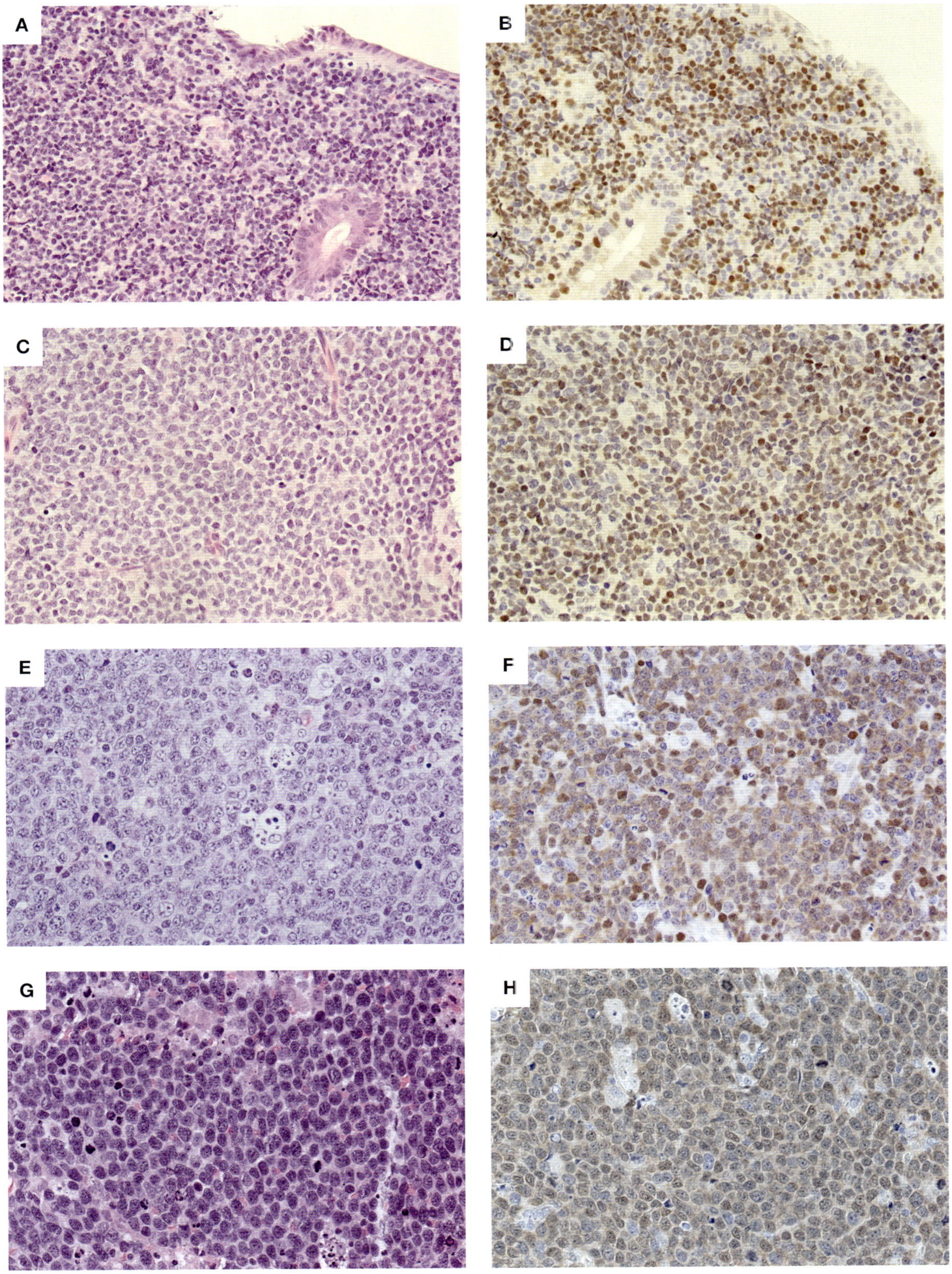

FIGURE 63.3 Cytological variants of mantle cell lymphoma (MCL). **A** and **B:** Small cell MCL localized in the colon mucosa. **C** and **D:** Classic MCL with centrocytic morphology. **E** and **F:** Pleomorphic MCL with starry sky pattern. **G** and **H**. Blastoid MCL with dispersed chromatin. **A, C, D,** and **G:** Hematoxylin and eosin staining. **B, D, F,** and **H:** Cyclin D1 staining.

particularly in nnMCL.[9] Some blastoid/pleomorphic MCL carrying *MYC* translocations may express TdT. These cases are usually SOX11 positive.[11] MCL usually contains a prominent meshwork of follicular dendritic cells. Ki67 staining is very relevant to define prognosis in MCL with a proposed cutoff of 30% defining more aggressive behavior.[12]

Cyclin D1 overexpression is essential for MCL diagnosis since it is negative in virtually all other lymphoid neoplasms (Figures 63.2 and 63.3). It is also detected in the nuclei of histiocytes, endothelial cells, and epithelial cells, providing an internal positive control. Cyclin D1 is expressed in 25% of multiple myelomas, hairy cell leukemia, and proliferation centers of CLL, but *CCND1* rearrangements are negative in the last two entities. SOX11 may be expressed in hairy cell leukemia but not in CLL or multiple myeloma.[13] Cyclin D1 expression has been identified in occasional diffuse large B-cell lymphomas (DLBCLs) with a variable number of cells. However, most of these cases are SOX11 negative and usually do not carry the t(11,14) translocation. However, occasional DLBCL may carry *CCND1* rearrangements as a secondary event.[14,15] The differential diagnosis of these cases may require additional genetic and molecular studies.

SOX11 is a neural transcription factor expressed in the nucleus of most MCLs, including blastoid/pleomorphic variants and cyclin D1–negative MCL carrying *CCND2/D3* rearrangements (Figure 63.4), but not in other B-cell lymphomas apart from weak expression in some Burkitt lymphomas and a proportion of T- and B-lymphoblastic lymphomas. SOX11 is not expressed or is very weak in nnMCL.[13]

Some tumors with morphological and phenotypic features identical to MCL are negative for cyclin D1 expression and rearrangement. SOX11 is highly expressed in these cases (Figure 63.4).[16] Most of these tumors carry *CCND2* and less frequently *CCND3* translocations with IG genes, sometimes cryptic including only the enhancer of kappa or lambda genes inserted in the vicinity of these cyclin genes. Immunohistochemistry is not discriminative enough to distinguish cyclin D2+ or cyclin D3+ MCL from other B-cell lymphomas, but reverse transcription quantitative polymerase chain reaction may reveal high *CCND2* and *CCND3* expression in these MCLs.[16]

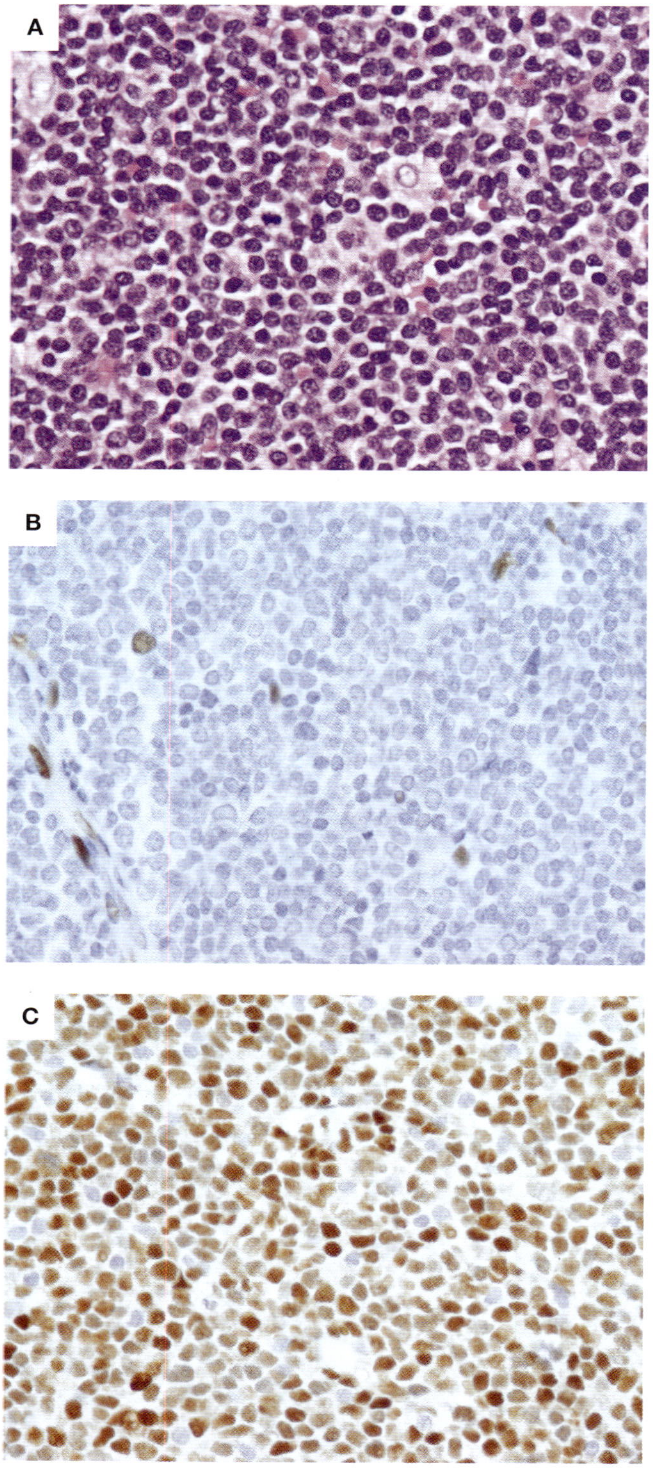

FIGURE 63.4 Cyclin D1–negative mantle cell lymphoma (MCL). **A:** MCL with classic morphology. **B:** Cyclin D1 is negative in tumor cells but positive in the nuclei of endothelial cells and histiocytes. **C:** SOX11 is strongly positive in the nuclei of tumor cells. This case carried a *CCND2* rearrangement.

In Situ Mantle Cell Neoplasia

Cells carrying the t(11;14) translocation have been detected at very low levels with sensitive techniques in the blood of approximately 8% of healthy individuals.[17] These clones can persist for long periods, but their potential to evolve into an overt lymphoma seems extremely low. Cyclin D1–positive cells carrying the

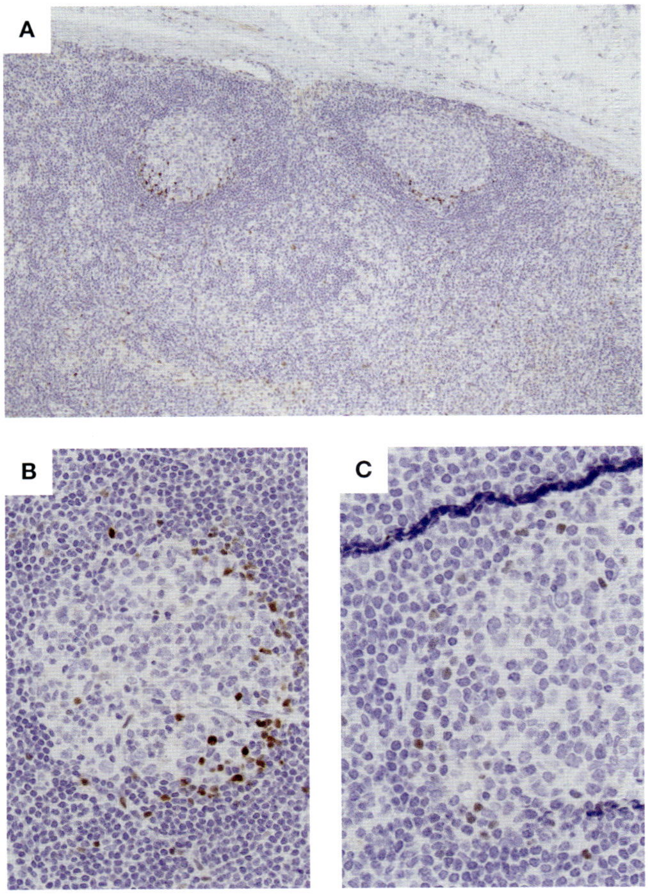

FIGURE 63.5 In situ mantle cell neoplasia. This lymph node was removed from a patient with atopic dermatitis and showed features compatible with dermatopathic lymphadenopathy. Cyclin D1 (**A and B**) staining showed a narrow rim of cyclin D1–positive lymphocytes surrounding germinal centers. These cells were also positive for SOX11 (**C**).

t(11;14) may be incidentally found in the mantle zones of otherwise reactive lymphoid tissue in healthy individuals (Figure 63.5).[18] These lesions are named "in situ MC neoplasia" (isMCN) to emphasize their very low malignant potential. The cells are seen within the inner layers of the mantle cuffs of normal-appearing follicles with preserved lymph node architecture. They may occupy a nonexpanded mantle zone usually intermingled with negative lymphocytes. In some patients, these lesions may be seen in different distant lymph nodes or associated with clonal lymphocytosis, but these findings have not been related to progressive disease, and patients should be managed conservatively.[18] The potential evolution to overt MCL seems very low and may precede development of overt lymphoma by 2 to 15 years.[18,19] Most in situ lesions express CD5 and SOX11, but they may also be negative for these markers. isMCN has been seen associated with other lymphoid neoplasms such as follicular lymphoma, CLL, and marginal zone lymphomas. isMCN must be differentiated from MCL with a mantle zone growth pattern in which the mantles are expanded and densely occupied by cyclin D1–positive cells focally extending to interfollicular areas.

Genetics

Antigen receptor genes and normal cell counterpart

IG genes are clonally rearranged with significantly higher identity with the germline in cMCL (98.7 ± 2.6) than in nnMCL (95.1 ± 1.5). However, a clear cutoff to distinguish both subtypes has not been well defined.[4] MCL has a biased use of several IGHV genes (IGHV4-34, IGHV5-21, IGHV3-51, IGHV3-21, IGHV3-23) and around 10% of MCLs have stereotyped heavy complementary-determining region 3 (VH CDR3) sequences, suggesting that antigen selection plays a role in the pathogenesis of at least a subset of MCL.[4] These findings together with DNA methylation profile support the relationship of cMCL with naïve-like B cells, whereas nnMCL seemed derived from germinal experience memory-like B cell (Figure 63.1).[20]

CCND1 and alternative *CCND2/D3* translocations

The characteristic cytogenetic alteration in MCL is the t(11;14)(q13;q32), which juxtaposes the 5′ region of *CCND1* with regulatory regions of the IG causing its overexpression. *CCND1* translocation with the kappa and lambda loci also occur. These translocations are detected by conventional cytogenetics in up to 65% of MCLs. However, they can be found in virtually all cases by fluorescence in situ hybridization. Break-apart probes for *CCND1* are recommended to identify translocations with the three IG loci.[21] These translocations occur in bone marrow precursors at the pre-B stage of differentiation during the recombination of the V(D)J segments of the IGH variable region mediated by recombination-activating genes (RAG enzymes) in both cMCL and nnMCL.[22] Some MCLs have a secondary translocation or point mutation in the 3′ region of *CCND1* that truncates and stabilizes the transcript leading to higher expression. This alteration is associated with higher proliferation and aggressive behavior. Cyclin D1–negative MCLs carry *CCND2* translocations with IGH in 75% of the cases.[16] The remaining carry *CCND2* or CCND3 translocations, which are usually cryptic including the enhancer regions of kappa and lambda. Cryptic translocations of IG near *CCND1* have been also reported.[23] The t(11;14) translocation is not specific for MCL since it has been found in 20% of multiple myelomas, in occasional DLBCL, and in the progression of other small B-cell neoplasms as a possible secondary event.[14,15]

The main function of cyclin D1 seems to be the deregulation of the cell cycle G1 phase by interactions with CDK4/CDK6 inactivating the suppressor effect of RB1 and possibly the cell cycle inhibitor CDKN1B (p27). Cyclin D1 may have an oncogenic potential independent of its catalytic function acting as a transcriptional modulator of multiple genes or participating in the DNA damage response pathway.[23]

SOX11

SOX11 is highly expressed in cMCL, including cyclin D1–negative variants, but not in nnMCL.[23] SOX11 acts as an oncogene in MCL regulating a broad transcriptional program that includes B-cell differentiation, proliferation, apoptosis, angiogenesis, motility, invasion, and BCR signaling. SOX11 seems to prevent terminal B-cell differentiation by promoting PAX5 expression and blocking BCL6, consistent with the lack of germinal center experience of the SOX11-positive MCL cells. The mechanisms leading to its specific upregulation in MCL are not well understood but seem to be mediated by altered epigenetic regulation.

Secondary genetic events and mutational profile

The most common secondary chromosomal alterations in MCL are losses of chromosomes 1p, 6q, 8p, 9p, 11q, 13q, and 17p and gains in 3q, 7p, 8q, and 18q (Table 63.1).[23] cMCL and particularly blastoid/pleomorphic variants have more complex karyotypes and high-level DNA amplifications than nnMCL and classic variants. Transformed blastoid MCLs display higher aneuploidy and poor outcome compared with de novo tumors.[26] The t(8;14)(q24;q32) targeting *MYC* has been identified in occasional blastoid MCLs with very aggressive clinical course. Copy neutral loss of heterozygosity is an alternative mechanism for the inactivation of mutated tumor suppressor genes such as *TP53*. nnMCL has significantly less chromosomal alterations, with t(11;14) being the sole alteration in some cases. 17p/*TP53* alterations are slightly more frequent in nnMCL than in cMCL. Chromoplexy, chromothripsis, and breakage-fusion-bridge cycles are more frequent in aggressive cMCL variants.[22]

Genomic studies have characterized the profile of alterations that target several pathways with different representation in cMCL and nnMCL (Table 63.1). The most altered pathway is DNA damage response with particular high frequency of *ATM* mutations and deletions (11q22.3), which seems to occur exclusively in cMCL. *TP53* is rarely mutated in low-proliferative-rate tumors but may reach 30% incidence in blastoid/pleomorphic variants and tumors with high proliferation rates. In addition to having mutations in *TP53*, highly proliferative and clinically aggressive MCLs carry frequent deletions of the *CDKN2A/B* locus (9p21) detected in 20% to 30% of blastoid/pleomorphic variants but in less than 5% of classical MCL and not in nnMCL. *CDK4* amplification and inactivating mutations of *RB1* have been found in some aggressive MCLs. Concomitant alterations in *TP53* and *CDKN2A/B* seem to have an additive prognostic effect independent of the Ki-67 index. *CCND1* mutations in the 5′ region are common in nnMCL, whereas truncations of the 3′ untranslated region are seen in both subtypes and associated with aggressive behavior. Activating mutations in different genes of the nuclear factor-κB (NF-κB) and BCR pathways have been observed including *NFKBIE, BIRC3,* and *CARD11* and have been associated with ibrutinib resistance. Activating mutations of *NOTCH1* and *NOTCH2* are usually detected in blastoid/pleomorphic cases. Mutations affecting chromatin modifier genes such as *KMT2D, NSD2,* and *MEF2B* (5%-8%) also occur in MCL. Other recurrent mutations occur in *HNRNPH1* involved in RNA regulation and *UBR5* in ubiquitinization mechanisms.

Prognosis and Clinical Comment

The clinical behavior of MCL is very heterogeneous, with some patients following a very rapid evolution, whereas approximately 20% to 40% may survive over 10 years (median overall survival >6 years with novel therapies). A subset of patients with MCL do not require treatment at diagnosis and may be maintained under a "watch and wait" approach for long periods without detriment to their overall survival.[27] These patients usually have stable disease for several months and are stage I/II with good performance status, no B symptoms, normal LDH levels, and no or limited nodal presentation compared with patients requiring early treatment. No validated biological markers are available to differentiate patients who would benefit of immediate treatment and those who could be expectantly observed. Pathology information should be combined with clinical features to decide the best management.

In cMCL, ongoing responses may be achieved with conventional therapies. Maintenance strategies after induction are improving long-term outcomes. After relapse, patients may again experience a relatively slow course for several months, which may evolve into a more rapid clinical course. In contrast, high-risk cases

TABLE 63.1 Profile of genomic mutations in MCL identified by whole genome/exome sequences

Pathway	Gene	All MCL (%)	cMCL/nnMCL (%)
DNA damage response and telomere maintenance	(11q23) *ATM*[a]	35-50	65/0
	(17p) *TP53*[a]	15-30	20/35
	SAMHD1	4-10	15/0
	TERT[a]	15	10/25
Cell proliferation and survival	5′ *CCND1*	17-21	5/80
	3′ UTR *CCND1*	17-21	20/15
	(8q24) *MYC*[a]	10-15	15/0
Chromatin remodelers	*KMT2D*	14-23	30/<5
	NSD2	11-18	15/0
	SMARCA4	7-9	10/0
	SP140	8-13	15/0
BCR/NFKB	*BIRC3*	5-10	5/<5
	CARD11	5	5/5
	NFKBIE	5	0
NOTCH	*NOTCH1*	5-3	5/<5
	NOTCH2	4-11	5/0
Other	*UBR5*[a]	5-10	5/0
	HNRNPH1	6-10	5/<5
	MEF2B	5-8	5/0
CNA	+3q25-q29	40-43	50/15
	−13q33-q34	33	40/<5
	−1p22	29	40/0
	−13q14	23-26	30/<5
	−6q	15-27	30/<5
	−8p	15-22	15/10
	(−9p21) *CDKN2A/B*[a]	15-20	25/<5
	18q21-q22	11-13	15/0
	+13q33 (*MIR17HG*)	10	10/0

The numbers are a summary of different studies.[22,24,25] Genes with at least 4% mutations have been considered.

CAN, copy number alterations; cMCL, conventional mantle cell lymphoma; MCL, mantle cell lymphoma; nnMCL, nonnodal mantle cell lymphoma; UTR, untranslated region.

[a]Combine mutations and structural alterations.

Nadeu F, Martin-Garcia D, Clot G, et al. Genomic and epigenomic insights into the origin pathogenesis, and clinical behavior of mantle cell lymphoma subtypes. *Blood.* 2020;136(12):1419-1432; Pararajalingam P, Coyle KM, Arthur SE, et al. Coding and noncoding drivers of mantle cell lymphoma identified through exome and genome sequencing. *Blood.* 2020;136(5):572-584; and Yi S, Yan Y, Jin M, et al. Genomic and transcriptomic profiling reveals distinct molecular subsets associated with outcomes in mantle cell lymphoma. *J Clin Invest.* 2022;132(3):e153283. doi:10.1172/JCI153283

(blastoid variants, high cell proliferation, or *TP53* alteration) already initially display a more aggressive clinical course and usually fail to obtain complete remissions.

The *MCL international prognostic index* (MIPI) is a highly informative clinical parameter. Based on four elements (age, Eastern Cooperative Oncology Group [ECOG] performance status, lactate dehydrogenase count, and leukocyte count), it stratifies patients with MCL into three groups—low-, intermediate-, and high-risk groups.

The *proliferative activity* is the most important biological prognostic factor in MCL. A high proliferative index recognized by Ki67 immunostaining (≥30%) results into adverse prognosis and has been validated in randomized trials.[12] Reproducibility of Ki67 assessment among pathologists is challenging, and therefore, standardization has been proposed.[12] Combining MIPI and Ki67 (MIPIc) improves the power of its prediction stratifying patients into four prognostic groups of low, low-intermediate, high-intermediate, and high risk.[12] A gene signature associated with proliferation (MCL35 assay) stratifies patients into high, standard, and low-risk groups, with median overall survival of 1.1, 2.6, and 8.6 years, respectively. This assay can use RNA extracted from routine formalin-fixed paraffin embedded tissue and is highly reproducible, and its prognostic value has been confirmed in different clinical trials.[28]

The main prognostic *genetic alterations* are *TP53*, *CDKN2A* inactivation and *MYC* amplification/rearrangement. The value of *TP53* and *CDKN2A* has been confirmed in numerous clinical trials.[16,29-31] Tumors with *complex karyotypes* (≥3 alterations) have a more aggressive course.[32] The combination of high MIPIc and *TP53* alterations identifies a subset of patients at high risk.[33] *Minimum residual disease* analysis, based on the evaluation of circulating residual lymphoma cells, has shown prognosis value in MCL and may be a parameter that may guide therapy, particularly with new agents.[34]

The management of MCL has changed in the past years owing to stratification of the patients according to stage, age, and particularly biological risk profile.[35] Some patients may be eligible for a watch and wait policy for a long period. In localized cases without additional risk factors, a shortened immunochemotherapy regimen followed by consolidating radiotherapy is considered appropriate. For young, fit patients with advanced disease requiring treatment, immunotherapy with cytarabine-based regimens in combination with ibrutinib (and optional autologous transplant) has produced a remarkable improvement in progression-free survival. Less intense regimens are recommended for patients who cannot tolerate these regimens, including immunotherapy combined with different chemotherapy regimens.[35] Subsequent rituximab maintenance is currently considered standard of care for younger and elderly patients. In relapsed disease, molecular targeted therapies, namely, Bruton tyrosine kinase inhibitors (BTKis), are preferred at least in early relapses. Lenalidomide in combination with rituximab achieves also high response rates.[35] New molecular targeted combinations and immunotherapeutic approaches (CAR-T cells) are available after BTKi failure.[34]

References

1. Swerdlow SH, Campo E, Harris NL, et al. WHO classification of tumours of haematopoietic and lymphoid tissues. World Health Organization Classification of Tumours. 4th ed, Vol 2. IARC; 2017:439.
2. Campo E, Jaffe ES, Cook JR, et al. The international consensus classification of mature lymphoid neoplasms: a report from the clinical advisory Committee. *Blood.* 2022;140(11):1229-1253. doi:10.1182/blood.2022015851
3. Sander B, Campo E, Hsi ED. Chronic lymphocytic leukaemia/small lymphocytic lymphoma and mantle cell lymphoma: from early lesions to transformation. *Virchows Arch.* 2023;482(1):131-145. doi:10.1007/s00428-022-03460-y
4. Puente XS, Jares P, Campo E. Chronic lymphocytic leukemia and mantle cell lymphoma: crossroads of genetic and microenvironment interactions. *Blood.* 2018;131(21):2283-2296. doi:10.1182/blood-2017-10-764373
5. Morello L, Rattotti S, Giordano L, et al. Mantle cell lymphoma of mucosa-associated lymphoid tissue: a European mantle cell lymphoma network study. *Hemasphere.* 2020;4(1):e302. doi:10.1097/HS9.0000000000000302
6. Cheah CY, George A, Giné E, et al. Central nervous system involvement in mantle cell lymphoma: clinical features, prognostic factors and outcomes from the European Mantle Cell Lymphoma Network. *Ann Oncol.* 2013;24(8):2119-2123. doi:10.1093/annonc/mdt139
7. Ferrer A, Salaverria I, Bosch F, et al. Leukemic involvement is a common feature in mantle cell lymphoma. *Cancer.* 2007;109(12):2473-2480. doi:10.1002/cncr.22715
8. Hu Z, Medeiros LJ, Chen Z, et al. Mantle cell lymphoma with MYC rearrangement: a report of 17 patients. *Am J Surg Pathol.* 2017;41(2):216-224. doi:10.1097/PAS.0000000000000758
9. Ribera-Cortada I, Martinez D, Amador V, et al. Plasma cell and terminal B-cell differentiation in mantle cell lymphoma mainly occur in the SOX11-negative subtype. *Mod Pathol.* 2015;28(11):1435-1447. doi:10.1038/modpathol.2015.99
10. Papathomas TG, Venizelos I, Dunphy CH, et al. Mantle cell lymphoma as a component of composite lymphoma: clinicopathologic parameters and biologic implications. *Hum Pathol.* 2012;43(4):467-480. doi:10.1016/j.humpath.2011.08.024
11. Aukema SM, Croci GA, Bens S, et al. Mantle cell lymphomas with concomitant MYC and CCND1 breakpoints are recurrently TdT positive and frequently show high-grade pathological and genetic features. *Virchows Arch.* 2021;479(1):133-145. doi:10.1007/s00428-021-03022-8
12. Hoster E, Rosenwald A, Berger F, et al. Prognostic value of Ki-67 index, cytology, and growth pattern in mantle-cell lymphoma: results from randomized trials of the European mantle cell lymphoma network. *J Clin Oncol.* 2016;34(12):1386-1394. doi:10.1200/JCO.2015.63.8387
13. Beekman R, Amador V, Campo E, et al. SOX11, a key oncogenic factor in mantle cell lymphoma. *Curr Opin Hematol.* 2018;25(4):299-306. doi:10.1097/moh.0000000000000434
14. Cheng J, Hashem MA, Barabe F, et al. CCND1 genomic rearrangement as a secondary event in high grade B-cell

lymphoma. *Hemasphere*. 2021;5(1):e505. doi:10.1097/HS9.0000000000000505

15. Özoğul E, Montaner A, Pol M, et al. Large B-cell lymphomas with CCND1 rearrangement have different immunoglobulin gene breakpoints and genomic profile than mantle cell lymphoma. *Blood Cancer J*. 2024;14(1):166. doi: 10.1038/s41408-024-01146-z
16. Martin-Garcia D, Navarro A, Valdes-Mas R, et al. CCND2 and CCND3 hijack immunoglobulin light-chain enhancers in cyclin D1(-) mantle cell lymphoma. *Blood*. 2019;133(9):940-951. doi:10.1182/blood-2018-07-862151
17. Lecluse Y, Lebailly P, Roulland S, Gac AC, Nadel B, Gauduchon P. t(11;14)-positive clones can persist over a long period of time in the peripheral blood of healthy individuals. *Leukemia*. 2009;23(6):1190-1193. doi:10.1038/leu.2009.31
18. Carvajal-Cuenca A, Sua LF, Silva NM, et al. In situ mantle cell lymphoma: clinical implications of an incidental finding with indolent clinical behavior. *Haematologica*. 2012;97(2):270-278.
19. Adam P, Schiefer AI, Prill S, et al. Incidence of preclinical manifestations of mantle cell lymphoma and mantle cell lymphoma in situ in reactive lymphoid tissues. *Mod Pathol*. 2012;25(12):1629-1636. doi:10.1038/modpathol.2012.117
20. Queiros AC, Beekman R, Vilarrasa-Blasi R, et al. Decoding the DNA methylome of mantle cell lymphoma in the light of the entire B cell lineage. *Cancer Cell*. 2016;30(5):806-821. doi:10.1016/j.ccell.2016.09.014
21. Sander B, Quintanilla-Martinez L, Ott G, et al. Mantle cell lymphoma—a spectrum from indolent to aggressive disease. *Virchows Arch*. 2016;468(3):245-257. doi:10.1007/s00428-015-1840-6
22. Nadeu F, Martin-Garcia D, Clot G, et al. Genomic and epigenomic insights into the origin, pathogenesis, and clinical behavior of mantle cell lymphoma subtypes. *Blood*. 2020;136(12):1419-1432. doi:10.1182/blood.2020005289
23. Navarro A, Bea S, Jares P, Campo E. Molecular pathogenesis of mantle cell lymphoma. *Hematol Oncol Clin North Am*. 2020;34(5):795-807. doi:10.1016/j.hoc.2020.05.002
24. Pararajalingam P, Coyle KM, Arthur SE, et al. Coding and noncoding drivers of mantle cell lymphoma identified through exome and genome sequencing. *Blood*. 2020;136(5):572-584. doi:10.1182/blood.2019002385
25. Yi S, Yan Y, Jin M, et al. Genomic and transcriptomic profiling reveals distinct molecular subsets associated with outcomes in mantle cell lymphoma. *J Clin Invest*. 2022;132(3):e153283. doi:10.1172/JCI153283
26. Jain P, Zhang S, Kanagal-Shamanna R, et al. Genomic profiles and clinical outcomes of de novo blastoid/pleomorphic MCL are distinct from those of transformed MCL. *Blood Adv*. 2020;4(6):1038-1050. doi:10.1182/bloodadvances.2019001396
27. Kumar A, Ying Z, Alperovich A, et al. Clinical presentation determines selection of patients for initial observation in mantle cell lymphoma. *Haematologica*. 2019;104(4):e163-e166. doi:10.3324/haematol.2018.201350
28. Scott DW, Abrisqueta P, Wright GW, et al. New molecular assay for the proliferation signature in mantle cell lymphoma applicable to formalin-fixed paraffin-embedded biopsies. *J Clin Oncol*. 2017;35(15):1668-1677. doi:10.1200/JCO.2016.70.7901
29. Delfau-Larue MH, Klapper W, Berger F, et al. High-dose cytarabine does not overcome the adverse prognostic value of CDKN2A and TP53 deletions in mantle cell lymphoma. *Blood*. 2015;126(5):604-611. doi:10.1182/blood-2015-02-628792
30. Eskelund CW, Dahl C, Hansen JW, et al. TP53 mutations identify younger mantle cell lymphoma patients who do not benefit from intensive chemoimmunotherapy. *Blood*. 2017;130(17):1903-1910. doi:10.1182/blood-2017-04-779736
31. Ferrero S, Rossi D, Rinaldi A, et al. KMT2D mutations and TP53 disruptions are poor prognostic biomarkers in mantle cell lymphoma receiving high-dose therapy: a FIL study. *Haematologica*. 2020;105(6):1604-1612.
32. Clot G, Jares P, Gine E, et al. A gene signature that distinguishes conventional and leukemic nonnodal mantle cell lymphoma helps predict outcome. *Blood*. 2018;132(4):413-422. doi:10.1182/blood-2018-03-838136
33. Scheubeck G, Jiang L, Hermine O, et al. Clinical outcome of mantle cell lymphoma patients with high-risk disease (high-risk MIPI-c or high p53 expression). *Leukemia*. 2023;37(9):1887-1894. doi:10.1038/s41375-023-01977-y
34. Giné E, de la Cruz F, Jiménez Ubieto A, et al. Ibrutinib in combination with Rituximab for indolent clinical forms of mantle cell lymphoma (IMCL-2015): a multicenter, open-label, single-arm, phase II trial. *J Clin Oncol*. 2022;40(11):1196-1205.
35. Silkenstedt E, Linton K, Dreyling M. Mantle cell lymphoma—advances in molecular biology, prognostication and treatment approaches. *Br J Haematol*. 2021;195(2):162-173. doi:10.1111/bjh.17419

Chapter 64

Diffuse Large B-Cell Lymphoma, Not Otherwise Specified

Elias Campo, Andrew Davies, Stefan Dirnhofer, George Lenz, John P. Leonard, Ari Melnick, Astrid Pavlovsky, Stefano A. Pileri, Gilles Salles, David W. Scott, Laurie H. Sehn, Margaret A. Shipp, Louis Staudt, Wyndham H. Wilson, and Jane N. Winter

Definition

Diffuse large B-cell lymphoma (DLBCL), not otherwise specified (NOS), is a neoplasm of large B lymphocytes whose nuclei are the same size or larger than those of normal macrophages, or more than twice the size of those of normal lymphocytes, with a diffuse growth pattern, without features of other specific entities also composed of large B cells (Table 64.1).[1] Therefore, it is a diagnosis of exclusion. It can arise de novo or as a transformation from a low-grade B-cell neoplasm, such as follicular lymphoma (FL) or chronic lymphocytic leukemia (CLL).

DLBCL, NOS is a heterogeneous disease. Different morphologic and phenotypic variants as well as molecular and genomic subtypes are recognized, although the clinical implication of many of these is an evolving area of study. The most well-established molecular subtypes are based on the cell of origin (COO) with germinal center B-cell-like (GCB) and activated B-cell-like (ABC) subtypes.

Synonyms

None.

Epidemiology

DLBCL is the most common lymphoma worldwide representing 30% to 40% of all adult lymphomas with an incidence of 6.9 cases per 100,000 in the United States, slightly higher in males than in females (rate 1.49) and in non-Hispanic whites than in other racial groups.[2] The frequency of this lymphoma is higher in developing countries.[1] The median patient age is in the seventh decade, but these tumors may also occur in children and young adults.

General Clinical Features

Most patients present with nodal disease, although any organ can be involved, and multiple sites are involved in 30% of patients.[1] Extranodal sites are involved in 25% to 40% with common locations including the gastrointestinal tract, liver, and lung. Lymphomas at specific topographic sites such as central nervous system (CNS), testis, mediastinum, or skin may correspond to distinct entities (Table 64.1). Approximately 50% of patients have localized disease (stage I/II), and some

TABLE 64.1 Large B-cell lymphomas with a diffuse growth pattern[a]

Predominantly nodal
Diffuse large B-cell lymphoma, NOS
Germinal center B-cell-like subtype
Activated B-cell-like subtype
Large B-cell lymphoma with 11q aberration[b]
T-cell/histiocyte-rich large B-cell lymphoma
Extranodal
Primary diffuse large B-cell lymphoma of the central nervous system
Primary diffuse large B-cell lymphoma of the testis[b]
Primary cutaneous diffuse large B-cell lymphoma, leg type
Intravascular large B-cell lymphoma
HHV-8 and Epstein-Barr virus–negative primary effusion-based lymphoma[b]
Primary mediastinal large B-cell lymphoma
Mediastinal gray-zone lymphoma[b]
Epstein-Barr virus related
Epstein-Barr virus–positive diffuse large B-cell lymphoma, NOS
Diffuse large B-cell lymphoma associated with chronic inflammation
Fibrin-associated diffuse large B-cell lymphoma
Large cell lymphoma with terminal B-cell differentiation
ALK-positive large B-cell lymphoma
Plasmablastic lymphoma
HHV-8-positive diffuse large B-cell lymphoma, NOS
Primary effusion lymphoma
High-grade B-cell lymphomas
High-grade B-cell lymphoma, with MYC and BCL2 rearrangements[b]
High grade B-cell lymphoma with MYC *and* BCL6 *rearrangements*[b]

[a]Other lymphomas with large cells (eg, nodular lymphocyte predominant B-cell lymphoma, large B-cell lymphoma with *IRF4* rearrangement) are not considered in this table because they frequently have a follicular pattern and their biological and clinical behavior are more indolent than most of the neoplasms with a diffuse growth pattern.
Italic font indicates provisional disease entities.
[b]Changes from the World Health Organization revised fourth edition classification.
HHV, human herpesvirus; NOS, not otherwise specified.

localized tumors may be bulky. Clinical presentation is heterogeneous, related to both the site of involvement and/or the presence of B symptoms.

Morphology

Nodal involvement by DLBCL, NOS may show partial or, more commonly, total architectural effacement by a diffuse proliferation of tumor cells that may extend beyond the capsule. Partial infiltration may respect reactive follicles and grow in interfollicular areas or have sinusoidal infiltration. Preexisting reactive follicles may be infiltrated by the tumor cells with destruction of the underlying follicular dendritic cell meshwork that should not be diagnosed as FL, grade 3B.[3] Extranodal involvement may efface the normal architecture of the organ, ulcerating mucosal surfaces, or may preserve preexisting structures. Sclerosis may be present.

The three common cytologic variants are centroblastic, immunoblastic, and anaplastic, although other rare variants and cases with variability may be seen.[1] They are not used for clinical decisions, but it is important to recognize them for the differential diagnosis. Centroblastic cytology is the most common and is composed of large cells with oval to round nuclei, with fine chromatin and two to four membrane-bound nucleoli with scant amphophilic or basophilic cytoplasm (Figure 64.1A). Some centroblastic tumors have multilobated nuclei (Figure 64.1B). The immunoblastic variant is considered when >90% of cells are immunoblasts having oval nuclei, vesicular chromatin, a single large central nucleolus and abundant basophilic cytoplasm (Figure 64.1C). Some cells may have plasmacytoid differentiation with an eccentric nucleus and paranuclear pale (Golgi) area[4] and must be distinguished from plasmablastic/plasma cell neoplasms by phenotyping. The anaplastic variant is characterized by very large cells with pleomorphic nuclei that may be multinucleated and mimic Reed-Sternberg cells or other neoplasms. The tumor cells may be very cohesive and have sinusoidal pattern mimicking metastatic carcinoma. Uncommon cytologic variants include tumors with myxoid or fibrillary stroma, pseudorosette formation, and spindle-shaped tumor cells or those with signet ring morphology.[1]

The tumor microenvironment may contain a variable number of inflammatory cells and evidence of angiogenesis. Some tumors have a stroma rich in T cells and histiocytes that may mimic T-cell/histocyte-rich large B-cell lymphoma, but the presence of sheets of tumor cells excludes this diagnosis. Epithelioid granulomas may be seen in some cases. Areas of necrosis may be focal to extensive. Some cases may have a nodal infarction obscuring the tumor cells.

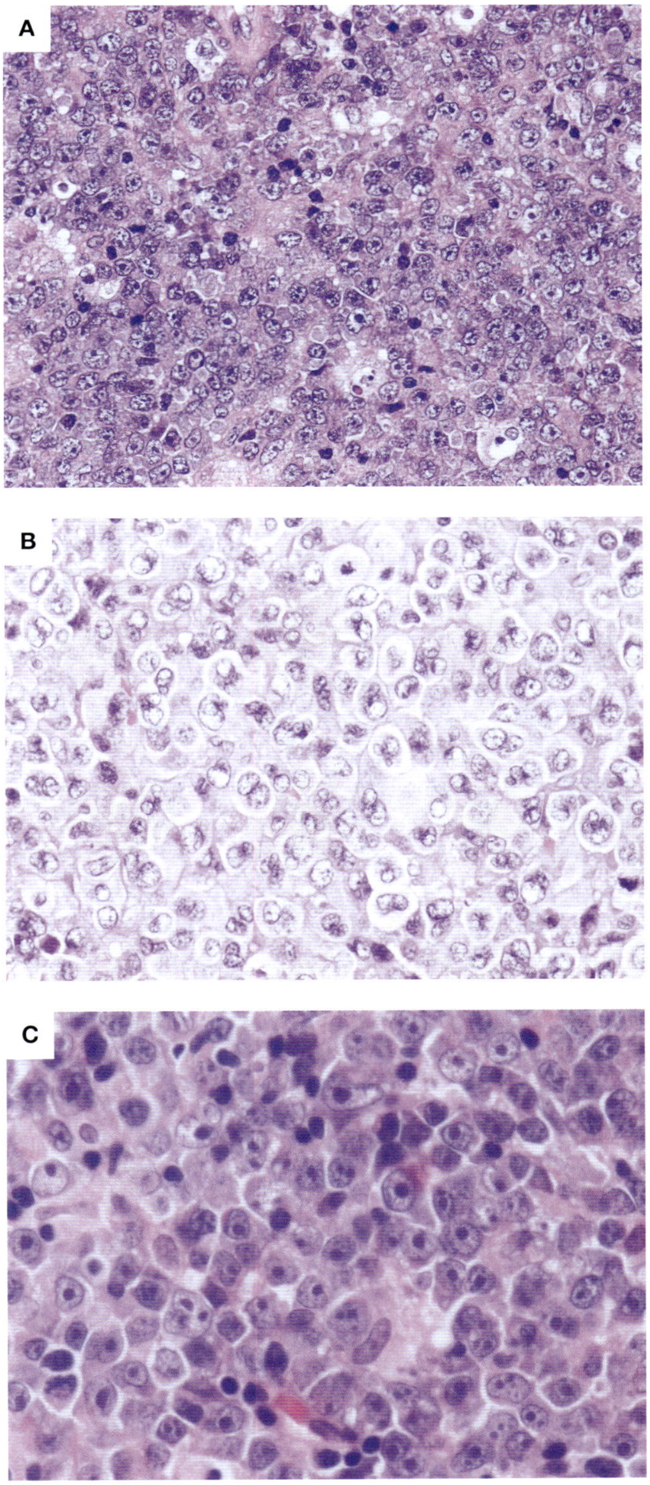

FIGURE 64.1 Diffuse large B-cell lymphoma, not otherwise specified, cytologic variants. **A:** Centroblastic polymorphic variant showing centroblast mixed with immunoblasts. **B:** Centroblastic variant with multilobated nuclei. **C:** Immunoblastic: The neoplastic cells have a large central nucleoli in most of the cells.

Some DLBCLs are transformed from small B-cell lymphomas that may still be present focally in the same biopsy. In these cases, the diagnosis should include the presence and estimated percent of the DLBCL and low-grade components in the biopsy. Establishing the clonal relationship between the low-grade and the DLBCL components may distinguish a real transformation from a second, unrelated malignancy.[5]

Bone marrow may be involved in 15% of patients. Two patterns are recognized: concordant when the tumor cells are large as in the primary tumor, and discordant when the infiltrating cells correspond to a small B-cell lymphoma. Concordant but not discordant involvement confers an adverse prognosis.[6]

Immunophenotype

The neoplastic cells express mature B-cell markers CD19, CD20, CD22, CD79a, CD79b, and PAX5 but may lose expression of some following anti-CD20 treatment or anti-CD19 CAR-T-cell therapy.[7] Surface and cytoplasmic immunoglobulins may be detected in 75% of the tumors, mainly IgM, and less commonly IgG or IgA. Cytoplasmic immunoglobulins are more frequently seen in tumors with plasmacytoid differentiation, but expression of plasma cell markers such as CD138 is uncommon and should raise diagnostic consideration of other, plasmablastic subtypes of lymphoma (Table 64.1).[4] CD30 is expressed in 15% to 25% of cases, particularly with anaplastic morphology. Ki67 proliferation index is usually high (>30%-80%) but can rarely be lower or higher. High Ki67 by itself is not a criterion to classify high-grade lymphoma.

Aberrant expression of T-cell markers may be seen in 5% to 15% of the patients. CD5 expression should prompt exclusion of underlying CLL or mantle cell lymphoma but can be seen in de novo DLBCL.[5] Cyclin D1 expression without *CCND1* rearrangements may be seen in 1% to 2% of DLBCL that are CD5 and SOX11 negative. However, occasional DLBCLs carry this translocation, usually as a secondary event.[8]

Immunohistochemistry (IHC) algorithms have been developed to identify the DLBCL COO subtypes, which provide prognostic and biologic information, in place of less practical gene expression profiling (GEP) assays (see later discussion).[8] The most widely accepted of these is the Hans algorithm, which uses CD10, BCL6, and IRF4/MUM1 stains.[9] Expression of CD10, BCL6, and MUM1/IRF4 is highly variable with positivity in 20% to 40%, 60% to 90%, and 35% to 65% of DLBCL, respectively (Figure 64.2). The cutoff for positivity using these markers is 30% of malignant cells. Using the Hans algorithm (Figure 64.3), DLBCL is divided into GCB and non-GCB (an approximation of the ABC

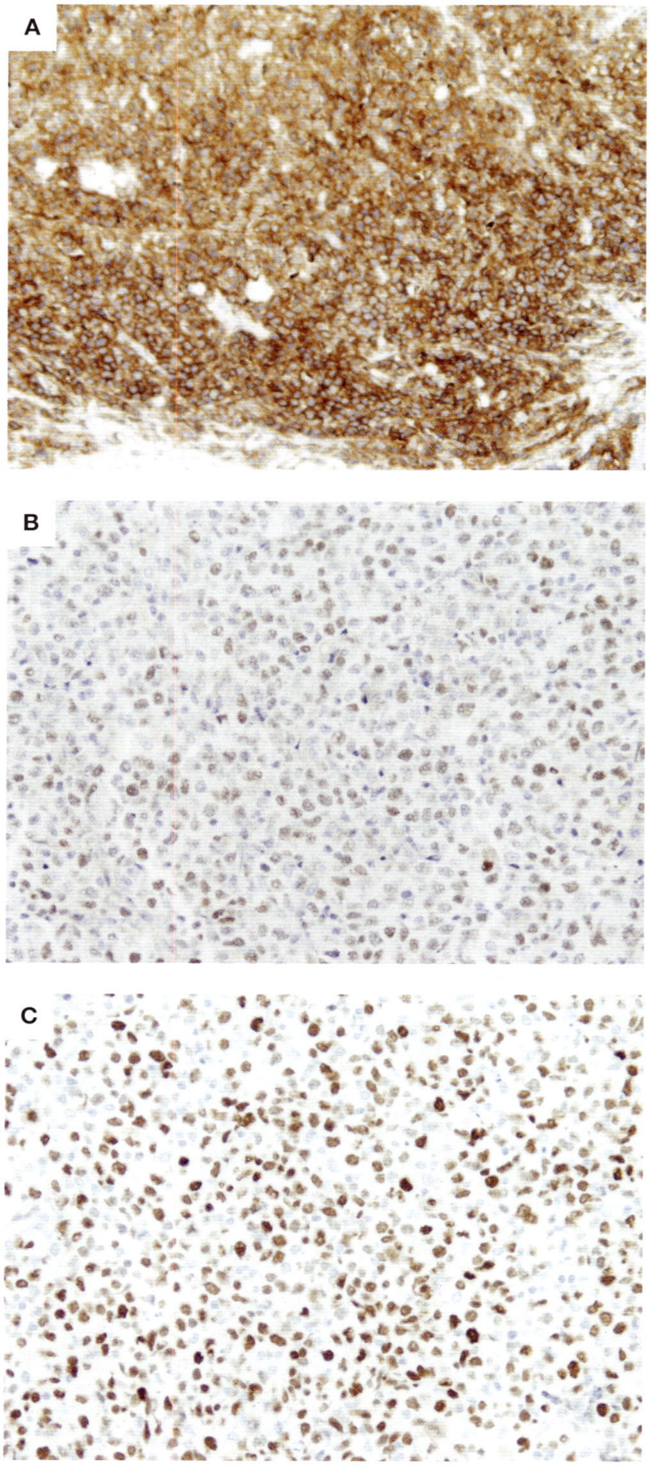

FIGURE 64.2 Immunophenotype of Diffuse large B-cell lymphoma (DLBCL), not otherwise specified (NOS). **A:** CD10 expression in GCB-like DLBCL, NOS. **B:** BCL6 expression in a GCB-like DLBCL. **C:** MUM1/IRF4 expression in an ABC-like DLBCL.

subtype) COO. By GEP, and to a more variable extent by IHC, GCB subtype DLBCLs have a more favorable prognosis than non-GCB/ABC cases (see later discussion). Cases expressing CD10, BCL6, and MUM1 should raise consideration of large B-cell lymphoma with *IRF4* rearrangement.[10]

BCL2 expression has been reported in 50% to 80% of the cases (Figure 64.4A). MYC expression is reported in a variable number of cases (10%-60%), depending on technical aspects, but an underlying translocation is detected only in 5% to 15% of tumors[11] (Figure 64.4B). Expression of both BCL2 and MYC (using cutoffs of 50% and 40%, respectively) without dual rearrangement of *MYC* and *BCL2* has been observed in 25% to 40% of tumors, and these have been called double protein expressers.[12] The reported association with an adverse prognosis of these cases has been related to their higher frequency in ABC subtype and association with other adverse factors, such as *TP53* alterations.[8] While these cases are consistently associated with poor prognosis, the International Consensus Classification (ICC) deemphasizes double protein expresser status within the classification, since this phenomenon most probably represents the final stage of different biological pathways.[13]

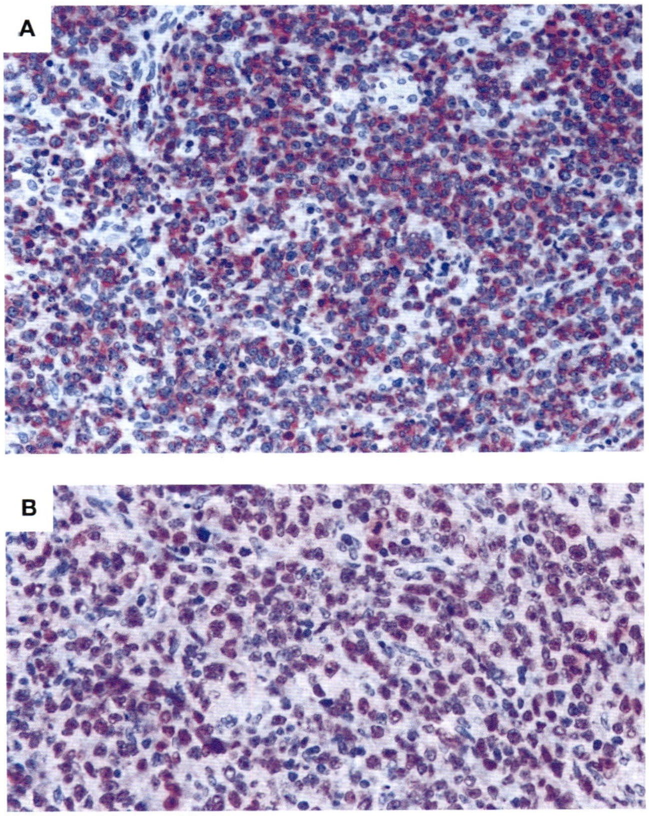

FIGURE 64.4 **A:** BCL2 cytoplasmic expression in a diffuse large B-cell lymphoma, not otherwise specified (DLBCL, NOS). **B:** MYC nuclear expression in a DLBCL, NOS.

Genetics

Molecular subtypes: cell of origin

GEP studies have identified two major DLBCL subtypes based on COO, with expression profile reminiscent of germinal center B cells (GCB-like) or that of post–germinal center B cells with overexpression of genes related to activation of the B cell (ABC-like) and plasmacytic differentiation.[12,14] The statistical models used to assign tumors to these categories recognize 50% to 60% GCB and 30% to 40% ABC and leave around 10% to 20% of cases unclassified. GCB and ABC DLBCLs differ in their basic pathogenic mechanisms. GCB lymphomas have activation of the PI3K/Akt/mTOR signaling pathway with absence of expression of the negative regulator PTEN in 50% of the cases and frequent expression of BCL6. Genetic alterations in these cases include the t(14;18) in around 40% of cases and frequent mutations in chromatin modifiers (*KMT2D*, *EZH2*, *CREBBP*) and other germinal center relevant genes such as *GNA13*, *FOXO1*, *TNFRSF14*, and *MEF2B*. ABC tumors have constitutive activation of the B-cell receptor (BCR) and NF-kB pathways and blockade of the terminal plasma cell differentiation. Frequently mutated genes in these cases are *MYD88*, *CD79B*, *CARD11*, *BCL10*, and *TNFAIP3* activating NFKB pathway and *PRMD1* blocking differentiation, among others. *BCL6* translocations are common.

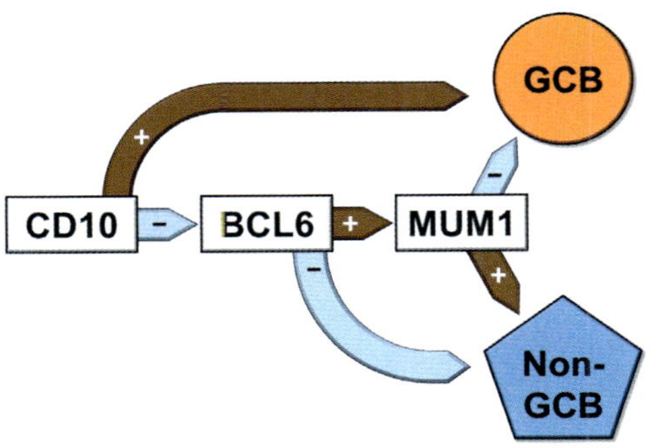

FIGURE 64.3 Hans algorithm for cell-of-origin determination by immunohistochemistry in Diffuse large B-cell lymphoma, not otherwise specified. GCB, germinal center B cell. (Utilized with permission from King et al. *Biopsy Interpretation of the Lymph Node*. Wolters Kluwer; 2023.)

GCB and ABC DLBCLs also differ in the clinical outcomes of patients treated with standard immunochemotherapy with 3-year overall survival of 80% and 60% for GCB and ABC, respectively. Although initial studies evaluating targeted therapies based on COO have shown disappointing results, a reanalysis of one of these studies suggested a benefit with a BTK inhibitor when specific genetic alterations were considered and when the ABC/GCB assignment was performed with GEP instead of IHC algorithms.[15] These findings suggest that the binary (GCB/ABC) molecular subclassification of DLBCL, NOS may not be sufficient to drive management decisions, which may require further discrimination of these categories. Despite this limitation, GCB/ABC molecular subtypes provide a basic biological division of DLBCL with prognostic impact. The ICC recommends maintaining the COO subtyping in the diagnosis of DLBCL, NOS using gene expression or IHC algorithms recognizing the limitations of the latter.[13]

Molecular subtypes: high-grade signatures

Recent studies have identified a novel gene expression signature in aggressive B-cell lymphomas related to the highly proliferative centroblastic cells of the dark zone of the germinal center.[16,17] This has been termed "dark-zone signature" or "molecular high grade" and is seen in Burkitt lymphoma (BL) and most tumors carrying rearrangements of *MYC* and *BCL2* (high-grade B-cell lymphoma with *MYC* and *BCL2* rearrangements [HGBCL-DH-*BCL2*]), as well as other GCB DLBCLs. Intriguingly, over 50% of the tumors expressing these high-grade signatures are not BL or HGBCL-DH-*BCL2,* although in some cases the rearrangements may be cryptic. These high-grade signatures are expressed in ~10% to 15% of DLBCL and 70% to 80% of HGBCL-DH-*BCL2*.[16] Phenotypically they are almost invariably GCB, frequently expressing CD10. Clinically, they are very aggressive. Interestingly a small subset of tumors carrying *MYC* and *BCL2* rearrangements but not expressing this signature have different molecular alterations and more favorable outcome. Therefore, this signature may identify a novel molecular subtype of aggressive B-cell lymphoma, divided between the categories of HGBCL-DH-*BCL2*, high-grade B-cell lymphoma, NOS and DLBCL, NOS in the current classification.[16] Future studies should clarify if this is a novel entity better defined by this molecular signature.

Functional subtypes

Transcriptional analysis of DLBCL has identified three subtypes with different functional characteristics that have been named BCR/proliferation, oxidative phosphorylation (OxPhos), and host response (HR) subgroups.[18] The BCR/proliferative subgroup is characterized by overexpression of genes involved in BCR signaling and frequent translocation of *BCL6*. It has been suggested that these tumors may be candidates for inhibitors of the BCR and BCL6 pathway. The OxPhos subgroup is significantly enriched in genes involved in mitochondrial function and elevated oxidative phosphorylation. Contrary to the BCR group, these tumors do not have active/functional BCR signaling. Interestingly, Richter transformation displays a similar pattern with low BCR signaling and high OxPhos activity.[19] The HR subgroup is characterized by a strong immune response with prominent T- and dendritic-cell signatures similar to those seen in T-cell/histiocyte-rich large B-cell lymphoma.

Antigen receptor genes

The IGH and light chains are clonally rearranged and carry somatic hypermutations in most cases with ongoing mutation in the GCB subtype.

Structural rearrangements

The most common recurrent translocations in DLBCL, NOS involve *BCL2 (*18q21*)*, *BCL6* (3q27*)*, and *MYC (*8q24*)* in approximately 20% to 30%, 30%, and 5% to 15% of tumors, respectively. *BCL2* is usually translocated with IGH, occurs almost exclusively in the GCB subtype, and is associated with high BCL2 expression levels. *BCL6* may be rearranged with IG (60%) and non-IG (40%) genes, and it is slightly more common in ABC (25%-30%) than in GCB (10%-15%) tumors. *MYC* is equally translocated to IG (mostly IGH) or non-IG genes, such as *PAX5*, *BCL6*, *BCL11A*, and *IKZF1*. *MYC* translocations usually occur in the context of complex karyotypes, and approximately 60% to 80% of the tumors also have *BCL2* and/or *BCL6* rearrangements. The presence of these double (or triple) genetic hits changes the diagnosis to HGBCL-DH-*BCL2* or "HGBCL with *MYC* and *BCL6* rearrangements" (HGBCL-DH-*BCL6*) (see Chapters 82 and 83). Isolated *MYC* translocation without *BCL2* or *BCL6* rearrangement may be seen in 30% of immunoblastic DLBCLs, which frequently express CD10,[20] and the prognostic impact of this finding remains controversial. These translocations are usually associated with high protein expression, but up to 30% of the tumors with *MYC* rearrangement may have low or nondetectable MYC protein by IHC. This is due to low mRNA expression in some cases or the presence of the *MYC* N11S polymorphism (8% cases) that renders the protein undetectable by certain antibodies.[11]

In clinical practice, fluorescence in situ hybridization (FISH) break-apart probes (BAPs) for *MYC*, *BCL2*, and *BCL6* are recommended due to the frequent use of partners other than IGH genes, especially in *MYC* and *BCL6* translocations. However, combining BAP and dual-fusion *MYC*-IGH probes diminishes the rate of false-negative cases. Given that no pathological clues can predict the presence of these rearrangements, the recommendation is to use FISH in all DLBCLs to detect tumors with these diagnostic rearrangements. IHC may not be fully reliable since there are cases carrying translocations, particularly *MYC*, with very low or negative expression and, vice versa, cases with strong MYC and BCL2 expression without the translocations. High Ki67, although frequently seen in HGBCL-DH-*BCL2* and HGBCL-DH-*BCL6* tumors, is not predictive of the presence of *MYC* translocations. If resources are limited, an acceptable approach may be to start with *MYC* probes and, if positive, follow with *BCL2* and *BCL6* probes and/or restrict the FISH analysis to tumors with a GCB phenotype, particularly CD10 positive. This later approach, however, may miss HGBCL-DH-*BCL6* that are phenotypically more heterogeneous.

Copy number alterations

DNA copy number alterations (CNAs) are common in DLBCL with differentially represented regions in GCB and ABC tumors and genomic subtypes.[21] Gain/amplifications and deletions can be associated with activating or inactivating mutations, respectively, of the target genes in these regions. *BCL2*, *BCL6*, and *MYC* may have gains/amplifications, but their significance is difficult to assess in the literature due to different definitions of these alterations. *MYC* gains (three to four copies)/high gains (≥5 copies) are detected in 20% of cases, but they are not associated with high *MYC* expression levels. Occasional cases, however, may show uncountable copies (amplification) of *MYC* with high levels of RNA expression.[11] Although *BCL2* CNA (30%) are associated with high expression, it is not currently clear whether they have similar biological significance to the translocation. Therefore, CNA of *BCL2* and *MYC* should not be considered equivalent to translocations for the definition of HGBCL-DH lymphomas.

GCB-DLBCLs carry recurrent deletions in 1p36 targeting *TNFRS14* (30%) facilitating immune escape, del(10q23) including *PTEN* (10%), and gains/amplifications of 13q31 (*MIR17HG*) involved in proliferation and antiapoptotic pathways. ABC-DLBCLs are characterized by frequent trisomy 3 and gains of 3q (*BCL6*, *FOXP1*) (20%), gains/amplifications of 19q13 (*SPIB*) (26%) involved in NF-kB activation with *CARD11*, and 18q21-q22 (*BCL2*) (55%). Common deletions affect 6q21-q22 (45%) targeting *TNFAIP3* and *PRDM1* activating the NF-kB pathway and blocking terminal differentiation, respectively. Other frequent CNAs in all subtypes of DLBCL are del(17p13) (*TP53*) and del(9p21) (*CDKN2A/B*) associated with adverse prognosis and deletions of 15q21 (*B2M* and *CD58*) and 19p13 (*CD70*) providing mechanisms of immune escape.

Genomic subtypes

The molecular heterogeneity of DLBCL has been further refined with the use of large-scale genomic studies that have identified up to seven subtypes in three independent studies (Table 64.2).[22-24] They expand the molecular COO classification of DLBCL providing new insights into pathogenic mechanisms and clinical features that may assist in future therapeutic decisions. Although the subtypes in the three models are relatively similar, there are also some differences. The Chapuy et al. system classifies all cases in any of their five clusters, whereas the models generated by Wright et al. and Lacy et al leave 27% to 37% of cases unclassified. Approximately 5% of cases may be classified in more than one subtype.

One of the subtypes is MCD/C5/MYD88, composed of tumors that virtually all have an ABC COO and carry frequent mutations in *MYD88*(L265P) and *CD79B*. Other common mutated genes are *ETV6*, *PIM1*, *PRDM1*, *TBL1XR1*, and *BTG1*. *CDKN2A/B* is frequently deleted, whereas *BCL2* and *SPIB* are commonly gained/amplified. Tumors of this subtype have activated BCR and NF-kB signaling. In addition, this group of lymphomas has frequent (70%) alterations that facilitate immune escape including inactivation of MHC class I and CD58 and overexpression of *CD274* (PD-L1) and *PDCD1LG2* (PD-L2). This genomic profile is shared by a group of extranodal DLBCL that arises in immune-privileged sites such as primary DLBCL of CNS and primary DLBCL of the testis, and also primary cutaneous DLBCL, leg type, intravascular large B-cell lymphoma, and primary DLBCL of other extranodal sites such as breast and adrenal. The outcome of these patients treated with conventional immunochemotherapy is unfavorable. Some studies suggest that these patients may respond to the inhibition of BCR signaling.[15]

BN2/C1/NOTCH2 is a frequent subtype of tumors with a heterogeneous COO. The most frequent mutated genes are *NOTCH2* and its negative regulator *SPEN* (50%) accompanied by *BCL6* translocations (70%). Other mutations target the BCR-dependent NF-kB pathway including *CD79B*, *BCL10*, *TNFAIP3*, cell cycle activation (*CCND3*), and immune escape (*B2M* and *CD70*). *MYD88* may be mutated but not with the canonical L265P. These tumors may represent transformation from marginal zone lymphomas. The outcome of these patients is more favorable.

EZB/C3/BCL2 is a subtype of GCB tumors with a mutational profile similar to FL with frequent *BCL2*

TABLE 64.2 Genomic subtypes of diffuse large B-cell lymphoma

Wright 2020[22]	Chapuy 2018[23]	Lacy 2020[24]	Hallmark drivers	COO	% of cases	Outcome 5-y OS (%)	Putative related small cell lymphoma
MCD	C5	MYD88	*MYD88/CD79B*	ABC	9-14-21	40-42	LPL
BN2	C1	NOTCH2	t*BCL6/NOTCH2*	GCB/ABC Unclassified	16-19	48-67	MZL
EZB-MYC-	C3	BCL2	*EZH2* t*BCL2*	GCB	13-18	63-82	FL
EZB-MYC+			*EZH2/* t*MYC*	GCB/DZ	6	48	FL
A53	C2		*TP53* Aneuploidy	All	7-21	63	
ST2	C4	SOCS1/SGK1 TET/SGK1	*SOCS1/TET2/ SGK1*	GCB	5-17	65-84	NLPBL
N1			*NOTCH1*	ABC	2	27	CLL
Other		UNCLASS		Unclass, GCB, ABC	27-37	66	

ABC, activated B-cell type; CLL, chronic lymphocytic leukemia; COO, cell of origin; DZ, dark zone signature; FL, follicular lymphoma, GCB, germinal center B-cell type; LPL, lymphoplasmacytic lymphoma, MZL, marginal zone lymphoma; NLPBL, nodular lymphocyte predominant B-cell lymphoma; t, translocation.

rearrangements, alterations in epigenetic regulators including activation of *EZH2*, and inactivation of *KMT2D*, *CREBBP*, *EP300*, and *ARID1A*. B-cell transcription factors such as *IRF8*, *MEF2B*, and *EBF1* are also mutated. The PI3K pathway may be activated by *PTEN* deletions/mutations and *MIR17HG* gain/amplification. Immune escape may be mediated by inactivation of *TNFRS14*. The outcome of these patients is relatively favorable.

EZB-MYC+ is a subtype with a similar mutational profile as the previous one defined by the expression of the dark-zone transcriptional signature and frequently carries *BCL2* and *MYC* translocations. Frequently mutated genes are *GNA13*, *DDX3X*, and *FOXO1*, which are uncommon in the EZB-MYC- group of tumors that do not express the dark-zone transcriptional signature. The outcome of these patients is poor.

A53/C2 defines a subset of DLBCL with frequent aneuploidy and inactivation of *TP53*, *CDKN2A*, and *RB1*. The COO may be not only ABC but also GCB, and this difference seems to confer a poor or more favorable outcome, respectively.

ST2/C4/SOCS1-TET-SGK1 are GCB tumors that differ from the EZB/C3 subtype by the absence of *BCL2* rearrangement and *PTEN* inactivation. The most common mutations inactivate *SGK1*, which may facilitate PI3K signaling. The JAK/STAT pathway is activated with mutations in *STAT3* and *SOCS1*. Alterations in chromatin modifiers are uncommon, but they have mutations in H1 linker and core histones that open the chromatin and facilitate the mutational effect of activation-induced cytidine deaminase. NF-kB may be activated with mutations in *NFKBIA*, *CARD11*, and *NFKBIE*. Some cases carry mutation in *TET2* and MAP kinases (*BRAF*, *MAP2K1*, *KRAS*). The mutational profile of these tumors is similar to that described in nodular lymphocyte predominant B-cell lymphoma. The outcome of these patients is significantly better than that of other GCB-derived tumors.

The N1 subtype is uncommon (2%) with activating mutations of *NOTCH1*. These tumors are mainly ABC and have been postulated to be related to CLL transformation, although this needs confirmation. The outcome of these patients is unfavorable.

These genomic subgroups represent a relevant advance in understanding the biological and clinical heterogeneity of DLBCL, NOS, and an important framework from which to implement precision medicine strategies. However, their application in the clinical practice has many challenges, mainly due to the requirement of genomic sequencing of whole exomes or large panels of genes and standardization of the methodological approaches. Additionally, although most of the subtypes overlap in the different models, a relatively large number of cases remain unclassifiable in some of them. One publicly available approach is the LymphGen algorithm, which has been validated in different cohorts and can assign subgroup on a biopsy-by-biopsy basis.[22] However, only about 60% of cases can be assigned to a specific molecular subgroup using LymphGen. In spite of these challenges, the incorporation of genomic profiling in future clinical trials, and eventually in routine practice, has the potential to provide improved biologic-based disease classification and open avenues for novel therapeutic strategies.

Tumor microenvironment

Interactions between tumor cells and their microenvironment play a role in the progression of DLBCL and may be targets for novel therapies. GEP studies have identified signatures related to extracellular matrix, myofibroblasts, dendritic cells, and $CD4^{+}$ T cells associated with better outcomes, whereas M2 macrophages and angiogenesis are associated with poorer outcomes.[12,25] Genomic studies described earlier have identified multiple alterations in genes modulating the interaction of tumor and host immune cells with certain differences between molecular subtypes. For example, tumor cells may have impaired antigen presentation by loss of MHC-I and II. Inactivation of *B2M* and *CIITA* also targets this mechanism. *CREBBP* and *EZH2* mutations downregulate the expression of MHC-II. Mutations in *CD58*, *CD70*, and *TNFRS14* may impair the antitumor activity of NK cells and subpopulations of T cells, respectively, via their interactions with CD27 (CD70) and HVEM (TNFRS14). PD-L1/PD-L2 are usually low expressed in DLBCL but are gained or translocated in some cases of genomic subtypes ST2/C1 and MCD/C5. Novel studies integrating bulk genomic and transcriptomic studies together with single cell analysis are opening new avenues to understand the role of microenvironment complexity in the progression of these tumors and response to novel therapies including CAR-T.[26,27]

Prognosis and Clinical Comment

DLBCL is an aggressive malignancy that requires treatment but can be cured even when widely disseminated at diagnosis. In addition to pathologic and genetic features discussed previously, clinical prognostic factors alone, and in combination, retain prognostic relevance. The International Prognostic Index combines five clinical and laboratory factors into a score that defines patient groups with distinct outcomes with standard immunochemotherapy. Staging is performed using positron emission tomography–computed tomography with ^{18}F-fluorodeoxyglucose using the Ann Arbor system. Bone marrow biopsy may contribute to staging, where appropriate, but is no longer required in all patients. Modern chemoimmunotherapy results in cure for 60% to 70% of patients, with the majority of progression/relapse occurring in the first 2 years. The overall survival of patients who are event free at 2 years is almost equivalent to the age- and sex-matched population. The outcomes for patients who experience progression during, or relapse shortly after, first-line therapy is poor. In contrast, those patients who experience late relapse, 2 years or more after diagnosis, typically respond to further chemotherapy-based therapy.[28] CNS involvement is rare at diagnosis, but relapse within the CNS occurs in 2% to 5% of patients, either in isolation or as part of systemic relapse.[12,29]

Upfront treatment with immunochemotherapy (R-CHOP: rituximab [an antibody against CD20], cyclophosphamide, doxorubicin, vincristine, and prednisone) has been the standard approach for over 2 decades, although other regimens incorporating novel agents have shown promise in trials. Historically, younger fit patients with progressive/relapsed disease were treated with second-line immunochemotherapy with a consolidative autologous stem cell transplant. However CAR-T-cell therapy has improved outcomes in this setting.[29]

References

1. Swerdlow SH, Campo E, Harris NL, et al. WHO classification of tumours of haematopoietic and lymphoid tissues. World Health Organization Classification of Tumours. 4th ed, Vol. 2. IARC; 2017:439.
2. Teras LR, DeSantis CE, Cerhan JR, Morton LM, Jemal A, Flowers CR. 2016 US lymphoid malignancy statistics by World Health Organization subtypes. *CA Cancer J Clin.* 2016;66(6):443-459. doi:10.3322/caac.21357
3. van Imhoff GW, Boerma EJ, van der Holt B, et al. Prognostic impact of germinal center-associated proteins and chromosomal breakpoints in poor-risk diffuse large B-cell lymphoma. *J Clin Oncol.* 2006;24(25):4135-4142. doi:10.1200/JCO.2006.05.5897
4. Simonitsch-Klupp I, Hauser I, Ott G, et al. Diffuse large B-cell lymphomas with plasmablastic/plasmacytoid features are associated with TP53 deletions and poor clinical outcome. *Leukemia.* 2004;18(1):146-155. doi:10.1038/sj.leu.2403206
5. Sander B, Campo E, Hsi ED. Chronic lymphocytic leukaemia/small lymphocytic lymphoma and mantle cell lymphoma: from early lesions to transformation. *Virchows Arch.* 2023;482(1):131-145. doi:10.1007/s00428-022-03460-y
6. Sehn LH, Scott DW, Chhanabhai M, et al. Impact of concordant and discordant bone marrow involvement on outcome in diffuse large B-cell lymphoma treated with R-CHOP. *J Clin Oncol.* 2011;29(11):1452-1457. doi:10.1200/JCO.2010.33.3419

7. Spiegel JY, Patel S, Muffly L, et al. CAR T cells with dual targeting of CD19 and CD22 in adult patients with recurrent or refractory B cell malignancies: a phase 1 trial. *Nat Med.* 2021;27(8):1419-1431. doi:10.1038/s41591-021-01436-0
8. Song JY, Dirnhofer S, Piris MA, Quintanilla-Martinez L, Pileri S, Campo E. Diffuse large B-cell lymphomas, not otherwise specified, and emerging entities. *Virchows Arch.* 2023;482(1):179-192. doi:10.1007/s00428-022-03466-6
9. Hans CP, Weisenburger DD, Greiner TC, et al. Confirmation of the molecular classification of diffuse large B-cell lymphoma by immunohistochemistry using a tissue microarray. *Blood.* 2004;103(1):275-282. doi:10.1182/blood-2003-05-1545
10. Frauenfeld L, Castrejon-de-Anta N, Ramis-Zaldivar JE, et al. Diffuse large B-cell lymphomas in adults with aberrant coexpression of CD10, BCL6, and MUM1 are enriched in IRF4 rearrangements. *Blood Adv.* 2022;6(7):2361-2372. doi:10.1182/bloodadvances.2021006034
11. Collinge B, Ben-Neriah S, Chong L, et al. The impact of MYC and BCL2 structural variants in tumors of DLBCL morphology and mechanisms of false-negative MYC IHC. *Blood.* 2021;137(16):2196-2208. doi:10.1182/blood.2020007193
12. Ennishi D, Hsi ED, Steidl C, Scott DW. Toward a new molecular taxonomy of diffuse large B-cell lymphoma. *Cancer Discov.* 2020;10(9):1267-1281. doi:10.1158/2159-8290.CD-20-0174
13. Campo E, Jaffe ES, Cook JR, et al. The international consensus classification of mature lymphoid neoplasms: a report from the clinical advisory committee. *Blood.* 2022;140(11):1229-1253. doi:10.1182/blood.2022015851
14. Roschewski M, Staudt LM, Wilson WH. Diffuse large B-cell lymphoma-treatment approaches in the molecular era. *Nat Rev Clin Oncol.* 2014;11(1):12-23. doi:10.1038/nrclinonc.2013.197
15. Wilson WH, Wright GW, Huang DW, et al. Effect of ibrutinib with R-CHOP chemotherapy in genetic subtypes of DLBCL. *Cancer Cell.* 2021;39(12):1643-1653 e3. doi:10.1016/j.ccell.2021.10.006
16. Alduaij W, Collinge B, Ben-Neriah S, et al. Molecular determinants of clinical outcomes in a real-world diffuse large B-cell lymphoma population. *Blood.* 2023;141(20):2493-2507. doi:10.1182/blood.2022018248
17. Sha C, Barrans S, Cucco F, et al. Molecular high-grade B-cell lymphoma: defining a poor-risk group that requires different approaches to therapy. *J Clin Oncol.* 2019;37(3):202-212. doi:10.1200/jco.18.01314
18. Caro P, Kishan AU, Norberg E, et al. Metabolic signatures uncover distinct targets in molecular subsets of diffuse large B cell lymphoma. *Cancer Cell.* 2012;22(4):547-560. doi:10.1016/j.ccr.2012.08.014
19. Nadeu F, Royo R, Massoni-Badosa R, et al. Detection of early seeding of Richter transformation in chronic lymphocytic leukemia. *Nat Med.* 2022;28(8):1662-1671. doi:10.1038/s41591-022-01927-8
20. Horn H, Staiger AM, Vohringer M, et al. Diffuse large B-cell lymphomas of immunoblastic type are a major reservoir for MYC-IGH translocations. *Am J Surg Pathol.* 2015;39(1):61-66. doi:10.1097/PAS.0000000000000319
21. Cascione L, Aresu L, Baudis M, Bertoni F. DNA copy number changes in diffuse large B cell lymphomas. *Front Oncol.* 2020;10:584095. 10.3389/fonc.2020.584095
22. Wright GW, Huang DW, Phelan JD, et al. A probabilistic classification tool for genetic subtypes of diffuse large B cell lymphoma with therapeutic implications. *Cancer Cell.* 2020;37(4):551-568 e14. doi:10.1016/j.ccell.2020.03.015
23. Chapuy B, Stewart C, Dunford AJ, et al. Molecular subtypes of diffuse large B cell lymphoma are associated with distinct pathogenic mechanisms and outcomes. *Nat Med.* 2018;24(5):679-690. doi:10.1038/s41591-018-0016-8
24. Lacy SE, Barrans SL, Beer PA, et al. Targeted sequencing in DLBCL, molecular subtypes, and outcomes: a Haematological Malignancy Research Network report. *Blood.* 2020;135(20):1759-1771. doi:10.1182/blood.2019003535
25. Ciavarella S, Vegliante MC, Fabbri M, et al. Dissection of DLBCL microenvironment provides a gene expression-based predictor of survival applicable to formalin-fixed paraffin-embedded tissue. *Ann Oncol.* 2018;29(12):2363-2370. doi:10.1093/annonc/mdy450
26. Steen CB, Luca BA, Esfahani MS, et al. The landscape of tumor cell states and ecosystems in diffuse large B cell lymphoma. *Cancer Cell.* 2021;39(10):1422-1437 e10. doi:10.1016/j.ccell.2021.08.011
27. Haradhvala NJ, Leick MB, Maurer K, et al. Distinct cellular dynamics associated with response to CAR-T therapy for refractory B cell lymphoma. *Nat Med.* 2022;28(9):1848-1859. doi:10.1038/s41591-022-01959-0
28. Hilton LK, Ngu HS, Collinge B, et al. Relapse timing is associated with distinct evolutionary dynamics in diffuse large B-cell lymphoma. *J Clin Oncol.* 2023;41(25):4164-4177. doi:10.1200/JCO.23.00570
29. Sehn LH, Salles G. Diffuse large B-cell lymphoma. *N Engl J Med.* 2021;384(9):842-858. doi:10.1056/NEJMra2027612

Chapter 65

Large B-Cell Lymphoma With 11q Aberration

Eric D. Hsi, Leticia Quintanilla-Martinez, and Jane N. Winter

Definition

Large B-cell lymphoma with 11q aberration (LBCL-11q) is a B-cell lymphoma of intermediate to large cells with a characteristic gain/loss pattern at chromosome 11q23.3 and 11q24-qter, respectively. These cases by definition lack *MYC* rearrangement. It is included as a provisional entity.

Synonyms

High-grade B-cell lymphoma with 11q aberration Burkitt-like lymphoma with 11q aberration (not recommended).

Epidemiology

LBCL-11q is rare, described in relatively small cases series and case reports. It has been reported frequently in posttransplant patients, in patients with HIV infection, and more recently in association with ataxia-telangiectasia.[1-3]

General Clinical Features

LBCL-11q occurs predominantly in children and young adults (YA) (median age 17 years, range 7-72 years) with a male predominance (M:F = 2.8). Lymphadenopathy in the head/neck region is the most common presentation, and disease tends to be localized; less frequently abdominal sites are involved. Extranodal sites such as tonsil, gastrointestinal tract, or ovary may also occur.[2-5]

Morphology

Most cases have a high grade B-cell lymphoma morphology with intermediate-sized cells, open chromatin, small indistinct nucleoli, and scant cytoplasm.[1,3] A starry-sky background with five to nine coarse apoptotic bodies within the tingible body macrophages is characteristic and a diagnostic clue as to the presence of the 11q aberration.[6] However, it is not observed in all cases and its absence does not preclude the diagnosis.[2,6] Several cases with morphologic features of diffuse large B-cell lymphoma have been reported.[1,2,6] Figure 65.1

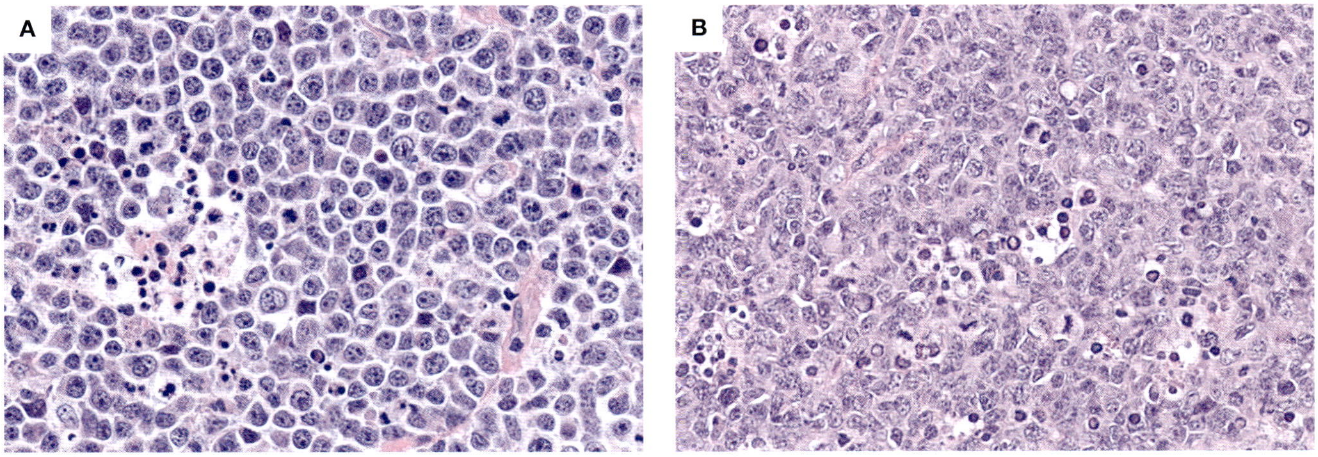

FIGURE 65.1 Histopathology of large B-cell lymphoma with 11q aberration. **A:** Hematoxylin and eosin (H&E) staining of a lymph node showing a case with Burkitt-like morphology and in the center a macrophage with coarse apoptotic bodies. **B:** Example of LBCL-11q with large cell morphology. This case had a starry-sky pattern with coarse apoptotic bodies as well; however, some cases may lack these features. (H&E stains, 400×).

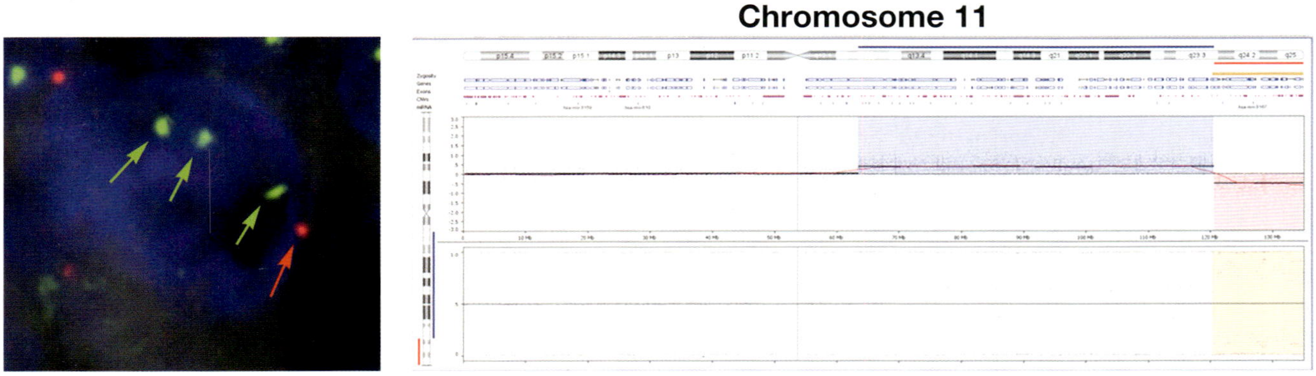

FIGURE 65.2 Fluorescence in situ hybridization (FISH) and comparative genomic hybridization array analyses in a case of large B-cell lymphoma with 11q aberration. FISH analysis was performed using a custom probe targeting the minimal regions of gain (RP11-414G21, spectrum green, 11q23.3, green arrows) and loss (RP11-629A20, spectrum red, 11q24.3, red arrow) combined with centromeric probe for chromosome 11 (CEP11, Spectrum aqua, Vysis, blue arrow). FISH analysis shows a hybridization pattern with 11q aberration, 1 centromere signal (blue), 1 loss (red), and 3 gains (green). Chromosomal microarray shows a copy number (CN) gain in 11q13.1-q23.3 with a CN loss in 11q23.3-q25. (Salaverria I, Martin-Guerrero I, Wagener R, et al. A recurrent 11q aberration pattern characterizes a subset of MYC-negative high-grade B-cell lymphomas resembling Burkitt lymphoma. *Blood.* 2014;123(8):1187-1198.)

illustrates cytologic features. The pattern is typically diffuse, but a vaguely nodular pattern with background disrupted follicular dendritic cell networks can be seen.[5]

Immunophenotype

LBCL-11q are mature B-cell lymphomas and express CD19 and CD20 but lack CD5. CD10 and BCL6 are each expressed in approximately 94% of cases while MUM1 is present in 12% to 15% of cases, and thus these lymphomas typically have a germinal center B-cell phenotype. MYC is weakly expressed (>40% of cells) in most cases tested while BCL2 expression (>50% of cells) occurs in approximately 20% of cases. The proliferative index is high (>90%).[2,3,5,6] Positive staining for LMO2 and lack of LEF1 expression support LBCL-11q over Burkitt lymphoma (BL).[2,5,7] By flow cytometry, expression of CD16/CD56 without bright CD38 expression may be present in up to 55% of cases and may help distinguish from BL, which lacks CD16/56 and has bright CD38.[8] Stains for Epstein-Barr virus are negative.[3]

Genetics

LBCL-11q is defined by the presence of chromosomal gain at 11q23.3 and telomeric loss at 11q24.1-qter, which can be detected by chromosomal microarray or fluorescence in situ hybridization strategies (Figure 65.2).[2,3,5] *MYC* translocation is absent by definition. This 11q abnormality is not entirely specific and may be found in *MYC*-R lymphomas, including BL.[4] Rare reported cases may lack the 11q23.3 gain. The presence of 11q23.3 gain alone is considered nonspecific.[1,2] Mutations in the ID3-TCF3 axis or the SWI/SNF complex, characteristic of BL, are not seen. It is unclear how genetic alterations in minimal regions of chromosomal gain and loss contribute to the pathogenesis of LBCL-11q. In the region of 11q23.3 gains, *PCSK7, DSCAML1,* and *TMEM25* were mutated in single cases. In the region of chromosomal loss, *ETS1* and *NFRKB* have been found to be recurrently mutated. Other reported frequently mutated genes include *GNA13, DDX3X, TTN, FAT4,* and *PKD1L2*, each found in >30% of cases.[9] Other less frequently reported mutations include *ATM*.[2,9] *TP53* mutations are observed in adult cases with dismal prognosis.[2]

Prognosis and Clinical Comment

The majority of reported cases are children or YA who have been treated with regimens typically used for BL. Outcomes have been excellent with high complete remission rates and durable remissions in those for whom long-term follow-up is reported.[3,5,10] Adult patients appear to have more disseminated disease at initial presentation and have received various aggressive B-cell lymphoma regimens.[2,3,5,10] Optimal treatment strategies require further investigation.

References

1. Gebauer N, Witte HM, Merz H, et al. Aggressive B-cell lymphoma cases with 11q aberration patterns indicate a spectrum beyond Burkitt-like lymphoma. *Blood Adv.* 2021;5(23):5220-5225. doi:10.1182/bloodadvances.2021004635

2. Quintanilla-Martinez L, Laurent C, Soma L, et al. Emerging entities: high-grade/large B-cell lymphoma with 11q aberration, large B-cell lymphoma with IRF4 rearrangement, and new molecular subgroups in large B-cell lymphomas—a report of the 2022 EA4HP/SH lymphoma workshop. *Virchows Arch*. 2023;483(3):281-298. doi:10.1007/s00428-023-03590-x
3. Salaverria I, Martin-Guerrero I, Wagener R, et al. A recurrent 11q aberration pattern characterizes a subset of MYC-negative high-grade B-cell lymphomas resembling Burkitt lymphoma. *Blood*. 2014;123(8):1187-1198. doi:10.1182/blood-2013-06-507996
4. Grygalewicz B, Woroniecka R, Rymkiewicz G, et al. The 11q-gain/loss aberration occurs recurrently in MYC-negative Burkitt-like lymphoma with 11q aberration, as well as MYC-positive Burkitt lymphoma and MYC-positive high-grade B-cell lymphoma, NOS. *Am J Clin Pathol*. 2017;149(1):17-28. doi:10.1093/ajcp/aqx139
5. Gonzalez-Farre B, Ramis-Zaldivar JE, Salmeron-Villalobos J, et al. Burkitt-like lymphoma with 11q aberration: a germinal center-derived lymphoma genetically unrelated to Burkitt lymphoma. *Haematologica*. 2019;104(9):1822-1829. doi:10.3324/haematol.2018.207928
6. Horn H, Kalmbach S, Wagener R, et al. A diagnostic approach to the identification of Burkitt-like lymphoma with 11q aberration in aggressive B-cell lymphomas. *Am J Surg Pathol*. 2021;45(3):356-364. doi:10.1097/PAS.0000000000001613
7. Hurwitz SN, Lockhart B, Onder O, et al. Proteogenomic profiling of high-grade B-cell lymphoma with 11q aberrations and Burkitt lymphoma reveals lymphoid enhancer binding factor 1 as a novel biomarker. *Mod Pathol*. 2023;36(7):100170. doi:10.1016/j.modpat.2023.100170
8. Rymkiewicz G, Grygalewicz B, Chechlinska M, et al. A comprehensive flow-cytometry-based immunophenotypic characterization of Burkitt-like lymphoma with 11q aberration. *Mod Pathol*. May 2018;31(5):732-743. doi:10.1038/modpathol.2017.186
9. Wagener R, Seufert J, Raimondi F, et al. The mutational landscape of Burkitt-like lymphoma with 11q aberration is distinct from that of Burkitt lymphoma. *Blood*. 2019;133(9):962-966. doi:10.1182/blood-2018-07-864025
10. Au-Yeung RKH, Arias Padilla L, Zimmermann M, et al. Experience with provisional WHO-entities large B-cell lymphoma with IRF4-rearrangement and Burkitt-like lymphoma with 11q aberration in paediatric patients of the NHL-BFM group. *Br J Haematol*. 2020;190(5):753-763. doi:10.1111/bjh.16578

Chapter 66

Nodular Lymphocyte Predominant B-Cell Lymphoma

Stefano A. Pileri, Ranjana Hira Advani, Astrid Pavlovsky and Lauren B. Smith

Definition

Nodular lymphocyte predominant B-cell lymphoma (NLPBL) was previously included in the category of Hodgkin lymphoma.[1,2] It is a rare lymphoma with distinct pathologic and clinical characteristics and an intact B-cell program, unlike classic Hodgkin lymphoma (CHL).[3] Based not only on its pathologic characteristics but also on its biology, clinical behavior, and treatment, which is similar to non-Hodgkin lymphoma (NHL), it has been renamed.[4,5] This lymphoma is characterized by a variably nodular proliferation of small, reactive B cells admixed with scattered larger cells that have lobated nuclei called lymphocyte predominant (LP) cells/popcorn cells.[1] Different architectural patterns exist that are believed to have some prognostic significance.[6,7]

Synonyms

Nodular lymphocyte predominant Hodgkin lymphoma (NLPHL) (not recommended).

Epidemiology

NLPBL has an incidence of 0.1 to 0.2/100,000/y. It is more common in males in the fourth to sixth decades but may be seen in all age groups, including children.[2]

General Clinical Features

NLPBL typically involves peripheral lymph nodes including cervical, axillary, and inguinal lymph nodes. Mediastinal or abdominal lymph nodes are rarely involved. The majority of patients present with early-stage disease. If spleen and bone marrow are involved, this raises concern for a more aggressive B-cell NHL such as T-cell/histiocyte-rich large B-cell lymphoma (THRLBCL). Most patients are asymptomatic, and patients often present with a clinical history of a lymph node that has been growing slowly over several months or years. B symptoms are rare. While the disease is typically indolent, late recurrence, even beyond 10 years, can be seen.

Morphology

NLPBL can have various morphologic patterns.[6] The classic or "B-cell rich nodular" pattern A is the most common pattern and shows large back-to-back nodules of reactive small lymphocytes, variable numbers of epithelioid histiocytes, and neoplastic LP cells. On low power, the large nodules tend to fit together like puzzle pieces and rarely have sclerosis (Figure 66.1A and B). The residual normal lymph node may be seen compressed at the edge of the neoplastic proliferation. Reactive germinal centers between the large nodules are rare, which helps distinguish it from follicular hyperplasia with progressive transformation of germinal centers, an important differential diagnosis, in which large nodules infiltrated by mantle zone cells are surrounded by reactive, smaller germinal centers (Figure 66.2A). If numerous admixed germinal centers are present, lymphocyte-rich CHL should also be considered. Another important differential diagnosis is the floral variant of follicular lymphoma, but this can typically be distinguished from NLPBL based on the immunophenotype of the small B cells (Figure 66.2B).

Beside the classic pattern, other patterns (Figure 66.3) include serpiginous nodules (pattern B) (Figure 66.4), numerous LP cells outside of the nodules (pattern C), nodules containing more T cells rather than B cells (pattern D), "diffuse areas" or "T-cell-rich large B-cell-like transformation" (pattern E), and a diffuse pattern with numerous admixed small B cells and a "moth-eaten" appearance (pattern F). Pattern E can be the most diagnostically challenging, as it can resemble THRLBCL. Extensive sampling of the lymph node should be performed to find areas with nodularity, as even a single "nodule" or area resembling the other NLPBL patterns excludes de novo THRLBCL. Other findings supporting NLPBL rather than THRLBCL include admixed

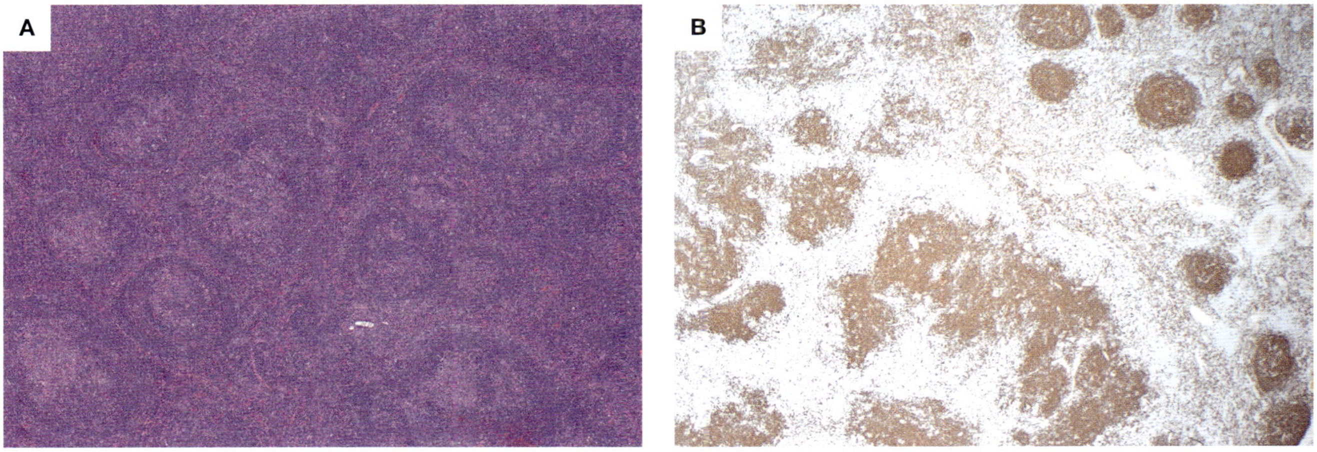

FIGURE 66.1 Nodular lymphocyte predominant B-cell lymphoma, the B-cell-rich nodular or classic pattern, with large expansile nodules. **A:** Hematoxylin and eosin and **(B)** CD20 showing the neoplastic nodules on the left and the reactive, compressed lymph node at the edge of the proliferation.

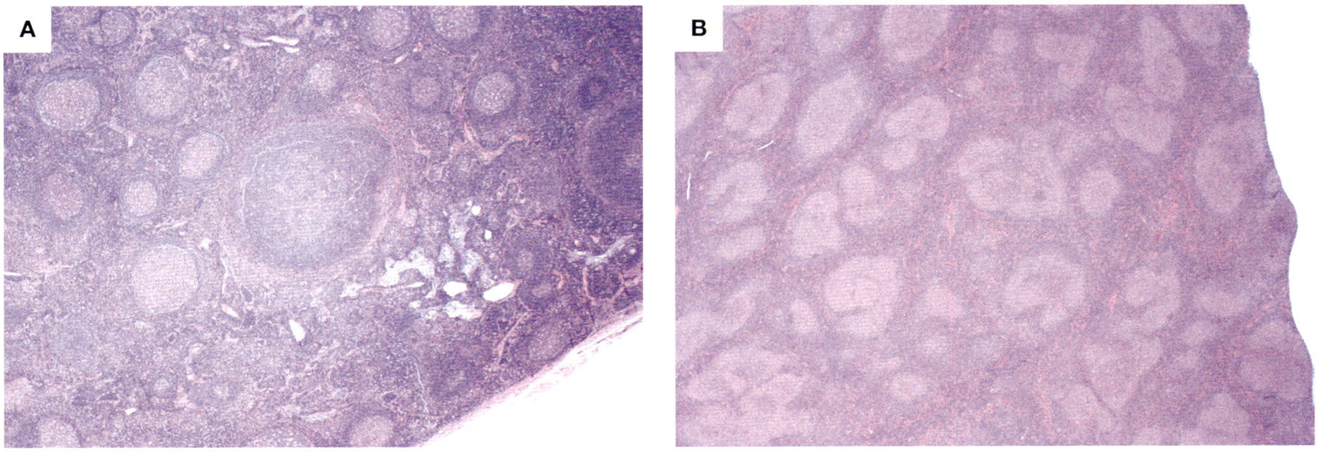

FIGURE 66.2 Low-magnification mimics of nodular lymphocyte predominant B-cell lymphoma (NLPBL). **A:** Follicular hyperplasia with progressive transformation of germinal centers. Unlike NLPBL, this reactive condition has large, transformed follicles surrounded by reactive germinal centers. **B:** Floral variant of follicular lymphoma. This pattern can mimic NLPBL, but the immunophenotype of small B cells positive for CD10 and BCL6 will allow it to be distinguished from NLPBL.

small B cells on immunohistochemistry and residual follicular dendritic cell meshworks. Owing to the difficulty distinguishing it from THRLBCL, a core biopsy may not be adequate to accurately diagnose NLPBL and an excisional biopsy of a lymph node is recommended.

The various patterns seen on low power have been correlated with prognosis and outcomes with typical patterns A/B associated with favorable outcomes.[7] The International Consensus Classification (ICC) suggests that patterns A-C (may be less aggressive) be termed grade 1 and patterns D-F (may be more aggressive) be termed grade 2.[8] The latter distinction will need to be studied further and validated using large data sets since overall prognosis is largely dependent on stage. A small fraction of cases (fewer than 5%) may transform to diffuse large B-cell lymphoma (DLBCL), further underscoring the relationship to other NHLs.[1,2] These cases behave similarly to de novo DLBCL. Pattern E (THRLBCL-like) can be seen at diagnosis or recurrence, but it should not be diagnosed as THRLBCL, as this may not be clinically as aggressive or identical to de novo THRLBCL.

The morphology of LP cells includes lobated/folded nuclei resembling a popped popcorn kernel (Figure 66.5), but other Hodgkin/Reed-Sternberg (HRS)-like cells including mummified cells or Hodgkin cells with prominent central nucleoli may also be seen.[1] The neoplastic cells may be difficult to distinguish from the admixed epithelioid histiocytes morphologically without careful study or immunohistochemistry. The LP cells are typically surrounded by small T cells, which

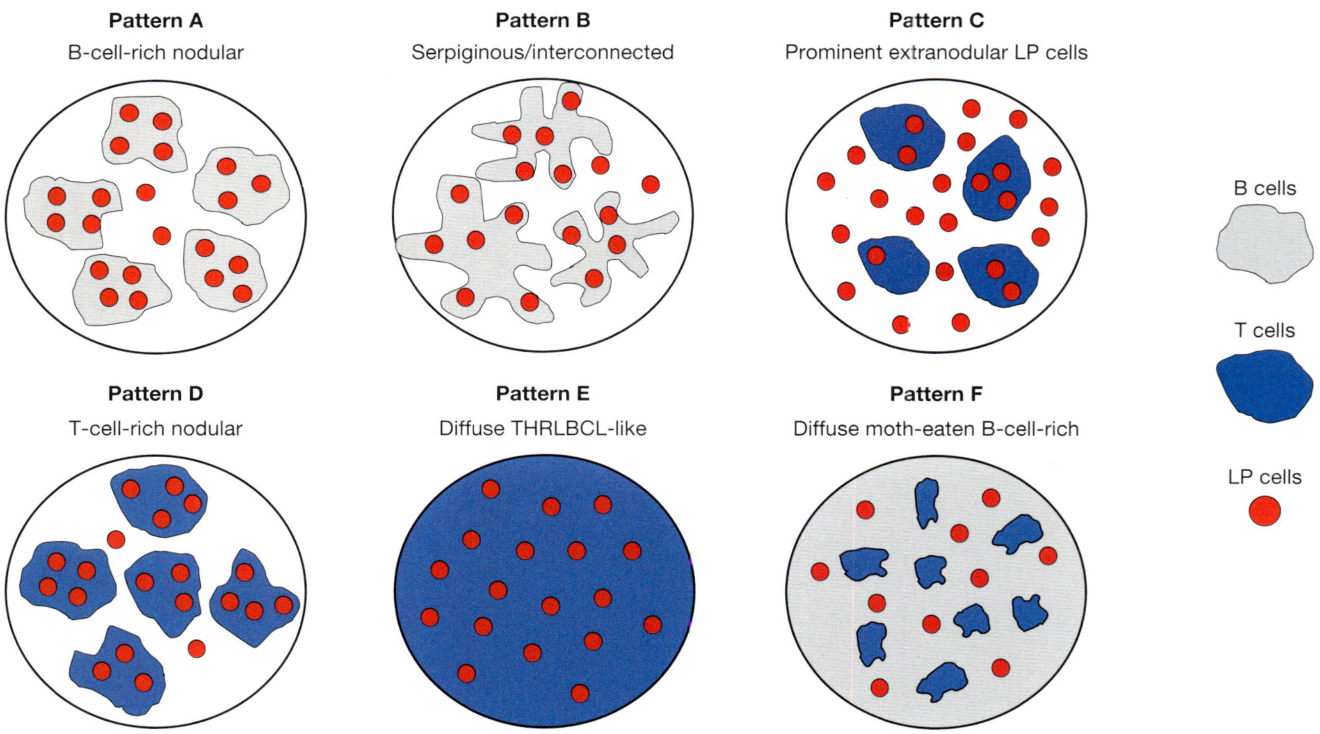

FIGURE 66.3 A schematic diagram showing the six patterns that can be seen in nodular lymphocyte predominant B-cell lymphoma.

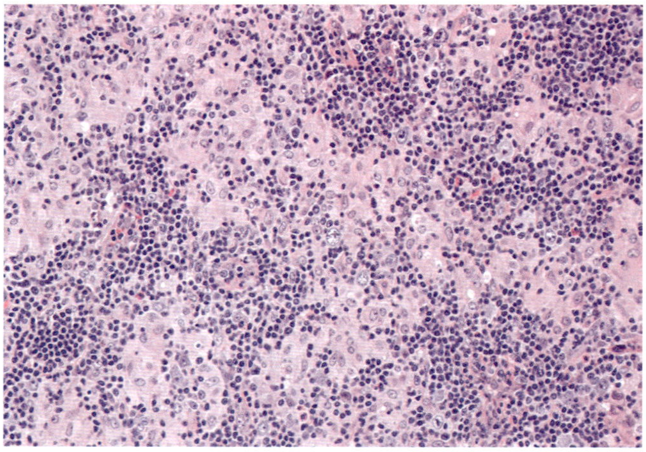

FIGURE 66.4 Nodular lymphocyte predominant B-cell lymphoma may have a serpiginous growth pattern in which the lymphocyte predominant cells are embedded in cords of histiocytes and small lymphocytes (pattern B).

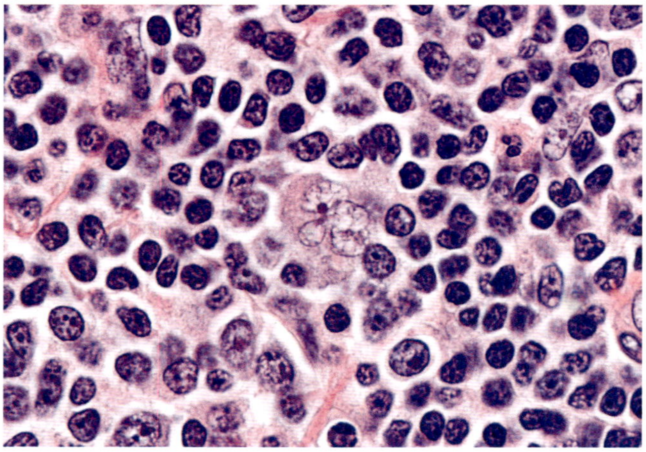

FIGURE 66.5 Lymphocyte predominant cell with multilobated nuclei (resembling popped popcorn) in a background of small lymphocytes and histiocytes.

form "T-cell rosettes," which can be seen by immunohistochemistry in the cases with large numbers of small B cells. Lymphocyte-rich (LR) CHL can also have Hodgkin-like Reed-Sternberg (HRS) cells that resemble LP cells and T-cell rosettes; therefore, immunohistochemistry becomes important in confirming the initial morphologic impression.[1,2] LR CHL is more likely to have HRS cells in the mantle zones of reactive follicles creating smaller nodules, which may have a moth-eaten appearance with a central regressed germinal center.

Immunophenotype

LP cells of NLPBL have an immunophenotype that is characteristic of a B-cell lymphoma with a preserved B-cell program (Figure 66.6A-D).[1,2] The LP cells are positive for B-cell markers including CD20 (typically

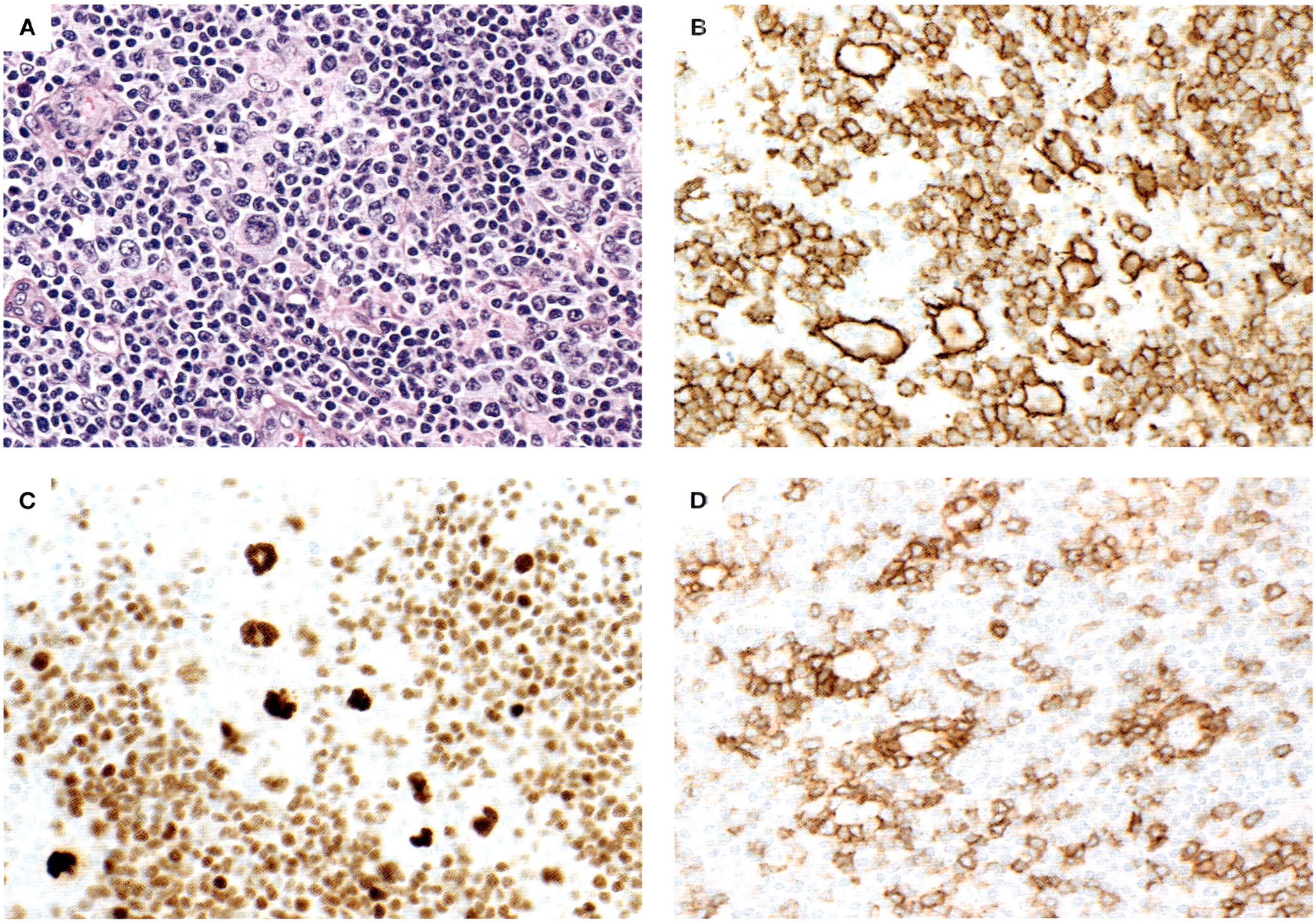

FIGURE 66.6 Immunophenotype of lymphocyte predominant (LP) cells. **A:** Hematoxylin and eosin stain showing large cells in a background of small lymphocytes and histiocytes. **B:** CD20 showing large lymphocyte predominant (LP) cells and small B cells (classic pattern). **C:** OCT2 highlights background B cells and large LP cells. **D:** PD-1/CD279 shows rosettes around LP cells.

strong and uniform), PAX5 (strong), CD79a, OCT2 (strong), and BOB1. Unlike in CHL, the LP cells are often positive for CD45 (leucocyte common antigen). CD30 may be positive in a small subset or may mark admixed immunoblasts between the nodules. CD15 is negative but can rarely be expressed. The LP cells are typically also positive for germinal center markers MEF2B and BCL6 and negative or only weakly positive for MUM1, features that can help distinguish it from CHL. CD10 is usually absent. EMA, PU.1, and J chain are positive in a substantial proportion of cases. Cases in young men, often with pattern C, are more likely to have IgD-positive LP cells.[9] EBER (in situ hybridization for Epstein-Barr virus) is usually negative on LP cells, but rare EBV-positive cases occur.[10] Follicular dendritic cell (FDC) markers including CD21 and CD23 may be helpful in demarcating the large expansile nodules of residual meshworks in diffuse areas.[1] However, FDC meshworks are not required to consider the pattern "nodular" and the underlying architecture may best be appreciated using stains for CD20/PAX5. T-cell rosettes are of T-follicular helper (TFH) type and may be identified using pan T-cell markers such as CD3. However, PD-1/CD279 is very helpful (and more sensitive than CD57) in highlighting the rosetting T cells.[11]

The background T cells in NLPBL are typically CD4 predominant and of TFH type, while THRLBCL is more likely to have a CD8 predominance. Flow cytometry may identify a population of T cells that express both CD4 and CD8 (double positive), which is reactive.[12]

Genetics

The LP cells in NLPBL have clonally rearranged immunoglobulin genes that are functional and have ongoing somatic hypermutation unlike the HRS cells in CHL. There are no clinically useful genetic hallmarks of NLPBL, although *BCL6* rearrangements are seen in a subset of cases and mutations/somatic hypermutations have also been reported in *MYC*, *PAX5*, *PIM1*, *RHOH (TTF)*, *SGK1*,

DUSP2, and *JUNB*.[13-16] Increased susceptibility to NLPBL has been reported to occur in patients with defective T and NK cells and mutations in *FS-7-associated surface antigen* (autoimmune lymphoproliferative syndrome).[2]

Gene expression profiling has found similarities between NLPBL and THRLBCL, suggesting that this may be a genetic continuum. Many of the mutations that have been found are similar between the two entities, and array comparative genomic hybridization studies have shown that THRLBCL has more genomic aberrations than NLPBL.[17]

Prognosis and Clinical Comment

NLPBL is typically an indolent disease, and late recurrences beyond 10 years can be seen.[18,19] Nevertheless, the prognosis of patients with NLPBL is excellent, with low excess mortality compared with the general population. In these patients, lymphoma does not represent the major cause of death. The management differs from that of CHL for both early and advanced stages and is similar to the approach used in indolent B-cell NHLs. Therapy for early-stage disease ranges from excision alone in selected cases, radiation therapy (RT), or combined modality therapy. Stage IA without risk factors can be treated with limited RT. Active surveillance can be an option in patients with complete remission (according to positron emission tomography) after lymph node resection.[20] Early stage with risk factors at diagnosis can also be treated with combined modality of rituximab plus chemotherapy with or without consolidation with RT.

Advanced-stage disease (if asymptomatic with low tumor burden) can be observed without any impact on outcomes. Single-agent rituximab has also been used.[21] If a high tumor burden is present or there is a concern for a transformation to an aggressive B-cell NHL, management is as for DLBCL with RCHOP-type therapy. Patients who have recurrence are more likely to have morphologic patterns D-F; however, clinical stage is more important than the morphology and it is unclear, at this time, whether a grade 2 pattern requires more aggressive initial treatment. Disease-related morbidity and mortality often result from therapy rather than from disease progression; thus, avoiding overtreatment is important. The hope is that the change in nomenclature from NLPHL to NLPBL might help achieve this goal.

References

1. Mason DY, Banks PM, Chan J, et al. Nodular lymphocyte predominance Hodgkin's disease. A distinct clinicopathological entity. *Am J Surg Pathol.* 1994;18(5):526-530.
2. Swerdlow S, Campo E, Harris NL, et al, eds. WHO Classification of Tumours of Haematopoietic and Lymphoid Tissues. 4th ed. International Agency for Research on Cancer (IARC); 2017.
3. Anagnostopoulos I, Hansmann ML, Franssila K, et al. European Task Force on Lymphoma project on lymphocyte predominance Hodgkin disease: histologic and immunohistologic analysis of submitted cases reveals 2 types of Hodgkin disease with a nodular growth pattern and abundant lymphocytes. *Blood.* 2000;96(5):1889-1899.
4. Campo E, Jaffe ES, Cook JR, et al. The international consensus classification of mature lymphoid neoplasms: a report from the Clinical Advisory Committee. *Blood* 2022;140(11):1229-1253.Tousseyn TA, King RL, Fend F, et al. Evolution in the definition and diagnosis of Hodgkin lymphomas and related entities. Virchows Archiv 2023;482:207-226.
5. Jaffe ES, Gale RP, Jaffe ES. Lymphoma nomenclature—what's in a name? *Br J Haematol.* 2022;197(5):539-543; Borchmann S, Joffe E, Moskowitz CH, et al. Active surveillance for nodular lymphocytes-predominant Hodgkin lymphoma. *Blood.* 2019;133:2121-2129.
6. Fan Z, Natkunam Y, Bair E, Tibshirani R, Warnke RA. Characterization of variant patterns of nodular lymphocyte predominant Hodgkin lymphoma with immunohistologic and clinical correlation. *Am J Surg Pathol.* 2003;27(10):1346-1356.
7. Hartmann S, Eichenauer DA, Plutschow A, et al. The prognostic impact of variant histology in nodular lymphocyte-predominant Hodgkin lymphoma: a report from the German Hodgkin Study Group (GHSG). *Blood.* 2013;122(26):4246-4292. quiz 4292.
8. Tousseyn TA, King RL, Fend F, Feldman AL, Brousset P, Jaffe ES. Evolution in the definition and diagnosis of the Hodgkin lymphomas and related entities. *Virchows Arch.* 2023;482(1):207-226.
9. Prakash S, Fountaine T, Raffeld M, Jaffe ES, Pittaluga S. IgD positive L&H cells identify a unique subset of nodular lymphocyte predominant Hodgkin lymphoma. *Am J Surg Pathol.* 2006;30(5):585-592.
10. Huppmann AR, Nicolae A, Slack GW, et al. EBV may be expressed in the LP cells of nodular lymphocyte-predominant Hodgkin lymphoma (NLPHL) in both children and adults. *Am J Surg Pathol.* 2014;38(3):316-324.
11. Nam-cha SH, Roncador G, Sanchez-Verde L, et al. PD-1, a follicular T-cell marker useful for recognizing nodular lymphocyte-predominant Hodgkin lymphoma. *Am J Surg Pathol.* 2008;32(8):1252-1257.
12. Rahemtullah A, Reichard KK, Preffer FI, Harris NL, Hasserjian RP. A double-positive CD4+CD8+ T-cell population is commonly found in nodular lymphocyte predominant Hodgkin lymphoma. *AJCP.* 2006;126(5):805-814.
13. Hartmann S, Schuhmacher B, Rausch T, et al. Highly recurrent mutations of SGK1, DUSP2 and JUNB in

nodular lymphocyte predominant Hodgkin lymphoma. *Leukemia*. 2016;30(4):844-853.

14. Hartmann S, Eichenauer DA. Nodular lymphocyte predominant Hodgkin lymphoma: pathology, clinical course and relation to T-cell/histiocyte rich large B-cell lymphoma. *Pathology*. 2020;52(1):142-153.
15. Schuhmacher B, Bein J, Rausch T, et al. JUNB, DUSP2, SGK1, SOCS1 and CREBBP are frequently mutated in T-cell/histiocyte-rich large B-cell lymphoma. *Haematologica*. 2019;104(2):330-337.
16. Weniger MA, Kuppers R. Molecular biology of Hodgkin lymphoma. *Leukemia*. 2021;35(4):968-981.
17. Hartmann S, Doring C, Vucic E, et al. Array comparative genomic hybridization reveals similarities between nodular lymphocyte predominant Hodgkin lymphoma and T cell/histiocyte rich large B cell lymphoma. *Br J Haematol*. 2015;169(3):415-422.
18. Nogova L, Reineke T, Brillant C, et al. Lymphocyte-predominant and classical Hodgkin's lymphoma: a comprehensive analysis from the German Hodgkin Study Group. *J Clin Oncol*. 2008;26(3):434-439.
19. Xing KH, Connors JM, Lai A, et al. Advanced-stage nodular lymphocyte predominant Hodgkin lymphoma compared with classical Hodgkin lymphoma: a matched pair outcome analysis. *Blood*. 2014;123(23):3567-3573.
20. Borchmann S, Joffe E, Moskowitz CH, et al. Active surveillance for nodular lymphocyte-predominant Hodgkin lymphoma. *Blood*. 2019;133(20):2121-2129.
21. Eichenauer DA, Fuchs M, Pluetschow A, et al. Phase 2 study of rituximab in newly diagnosed stage IA nodular lymphocyte-predominant Hodgkin lymphoma: a report from the German Hodgkin Study Group. *Blood*. 2011;118(16):4363-4365.

Chapter 67

T-Cell/Histiocyte-Rich Large B-Cell Lymphoma

Stefano A. Pileri, Ranjana Hira Advani, Margaret A. Shipp, and Lauren B. Smith

Definition

T-cell/histiocyte-rich large B-cell lymphoma (THRLBCL) is a distinct entity within the broader category of diffuse large B-cell lymphoma (DLBCL).[1,2] The neoplastic cells, which range from 1% to <10% of the infiltrate, are embedded within an extensive reactive background of cytotoxic T cells and histiocytes.[1,3] THRLBCL and nodular lymphocyte predominant B-cell lymphoma (NLPBL), especially in the variant E subtype, are often difficult to distinguish.[1-3] A possible transition from one tumor type to the other has been suggested, which underscores the importance of adequate tissue at diagnosis. In this setting, remnants of nodularity favor the diagnosis of NLPBL. The distinction between these two neoplasms is relevant, as de novo THRLBCL is characterized by a more aggressive clinical course.[1,4]

Synonyms

None.

Epidemiology

Data are sparse on the epidemiology of this disease due to its rarity and challenge in its definitive diagnosis. THRLBCL accounts for <10% of all DLBCLs. It may affect patients at any age but has a median age of 57 years and a male:female ratio of 2.7:1.[1-4] Incidence is higher in blacks compared with whites in the United States.[4]

General Clinical Features

THRLBCL has an aggressive presentation with widespread lymphadenopathy, fever, malaise, and frequent involvement of the bone marrow, spleen, and/or liver.[1,3,5] In contrast to NLPBL, most patients with THRLBCL have advanced stage, positron emission tomography–avid disease, and an intermediate or high International Prognostic Index (IPI) score at diagnosis.

Morphology

The lymph node shows almost complete effacement of the normal architecture due to diffuse, or rarely vaguely nodular, growth that lacks follicular dendritic cell (FDC) networks. Because any remaining truly nodular growth within background follicular structures (FDCs or small B cells) supports a diagnosis of NLPBL, a diagnosis of THRLBCL should not be made on core biopsy. In THRLBCL the neoplastic large B cells, which can have variable morphology (centroblastic, immunoblastic, Reed-Sternberg-like, popcorn-like), are present within an extensive reactive background with variable proportions of small T cells and clusters of benign histiocytes (Figure 67.1). The reactive infiltrate can include only rare, scattered B cells, but not remnants of IgM/IgD$^+$ mantle zone B cells, which suggests NLPBL. Plasma cells and eosinophils are not seen. Importantly, in THRLBCL the neoplastic cells are singly scattered without clustering or sheet-like growth seen in DLBCL. DLBCL can have abundant background T cells and/or histiocytes, but classification as THRLBCL should be restricted to cases in which tumor cells are sparse and singly distributed.

A subset of cases present with splenic involvement and show multifocal or micronodular involvement of the white pulp without a small reactive B-cell component to suggest NLPBL. In the liver, foci of infiltration occur in the portal tracts. The bone marrow may be variably affected, from diffuse replacement to paratrabecular foci of infiltration with a cellular composition similar to that in involved lymph nodes.

Immunophenotype

The neoplastic large cells have a complete B-cell phenotype, which is derived from germinal centers. Malignant cells are positive for CD45, CD19, CD20, CD22, CD79a

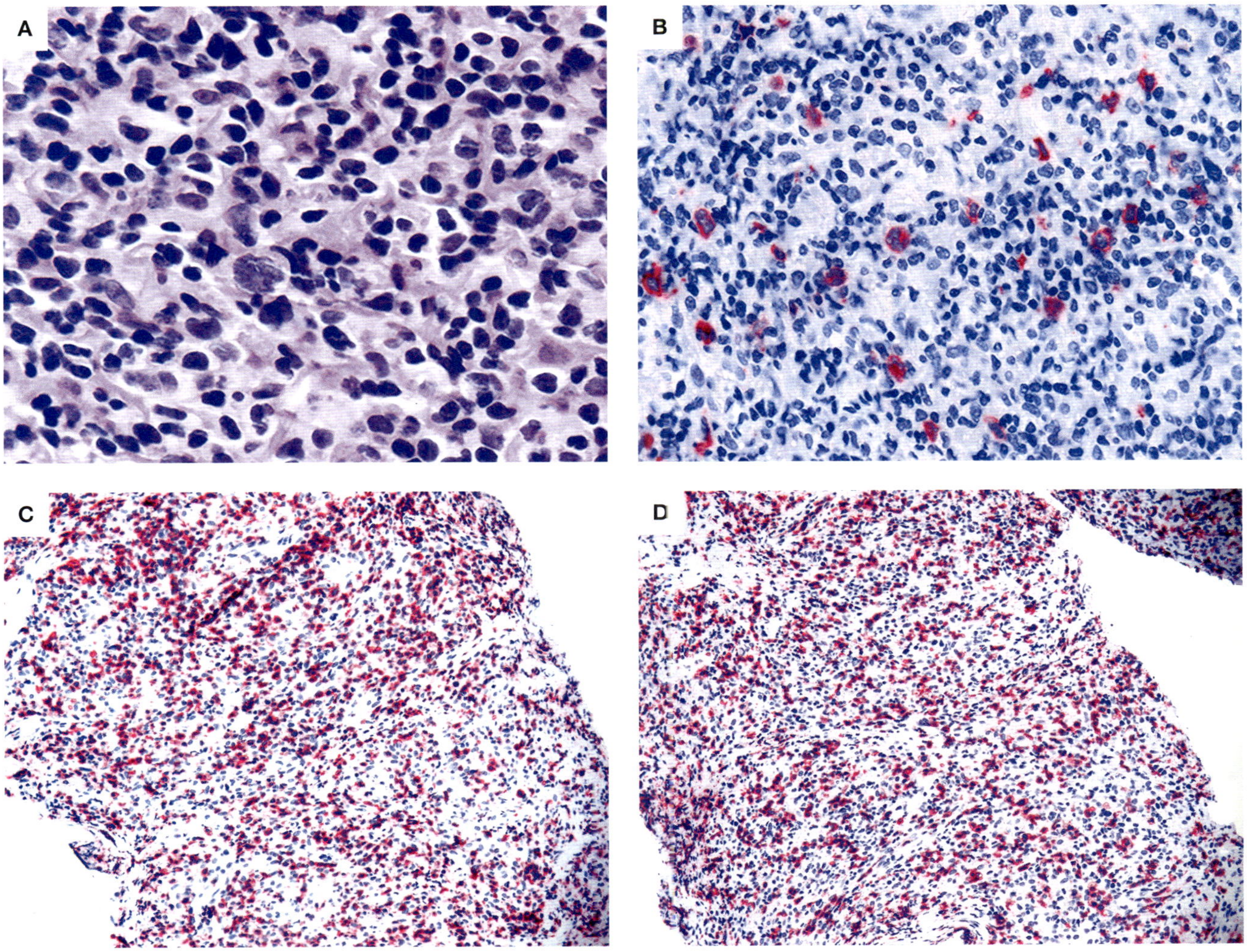

FIGURE 67.1 **A:** Neoplastic cells, one of them with Reed-Sternberg-like features, are present within a milieu consisting of lymphocytes and histiocytes (hematoxylin and eosin); **B:** scattered neoplastic large B cells strongly express CD79a; **C:** reactive T lymphocytes are positive for CD3 (**D**) and positive for CD8 (b-d: immunoalkaline phosphatase technique; Gill hematoxylin counterstaining).

(Figure 67.1), CD79b, PAX5/BSAP, BCL6, BOB-1, and OCT2. PU.1 is more often negative.[1,3] Variable/occasional staining for BCL2, EMA, CD10, and CD30 can be seen. LSP1, CD15, and CD138 are usually negative.[1,3] Most neoplastic cells are in the cell cycle, as shown by high Ki-67 staining. The above-reported phenotypic profile of large B cells allows the easy distinction of THRLBCL from classic Hodgkin lymphoma. One marker that may differentiate THRLBCL from NLPBL is the insulin-like growth factor II mRNA-binding protein 3 (IMP3), which is reported to be positive in THRLBCL and negative or weak in NLPBL, a finding that needs further confirmation.[6] In contrast to NLPBL, antibodies against CD21, CD23, CD35, and CXCL13 do not reveal FDCs in the background.[1,3,5]

In THRLBCL, the overwhelming reactive component consists of histiocytes and T cells (Figures 67.1 and 67.2). The secretion of proinflammatory factors by histiocytes in THRLBCL might represent an important factor for tumor survival. Histiocytes show strong expression of CD68 and CD163. Unlike histiocytes in NLPBL, they have been shown to overexpress the metal-binding protein, MT2A, which may help in the differential diagnosis.[7] Additionally, the expression of PD-L1 by tumor-associated histiocytes may contribute to immune escape in THRLBCL.[8,9] The infiltrating CD3-positive T cells in THRLBCL have a cytotoxic CD8+ phenotype and often express PD1.[9] TFH markers are largely negative.[3] Immunohistochemical analysis of TCF1 may be warranted to identify the percentage of progenitors of exhausted T cells as a higher percentage may predict response to PD-1/PD-L1 blockade.[9] Finally, if the neoplastic cells are positive by Epstein–Barr virus–encoded small RNAs in situ hybridization, the tumor should not be classified as THRLBCL but instead as EBV-positive DLBCL.[1,3]

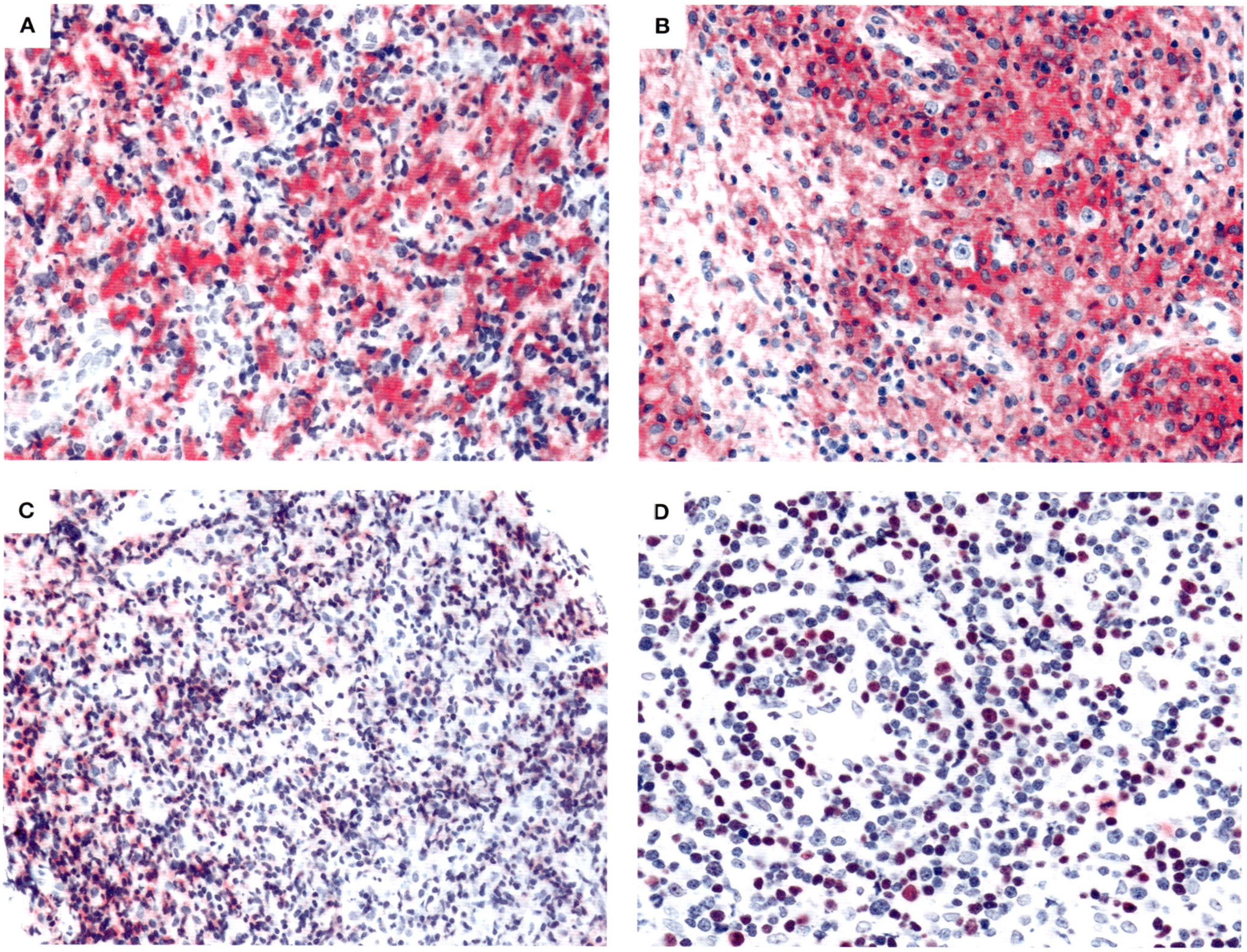

FIGURE 67.2 **A:** CD163 expression by the histiocytic component; **B:** reactive histiocytes express PD-L1; **C:** content of reactive T lymphocytes positive for PD-1; **D:** reactive T cells carry TCF1 (immunoalkaline phosphatase technique; Gill hematoxylin counterstaining).

Genetics

The neoplastic cells carry clonal IGHV gene rearrangements with a high load of somatic mutations and intraclonal diversity, further supporting a germinal center cell derivation.[1,3] Such a finding is easily detected by single cell microdissection. TCR gene analysis shows a polyclonal pattern. Karyotypic studies are limited. While early comparative genomic hybridization (CGH) of microdissected neoplastic cells found that the average genome imbalance was higher in NLPBL than in THRLBCL, more recent studies have found the opposite, thus raising further question as to whether de novo THRLBCL is a form of NLPBL progression.[10] Recent CGH array studies suggest that THRLBCL has more genomic aberrations compared with typical and THRLBCL-like variants of NLPBL. There is also mutational overlap between the two diseases, and the median number of mutated genes in these entities is similar. In both THRLBCL and NLPBL, the genes with the highest overall mutation frequency are *JUNB*, *DUSP2*, *SGK1*, *SOCS1*, *CREBBP*, *FN1*, and *TRRAP*; *SOCS1* is the only gene in which mutations occur more frequently in THRLBCL than in NLPBL.[11] Recently, spatial signatures have revealed the occurrence of *PD-L1/PD-L2* copy number alterations and increased expression of PD-1 ligands in a subset of THRLBCLs.[8] These findings highlight the potential importance of the PD1/PDL1 axis and possible sensitivity to immune checkpoint inhibitors.[8,9] The latter is further supported by targeted GEP of the tissue microenvironment, which reveals overexpression of genes related to the functional exhaustion of T cells. Cases enriched in progenitors of exhausted T cells that overexpress *TCF7* (encodes for TCF1, see earlier discussion), may be particularly amenable to anti-PD-1 therapy.[9]

Prognosis and Clinical Comment

THRLBCL is more aggressive than DLBCL, not otherwise specified, and the IPI is prognostic. Treatment is standard chemoimmunotherapy; however, a significant percentage of patients have an aggressive clinical course, refractory disease, and a median overall survival of ~5 years.[12] Importantly, relapsed/refractory (r/r) THRLBCL also appears to be resistant to CD19-directed chimeric antigen receptor T-cell therapy.[13] Anti-PD-1 therapy may represent an attractive option for a subset of r/r patients, and tests that can predict a higher response probability to immune checkpoint inhibitors are of interest.[8,9,14]

References

1. Swerdlow S, Campo E, Harris NL, et al, eds. WHO Classification of Tumours of Haematopoietic and Lymphoid Tissues. 4th ed. International Agency for Research on Cancer (IARC); 2017.
2. Campo E, Jaffe ES, Cook JR, et al. The international consensus classification of mature lymphoid neoplasms: a report from the Clinical Advisory Committee. *Blood*. 2022;140(11):1229-1253.
3. Pittaluga S, Jaffe ES. T-cell/histiocyte-rich large B-cell lymphoma. *Haematologica*. 2010;95(3):352-356.
4. Kommalapati A, Tella SH, Go RS, Nowakowski GS, Goyal G. T cell/histiocyte-rich large B cell lymphoma: incidence, demographic disparities, and long-term outcomes. *Br J Haematol*. 2019;185(1):140-142.
5. Mourad WA, Al Tani S, Tbakhi A, et al. Morphologic, immunphenotypic and clinical discriminators between T-cell/histiocyte-rich large B-cell lymphoma and lymphocyte-predominant Hodgkin lymphoma. *Hematol Oncol Stem Cell Ther*. 2008;1:22-27.
6. Kosari F, Bakhshi T, Ameli F, Mokhtari M. The utility of IMP3 immunohistochemical staining in differentiating nodular lymphocyte predominant Hodgkin lymphoma from T-cell/histiocyte-rich large B-cell lymphoma. *BMC Cancer*. 2022;22(1):1359-1368.
7. Hartmann S, Tousseyn T, Döring C, et al. Macrophages in T cell/histiocyte rich large B cell lymphoma strongly express metal-binding proteins and show a bi-activated phenotype. *Int J Cancer*. 2013;133(11):2609-2618.
8. Griffin GK, Weirather JL, Roemer MGM, et al. Spatial signatures identify immune escape via PD-1 as a defining feature of T-cell/histiocyte-rich large B-cell lymphoma. *Blood*. 2021;137(10):1353-1364.
9. Tabanelli V, Melle F, Motta G, et al. The identification of TCF1+ progenitor exhausted T cells in THRLBCL may predict a better response to PD-1/PD-L1 blockade. *Blood Adv*. 2022;6(15):4634-4644.
10. Hartmann S, Doring C, Vucic E, et al. Array comparative genomic hybridization reveals similarities between nodular lymphocyte predominant Hodgkin lymphoma and T cell/histiocyte rich large B cell lymphoma. *Br J Haematol*. 2015;169(3):415-422.
11. Schuhmacher B, Bein J, Rausch T, et al. *JUNB, DUSP2, SGK1, SOCS1* and *CREBBP* are frequently mutated in T-cell/histiocyte rich large B-cell lymphoma. *Haematologica*. 2019;104(2):330-337.
12. Kim YS, Ji JH, Ko YH, Kim SJ, Kim WS. Matched-pair analysis comparing the outcomes of T cell/histiocyte-rich large B cell lymphoma and diffuse large B cell lymphoma in patients treated with rituximab-CHOP. *Acta Haematol*. 2014;131(3):156-161.
13. Trujillo JA, Godfrey J, Hu Y, et al. Primary resistance to CD19-directed chimeric antigen receptor T-cell therapy in T-cell/histiocyte-rich large B-cell lymphoma. *Blood*. 2021;137(24):3454-3459.
14. Chong EA, Alanio C, Svoboda J, et al. Pembrolizumab for B-cell lymphomas relapsing after or refractory to CD19-directed CAR T-cell therapy. *Blood*. 2022;139(7):1026-1038.

Chapter 68

Primary Diffuse Large B-Cell Lymphoma of the Central Nervous System

Lorinda A. Soma, Andrew Davies, Stefan Dirnhofer, and Gilles Salles

Definition

Primary diffuse large B-cell lymphoma of the central nervous system (PCNS-DLBCL) is a DLBCL involving the brain, leptomeninges, spinal cord, and/or intraocular/vitreoretinal space in immunocompetent patients without systemic involvement. Primary vitreoretinal DLBCL is included here. While rare cases of systemic relapse have been reported,[1,2] these may represent an occult systemic primary tumor.[2] Excluded from this category are intravascular large B-cell lymphoma, systemic lymphoma involving the central nervous system (CNS), dural-based lymphoma, high-grade B-cell lymphoma with *MYC*, *BCL2*, and/or *BCL6* rearrangements, and lymphomas associated with immunodeficiency.[1]

Synonyms

Diffuse large B-cell lymphoma of immune privileged sites (not recommended).

Epidemiology

There are no confirmed risk factors for PCNS-DLBCL. Overall incidence is challenging to define given that many of the large studies include immunocompromised patients and/or non-DLBCL primary CNS lymphomas. However, considering the limitations, the incidence is about 0.4 per 100,000, which has increased over the past 50 years (particularly in the elderly).[1,3,4] PCNS-DLBCL accounts for less than 4% of all intracranial neoplasms and ~4% to 6% of all extranodal lymphomas, with a median age of ~65 years. Although any age group can be affected, most cases occur in patients 60 to 79 years of age. Men are affected at a slightly higher rate than women.[1,3,4]

General Clinical Features

Diagnosing PCNS-DLBCL can be challenging due to diverse clinical presentations.[5] Approximately 50% to 70% of patients exhibit focal neurologic deficits. Another 40% to 50% experience cognitive or behavioral changes. Some may have elevated intracranial pressure symptoms like headaches, vomiting, or nausea (~30%). Rarely the initial signs may manifest as subtle visual abnormalities. When isolated to the eye, symptoms often resemble uveitis. B symptoms are uncommon in PCNS-DLBCL.

Magnetic resonance imaging (MRI) with contrast shows characteristic features including T2 hyperintensity, homogeneous enhancement, and mild edema often involving periventricular or deep brain structures. While rare, PCNS-DLBCL can present with isolated leptomeningeal or ocular involvement, so lumbar puncture and ocular examinations are needed even with a normal MRI. Dissemination outside the CNS is uncommon but shows a predilection for the testes.

Morphology

Similar to DLBCL at other sites, the neoplastic cells may have an immunoblastic, centroblastic, or potentially pleomorphic appearance (Figure 68.1) with scant cytoplasm, round/oval to irregular nuclear contours, open to vesicular chromatin, and variably prominent nucleoli. Tumor cells typically grow in diffuse sheets, with an infiltrative or pushing margin, often associated with mixed inflammatory cells and reactive glial atypia. On occasion the infiltrate is more subtle with isolated neoplastic cells infiltrating in an interstitial pattern. In these cases the cells often appear more intermediate in size on hematoxylin and eosin staining and require immunohistochemistry to highlight their presence and nuclear atypia. A perivascular growth pattern, as well as perivascular T cells associated with and without neoplastic cells, may also be observed. Necrosis may be prominent, leaving only perivascular tumor islands. Necrosis may be amplified after steroid therapy, so knowledge of prebiopsy treatment is critical.[1]

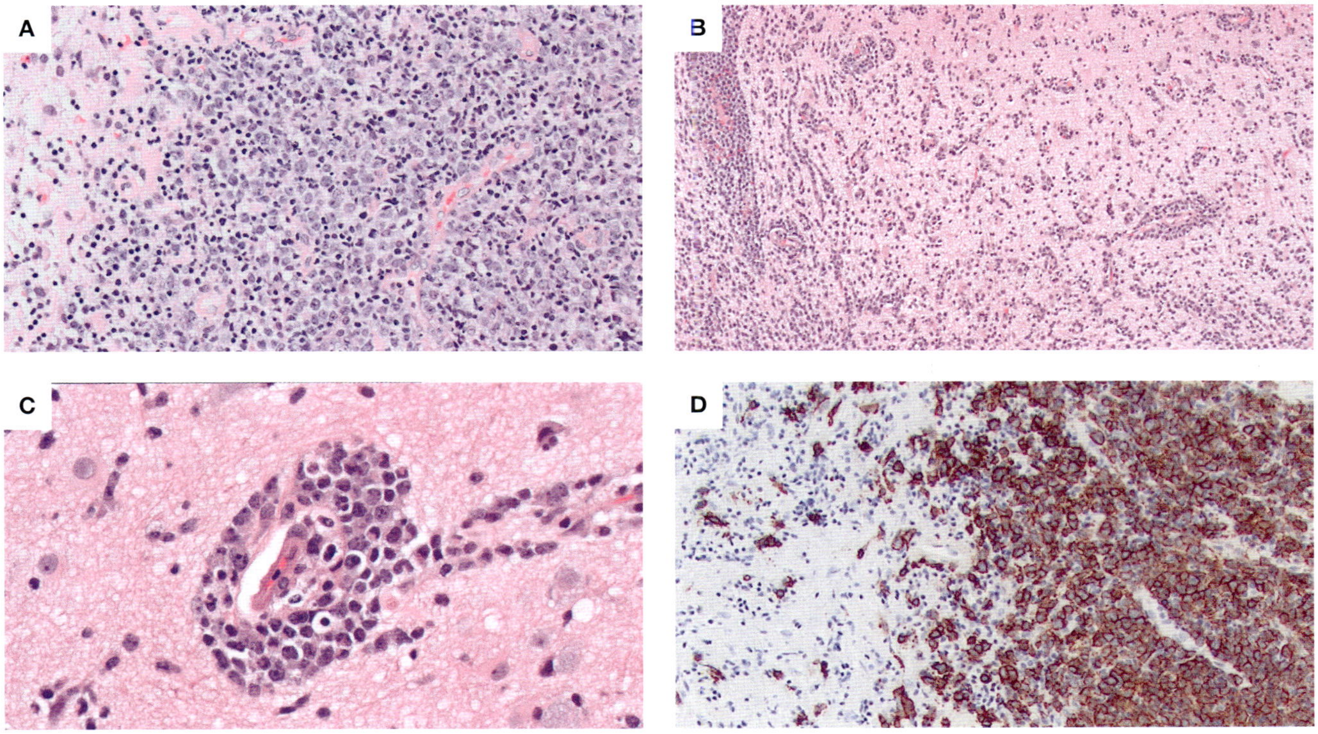

FIGURE 68.1 **A:** Hematoxylin and eosin (H&E) section demonstrates large atypical lymphoid cells infiltrating glial tissue with a pushing margin and associated small reactive lymphocytes. The neoplastic cells have scant cytoplasm, predominantly round nuclear contours, open to vesicular chromatin and most with prominent nucleoli. **B** and **C:** H&E sections demonstrating the perivascular growth pattern. **D:** The lymphoma is positive for CD20 by immunohistochemistry.

Immunophenotype

Tumor cells express B-lineage markers (CD19, CD20, CD79a, PAX5, OCT2, BOB.1) and commonly express BCL2, BCL6, MYC, and MUM1. CD5 is expressed in a subset (~30%) while CD10 expression is uncommon (≤10%) and should raise consideration of systemic lymphoma if present.[1,6] Tumor cells are negative for markers of immaturity (CD34 and TdT), CD138, cyclin D1, and EBER.[1] Similar to primary testicular diffuse large B-cell lymphoma (PT-DLBCL), the neoplastic cells often show decreased or absent expression of HLA-A and HLA-DR.[7] PD-L1 is expressed in a subset of tumors.[5] In the small numbers studied, PCNS-DLBCL exclusively expressed IgM and not IgG.[8] Of note, flow cytometry can be a useful adjunct to diagnosis in cerebrospinal or vitreoretinal fluid samples if cell blocks and tissue biopsy are unavailable.

Genetics

PCNS-DLBCL is typically activated B-cell (ABC) type by cell of origin studies and demonstrates preferential usage of the IGHV4-34 gene segment.[1,9] Although somatically hypermutated, they have not shown successful class switch secondary to deletion of the S-mu region and express IgM and IgD mRNA in the absence of IgG, IgA, and IgE.[8,9] The tumor cells are thought to be derived from late germinal center or non-class-switched IgM memory B cells (*TBL1XR1* mutation impairs terminal B-cell differentiation).[1,9] There is ongoing, aberrant somatic hypermutation, typically 2- to 5-fold higher than systemic DLBCL (Table 68.1).[1,9-11] *BCL6* translocation is common (17%-47%), with *MYC* rearrangements rare and *BCL2* rearrangement essentially absent.[1,9]

Many PCNS-DLBCLs demonstrate a genetic profile similar to the MCD/C5/MYD88 cluster (Table 68.2), resulting in deregulation of the cell cycle, apoptosis inhibition, immune evasion, and blocked terminal B-cell differentiation.[9-13,16] There are frequent recurrent mutations that affect the B-cell receptor, Toll-like receptor, and NF-kB pathway such as *MYD88* (typically L265P), *CD79B* (hot spot Y196), *PIM1, TBL1XR1,* and gains of *BCL2* (Table 68.1).[9-13] Although some have suggested restricting PCNS-DLBCL to the MCD/C5/MYD88 cluster tumors,[9]

TABLE 68.1 Genetic features of primary central nervous system diffuse large B-cell lymphoma[1,3,7,9-15]

	PCNS-DLBCL
Mutations	*MYD88*[a,b] (mostly L265P), *CD79B*[a,c](mostly Y196N, Y196D, Y196C, Y196H, Y196S), *PIM1*[c], *CARD11, ETV6, TBL1XR1,*[b] *KMT2D, PRDM1, SLIT2, TERT, HLA-A/B/C, B2M, CD58, PAX5,*[c] *MYC,*[c] *RHOH,*[c] *HIST1H1E,*[c] *KLHL14,*[c] *BTG2,*[d] *SUSD2,*[c] *IRF4,*[c] *GRHPR,*[d] *OSBPL10,*[d] *TOX, CDKN2A, BCL11A, DAZAP1, FOXC1, DTX1,*[c] *ZNF860,*[d] *BCL2,*[c] *BCL6,*[c] *CXCR4,*[c] *BACH2,*[c] *MPEG1, BTG1, IGLL5*
Rearrangements	*BCL6* (17%-47%), *Ig* genes (38%), *ETV6* (13%-33%), *PD-L1/PDL-2* (13%)
Gains or amplifications	1q32.1 (*IL10*), 3q12 (*NFKBIZ*), 9p24.1 (*PD-L1/PD-L2*), 11q23.3 (*CD3G*), 18q21 (*BCL2, MALT*), 19q13 (*EPN1, FIZ1, ZNF579*)
Losses	3p14 (*FHIT*), 4q35.2, 6p21.32 (*HLA*), 6q21 (*PRDM1, TNFAIP3*), 6q27, 6p25.3 (*IRF4*), 8q12 (*TOX*), 9p21.3 (*CDKN2A*, often biallelic), 10q23.1, 12p13.2, 14q32.33 (*IGH*), 15q21 (*B2M*), 22q11.2 (*GGTLC2)*

[a]Often occurs as comutations.
[b]Often occurs as comutations.
[c]Aberrant somatic hypermutation (ASHM).
[d]ASMH significantly more frequent in PCNS-DLBCL than in ABC DLBCL; note that study[14] included primary and secondary vitreoretinal lymphoma; however, it noted few differences (only six cases were not subsequent to PCNS-DLBCL, three of which were extranodal DLBCL).

Swerdlow SH, Campo E, Harris NL, et al. eds. *WHO classification of Tumours of Haematopoietic and Lymphoid Tissue.* 4th ed. Lyon: International Agency for Research on Cancer, 2017; Ferreri AJM, Calimeri T, Cwynarski K, et al. Primary central nervous system lymphoma. *Nat Rev Disease Primers.* 2023:9(29):1-19; Riemersma SA, Jordanova ES, Schop RFJ, et al. Extensive genetic alterations of the HLA region, including homozygous deletions of HLA class II genes in B-cell lymphomas arising in immune-privileged sites. *Blood.* 2000;96(10):3569-3577; Bertoni F, Montesinos-Rongen M. Primary diffuse large B cell lymphoma of the central nervous system: molecular and biological features of neoplastic cells. *Ann Lymphoma.* 2022;6:1-22; Hernandez-Verdin I, Kirasic E, Wienand K, et al. Molecular and clinical diversity in primary central nervous system lymphoma. *Annals Oncol.* 2023;34(2):186-199; Radke J, Ishaque N, Koll R, et al. The genomic and transcriptional landscape of primary central nervous system lymphoma. *Nat Commun.* 2022;13:2558-2577; Chapuy B, Roemer MGM, Stewart C, et al. Targetable genetic features of primary testicular and primary central nervous system lymphomas. *Blood.* 2016;127(7):869-881; Schmitz R, Wright GW, Huang DW, et al. Genetics and pathogenesis of diffuse large B cell lymphoma. *NEJM.* 2018;378:1396-1407; Bonzheim I, Sander P, Salmeraon-Villalobos J, et al. The molecular hallmarks of primary and secondary vitreoretinal lymphoma. *Blood Adv.* 2022;6(5):1598-1607; and Schwindt H, Vater I, Kreuz M, et al. Chromosomal imbalances and partial uniparental disomies in primary central nervous system lymphoma. *Leukemia.* 2009;23:1875-1884.

a recent large multi-institutional study[10] reported only 40% MCD, with 39% classified as "other," 13% as A53, and 8% as BN2 subgroups using the LymphGen algorithm and genetic subtype described by Wright et al.[17]

Although there are similarities between PCNS-DLBCL, PT-DLBCL, and the MCD/M5/MYD88 DLBCL cluster, which contains predominantly ABC-type tumors (Table 68.2), genetic alterations and gene expression profiling studies have shown PCNS-DLBCL to be distinct from systemic ABC-type DLBCL.[11,12] Additionally, a recent study using a "multiomic" data consensus clustering approach reports that PCNS-DLBCL can be separated into four subtypes with differences in prognosis and genetic clusters, with meningeal infiltration having the worst prognosis.[10] Interestingly, a small cohort of PCNS-DLBCL with meningeal manifestation was found to have RNA expression signature more similar to systemic DLBCL (and one with *BCL2* rearrangement), also suggesting meningeal involvement may represent a distinct subtype.[11]

Highlighting their distinct biology from PCNS-DLBCL, CNS lymphomas arising in immunocompromised patients essentially lack mutations in *MYD88* L265P, *CD79B* Y196, and *PIM1*; and lack loss of *CDKN2A*, with rare *HLA* loss, and lower incidence of ABC subtype.[11,12,18,19]

Of note, molecular studies to either establish clonality or identify common mutations such as MYD88 L265P can be a useful diagnostic adjunct in cases with sparse material (such as cerebrospinal or vitreous fluids).[14] However, tissue biopsy assessment remains the gold standard as other B-cell lymphomas can involve the CNS.

Prognosis and Clinical Comment

Prognostic factors in PCNS-DLBCL include age, performance status, deep brain structure involvement, serum lactate dehydrogenase, and cerebrospinal fluid protein concentration.[5] Corticosteroid use should be deferred until after pathologic confirmation to avoid reducing diagnostic yield. High-dose methotrexate is the mainstay of treatment, often combined with agents like high-dose cytarabine, procarbazine, thiotepa, and rituximab to enhance response rates. Whole-brain or focal radiation, previously used for consolidation, is now being replaced by high-dose chemotherapy with autologous stem cell transplant, particularly in younger patients.[20] Although sensitive to chemoradiation, relapse rates are high, with a 30% to 40% 5-year survival.[5] Given the prevalence of B-cell receptor signaling pathway alterations in PCNS-DLBCL, targeted therapies like Bruton tyrosine kinase inhibitors or lenalidomide have shown efficacy in relapse cases. CD19-directed chimeric antigen receptor T cells have also demonstrated effectiveness in patients with PCNS-DLBCL. Ongoing research aims to determine the optimal combinations or sequencing of these modalities.[5,21] Recent studies have also explored the integration of plasma ctDNA profiling for diagnosing and monitoring patients with PCNS-DLBCL.[14,22]

TABLE 68.2 Comparison of the incidence of genetic alterations in primary central nervous system diffuse large B-cell lymphoma (PCNS-DLBCL), primary testicular diffuse large B-cell lymphoma (PT-DLBCL), diffuse large B-cell lymphoma, not otherwise specified (DLBCL, NOS), MCD/C5/MYD88 cluster[1,7,9,11-13,16,17]

	PCNS-DLBCL	PT-DLBCL	MCD/C5/MYD88	DLBCL, NOS
BCL6 translocation	Low to moderate	Moderate	Low	- GCB: Low - ABC: Moderate
HLA class 1 (6p21.32) inactivation	Moderate to high[a]	Moderate (deletion)	Moderate to high[a]	- GCB: Very low to low[a] - ABC: Low to moderate[a]
CDKN2A (9p21.3) loss	High (often biallelic)	Very high (often biallelic)	Very high	- GCB: Very low - ABC: Moderate
TP53 mutation	Very low[b]	Very low	Very low	- GCB: Moderate - ABC: Moderate
NFKBIZ (3q12) copy gain	Moderate to high	Moderate	NR	- GCB: Very low - ABC: Very low to moderate
MYD88	Moderate to high	High	High	- GCB: Very low - ABC: Moderate
CD79B	Moderate to high	Moderate	High	- GCB: Very low - ABC: Low to moderate
PIM1	Moderate to high[a]	Moderate	Very high	- GCB: Low - ABC: Moderate
COO	High ABC	High ABC	Very high ABC	- GCB: ~60% - ABC: ~30% - Unclassifiable: ~10%

Incidence: Very low (<10%), low (10%-19%), moderate (20%-49%), high 50% to 79%, very high >80%.
ABC, germinal center exit/post–germinal center origin; COO, cell of origin; GCB, germinal center origin; NR, not reported.
[a]Includes mutations in addition to deletions.
[b]Although most studies show a very low incidence (<10%), there is variation in the literature.
Swerdlow SH, Campo E, Harris NL, et al. eds. *WHO classification of Tumours of Haematopoietic and Lymphoid Tissue.* 4th ed. Lyon: International Agency for Research on Cancer, 2017; Riemersma SA, Jordanova ES, Schop RFJ, et al. Extensive genetic alterations of the HLA region, including homozygous deletions of HLA class II genes in B-cell lymphomas arising in immune-privileged sites. *Blood.* 2000;96(10):3569-3577; Bertoni F, Montesinos-Rongen M. Primary diffuse large B cell lymphoma of the central nervous system: molecular and biological features of neoplastic cells. *Ann Lymphoma.* 2022;6:1-22; Radke J, Ishaque N, Koll R, et al. The genomic and transcriptional landscape of primary central nervous system lymphoma. Nat Commun. 2022;13:2558-2577; Chapuy B, Roemer MGM, Stewart C, et al. Targetable genetic features of primary testicular and primary central nervous system lymphomas. *Blood.* 2016;127(7):869-881; Schmitz R, Wright GW, Huang DW, et al. Genetics and pathogenesis of diffuse large B cell lymphoma. *NEJM.* 2018;378:1396-1407; Chapuy B, Stewart C, Dunford AJ, et al. Molecular subtypes of diffuse large B cell lymphoma are associated with distinct pathogenic mechanisms and outcomes. *Nat Med.* 2018;24:679-690; and Wright GW, Huang DW, Phelan JD, et al. A probabilistic classification tool for genetics subtypes of diffuse large B cell lymphoma with therapeutic implications. *Cancer Cell.* 2020;37:551-568.

References

1. Kluin PM, Deckert M, Ferry FA. Primary diffuse large B cell lymphoma of the CNS. In: Swerdlow SH, Campo E, Harris NL, et al, eds. *WHO Classification of Tumours of Haematopoietic and Lymphoid Tissue.* 4th ed. International Agency for Research on Cancer; 2017:300-302.
2. Provencher S, Ferlay C, Alaoui-Slimani K, et al. Clinical characteristics and outcome of isolated extracerebral relapses of primary central nervous system lymphoma: a case series. *Hematol Oncol.* 2011;29(1):10-16. doi:10.1002/hon.944
3. Ferreri AJM, Calimeri T, Cwynarski K, et al. Primary central nervous system lymphoma. *Nat Rev Dis Primers.* 2023;9(1):29-19. doi:10.1038/s41572-023-00439-0

4. Mendez JS, Ostrom QT, Gittleman H, et al. The elderly left behind – changes in survival trends of primary central nervous system lymphoma over the past 4 decades. *Neuro Oncol.* 2018;20(5):687-694. doi:10.1093/neuonc/nox187
5. Schaff LR, Grommes C. Primary central nervous system lymphoma. *Blood.* 2022;140(9):971-979. doi:10.1182/blood.2020008377
6. Imai H, Shimada K, Shimada S, et al. Comparative clinicopathological study of primary CNS diffuse large B-cell lymphoma and intravascular large B-cell lymphoma. *Pathol Int.* 2009;59(7):431-437. doi:10.1111/j.1440-1827.2009.02390.x
7. Riemersma SA, Jordanova ES, Schop RFJ, et al. Extensive genetic alterations of the HLA region, including homozygous deletions of HLA class II genes in B-cell lymphomas arising in immune-privileged sites. *Blood.* 2000;96(10):3569-3577.
8. Montesinos-Rongen M, Schmitz R, Courts C, et al. Absence of immunoglobulin class switch in primary lymphomas of the central nervous system. *Aust J Pharm.* 2005;166(6):1773-1779. doi:10.1016/S0002-9440(10)62487-X
9. Bertoni F, Montesinos-Rongen M. Primary diffuse large B cell lymphoma of the central nervous system: molecular and biological features of neoplastic cells. *Ann Lymphoma.* 2022;6:1-22. doi:10.21037/aol-21-38
10. Hernandez-Verdin I, Kirasic E, Wienand K, et al. Molecular and clinical diversity in primary central nervous system lymphoma. *Ann Oncol.* 2023;34(2):186-199. doi:10.1016/j.annonc.2022.11.002
11. Radke J, Ishaque N, Koll R, et al. The genomic and transcriptional landscape of primary central nervous system lymphoma. *Nat Commun.* 2022;13(1):2558-2577. doi:10.1038/s41467-022-30050-y
12. Chapuy B, Roemer MGM, Stewart C, et al. Targetable genetic features of primary testicular and primary central nervous system lymphomas. *Blood.* 2016;127(7):869-881. doi:10.1182/blood-2015-10-673236
13. Schmitz R, Wright GW, Huang DW, et al. Genetics and pathogenesis of diffuse large B cell lymphoma. *NEJM.* 2018;378(15):1396-1407. doi:10.1056/NEJMoa1801445
14. Bonzheim I, Sander P, Salmeraon-Villalobos J, et al. The molecular hallmarks of primary and secondary vitreoretinal lymphoma. *Blood Adv.* 2022;6(5):1598-1607. doi:10.1182/bloodadvances.2021004212
15. Schwindt H, Vater I, Kreuz M, et al. Chromosomal imbalances and partial uniparental disomies in primary central nervous system lymphoma. *Leukemia.* 2009;23(10):1875-1884. doi:10.1038/leu.2009.120
16. Chapuy B, Stewart C, Dunford AJ, et al. Molecular subtypes of diffuse large B cell lymphoma are associated with distinct pathogenic mechanisms and outcomes. *Nat Med.* 2018;24(5):679-690. doi:10.1038/s41591-018-0016-8
17. Wright GW, Huang DW, Phelan JD, et al. A probabilistic classification tool for genetic subtypes of diffuse large B cell lymphoma with therapeutic implications. *Cancer Cell.* 2020;37(4):551-568.e14. doi:10.1016/j.ccell.2020.03.015
18. Kaulen LD, Denisoa E, Hinz F, et al. Integrated genetic analyses of immunodeficiency-associated Epstein-Barr virus- (EBV) positive primary CNS lymphomas. *Acta Neuropathol.* 2023;146(3):499-514. doi:10.1007/s00401-023-02613-w
19. Gandhi MK, Hoang T, Law SC, et al. EBV-associated primary CNS lymphoma occurring after immunosuppression is a distinct immunobiological entity. *Blood.* 2021;137(11):1468-1477. doi:10.1182/blood.2020008520
20. Ferreri AJM, Cwynarski K, Pulczynski E, et al. Long-term efficacy, safety and neurotolerability of MATRix regimen followed by autologous transplant in primary CNS lymphoma: 7-year results of the IELSG32 randomized trial. *Leukemia.* 2022;36(7):1870-1878. doi:10.1038/s41375-022-01582-5
21. Roschewski M, Hodson DJ. Diffuse large B-cell lymphoma involving the central nervous system: biologic rationale for targeted therapy. *Haematologica.* 2023;109(2):388-400. doi:10.3324/haematol.2021.278613
22. Mutter JA, Alig SK, Esfahani MS, et al. Circulating tumor DNA profiling for detection, risk stratification, and classification of brain lymphomas. *J Clin Oncol.* 2023;41(9):1684-1694. doi:10.1200/JCO.22.00826

Chapter 69

Primary Diffuse Large B-Cell Lymphoma of the Testis

Lorinda A. Soma, Andrew Davies, Stefan Dirnhofer, and Gilles Salles

Definition

Primary diffuse large B-cell lymphoma of the testis (PT-DLBCL) is a lymphoma composed of large B cells arising in the testis. It is a lymphoma of an immune-privileged, or sanctuary, site given the blood-testis barrier. The majority of cases are limited to the testes (a small percentage with bilateral involvement), although a subset presents with systemic disease.[1-3] Spread at presentation is typically to extranodal sites (commonly central nervous system [CNS]), and locoregional lymph nodes, with relapse more often extranodal (particularly CNS and contralateral testis) than nodal.[3,4] Excluded are other lymphoma subtypes, such as immunodeficiency-associated lymphoma, mantle cell lymphoma, Burkitt lymphoma, high-grade B-cell lymphomas with *MYC* and *BCL2* and/or *BCL6* rearrangement, systemic DLBCL involving the testis, and follicular lymphoma of the testis.

Synonyms

Diffuse large B-cell lymphoma of immune-privileged sites (not recommended).

Epidemiology

Primary diffuse large B-cell lymphoma of the testis (PT-DLBCL) is uncommon, comprising <1% of all lymphomas and <3% of all testicular neoplasms; however, it is the most common primary lymphoma of the genitourinary tract.[5] A Surveillance, Epidemiology, and End Results data study reported an annual incidence that has increased from the early 1980s to the early 2000s (0.06-0.09 per 100,000).[6] Note that many epidemiologic studies evaluate all testicular lymphomas as a whole[5]; however, DLBCL accounts "only" for ~80% of all histologic types, skewing the data toward PT-DLBCL. The median age of diagnosis is 68 to 71 years (range 26-93),[1,5-7] typically being a disease of older men compared with germ cell tumors which affect a younger age group (median 34 years).[5] PT-DLBCL is the most common testicular malignancy in patients >60 years of age, which may be related to Sertoli cell loss with age, a cell type that plays an essential role in the blood-testis barrier.[8,9] Whites are most commonly affected (81%-86% of cases),[5,6] with a higher incidence (0.1 per 100,000) than Hispanics, Asians, Pacific Islanders, or blacks (0.08-0.05 per 100,000).[6]

General Clinical Features

PT-DLBCL presents as a firm mass, most commonly painless, discovered by the patient on either testicular side.[3,6] An orchiectomy is optimal for diagnosis. Systemic symptoms are rare (~10%), but elevation of serum lactate dehydrogenase is encountered in ~25% of the patients. Staging (including thorough investigations for CNS dissemination) may reveal satellite iliac nodes, and while bilateral cases occur in less than 10% of patients, other extranodal disease sites can be involved at initial staging in 10% to 20% of the cases.[3,6,8]

Morphology

PT-DLBCL comprises a diffuse proliferation of discohesive, atypical lymphoid cells that infiltrate the testicular parenchyma, surrounding, distorting, and/or obliterating the normal structures, which may also include the epididymis and spermatic cord. The cells are intermediate to large in size with scant cytoplasm, typically with centroblastic cytomorphology (Figure 69.1).[7]

Immunophenotype

Immunophenotypic characteristics are similar to nodal DLBCL, with expression of B-lineage antigens (CD19, CD20, CD79a, PAX5) with CD79a being the most commonly expressed at 100%.[7] Unlike nodal DLBCL (but similar to primary CNS diffuse large B-cell lymphoma, PCNS-DLBCL), the majority are non-germinal center

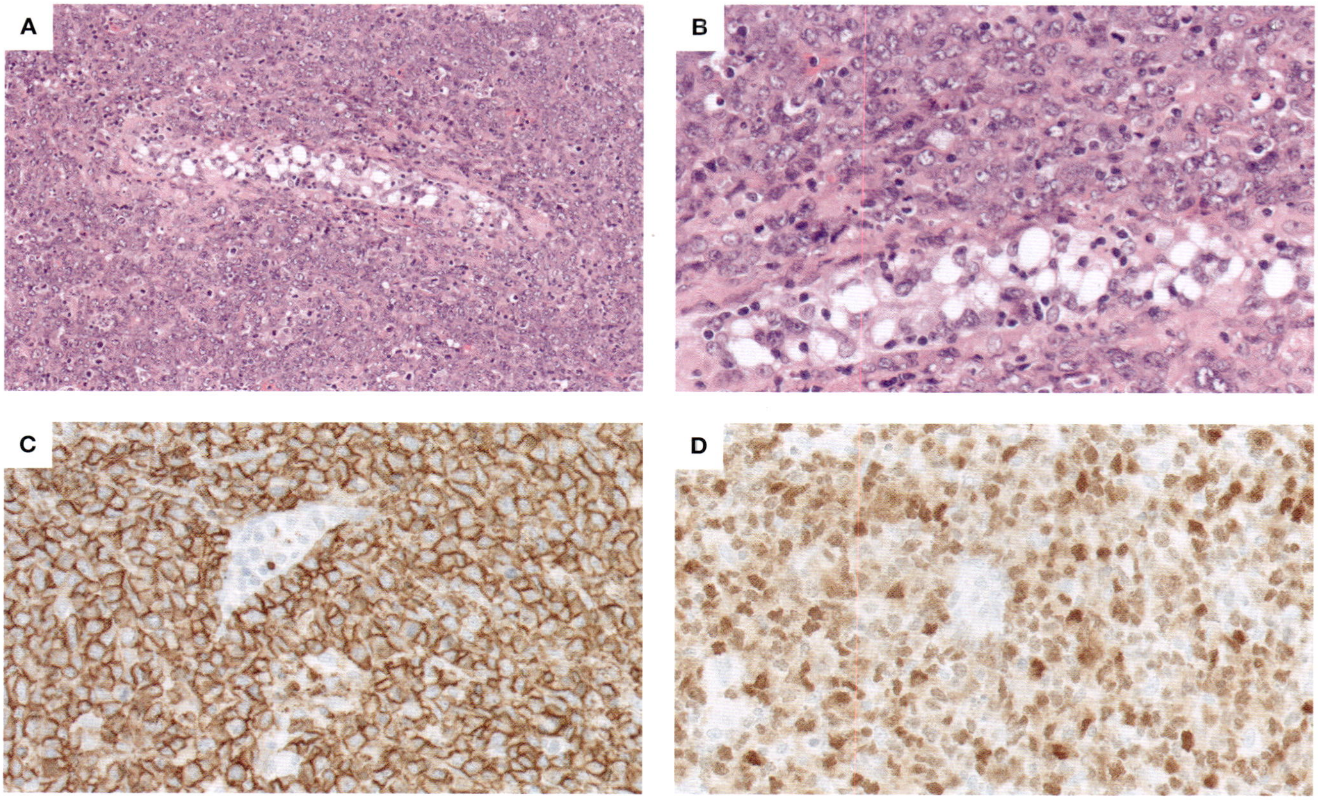

FIGURE 69.1 Primary diffuse large B-cell lymphoma of the testis showing a diffuse proliferation of large pleomorphic cells with prominent nucleoli. There is destructive intertubular spread associated with obliteration of the seminiferous tubules (**A** and **B**). Tumor cells are positive for CD20 (**C**) and MUM1/IRF4 (**D**).

B-cell subtype (>75%)[1,4,7] and GCB versus non-GCB does not appear to impact prognosis.[4] PT-DLBCL is typically IgM and BCL2 positive (70%), with a small number expressing MYC (13%) and fewer double expressers than nodal DLBCL.[7,9] There is variable expression of CD5 (22%), CD10 (20%-29%), BCL6 (5%-40%) and MUM1 (23%-78%), with GCET and LMO2 being uncommon (<10%) and CD138 rare (5%).[7,9] TCL1, FOXP1, and PD-L1/L2 are often expressed (67%, 53%-78%, and 35%-47%, respectively).[4,7,9,10] The majority of cases show active STAT and CXCR4 signaling, with expression of phosphorylated proteins.[7] CyclinD1, HHV8, and EBER are negative in this entity. Considering markers that can be expressed in germ cell tumors, CD30 is uncommon with absence of SALL4, PLAP, NUT1, and CD117 and with rare cases reporting OCT4 expression.[7,9]

Genetics

There are many similarities between PT-DLBCL and PCNS-DLBCL, such as common assignment to the MCD/C5/MYD88 subgroup,[2,10] with alterations of the NF-kB pathway, increased Toll-like receptor and B-cell receptor signaling, and predominantly activated B-cell type by gene expression profiling[4] (please refer to Table 68.2). PT-DLBCL demonstrates a high level of somatic hypermutation[4,8] and increased incidence of mutations in *MYD88* L265P (67%-82%),[1,2,9,10] *PIM1* (66%),[2] and *CD79B* (16%-50%; hotspot Y196).[2,10] Of note, a similar incidence in *MYD88* L265P and other genetic alterations have been reported in both limited and advanced-stage disease, supporting the concept that patients presenting with extratesticular involvement can represent PT-DLBCL.[1,2] Gains of *NFKBIZ* (3q12.3; 42%), *FIZ1* (19q13; 70%), and *BLC2* (18q21; 47%), as well as loss of *CDKN2A* (9p21.3 88%; 77% biallelic) and *TNFAIP3* (6p23.3; 50%), are frequently seen copy number alterations.[10] Unlike in systemic DLBCL, *TP53* mutations are infrequent, with loss of upstream *CDKN2A* instead causing perturbations of the *TP53* pathway.[10] *BCL6* rearrangement is common (30%),[1,2,7,9,10] whereas *BCL2* and *MYC* rearrangements are much less (<5% and ≤10%, respectively).[1,7,9] Gains, amplification, or rearrangement of 9p24.1 (*PD-L1/L2* locus, with associated overexpression); copy loss of 6p21 (*HLA*); deletion 15q21.1 (*B2M*); and rearrangements of *CIITA* (transcription factor regulating MHC class II expression) may contribute to immune evasion and disease spread.[1,8,10]

Prognosis and Clinical Comment

This extranodal disease is highly curable with a classical modern immunochemotherapy approach, including rituximab and anthracycline, but the risk of contralateral testis or CNS recurrence is particular to this entity.[8] Hence, after orchiectomy and completion of systemic therapy, prophylactic contralateral testis irradiation and CNS-directed prophylaxis are highly recommended, with the respective merits of high-dose intravenous versus local intrathecal methotrexate/cytarabine being unclear.[8] A phase II prospective study of stage I-II PT-DLBCL reported 5-year progression-free and overall survival of 74% and 85%, respectively,[11] but real-world reports indicate that patients with advanced age, disseminated disease, or high international prognostic index score at diagnosis have a less favorable outcome.[12,13] The prognosis of patients with recurrent disease is poor. Given the rarity of the disease, approaches relying on molecular features or cellular therapies have not yet been reported.

References

1. Twa DDW, Lee DG, Tan KL, et al. Genomic predictors of central nervous system relapse in primary testicular diffuse large B cell lymphoma. *Blood.* 2021;137(9):1256-1259. doi:10.1182/blood.2020006338
2. Wong J, Collinge B, Hilton LK, et al. Genetic determinants of isolated and systemic testicular diffuse large B-cell lymphoma highlight a disease spectrum. *Blood.* 2022;140(suppl 1):6374-6375. doi:10.1182/blood-2022-165546.
3. Zucca E, Conconi A, Mughal TI, et al. Patterns of outcome and prognostic factors in primary large-cell lymphoma of the testis in a survey by the International Extranodal Lymphoma Study Group. *J Clin Oncol.* 2003;21(1):20-27. doi:10.1200/JCO.2003.11.141
4. Deng L, Xu-Monette ZY, Longhavi S, et al. Primary testicular diffuse large B cell lymphoma displays distinct clinical and biological features for treatment failure in rituximab era: a report from the International PTL Consortium. *Leukemia.* 2016;30(2):361-372. doi:10.1038/leu.2015.237
5. Palumbo C, Mazzone E, Mistretta FA, et al. Primary lymphomas of the genitourinary tract: a population-based study. *Asian J Urol.* 2020;7(4):332-339. doi:10.1016/j.ajur.2019.11.002
6. Gundrum JD, Mathiason MA, Moore DB, Go RS. Primary testicular diffuse large B-cell lymphoma: a population-based study on the incidence, natural history, and survival comparison with primary nodal counterpart before and after the introduction of rituximab. *AJCO (Am J Clin Oncol).* 2009;27(31):5227-5232. doi:10.1200/JCO.2009.22.5896
7. Mentor T, Ernst M, Drachneris J, et al. Phenotype profiling of primary testicular diffuse large B-cell lymphomas. *Hematol Oncol.* 2014;32(2):72-81. doi:10.1002/hon.2090
8. Cheah CY, Wirth A, Seymour JF. Primary testicular lymphoma. *Blood.* 2014;123(4):486-493. doi:10.1182/blood-2013-10-530659
9. Twa DDW, Mottok A, Savage KJ, Steidl C. The pathobiology of primary testicular diffuse large B cell lymphoma: implications for novel therapies. *Blood Rev.* 2018;32(3):249-255. doi:10.1016/j.blre.2017.12.001
10. Chapuy B, Roemer MGM, Stewart C, et al. Targetable genetic features of primary testicular and primary central nervous system lymphomas. *Blood.* 2016;127(7):869-881. doi:10.1182/blood-2015-10-673236
11. Vitolo U, Chiappella A, Ferreri AJ, et al. First-line treatment for primary testicular diffuse large B-cell lymphoma with rituximab-CHOP, CNS prophylaxis, and contralateral testis irradiation: final results of an international phase II trial. *J Clin Oncol.* 2011;29(20):2766-2772. doi:10.1200/JCO.2010.31.4187
12. Kridel R, Telio D, Villa D, et al. Diffuse large B-cell lymphoma with testicular involvement: outcome and risk of CNS relapse in the rituximab era. *Br J Haematol.* 2017;176(2):210-221. doi:10.1111/bjh.14392
13. Mannisto S, Vähämurto P, Pollari M, et al. Intravenous but not intrathecal central nervous system-directed chemotherapy improves survival in patients with testicular diffuse large B-cell lymphoma. *Eur J Cancer.* 2019;115:27-36. doi:10.1016/j.ejca.2019.04.004

Chapter 70

Primary Cutaneous Diffuse Large B-Cell Lymphoma, Leg Type

John R. Goodlad, Steven T. Rosen, and Anne-Roos Schrader

Definition

Primary cutaneous diffuse large B-cell lymphoma, leg type (PCDLBCL-LT) is a B-cell neoplasm arising primarily in and confined to the skin at presentation. It is composed of large centroblasts and/or immunoblasts. While it most frequently arises on the legs it is not limited to this site. "Primary cutaneous diffuse large B-cell lymphoma other" is no longer recognized as an entity, most cases fulfilling criteria for PCDLBCL-LT or primary cutaneous follicle center lymphoma with a diffuse growth pattern.

Synonyms

None.

Epidemiology

PCDLBCL-LT accounts for around 20% of primary cutaneous B-cell lymphomas but only 4% of all primary cutaneous lymphomas. Most patients are elderly with a median age of >70 years at presentation. There is a pronounced female bias (F:M ratio = 3-4:1).

General Clinical Features

The majority of PCDLBCL-LT present with lesions in the skin of the lower leg, although non-leg sites are involved in 10% to 15% of cases. Disease usually presents as multiple, or less frequently solitary, red or reddish-blue nodules and tumors (Figure 70.1).

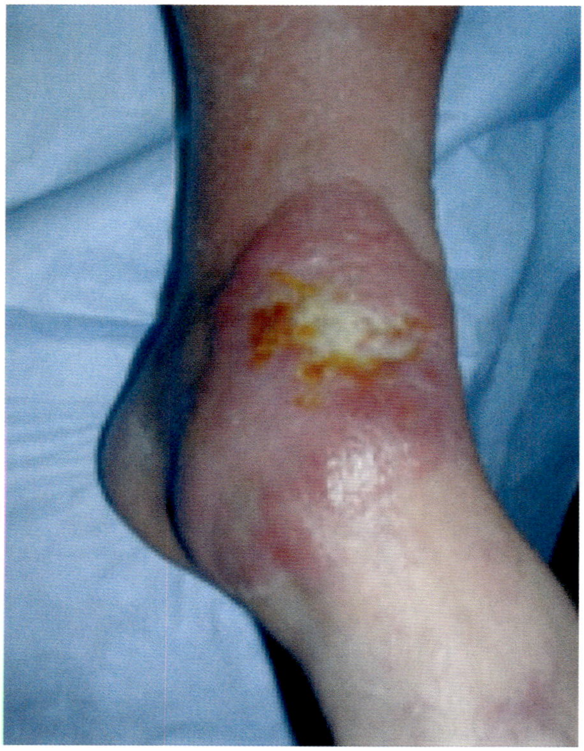

FIGURE 70.1 Primary cutaneous diffuse large B-cell lymphoma, leg type presenting as an ulcerated tumor on the lower leg.

Morphology

PCDLBCL-LT manifests as diffuse sheets of large B cells with centroblast-like and/or immunoblast-like morphology that often fill the dermis and may extend into subcutis but with epidermal sparing (Figure 70.2). Background small reactive T cells are generally sparse.

Immunophenotype

The neoplastic B cells most often display a post–germinal center phenotype. Typically, they express CD20, CD79A, and PAX5, with strong coexpression of BCL2 (95%), IRF4/MUM1 (84%), and FOXP1, usually with BCL6 (67%) and MYC, and absence of CD10 and cyclin D1[11] (Figure 70.3). In contrast to primary cutaneous follicle center lymphoma, PCDLBCL-LT is typically positive for IgM, and this may be useful for discriminating between the two entities[7] (Figure 70.3). However, the phenotype is not entirely uniform. Some cases are negative for BCL6, IRF4/MUM1, and/or BCL2, and a small

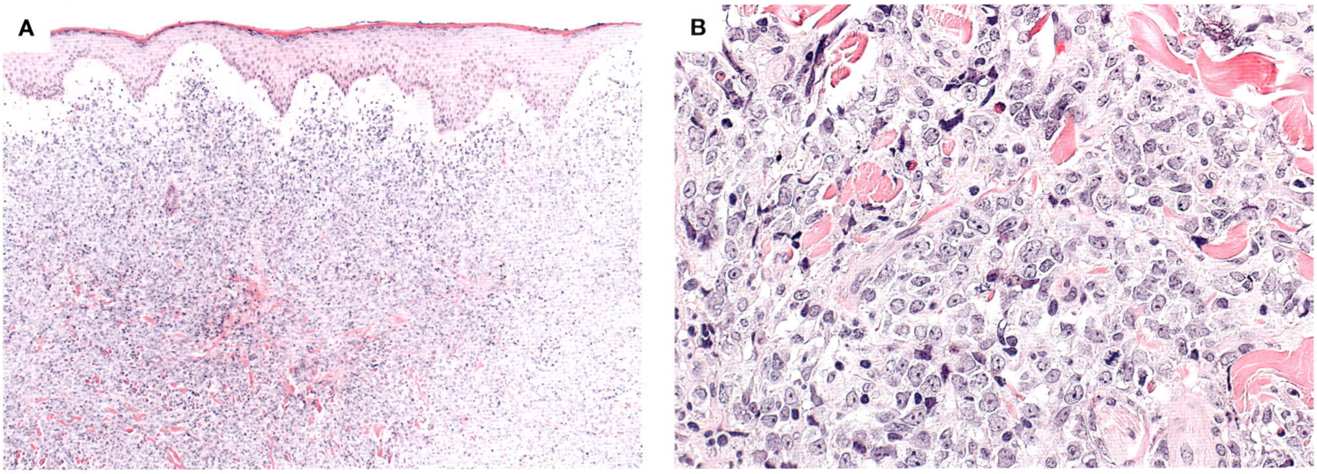

FIGURE 70.2 Primary cutaneous diffuse large B-cell lymphoma, leg type. **A:** The dermis is filled by a diffuse infiltrate of large lymphoid cells. **B:** The tumor cells possess oval to round nuclei, finely dispersed nuclear chromatin, and prominent nucleoli.

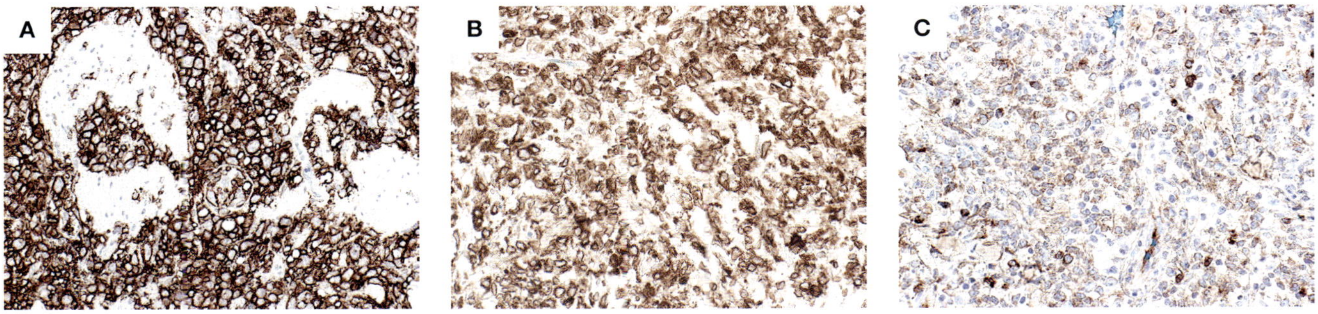

FIGURE 70.3 Primary cutaneous diffuse large B-cell lymphoma, leg type. **A:** The tumor cells are positive for CD20. **B:** Strong expression of BCL2. **C:** Cytoplasmic expression of IgM; this can help differentiate from large cell variant of primary cutaneous follicle center lymphoma with diffuse growth.

percentage of cases express CD10 (10%).[4,11] A diagnosis of PCDLBCL-LT is still tenable in such a situation provided other findings are typical. Rare TdT-positive cases have been reported, raising a diagnostic dilemma with B-lymphoblastic leukemia/lymphoma, which may also present in the skin.[3] Absent or weak expression of CD20 is a clue to the latter.

Genetics

Rearrangements of *MYC*, usually with an immunoglobulin gene partner, are found in 5% to 44% of cases, and *BCL6* rearrangements in 12% to 50%.[12] Occasional cases with both *MYC* and *BCL6* rearrangements are described. Amplification of 18q21.3, housing *BCL2* and *MALT1*, is present in 60% to 70% of PCDLBCL-LT, and this may account for the high levels of *BCL2* expression associated with this neoplasm.[1] *BCL2* rearrangements are extremely rare. Inactivation of *CDKN2A* and *CDKN2B* due to promoter methylation or loss of 9p21.3 is found in two-thirds of cases, and there is frequent loss of *PRDM1* (15%) and *TNFAIP3* (25%).[1,8,10]

Gene expression profiling is inconsistent with respect to assigning cell of origin in PCDLBCL-LT. Early studies classified all cases as activated B-cell type of diffuse large B-cell lymphoma (DLBCL), but other more recent investigations show a much more mixed picture, with many cases classifying as germinal center B-cell type.[6,11] Consequently, this technique has little diagnostic value. Irrespective of cell of origin, PCDLBCL-LT has a distinctive mutational profile with many similarities to that of other extranodal DLBCL arising in immune-privileged sites, including primary central nervous system DLBCL, primary testicular DLBCL, and intravascular large B-cell lymphoma, as well as with the C5/MCD subtype of DLBCL.[8,13,16] There is frequent mutation of the Toll-like receptor *MYD88* (60%-75% of cases), B-cell signaling pathway components *CD79B* (30%-40%), and *CARD11*, as well as *PIM1* (37%-70%), *IRF4* (16%), and *MYC* (20%). Loss of TNFAIP and mutations of B-cell signaling pathway genes, as well as *IRF4*, implicate constitutive activation of NFkB in the pathogenesis of PCDLBCL-LT and may provide an explanation for poor response to treatment in some cases.[2,10,16]

Prognosis and Clinical Comment

Systemic chemotherapy with R-CHOP is the treatment of choice for patients with PCDLBCL-LT, combined with involved field radiotherapy for those with localized disease. Patients unable to tolerate systemic chemotherapy may benefit from single-agent rituximab plus radiotherapy in appropriate cases.[15]

For relapse/refractory disease, drug conjugates, bispecific monoclonal antibodies, and CAR-T-cell treatments can be considered in appropriate patients. Disease-specific 5-year survival is 74% for patients receiving polychemotherapy and rituximab but lower when this approach is not feasible.[5,14] Factors reported to predict a poorer outcome in terms of survival include presence of multiple skin lesions at diagnosis, inactivation of *CDKN2A*, rearrangement of *MYC*, and *MYD88* mutation.[1,9,12,14]

References

1. Dijkman R, Tensen CP, Jordanova ES, et al. Array-based comparative genomic hybridization analysis reveals recurrent chromosomal alterations and prognostic parameters in primary cutaneous large B-cell lymphoma. *J Clin Oncol.* 2006;24(2):296-305. doi:10.1200/JCO.2005.02.0842.
2. Ducharme O, Beylot-Barry M, Pham-Ledard A, et al. Mutations of the B-cell receptor pathway confer chemoresistance in primary cutaneous diffuse large B-cell lymphoma leg type. *J Invest Dermatol.* 2019;139(11):2334-2342.e8. doi:10.1016/j.jid.2019.05.008.
3. Endo M, Ohtsuka M, Watanabe Y, et al. TdT-positive primary cutaneous diffuse large B-cell lymphoma, leg type phenotypically mimicking B-lymphoblastic lymphoma. *J Cutan Pathol.* 2021;48(5):721-724. doi:10.1111/cup.13955.
4. Goodlad JR, Krajewski AS, McKay P, et al. Site and disease extent as prognostic indicators in primary cutaneous diffuse large B-cell lymphoma. *J Pathol.* 2002;198:13A-13A.<Go to ISI>://WOS:000177903200052.
5. Grange F, Joly P, Barbe C, et al. Improvement of survival in patients with primary cutaneous diffuse large B-cell lymphoma, leg type, in France. *JAMA Dermatol.* 2014;150(5):535-541. doi:10.1001/jamadermatol.2013.7452.
6. Hoefnagel JJ, Dijkman R, Basso K, et al. Distinct types of primary cutaneous large B-cell lymphoma identified by gene expression profiling. *Blood.* 2005;105(9):3671-3678. doi:10.1182/blood-2004-04-1594.
7. Koens L, Vermeer MH, Willemze R, Jansen PM. IgM expression on paraffin sections distinguishes primary cutaneous large B-cell lymphoma, leg type from primary cutaneous follicle center lymphoma. *Am J Surg Pathol.* 2010;34(7):1043-1048. doi:10.1097/PAS.0b013e3181e5060a.
8. Mareschal S, Pham-Ledard A, Viailly PJ, et al. Identification of somatic mutations in primary cutaneous diffuse large B-cell lymphoma, leg type by massive parallel sequencing. *J Invest Dermatol.* 2017;137(9):1984-1994. doi:10.1016/j.jid.2017.04.010.
9. Pham-Ledard A, Beylot-Barry M, Barbe C, et al. High frequency and clinical prognostic value of MYD88 L265P mutation in primary cutaneous diffuse large B-cell lymphoma, leg-type. *JAMA Dermatol.* 2014;150(11):1173-1179. doi:10.1001/jamadermatol.2014.821.
10. Schrader AMR, de Groen RAL, Willemze R, et al. Genetic stability of driver alterations in primary cutaneous diffuse large B-cell lymphoma, leg type and their relapses: a rationale for the use of molecular-based methods for more effective disease monitoring. *Cancers.* 2022;14(20):5152. doi:10.3390/cancers14205152.
11. Schrader AMR, de Groen RAL, Willemze R, et al. Cell-of-origin classification using the Hans and Lymph2Cx algorithms in primary cutaneous large B-cell lymphomas. *Virchows Arch.* 2022;480(3):667-675. doi:10.1007/s00428-021-03265-5.
12. Schrader AMR, Jansen PM, Vermeer MH, Kleiverda JK, Vermaat JSP, Willemze R. High incidence and clinical significance of MYC rearrangements in primary cutaneous diffuse large B-cell lymphoma, leg type. *Am J Surg Pathol.* 2018;42(11):1488-1494. doi:10.1097/pas.0000000000001132.
13. Schrader AMR, Jansen PM, Willemze R, et al. High prevalence of MYD88 and CD79B mutations in intravascular large B-cell lymphoma. *Blood.* 2018;131(18):2086-2089. doi:10.1182/blood-2017-12-822817.
14. Senff NJ, Hoefnagel JJ, Jansen PM, et al. Reclassification of 300 primary cutaneous B-Cell lymphomas according to the new WHO-EORTC classification for cutaneous lymphomas: comparison with previous classifications and identification of prognostic markers. *J Clin Oncol.* 2007;25(12):1581-1587. doi:10.1200/JCO.2006.09.6396.
15. Willemze R, Hodak E, Zinzani PL, Specht L, Ladetto M; ESMO Guidelines Committee. Primary cutaneous lymphomas: ESMO Clinical Practice Guidelines for diagnosis, treatment and follow-up. *Ann Oncol.* 2018;29(suppl 4):iv30-iv40. doi:10.1093/annonc/mdy133.
16. Wright GW, Huang DW, Phelan JD, et al. A probabilistic classification tool for genetic subtypes of diffuse large B cell lymphoma with therapeutic implications. *Cancer Cell.* 2020;37(4):551-568.e14. doi:10.1016/j.ccell.2020.03.015.

Chapter 71
Intravascular Large B-Cell Lymphoma

Shigeo Nakamura and Girish Venkataraman

Definition

Intravascular large B-cell lymphoma (IVLBCL) is a rare subtype of extranodal large B-cell lymphoma characterized by the selective growth of lymphoma cells within the lumina of vessels, particularly in capillaries, and with the exception of large arteries and veins.

Synonyms

None.

Epidemiology

IVLBCL occurs in adults, with a median patient age of 67 years (range: 13-85 years) and a male-to-female ratio of 1.1. The frequency and clinical presentation differ according to patients' geographical origin (West vs Far East).

General Clinical Features

Clinical manifestation is quite variable, mostly exemplified by single case reports. Three major variants are recognized. The first is the "classic" variant—occurring predominantly in Western countries with predominant neurological or cutaneous involvement. The second is a "hemophagocytic syndrome–associated" variant (Figure 71.1F), originally documented as an Asian variant, in which patients present with multiorgan failure, hepatosplenomegaly, and pancytopenia. The third is an isolated cutaneous variant, occurring frequently in Western populations with female predilection, characterized by skin-limited disease and better prognosis relative to the other variants.[1,2]

Conventional staging procedures are generally associated with a high proportion of false negatives due to the lack of detectable tumor masses. Hence, a random skin biopsy of normal-looking skin, bone marrow biopsy (when presenting with pyrexia of unknown origin and/or pancytopenia), or transbronchial lung biopsy is often helpful for a timely diagnosis. In skin biopsies, tumor cells are often seen in subcutaneous tissue irrespective of any skin eruption, even in the hemophagocytic syndrome–associated form. Genetic analysis of peripheral blood cell-free DNA may potentially assist in diagnosis when there are sufficient circulating tumor cells.[3]

Morphology

The neoplastic lymphoid cells are mainly present in the lumina of small or intermediate vessels in many organs (Figure 71.1A). Fibrin thrombi, hemorrhage, and necrosis may be observed in some cases. The neoplastic cells are large, with prominent nucleoli and frequent mitotic figures. Rare cases have cells with anaplastic features or smaller size. Minimal extravascular location of neoplastic cells may be seen. In the central nervous system (CNS), recurrences may be associated with extravascular brain masses.[4] Sinusoidal involvement occurs in the liver, spleen, bone marrow, and infrequently lymph node where a high degree of suspicion is needed to get to a timely diagnosis. Circulating large lymphoma cells are occasionally detected in peripheral blood (Figure 71.1D and E).

Immunophenotype

Tumor cells express mature B cell antigens (Figure 71.1B). CD5 and CD10 coexpression is seen in 38% and 13% of the cases, respectively. Almost all CD10-negative cases are positive for MUM1. PD-L1 expression is detected in 34% to 45% across all IVLBCL variants[4,5] (Figure 71.1C).

The differential diagnosis includes intravascular NK/T-cell lymphomas with Epstein-Barr virus–positive tumor cells[6] and (rarely) intralymphatic anaplastic large cell lymphoma.[1] Rarely HHV8+ lymphomas may also exhibit intravascular predilection.[7] These can be excluded using immunohistochemistry panels.

The intravascular growth pattern is thought to be secondary to a defect in homing receptors, CD29 (integrin beta-1) and CD54 (ICAM1) adhesion beta-molecules on the neoplastic cells.[1]

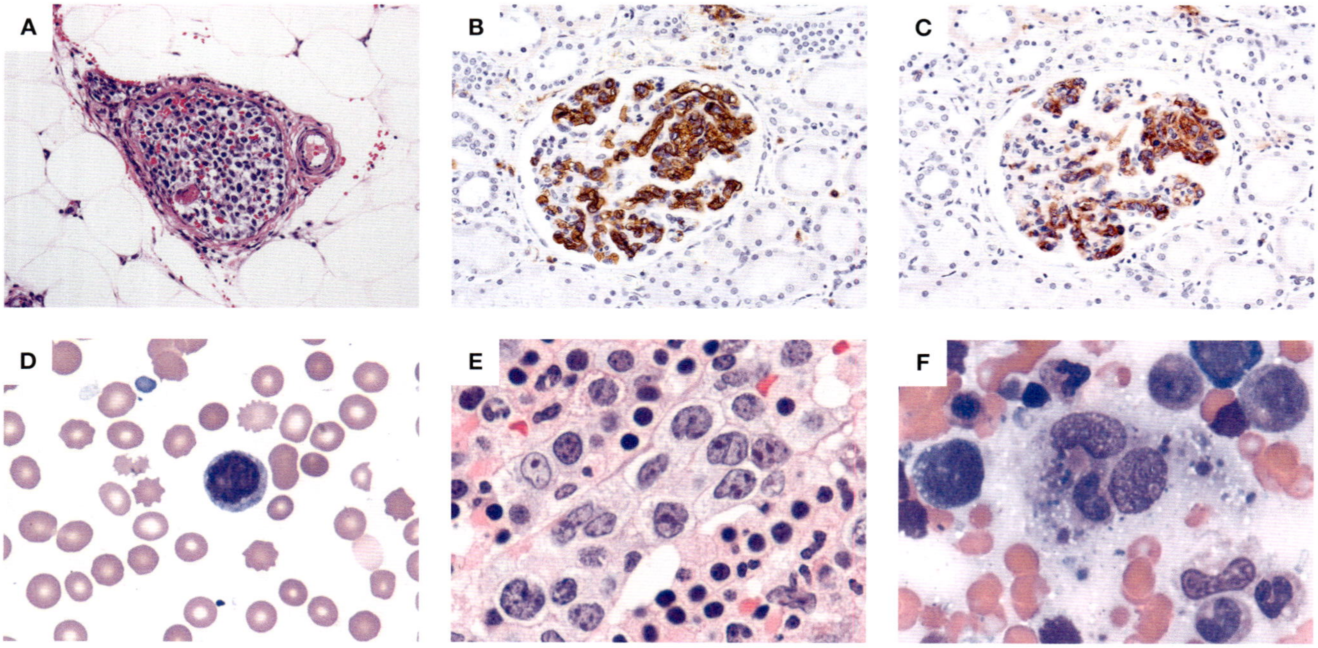

FIGURE 71.1 Intravascular large B-cell lymphoma (IVLBCL). **A:** A random skin biopsy shows large lymphoma cells filling the capillary. **B:** CD20 and **(C)** PD-L1 stains highlight tumor cells in glomerular capillaries of the kidney. **D:** Circulating atypical large lymphoma cells in an Asian-Indian patient. (Wright-Giemsa). **E:** Extensive sinusoidal bone marrow involvement by large lymphoid cells consistent with IVLBCL. **F:** Marrow aspirate smears showing prominent hemophagocytosis in the patient depicted in **D/E**. Serum ferritin levels tested shortly thereafter were markedly elevated supporting a diagnosis of hemophagocytic lymphohistiocytosis.

Genetics

IVLBCL shows a high frequency of mutations in *MYD88* (26%-57%), *CD79B* (25%-67%), *SETD1B* (57%), *HLA-B* (57%), *HLA-A* (33%), *HLA-C* (33%), and *CD58* (29%), similar to ABC-type and/or MCD-type DLBCL. Loss of *CDKN2A/2B* is found in 86% of patients. Structural variants affecting the *CD274* (PD-L1) and *PDCD1LG2* (PD-L2) genes are seen in 38%.[4,8,9]

Prognosis and Clinical Comment

IVLBCL is generally aggressive, except for cases with disease limited to the skin. The poor prognosis is due in part to the delay of timely and accurate diagnosis related to the protean presentation of this lymphoma. Chemotherapeutic regimens with rituximab have significantly improved the clinical outcomes of these patients, with a 3-year overall survival rate of 60% to 81%.[2,10] However, CNS relapse (occurring in ~25% of cases) and neurolymphomatosis remain a cause of mortality and morbidity in the rituximab era. Neither the clinical type of presentation nor clinical parameters predict CNS relapse.

In cases with CNS involvement, methotrexate-based chemotherapy may improve outcome.[10] More recently, among IVLBCL treated with standard chemotherapy, PD-L1 expression portended significantly worse outcome in the Japanese population, indicating that adding checkpoint inhibitors will likely be beneficial.

References

1. Ponzoni M, Campo E, Nakamura S. Intravascular large B-cell lymphoma: a chameleon with multiple faces and many masks. *Blood*. 2018;132(15):1561-1567. doi:10.1182/blood-2017-04-737445
2. Shimada K, Kiyoi H. Current progress and future perspectives of research on intravascular large B-cell lymphoma. *Cancer Sci*. 2021;112(10):3953-3961. doi:10.1111/cas.15091
3. Sakakibara A, Suzuki Y, Kato H, et al. Follicular T-cell lymphoma mimicking lymphocyte-rich classic Hodgkin lymphoma: a case report of a diagnostic pitfall. *J Clin Exp Hematop*. 2021;61(2):97-101. doi:10.3960/jslrt.20052
4. Patel N, Slack GW, Bodo J, et al. Immune escape mechanisms in intravascular large B-cell lymphoma: a molecular cytogenetic and immunohistochemical study. *Am J Clin Pathol*. 2022;157(4):578-585. doi:10.1093/ajcp/aqab154
5. Gupta GK, Jaffe ES, Pittaluga S. A study of PD-L1 expression in intravascular large B cell lymphoma: correlation with clinical and pathological features. *Histopathology*. 2019;75(2):282-286. doi:10.1111/his.13870

6. Zanelli M, Parente P, Sanguedolce F, et al. Intravascular NK/T-Cell lymphoma: what we know about this diagnostically challenging, aggressive disease. *Cancers*. 2022;14(21):5458. doi:10.3390/cancers14215458
7. Ferry JA, Sohani AR, Longtine JA, Schwartz RA, Harris NL. HHV8-positive, EBV-positive Hodgkin lymphoma-like large B-cell lymphoma and HHV8-positive intravascular large B-cell lymphoma. *Mod Pathol*. 2009;22(5):618-626. doi:10.1038/modpathol.2009.36
8. Shimada K, Yoshida K, Suzuki Y, et al. Frequent genetic alterations in immune checkpoint-related genes in intravascular large B-cell lymphoma. *Blood*. 2021;137(11):1491-1502. doi:10.1182/blood.2020007245
9. Gonzalez-Farre B, Ramis-Zaldivar JE, Castrejon de Anta N, et al. Intravascular large B-cell lymphoma genomic profile is characterized by alterations in genes regulating NF-κB and immune checkpoints. *Am J Surg Pathol*. 2023;47(2):202-211. doi:10.1097/PAS.0000000000001978
10. Yoon SE, Kim WS, Kim SJ. Asian variant of intravascular large B-cell lymphoma: a comparison of clinical features based on involvement of the central nervous system. *Korean J Intern Med*. 2020;35(4):946-956. doi:10.3904/kjim.2018.396

Chapter 72

HHV8- and EBV-Negative Primary Effusion-Based Lymphoma

Lorinda A. Soma, George Lenz, and Leticia Quintanilla-Martinez

Definition

This provisional entity is an effusion-based large B-cell lymphoma that is both HHV8 and EBV negative and confined to a body cavity without adenopathy or solid tumor. Nodal or extranodal diffuse large B-cell lymphoma with an associated effusion must be excluded. Cases otherwise classified as Burkitt lymphoma, mantle cell lymphoma, plasmablastic lymphoma, multiple myeloma, transformed lymphomas, and posttransplant lymphomas are excluded.

Synonyms

Fluid overload associated large B-cell lymphoma (not recommended).

Epidemiology

Typical presentation is in elderly patients (median age 80 years) with a clinical predisposition to chronic fluid overload (eg, congestive heart failure, renal failure, hepatic disorders, protein losing enteropathy).[1-4] There is a male predominance in the Japanese literature and no gender predisposition in the Western literature.[1,3,4] Immunosuppressed patients (such as HIV-positive and posttransplant patients) should be excluded from this entity.[2]

General Clinical Features

Patients present with signs or symptoms related to the effusion (dyspnea, abdominal fullness), and multiple body cavities may be involved with pleural the most common site.[1-4] B symptoms are uncommon.

Morphology

Cytologically the large cells are typically immunoblastic or centroblastic, but rarely tumor cells may be pleomorphic/anaplastic (Figure 72.1).[1-4]

Immunophenotype

Tumor cells show positivity for at least one B-cell marker (CD19, CD20, CD22, PAX5, CD79a) and CD45. The majority are positive for BCL6, MUM1, and BCL2 with fewer cases expressing MYC and/or CD30. CD10 expression is uncommon (majority are non–germinal center).[1-4] The neoplasm is negative for EBER, HHV8, CD3, and cyclinD1.[2,4] CD138 expression is typically negative, and if expressed, it should be limited to cases that are CD20 and/or PAX5 positive (cases that otherwise would not suggest plasmablastic lymphoma).[2]

Genetics

The few cases analyzed demonstrate complex genetic findings, including complex karyotype and high copy number alterations (mean of 33.6), with gains of 1q31 and deletions of 3p14.2 and 6q21 being common. High numbers of mutations have also been reported, most commonly including *HIST1HE1*, *MYD88*, *BTG1/2*, *IRF4*, *SYNE1*, and *PIM1*.[5] These cases may have *BCL6*, *MYC*, or *BCL2* rearrangement; however, cases with *MYC* and *BCL2* (or *BCL6*) rearrangement are excluded.[2]

Prognosis and Clinical Comment

Prognosis is difficult to establish due to limited data from retrospective cohorts with variable inclusion criteria and confounding clinical factors. Median survival of Western cohorts is reported as 14.9 months versus 63.6 for Japanese cohorts, with some Japanese cohorts demonstrating a more favorable prognosis after anthracycline-based chemotherapy.[3,4] Some patients achieve complete remission with drainage alone.[1,3,4] Although it is believed to be a lymphoma with a more favorable prognosis, more studies are required.

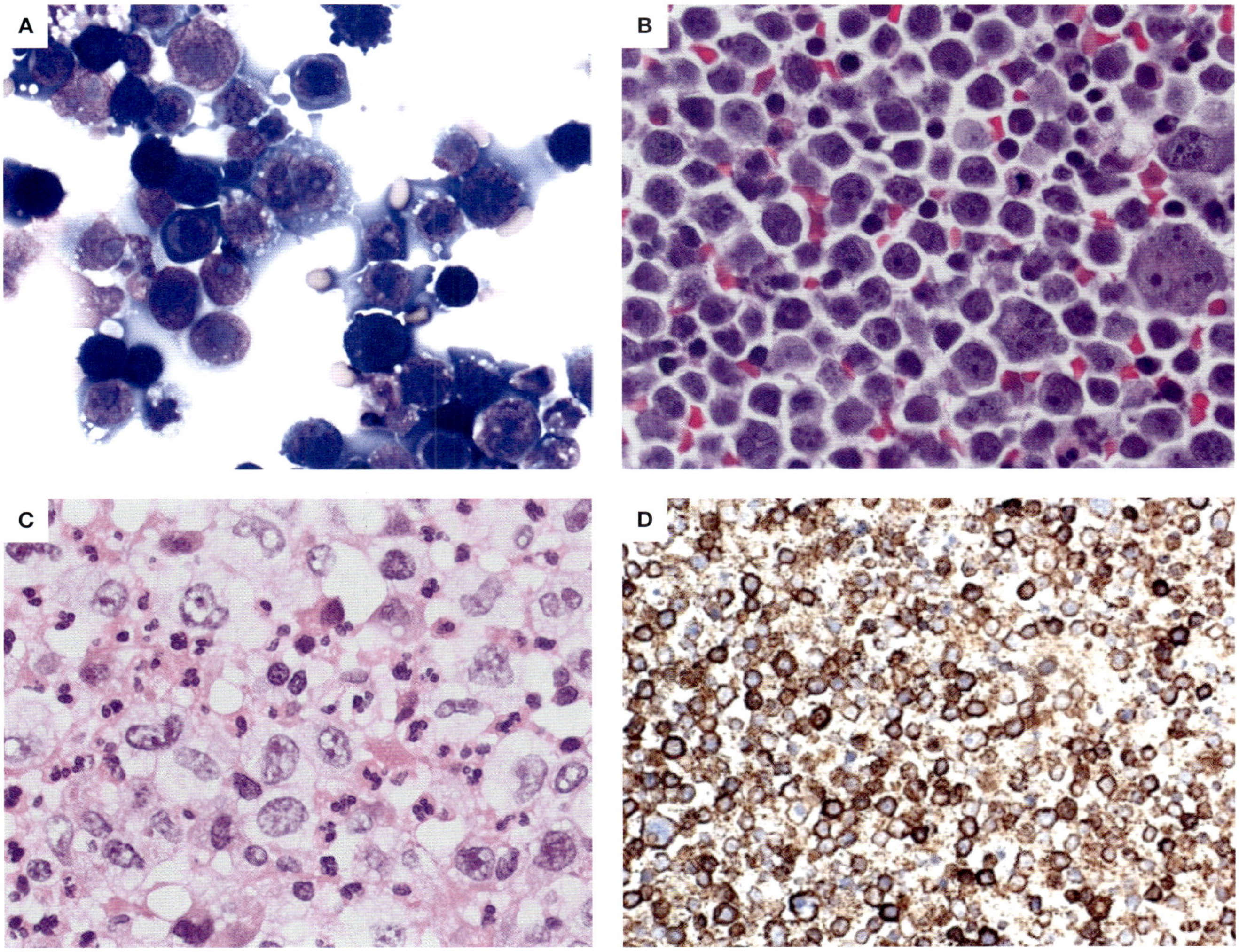

FIGURE 72.1 Three cases of HHV8- and EBV-negative primary effusion-based lymphoma. Two cases demonstrate numerous neoplastic cells (**A** and **B**). The majority of cells in case **A** (Giemsa, cytospin) have an immunoblastic appearance; however, they include subsets with plasmacytoid/plasmablastic cytomorphology. Case **B** (hematoxylin and eosin [H&E], cell block) demonstrates anaplastic morphology. Case **C** demonstrates fewer neoplastic cells (immunoblastic and centroblastic) with associated inflammatory cells (H&E, cell block). The neoplastic cells from case **A** are positive for CD20 (**D:** CD20 immunohistochemistry). (Images A and D were kindly provided by Dr. John Goodlad.)

References

1. Alexanian S, Said J, Lones M, Pullarkat ST. KSHV/HHV8-negative effusion-based lymphoma, a distinct entity associated with fluid overload states. *AJSP*. 2013;37(2):241-249.doi:10.1097/PAS.0b013e318267fabc
2. DiNapoli A, Soma L, Quintenella-Martinez L, et al. Cavity-based lymphomas: challenges and novel concepts. A report of the 2022 EA4HP/SH lymphoma workshop. *Virchows Arch*. 2023;483(3):299-316. doi:10.1007/s00428-023-03599-2
3. Kaji D, Ota Y, Sato Y, et al. Primary human herpesvirus 8-negative effusion-based lymphoma: a large B cell lymphoma with favorable prognosis. *Blood Adv*. 2020;4(18):4442-4450. doi:10.1182/bloodadvances.2020002293
4. Gisriel SD, Yuan J, Braunberger RC, et al. Human herpesvirus 8-negative effusion-based large B-cell lymphoma: a distinct entity with unique clinicopathologic characteristics. *Mod Pathol*. 2022;35(10):1411-1422. doi:10.1038/s41379-022-01091-x
5. Mendeville M, Roemer MGM, van den Hout MFCM, et al. Aggressive genomic features in clinically indolent primary HHV8-negative effusion-based lymphoma. *Blood*. 2019;133(4):377-380. doi:10.1182/blood-2017-12-822171

Chapter 73
Epstein-Barr Virus–Positive Mucocutaneous Ulcer

Stefan Dojcinov, Jeffrey I. Cohen, and Elaine S. Jaffe

Definition

Epstein-Barr virus (EBV)-positive mucocutaneous ulcer (EBV MCU) is a clinicopathological entity affecting patients with primary or age-related immunodeficiency (immunosenescence), iatrogenic immunosuppression, or HIV infection. It presents as a localized mucosal or skin lesion, most commonly involving the oropharynx.[1,2] Preexisting local injury likely generates an environment of immune sequestration, contributing to the development of localized EBV-driven B-cell lymphoproliferation.[3] The EBV-positive cells may resemble the Reed-Sternberg cells of classic Hodgkin lymphoma, but the clinical course is distinctly different, and lesions may show spontaneous regression.

Synonyms

None.

Epidemiology

EBV MCU is rare, with the incidence being difficult to establish due to common spontaneous regression.[1,2] It may arise not only in the context of iatrogenic immunosuppression for autoimmune diseases, solid organ, and allogeneic bone marrow transplantation but also as a result of immunosenescence, HIV infection, or primary immunodeficiencies.[1,2] The immunosuppressive agents associated with EBV MCU are varied, including methotrexate, cyclosporin A, azathioprine, mycophenolate, tumor necrosis factor inhibitors, tacrolimus, and systemic and topical steroids.[1,2] EBV MCU mostly affects the elderly (median age, 77 years), with no sex predilection. The patients with iatrogenic immunosuppression, primary immunodeficiency, or HIV infection are younger (median age, 63 years).[1,4] There are incidental reports of EBV MCU in children.[5]

General Clinical Features

EBV MCU presents as a circumscribed, solitary ulcer most often in the oropharyngeal mucosa (tonsil, tongue, palate, buccal mucosa, and gingiva) but also in the esophagus, stomach, small and large intestine, rectum, gallbladder, trachea, and skin.[1,2] It appears to arise at sites of preexisting local injury. The preceding tissue damage, necrosis, and fibrinous exudate likely form an immune-sequestered environment resulting in a circumscribed EBV+ B-cell lymphoproliferative disorder.[3] The lesions vary in size, have a circumferential peripheral ridge, and are often clinically suspected to be nonhematological cancers. They do not breach anatomical compartmental boundaries on imaging studies. Lymphadenopathy should be absent, without evidence of systemic spread. Occasionally, enlarged neck lymph nodes have been seen with oropharyngeal disease, which regress upon resolution of EBV MCU.[1] The symptoms relate to the ulcer and depend on the site of involvement. Systemic symptoms are uncommon and may reflect general frailty often seen in the elderly with EBV MCU. Most patients have serological evidence of prior EBV infection, which may be lacking in younger subjects in the posttransplant setting.[6] Elevated levels of circulating viral DNA are not detectable and there is no lactate dehydrogenase elevation.[7] The existence of more than a single lesion should prompt consideration of other diagnoses, including EBV+ diffuse large B-cell lymphoma (EBV DLBCL) or EBV+ polymorphic B-cell lymphoproliferative disorder (EBV PLPD), not otherwise specified.[2]

Morphology

EBV MCU displays a characteristic histological architecture. The lesions are circumscribed ulcers, sharply demarcated from the underlying structures, without infiltrative spread. Lesions arising in squamous epithelium–lined mucosa or skin may show adjacent pseudoepitheliomatous hyperplasia (Figure 73.1). Underlying

FIGURE 73.1 Epstein-Barr virus (EBV)-positive mucocutaneous ulcer—architectural features. **A:** Gingival lesion showing ulcerated surface with necrotic debris. The adjacent squamous epithelium shows irregular acanthosis and pseudoepitheliomatous features. The entire lesion is well circumscribed at the base. The lesional lymphoid proliferation forms a band which follows the contour of the ulcerated surface. **B:** Immunohistochemistry for CD3 shows a small lymphocytic T-cell infiltrate at the base. **C:** In situ hybridization for EBV-encoded small RNA highlights a "bandlike" distribution of the EBV-positive infiltrate, which also follows the contour of the ulcerated surface and appears well circumscribed.

the ulcerated surface and granulation tissue, there is a polymorphous infiltrate with a variable content of lymphocytes, plasma cells, histiocytes, and occasionally prominent eosinophils. There are scattered immunoblasts and variably pleomorphic, large, mononuclear, bi- or multinucleated cells with Hodgkin/Reed-Sternberg (HRS) cell features, which may be particularly prominent within the overlying necrotic debris. Scattered apoptotic cells with basophilic cytoplasm ("plasmacytoid apoptotic cells") can be seen (Figure 73.2). This mixed infiltrate forms a band following the contour of the ulcerated surface, rimmed off at the base by a layer of small lymphocytes. The entrapped blood vessels may show thrombosis and angioinvasion in the form of intramural lymphocytes, immunoblasts, and HRS-like cells (Figure 73.2). The proportion of large and HRS-like cells is variable and they may occasionally predominate but the overall architectural features are retained. Some lesions are particularly rich in plasma cells, often seen in small and shallow ulcers.[1,3]

Immunophenotype

The large, atypical EBV-positive cells in EBV MCU show a postgerminal center phenotype with at least partial retention of the B-cell program including expression of CD45, CD20, CD79a, PAX5, OCT2, and BOB1 (Figure 73.3). The extent and intensity of CD20 expression is variable and occasionally may be completely lacking. MUM1 is positive, there is variable

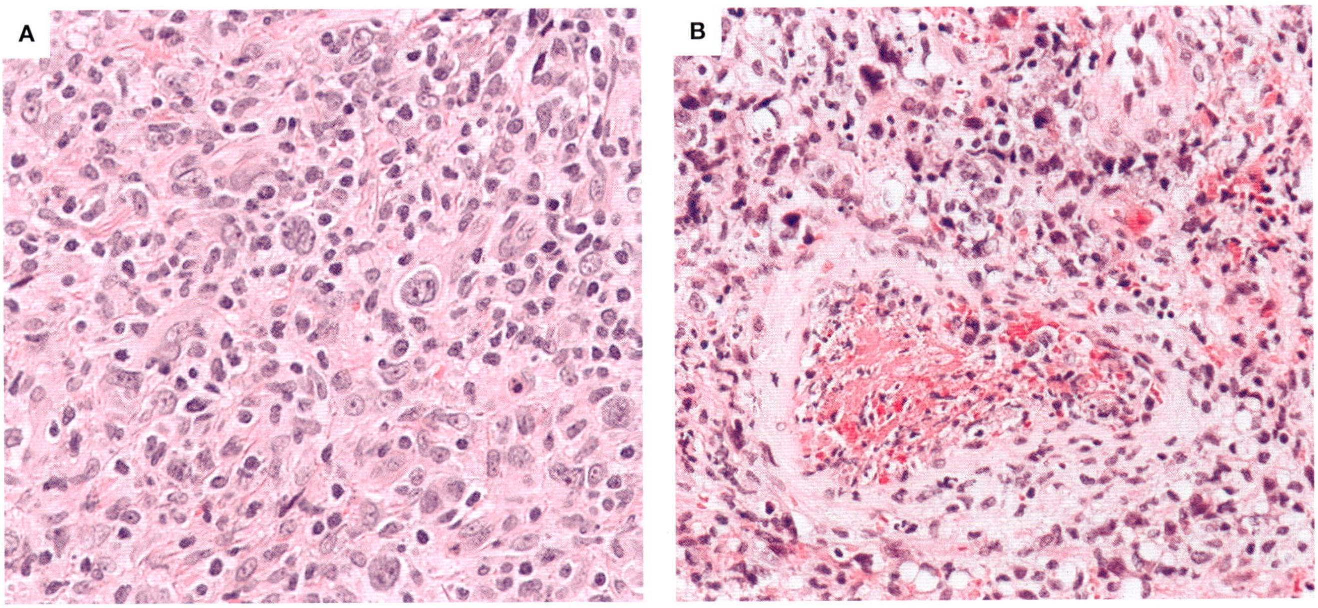

FIGURE 73.2 Epstein-Barr virus–positive mucocutaneous ulcer—histological features. **A:** The infiltrate is polymorphic, comprising lymphocytes, histiocytes, immunoblasts, and pleomorphic cells with Hodgkin and Reed-Sternberg cell features. Apoptotic bodies can be seen. **B:** Rarely, angioinvasion could be observed.

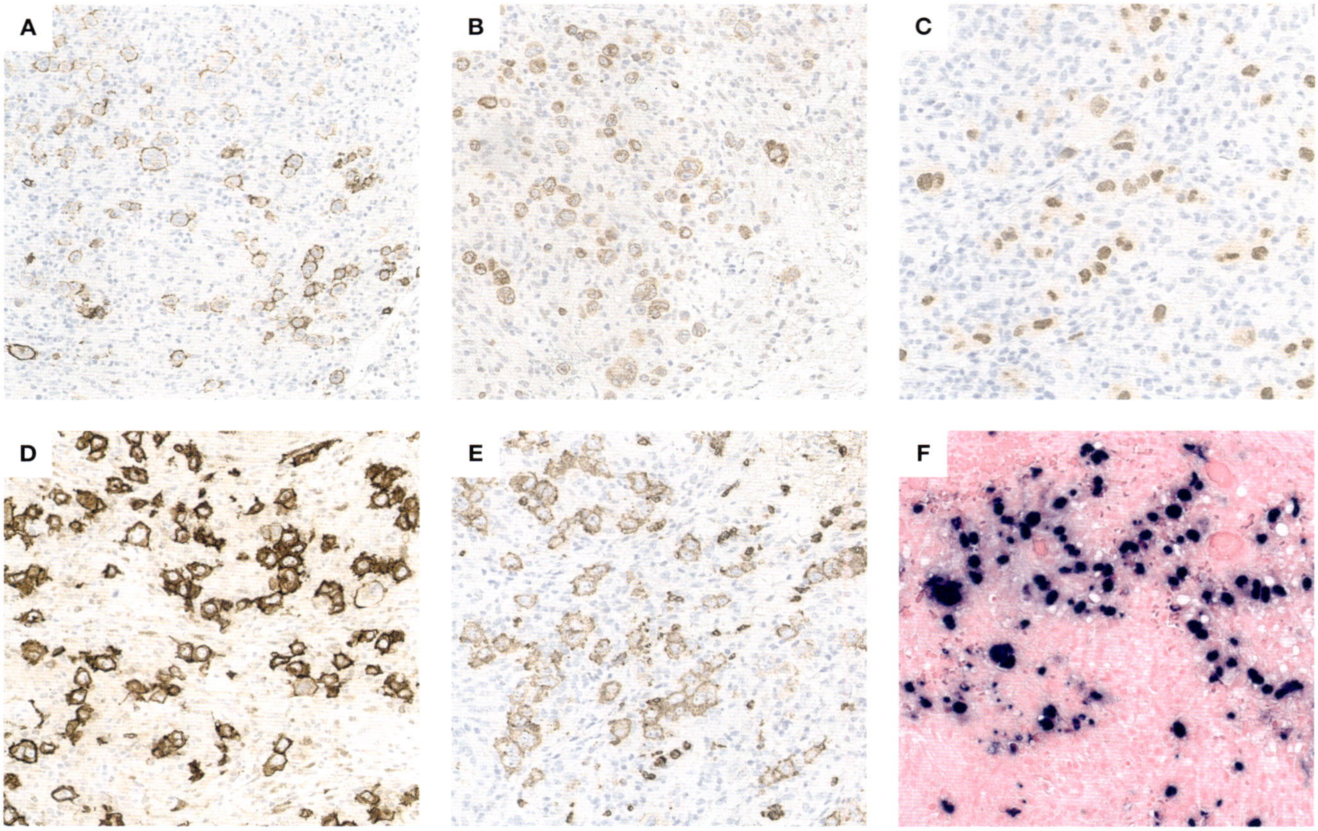

FIGURE 73.3 Epstein-Barr virus (EBV)-positive mucocutaneous ulcer—immunophenotype. **A:** The immunoblasts and Hodgkin/Reed-Sternberg–like cells show variable expression of CD20. **B:** Expression of CD79a is retained as well as that of PAX5 **(C)**. The lesional B cells show strong expression of CD30 **(D)** and are frequently positive for CD15 **(E)**. EBV-encoded small RNA is positive in the lesional B cells **(F)**. All the immunostains **(A-F)** highlight a range of cell sizes.

expression of BCL6, but CD10 is negative. CD30 is strongly expressed, with coexpression of CD15 in up to 50% of cases (Figure 73.3).[1] In situ hybridization for EBV-encoded small RNA (EBER) highlights bandlike or vaguely nodular positivity underlying the ulcerated surface, colocalizing with the CD30/PAX5/CD20-positive cells (Figure 73.1). In a minority of cases, the EBER-positive nuclei are variably sized, including both those of small lymphoid cells as well as large and pleomorphic blasts (Figure 73.3). Full characterization of EBV status with EBER, LMP1, and EBNA2 reveals EBV latency II or III.[4] There is abundant small lymphocytic EBV-negative T-cell background (CD8 > CD4), with a prominent band of T cells at the base of the lesion (Figure 73.1). Recent studies indicate absence of expression of PD-L1 on cells in EBV MCU compared to extranodal EBV DLBCL and EBV+ classic Hodgkin lymphoma (EBV CHL), which show intermediate and high expression, respectively. Immune evasion mechanisms, therefore, most likely do not play a role in the pathogenesis of EBV MCU.[8] The morphophenotypic features of EBV MCU overlap with other EBV-positive disease. The main differential diagnoses include EBV DLBCL, EBV CHL, and EBV PLPD (Table 77.1). Extranodal presentation, typical histological architecture, at least partial expression of B-cell markers, cellular polymorphism, EBV latency III, and no evidence of systemic disease distinguish EBV MCU from EBV CHL. Lesions breaching anatomical boundaries and lacking typical architecture may represent EBV DLBCL.[1,2] In cases of lymphomatoid granulomatosis (LYG) with extrapulmonary involvement, the differential diagnosis could be difficult. These cases are exceptionally rare at sites affected by EBV MCU. For diagnosis of LYG, lung involvement is an essential diagnostic feature.

Genetics

Immunoglobulin gene rearrangements by polymerase chain reaction (PCR) are detectable in less than half of the cases. Oligoclonal or restricted patterns of T-cell receptor gene rearrangements are frequently encountered.[1] This is a consequence of the reduction of the EBV-specific CD8+ cytotoxic T-cell repertoire because of immunosuppression from any source, resulting in diminished ability to react to EBV-related antigens with the full spectrum of epitope specificities. Therefore, the EBV infected B-cell population cannot be efficiently controlled and kept at very low or undetectable numbers.[1] In patients with EBV MCU, it is postulated that their EBV-related T-cell immune competence is at the threshold and marginally able to prevent B-cell proliferation from reactivated EBV. Other molecular features of EBV MCU are not well understood. Recent whole genome spatial expression profiling suggests that antiviral response signatures from the HRS-like cells and macrophages distinguish EBV MCU from both EBV DLBCL and EBV CHL.[9]

Prognosis and Clinical Comment

In cases associated with iatrogenic immunosuppression, reduction or withdrawal of immunosuppression results in complete resolution, usually achieved within 8 weeks. In elderly patients with postulated underlying immunosenescence which cannot be therapeutically modulated, the lesions may pursue a self-remitting and relapsing course with an overall indolent behavior. Particularly symptomatic or destructive lesions may benefit from rituximab monotherapy, local irradiation, or combined immunochemotherapy.[1,2,4] EBV MCU may complicate checkpoint inhibitor–associated colitis. Administration of steroids in these patients should be considered with extreme caution as it further impairs cellular immunity, which can result in expansion of lesions and bowel perforation.[3] Very rare instances of progression to aggressive disease have been recorded.[7,10]

References

1. Dojcinov SD, Venkataraman G, Raffeld M, Pittaluga S, Jaffe ES. EBV positive mucocutaneous ulcer—a study of 26 cases associated with various sources of immunosuppression. *Am J Surg Pathol*. 2010;34(3):405-417.
2. Quintanilla-Martinez L, Swerdlow SH, Tousseyn T, Barrionuevo C, Nakamura S, Jaffe ES. New concepts in EBV-associated B, T, and NK cell lymphoproliferative disorders. *Virchows Arch*. 2023;482(1):227-244.
3. Pugh MR, Leopold GD, Morgan M, et al. Epstein-Barr virus-positive mucocutaneous ulcers complicate Colitis caused by immune checkpoint regulator therapy and associate with colon perforation. *Clin Gastroenterol Hepatol*. 2020;18(8):1785-1795.e3.
4. Natkunam Y, Goodlad JR, Chadburn A, et al. EBV-positive B-cell proliferations of varied malignant potential: 2015 SH/EAHP workshop report-Part 1. *Am J Clin Pathol*. 2017;147(2):129-152.
5. Coelho KMPA, Bublitz GS, Condeixa de França PH, Stall J, Hanauer AD, Sangueza JM. Epstein-Barr virus-positive mucocutaneous ulcer in a pediatric patient-case report. *Am J Dermatopathol*. 2020;42(4):e49-e52.
6. Prieto-Torres L, Eraña I, Gil-Redondo R, et al. The spectrum of EBV-positive mucocutaneous ulcer: a study of 9 cases. *Am J Surg Pathol*. 2019;43(2):201-210.
7. Gaulard P, Swerdlow SH, Harris NL, Sundstrom C, Jaffe ES. EBV-positive mucocutaneous ulcer. In: Swerdlow SH, campo E, Harris NL, Jaffe ES, Pileri S, stein H, et al, eds. WHO Classification of Tumours of Haematopoietic and Lymphoid Tissues. IARC; 2017:307-308.
8. Sakakibara A, Kohno K, Ishikawa E, et al. Age-related EBV-associated B-cell lymphoproliferative disorders and other EBV+ lymphoproliferative diseases: new insights into immune escape and immunodeficiency through staining with anti-PD-L1 antibody clone SP142. *Pathol Int*. 2020;70(8):481-492.
9. Pugh MR, Fennel E, Leopold G, Murray PG, Dojcinov SD. Spatial transcriptomic profiling: the "Next Generation Diagnosis" distinguishing between EBV+ lymphoproliferations with Hodgkin-like features. *Hematol Oncol*. 2023;41(suppl 2):262-263.
10. Daroontum T, Kohno K, Inaguma Y, et al. Epstein-Barr virus (EBV)-positive diffuse large B-cell lymphoma arising in patient with a history of EBV-positive mucocutaneous ulcer and EBV-positive nodal polymorphous B-lymphoproliferative disorder. *Pathol Int*. 2019;69(1):37-41.

Chapter 74

Epstein-Barr Virus–Positive Diffuse Large B-Cell Lymphoma, Not Otherwise Specified

Elaine S. Jaffe, Stefania Pittaluga, and Wyndham H. Wilson

Definition

Epstein-Barr virus (EBV)-positive diffuse large B-cell lymphoma (DLBCL), not otherwise specified (NOS), is an EBV-positive clonal B-cell lymphoid proliferation not conforming to any of the other EBV-driven B-cell neoplasms defined as distinct entities. Among others, it excludes lymphomatoid granulomatosis, plasmablastic lymphoma, and posttransplant lymphoproliferative disorders. It can present in extranodal or nodal sites. It is most common in elderly patients, associated with a decrease in immune surveillance, but occurs sporadically in younger patients, under the age of 45 years.[1-3] Although many cases have a distinctive histological appearance, routine testing for EBV by EBER in situ hybridization is generally required for diagnosis. The majority of the tumor cells should be demonstrably EBV positive, more than 80%, as admixed EBV-positive cells can be encountered in other benign and malignant lesions of either B-cell or T-cell origin. The clinical outcome is variable.

Synonyms

None.

Epidemiology

Previously, this disease was termed EBV-positive DLBCL of the elderly, but limitation to elderly patients was removed in the revised fourth edition World Health Organization classification. Its frequency ranges from 2.5% to 14% of DLBCL with a higher incidence in East Asians. Incidence increases with age, with peak incidence beyond the seventh decade of life. A smaller peak is seen in younger patients, less than 30 years.[2,4] It is more frequent in males than in females, approximately 2:1.

General Clinical Features

EBV+ DLBCL is more common in extranodal than nodal sites.[5,6] Common anatomic sites of involvement include gastrointestinal tract, lung, adrenal glands, and skin. The presentation is often acute with a rapidly enlarging mass lesion, advanced clinical stage, and poor performance status. Elevated EBV viral load may be detected in blood or serum.[7] B symptoms are commonly present.

Morphology

The morphological spectrum is very broad.[1,3,8] The lesions fall into two broad categories: polymorphic and monomorphic. However, these are not distinct subtypes, and a spectrum of morphological appearances is often present. Polymorphic lesions have a significant background of reactive cells including lymphocytes and histiocytes. Eosinophils and plasma cells are distinctly less common. Necrosis is commonly present and may be accompanied by increased neutrophils. The tumor cells often show marked pleomorphism (Figure 74.1) and may contain multinucleated forms. Cases occurring in young patients are often rich in histiocytes and may resemble T-cell/histiocyte-rich large B-cell lymphoma (Figure 74.2).[2] The neoplastic cells often have an immunoblastic appearance with prominent central nucleoli.

Immunophenotype

The neoplastic cells express pan B-cell markers including CD20, CD79, CD19, PAX5, OCT2, and Bob.1 (see Figures 74.1 and 74.2).[6] Most cases have a non-GCB phenotype with the Hans algorithm and are positive for MUM1/IRF4 and negative for CD10. BCL6 is usually positive, at least in a subset of the neoplastic cells. Most cases are positive for CD30, but CD15 is less often present.[3] The presence of pleomorphic cells with expression of CD30 and CD15 may prompt consideration for a diagnosis of gray zone lymphoma. However,

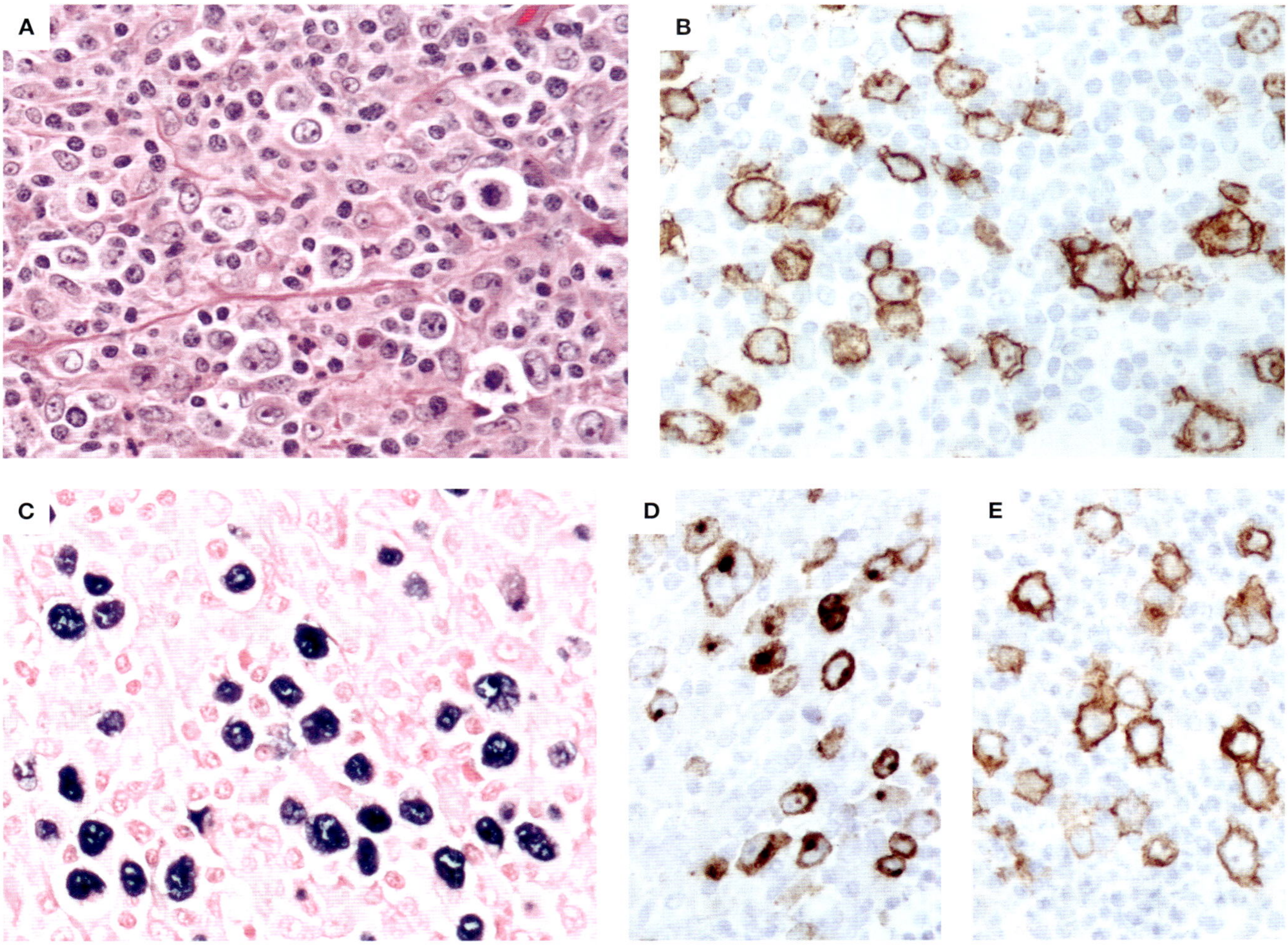

FIGURE 74.1 This case of EBV+ diffuse large B-cell lymphoma presented in the axillary lymph node of a 74-year-old woman. **A:** Atypical large lymphoid cells with vesicular chromatin and prominent nucleoli are present in a background of small lymphocytes and histiocytes with occasional neutrophils. **B:** The neoplastic cells are strongly positive for CD20. **C:** EBER highlights the neoplastic cells, but small B cells positive for EBV are rare. **D:** The neoplastic cells show strong expression of LMP-1, indicative of latency II; EBNA2 was negative. **E:** Neoplastic cells are positive for CD30, but CD15 was negative, helping to rule out classic Hodgkin lymphoma.

although rare cases of EBV-positive mediastinal gray zone lymphoma (MGZL) are reported, EBV positivity is generally an exclusion for MGZL and a diagnosis of MGZL should be limited to those cases arising in the thymic niche.[9] PD-L1/PD-L2 are often positive.[10] Other markers may show evidence of defective immune surveillance.[2] The EBV-positive tumor cells usually have a latency II phenotype (LMP1+) (see Figure 74.1), with a subset of patients (less than 30%) having latency III with expression of EBNA-2.[2]

Genetics

Clonal immunoglobulin gene rearrangement is demonstrable in most cases.[3] The presence of clonal T-cell gene rearrangement should prompt consideration of a diagnosis of peripheral T-cell lymphoma with expansion of an EBV-driven B-cell population masking the underlying malignancy. Translocations involving *MYC, BCL2,* and *BCL6* are uncommon, in comparison with sporadic DLBCL.[11] Most cases do not fall into one of the genomic categories that have been recognized in EBV-negative DLBCL.[12] While the tumors may have an activated B-cell gene expression profile, mutations in *MYD88* and *CD79B* are rare.[11,13] Among the genes involved, there is a significant enrichment in alterations in *NF-κB, WNT*, and the IL6/JAK/STAT pathways as well as in epigenetic modifiers.[11,12] Mutations in NOTCH pathway genes have been reported. Amplification of 9p24.1 contributes to the expression of PD-L1/PD-L2, which may contribute to immune escape.[10,12,14]

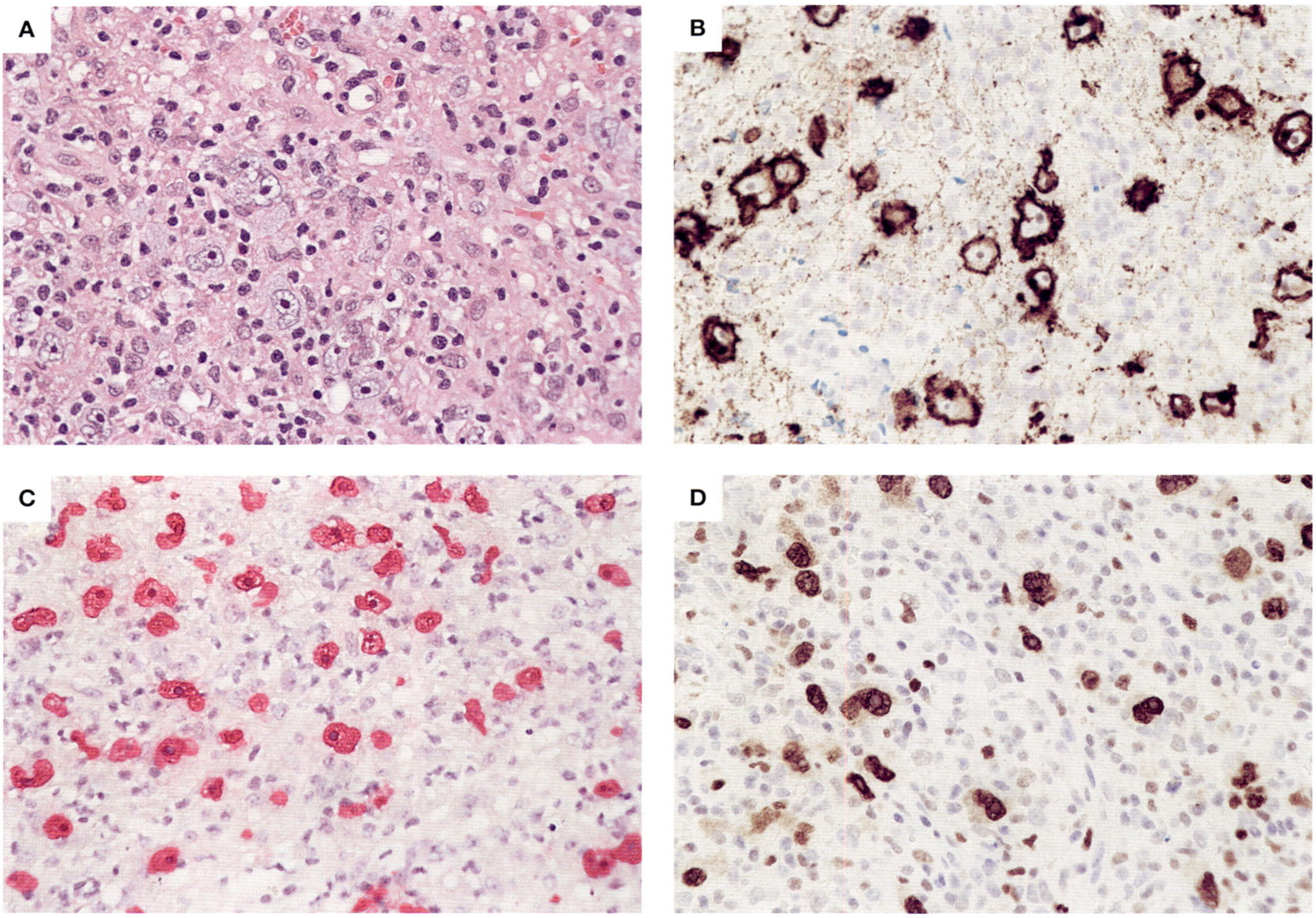

FIGURE 74.2 EBV+ diffuse large B-cell lymphoma is less common in patients under the age of 40 years. This case presented in the cervical lymph nodes of a 16-year-old boy. **A:** Large neoplastic cells have lobulated nuclei and prominent nucleoli. The background is rich in histiocytes. The neoplastic cells can resemble classic Reed-Sternberg cells or lymphocyte predominant cells in some cases. **B:** The tumor cells are strongly and uniformly positive for CD20 and EBER (**C**). D. OCT2 is strongly positive, in keeping with the full expression of the B-cell program.

Prognosis and Clinical Comment

Similarly to DLBCL, the standard treatment of EBV-positive DLBCL is immunochemotherapy with rituximab, cyclophosphamide, doxorubicin hydrochloride (hydroxydaunomycin), and vincristine sulfate (Oncovin), and prednisone or DA-etoposide phosphate (E), prednisone (P), vincristine sulfate (Oncovin), cyclophosphamide (C), and doxorubicin hydrochloride (H) (hydroxydaunorubicin), and rituximab (R). In general, patients should receive six cycles of treatment as tolerated. There is no clear role for radiation therapy. The prognosis is poorer compared with EBV-negative DLBCL, especially among older patients, with approximately half of patients free of disease at 5 years.[6,15] In general, younger patients usually achieve long-term survival with systemic chemotherapy. The role of EBV-specific adoptive immunotherapy and antibody-drug conjugates such as brentuximab vedotin is unknown.

References

1. Oyama T, Yamamoto K, Asano N, et al. Age-related EBV-associated B-cell lymphoproliferative disorders constitute a distinct clinicopathologic group: a study of 96 patients. *Clin Cancer Res*. 2007;13(17):5124-5132.
2. Nicolae A, Pittaluga S, Abdullah S, et al. EBV-positive large B-cell lymphomas in young patients: a nodal lymphoma with evidence for a tolerogenic immune environment. *Blood*. 2015;126(7):863-872.
3. Dojcinov SD, Venkataraman G, Pittaluga S, et al. Age-related EBV-associated lymphoproliferative disorders in the Western population: a spectrum of reactive lymphoid hyperplasia and lymphoma. *Blood*. 2011;117(18):4726-4735.
4. Hong JY, Yoon DH, Suh C, et al. EBV-positive diffuse large B-cell lymphoma in young adults: is this a distinct disease entity? *Ann Oncol*. 2015;26(3):548-555.
5. Oyama T, Ichimura K, Suzuki R, et al. Senile EBV+ B-cell lymphoproliferative disorders: a clinicopathologic study of 22 patients. *Am J Surg Pathol*. 2003;27(1):16-26.

6. Bourbon E, Maucort-Boulch D, Fontaine J, et al. Clinicopathological features and survival in EBV-positive diffuse large B-cell lymphoma not otherwise specified. *Blood Adv*. 2021;5(16):3227-3239.
7. Okamoto A, Yanada M, Inaguma Y, et al. The prognostic significance of EBV DNA load and EBER status in diagnostic specimens from diffuse large B-cell lymphoma patients. *Hematol Oncol*. 2017;35(1):87-93.
8. Hofscheier A, Ponciano A, Bonzheim I, et al. Geographic variation in the prevalence of Epstein-Barr virus-positive diffuse large B-cell lymphoma of the elderly: a comparative analysis of a Mexican and a German population. *Mod Pathol*. 2011;24(8):1046-1054.
9. Sarkozy C, Hung SS, Chavez EA, et al. Mutational landscape of gray zone lymphoma. *Blood*. 2021;137(13):1765-1776.
10. Chen BJ, Chapuy B, Ouyang J, et al. PD-L1 expression is characteristic of a subset of aggressive B-cell lymphomas and virus-associated malignancies. *Clin Cancer Res*. 2013;19(13):3462-3473.
11. Gebauer N, Gebauer J, Hardel TT, et al. Prevalence of targetable oncogenic mutations and genomic alterations in Epstein-Barr virus-associated diffuse large B-cell lymphoma of the elderly. *Leuk Lymphoma*. 2015;56(4):1100-1106.
12. Frontzek F, Staiger AM, Wullenkord R, et al. Molecular profiling of EBV associated diffuse large B-cell lymphoma. *Leukemia*. 2023;37(3):670-679.
13. Vermaat JS, Somers SF, de Wreede LC, et al. MYD88 mutations identify a molecular subgroup of diffuse large B-cell lymphoma with an unfavorable prognosis. *Haematologica*. 2020;105(2):424-434.
14. Kataoka K, Miyoshi H, Sakata S, et al. Frequent structural variations involving programmed death ligands in Epstein-Barr virus-associated lymphomas. *Leukemia*. 2019;33(7):1687-1699.
15. Malpica L, Marques-Piubelli ML, Beltran BE, Chavez JC, Miranda RN, Castillo JJ. EBV-positive diffuse large B-cell lymphoma, not otherwise specified: 2022 update on diagnosis, risk-stratification, and management. *Am J Hematol*. 2022;97(7):951-965.

Chapter 75

Diffuse Large B-Cell Lymphoma Associated With Chronic Inflammation

Philippe Gaulard, Ellen D. McPhail, and Ari Melnick

Definition

Diffuse large B-cell lymphoma (DLBCL) associated with chronic inflammation (CI-DLBCL) is an Epstein-Barr virus (EBV)-associated large B-cell lymphoma occurring in the context of long-standing chronic inflammation involving confined natural or acquired body spaces.[1] CI-DLBCL can present as a tumor mass, the prototypic form being pyothorax-associated lymphoma (PAL), which develops in the pleural cavity of patients with pyothorax secondary to artificial pneumothorax as therapy for tuberculosis,[2] but other cases may occur within bone, joint, and skin in the settings of chronic osteomyelitis, metallic implants, surgical mesh, and chronic stasis ulcer.[1,3] Fibrin-associated DLBCL (FA-DLBCL) is currently considered a subtype of CI-DLBCL, although it has distinct features and is discussed separately later (Table 75.1).[4-6]

Synonyms

Pyothorax-associated lymphoma.

Epidemiology

CI-DLBCL (PAL) affects adult patients (median age, 70 years; range, 50-80) with a marked male predominance (M:F 12:1).[2] Artificial pneumothorax, used in the past as a form of surgical therapy for pulmonary tuberculosis,

TABLE 75.1 Comparison of clinical, pathologic, and genetic features between diffuse large B-cell lymphoma (DLBCL) associated with chronic inflammation (CI-DLBCL) and fibrin-associated DLBCL (FA-DLBCL)

	CI-DLBCL (tumor mass)	FA-DLBCL
Sites of involvement	Pleura, lung, bone, joints, soft tissue	Confined to natural or acquired spaces including foreign body cavity
M/F ratio	12:1	2:1 (except those associated with BI)
Median age (range)	70 y (50->80 y)	56 y (25-96 y)
Median time from presumed etiologic conditions to lymphoma	37 y (1.5-64 y)	10 y (4-26 y)
Clinical context/setting	Artificial pneumothorax for tuberculosis (PAL), chronic osteomyelitis, metallic implants	Cardiac valves or myxomas, preexisting cysts and pseudocyst cavities (including around breast implants), chronic hematomas or thrombi
Clinical features/symptoms	Tumor mass and pain	Asymptomatic
Morphology	Centroblastic, immunoblastic, or plasmablastic, necrosis, angiocentric growth	Centroblastic, immunoblastic, or plasmablastic within superficial layers of fibrinous material, as single cells or small aggregates
Phenotype	$CD20^{+/-}$, $CD79a^{+/-}$, $CD138^{-/+}$, CD30 var, non-GC, expression of T-cell markers possible	$CD20^{+/-}$, $CD79a^{+/-}$, PAX5 var, $CD138^{-/+}$, CD30 frequent, non-GC, expression of T-cell markers possible, PD-L1 expression
EBV	+ (EBER ISH), latency type III (LMP1+, EBNA2+)	+ (EBER ISH), latency type III (LMP1+, EBNA2+)
Genetic features	*MYC* rearrangement or amplification, *TP53* mutation	Mutations in genes related to immune surveillance (*HLA* genes), in *PTEN, JAK2, STAT5B*
Prognosis, treatment	Dismal prognosis (20%-35% OS at 5 y for PAL) with polychemotherapy (R-CHOP)	Indolent, good prognosis with surgical excision alone

BI, breast implant; EBER, EBV-encoded small RNA; ISH, in situ hybridization; non-GC, non–germinal center phenotype; OS, overall survival; PAL, pyothorax-associated lymphoma; R-CHOP, rituximab-cyclophosphamide, Adriamycin (doxorubicin), oncovin, prednisone.

is the only significant risk factor for development of PAL. As this therapy has become rare, PAL is less frequent. Most cases of PAL have been reported in Japan, with rare cases described in the West.[1,2,7] For DLBCLs arising in other settings of chronic inflammation, such as chronic osteomyelitis, metallic implant insertion, surgical mesh implant, and chronic skin venous ulcer, the interval between the predisposing event and lymphoma is usually over 10 years, ranging from 1.2 to 57 years.[1] CI-DLBCL is strongly associated with EBV usually with type III latency.[7] Patients with CI-DLBCL do not have any known predisposing systemic immunodeficiency. Chronic inflammation in a confined space is thought to play a role in the proliferation of EBV-transformed B cells by enabling them to escape from the host immune surveillance through production of IL-10, an immunosuppressive cytokine, and providing autocrine to paracrine growth via IL-6 and IL-6 receptor.[1] In addition to IL-10, expression of high levels of TGF-β1, IL-35, and PD-L1 by EBV latency type III–immortalized B cells support this hypothesis.[3,8] Accumulation of CCR4-expressing Treg cells in primary PAL tissues, as a consequence of secretion of CCL17 and CCL22 chemokines by PAL lymphoma cells, has been demonstrated.[9]

General Clinical Features

CI-DLBCL presents as an often painful tumor mass, most commonly involving the pleural cavity (PAL), bone (especially femur), joints, and periarticular soft tissue. Patients with PAL present with chest pain, back pain, fever, or tumorous swelling in the chest wall or with respiratory symptoms such as productive cough, hemoptysis, and dyspnea. Radiological examination reveals a tumor mass in the pleura (in 80% of cases), pleura and lung (in 10%), or lung near the pleura (in 7%). The serum lactate dehydrogenase (LDH) level is commonly elevated.[2,7,10] In more than 50% of PAL, the tumor mass is >10 cm. The involved bone in CI-DLBCL arising in the context of osteomyelitis typically shows lytic lesions on radiological examination.

Morphology

The morphological features are those of a large B-cell lymphoma with centroblastic or immunoblastic cells (Figure 75.1). Plasmacytoid differentiation or plasmablastic features are frequent.[7] Necrosis and angiocentric growth may be present.

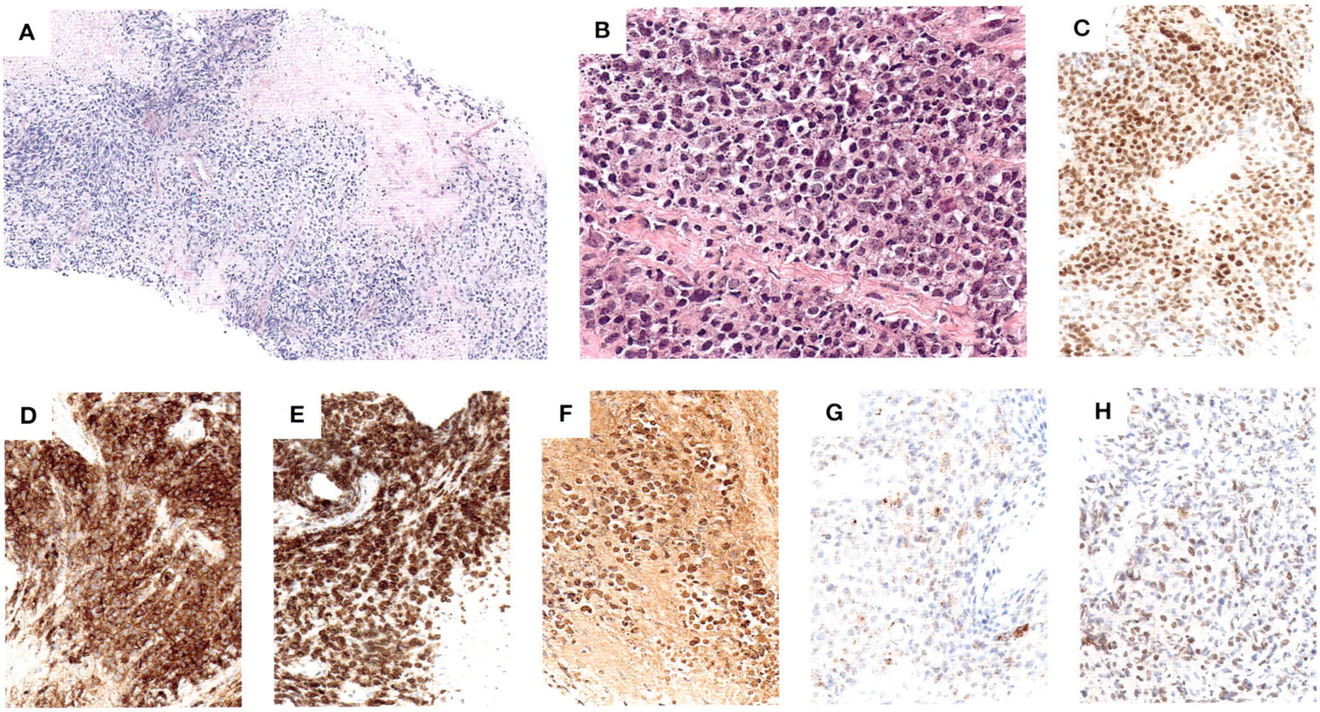

FIGURE 75.1 Pyothorax-associated lymphoma in an 87-year-old man with a past history of artificial pneumothorax for tuberculosis: Pleural biopsy shows a large proliferation with necrosis (**A** and **B:** hematoxylin and eosin); neoplastic cells are large B cells expressing PAX5 (**C**), with aberrant coexpression of CD2 (**D**) and CD3 (**E**). Virtually all cells are positive for EBER by in situ hybridization (**F**). By immunohistochemistry, they are LMP1+ (**G**) and EBNA2+ (**H**).

Immunophenotype

Most cases express CD20 and CD79a. However, a proportion of cases may show plasmacytic differentiation, with loss of CD20 and/or CD79a and expression of MUM1 and CD138. CD30 can be expressed. Aberrant expression of T-cell markers has been reported (Figure 75.1).[1,7] EBER, LMP1, and EBNA-2 are positive in most cases (latency III). Human herpesvirus-8 is negative.[7]

Genetics

Immunoglobulin (IG) genes are clonally rearranged and hypermutated but lack ongoing mutations. CI-DLBCL demonstrates a complex karyotype, and *MYC* amplification and *TP53* mutations are found in up to 70% of cases.[3] *TNFAIP3* is deleted in a proportion of cases. Downregulation of HLA class I expression, which is essential for efficient induction of host cytotoxic T lymphocytes, and mutations in EBNA3B might also contribute to escape of PAL cells from host cytotoxic T lymphocytes.[1]

Prognosis and Clinical Comment

CI-DLBCL is an aggressive lymphoma. Clinical outcome is mostly available for PAL cases, which have a dismal prognosis (20%-35% 5-year overall survival rate).[2,10] For patients achieving complete remission with chemotherapy and/or radiotherapy, the 5-year survival rate is 50%.[10] Poor performance status, high serum LDH, and high clinical stage are unfavorable prognostic factors.[2]

FIBRIN-ASSOCIATED DIFFUSE LARGE B-CELL LYMPHOMA

Definition

FA-DLBCL has historically been considered a subtype of CI-DLBCL, although it has distinct features that may warrant reconsideration of this placement in the future. FA-DLBCL is not mass forming and does not directly produce symptoms. It is discovered incidentally on histologic examination of specimens excised for various pathologies other than lymphoma, and it arises in confined, natural, or acquired spaces such as cardiac valves or myxomas, preexisting cysts and pseudocyst cavities (including those forming around breast implants),[3-6] chronic hematomas, or thrombi. Some FA-DLBCLs arise in association with foreign bodies, such as prosthetic cardiovascular devices, pacemakers, surgical mesh, or breast implants, whereas others arise in the context of native tissue.[1,3,11-14]

Synonyms

None.

Epidemiology

Prevalence of this condition cannot be established, but FA-DLBCL accounts for the majority of cases of CI-DLBCL reported in the last 10 years, with those occurring in the setting of atrial myxoma and breast implants being the most frequent. Median age for FA-DLBCL is 56 years (range, 25-96), with a slight male predominance (M:F ratio 2:1), with the exception of those associated with breast implants. In FA-DLBCL associated with breast implants, the mean time from implantation to lymphoma is 10 years (range, 4-26 years).[3-5] FA-DLBCL is strongly associated with EBV; however, rare EBV-negative cases have been reported.[3,15] Similar to PAL, local immunodeficiency induced by chronic inflammation is thought to favor immune evasion of EBV-transformed B cells. Upregulation of PD-L1 may also support immune evasion.[3,12]

General Clinical Features

By definition, the disease is localized, is non–mass forming, does not directly produce symptoms, and is incidentally discovered. Rare cases presenting with tumor masses but otherwise characteristic of FA-DLBCL have been reported and are difficult to differentiate from CI-DLBCL.[16]

Morphology

Large lymphoma cells, which are singly placed or form small aggregates, are found within fibrinous acellular material, which can be abundant and is typically present at the edge of normal tissue or foreign material (Figure 75.2). Cytology is as described earlier. Tumor cells may focally infiltrate adjacent fibrotic stroma but not the preexisting normal tissue.[3,4]

Phenotype

The immunophenotypic features are similar to those of CI-DLBCL as described earlier.

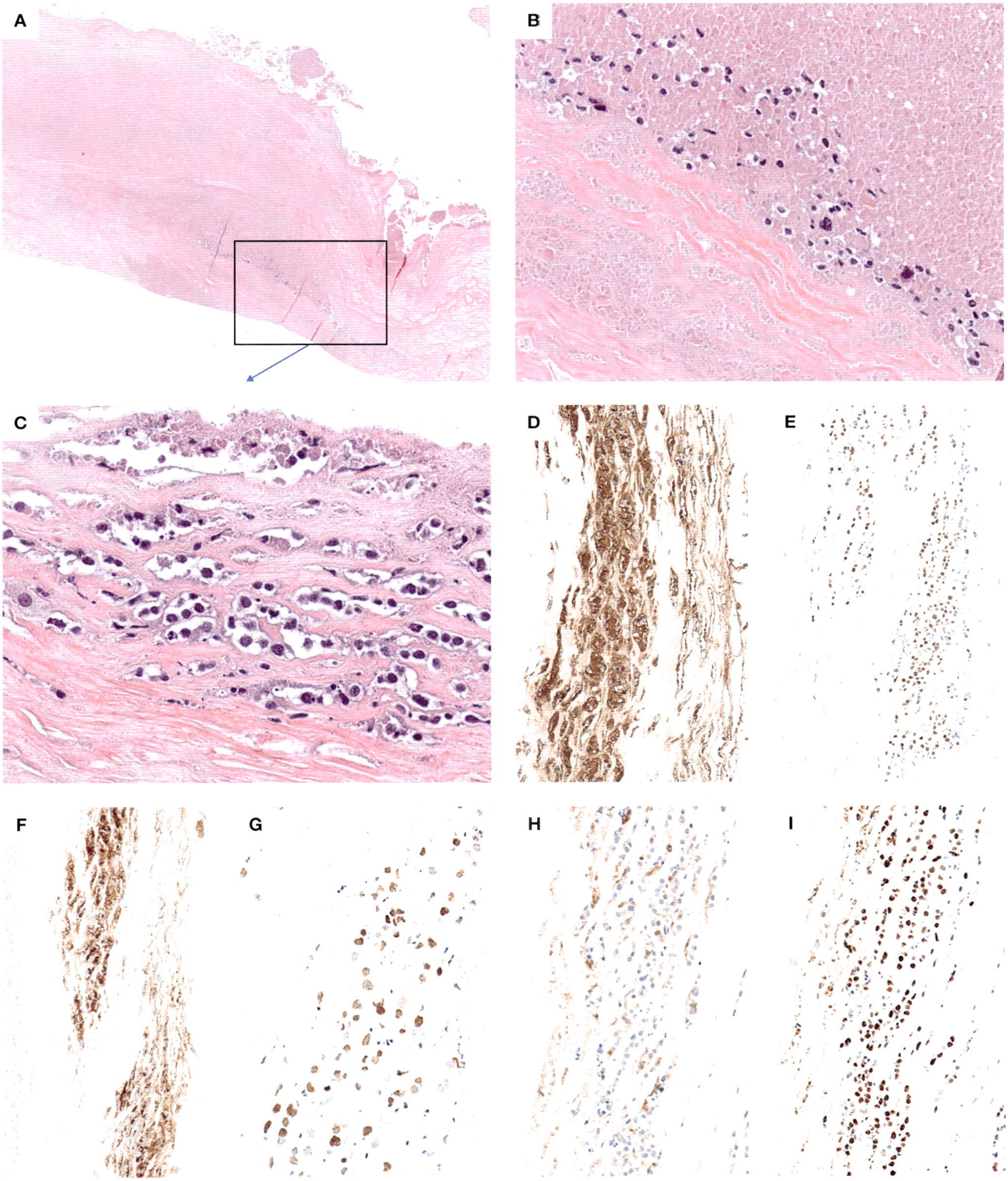

FIGURE 75.2 A case of a fibrin-associated diffuse large B-cell lymphoma discovered incidentally during surgery for breast invasive carcinoma in a 56-year-old woman with macrotextured breast implant. The surface of the capsule shows a fibrinous material (hematoxylin and eosin [H&E], **A**) containing large lymphoma cells (H&E, **B** and **C**), which are CD20 positive **(D)** and express PAX5 **(E)** and CD30 **(F)**. They are EBER positive by in situ hybridization **(G)** and express LMP1 **(H)** and EBNA-2 **(I)**.

Genetics

IG genes are clonally rearranged, and *MYC* rearrangement has been rarely reported.[3,4] Only few cases have been the subject of mutation analysis.[3,4,11] In a recent analysis of six FA-DLBCL cases involving diverse anatomic sites, recurrent mutations in genes related to immune surveillance (including *HLA* genes) in the tumor suppressor gene *PTEN* and in genes of the JAK-STAT pathway (*JAK2, STAT5B*) were found.[11]

Prognosis and Clinical Comment

Unlike PAL/CI-DLBCL, the clinical outcome is highly favorable, even with surgical excision alone. However, some studies suggested that the prognosis could be influenced by the site of origin, with the vascular compartment potentially having the highest risk for systemic involvement and complications.[3,12] Single cases presenting as a solid mass or showing infiltration of the adjacent tissue or progressive disease have been reported,[3,12,13,16] raising the possibility of progression in rare cases. Whether targeted therapies, for example, PI3/STAT pathway inhibition, could be a therapeutic option when surgical excision is incomplete is questionable.[11]

References

1. Chan JCK, Aozasa K, Gaulard P. Diffuse large B-cell lymphoma associated with chronic inflammation. In: Swerdlow SH, Campo E, Harris NL, eds. *WHO Classification of Tumours of Haematopoietic and Lymphoid Tissues*. 4th ed. International Agency for Research on Cancer; 2017.
2. Narimatsu H, Ota Y, Kami M, et al. Clinicopathological features of pyothorax-associated lymphoma; a retrospective survey involving 98 patients. *Ann Oncol.* 2007;18(1):122-128. doi:10.1093/annonc/mdl349
3. Di Napoli A, Soma L, Quintanilla-Martinez L, et al. Cavity-based lymphomas: challenges and novel concepts. A report of the 2022 EA4HP/SH lymphoma workshop. *Virchows Arch.* 2023;483(3):299-316. doi:10.1007/s00428-023-03599-2
4. Mescam L, Camus V, Schiano JM, et al. EBV+ diffuse large B-cell lymphoma associated with chronic inflammation expands the spectrum of breast implant-related lymphomas. *Blood.* 2020;135(22):2004-2009. doi:10.1182/blood.2019003408
5. Medeiros LJ, Marques-Piubelli ML, Sangiorgio VFI, et al. Epstein-Barr-virus-positive large B-cell lymphoma associated with breast implants: an analysis of eight patients suggesting a possible pathogenetic relationship. *Mod Pathol.* 2021;34(12):2154-2167. doi:10.1038/s41379-021-00863-1
6. Rodríguez-Pinilla SM, García FJS, Balagué O, Rodríguez-Justo M, Piris MÁ. Breast implant-associated Epstein-Barr virus-positive large B-cell lymphomas: a report of three cases. *Haematologica.* 2020;105(8):e412-e414. doi:10.3324/haematol.2019.232355
7. Petitjean B, Jardin F, Joly B, et al. Pyothorax-associated lymphoma: a peculiar clinicopathologic entity derived from B cells at late stage of differentiation and with occasional aberrant dual B- and T-cell phenotype. *Am J Surg Pathol.* 2002;26(6):724-732. doi:10.1097/00000478-200206000-00005
8. Auclair H, Ouk-Martin C, Roland L, et al. EBV latency III-transformed B cells are inducers of conventional and unconventional regulatory T cells in a PD-L1-dependent manner. *J Immunol.* 2019;203(6):1665-1674. doi:10.4049/jimmunol.1801420
9. Higuchi T, Matsuo K, Hashida Y, et al. Epstein-Barr virus-positive pyothorax-associated lymphoma expresses CCL17 and CCL22 chemokines that attract CCR4-expressing regulatory T cells. *Cancer Lett.* 2019;453:184-192. doi:10.1016/j.canlet.2019.03.053
10. Nakatsuka SI, Yao M, Hoshida Y, Yamamoto S, Iuchi K, Aozasa K. Pyothorax-associated lymphoma: a review of 106 cases. *J Clin Oncol.* 2002;20(20):4255-4260. doi:10.1200/JCO.2002.09.021
11. Boyer DF, Perry A, Wey E, et al. Fibrin-associated large B-cell lymphoma shows frequent mutations related to immune surveillance and PTEN. *Blood.* 2023;142(11):1022-1025. doi:10.1182/blood.2023020349
12. Boyer DF, McKelvie PA, de Leval L, et al. Fibrin-associated EBV-positive large B-cell lymphoma: an indolent neoplasm with features distinct from diffuse large B-cell lymphoma associated with chronic inflammation. *Am J Surg Pathol.* 2017;41(3):299-312. doi:10.1097/PAS.0000000000000775
13. Kameda K, Shono T, Takagishi S, et al. Epstein-Barr virus-positive diffuse large B-cell primary central nervous system lymphoma associated with organized chronic subdural hematoma: a case report and review of the literature. *Pathol Int.* 2015;65(3):138-143. doi:10.1111/pin.12242
14. Miller DV, Firchau DJ, McClure RF, Kurtin PJ, Feldman AL. Epstein-Barr virus-associated diffuse large B-cell lymphoma arising on cardiac prostheses. *Am J Surg Pathol.* 2010;34(3):377-384. doi:10.1097/PAS.0b013e3181ce9128
15. Baugh L, Brown N, Song JY, Pandya S, Montoya V, Perry AM. Fibrin-associated, EBV-negative diffuse large B-cell lymphoma arising in atrial myxoma: expanding the spectrum of the entity. *Int J Surg Pathol.* 2022;30(1):39-45. doi:10.1177/10668969211014959
16. Vets J, Marcelis L, Schepers C, et al. Breast implant associated EBV-positive Diffuse Large B-cell lymphoma: an underrecognized entity? *Diagn Pathol.* 2023;18(1):52. doi:10.1186/s13000-023-01337-5

Chapter 76
Lymphomatoid Granulomatosis

Elaine S. Jaffe, Christopher Melani, and Stefania Pittaluga

Definition

Lymphomatoid granulomatosis (LYG) is a rare Epstein-Barr virus (EBV)-associated B-cell lymphoproliferative disorder (LPD) with unique histopathologic and clinical features that traditionally distinguish it from other EBV-positive B-cell LPDs and lymphomas.[1,2] Pulmonary involvement is considered an essential feature.[3] It is characterized by angiocentric and angiodestructive growth, and a population of EBV-positive B cells that are admixed with numerically predominant reactive T lymphocytes.

Synonyms

Angiocentric lymphoproliferative lesion (obsolete) (not recommended).

Epidemiology

There are no predisposing racial or ethnic features. However, most cases have been reported in the Western world.[4] Some EBV-positive LPDs arising in the setting of immune deficiency can show marked phenotypic and genotypic similarity.[4,5] In most patients with LYG, laboratory findings show subtle defects in immune function without overt immune deficiency.

General Clinical Features

LYG typically presents in adults in the fourth to sixth decade of life and shows a 2:1 male predominance.[3] Involvement of the lung is a universal finding, with common involvement of other extranodal sites including the central nervous system (CNS; 40%), skin (40%), kidney (20%), and liver (15%-20%) (Figure 76.1). Radiologically, pulmonary involvement is often bilateral, with most lesions concentrated in the lower lobes. Cutaneous manifestations are very common (33% of patients), but do not usually contain EBV-positive B cells.[6] Involvement of hematolymphoid tissues, including lymph nodes, spleen, or bone marrow, is exceedingly rare and suggests an alternative diagnosis.

Most patients present with pulmonary symptoms related to lung involvement. Laboratory studies show evidence of prior infection by EBV, but the EBV viral load is generally found at low levels in the plasma or blood. Flow cytometry of peripheral blood often shows a modest decrease in CD3-positive T cells, mostly in CD8-positive T cells with frequently normal CD4-positive T cells, as well as reduction in CD56-positive natural killer cells. However, evidence of overt immune deficiency is generally absent. Similar lesions may be seen in extranodal sites in patients with immune deficiency, and in some instances, it can be challenging to distinguish LYG from EBV-positive polymorphic B-cell LPDs in other clinical settings.

Morphology

The essential histological findings in LYG include an angiocentric and angiodestructive lymphoid infiltrate.[1,2,4] Lung biopsies show a perivascular lymphoid infiltrate with lymphoid cells often extending into the vascular wall. The lymphoid infiltrate may lead to vascular destruction, obliteration of the vascular lumen, and tissue necrosis (Figure 76.2). The infiltrates have a nodular pattern, with larger pulmonary nodules more likely to be associated with necrosis. The lesions in the lung are often sharply circumscribed, and the adjacent pulmonary parenchyma may appear largely normal. Interstitial lymphocytic infiltration of the lung is not common.

The lymphoid infiltrate usually has a polymorphous cytological composition with admixed plasma cells and histiocytes. Lymphoid cells are generally small with admixed larger immunoblastic-appearing cells, and occasional pleomorphic lymphoid cells resembling Hodgkin/Reed-Sternberg (HRS) cells. The cytological composition reflects the immunophenotype. The larger atypical lymphoid cells are of B-cell lineage, while the background small lymphocytes are mostly T cells. Increased eosinophils are not usually

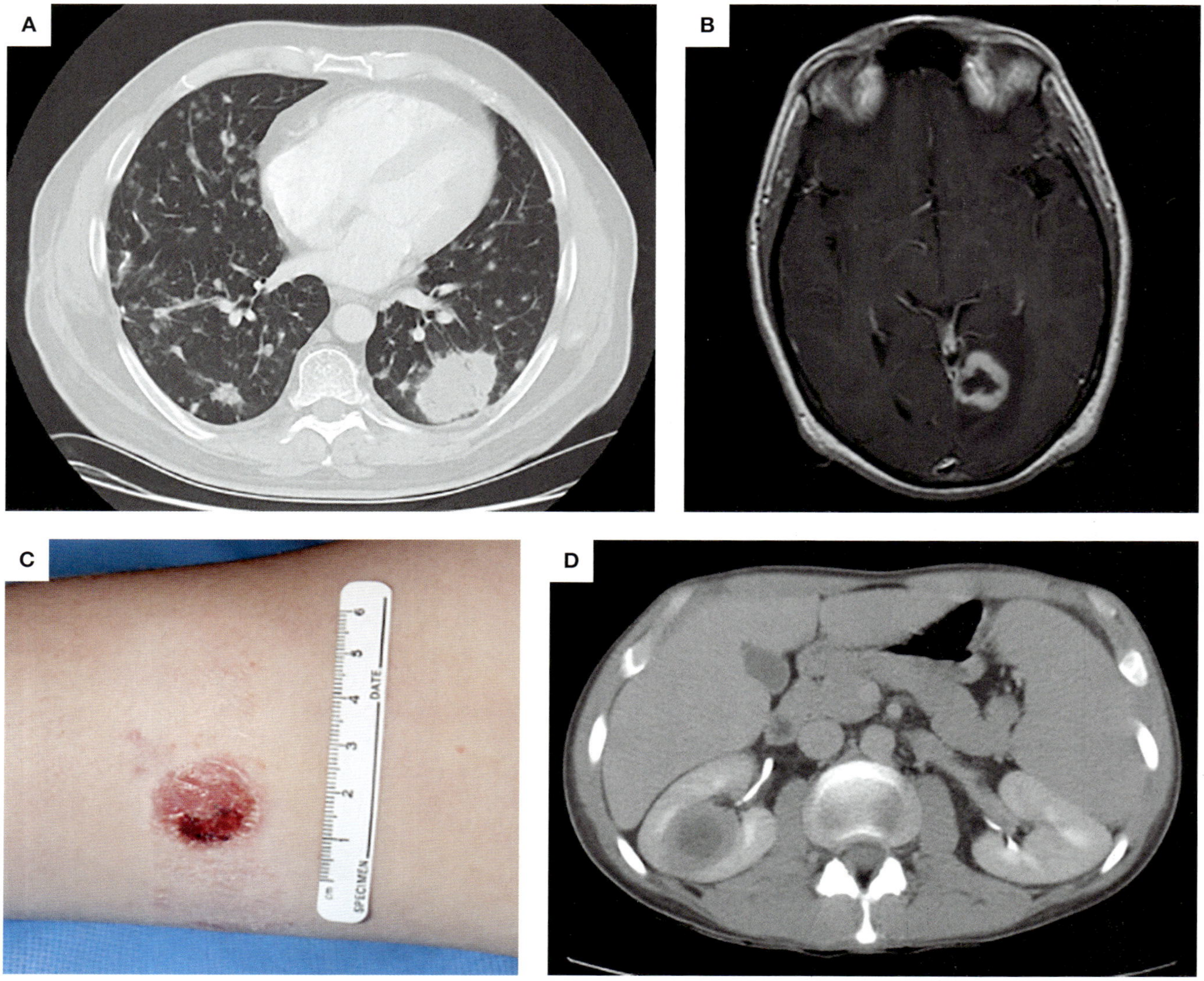

FIGURE 76.1 Radiological and clinical features of disease. **A:** Computed tomography scan of the chest in a 62-year-old patient with grade 1 lymphomatoid granulomatosis (LYG) showing multiple pulmonary nodules in the bilateral lower lobes of the lungs. **B:** Axial T1 post-contrast magnetic resonance image of the brain in a 38-year-old patient with grade 3 LYG showing a ring-enhancing lesion with central necrosis and surrounding vasogenic edema in the left medial temporal lobe of the brain. **C:** Photograph of the right forearm in a 14-year-old patient with grade 2 LYG showing an erythematous slightly raised macule with associated ulceration. **D:** Computed tomography scan of the abdomen in a 27-year-old patient with grade 3 LYG showing a large low-density mass in the right kidney with a rim of associated higher density surrounding the mass.

seen, but necrosis may lead to some admixed neutrophils. However, many of the necrotic lesions are poorly cellular.

Involvement of the CNS, kidney, or other extranodal sites by LYG is similar to that seen in the lung. However, cutaneous lesions are histologically diverse, and often show granulomatous panniculitis with absence of EBV-positive cells.[6]

Immunophenotype

The atypical lymphoid cells are EBV-positive B cells that are associated with a numerically predominant population of T cells (Figure 76.2). LYG is generally graded according to the number of EBV-positive cells as determined by EBV-encoded small RNA (EBER) in situ hybridization. Grade 1 contains infrequent

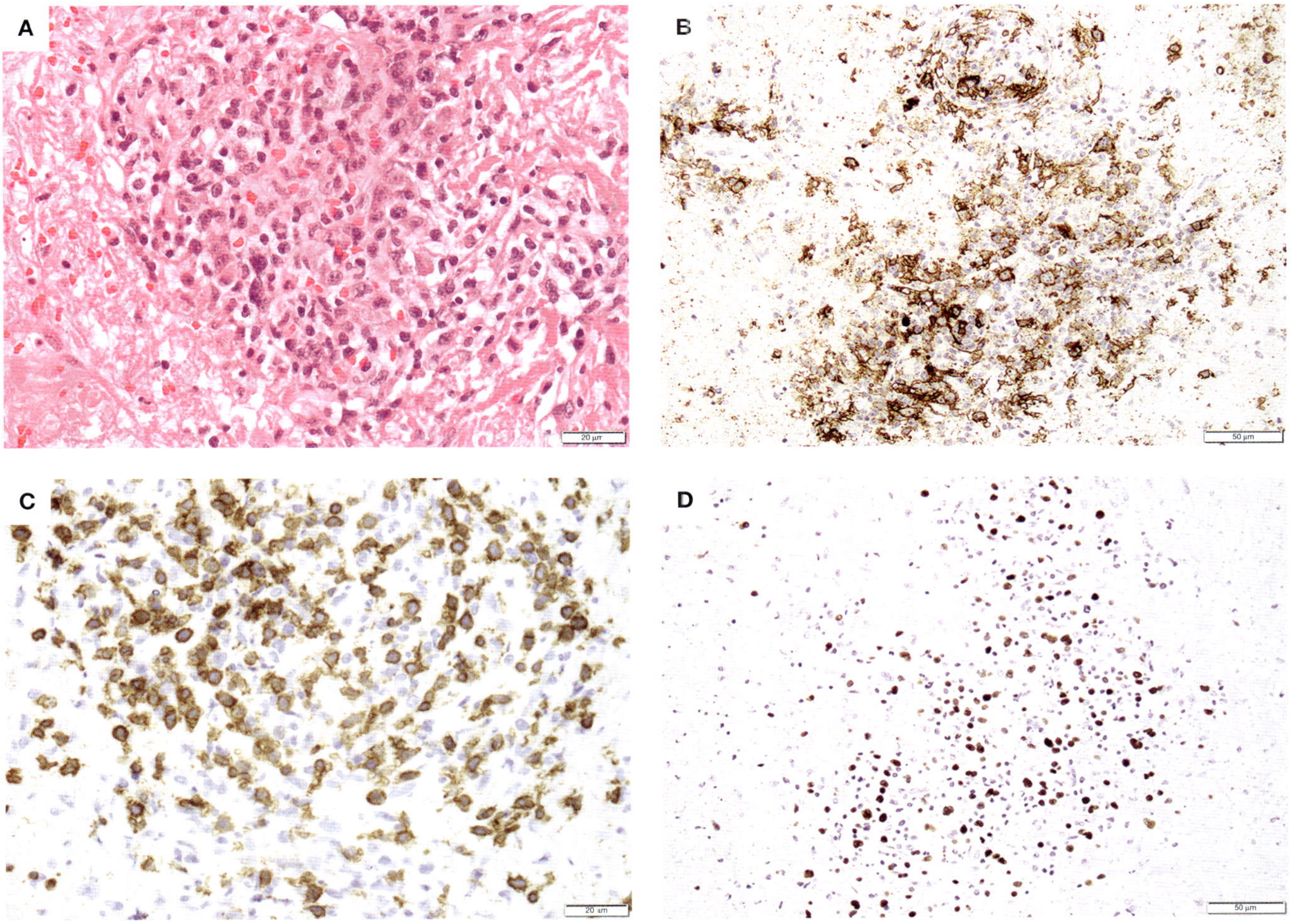

FIGURE 76.2 Pathological features of disease. **A:** Lung biopsy shows an angiocentric atypical lymphoid infiltrate. The cells infiltrate the vascular wall. The surrounding parenchyma is necrotic. **B:** CD20 immunostain highlights the large atypical cells, which focally disrupt the vascular wall. **C:** Numerous small CD3-positive T cells are present, and show infiltration of the vessel wall. **D:** The atypical B cells are positive for Epstein-Barr virus (EBV) with EBV-encoded small RNA (EBER) in situ hybridization, with more than 20 positive cells/hpf.

EBV-positive B cells, less than 5/high-power field (hpf). Grade 2 contains more frequent EBV-positive cells, overall from 5 to 20/hpf. Grade 3 LYG should still have a rich T-cell background, but has more numerous EBV-positive cells, more than 20 and focally more than 50/hpf. However, the presence of confluent sheets of EBV-positive cells should raise concern for a diagnosis of EBV-positive diffuse large B-cell lymphoma, not otherwise specified.[7]

The atypical EBV-positive cells generally show expression of CD20, CD79a, and MUM1/IRF-4. BCL-6 is often negative or seen in a minor subset. The atypical B cells show expression of LMP1, usually in a subset of the EBER-positive cells. Further studies of EBV latency have shown expression of EBNA2, consistent with latency III.[4] This finding is in keeping with defective immune surveillance as an essential feature of LYG.

The atypical B cells may show evidence of plasmacytoid differentiation, with cytoplasmic light chain expression seen in a subset of cases. The larger HRS-like cells may show expression of CD30, but CD15 is usually negative. There may be partial loss of CD20 and PAX5, consistent with plasmacytoid differentiation. Background T cells are abundant with CD4 usually greater than CD8. One study suggested the presence of increased Treg cells, as evidenced by the expression of CD25 and FOXP3.[4] The vascular lesions are the hallmark of LYG. T cells comprise a significant proportion of the vasculitic cells. Release of chemokines contribute to the angiodestruction, with EBV playing a major role in the pathogenesis.[8]

Genetics

Polymerase chain reaction (PCR) studies for clonal immunoglobulin rearrangement show evidence of a monoclonal B-cell proliferation in a subset. PCR studies are more likely to be clonal in higher grade lesions. In one study, positive PCR was seen in 69% of grade 3, 50% of grade 2, and only 8% of grade 1 lesions.[4] PCR for T-cell receptor gamma gene rearrangement usually shows a polyclonal pattern, or in some cases a restricted or abnormal pattern, perhaps suggesting an altered reactive T-cell repertoire. Genomic alterations in either the EBV-positive cells or the reactive cells have not been reported, but studies are limited.

Prognosis and Clinical Comment

Historic studies have noted an overall poor prognosis for most patients with LYG, with a median survival of under 2 years, and a high rate of mortality secondary to progression to high-grade disease or overt malignant lymphoma.[1] Early prospective studies utilized corticosteroid therapy and/or single-agent chemotherapy, modeled after regimens used in pulmonary vasculitis, which leads to only transient disease control in a subset of patients. Modern therapeutic approaches have focused on restoration of antiviral immunity given that defective immune surveillance of EBV is thought to play a major role in disease pathogenesis.[3,9] Immunotherapies, most commonly with interferon alfa-2b, have been used in patients with low-grade LYG in an effort to control disease and inhibit the progression to high-grade disease and overt lymphoma. Systemic combination cytotoxic chemotherapy with the addition of rituximab immunotherapy has been the mainstay of therapy for patients with high-grade LYG or low-grade patients with advanced and symptomatic disease requiring a more rapid clinical response, similar to the treatments used in other aggressive B-cell lymphomas. Given the frequent unbated defective immune surveillance of EBV following therapy, disease relapse with alternate grade disease is commonly encountered and can be successfully treated with crossover therapy (ie, immunotherapy to chemotherapy or chemotherapy to immunotherapy). Utilization of this treatment approach based on underlying pathologic grade of disease has led to significantly improved survival in LYG patients with a current median overall survival of over 2 decades.[9]

References

1. Katzenstein AL, Doxtader E, Narendra S. Lymphomatoid granulomatosis: insights gained over 4 decades. *Am J Surg Pathol.* 2010;34(12):e35-e48. 00000478-201012000-00028 [pii]. doi:10.1097/PAS.0b013e3181fd8781
2. Guinee D Jr, Jaffe E, Kingma D, et al. Pulmonary lymphomatoid granulomatosis. Evidence for a proliferation of Epstein-Barr virus infected B-lymphocytes with a prominent T-cell component and vasculitis. *Am J Surg Pathol.* 1994;18(8):753-764. doi:10.1097/00000478-199408000-00001
3. Melani C, Jaffe ES, Wilson WH. Pathobiology and treatment of lymphomatoid granulomatosis, a rare EBV-driven disorder. *Blood.* 2020;135(16):1344-1352. doi:10.1182/blood.2019000933
4. Song JY, Pittaluga S, Dunleavy K, et al. Lymphomatoid granulomatosis—a single institute experience: pathologic findings and clinical correlations. *Am J Surg Pathol.* 2015;39(2):141-156. doi:10.1097/pas.0000000000000328
5. Jaffe ES, Wilson WH. Lymphomatoid granulomatosis: pathogenesis, pathology and clinical implications. *Cancer Surv.* 1997;30:233-248.
6. Beaty MW, Toro J, Sorbara L, et al. Cutaneous lymphomatoid granulomatosis: correlation of clinical and biologic features. *Am J Surg Pathol.* 2001;25(9):1111-1120.
7. Quintanilla-Martinez L, Swerdlow SH, Tousseyn T, Barrionuevo C, Nakamura S, Jaffe ES. New concepts in EBV-associated B, T, and NK cell lymphoproliferative disorders. *Virchows Arch.* 2023;482(1):227-244. doi:10.1007/s00428-022-03414-4
8. Teruya-Feldstein J, Jaffe ES, Burd PR, et al. The role of Mig, the monokine induced by interferon-gamma, and IP-10, the interferon-gamma-inducible protein-10, in tissue necrosis and vascular damage associated with Epstein-Barr virus-positive lymphoproliferative disease. *Blood.* 1997;90(10):4099-4105.
9. Melani C, Dowdell K, Pittaluga S, et al. Interferon alfa-2b in patients with low-grade lymphomatoid granulomatosis and chemotherapy with DA-EPOCH-R in patients with high-grade lymphomatoid granulomatosis: an open-label, single-centre, phase 2 trial. *Lancet Haematol.* 2023;10(5):e346-e358. doi:10.1016/s2352-3026(23)00029-7

Chapter 77

Epstein-Barr Virus–Positive Polymorphic B-Cell Lymphoproliferative Disorder, Not Otherwise Specified

Stefan Dojcinov, Genevieve M. Crane, Elaine S. Jaffe, Leticia Quintanilla-Martinez, and Wyndham H. Wilson

Definition

EBV-positive polymorphic B-cell lymphoproliferative disorder, not otherwise specified (EBV+ polymorphic B-LPD, NOS) is a new provisional category, introduced to provide a unifying diagnostic term that can be used in a variety of clinical settings. Morphologically, it is defined as an EBV-associated proliferation of B cells displaying a full range of maturation that alters tissue architecture in extranodal sites or lymph nodes. Such polymorphic proliferations of EBV-positive B cells may be seen in patients without known cause for decreased immune surveillance but may include cases that arise as a consequence of presumed immune senescence. They are also encountered in patients with known immunodeficiency, such as congenital immunodeficiency or HIV infection. However, morphologically similar lesions arising in the context of immunomodulatory drug therapy for autoimmune disease or in a posttransplant setting should be categorized as either iatrogenic immunosuppression-associated lymphoproliferative disorders (see Chapter 114) or posttransplant lymphoproliferative disorders (see Chapter 113), respectively. In addition, the infiltrate should **not** fulfill diagnostic criteria for any other EBV-related lymphoproliferative entity, such as EBV-positive mucocutaneous ulcer, lymphomatoid granulomatosis, and EBV-positive diffuse large B-cell lymphoma, NOS.[1-3] Lack of detection of EBV by in situ hybridization for EBV encoded small RNA (EBER) excludes this diagnosis.[4,5]

Synonyms

None.

Epidemiology

EBV+ polymorphic B-LPD, NOS affects patients over a wide age range without gender predilection. It may be seen in patients without a known cause for immunosuppression but with presumed immune senescence. These patients tend to be older.[1-4] It may also be seen in the setting of primary immunodeficiency and HIV infection. These patients are younger (median age 38 years) and, in the context of primary immunodeficiency, it is particularly common in children.

General Clinical Features

Most patients present with localized lymphadenopathy or, less commonly, extranodal lesions. Extranodal sites of involvement may include lung, central nervous system, gastrointestinal tract, skin, and liver. The symptoms are varied, depending on the presenting site and extent of disease. Most patients have high EBV copy numbers in peripheral blood.[1-3]

Morphology

The pathologic features are the same regardless of the underlying etiology. Partial architectural effacement should be seen, but large mass lesions with extensive tissue destruction are uncommon. The polymorphic infiltrate comprises the full B-cell maturation range, including lymphocytes, plasma cells, immunoblasts, and "transitional" medium-sized cells. Scattered more pleomorphic Hodgkin/Reed-Sternberg (HRS)-like cells may rarely be seen, but a high content of large pleomorphic cells should raise consideration of an alternative diagnosis (Figure 77.1) (Table 77.1). A proportion of cases may also show prominence of eosinophils, histiocytes, nonnecrotizing granulomas, angioinvasion, and necrosis.[1-3,6] EBV+ polymorphic B-LPD, NOS should

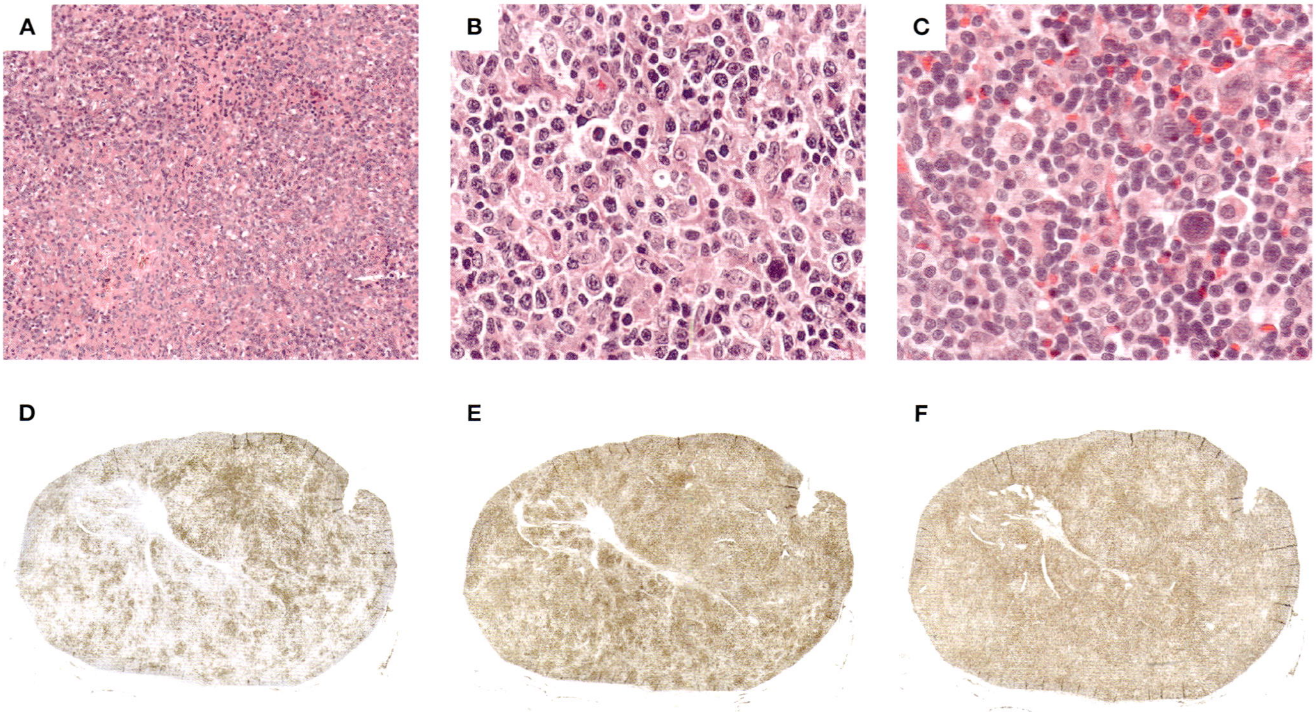

FIGURE 77.1 EBV-positive polymorphic B-cell lymphoproliferative disorder—Histological features. **A:** The lymph node tissue or extranodal sites display a vaguely nodular infiltrate altering lymph node architecture. **B:** The infiltrate is markedly polymorphic including lymphocytes, histiocytes, plasma cells, immunoblasts, and "transitional" medium-sized cells. Compared with diffuse large B-cell lymphoma, pleomorphism is less marked. **C:** The infiltrate also contains a very rare Hodgkin and Reed-Sternberg-like cell. **D-F:** Low-power views of immunostaining for CD20 (**D**), CD79a (**E**), and CD3 (**F**) highlight altered architecture, with a prominent plasmacytic component highlighted by CD79a (**E**) and not staining with CD20 (**D**).

be distinguished from lymphoid hyperplasias that result from reactivation of the latent EBV infection, in which EBV-positive cells are only focally distributed, constitute a minority of the cells present, and do not typically destroy tissue architecture.[2,4]

Immunophenotype

The infiltrate is polymorphous and contains EBV-positive B cells that may have variable phenotypes due to the spectrum of cell types and maturation stages present. The majority of cells usually have retained B-cell marker expression including CD45, CD20, CD79a, PAX5, OCT2, and BOB1 (Figure 77.1 and Figure 77.2). Cells in the infiltrate with plasmacytic features may show loss of CD20, show staining for CD79a, and express plasma cell markers including CD138 and MUM1 (see Figure 77.2). Rare cells with immunoblastic and occasional HRS-cell morphology are CD30 positive and may also coexpress CD15. These cases can be distinguished from classic Hodgkin lymphoma by their expression of B cell–associated antigens and the presence of EBV in cells of varying size. Immunoglobulin light chain expression is often polytypic, but light chain restriction can be observed. In situ hybridization for EBER is positive in all cases, with variable expression of LMP1 and EBNA2 indicating latency II or III. Type III latency is seen more frequently in EBV+ polymorphic B-LPD, NOS than in EBV-positive diffuse large B-cell lymphoma, NOS. There is a variably prominent background T-cell infiltrate, which may contain populations of T-follicular helper (PD-1-positive) cells mimicking T-cell lymphoma.[2,4] Expression of PD-L1 is noted in approximately 30% of cases, indicating pathogenetic heterogeneity and a potential role of immune evasion in a proportion of cases.[7]

TABLE 77.1 Differential diagnosis of EBV-positive B-cell lymphoproliferations with Hodgkin-like features

	EBV-positive polymorphic lymphoproliferative disorder	EBV-positive mucocutaneous ulcer	EBV-positive diffuse large b-cell lymphoma	Lymphomatoid granulomatosis	EBV-positive classic hodgkin lymphoma
Clinical features	• Nodal more common than extranodal • Usually localized without systemic symptoms	• Mucosal and cutaneous • Solitary lesion • Circumscribed • No systemic disease	• Nodal and extranodal • Often advanced stage • Systemic symptoms common	• Lung lesions essential for diagnosis • Extrapulmonary lesions diagnostic of LYG if lung lesions present • No lymph node/ BM involvement	• Primarily nodal lymphoma • No primary extranodal disease
Morphology	• Altered architecture but complete effacement uncommon • Focal necrosis may be present • Polymorphic; little pleomorphism; plasmacytoid features common; rare HRS-like cells • Marked cell size variation	• Distinctive architecture • No breach of anatomical compartments • Polymorphic Hodgkin-like infiltrate; could be markedly pleomorphic • Major large cell component • Polymorphic background rich in reactive cells	• Effaced architecture • Destructive lesions breaching anatomical compartments • Pleomorphic infiltrate often Hodgkin-like • Less variation in cell size	• Dominantly angiocentric/ angiodestructive with copious necrosis • Vasculitic changes associated with T-cell infiltration	• Effaced architecture • Large lesional cells only; no variation • Histiocyte-rich background in EBV+ cases
Immunophenotype	• B-cell program retained • Prominent plasma cell/terminally differentiated B-cell component • EBV latency II/III	• B-cell program retained • >50% cells CD20+ • EBV latency II/III	• B-cell program retained • >50% cells CD20+ • EBV latency II/III	• B-cell program retained • EBV latency II	• B-cell program not retained • CD20- • EBV latency II (latency III excludes CHL)
Genetics/Molecular	• Polyclonal or monoclonal B cells • Frequent "restricted" clonality T-cell patterns • No stable genetic markers	• Polyclonal or monoclonal B cells • Frequent "restricted" clonality T-cell patterns • No stable genetic markers	• Monoclonal B cells • Frequent "restricted" T-cells • No stable genetic markers	• Monoclonal B cells (grade 2/3) • No stable genetic markers	• Monoclonal B cell • A proportion with *CIITA* and *PD-L1/L2* gene loci abnormalities • Common mutations of the JAK-STAT and NOTCH pathways • Most do not correspond to established molecular DLBCL subtypes

BM, bone marrow; CHL, classic Hodgkin lymphoma; DLBCL, diffuse large B-cell lymphoma; EBV, Epstein-Barr virus; HRS, Hodgkin/Reed-Sternberg; LYG, lymphomatoid granulomatosis.

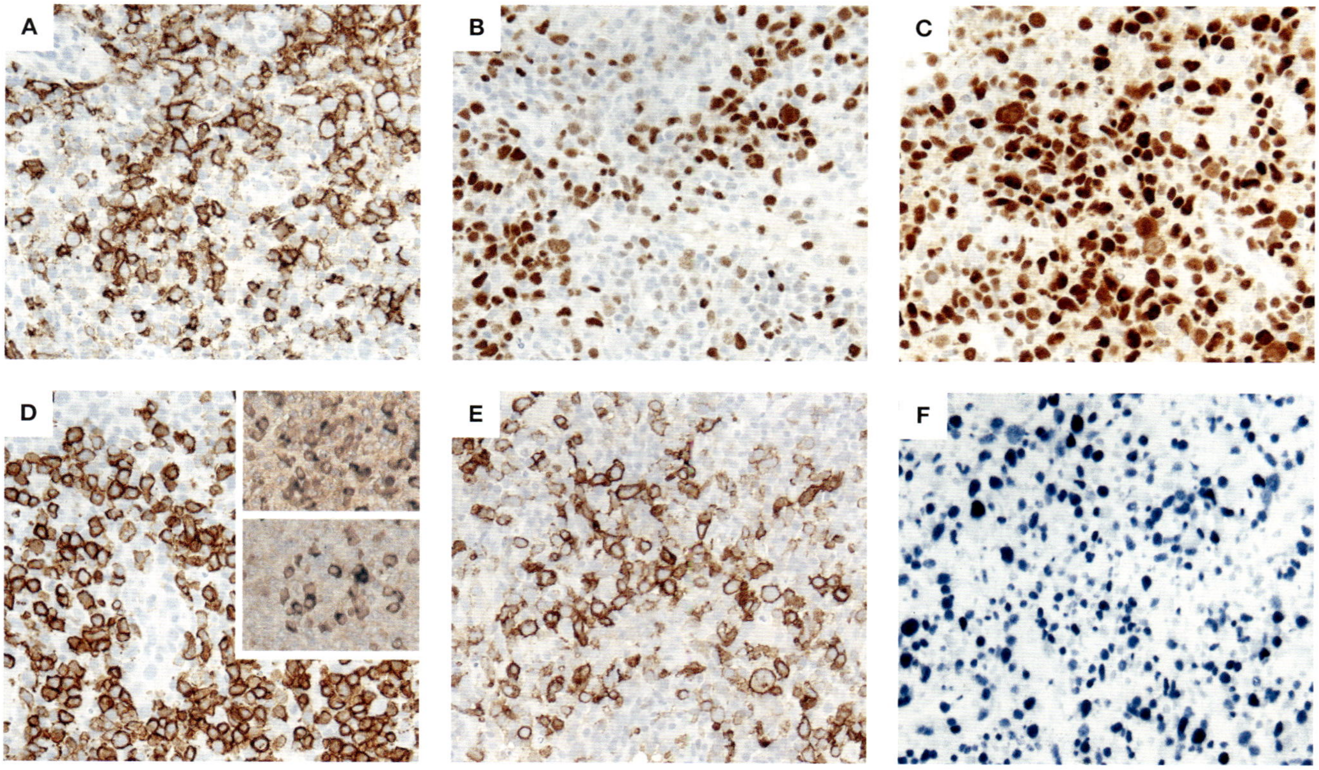

FIGURE 77.2 EBV-positive polymorphic B-cell lymphoproliferative disorder—Immunophenotype. **A-C:** A proportion of the infiltrate shows retention of the B-cell phenotype with expression of CD20 **(A)**, PAX5 **(B)**, and OCT2 **(C)**. These immunostains also highlight the polymorphous nature of the infiltrate with variably sized cells including lymphocytes and immunoblasts. **D:** The plasmacytic component is highlighted by CD138 and in this case shows polytypic light chain expression (inset top, lambda; inset bottom kappa). **E:** There is widespread expression of CD30, colocalizing with the expression of B-cell markers, also highlighting the polymorphic range of cell sizes. **F:** EBER shows patchy positivity, highlighting the wide range of nuclear sizes of the lesional cells.

Genetics

B-cell clonality is seen in 50% to 70% of cases of EBV+ polymorphic B-LPD, NOS.[4] Most cases lack gross genetic abnormalities, with no characteristic genetic alterations.[8,9] However, the mutational profile is poorly characterized and has not been systematically studied. Diminished specific T-cell response to EBV because of immunodeficiency in some cases may result in oligoclonal or restricted T-cell clonality results.[1,4,5]

Prognosis and Clinical Comment

Therapeutic approach to EBV+ polymorphic B-LPD, NOS has not been standardized and is variable. It depends on the clinical aspects of the disease and the context. Some cases are self-limited and will regress without therapy. Patients with symptomatic disease may benefit from single-agent rituximab, other means of immunomodulation, or immunochemotherapy. Outcomes are also variable and depend on the underlying immunosuppression and the therapeutic ability to modulate it.[2,4]

References

1. Natkunam Y, Goodlad JR, Chadburn A, et al. EBV-positive B-cell proliferations of varied malignant potential: 2015 SH/EAHP workshop report-part 1. *Am J Clin Pathol*. 2017;147(2):129-152.
2. Quintanilla-Martinez L, Swerdlow SH, Tousseyn T, Barrionuevo C, Nakamura S, Jaffe ES. New concepts in EBV-associated B, T, and NK cell lymphoproliferative disorders. *Virchows Arch*. 2023;482(1):227-244.
3. Campo E, Jaffe ES, Cook JR, et al. The international consensus classification of mature lymphoid neoplasms: a report from the clinical advisory committee. *Blood*. 2022;140(11):1229-1253.
4. Dojcinov SD, Venkataraman G, Pittaluga S, et al. Age-related EBV-associated lymphoproliferative disorders in the Western population: a spectrum of reactive lymphoid hyperplasia and lymphoma. *Blood*. 2011;117(18):4726-4735.

5. Munz C. Latency and lytic replication in Epstein-Barr virus-associated oncogenesis. *Nat Rev Microbiol.* 2019;17(11):691-700.
6. Kurita D, Miyoshi H, Ichikawa A, et al. Methotrexate-associated lymphoproliferative disorders in patients with rheumatoid arthritis: clinicopathologic features and prognostic factors. *Am J Surg Pathol.* 2019;43(7):869-884.
7. Schiefer AI, Salzer E, Fureder A, et al. PD-L1 and PD1 expression in post-transplantation lymphoproliferative disease (PTLD) of childhood and adolescence: an inter- and intra-individual descriptive study covering the whole spectrum of PTLD categories. *Cancer Med.* 2019;8(10):4656-4668.
8. Djokic M, Le Beau MM, Swinnen LJ, et al. Post-transplant lymphoproliferative disorder subtypes correlate with different recurring chromosomal abnormalities. *Genes Chromosomes Cancer.* 2006;45(3):313-318.
9. Poirel HA, Bernheim A, Schneider A, et al. Characteristic pattern of chromosomal imbalances in posttransplantation lymphoproliferative disorders: correlation with histopathological subcategories and EBV status. *Transplantation.* 2005;80(2):176-184.

Chapter 78
ALK-Positive Large B-Cell Lymphoma

Eric D. Hsi, Philippe Gaulard, and Astrid Pavlovsky

Definition

ALK-positive large B-cell lymphoma (ALK+ LBCL) is an LBCL with a plasmablastic phenotype characterized by ALK expression due to an activating *ALK* rearrangement.

Synonyms

None.

Epidemiology

This is a very rare lymphoma with cases described in small, retrospective series or case reports. The median age at diagnosis is 38 years with a broad age range (9-90). Only 10% of cases occur in the pediatric population. There is a male predominance (M:F = 4.2:1).

General Clinical Features

ALK + LBCL is a rare and aggressive B-cell lymphoma; 61% of patients present with advanced-stage disease. The most common extranodal sites include the upper airway, gastrointestinal tract, spleen, liver, and bone marrow. Elevated lactate dehydrogenase and B symptoms at presentation are common.[1]

Morphology

The lymph node architecture is usually effaced, but preserved sinuses can sometimes be seen. A sinusoidal pattern of infiltration is common. In less involved lymph nodes this sinusoidal pattern can be quite prominent and raise the possibility of metastatic carcinoma or melanoma. The large lymphoma cells are immunoblastic, with round nuclei and prominent central nucleoli. Plasmablastic cells are also present with eccentric nuclei, amphophilic-to-basophilic cytoplasm, and sometimes a paranuclear hof (Figure 78.1). Reed-Sternberg-like binucleated cells may be seen.[1,2]

Immunophenotype

Tumor cells generally lack CD20 but express CD138, VS38c, EMA, and MUM1. CD45 is expressed in 80% of cases. PAX5, CD79a, and BCL6 each may be expressed in approximately 20% of cases, and CD10 may be seen in a minority (30%-50%) of cases. OCT2 and BOB1 are expressed in most cases studied. While CD30 is absent in 85% of cases, CD15 may be weakly expressed in 20% of cases. ALK is expressed and, like anaplastic large cell lymphoma, the particular rearrangement dictates the expression patten of ALK. The most common translocation (see later discussion) results in ALK expression with a cytoplasmic granular staining pattern (Figure 78.1).[1] Other rare patterns can be seen (Table 78.1).

Cytoplasmic IgA is expressed in approximately 90% of cases, and immunoglobulin light chain restriction may be identified in a subset of cases, with lambda being more frequent than kappa. T cell–associated markers such as CD2, CD3, CD5, CD7, and CD8 are not expressed, but CD4 can be expressed in 50% of cases and 10% may express CD56. Expression of cytotoxic markers such as TIA1, granzyme B, and perforin may occur. Although the number of cases studied is low, phospo-STAT3 has been reported to be present in most studied cases, likely a consequence of ALK kinase activation. HHV8 and EBV stains are negative. Of note, cytokeratin has been reported in approximately 15% of cases, which may cause confusion with metastatic carcinoma. The Ki67 index varies (10%-95%) but is usually elevated (median 70%).[1,3-5]

Genetics

ALK+ LBCLs harbor an *ALK* translocation resulting in ligand-independent activation of the ALK kinase. By far the most common partner gene is *CLTC* resulting from a t(2;17)(p23;q23), resulting in expression of ALK by immunohistochemistry.[1,6] Other reported partner genes include *EML4, GORASP2, NPM1, RANBP2, SEC31A,* and *SQSTM1* (Table 80.1).[1] The exact mechanisms of transformation are not fully elucidated, but

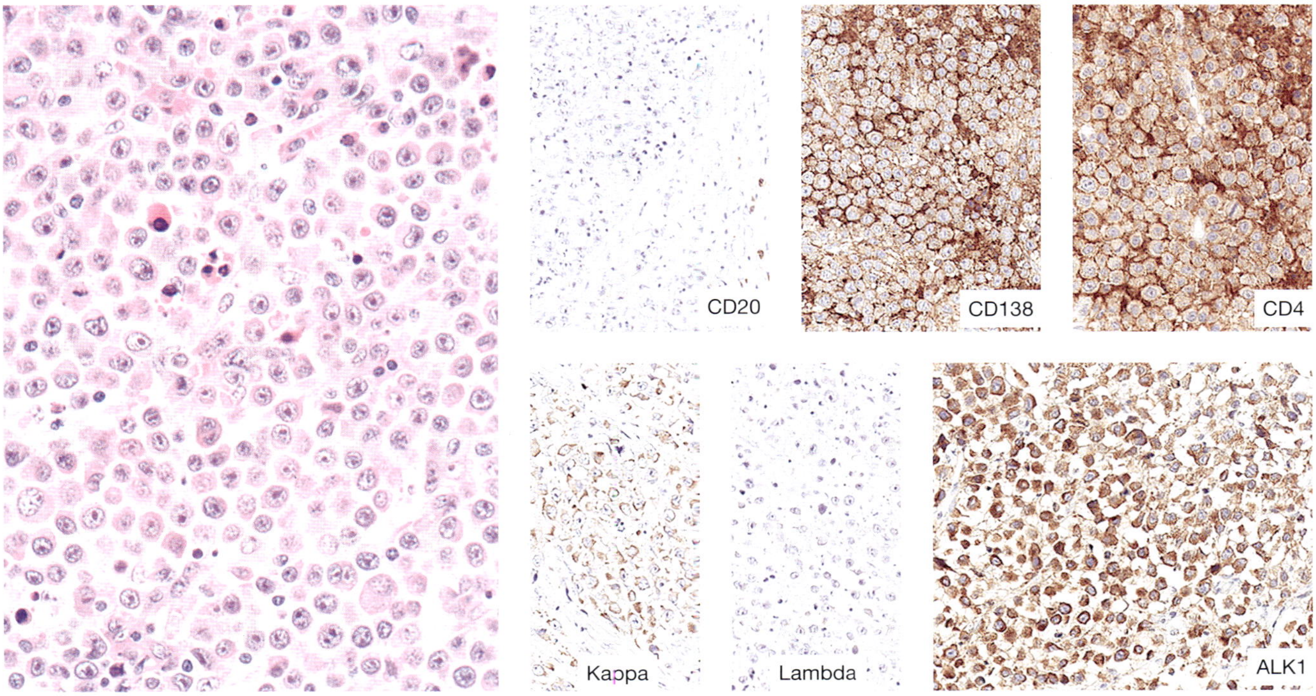

FIGURE 78.1 ALK-positive large B-cell lymphoma. The hematoxylin and eosin stain (left) shows a diffuse proliferation of immunoblasts with open, vesicular chromatin, prominent central nucleoli, and moderate to abundant amounts of pink cytoplasm. A rare binucleated cell is present. Immunophenotyping shows a plasmablastic phenotype with expression of CD138 and kappa but lacking CD20 and lambda. A characteristic granular cytoplasmic pattern of ALK staining is shown, which is associated with the common *CLTC::ALK* rearrangement. This case aberrantly expresses CD4.

TABLE 78.1 *ALK* rearrangements and ALK IHC pattern

Rearrangement	ALK IHC pattern
CLTC::ALK[a]	Granular cytoplasmic staining
NPM1::ALK	Nuclear and diffuse cytoplasmic staining
SQSTM1::ALK	Diffuse cytoplasmic with few fine granules
EML4::ALK	Diffuse cytoplasmic
SEC31A::ALK	Granular cytoplasmic staining
RANBP2::ALK	Nuclear membrane with perinuclear dot
GORASP2::ALK	Diffuse cytoplasmic with perinuclear accentuation
TFG::ALK	Diffuse cytoplasmic with few fine granules

IHC, immunohistochemistry.
[a]Most common.

activation of STAT3 and the PI3K, PLCγ, and RAS pathways may be important.[1]

Prognosis and Clinical Comment

ALK+ LBCL has a dismal prognosis with an overall survival of less than 12 months. Few patients achieve durable remissions following frontline chemotherapy. Treatment of these relapsed/refractory patients with salvage chemotherapy or crizotinib (an ALK inhibitor) was reported to induce short-term remissions in some patients, and only a rare long-term survivor has been reported in the literature.[7-9] A better understanding of the biology of this entity may lead to development of novel therapeutic approaches for these high-risk patients.

References

1. Castillo JJ, Beltran BE, Malpica L, Marques-Piubelli ML, Miranda RN. Anaplastic lymphoma kinase-positive large B-cell lymphoma (ALK + LBCL): a systematic review of clinicopathological features and management. *Leuk Lymphoma*. 2021;62(12):2845-2853. doi:10.1080/10428194.2021.1941929

2. Pan Z, Hu S, Li M, et al. ALK-positive large B-cell lymphoma: a clinicopathologic study of 26 cases with review of additional 108 cases in the literature. *Am J Surg Pathol.* 2017;41(1):25-38. doi:10.1097/PAS.0000000000000753
3. Stachurski D, Miron PM, Al-Homsi S, et al. Anaplastic lymphoma kinase-positive diffuse large B-cell lymphoma with a complex karyotype and cryptic 3' ALK gene insertion to chromosome 4 q22-24. *Hum Pathol.* 2007;38(6):940-945. doi:10.1016/j.humpath.2006.12.019
4. Momose S, Tamaru J, Kishi H, et al. Hyperactivated STAT3 in ALK-positive diffuse large B-cell lymphoma with clathrin-ALK fusion. *Hum Pathol.* 2009;40(1):75-82.
5. Petronilho S, Gournay V, Tauziede-Espariat A, et al. ALK+ large B cell lymphoma presenting as multiple bowel-obstructing, cytokeratin-positive tumours. *Histopathology.* 2022;80(7):1128-1130. doi:10.1111/his.14635
6. De Paepe P, Baens M, van Krieken H, et al. ALK activation by the CLTC-ALK fusion is a recurrent event in large B-cell lymphoma. *Blood.* 2003;102(7):2638-2641. doi:10.1182/blood-2003-04-1050
7. Li J, Ouyang J, Zhou R, Chen B, Xu Y. Promising response of anaplastic lymphoma kinase-positive large B-cell lymphoma to crizotinib salvage treatment: case report and review of literature. *Int J Clin Exp Med.* 2015;8(5):6977-6985.
8. Soumerai JD, Rosenthal A, Harkins S, et al. Next-generation ALK inhibitors are highly active in ALK-positive large B-cell lymphoma. *Blood.* 2022;140(16):1822-1826. doi:10.1182/blood.2022015443
9. Takiar R, Phillips TJ. Durable responses with ALK inhibitors for primary refractory anaplastic lymphoma kinase-positive large B cell lymphoma. *Blood Adv.* 2023;7(12):2912-2916. doi:10.1182/bloodadvances.2022007537

Chapter 79
Plasmablastic Lymphoma

Camille Laurent, Stefan Dirnhofer, and George Lenz

Definition

Plasmablastic lymphoma (PBL) is an aggressive subtype of large B-cell lymphoma with a predominant morphology of immunoblasts or plasmablasts that have a plasmacytic phenotype. PBL was first described in the oral cavity/jaw of HIV-positive patients[1] but may occur in other sites, mostly extranodal, and in association with other immunodeficiency states and/or in advanced age.

Synonyms

None.

Epidemiology

PBL is rare in immunocompetent settings but accounts for 2% of HIV-related lymphomas. Patients are typically adults with a male predominance (~4:1). Median age at diagnosis is 42 years in HIV-positive patients and ~55 years in HIV-negative patients. In addition to occurring in patients with HIV infection, PBL may also occur in patients with iatrogenic immunosuppression (posttransplantation, autoimmune disease). Some cases arise in HIV-negative patients without an apparent cause of immunodeficiency, which is presumed to be due to age-related immune senescence. Of note, rare cases of PBL transformation from low-grade B cell lymphoma (chronic lymphocytic leukemia/small lymphocytic lymphoma and follicular lymphoma) have been reported.

General Clinical Features

PBL typically presents as a mass in one or more extranodal sites. It usually involves the oral cavity/jaw, especially in HIV-positive patients. Other sites are gastrointestinal tract, skin, lymph node, soft tissue, bone, and lung. Nodal involvement is more frequent in HIV-negative PBL. Disseminated stages III/IV (including bone marrow involvement) with B symptoms are present at diagnosis in 75% of HIV-positive patients and 50% of posttransplant disease but only in 25% of patients without apparent immunodeficiency.[2]

Morphology

PBL is composed of diffuse and cohesive large cells resembling immunoblasts to plasmablastic cells (Figure 79.1A and B). Immunoblasts are large cells with an abundant cytoplasm and vesicular chromatin containing prominent nucleoli (Figure 79.1A). Large plasmablastic cells have basophilic cytoplasm, paranuclear hof, and eccentric large nuclei (Figure 79.1B). A "starry-sky" pattern with tingible body macrophages is common, and necrosis is seen in over half of cases. These last two features may be useful in distinguishing PBL from plasmacytomas.[3]

Immunophenotype

Neoplastic cells show a plasma cell–like immunophenotype, positive for CD38, CD138, IRF4/MUM1, BLIMP1, and XBP1 (Figure 79.2A and B). Cytoplasmic immunoglobulin is commonly expressed, most frequently IgG, and light chain expression (either kappa or lambda) occurs in ~50% of cases (Figure 79.2C).[2-4] Variable expression of CD30, EMA, CD79a, and CD56 is reported. PBL cells are usually negative for CD19, CD20, and PAX5; however, they may be weakly positive. Rare cases can express T-cell markers, including CD3, causing diagnostic confusion. MYC is expressed in 50% of cases correlated to *MYC* translocation/amplification as well as constitutive activation of STAT3.[4] BCL2 and BCL6 are usually negative, whereas CD10 is expressed in 20% of cases. Ki67 proliferation index is typically 75% to 100%. In situ hybridization for EBER is positive in 50% to 70% of cases (Figure 79.2D), most frequently in HIV-positive and posttransplant patients. LMP1 and EBNA2 are typically negative (Latency 0/1 pattern). PD-L1 is expressed in most cases. ALK, Cyclin D1, and HHV8 are negative. Up to 15% of PBL can show cytokeratin expression, which may represent a pitfall in the routine diagnostic setting.[5]

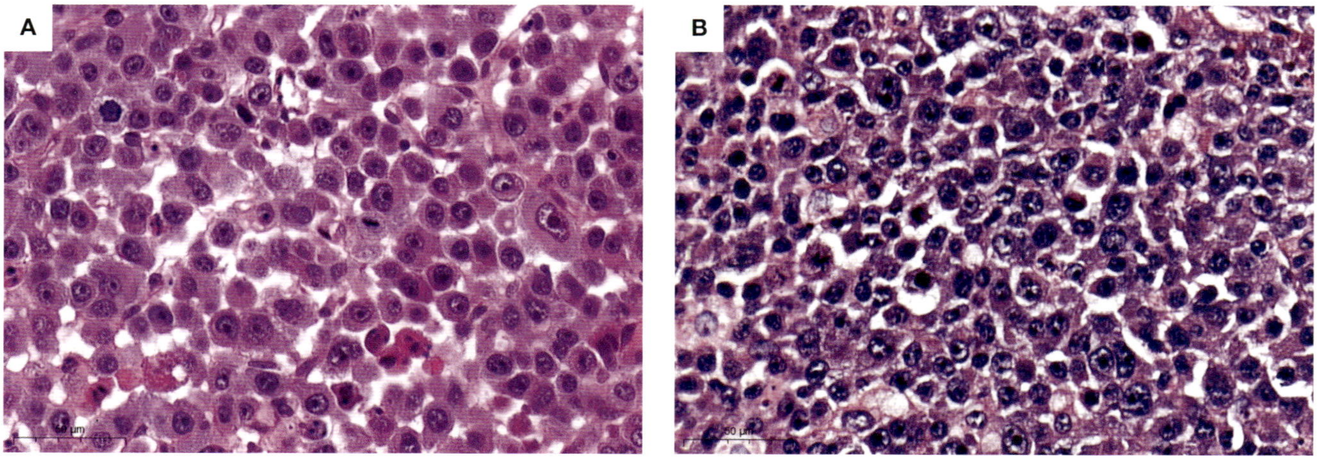

FIGURE 79.1 Plasmablastic lymphoma (PBL). **A:** PBL case showing a proliferation of large immunoblastic cells with prominent nucleoli. **B:** PBL case with monomorphic plasmablastic cytology.

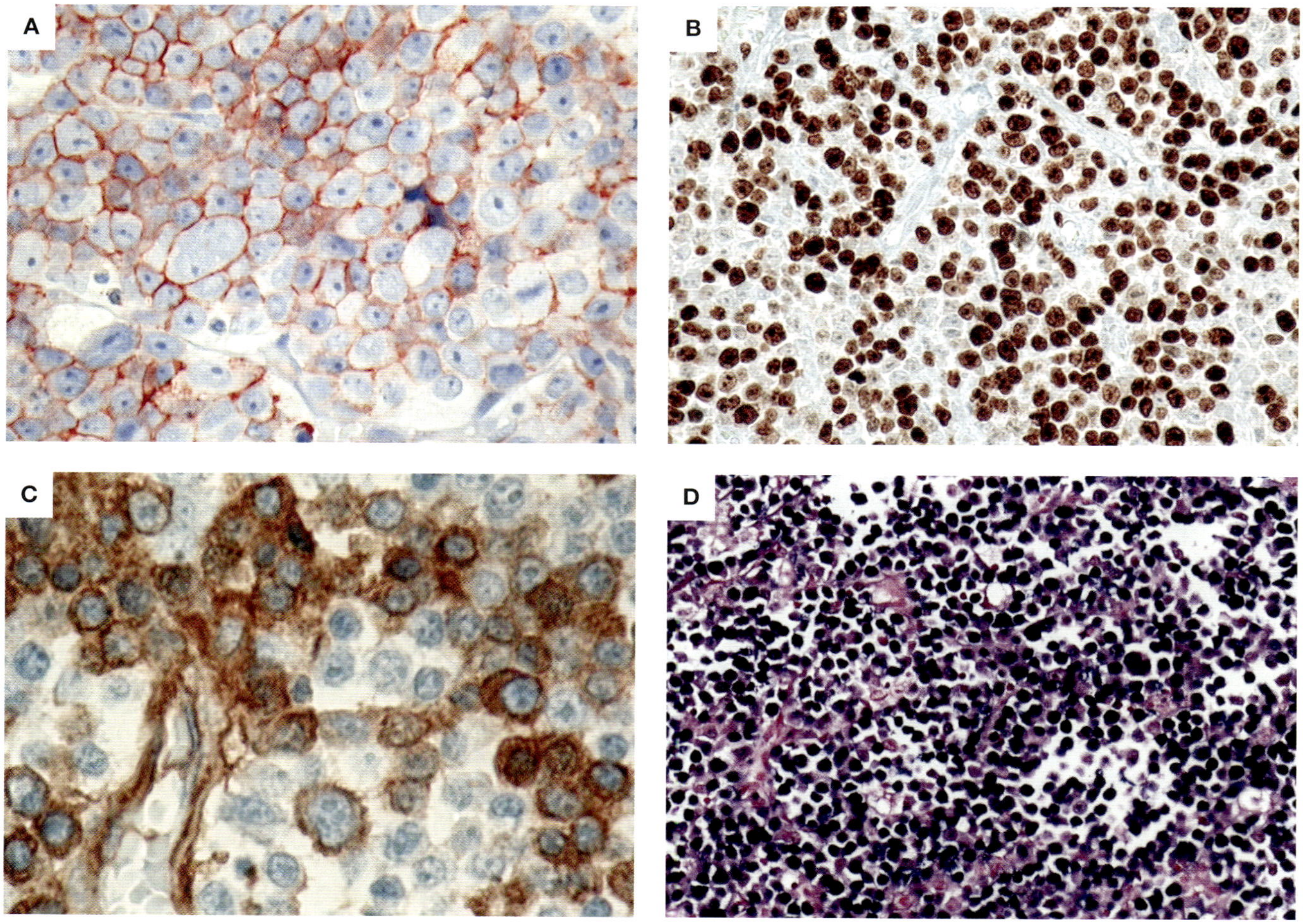

FIGURE 79.2 Plasmablastic lymphoma (PBL) phenotype. Tumor cells are positive for CD138 **(A)**, MUM1 **(B)**, with some expressing cytoplasmic IgG **(C)**. PBL cells are positive for EBV-encoded small RNA (EBER) **(D)**.

Genetics

PBL shows a complex karyotype. *MYC* (8q24) rearrangement (*MYC*-R) (often involving the IGH gene [14q32]) is frequently detected, especially in EBV-positive/HIV-positive cases (>70%) as compared with EBV-negative or HIV-negative cases (40%-50%). Recurrent mutations affecting JAK-STAT, ERK-MAPK, and NOTCH signaling are commonly observed.[6,7] Among them, *STAT3* and *NRAS* are the most frequently mutated genes. Additional mutations in epigenetic modifiers such as *TET2* and *EP300*, *CARD11*, and *MYC* and *TP53* have been also described. EBV-positive PBL, especially in HIV-positive patients, shows high frequency of mutations in *STAT3*, whereas *TP53*, *CARD11*, and *MYC* mutations are more frequent in EBV-negative PBL cases.[6,7]

Prognosis and Clinical Comment

The prognosis is poor with 75% of patients dying of the disease at a median interval time of 6 to 7 months. EBV positivity is associated with better survival,[8] whereas *MYC*-R may be associated with poor prognosis.[4,9] The optimal treatment of PBL has not yet been established due to the rarity of the disease. By default, most experts use EPOCH to treat PBL.[10]

References

1. Delecluse HJ, Anagnostopoulos I, Dallenbach F, et al. Plasmablastic lymphomas of the oral cavity: a new entity associated with the human immunodeficiency virus infection. *Blood*. 1997;89(4):1413-1420.
2. Castillo JJ, Bibas M, Miranda RN. The biology and treatment of plasmablastic lymphoma. *Blood*. 2015;125(15):2323-2330.
3. Zhou T, Cheng J, Karrs J, et al. Clinicopathologic and molecular characterization of Epstein-Barr virus-positive plasmacytoma. *Am J Surg Pathol*. 2022;46(10):1364-1379.
4. Bailly J, Jenkins N, Chetty D, Mohamed Z, Verburgh ER, Opie JJ. Plasmablastic lymphoma: an update. *Int J Lab Hematol*. 2022;44(suppl 1):54-63.
5. Huettl KS, Staiger AM, Horn H, et al. Cytokeratin expression in plasmablastic lymphoma—a possible diagnostic pitfall in the routine work-up of tumours. *Histopathology*. 2021;78(6):831-837.
6. Ramis-Zaldivar JE, Gonzalez-Farre B, Nicolae A, et al. MAPK and JAK-STAT pathways dysregulation in plasmablastic lymphoma. *Haematologica*. 2021;106(10):2682-2693.
7. Frontzek F, Staiger AM, Zapukhlyak M, et al. Molecular and functional profiling identifies therapeutically targetable vulnerabilities in plasmablastic lymphoma. *Nat Commun*. 2021;12(1):5183.
8. Laurent C, Fabiani B, Do C, et al. Immune-checkpoint expression in Epstein-Barr virus positive and negative plasmablastic lymphoma: a clinical and pathological study in 82 patients. *Haematologica*. 2016;101(8):976-984.
9. Valera A, Balagué O, Colomo L, et al. IG/MYC rearrangements are the main cytogenetic alteration in plasmablastic lymphomas. *Am J Surg Pathol*. 2010;34(11):1686-1694.
10. Horwitz SM, Zelenetz AD, Gordon LI, et al. NCCN guidelines insights: non-Hodgkin's lymphomas, version 3.2016. *J Natl Compr Canc Netw*. 2016;14(9):1067-1079.

Chapter 80

Human Herpesvirus 8–Associated Lymphoproliferative Disorders

Miguel A. Piris, Elias Campo, and Antonino Carbone

Human herpesvirus 8 (HHV8), also known as Kaposi sarcoma (KS) herpesvirus (KSHV), in addition to being the causative agent of KS, is a lymphotropic virus that is involved in the pathogenesis of a family of lymphoproliferative disorders (LPDs), including highly aggressive tumors as well as indolent conditions. HHV8 infection often co-occurs with human immunodeficiency virus (HIV) and Epstein-Barr virus (EBV), thus partially explaining this diversity of conditions. Most HHV8-related LPDs affect immunosuppressed patients, with the exception of germinotropic lymphoproliferative disorder (GLPD). This chapter will discuss the HHV8-related LPDS including HHV8-positive multicentric Castleman disease (CD) (HHV8+ MCD), HHV8+ GLPD, HHV8+ diffuse large B-cell lymphoma, not otherwise specified (NOS) (HHV8+ DLBCL), and primary effusion lymphoma (PEL) (Table 80.1).

TABLE 80.1 Lymphoproliferative diseases associated with HHV8

Disease	Clinical context	HHV8/LANA-1	HIV	EBV	Ig clonality	Other genetic events
GLPD	Immunocompetent patients Indolent disorder	+	-	+ (>90%)	Polyclonal or oligoclonal, despite the frequent light-chain restriction	Plasmablasts show somatic mutation and intraclonal variation in the rearranged Ig genes
PEL/EC-PEL	Immunodeficient patients or living in HHV8-endemic regions	+	+ (>90%)	+ (90%)	Immunoglobulin heavy chain (IGH) gene is clonally rearranged and hypermutated, with a subset also having clonal T-cell receptor gene rearrangement	Karyotype is often complex, lacking *MYC* rearrangements.Mutations in *BCL6*, *MYC*, *PAX5*, and *RHOH/TTF* have been described. APOBEC3 family members are involved in PEL pathogenesis.
HHV8+ MCD	Immunodeficient patients or living in HHV8-endemic regions	+	+ (>90%)	-	Plasmablasts in HHV8+ MCD are polyclonal or oligoclonal B cells with unmutated Ig genes, despite being lambda restricted	
HHV8+ DLBCL	Often associated with HHV8+ MCD	+	+ (>90%)	-	Monoclonal B cells that do not contain somatic hypermutations, consistent with a naïve B-cell derivation	

HHV8-induced lymphoid transformation in most cases leads to a plasmablastic phenotype, where B cells lose B cell–specific markers (PAX5, CD19, CD20, CD79a) and display terminal B-cell differentiation antigens (CD138, MUM1, BLIMP1, XBP1, cytoplasmatic immunoglobulins). Occasionally these B cells may also acquire some T- or NK-cell markers.

Cell transformation by HHV8 is caused by the action of different viral oncogenes and microRNAs, including viral analogues for human interleukin 6 (IL-6), together with other HHV8-encoded genes (latency-associated nuclear antigen [LANA-1], viral interferon regulatory factor 3 [vIRF3], viral cyclin [vCYC], viral FLICE-inhibitory protein [vFLIP], v-GPCR, v-CCL, v-MIP, v-IRF, kaposin proteins, etc.) that induce apoptosis inhibition, cell proliferation, angiogenesis, inflammation, and immune escape.[1]

In the definition of these disorders, the scientific community has used a combination of clinical, histologic, and molecular data, which has helped identify the distinct HHV8-related LPDs and has begun to reveal potential therapeutic targets. Nevertheless, some HHV8-associated LPDs may not precisely fulfill the criteria for these previously recognized entities, thus highlighting our continuously expanding knowledge on the clinical and pathological spectrum of HHV8-related lymphoid proliferations.[2] Cases with overlapping features of the entities discussed later have also been described, for instance, for HHV8-positive large B-cell lymphoma (LBCL) and extracavitary primary effusion lymphoma (EC-PEL) and also for EC-PEL and GLPD.[3-5] The specific HHV8-associated disease entities currently recognized by the International Consensus Classification (ICC) are each discussed in the following pages.

HHV8-POSITIVE MULTICENTRIC CASTLEMAN DISEASE

Definition

HHV8+ MCD is a systemic LPD, associated with HHV8 infection, characterized by multifocal lymphadenopathy and hypercytokinemia. Although largely associated with HIV infection, it can also be seen in the setting of other types of immune compromise.[6]

Pathologically, CD is divided into two subtypes: plasma cell and hyaline vascular (HV), although cases with overlapping features occur. Clinically CD may be unicentric (UCD) or multicentric (MCD). Most cases of MCD are associated with plasma cell variant histology, and most cases of UCD are associated with HV CD, although variation can occur.

HHV8+ MCD has distinct features from both UCD and idiopathic, HHV8-negative, MCD (iMCD), although both HHV8+ MCD and iMCD share a common pathogenic role for either cellular or viral IL-6. As a nonneoplastic entity, iMCD is not otherwise discussed in the ICC and so will be briefly reviewed here for context. iMCD includes cases of MCD that occur in people who are not infected with KSHV/HHV8 or HIV. Although the precise etiology is still unknown, iMCD involves polyclonal lymphoproliferation and hypercytokinemia driven by autoimmune or paraneoplastic mechanisms. iMCD may be associated with an increasingly broad spectrum of clinical syndromes, including the most well-documented TAFRO syndrome, in which patients present with Thrombocytopenia, Ascites, Fever, Reticulin fibrosis, and Organomegaly.

iMCD lacks pathognomonic histologic features, and the diagnosis is made by the integration of clinical, imaging, and pathologic features. Clinical history and staining for HHV8 LANA-1 are essential for distinction from HHV8+ MCD. Histologic features are nonspecific. In iMCD, the common lymph node histologic features are those described in the plasma cell variant of CD and include sheets of plasma cells present in the interfollicular zones along with follicular hyperplasia. Hyaline vascular features seen more commonly in UCD are variable and may be absent entirely.[7] These features are similar to what is seen in HHV8+ MCD (described later), except without HHV8+ plasmablasts.

Synonyms

None.

Epidemiology

HHV8+ MCD is typically seen in the setting of HIV infection and frequently coexists with other HHV8-induced disorders such as KS and PEL.[6,8,9] It can also be found in immunocompetent patients in HHV8-endemic areas (East and Central Africa and Mediterranean countries).

General Clinical Features

Patients with HHV8+ MCD present with florid clinical symptoms related to hypercytokinemia, multifocal lymphadenopathy, and splenomegaly.[8] Common constitutional symptoms include fever, night sweats, fatigue, weight loss, rash, and respiratory compromise. Anemia and thrombocytopenia are common, as are hypoalbuminemia and polyclonal hypergammaglobulinemia.

Morphology

Involved lymph nodes show the pathology described as the plasma cell variant of CD with reactive follicular hyperplasia, interfollicular plasmacytosis, and the presence of scattered HHV8-positive plasmablasts and plasmacytoid cells distributed in a perifollicular concentric pattern, occupying the outer mantle zone or the marginal zone (Figure 80.1).[1]

Reactive secondary follicles show variably sized germinal centers, some with hyperplastic appearance and some with variable degrees of germinal center regression and hyalinization. Mantle zones may be prominent with variable "concentric ring" appearance more typical of HVCD. Interfollicular vascular proliferation with variable degrees of hyalinization can be seen but is typically not as prominent as in HVCD and is not required for the diagnosis. Sheets of mature plasma cells occupy the interfollicular areas. Singly scattered or small clusters of large

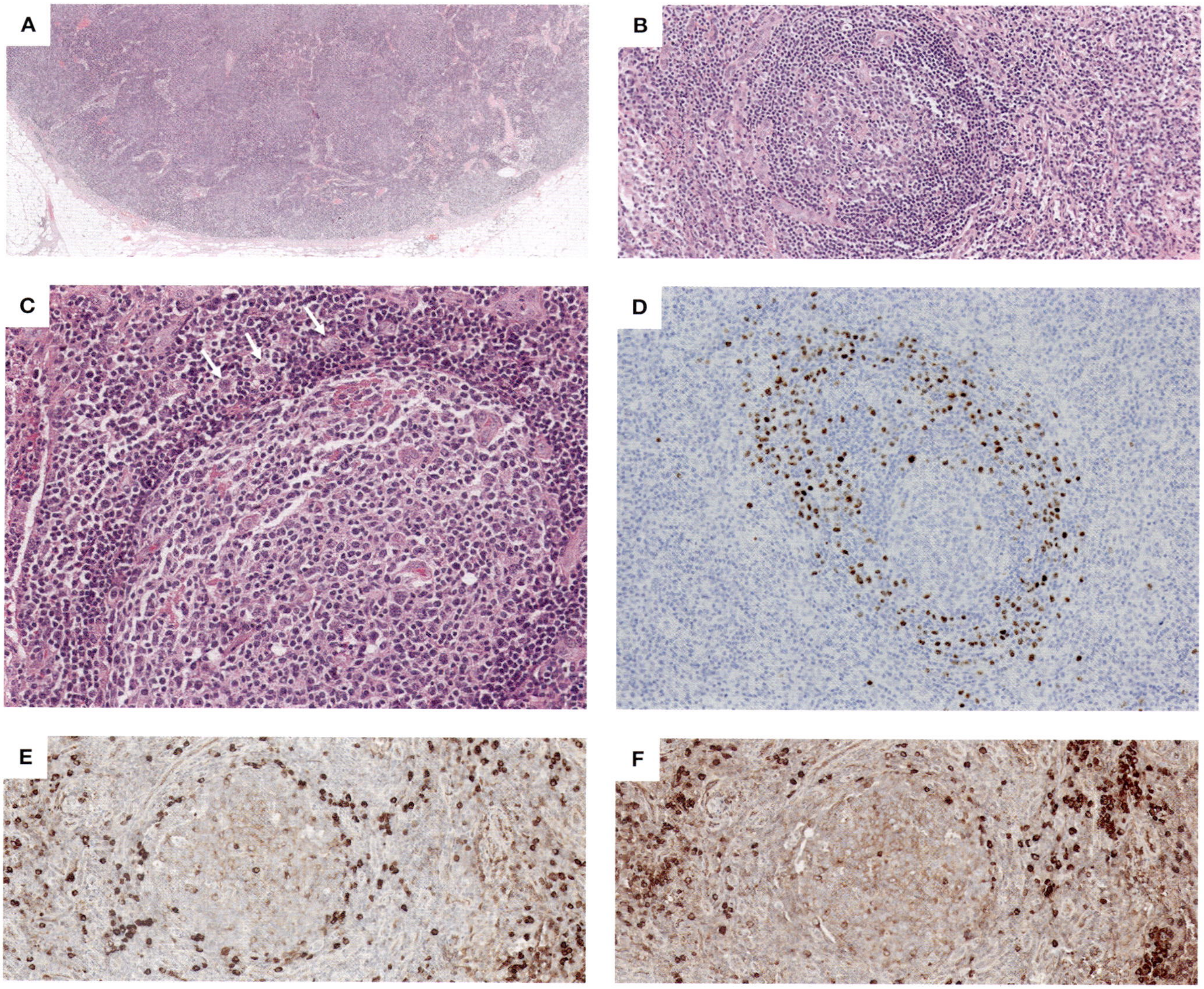

FIGURE 80.1 HHV8-associated multicentric Castleman disease (HHV8+MCD). **A:** At low power the lymph node shows increased numbers of small lymphoid follicles and interfollicular expansion. **B:** At higher power a lymphoid follicle shows regressed germinal center with a prominent mantle zone surrounded by several hyalinized vessels. **C:** Plasmablasts (arrows) surround a hyperplastic germinal center. **D:** In the follicular mantle several large atypical cells, consistent with plasmablasts, are positive for KSHV/HHV8-encoded LANA-1/ORF73. **E:** These cells are lambda light chain positive and **(F)** kappa light chain negative while the interfollicular plasma cells are polytypic.

"plasmablasts" are found in the mantle zones or marginal zones. These plasmablasts are typically larger than the interfollicular mature plasma cells, with more amphophilic cytoplasm and distinct nucleoli. In some cases they may coalesce forming larger aggregates.[7] These clusters are polyclonal or oligoclonal, in contrast with the monoclonal nature of the LBCL that eventually may develop in these cases (Figure 80.1).[1] KS is a frequent finding in lymph nodes of HHV8+ MCD, occasionally only recognizable after HHV8 immunostaining.[2]

Immunophenotype

Perifollicular plasmablasts express HHV8 LANA-1, with most cases being negative for EBV (EBER). They additionally are positive for viral interleukin 6 (vIL-6) and cytoplasmic IgM and always show lambda restriction (Figure 80.1). Plasmablasts exhibit variable, often weak to negative, expression of B-cell markers such as CD20, CD79a, and PAX5 and lack expression of germinal center markers (CD10 and BCL6), but they are uniformly positive for MUM1/IRF4 and terminal B-cell markers such as BLIMP1 and XBP1, although CD138 is usually negative.[7] This phenotype contrasts with the more numerous interfollicular HHV8-negative plasma cells, which are CD138 positive, typically IgA positive, and usually polytypic for kappa and lambda light chains.

Follicular dendritic cells may show cytoplasmatic or surface expression of HHV8/LANA-1, presumably due to antigen trapping by the interconnected follicular dendritic cell meshwork.[2] Scattered EBER-positive B cells are also frequently observed in these lymph nodes (in keeping with the immune-compromised nature of the patients), although these are distinct from the HHV8-positive cells.

Genetics

Molecular studies have demonstrated that the plasmablasts in HHV8+ MCD are polyclonal or oligoclonal B cells with unmutated Ig genes despite being lambda restricted.

Prognosis and Clinical Comment

Properly treated cases have a 5-year overall survival of 90%. Coexistence of KS and PEL is associated with a much lower survival probability.[8] Treatment options include rituximab, antiviral agents, and liposomal doxorubicin, depending on the combination of disorders. The simultaneous occurrence of PEL may require combination cytotoxic chemotherapy.[9]

HHV8-POSITIVE GERMINOTROPIC LYMPHOPROLIFERATIVE DISORDER

Definition

HHV8-positive GLPD is a rare disorder that typically occurs in HIV-negative individuals, and is characterized by the intrafollicular presence of HHV8/EBV double-positive plasmablasts.[3,10]

Synonyms

None.

Epidemiology

HIV-negative patients, although exceptional cases have been described in patients with HIV,[2] with more frequent IGH monoclonal rearrangements.

General Clinical Features

This is a rare disease. Patients most often present with localized lymphadenopathy; HIV-positive patients may have atypical features such as generalized lymphadenopathy and B symptoms.[2]

Morphology

Preserved lymph node architecture with follicular hyperplasia is typical. Germinal centers are replaced/colonized by plasmablastic cells forming confluent aggregates (Figure 80.2).[10]

Immunophenotype

Plasmablastic cells are negative for CD20, CD79a, CD138, BCL6, and CD10 but may express MUM1/IRF4. In most cases they show monotypic kappa or lambda light chain. Clusters of $CD10^+$ $CD20^+$ residual germinal center B cells can be identified in some of the follicles. The plasmablasts are positive for both HHV8/LANA-1 and EBV (EBER) with latency I (negative for LMP1 and EBNA2), and most also express vIL-6 (Figure 80.2).[5] Some cases may coexpress CD3 or be EBV negative.

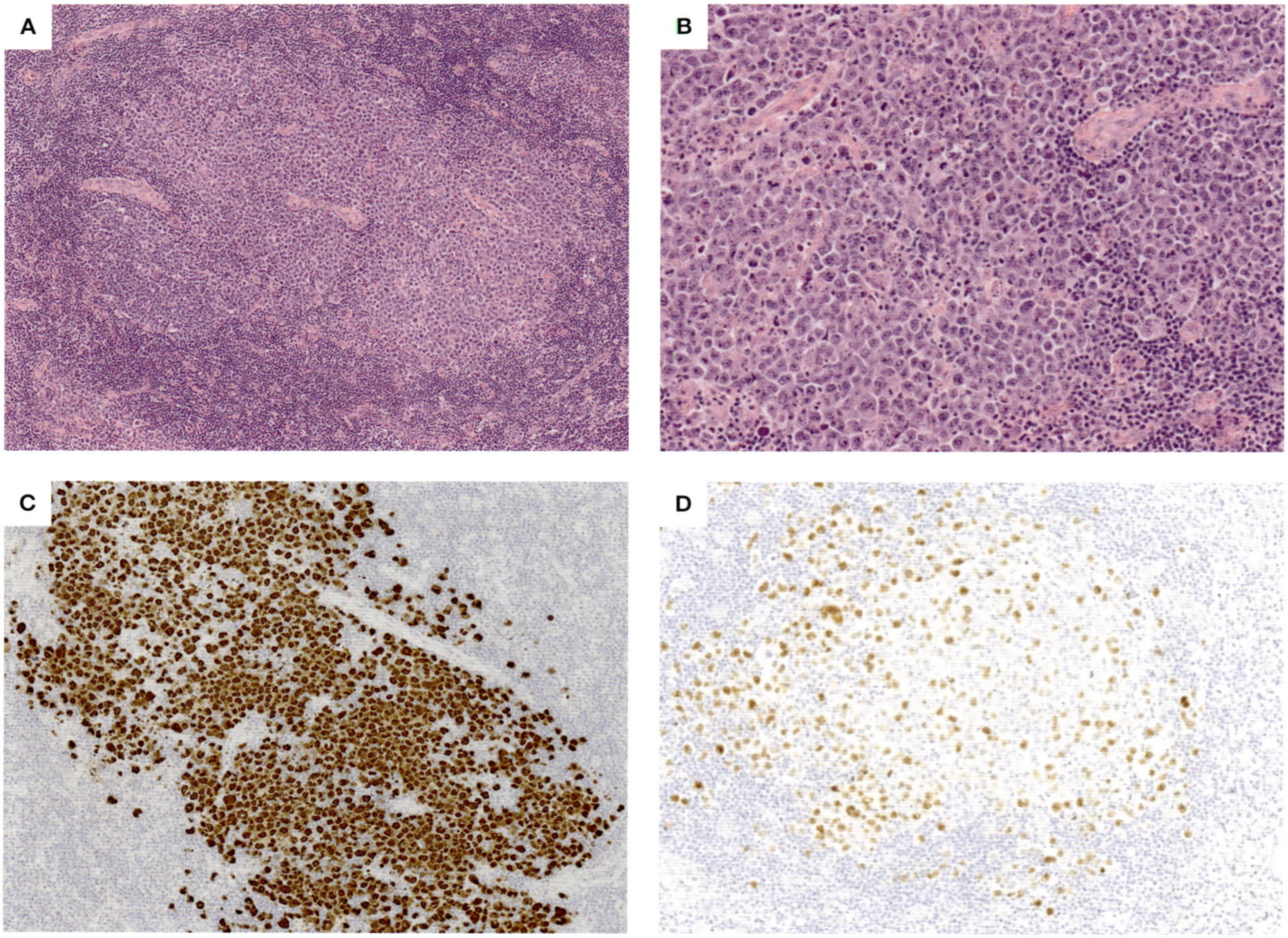

FIGURE 80.2 HHV8-positive germinotropic lymphoproliferative disorder. On low power **(A)** germinal centers of lymphoid follicles are replaced by large cells that at higher power **(B)** show a moderate amount of cytoplasm and a large vesicular nucleus containing one or 2 prominent nucleoli. **(C)** These cells are positive for both KSHV/HHV8 and **(D)** EBV/EBER.

Genetics

Molecular studies have shown GLPD to be polyclonal or oligoclonal, in spite of the frequent light-chain restriction.[5] Plasmablasts show somatic mutation and intraclonal variation in the rearranged Ig genes, suggesting that they originate from germinal center B cells.

Prognosis and Clinical Comment

This disease has an indolent clinical course, with favorable response to therapy.[5,11]

HHV8-POSITIVE DIFFUSE LARGE B-CELL LYMPHOMA, NOS

Definition

HHV8+ diffuse large B-cell lymphoma, NOS (HHV8+ DLBCL) is a LBCL with plasmablastic/anaplastic cytology that is positive for HHV8/LANA-1 and negative for EBV. It is usually associated with HHV8+ MCD, although some cases may be independent of MCD.[6] It is essential to exclude PEL and EC-PEL. HHV8+ DLBCL should be favored in EBV-negative cases with cytoplasmic IgM, lambda, and/or associated with MCD. Nevertheless, in occasional cases some overlapping features between HHV8+ DLBCL and EC-PEL may be seen.[4]

Synonyms

None.

Epidemiology

This is a rare disease. Similar to HHV8+ MCD, patients typically have HIV.

General Clinical Features

HHV8+ DLBCL typically presents as disease progression in patients with HHV8+ MCD. Patients have diffuse lymphadenopathy as well as massive splenomegaly. Lymphoma can involve extranodal organs such as liver, lung, and gastrointestinal tract as well as the bone marrow.

Morphology

Aggregates or sheets of large tumor cells are characteristic. Cells have plasmablastic cytology with eccentric nuclei, prominent nucleoli, and amphophilic cytoplasm.

Immunophenotype

HHV8/LANA-1 positivity is required for diagnosis, along with negativity for EBV. Tumor cells are vIL-6, MUM1/IRF4, and cytoplasmic IgM positive with lambda restriction. Some cases of HHV8+ DLBCL may show weak or focal expression of B-cell markers such as CD20 and/or CD79a and are usually CD138 negative. Aberrant T-cell antigen expression has been described.[1]

Genetics

HHV8+ DLBCL is composed of monoclonal B cells that do not contain somatic immunoglobulin gene hypermutations, consistent with a naïve B-cell derivation.

Prognosis and Clinical Comment

Outcome of patients with HHV8+ DLBCL is very poor, especially in persons with HIV/AIDS. Treatment strategy includes immune restoration, high-dose chemotherapy, and antivirals.[1]

PRIMARY EFFUSION LYMPHOMA

Definition

PEL is an effusion-based B-cell lymphoma with plasmablastic/anaplastic phenotype and morphology.[12] Presentation is typically effusion based, without a solid component (although EC-PEL is also included). By definition, PEL is always associated with HHV8, usually with coinfection by EBV.

Synonyms

None.

Epidemiology

PEL was initially described in the setting of HIV, but it can also be seen in other settings of immune suppression and in immune-competent elderly patients, especially from HHV8-endemic regions.[13] Median patient age is in the 5th decade, distinct from HHV8-negative, EBV-negative primary effusion-based lymphoma, which typically presents in elderly, immunocompetent individuals (see Chapter 72).

General Clinical Features

PEL classically occurs in pleural, peritoneal, and pericardial effusions, but it can occur in other cavities, including blood vessels and the subarachnoid space. EBV-negative cases more often occur in HIV-negative elderly men from HHV8-endemic regions.[4,13] EC-PEL is typically EBV+, helping to distinguish from HHV8+ DLBCL. EC-PEL is most common in HIV-positive males with a younger median age than typical PEL.

Morphology

PEL exhibits plasmablastic, immunoblastic, or anaplastic cytology in cytospin or cell block preparations (Figures 80.3 and 80.4) Nuclei are large, often with prominent nucleoli. Basophilic or amphophilic cytoplasm is typical, and cells may have a perinuclear hof. EC-PEL resembles plasmablastic lymphoma, ALK+ LBCL, and HHV8+ DLBCL and can be mistaken for other poorly differentiated, nonhematolymphoid tumors. Sinusoidal involvement of lymph nodes can mimic metastatic disease.

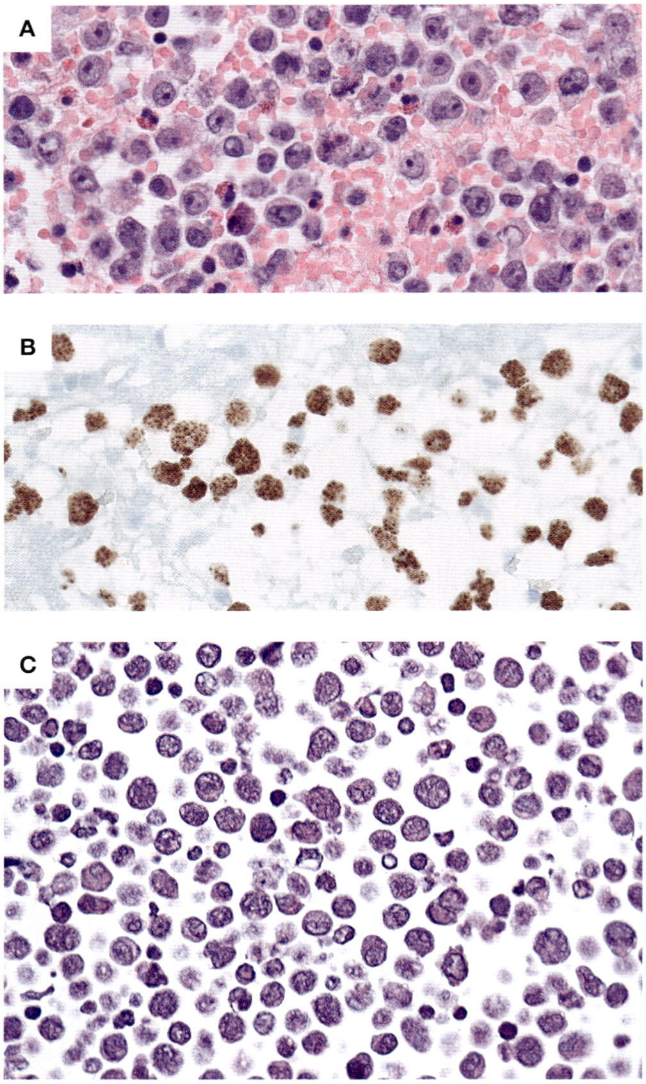

FIGURE 80.3 Primary effusion lymphoma (PEL). **(A).** Cell block of a pleural effusion containing large-sized tumor cells with immunoblastic/plasmablastic features. **(B)** By immunohistochemistry they are consistently positive for HHV8-encoded LANA-1. The staining pattern is "speckled" (punctuate nuclear). PEL tumor cells are often positive for EBV-encoded small RNAs (EBERs) (not shown). **(C)** Cytospin staining showing the plasmablastic/pleomorphic cytology.

Immunophenotype

Neoplastic cells are of B-cell lineage and express HHV8 (LANA-1) typically with coexpression of EBV (EBER) (Figures 80.3 and 80.4). They are often negative for pan-B-cell antigens such as PAX5, CD19, CD20, and CD79a and may be CD45 negative. Surface and cytoplasmic immunoglobulins are often negative. While they may express CD30, CD38, CD138, EMA, MUM1, XBP1, BLIMP1, and HLA-DR, a null cell phenotype with loss of lineage-defining markers is not uncommon.[12] Aberrant expression of T/NK-cell markers (CD3, CD4, CD56) has been described, more frequently in EC-PEL, making distinction from T-cell lymphoma a challenge. Identification of HHV8 and EBV coexpression is key for avoiding misdiagnosis.

Genetics

Immunoglobulin heavy chain (IGH) gene is clonally rearranged and hypermutated, with a subset also having clonal T-cell receptor gene rearrangement.

No specific chromosomal abnormalities have been described[14]; however, the karyotype is often complex and notably lacking *MYC* rearrangements. Mutations in *BCL6*, *MYC*, *PAX5*, and *RHOH/TTF* have been described.[1]

Mutational studies performed in a panel of PEL cell lines have shown that APOBEC3 family members are involved in the pathogenesis of PEL, in contrast with other aggressive B-cell lymphoma cell lines.[15]

Prognosis and Clinical Comment

PEL is an aggressive lymphoma with a poor prognosis. Reported median overall survival has ranged from 6 to 42.5 months, with antiretroviral therapy being an important component in achieving better survival rates.

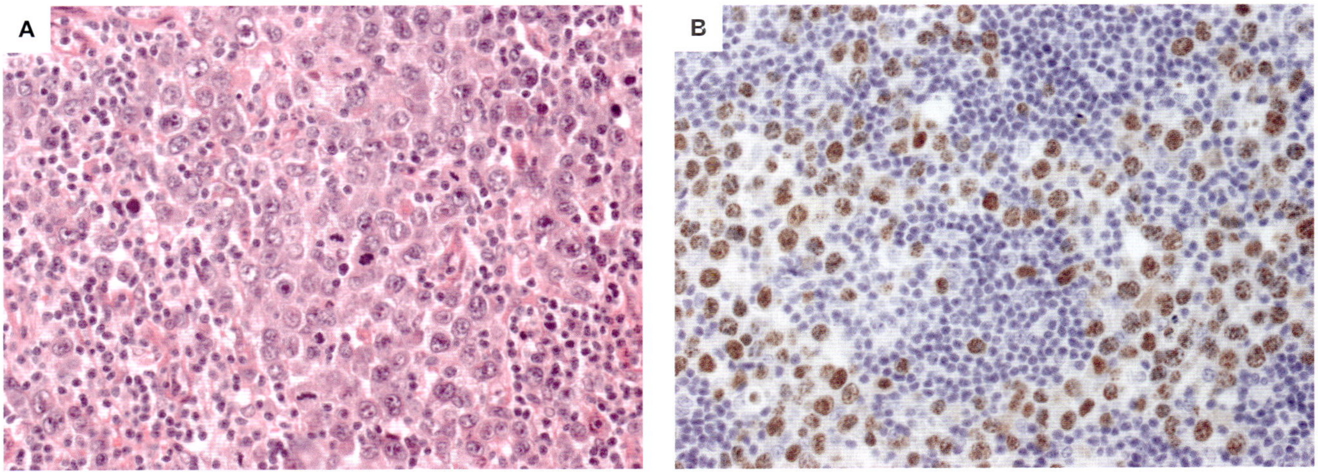

FIGURE 80.4 Extracavitary primary effusion lymphoma (EC-PEL). **(A)** Lymph node showing infiltration by large plasmablastic/immunoblastic cells with abundant amphophilic cytoplasm, eccentric round large nuclei, and prominent single macronucleoli. **(B)** Tumor cells are positive for HHV8-encoded LANA-1; the staining pattern is characteristically punctuate nuclear. HHV8 immunostaining highlights the sinus involvement by the lymphoid tumor cells.

References

1. Cesarman E, Chadburn A, Rubinstein PG. KSHV/HHV8-mediated hematologic diseases. *Blood*. 2022;139(7):1013-1025.
2. Gonzalez-Farre B, Martinez D, Lopez-Guerra M, et al. HHV8-related lymphoid proliferations: a broad spectrum of lesions from reactive lymphoid hyperplasia to overt lymphoma. *Mod Pathol*. 2017;30(5):745-760.
3. Chadburn A, Said J, Gratzinger D, et al. HHV8/KSHV-Positive lymphoproliferative disorders and the spectrum of plasmablastic and plasma cell neoplasms: 2015 SH/EAHP workshop report-Part 3. *Am J Clin Pathol*. 2017;147(2):171-187.
4. Dotlic S, Gibson SE, Hartmann S, et al. Lymphomas with plasmablastic features: a report of the lymphoma workshop of the 20th meeting of the European Association for Haematopathology. *Virchows Arch*. 2023;483(5):591-609. doi:10.1007/s00428-023-03585-8
5. Di Napoli A, Soma L, Quintanilla-Martinez L, et al. Cavity-based lymphomas: challenges and novel concepts. *Virchows Arch*. 2023;483:299-316. doi:10.1007/s00428-023-03599-2
6. Oksenhendler E, Boulanger E, Galicier L, et al. High incidence of Kaposi sarcoma-associated herpesvirus-related non-Hodgkin lymphoma in patients with HIV infection and multicentric Castleman disease. *Blood*. 2002;99(7):2331-2336.
7. Carbone A, Borok M, Damania B, et al. Castleman disease. *Nat Rev Dis Primers*. 2021;7(1):84.
8. Ramaswami R, Lurain K, Polizzotto MN, et al. Characteristics and outcomes of KSHV-associated multicentric Castleman disease with or without other KSHV diseases. *Blood Adv*. 2021;5(6):1660-1670.
9. Lurain K, Polizzotto MN, Aleman K, et al. Viral, immunologic, and clinical features of primary effusion lymphoma. *Blood*. 2019;133(16):1753-1761.
10. Du MQ, Diss TC, Liu H, et al. KSHV- and EBV-associated germinotropic lymphoproliferative disorder. *Blood*. 2002;100(9):3415-3418.
11. Zanelli M, Zizzo M, Bisagni A, et al. Germinotropic lymphoproliferative disorder: a systematic review. *Ann Hematol*. 2020;99(10):2243-2253.
12. Hu Z, Pan Z, Chen W, et al. Primary effusion lymphoma: a clinicopathological study of 70 cases. *Cancers*. 2021;13(4):878.
13. Zanelli M, Sanguedolce F, Zizzo M, et al. Primary effusion lymphoma occurring in the setting of transplanted patients: a systematic review of a rare, life-threatening post-transplantation occurrence. *BMC Cancer*. 2021;21(1):468.
14. Wilson KS, McKenna RW, Kroft SH, Dawson DB, Ansari Q, Schneider NR. Primary effusion lymphomas exhibit complex and recurrent cytogenetic abnormalities. *Br J Haematol*. 2002;116(1):113-121.
15. Wagener R, Alexandrov LB, Montesinos-Rongen M, et al. Analysis of mutational signatures in exomes from B-cell lymphoma cell lines suggest APOBEC3 family members to be involved in the pathogenesis of primary effusion lymphoma. *Leukemia*. 2015;29(7):1612-1615.

Chapter 81
Burkitt Lymphoma

Eric D. Hsi, Jonathan W. Friedberg, Michael Link, and Anamarija M. Perry

Definition

Burkitt lymphoma (BL) is a high-grade, aggressive, mature B-cell lymphoma (BCL) characterized by monotonous medium-sized cells, high proliferative index, germinal center B-cell phenotype, and *MYC* rearrangement (*MYC*-R) to an immunoglobulin (IG) gene (IG::*MYC*).

Synonyms

None.

Epidemiology

BL manifests in three clinicopathologic variants: endemic (eBL), sporadic (sBL), and immunodeficiency-associated (iBL) (Table 81.1). eBL occurs in equatorial Africa and Papua New Guinea correlating with the distribution of *Plasmodium falciparum* (PF) infection.[1,2] Patients with eBL are young with a median age of 6 to 9 years. In eBL, children have increased incidence of mixed PF infection, as indicated by genetic diversity of the *Pfsera5* gene. Chronic PF infection stimulates activation-induced cytidine deaminase (AICDA) activity, resulting in increased opportunity for DNA damage and chromosomal translocations.[3-5] sBL and iBL have a worldwide distribution. sBL has onset ages distributed across peaks at 10, 40, and 70 years, with a male predominance (2-3:1).[6,7] iBL has a median age of 40 to 45 years with equal sex distribution. Notably, the use of highly active antiretroviral therapy (HAART) has not decreased the risk of iBL. Epstein-Barr virus (EBV) is present in over 90% of eBL, 20% to 30% of sBL, and 25% to 40% of iBL. Recent data suggest EBV status associates better with distinct molecular subtypes than traditional clinicopathologic/geographic classification.[2,8]

General Clinical Features

In eBL, extranodal presentations are frequent (32%) including abdominal sites and less commonly jaw and orbit. The central nervous system (CNS) is involved in less than 10% of cases. sBL frequently involves the abdomen (Figure 81.1) or head/neck, whereas iBL is more often nodal. In a combined series of over 600 cases of BL (sBL and iBL), most patients (78%) had advanced-stage disease (Ann Arbor stage III or IV), 47% had B symptoms, and 43% had involvement of more than one extranodal site. Bone marrow (BM) involvement

TABLE 81.1 Epidemiologic and clinical features of three recognized variants of Burkitt lymphoma (BL)

	Endemic BL	Sporadic BL	Immunodeficiency-associated BL
Incidence	50% of childhood lymphomas in endemic areas	30%-50% of childhood lymphomas 2% of adult lymphomas	40% of HIV-associated lymphomas
Geographic distribution	Equatorial Africa and Papua New Guinea (areas endemic for *Plasmodium falciparum*)	Worldwide	Worldwide
Association with EBV	>90% of cases	20%-30% of cases	25%-40% of cases
Age of diagnosis and male-to-female ratio	Median 6-9 y M:F = 2-3:1	Peaks at 10, 40, and 70 y M:F = 2-3:1	Median 40-45 y M:F = 1:1
Sites of involvement	Abdomen, jaw and orbit (less common now), ovaries, breasts, kidneys, and adrenal glands CNS, <10% BM, occasional	Abdominal masses with frequent ileocecal involvement, head and neck, ovaries, breasts (rarely bilateral in pregnant or lactating women), kidneys CNS, 15% BM, 20%-30%	Lymph nodes (nodal presentation most frequent in this variant), gastrointestinal tract, and frequently bone marrow CNS, 30%

BM, bone marrow; CNS, central nervous system; EBV, Epstein-Barr virus; HIV, human immunodeficiency virus.

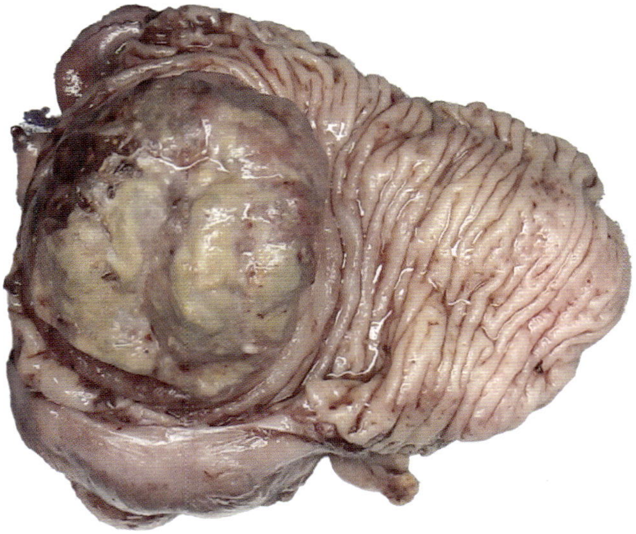

FIGURE 81.1 Sporadic Burkitt lymphoma involving the ileocecal valve, presenting as fungating mass.

was reported in up to 35% of patients. Compared with sBL, patients with iBL were more likely to have CNS involvement (30% vs 16%), poor performance status (32% vs 22%), more than two extranodal sites (59% vs 40%), and stage IV disease (89% vs 69%).

Morphology

BL obliterates the normal tissue architecture with diffuse, monotonous sheets of medium-sized lymphocytes with round nuclear contours, open chromatin, multiple small paracentric nucleoli, and scant cytoplasm. Nuclei are similar in size to that of histiocytes, and cytoplasm is scant to moderate. Rare cases with a nodular pattern have been reported, but true follicle formation with follicular dendritic cell networks is absent. Necrosis is common. Numerous mitotic figures and tingible body macrophages are seen; the latter impart a characteristic but nonspecific moth eaten or "starry sky" pattern (Figure 81.2A and B). Background

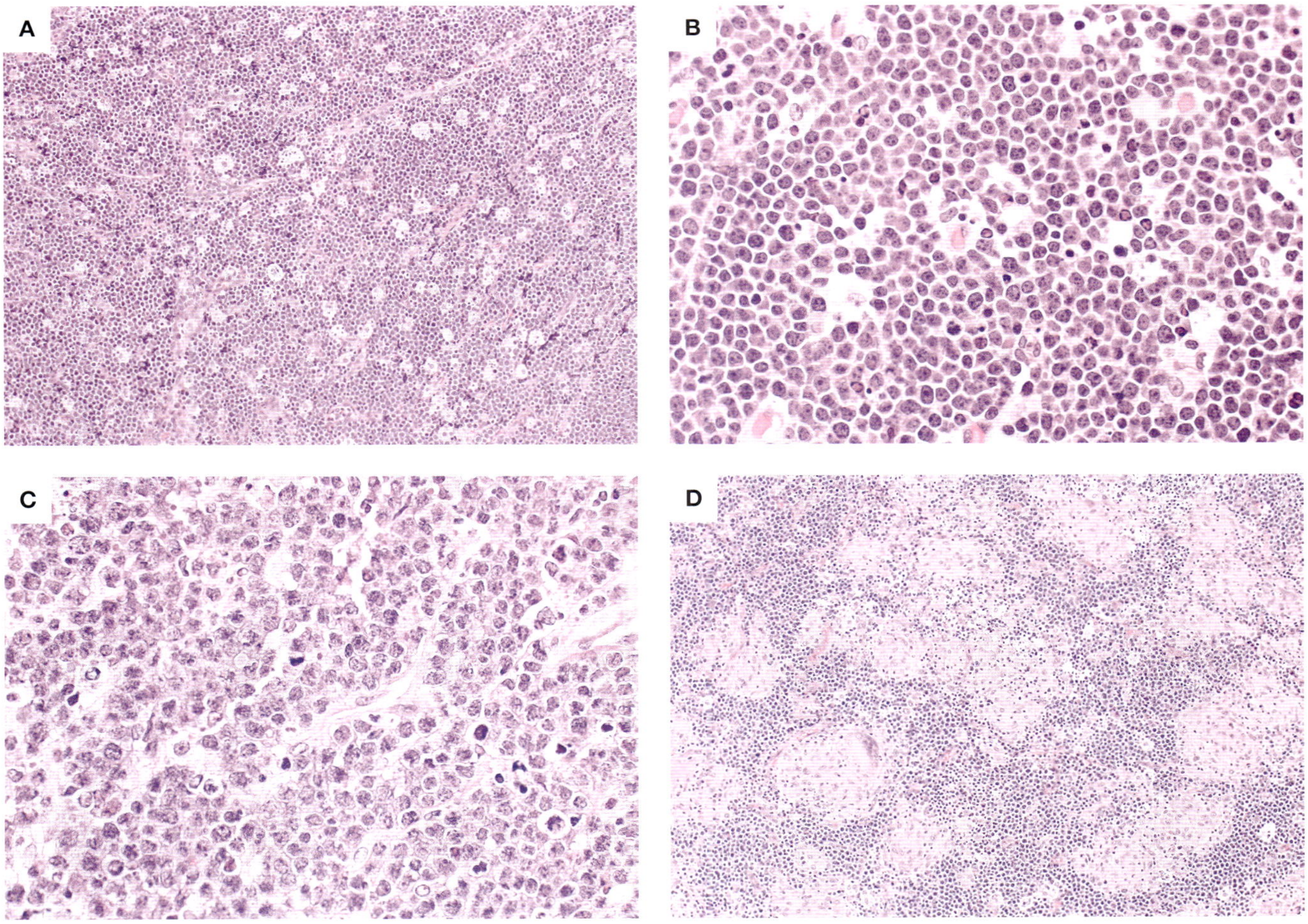

FIGURE 81.2 Burkitt lymphoma (BL). **A:** Diffuse obliteration of tissue architecture by monotonous lymphoma cells with scattered tingible body macrophages imparting a "starry sky" pattern. **B:** Lymphoma cells are intermediate sized with round nuclear contours, open chromatin, multiple small paracentric nucleoli, and scant cytoplasm. **C:** Another case of BL shows mildly irregular nuclear borders or small nucleoli in some cells. **D:** A case of BL with extensive granulomatous inflammation.

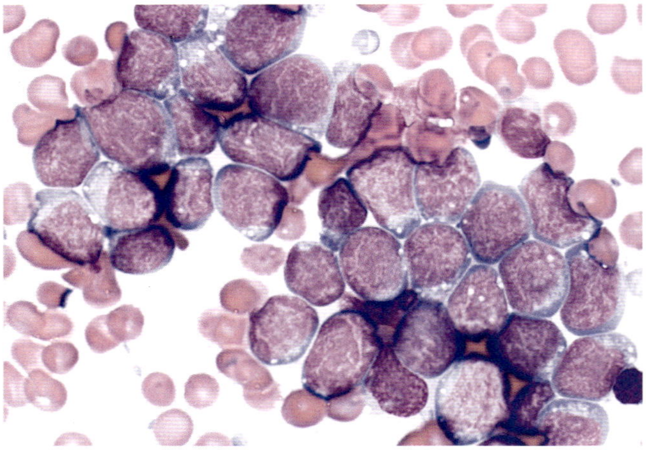

FIGURE 81.3 Burkitt lymphoma, bone marrow aspirate smear. Cytoplasm is deeply basophilic and contains lipid vacuoles.

reactive lymphocytes are often sparse. In some cases one may see a fixation-related retraction artifact, causing characteristic squared-off spaces around cells ("cobblestone" appearance). On Wright-stained touch imprint or blood/BM smears the cytoplasm is basophilic and cytoplasmic vacuoles containing lipid are commonly seen (Figure 81.3). Some cases will have modest variation in size, with slightly more prominent small nucleoli (Figure 81.2C).[9] iBL cases may show some degree of plasmacytoid differentiation with slightly eccentric nuclei, basophilic cytoplasm, and small central nucleoli.[10,11] Rare BL cases may have a marked inflammatory background with granuloma formation and necrosis that may obscure the lymphoma (Figure 81.2D). Such cases are usually EBV+, present with low-stage disease, and have a favorable prognosis. Spontaneous regression is rare but well documented.[12]

Cases of suspected BL with a starry sky pattern that have a more varied and pleomorphic cytologic appearance should be characterized immunophenotypically and genetically for the possibility of a non-BL, high-grade, or large BCL.

Immunophenotype

BL expresses the pan-B-cell markers CD19, CD20, CD22, PAX5, and CD79a as well as germinal center B-cell markers CD10, BCL6, CD38, HGAL, and MEF2B. It shows variable or low expression of LMO2 and GCET1. BCL2 is absent or weakly expressed, and the Ki67 index is high (≥95%) (Figure 81.4A-C). CD43 is often positive. As mature B cells, they express sIg (IgM) and lack TdT.[2,9,13-15] MYC immunohistochemistry (IHC) generally shows high expression (>50%), but this varies and IHC cannot be reliably used to predict *MYC*-R. Mutations in *MYC* that affect the epitope of MYC IHC antibodies may account for IHC-negative cases that harbor a *MYC*-R.[16]

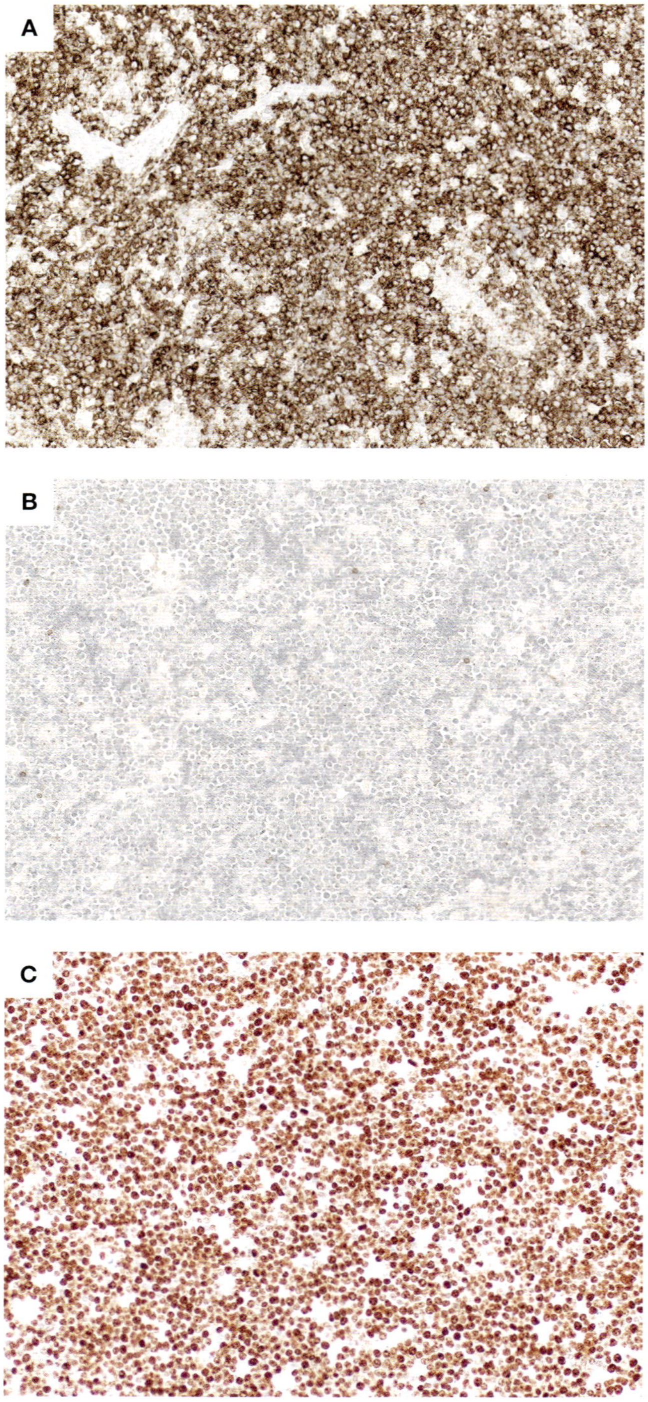

FIGURE 81.4 Burkitt lymphoma with typical immunophenotype, positive for CD10 (**A**) and negative for BCL2 (**B**), with Ki67 (**C**) showing very high proliferative index (>95%).

Genetics

The hallmark of BL is an IG::*MYC*. IGH (14q32) is the most common *MYC* (8q24) partner (70%-80%), followed by IGL (22q11) and IGK (2p12) (Figure 81.5A and B). IG::*MYC* are present in over 95% of cases with the remaining cases harboring *MYC*-R with non-IG partners, although inclusion of these cases in the category of BL is controversial. Recent studies applying whole genome sequencing to "*MYC*-negative" BL have found cryptic insertion of *MYC* into an IG locus.[17]

Genomic and transcriptomic studies have identified abnormalities in several key pathways regulating proliferation, B-cell receptor (BCR) signaling, and protein synthesis/growth, cell survival, cell motility, and epigenetics (Figure 81.6). Mutations in *TCF3*, its negative regulator *ID3*, and *CCND3* promote proliferation. BCR signaling and cell growth are also promoted through *TCF3/ID3* alterations. The p53 pathway may be altered through *TP53* mutation and deletion, or loss of function of the tumor suppressors *CDKN2A(ARF4)* and *USP7* that facilitate MDM2-mediated inactivation of p53. Loss-of-function mutations in *PDRY8* and *GNA13* affect migration of germinal center B cells and promote lymphomagenesis. AICDA activity is variable in BL, is elevated in EBV+ BL, and correlates with IGHV and aberrant genome-wide somatic hypermutation. These lymphomas appear to have fewer driver mutations compared with EBV-negative BL, particularly in the *TCF3/ID3* and apoptosis-related genes (*TP53/USP7/CDKN2A*[*ARF4*]) that track with EBV status.[2,18,19] Expression profiling has identified molecular BL signatures that converge around a signature of dark-zone germinal center B cells.[20]

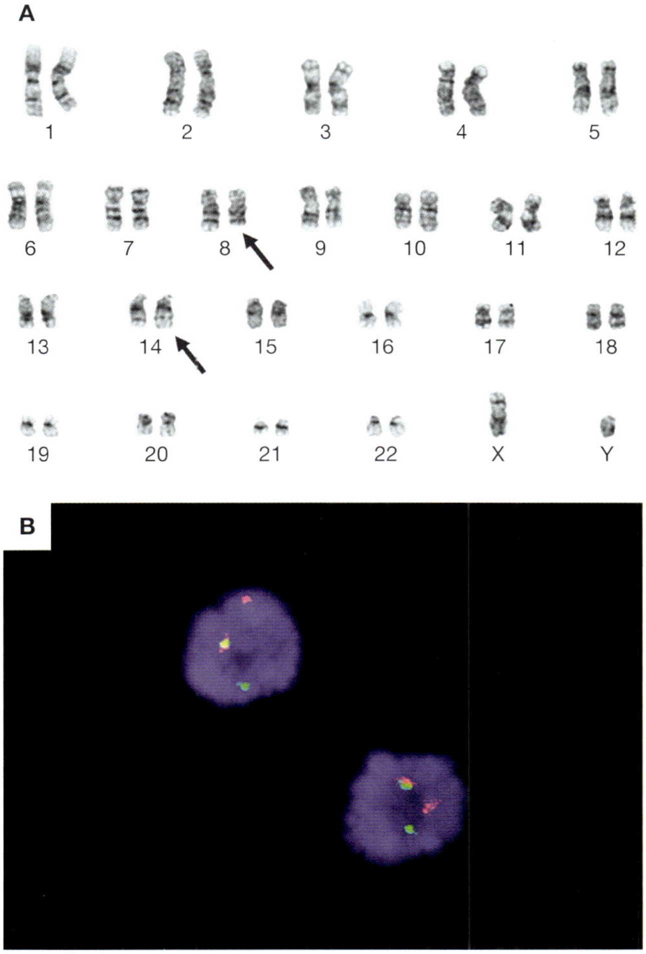

FIGURE 81.5 Burkitt lymphoma shows simple karyotype (**A**) with t(8;14)(q24.1;q32) as the sole abnormality (arrows). Break-apart fluorescence in situ hybridization study for *MYC* (**B**) shows one allele with separation of the probes (green and red) consistent with *MYC* rearrangement. (Figures courtesy of Dr. Lina Shao, University of Michigan, Ann Arbor, MI.)

Prognosis and Clinical Comment

Most patients with BL are cured when treated aggressively. A recent clinical prognostic index included age ≥40 years, lactate dehydrogenase >3× the upper limit of normal, performance status ≥2, and CNS involvement as risk factors and delineated groups with low- (no risk factors, 3-year progression-free survival [PFS] = 92%), intermediate- (one factor, PFS = 72%), and high-risk (≥2 factors, PFS = 53%) BL.[21] Older patients have been understudied and have inferior outcomes. When treated in the setting of HAART, outcomes in patients with HIV are similar to those in patients without HIV.[22]

Principles of therapy include the use of multiple non-cross-resistant systemic chemotherapy agents administered in high doses in a continuous or hyperfractionated manner, short-duration therapy, and central nervous system prophylaxis (or treatment). In the only phase III randomized trial in adult BL, addition of rituximab to chemotherapy showed significant event-free survival benefit.[23] These results were confirmed in a study of over 600 "real-world" patients with BL treated in the United States.[24] There are several intensive regimens that adhere to the aforementioned treatment principles with high cure rates.[25] Recent prospective and retrospective experiences of the dose-adjusted infusional EPOCH-R regimen (etoposide, prednisone, vincristine, cyclophosphamide, doxorubicin, rituximab, and intrathecal methotrexate) suggest high cure rates and improved tolerability over historic more aggressive regimens.[26] Patients with relapsed or refractory BL have a very poor prognosis, and stem cell transplantation has very limited efficacy. Anecdotal experiences

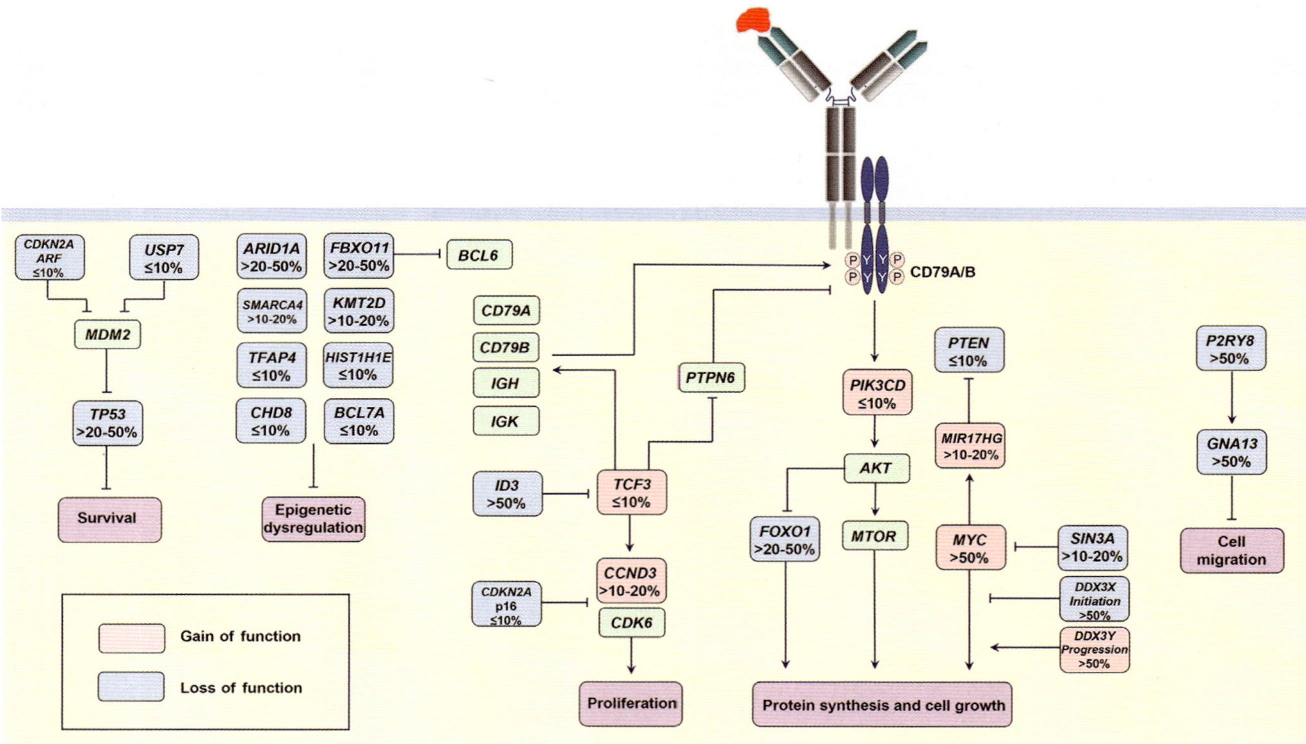

FIGURE 81.6 Summary of genetic alterations in Burkitt lymphoma and their prevalence. Genomic and transcriptomic studies have identified abnormalities in pathways regulating cell survival, proliferation, B-cell receptor signaling, protein synthesis/growth, cell migration, and epigenetics.

with chimeric antigen receptor–engineered T cells and bispecific antibodies show promise, but new strategies are needed for this small group of patients.

References

1. Hammerl L, Colombet M, Rochford R, Ogwang DM, Parkin DM. The burden of Burkitt lymphoma in Africa. *Infect Agent Cancer*. 2019;14:17. doi:10.1186/s13027-019-0236-7
2. Roschewski M, Staudt LM, Wilson WH. Burkitt's lymphoma. *N Engl J Med*. 2022;387(12):1111-1122. doi:10.1056/NEJMra2025746
3. Johnston WT, Mutalima N, Sun D, et al. Relationship between Plasmodium falciparum malaria prevalence, genetic diversity and endemic Burkitt lymphoma in Malawi. *Sci Rep*. 2014;4:3741. doi:10.1038/srep03741
4. Robbiani DF, Deroubaix S, Feldhahn N, et al. Plasmodium infection promotes genomic instability and AID-dependent B cell lymphoma. *Cell*. 2015;162(4):727-737. doi:10.1016/j.cell.2015.07.019
5. Arisue N, Chagaluka G, Palacpac NMQ, et al. Assessment of mixed Plasmodium falciparum sera5 infection in endemic Burkitt lymphoma: a case-control study in Malawi. *Cancers*. 2021;13(7):1692. doi:10.3390/cancers13071692
6. Negahban S, Ahmadi N, Oryan A, et al. Primary bilateral Burkitt lymphoma of the lactating breast: a case report and review of the literature. *Mol Diagn Ther*. 2010;14(4):243-250. doi:10.1007/BF03256380
7. Altshuler E, Wheeler S, Daily K. Bilateral primary breast Burkitt's lymphoma in pregnancy. *BMJ Case Rep*. 2023;16(1):e251896. doi:10.1136/bcr-2022-251896
8. Carbone A, Vaccher E, Gloghini A. Hematologic cancers in individuals infected by HIV. *Blood*. 2022;139(7):995-1012. doi:10.1182/blood.2020005469
9. Leoncini L, Campo E, Stein H, Harris NL, Jaffe ES, Kluin PM. Burkitt lymphoma. In: Swerdlow SH, Campo E, Harris NL, eds. WHO Classification of Tumours of Haematopoietic and Lymphoid Tissues. WHO Press; 2016:300-334.
10. Carbone A, Gloghini A, Gaidano G, et al. AIDS-related Burkitt's lymphoma. Morphologic and immunophenotypic study of biopsy specimens. *Am J Clin Pathol*. 1995;103(5):561-567. doi:10.1093/ajcp/103.5.561
11. Davi F, Delecluse HJ, Guiet P, et al. Burkitt-like lymphomas in AIDS patients: characterization within a series of 103 human immunodeficiency virus-associated non-Hodgkin's lymphomas. Burkitt's Lymphoma Study Group. *J Clin Oncol*. 1998;16(12):3788-3795. doi:10.1200/JCO.1998.16.12.3788

12. Granai M, Lazzi S, Mancini V, et al. Burkitt lymphoma with a granulomatous reaction: an M1/Th1-polarised microenvironment is associated with controlled growth and spontaneous regression. *Histopathology*. 2022;80(2):430-442. doi:10.1111/his.14391
13. King RL, Hsi ED, Chan WC, et al. Diagnostic approaches and future directions in Burkitt lymphoma and high-grade B-cell lymphoma. *Virchows Arch*. 2023;482(1):193-205. doi:10.1007/s00428-022-03404-6
14. Menter T, Gasser A, Juskevicius D, Dirnhofer S, Tzankov A. Diagnostic utility of the germinal center-associated markers GCET1, HGAL, and LMO2 in hematolymphoid neoplasms. *Appl Immunohistochem Mol Morphol*. 2015;23(7):491-498. doi:10.1097/PAI.0000000000000107
15. Moore EM, Swerdlow SH, Gibson SE. Comparison of myocyte enhancer factor 2B versus other germinal center-associated antigens in the differential diagnosis of B-cell non-Hodgkin lymphomas. *Am J Surg Pathol*. 2018;42(3):342-350. doi:10.1097/PAS.0000000000001015
16. Mundo L, Ambrosio MR, Raimondi F, et al. Molecular switch from MYC to MYCN expression in MYC protein negative Burkitt lymphoma cases. *Blood Cancer J*. 2019;9(12):91. doi:10.1038/s41408-019-0252-2
17. Woroniecka R, Rymkiewicz G, Szafron LM, et al. Cryptic MYC insertions in Burkitt lymphoma: new data and a review of the literature. *PLoS One*. 2022;17(2):e0263980. doi:10.1371/journal.pone.0263980
18. Leventaki V, Rodic V, Tripp SR, et al. TP53 pathway analysis in paediatric Burkitt lymphoma reveals increased MDM4 expression as the only TP53 pathway abnormality detected in a subset of cases. *Br J Haematol*. 2012;158(6):763-771. doi:10.1111/j.1365-2141.2012.09243.x
19. Grande BM, Gerhard DS, Jiang A, et al. Genome-wide discovery of somatic coding and noncoding mutations in pediatric endemic and sporadic Burkitt lymphoma. *Blood*. 2019;133(12):1313-1324. doi:10.1182/blood-2018-09-871418
20. Sha C, Barrans S, Cucco F, et al. Molecular high-grade B-cell lymphoma: defining a poor-risk group that requires different approaches to therapy. *J Clin Oncol*. 2019;37(3):202-212. doi:10.1200/jco.18.01314
21. Olszewski AJ, Jakobsen LH, Collins GP, et al. Burkitt lymphoma international prognostic index. *J Clin Oncol*. 2021;39(10):1129-1138. doi:10.1200/JCO.20.03288
22. Atallah-Yunes SA, Murphy DJ, Noy A. HIV-associated Burkitt lymphoma. *Lancet Haematol*. 2020;7(8):e594-e600. doi:10.1016/S2352-3026(20)30126-5
23. Ribrag V, Koscielny S, Bosq J, et al. Rituximab and dose-dense chemotherapy for adults with Burkitt's lymphoma: a randomised, controlled, open-label, phase 3 trial. *Lancet*. 2016;387(10036):2402-2411. doi:10.1016/S0140-6736(15)01317-3
24. Evens AM, Danilov A, Jagadeesh D, et al. Burkitt lymphoma in the modern era: real-world outcomes and prognostication across 30 US cancer centers. *Blood*. 2021;137(3):374-386. doi:10.1182/blood.2020006926
25. Crombie J, LaCasce A. The treatment of Burkitt lymphoma in adults. *Blood*. 2021;137(6):743-750. doi:10.1182/blood.2019004099
26. Roschewski M, Dunleavy K, Abramson JS, et al. Multicenter study of risk-adapted therapy with dose-adjusted EPOCH-R in adults with untreated Burkitt lymphoma. *J Clin Oncol*. 2020;38(22):2519-2529. doi:10.1200/JCO.20.00303

Chapter 82

High-Grade B-Cell Lymphoma With *MYC* and *BCL2* Rearrangements

Rebecca L. King, Ellen D. McPhail, David W. Scott, and John F. Seymour

Definition

High-grade B-cell lymphoma (HGBCL) with *MYC* and *BCL2* rearrangements, commonly referred to as double-hit lymphoma (HGBCL-DH-BCL2), is an aggressive, mature B-cell malignancy that requires a diffuse growth pattern, either large cell or high-grade morphology, and the presence of both *MYC* and *BCL2* gene rearrangements for diagnosis. This disease may occur de novo or as transformation from follicular lymphoma (FL). Cases of true B-lymphoblastic leukemia/lymphoma harboring these rearrangements are exceedingly rare but are excluded from this category. In addition, approximately 2% of FL, without evidence of morphologic transformation to large cell or high-grade lymphoma, also harbor both *MYC* and *BCL2* rearrangements but are also excluded from this category as their clinical behavior is more variable and their biology is not well understood.[1,2]

Synonyms

- Diffuse large B-cell lymphoma/high-grade B-cell lymphoma with *MYC* and *BCL2* rearrangements
- Double-hit lymphoma
- High-grade B-cell lymphoma with *MYC*, *BCL2*, and *BCL6* rearrangements
- Triple-hit lymphoma

Epidemiology

HGBCL with *MYC* and *BCL2* rearrangements (HGBCL-DH-BCL2) accounts for approximately 2% of non-Hodgkin lymphomas overall, 4% to 9% of diffuse large B-cell lymphoma (DLBCL), and approximately 50% of lymphomas with high-grade morphology.[3-8] Among cases categorized as high-grade B-cell lymphoma with *MYC* and *BCL2* and/or *BCL6* rearrangements by the WHO revised fourth edition, 80% to 90% are HGBCL-DH-BCL2.[7,9]

General Clinical Features

HGBCL-DH-BCL2 are aggressive lymphomas that require prompt treatment. The majority of patients present with widely disseminated disease with ~80% having Ann Arbor stage III/IV. In those with early-stage disease, bulky disease is frequent. Median age at presentation is approximately 60 years with a male predominance (~1.5:1). Cases in children and adults less than 30 years old are exceptionally rare. Bone marrow involvement may be as frequent as 50%, higher than the ~15% in DLBCL, not otherwise specified (NOS); the proportions involved with concordant (ie, aggressive lymphoma) versus discordant (ie, indolent lymphoma) is not certain. Involvement of the central nervous system (CNS) at both diagnosis and relapse appears to be higher than in DLBCL, NOS. Overall, the proportion of patients with extranodal involvement is ~60%.[10]

Morphology

Microscopic appearance of HGBCL-DH-BCL2 generally fits into one of two categories: those with standard diffuse large B-cell lymphoma morphology (more common, at least 60% of cases) (Figure 82.1) and those with high-grade B-cell lymphoma morphology (Figure 82.2). As in the WHO revised fourth edition, the International Consensus Classification (ICC) continues to recommend commenting on tumor morphology in the pathology report as some studies describe more aggressive clinical behavior with high-grade morphology.[4,7,11] Both morphologic variants have diffuse growth of tumor cells and may have tingible body macrophages, starry-sky appearance, and/or abundant mitotic figures. Chromatin pattern in DLBCL-like cases can range from fine, blastic chromatin to more coarse, vesicular chromatin with nucleoli resembling centroblasts or immunoblasts. High-grade morphology is defined as intermediate-sized cells that are typically uniform and may have open chromatin (blastoid)

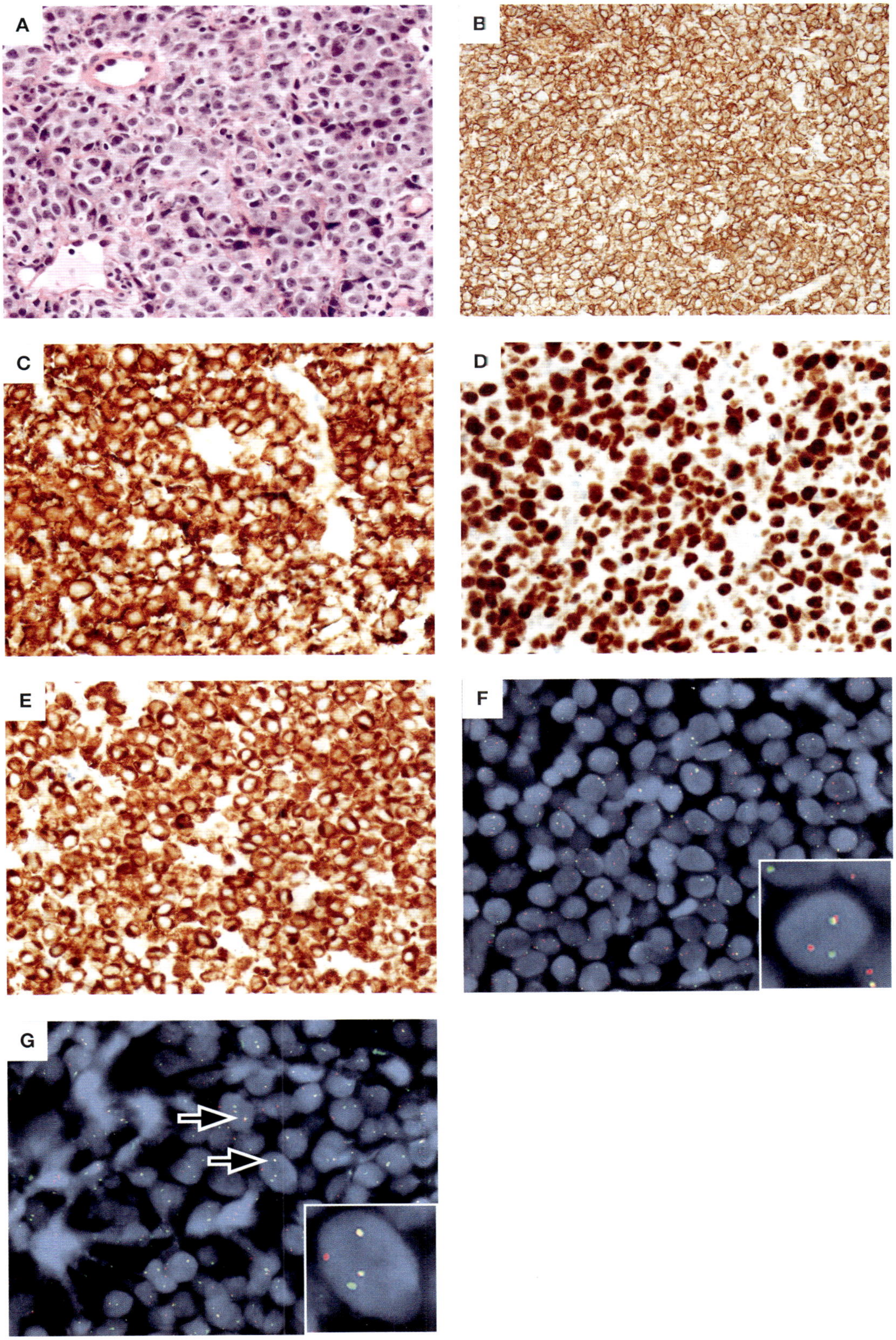

FIGURE 82.1 High-grade B-cell lymphoma with *MYC* and *BCL2* rearrangements and diffuse large B-cell lymphoma morphology. Diffuse proliferation of large, atypical lymphocytes with vesicular chromatin, small nucleoli, and brisk mitotic activity **(A)**. The malignant cells are positive for CD20 **(B)**, CD10 **(C)**, BCL6 **(D)**, and BCL2 **(E)**. *MYC* rearrangement, 1R1G1F signal pattern, *MYC* break-apart probe **(F)**. IGH::*BCL2* fusion, 1R1G2F signal pattern, IGH::*BCL2* dual-fusion probe **(G)** arrows indicate yellow fusion signals.

or more finely clumped chromatin resembling cells of Burkitt lymphoma. Lymphomas with an entirely follicular growth pattern are not considered as part of this entity, although follicular lymphoma can acquire *MYC* rearrangement and undergo transformation to HGBCL-DH-BCL2, which requires at least a component of diffuse growth for diagnosis.

Immunophenotype

HGBCL-DH-BCL2 are mature B-cell lymphomas that virtually always express the pan-B-cell markers CD20, PAX5, CD79a, and CD19 and show surface light chain expression in up to 80% of cases. Bright CD38 is often seen by flow cytometry. CD34 is absent, helping to distinguish from B-lymphoblastic leukemia/lymphoma (B-ALL). TdT expression, in contrast, can be seen in 2% to 14% of cases.[12,13] Recent data support that the majority of these TdT-positive cases have a phenotypic and genetic profile of a mature B cell, and thus expression of TdT does not require reclassification to B-ALL. In these cases, TdT expression is acquired as a secondary event, usually in the process of clonal evolution of a neoplastic mature B cell, as evidenced by somatic hypermutation in the TdT-positive clone.[11-14] Many of these cases are transformations of prior, often subclinical, follicular lymphomas or DLBCLs that have acquired additional genetic changes. They do not have CD34, and many retain surface Ig expression. Cases with both TdT and CD34 expression should prompt careful clinicopathologic examination as very rare cases of true B-ALL with *MYC* and *BCL2* rearrangements have been described.[15]

At least 90% of HGBCL-DH-BCL2 are of germinal center B-cell (GCB) origin by Hans algorithm immunohistochemistry (IHC) and gene expression profiling methods.[9] CD10 and BCL6 are positive in greater than 90% of cases. MUM1 is usually negative but has been reported in up to 42% of cases.

BCL2 and MYC proteins are expressed in most cases, in keeping with upregulation of both genes by the respective rearrangements; however, IHC positivity is neither required nor should it be used as a selection criterion for performance of fluorescence in situ hybridization (FISH) testing. Thresholds of 40% positivity for MYC and 50% positivity for BCL2 have been used in the majority of studies to consider a case positive, and these thresholds are recommended for clinical practice.[9] However, lack of expression of either MYC or BCL2 does not preclude the diagnosis, as both biologic and technical factors can affect protein expression by IHC.[9] Mechanisms explaining MYC negativity in tumors with *MYC* rearrangement have been elucidated and include low *MYC* mRNA levels and a *MYC* polymorphism (NS11S), which disrupts the epitope bound by the antibody used for IHC.[16] Detection of BCL2 protein expression can also be affected by *BCL2* point mutations, which may affect detection by some antibodies used for IHC. Regardless, IHC results should not be used to screen for the presence of *MYC* or *BCL2* rearrangements. Ki-67 proliferation index is variable and cannot be used to predict the presence of the diagnostic rearrangements.

Genetics

HGBCL-DH-BCL2 is defined by structural rearrangement of the *MYC* gene on chromosome 8q24 and separate, concurrent rearrangement of the *BCL2* gene on chromosome 18q21. Cases with *MYC*, *BCL2*, and also *BCL6* rearrangements (triple hit lymphomas) are also included in this category as they are biologically and clinically similar. HGBCLs with *MYC* and *BCL6* rearrangement but without *BCL2* (HGBCL-DH-BCL6) are now considered a separate provisional entity, representing a change from the WHO revised fourth edition. Cases with copy number alterations of these loci without rearrangement are not considered in this category, as data remain inadequate to support their biologic and clinical equivalence.[16-21]

All lymphomas with diffuse large B-cell or high-grade B-cell morphology should be screened by sensitive FISH techniques for the presence of these rearrangements, as screening by morphologic features, Ki-67 index, or protein expression of MYC and BCL2 is not sensitive enough to detect all cases. Since the vast majority of HGBCL-DH-BCL2 cases are of GCB origin, screening only GCB cases can be considered. However, since a small number of HGBCL-DH-BCL2 cases will be misclassified by the Hans algorithm, this method is also imperfect.

FISH is more sensitive and specific compared with conventional karyotyping for detecting *MYC* and *BCL2* rearrangements. Depending on cost and time considerations, screening for *BCL2* rearrangement can be performed concurrently with, or as a reflex following, FISH for *MYC* rearrangement. *MYC* FISH should be ideally performed using a break-apart probe, as its sensitivity far exceeds that of a *MYC*::IGH dual fusion probe alone. However, *MYC* break-apart probe alone will miss 4% to 12% of *MYC* rearrangements, many of which will be detected by the *MYC*::IGH probe set, and thus additional testing with *MYC*::IGH dual-fusion probe may be considered.[22-25]

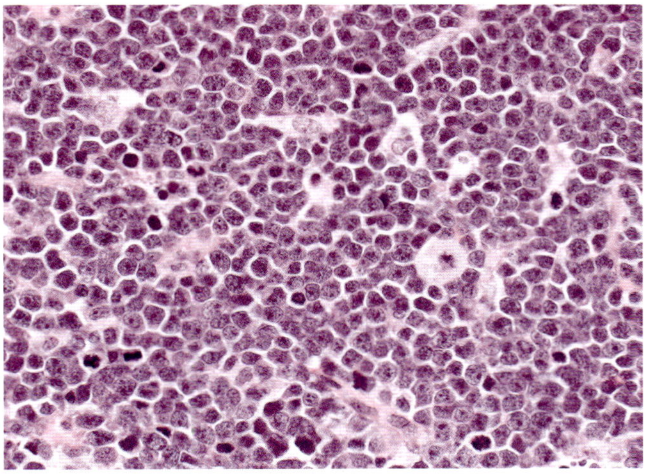

FIGURE 82.2 High-grade B-cell lymphoma with *MYC* and *BCL2* rearrangements and high-grade B-cell lymphoma morphology. Diffuse proliferation of intermediate-sized lymphocytes with blastoid chromatin, inconspicuous nucleoli, and scant cytoplasm.

Unlike in Burkitt lymphoma in which the *MYC* partner is virtually always IGH, IGL, or IGK, only 50% to 60% of HGBCL-DH-BCL2 cases have a *MYC*-IG rearrangement. The remaining 40% include various partner genes such as *BCL6, PAX5, IRF4, BCL11A, IKZF1, IMMP2L*, and *RFTN1*. The significance of the *MYC* partner gene in HGBCL-DH-BCL2 has been the subject of much study and debate in recent years. Classically, overexpression of MYC secondary to juxtaposition of IG enhancers to the *MYC* gene is considered to be a major driver of the aggressive biology seen in HGBCL-DH-BCL2, and it is uncertain whether a similar degree of overexpression results from juxtaposition to non-IG genes. While mounting data suggest that, in cases with DLBCL morphology, the prognosis of HGBCL-DH-BCL2 with *MYC*::IG translocations is inferior to those with *MYC*-non-IG translocations, others have shown discrepant results.[4,7,26] Thus, the significance of the *MYC* partner gene remains an unresolved question. Importantly, the lack of widespread availability of IGK and IGL probes precludes routine testing for all IG rearrangements in clinical practice, and, as such, the ICC does not require identification of the *MYC* partner or exclude non-IG cases from this category.

HGBCL-DH-BCL2 typically have a complex karyotype highlighting biologic complexity beyond the defining rearrangements. In addition to rearrangements, *MYC* mutations are frequently seen (~40%).[27] The mutation profile of HGBCL-DH-BCL2 overlaps with other GCB tumors and includes recurrent mutations in *BCL2* (~80%), *KMT2D* (~60%), *CREBBP* (~50%), *EZH2* (~50%), and *TNFRSF14* (~45%).[27-30] There is also some mutational overlap with Burkitt lymphoma, with recurrent mutations in *CCND3* (10%-20%), as well as *FOXO1* (~25%).[27-30] HGBCL-DH-BCL2 that also have *BCL6* rearrangements in general show mutational similarity.[27,28]

RNA sequencing studies have shown that HGBCL-DH-BCL2 have a unique germinal center dark-zone signature shared by not only these cases but also Burkitt lymphoma and a subset of GCB-DLBCLs with aggressive biology.[31,32] Although assays have not been adapted into clinical practice, they highlight the potential future of molecular testing to improve upon our ability to detect high-grade biology and clinical behavior.

Prognosis and Clinical Comment

The prognosis of HGBCL-DH-BCL2 is inferior compared with DLBCL, NOS when standard-of-care R-CHOP immunochemotherapy is used. The initial reports, where these patients were identified using selective FISH strategies based on unusual morphology and/or clinical behavior, indicated a dismal prognosis, but these studies are flawed by these screening biases. Meanwhile, more recent studies, where routine FISH was applied, observed a 2-year progression-free survival of ~50%.[4] Although not universally supported by the published literature, inferior prognosis has been associated with high-grade morphology and IG (vs non-IG) *MYC* translocation partner in some studies. Limited-stage HGBCL-DH-BCL2 is uncommon, and the outcomes appear comparable with DLBCL, NOS, with a suggestion of potential utility for inclusion of local radiation therapy,[33] albeit based on very small numbers of patients. The prognostic impact of a preceding diagnosis of FL is not clear, often being confounded by previous treatment for the indolent disease.

Based on the poor outcomes with R-CHOP, many centers have adopted escalated intensity immunochemotherapy regimens, including DA-EPOCH-R, McGrath, or early consolidative autologous stem cell transplantation, based on superior outcomes in observational studies.[10] Incorporation of novel agents, including BCL2 inhibitor (venetoclax) and antibody-drug conjugates (polatuzumab vedotin–anti-CD79b), into upfront treatment has not resulted in improved outcomes. Staging of the CNS may be considered based on the historically observed higher rate of CNS involvement at diagnosis.

Progression and relapse occur earlier than in DLBCL, NOS, with the vast majority occurring in the first year after diagnosis and relapses beyond this being rare. Based on a very small number of cases, the rare relapses beyond 2 years represent new DLBCL, transformed from a persistent common precursor cell harboring *BCL2* rearrangement. When chemotherapy-based strategies, including consolidative autologous stem cell transplantation, have been employed, the outcomes of progression/relapse are very poor. Subgroup analyses of larger trials show improved outcomes when chimeric antigen receptor T-cell (CAR-T) therapy is used at this juncture.

References

1. Miyaoka M, Kikuti YY, Carreras J, et al. Clinicopathological and genomic analysis of double-hit follicular lymphoma: comparison with high-grade B-cell lymphoma with MYC and BCL2 and/or BCL6 rearrangements. *Mod Pathol.* 2018;31(2):313-326. doi:10.1038/modpathol.2017.134
2. Miao Y, Hu S, Lu X, et al. Double-hit follicular lymphoma with MYC and BCL2 translocations: a study of 7 cases with a review of literature. *Hum Pathol.* 2016;58:72-77. doi:10.1016/j.humpath.2016.07.025
3. Savage KJ, Johnson NA, Ben-Neriah S, et al. MYC gene rearrangements are associated with a poor prognosis in diffuse large B-cell lymphoma patients treated with R-CHOP chemotherapy. *Blood.* 2009;114(17):3533-3537. doi:10.1182/blood-2009-05-220095
4. Rosenwald A, Bens S, Advani R, et al. Prognostic significance of MYC rearrangement and translocation partner in diffuse large B-cell lymphoma: a study by the Lunenburg lymphoma biomarker consortium. *J Clin Oncol.* 2019;37(35):3359-3368. doi:10.1200/jco.19.00743
5. Horn H, Ziepert M, Becher C, et al. MYC status in concert with BCL2 and BCL6 expression predicts outcome in diffuse large B-cell lymphoma. *Blood.* 2013;121(12):2253-2263. doi:10.1182/blood-2012-06-435842
6. Klapper W, Stoecklein H, Zeynalova S, et al. Structural aberrations affecting the MYC locus indicate a poor prognosis independent of clinical risk factors in diffuse large B-cell lymphomas treated within randomized trials of the German High-Grade Non-Hodgkin's Lymphoma Study Group (DSHNHL). *Leukemia.* 2008;22(12):2226-2229. doi:10.1038/leu.2008.230
7. McPhail ED, Maurer MJ, Macon WR, et al. Inferior survival in high-grade B-cell lymphoma with MYC and BCL2 and/or BCL6 rearrangements is not associated with MYC/IG gene rearrangements. *Haematologica.* 2018;103(11):1899-1907. doi:10.3324/haematol.2018.190157
8. Oki Y, Noorani M, Lin P, et al. Double hit lymphoma: the MD Anderson Cancer Center clinical experience. *Br J Haematol.* 2014;166(6):891-901. doi:10.1111/bjh.12982
9. Scott DW, King RL, Staiger AM, et al. High-grade B-cell lymphoma with MYC and BCL2 and/or BCL6 rearrangements with diffuse large B-cell lymphoma morphology. *Blood.* 2018;131(18):2060-2064. doi:10.1182/blood-2017-12-820605
10. Petrich AM, Gandhi M, Jovanovic B, et al. Impact of induction regimen and stem cell transplantation on outcomes in double-hit lymphoma: a multicenter retrospective analysis. *Blood.* 2014;124(15):2354-2361. doi:10.1182/blood-2014-05-578963
11. Moore EM, Aggarwal N, Surti U, Swerdlow SH. Further exploration of the complexities of large B-cell lymphomas with MYC abnormalities and the importance of a blastoid morphology. *Am J Surg Pathol.* 2017;41(9):1155-1166. doi:10.1097/pas.0000000000000818
12. Bhavsar S, Liu YC, Gibson SE, Moore EM, Swerdlow SH. Mutational landscape of TdT+ large B-cell lymphomas supports their distinction from B-lymphoblastic neoplasms: a multiparameter study of a rare and aggressive entity. *Am J Surg Pathol.* 2022;46(1):71-82. doi:10.1097/pas.0000000000001750
13. Khanlari M, Medeiros LJ, Lin P, et al. Blastoid high-grade B-cell lymphoma initially presenting in bone marrow: a diagnostic challenge. *Mod Pathol.* 2022;35(3):419-426. doi:10.1038/s41379-021-00909-4
14. Ok CY, Medeiros LJ, Thakral B, et al. High-grade B-cell lymphomas with TdT expression: a diagnostic and classification dilemma. *Mod Pathol.* 2019;32(1):48-58. doi:10.1038/s41379-018-0112-9
15. Wagener R, López C, Kleinheinz K, et al. IG-MYC (+) neoplasms with precursor B-cell phenotype are molecularly distinct from Burkitt lymphomas. *Blood.* 2018;132(21):2280-2285. doi:10.1182/blood-2018-03-842088
16. Collinge B, Ben-Neriah S, Chong L, et al. The impact of MYC and BCL2 structural variants in tumors of DLBCL morphology and mechanisms of false-negative MYC IHC. *Blood.* 2021;137(16):2196-2208. doi:10.1182/blood.2020007193
17. Yoon SO, Jeon YK, Paik JH, et al. MYC translocation and an increased copy number predict poor prognosis in adult diffuse large B-cell lymphoma (DLBCL), especially in germinal centre-like B cell (GCB) type. *Histopathology.* 2008;53(2):205-217. doi:10.1111/j.1365-2559.2008.03076.x
18. Landsburg DJ, Falkiewicz MK, Petrich AM, et al. Sole rearrangement but not amplification of MYC is associated with a poor prognosis in patients with diffuse large B cell lymphoma and B cell lymphoma unclassifiable. *Br J Haematol.* 2016;175(4):631-640. doi:10.1111/bjh.14282
19. Testoni M, Kwee I, Greiner TC, et al. Gains of MYC locus and outcome in patients with diffuse large B-cell lymphoma treated with R-CHOP. *Br J Haematol.* 2011;155(2):274-277. doi:10.1111/j.1365-2141.2011.08675.x
20. Schieppati F, Balzarini P, Fisogni S, et al. An increase in MYC copy number has a progressive negative prognostic impact in patients with diffuse large B-cell and high-grade lymphoma, who may benefit from intensified treatment

regimens. *Haematologica.* 2020;105(5):1369-1378. doi:10.3324/haematol.2019.223891

21. Sermer D, Bobillo S, Dogan A, et al. Extra copies of MYC, BCL2, and BCL6 and outcome in patients with diffuse large B-cell lymphoma. *Blood Adv.* 2020;4(14):3382-3390. doi:10.1182/bloodadvances.2020001551
22. Muñoz-Mármol AM, Sanz C, Tapia G, Marginet R, Ariza A, Mate JL. MYC status determination in aggressive B-cell lymphoma: the impact of FISH probe selection. *Histopathology.* 2013;63(3):418-424. doi:10.1111/his.12178
23. Bertrand P, Bastard C, Maingonnat C, et al. Mapping of MYC breakpoints in 8q24 rearrangements involving non-immunoglobulin partners in B-cell lymphomas. *Leukemia.* 2007;21(3):515-523. doi:10.1038/sj.leu.2404529
24. Chong LC, Ben-Neriah S, Slack GW, et al. High-resolution architecture and partner genes of MYC rearrangements in lymphoma with DLBCL morphology. *Blood Adv.* 2018;2(20):2755-2765. doi:10.1182/bloodadvances.2018023572
25. King RL, McPhail ED, Meyer RG, et al. False-negative rates for MYC fluorescence in situ hybridization probes in B-cell neoplasms. *Haematologica.* 2019;104(6):e248-e251. doi:10.3324/haematol.2018.207290
26. Copie-Bergman C, Cuillière-Dartigues P, Baia M, et al. MYC-IG rearrangements are negative predictors of survival in DLBCL patients treated with immunochemotherapy: a GELA/LYSA study. *Blood.* 2015;126(22):2466-2474. doi:10.1182/blood-2015-05-647602
27. Cucco F, Barrans S, Sha C, et al. Distinct genetic changes reveal evolutionary history and heterogeneous molecular grade of DLBCL with MYC/BCL2 double-hit. *Leukemia.* 2020;34(5):1329-1341. doi:10.1038/s41375-019-0691-6
28. Künstner A, Witte HM, Riedl J, et al. Mutational landscape of high-grade B-cell lymphoma with MYC-BCL2 and/or BCL6 rearrangements characterized by whole-exome sequencing. *Haematologica.* 2022;107(8):1850-1863. doi:10.3324/haematol.2021.279631
29. Gebauer N, Bernard V, Feller AC, Merz H. ID3 mutations are recurrent events in double-hit B-cell lymphomas. *Anticancer Res.* 2013;33(11):4771-4778.
30. Momose S, Weißbach S, Pischimarov J, et al. The diagnostic gray zone between Burkitt lymphoma and diffuse large B-cell lymphoma is also a gray zone of the mutational spectrum. *Leukemia.* 2015;29(8):1789-1791. doi:10.1038/leu.2015.34
31. Ennishi D, Jiang A, Boyle M, et al. Double-hit gene expression signature defines a distinct subgroup of germinal center B-cell-like diffuse large B-cell lymphoma. *J Clin Oncol.* 2019;37(3):190-201. doi:10.1200/jco.18.01583
32. Sha C, Barrans S, Cucco F, et al. Molecular high-grade B-cell lymphoma: defining a poor-risk group that requires different approaches to therapy. *J Clin Oncol.* 2019;37(3):202-212. doi:10.1200/jco.18.01314
33. Grass GD, Mills MN, Ahmed KA, et al. Radiotherapy for early stage diffuse large B-cell lymphoma with or without double or triple hit genetic alterations. *Leuk Lymphoma.* 2019;60(4):886-893. doi:10.1080/10428194.2018.1506586

Chapter 83

High-Grade B-Cell Lymphoma With *MYC* and *BCL6* Rearrangements

Rebecca L. King, Ellen D. McPhail, David W. Scott, and John F. Seymour

Definition

High-grade B-cell lymphoma (HGBCL) with *MYC* and *BCL6* rearrangements, commonly referred to as double-hit lymphoma (HGBCL-DH-BCL6), is an aggressive, mature B-cell malignancy. Diagnosis of HGBCL-DH-BCL6 requires a diffuse growth pattern, either large cell or high-grade morphology, and the presence of rearrangements of both *MYC* and the germinal center B-cell transcriptional repressor *BCL6*. If a *BCL2* rearrangement is also present, such cases are classified as HGBCL-DH-BCL2 (see Chapter 82). This disease may occur de novo or as transformation from low-grade B-cell lymphoma, which may be either follicular lymphoma or less commonly marginal zone lymphoma.[1] Very rarely, histologic low-grade lymphomas such as follicular lymphomas, without evidence of morphologic transformation to large cell or high-grade lymphoma, harbor both *MYC* and *BCL6* rearrangements but are excluded from this category as their clinical behavior is more variable and their biology is not well understood. HGBCL-DH-BCL6 is considered a provisional entity.

Synonyms

Double-hit lymphoma.

Epidemiology

HGBCL-DH-BCL6 accounts for less than 1% of non-Hodgkin lymphomas overall and less than 5% of diffuse large B-cell lymphoma (DLBCL).[2,3] Among cases categorized as HGBCL with *MYC* and *BCL2* and/or *BCL6* rearrangements by the World Health Organization (WHO) revised fourth edition, 10% to 20% are HGBCL-DH-BCL6.[4,5] The median age at presentation is approximately 66 years.[1] Cases in children and adults less than 30 years old are rare but more common than HGBCL-DH-BCL2 in this age group. There is a slight male predominance.

General Clinical Features

Natural history is somewhat variable, but these tumors generally have aggressive clinical behavior requiring prompt treatment. However, they are potentially curable even when widely disseminated at presentation. The rarity of this lymphoma entity and prior reports grouping these cases together with HGBCL-DH-BCL2 have resulted in uncertainty regarding patient characteristics. Based on available information, it appears that the median age at presentation and the gender distribution are similar to DLBCL, not otherwise specified (NOS). It may be associated with more frequent Ann Arbor stage III/IV, higher number of extranodal sites, and higher International Prognostic Index than DLBCL, NOS.[2,3]

Morphology

Like HGBCL-DH-BCL2, the microscopic appearance of HGBCL-DH-BCL6 generally fits into one of two categories: those with DLBCL morphology (Figure 83.1) and those with high-grade B-cell lymphoma morphology (see Chapter 82 for details). In HGBCL-DH-BCL6, a higher percentage have large cell morphology[6] than in HGBCL-DH-BCL2. As in the WHO-4R, the International Consensus Classification (ICC) continues to recommend commenting on the type of morphology in the pathology report as some studies support more aggressive behavior with high-grade morphology, although these data are for cohorts of patients with both types of HGBCL-DH and data on prognostic factors in HGBCL-DH-BCL6 specifically are lacking. Lymphomas with an entirely follicular growth pattern are not considered as part of this entity.

Immunophenotype

HGBCL-DH-BCL6 are mature B-cell lymphomas that virtually always express pan-B-cell markers CD20, PAX5, CD79a, and CD19 and are expected to show

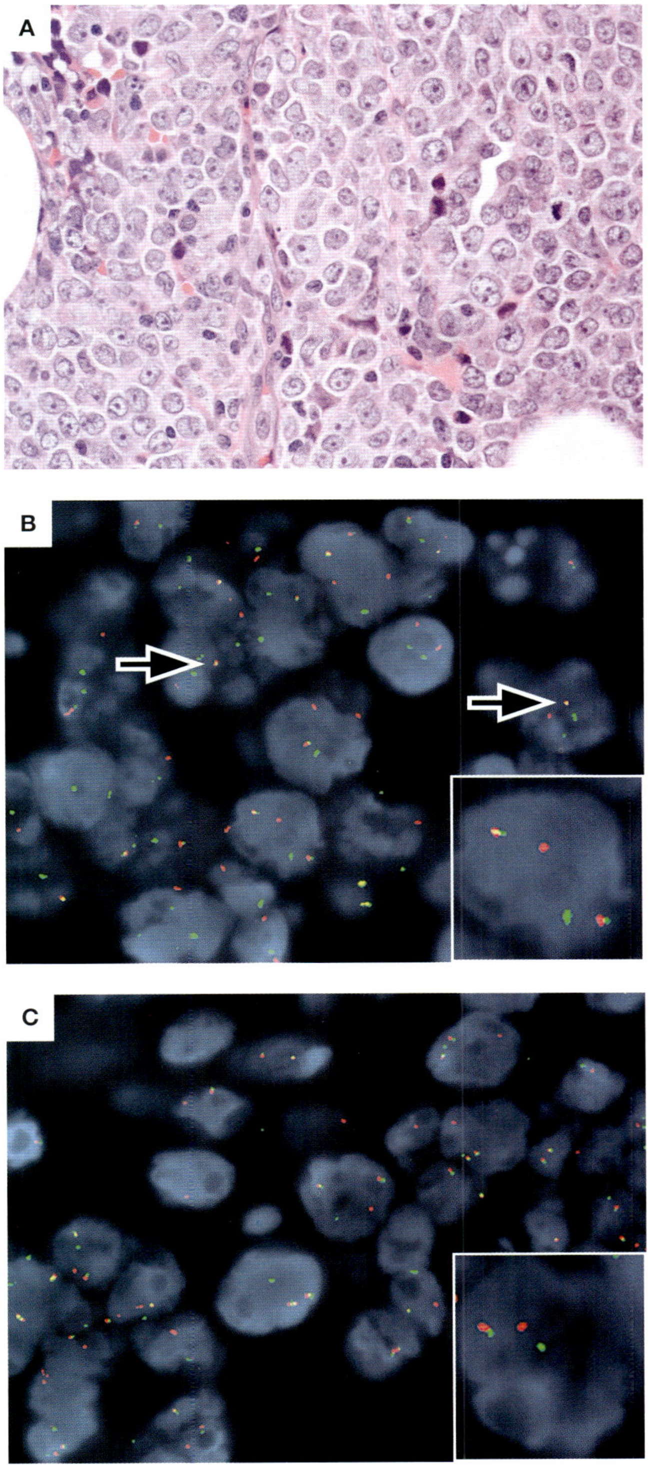

FIGURE 83.1 High-grade B-cell lymphoma with *MYC* and *BCL6* rearrangements with large cell morphology. Diffuse proliferation of large, atypical lymphocytes with vesicular chromatin, small nucleoli and brisk mitotic activity (**A**). IGL::*MYC* fusion, 1R1G2F signal pattern, IGL::*MYC* dual fusion probe (**B**) arrows indicate yellow fusion signals. *BCL6* rearrangement, 1R1G1F signal pattern, *BCL6* break-apart probe (**C**).

surface light chain expression. TdT is virtually always absent, although its expression, as in HGBCL-DH-BCL2, does not independently preclude the diagnosis. CD34 expression should prompt strong consideration for an immature B-cell neoplasm.

Unlike HGBCL-DH-BCL2, HGBCL-DH-BCL6 are evenly split between germinal center B-cell-like (GCB) and activated B-cell-like (or non-GCB) cell of origin by gene expression studies, highlighting the more heterogeneous nature of this disease.[1,3-7] CD10 is less commonly expressed than in HGBCL-DH-BCL2 cases, and IRF4/MUM1 expression is seen in up to 90% of cases. MYC and BCL2 coexpression by IHC is less commonly seen than in HGBCL-DH-BCL2.[1] Ki-67 proliferation index is variable and cannot be used to predict the presence of the diagnostic rearrangements.

Genetics

HGBCL-DH-BCL6 is defined by structural rearrangement of the *MYC* gene on chromosome 8q24 and concurrent rearrangement of the BCL6 gene on chromosome 3q27 without concurrent rearrangement of *BCL2*. As in HGBCL-DH-*BCL2*, cases with copy number alterations of these loci without rearrangement are not considered to fulfill diagnostic criteria for inclusion in this category.

Although the WHO fifth edition has removed this diagnostic category, the ICC recommends that all lymphomas with DLBCL or HGBCL morphology should be screened by sensitive fluorescence in situ hybridization (FISH) techniques for the presence of these rearrangements. Screening by morphologic features, Ki-67 index, or protein expression of MYC and BCL6 is not sensitive enough to detect all cases. Since approximately half of HGBCL-DH-BCL6 cases are of activated B cell origin, screening only GCB tumors will miss a significant proportion of cases and is not recommended.

FISH studies for *MYC* and *BCL6* should proceed with the same considerations discussed in Chapter 82 on HGBCL-DH-BCL2.

As in HGBCL-DH-BCL2, *MYC* gene partners include both IG and various non-IG loci, one of which is the *BCL6* gene itself. These cases harbor the t(3;8)(q27;q24) and have been referred to as a "pseudo-double-hit lymphomas."[8] This *BCL6*::*MYC* translocation has been found to account for up to 30% of cases of HGBCL-DH-BCL6. Since most laboratories do not utilize *BCL6*::*MYC* dual fusion probes, these cases remain within the HGBCL-DH-BCL6 category and FISH to determine the *MYC* partner is not required for diagnosis.

Mutational studies of HGBCL-DH-BCL6 cases are limited, but data suggest more heterogeneity than in HGBCL-DH-BCL2. Recurrent GCB-associated mutations such as *CREBBP* (~14%), *KMT2D* (~18%), and *EZH2* (~5%) are seen at lower frequencies than in HGBCL-DH-BCL2.[9] *BCL2* mutations are exceptionally rare in comparison with HGBCL-DH-BCL2[4] and when present may indicate a cryptic *BCL2* rearrangement.[9,10] Mutations in CCND3 are observed in ~25% of tumors.[9] While some HGBCL-DH-BCL6 tumors cluster with DLBCL genetically related to follicular lymphoma (EZB subgroup) in large-scale genomic classifiers of DLBCL, others cluster with the BN2 subgroup, which is genetically related to marginal zone lymphomas, and many others remain unclassified, suggesting multiple pathways of evolution and biologic heterogeneity in HGBCL-DH-BCL6.[9] *TP53* mutations are reported at a lower incidence than in HGBCL-DH-BCL2.[2]

Prognosis and Clinical Comment

The largest study of prognosis of HGBCL-DH-BCL6, involving 31 R-CHOP-treated patients and limited to DLBCL morphology, showed inferior outcomes compared with DLBCL, NOS, with a 2-year progression-free survival of ~50%.[11] This prognostic impact is not consistent across all studies with other cohorts reporting no adverse impact of HGBCL-DH-BCL6 status relative to DLBCL, NOS and a more favorable outcome than HGBCL-DH-BCL2.[2,3] There are insufficient data on the impact of either morphology or use of regimens other than R-CHOP on outcomes in this disease. As such, it is difficult to draw firm conclusions or recommend deviation from standard DLBCL, NOS chemoimmunotherapy approaches. In contrast to HGBCL-DH-BCL2, there are no data describing any specific impact of HGBCL-DH-BCL6 on risk of central nervous system involvement or relapse.

References

1. Do HKGT, Lin P, Xu J, et al. USCAP 2023 abstracts hematopathology. *Lab Invest*. 2023;103(3 suppl):1167-1168. doi:10.1016/j.labinv.2023.100106
2. Ye Q, Xu-Monette ZY, Tzankov A, et al. Prognostic impact of concurrent MYC and BCL6 rearrangements and expression in de novo diffuse large B-cell lymphoma. *Oncotarget*. 2016;7(3):2401-2416. doi:10.18632/oncotarget.6262
3. Tsai CC, Su YC, Bamodu OA, et al. High-grade B-cell lymphoma (HGBL) with MYC and BCL2 and/or BCL6 rearrangements is predominantly BCL6-rearranged and BCL6-expressing in Taiwan. *Cancers*. 2021;13(7):1620. doi:10.3390/cancers13071620
4. McPhail ED, Maurer MJ, Macon WR, et al. Inferior survival in high-grade B-cell lymphoma with MYC and BCL2 and/or BCL6 rearrangements is not associated with MYC/IG gene rearrangements. *Haematologica*. 2018;103(11):1899-1907. doi:10.3324/haematol.2018.190157
5. Scott DW, King RL, Staiger AM, et al. High-grade B-cell lymphoma with MYC and BCL2 and/or BCL6 rearrangements with diffuse large B-cell lymphoma morphology. *Blood*. 2018;131(18):2060-2064. doi:10.1182/blood-2017-12-820605
6. Li S, Desai P, Lin P, et al. MYC/BCL6 double-hit lymphoma (DHL): a tumour associated with an aggressive clinical course and poor prognosis. *Histopathology*. 2016;68(7):1090-1098. doi:10.1111/his.12884
7. Pillai RK, Sathanoori M, Van Oss SB, Swerdlow SH. Double-hit B-cell lymphomas with BCL6 and MYC translocations are aggressive, frequently extranodal lymphomas distinct from BCL2 double-hit B-cell lymphomas. *Am J Surg Pathol*. 2013;37(3):323-332. doi:10.1097/PAS.0b013e31826cebad
8. Johnson SM, Umakanthan JM, Yuan J, et al. Lymphomas with pseudo-double-hit BCL6-MYC translocations due to t(3;8)(q27;q24) are associated with a germinal center immunophenotype, extranodal involvement, and frequent BCL2 translocations. *Hum Pathol*. 2018;80:192-200. doi:10.1016/j.humpath.2018.06.006
9. Künstner A, Witte HM, Riedl J, et al. Mutational landscape of high-grade B-cell lymphoma with MYC-BCL2 and/or BCL6 rearrangements characterized by whole-exome sequencing. *Haematologica*. 2022;107(8):1850-1863. doi:10.3324/haematol.2021.279631
10. Stengel A, Kern W, Meggendorfer M, Haferlach T, Haferlach C. Detailed molecular analysis and evaluation of prognosis in cases with high grade B-cell lymphoma with MYC and BCL2 and/or BCL6 rearrangements. *Br J Haematol*. 2019;185(5):951-954. doi:10.1111/bjh.15653
11. Rosenwald A, Bens S, Advani R, et al. Prognostic significance of MYC rearrangement and translocation partner in diffuse large B-cell lymphoma: a study by the Lunenburg lymphoma biomarker consortium. *J Clin Oncol*. 2019;37(35):3359-3368. doi:10.1200/jco.19.00743

Chapter 84

High-Grade B-Cell Lymphoma, Not Otherwise Specified

Anamarija M. Perry, Rebecca L. King, and David W. Scott

Definition

High-grade B-cell lymphoma, not otherwise specified (HGBCL, NOS) is an aggressive, mature B-cell lymphoma that does not fulfill criteria for HGBCL with *MYC* and *BCL2* and/or *BCL6* rearrangements (ie, genetic "double-hit" [HGBCL-DH]). These cases likely do not represent a uniform biologic entity but rather a heterogeneous group of aggressive B-cell lymphomas. Prior to the World Health Organization (WHO) revised fourth edition, these cases were typically placed into the category of B-cell lymphoma, unclassifiable with features intermediate between diffuse large B-cell lymphoma (DLBCL) and Burkitt lymphoma (BL)—BCLU. The BCLU category was removed in the WHO revised fourth edition in 2017, but there remained cases, which in addition to lacking double-hit genetics, did not neatly fit into the DLBCL, NOS; BL; or other specific disease categories. For these cases, the WHO revised fourth edition introduced the category of HGBCL, NOS, which remains, essentially unchanged, in the current International Consensus Classification. It must be emphasized that HGBCL, NOS is a diagnosis of exclusion, should be used sparingly, and is only for cases that cannot be confidently classified as either BL or DLBCL, NOS. Published studies on this entity are few, retrospective, and limited by poor reproducibility in rendering this diagnosis.

Synonyms

None.

Epidemiology

These lymphomas usually occur in elderly patients, with a median age of diagnosis in the seventh decade. They have been reported in younger patients and are very rarely seen in children. Males are more commonly affected than females with a male-to-female ratio of approximately 2:1.[1-4]

General Clinical Features

Most patients present with advanced clinical stage (III/IV) by Ann Arbor Staging Classification (56%-77%), with lymph node involvement, as well as frequent involvement of multiple extranodal sites (42%-66%), high or intermediate International Prognostic Index, and elevated lactate dehydrogenase.[1,2,4] The most commonly involved extranodal sites include bone marrow (24%-32%) and gastrointestinal tract (22%), with variable rates of central nervous system involvement (7%-26%) reported.[2,4] Some cases represent progression/transformation from a low-grade B-cell lymphoma, most commonly follicular lymphoma.[2,4]

Morphology

Morphologic diagnosis of HGBCL, NOS is subjective and poorly reproducible among pathologists. This diagnosis should only be made on a well-fixed tissue biopsy where reliable assessment of cell size can be performed. These cases show diffuse proliferation of intermediate-sized lymphoma cells with many having tingible-body macrophages imparting a starry-sky appearance, as well as increased mitotic figures and apoptotic bodies. Cases of large cell lymphoma with starry-sky morphology or a high proliferation index should not be placed into this category. Cases of HGBCL, NOS generally show two main morphologic appearances—Burkitt-like (more common) and blastoid. In cases with Burkitt-like morphology, the lymphoma cells are medium sized, usually with some larger cells admixed, and show greater degree of nuclear irregularity than is usually seen in BL (Figure 84.1). Nuclear and nucleolar features are otherwise similar to BL, and cytoplasmic vacuoles are variably present. Cases that morphologically resemble BL should only be classified as HGBCL, NOS if they have phenotypic and/or genetic features incompatible with BL. A diagnosis of large B cell lymphoma with 11q aberration must also be excluded in cases that closely resemble

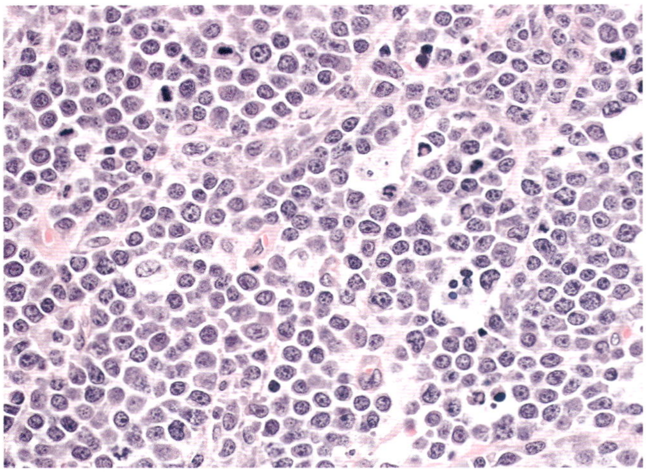

FIGURE 84.1 High-grade B-cell lymphoma, NOS with Burkitt-like morphology. The lymphoma cells are medium sized with fine chromatin and inconspicuous to small nucleoli. Tingible body macrophages are present.

BL but lack *MYC* rearrangement. The other, relatively rare, morphologic appearance is blastoid, where the lymphoma cells are reminiscent of lymphoblasts: medium sized with round to slightly irregular nuclei, finely dispersed chromatin and variably prominent nucleoli (Figure 84.2).[2,4,5]

Immunophenotype

The lymphoma cells express pan B-cell markers (CD20, CD19, PAX5, CD79A). Many cases express CD10 (65%-77%) and BCL6 (80%-91%), while the expression of MUM1 is slightly less common (46%-63%). As a result, most cases are classified as germinal center B-cell-like (GCB), with the minority being non-GCB phenotype by the Hans algorithm. MYC expression is variable and reported in around 70% of cases, while BCL2 expression varies in different studies (54%-75%).[1,2,4,6] In one study, BL-like immunophenotype ($CD10^+/BCL6^+/BCL2^-$) was seen in 30% of cases.[4] Median Ki-67 is >85% but can be variable. CD5 expression is occasionally seen.[4,5] TdT can be rarely expressed (in around 10% of cases or less), typically in cases with blastoid morphology, and expression is usually variable and in a subset of cells.[2,4]

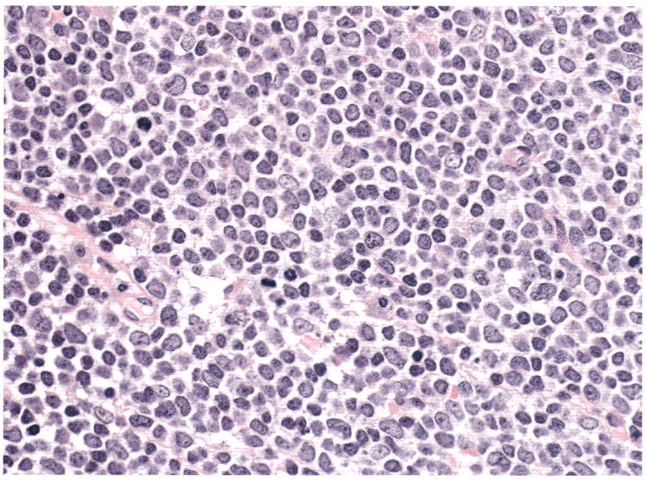

FIGURE 84.2 High-grade B-cell lymphoma, NOS with blastoid morphology. Lymphoma cells are reminiscent of lymphoblasts, medium sized with round to slightly irregular nuclei, finely dispersed chromatin, and small nucleoli.

Genetics

By conventional cytogenetic study, cases of HGBCL, NOS frequently have complex karyotype with multiple (≥3) structural/numerical abnormalities.[2,5,7] By definition, cases with *MYC* and *BCL2* and/or *BCL6* rearrangements are excluded from this category. However, *MYC* rearrangement (*MYC*-R) is seen in 13% to 46% of cases in different studies with most series showing >25%. *BCL2* rearrangement (without *MYC*-R) is seen in 5% to 13% of cases, while *BCL6* rearrangement (without *MYC*-R) is reported in 7% to 12% of cases.[1-4,6,8] As gains/amplification of *MYC*, *BCL2*, and *BCL6* are not equivalent to translocation for the purposes of defining HGBCL-DH, these alterations are allowed in cases of HGBCL, NOS.

Limited genetic data are available on these cases due to their rarity and relatively recent introduction into the classification scheme. In one study of HGBCL, NOS, 56% of cases were classified as GCB, 28% were classified as activated B cell, and 16% were unclassified by cell-of-origin gene expression profiling (GEP). In this series, 54% of cases showed a dark zone signature profile. Moreover, there were no significant differences in cytogenetic, GEP, or genomic features between HGBCL, NOS cases and cases that were reclassified as DLBCL (53% of cases) upon central review.[8]

Next-generation sequencing studies have detected recurrent mutations in *KMT2D*, *TP53*, *MYC*, *TNFRSF14*, *CXCR4*, and *TET2* each in >25% of cases.[2,8]

Prognosis and Clinical Comment

In the largest study of HGBCL, NOS, where current diagnostic criteria are used, progression-free survival at 2 years following immunochemotherapy was 55%. Most of the progression events occurred within the first 6 months. The optimal therapy for this group is uncertain, reflecting the biological heterogeneity encompassed therein. While the majority of patients in that cohort received escalated treatment regimens, eg dose adjusted etoposide, prednisolone, vincristine, cyclophosphamide, doxorubicin, and rituximab (DA-EPOCH-R) superiority of these regimens over rituximab, cyclophosphamide, doxorubicin, vincristine, and prednisolone (R-CHOP) was not demonstrated.

References

1. Li J, Liu X, Yao Z, Zhang M. High-grade B-cell lymphomas, not otherwise specified: a study of 41 cases. *Cancer Manag Res*. 2020;12:1903-1912.
2. Li S, Qiu L, Xu J, et al. High-grade B-cell lymphoma (HGBL)-NOS is clinicopathologically and genetically more similar to DLBCL/HGBL-DH than DLBCL. *Leukemia*. 2023;37(2):422-432.
3. Olszewski AJ, Kurt H, Evens AM. Defining and treating high-grade B-cell lymphoma, NOS. *Blood*. 2022;140(9):943-954.
4. Zayac AS, Landsburg DJ, Hughes ME, et al. High-grade B-cell lymphoma, not otherwise specified: a multi-institutional retrospective study. *Blood Adv*. 2023;7(21):6381-6394.
5. Kanagal-Shamanna R, Medeiros LJ, Lu G, et al. High-grade B cell lymphoma, unclassifiable, with blastoid features: an unusual morphological subgroup associated frequently with BCL2 and/or MYC gene rearrangements and a poor prognosis. *Histopathology*. 2012;61(5):945-954.
6. Huttl KS, Staiger AM, Richter J, et al. The "Burkitt-like" immunophenotype and genotype is rarely encountered in diffuse large B cell lymphoma and high-grade B cell lymphoma, NOS. *Virchows Arch*. 2021;479(3):575-583.
7. Perry AM, Crockett D, Dave BJ, et al. B-cell lymphoma, unclassifiable, with features intermediate between diffuse large B-cell lymphoma and burkitt lymphoma: study of 39 cases. *Br J Haematol*. 2013;162(1):40-49.
8. Collinge BJH LK, Wong J, Ben-Neriah S, et al. Characterization of the genetic landscape of high-grade B-cell lymphoma, NOS - an LLMPP project. *Hematol Oncol*. 2021;39:S2.

Chapter 85

Primary Mediastinal Large B-Cell Lymphoma

Sarah L. Ondrejka, Adam Bagg, and Kerry J. Savage

Definition

Primary mediastinal large B-cell lymphoma (PMBL) is an aggressive neoplasm of mature B cells that arises within the thymic niche of the mediastinum, with the thymic medullary B cell as its postulated normal counterpart. PMBL has distinctive morphologic, immunophenotypic, and genetic features that establish it as a separate entity from diffuse large B-cell lymphoma, not otherwise specified. Gene expression profiling established that PMBL shares biologic and genetic features with classic Hodgkin lymphoma (CHL), with mediastinal gray zone lymphoma displaying features intermediate between the two.[1,2] Rarely, diffuse large B-cell lymphoma cases with a nonmediastinal location can have a molecular signature reminiscent of PMBL, which may become more relevant as gene expression becomes more available in routine practice.[3]

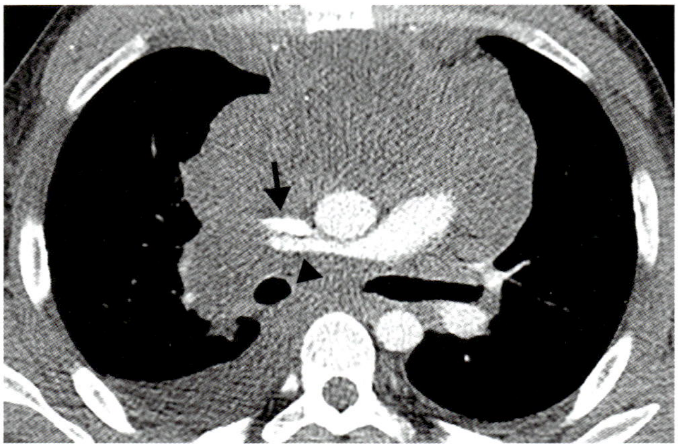

FIGURE 85.1 Axial contrast-enhanced computed tomography image from a 29-year-old with newly diagnosed primary mediastinal large B-cell lymphoma. There is a large anterior mediastinal soft tissue mass encasing and displacing the aorta and pulmonary trunk dorsally, with encasement and narrowing of the superior vena cava (arrow) and right pulmonary artery (arrowhead). There is associated right hilar lymphadenopathy and a small right pleural effusion. (Image courtesy of Ruchi Yadav, MD, Cleveland Clinic, Ohio, USA.)

Synonyms

Primary mediastinal (thymic) large B-cell lymphoma.

Epidemiology

PMBL accounts for approximately 6% to 10% of large B-cell lymphomas. The median age at presentation is in the third to fourth decade, and there is a female predominance. There is no established environmental exposure or geographic/ethnic tendency for development of PMBL, and there is limited information regarding genetic susceptibility.

General Clinical Features

By definition, patients present with an anterior mediastinal mass often with compressive symptoms including superior vena cava syndrome and rare vascular thrombosis (Figure 85.1). There is a propensity to invade adjacent thoracic structures including lung and pleura and pericardium, with associated effusions. Rarely, extrathoracic disease can occur at presentation, or at relapse including involvement of the kidneys, adrenal glands, liver, and central nervous system.[4,5]

Morphology

PMBL exhibits a diffuse growth pattern of medium- to large-sized neoplastic cells embedded in fine strands of fibrosis that may surround groups of cells forming a compartmentalizing or alveolar pattern. The cytologic features are varied, ranging from centroblast-like cells with round to ovoid nuclei to cells with variability in size and nuclear contours to cells with lobated nuclei and a higher degree of pleomorphism including Reed-Sternberg-like cells and variants (Figure 85.2). The cytoplasm is moderate to abundant and may be clear or faintly eosinophilic. There can be zonal necrosis, particularly in large tumors. If sampling is generous, a distorted thymic epithelial meshwork may be apparent, and this can form cystic structures (Figure 85.3).[5-7] The diagnosis of PMBL is challenging in small biopsy samples or in the presence of crush artifact. Adequate sampling of these specimens is essential to evaluate the growth pattern and cytologic characteristics and for full immunohistochemical analysis.

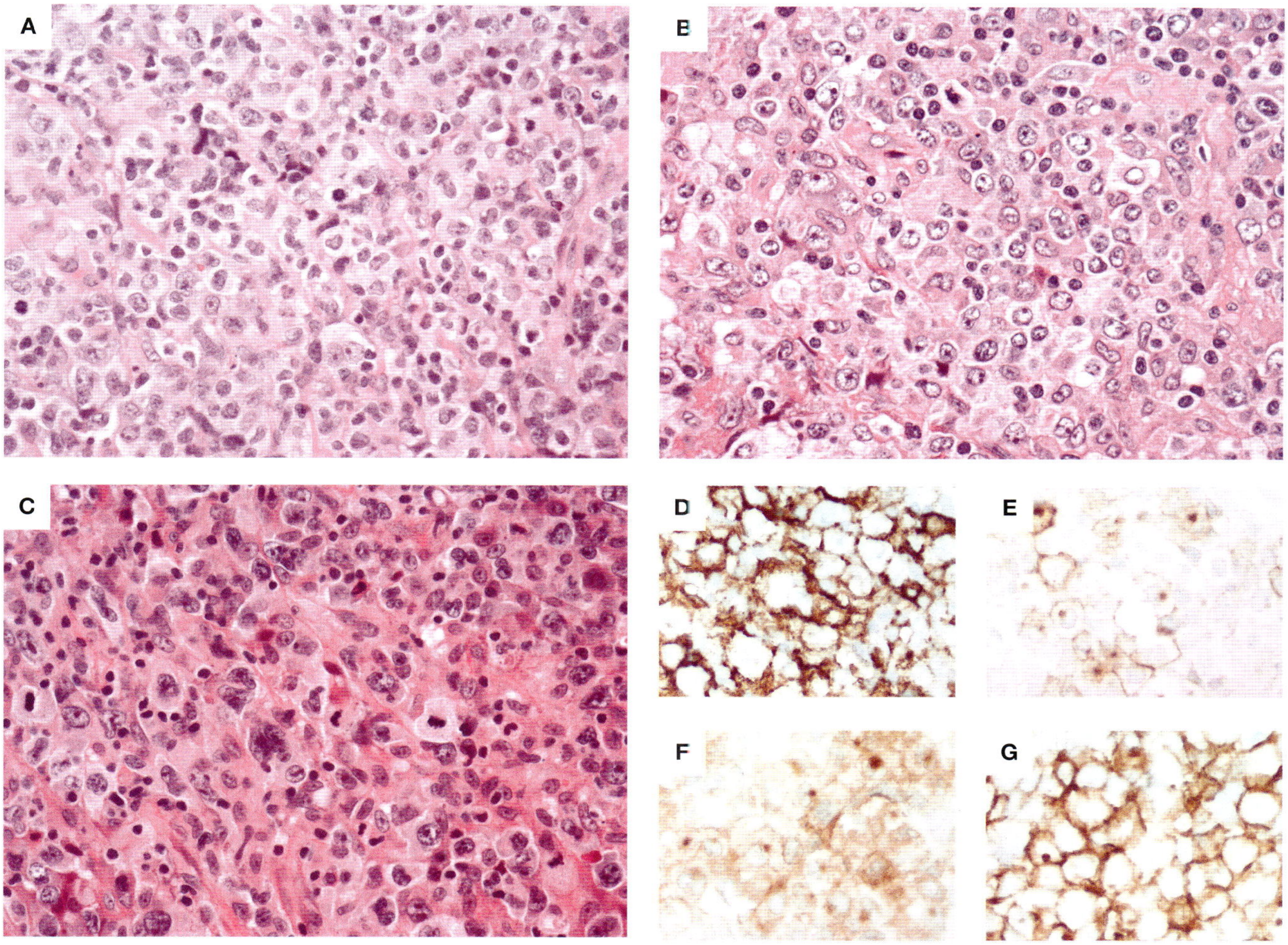

FIGURE 85.2 Primary mediastinal large B-cell lymphoma with delicate interstitial fibrosis and increasing degrees of pleomorphism **(A-C)**. Variable cellular morphology including **(A)** intermediate-sized cells with ovoid nuclei and nuclear irregularity, **(B)** moderate eosinophilic cytoplasm and prominent nucleoli, and **(C)** occasional Hodgkin/Reed-Sternberg-like variants. PMBL with positivity for CD20 **(D)**, heterogeneous CD30, **(E)**, MAL **(F)**, and CD23 **(G)**.

Immunophenotype

PMBL expresses B-cell lineage antigens including CD19, CD20, CD22, and PAX5, as well as the transcription factors OCT2, BOB.1, and PU.1. CD79a, which forms a component of the B-cell receptor heterodimer complex with immunoglobulin, is positive in PMBL despite a frequent lack of surface or cytoplasmic light chain immunoglobulin. CD30 is positive in most cases, but in contrast to CHL, it typically shows weak intensity and sometimes heterogeneous distribution. BCL2, MUM1, CD23, MAL, CD200, PDL1, and PDL2 are positive in ≥70% of cases. Nuclear c-Rel and cytoplasmic TRAF expression is seen in slightly over 60% of cases. CD15 may be expressed in a minority of cases and demonstrates a perinuclear dot-like pattern.[7,8] Positivity rates for BCL6 (45%-100%) and CD10 (20%-30%), together with a high frequency of somatically mutated IGHV genes, suggest derivation from a germinal center (GC) B-cell, noting that it is nevertheless distinct from DLBCL, NOS, GCB.[9]

Genetics

Immunoglobulin genes are clonally rearranged and class switched. *BCL6* rearrangement is uncommon (approximately 5% of cases), although *BCL6* mutations can be seen in more than 70% of cases. *BCL2* or *MYC* rearrangements are absent or rare. Copy number

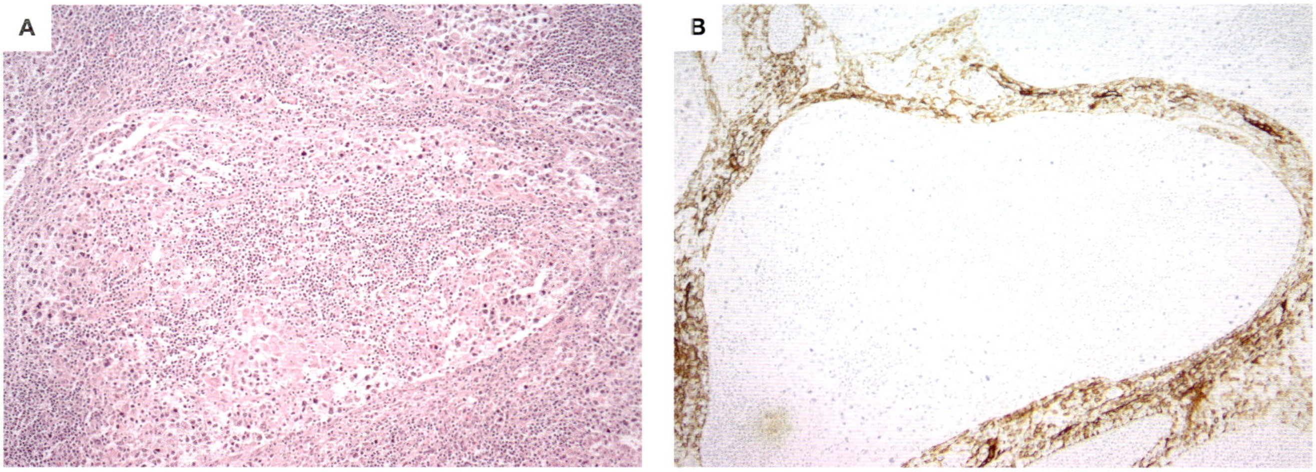

FIGURE 85.3 Primary mediastinal large B-cell lymphoma with altered thymic epithelium and growth of large tumor cells (**A**) around expanded cytokeratin AE1/AE3-positive epithelial networks (**B**).

gains are seen at 2p16.1/*REL* (leading to constitutive NF-κB signaling) and at 9p24.1 with amplifications of *JAK2*, *PDL1*, and *PDL2* (contributing to JAK-STAT activation and T-cell anergy).[10-12] A rearrangement or mutation of the class II MHC transactivator *CIITA* contributes to an immune escape mechanism and is seen in >50% of cases.[13] Gains involving other chromosomal loci including Xp11.4-21, Xq24-26, 7q22, 12q31, and 9q34 have also been reported in up to one-third of cases.[14]

The gene expression profile of PMBL is distinct from that of DLBCL but overlaps with that of CHL. There is increased expression of cytokine pathway members associated with JAK-STAT and NF-κB activation and effectors of IL-13 signaling and decreased expression of B-cell receptor signaling cascade components (Figure 85.4).[15,16] Recently developed gene expression–based tests, although not widely available, can differentiate PMBL from DLBCL, NOS.[17]

Characteristic mutations include those that inactivate negative regulators of NF-κB including *TNFAIP3* (~60%) and *NFKBIE* (~30%). Those impacting the JAK-STAT pathway include loss-of-function mutations in *SOCS1* (~60%) and *PTPN1* (~25%) and gain-of-function mutations in *STAT6* (~70%) and *IL4R*. The landscape also includes mutations involved in escape from T-cell immunity (*B2M*, *CD58*, *CIITA*) and mutations in *XPO1* and *ITPKB*.[18]

Prognosis and Clinical Comment

PMBL is associated with a more favorable survival than DLBCL, NOS. The standard prognostic index in DLBCL, the International Prognostic Index, has more limited utility in PMBL given the young age of presentation and often localized disease. Owing to relative disease rarity, there are no randomized controlled studies specifically in PMBL. However, rituximab and CHOP/CHOP-like chemotherapy regimen or dose-adjusted etoposide, prednisone, vincristine, cyclophosphamide, doxorubicin, and rituximab (DA-EPOCH-R) are considered standard, with the latter preferred in recent years as dose intensity may be important in some patients and most patients do not require radiotherapy.[19,20] More recently, the checkpoint inhibitor pembrolizumab has been explored given abundant PDL expression with long-term remissions with studies ongoing integrating them into the frontline setting.[21]

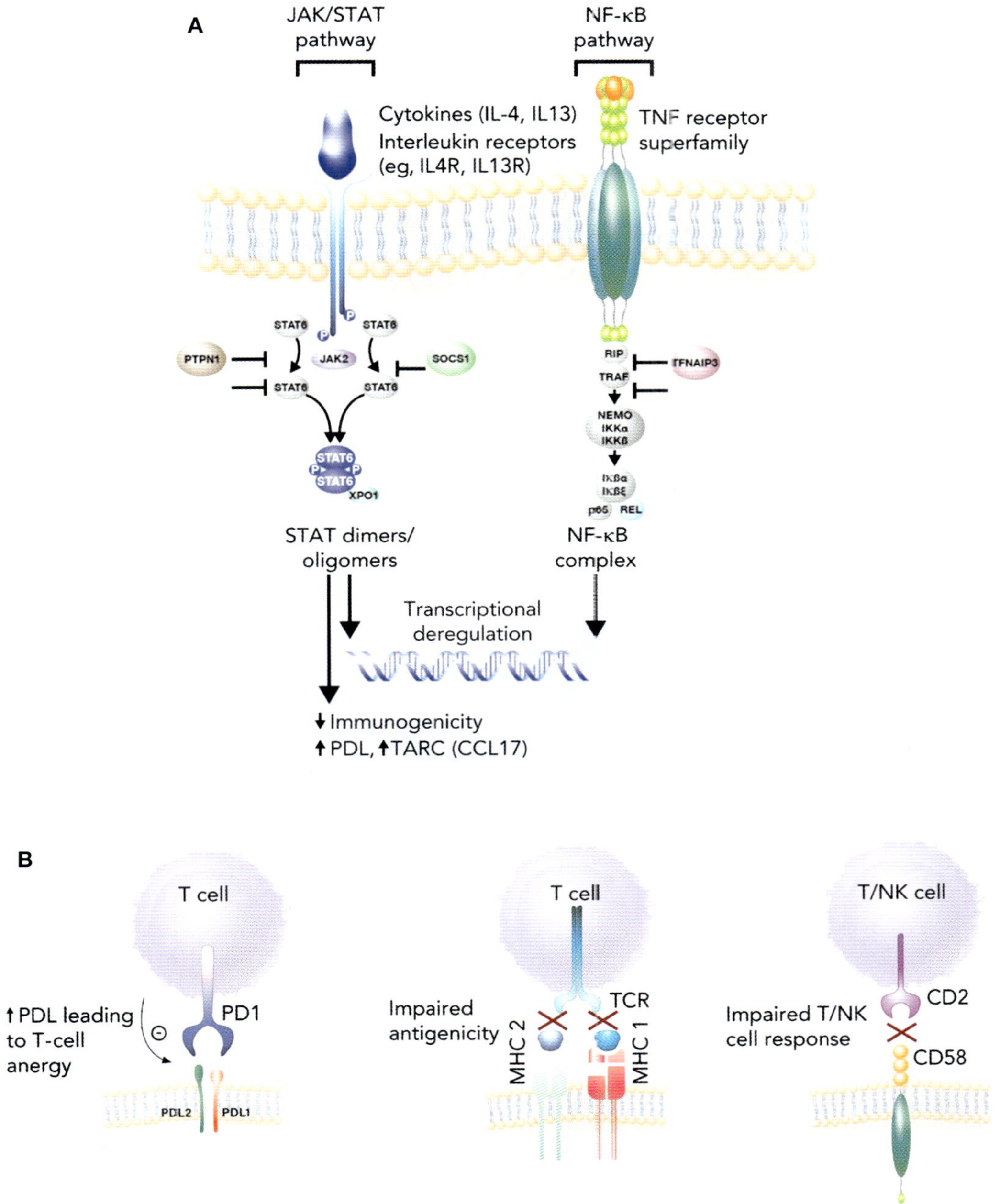

FIGURE 85.4 Key pathogenic hallmarks of primary mediastinal large B-cell lymphoma (PMBL) and pathway perturbation. **A:** JAK-STAT and NF-κB are key activation pathways in PMBL leading to transcriptional deregulation and impaired immunogenicity. **B:** Mechanisms of immune evasion in PMBL, including PDL1/2 expression with resultant T-cell anergy, reduced antigenicity through MHC class 2 down-regulation (in part, due to CIITA rearrangements and mutations), MHC class 1 defects caused by B2M mutations, and CD58 mutations/microdeletions leading to impaired T- and NK-cell interactions. (Reproduced from Savage KJ. Primary mediastinal large B-cell lymphoma (Figure 3). *Blood*. 2022;140(9):955-970.)

References

1. Rosenwald A, Wright G, Leroy K, et al. Molecular diagnosis of primary mediastinal B cell lymphoma identifies a clinically favorable subgroup of diffuse large B cell lymphoma related to Hodgkin lymphoma. *J Exp Med*. 2003;198(6):851-862.
2. Savage KJ, Monti S, Kutok JL, et al. The molecular signature of mediastinal large B-cell lymphoma differs from that of other diffuse large B-cell lymphomas and shares features with classical Hodgkin lymphoma. *Blood*. 2003;102(12):3871-3879.
3. Duns G, Viganò E, Ennishi D, et al. Characterization of DLBCL with a PMBL gene expression signature. *Blood*. 2021;138(2):136-148.

4. Abou-Elella AA, Weisenburger DD, Vose JM, et al. Primary mediastinal large B-cell lymphoma: a clinicopathologic study of 43 patients from the Nebraska Lymphoma Study Group. *J Clin Oncol.* 1999;17(3):784-790.
5. Cazals-Hatem D, Lepage E, Brice P, et al. Primary mediastinal large B-cell lymphoma. A clinicopathologic study of 141 cases compared with 916 nonmediastinal large B-cell lymphomas, a GELA ("Groupe d'Etude des Lymphomes de l'Adulte") study. *Am J Surg Pathol.* 1996;20(7):877-888.
6. Oschlies I, Burkhardt B, Salaverria I, et al. Clinical, pathological and genetic features of primary mediastinal large B-cell lymphomas and mediastinal gray zone lymphomas in children. *Haematologica.* 2011;96(2):262-268.
7. Gibson SE, Dojcinov S, Dotlic S, et al. Mediastinal large B cell lymphoma and surrounding gray areas: a report of the lymphoma workshop of the 20th meeting of the European Association for Haematopathology. *Virchows Arch.* 2023;483(6):733-749.
8. Pileri SA, Zinzani PL, Gaidano G, et al. Pathobiology of primary mediastinal B-cell lymphoma. *Leuk Lymphoma.* 2003;44:S21-S26.
9. de Leval L, Ferry JA, Falini B, Shipp M, Harris NL. Expression of bcl-6 and CD10 in primary mediastinal large B-cell lymphoma: evidence for derivation from germinal center B cells? *Am J Surg Pathol.* 2001;25(10):1277-1282.
10. Shi M, Roemer MG, Chapuy B, et al. Expression of programmed cell death 1 ligand 2 (PD-L2) is a distinguishing feature of primary mediastinal (thymic) large B-cell lymphoma and associated with PDCD1LG2 copy gain. *Am J Surg Pathol.* 2014;38(12):1715-1723.
11. Twa DD, Chan FC, Ben-Neriah S, et al. Genomic rearrangements involving programmed death ligands are recurrent in primary mediastinal large B-cell lymphoma. *Blood.* 2014;123(13):2062-2065.
12. Joos S, Otaño-Joos MI, Ziegler S, et al. Primary mediastinal (thymic) B-cell lymphoma is characterized by gains of chromosomal material including 9p and amplification of the REL gene. *Blood.* 1996;87(4):1571-1578.
13. Mottok A, Woolcock B, Chan FC, et al. Genomic alterations in CIITA are frequent in primary mediastinal large B cell lymphoma and are associated with diminished MHC class II expression. *Cell Rep.* 2015;13(7):1418-1431.
14. Wessendorf S, Barth TF, Viardot A, et al. Further delineation of chromosomal consensus regions in primary mediastinal B-cell lymphomas: an analysis of 37 tumor samples using high-resolution genomic profiling (array-CGH). *Leukemia.* 2007;21(12):2463-2469.
15. Feuerhake F, Kutok JL, Monti S, et al. NFkappaB activity, function, and target-gene signatures in primary mediastinal large B-cell lymphoma and diffuse large B-cell lymphoma subtypes. *Blood.* 2005;106(4):1392-1399.
16. Savage KJ. Primary mediastinal large B-cell lymphoma. *Blood.* 2022;140(9):955-970.
17. Mottok A, Wright G, Rosenwald A, et al. Molecular classification of primary mediastinal large B-cell lymphoma using routinely available tissue specimens. *Blood.* 2018;132(22):2401-2405.
18. Dubois S, Viailly PJ, Mareschal S, et al. Next-generation sequencing in diffuse large B-cell lymphoma highlights molecular divergence and therapeutic opportunities: a LYSA study. *Clin Cancer Res.* 2016;22(12):2919-2928.
19. Hayden AR, Tonseth P, Lee DG, et al. Outcome of primary mediastinal large B-cell lymphoma using R-CHOP: impact of a PET-adapted approach. *Blood.* 2020;136(24):2803-2811.
20. Dunleavy K, Pittaluga S, Maeda LS, et al. Dose-adjusted EPOCH-rituximab therapy in primary mediastinal B-cell lymphoma. *N Engl J Med.* 2013;368(15):1408-1416.
21. Zinzani PL, Thieblemont C, Melnichenko V, et al. Pembrolizumab in relapsed or refractory primary mediastinal large B-cell lymphoma: final analysis of KEYNOTE-170. *Blood.* 2023;142(2):141-145.

Chapter 86

Mediastinal Gray Zone Lymphoma

Elaine S. Jaffe, Kieron Dunleavy, and Stefania Pittaluga

Definition

Mediastinal gray zone lymphoma (MGZL) is an aggressive B-cell lymphoma with immunopathological features intermediate between mediastinal classic Hodgkin lymphoma (CHL) and primary mediastinal large B-cell lymphoma (PMBL), with a close biological relationship to both parent entities.[1] Cases with overlapping features between CHL and diffuse large B-cell lymphoma (DLBCL) and presenting without involvement of the thymic niche are generally excluded from this category and share genomic features with DLBCL, NOS.

Synonyms

B-cell lymphoma, unclassifiable, with features intermediate between diffuse large B-cell lymphoma and classic Hodgkin lymphoma.

Epidemiology

This tumor is most common in adolescents and young adults, between the ages of 20 and 40 years.[2] It is more common in males than females. Most cases have been reported in Western countries. MGZL parallels the prevalence of the parent entities, CHL, nodular sclerosis subtype (NS), and PMBL, in terms of populations at greatest risk. It is rare in the elderly.

General Clinical Features

Most patients present with a bulky anterior mediastinal mass, sometimes leading to superior vena cava syndrome. Lesions demonstrate hypermetabolism on positron emission tomography imaging, which is helpful for disease response assessment and posttreatment surveillance. Regional lymph node involvement may be seen, but distant lymph node involvement at presentation is uncommon. Pleural and sometimes pericardial effusions may be present. B symptoms are common.

Morphology

MGZL is typically composed of a confluent, sheet-like growth of pleomorphic tumor cells with a variably fibrotic stromal background.[1] Well-formed fibrous bands are less common than in CHL, NS. A key feature for diagnosis is high tumor cell density, and focal necrosis is common. The cells are larger and more pleomorphic than in the typical case of PMBL, although some centroblast-like cells may be present (Figure 86.1). Some cells may resemble Hodgkin/Reed Sternberg cells or lacunar variants. However, the cells typically show a broad spectrum of cytologic appearances, including a range in cell size and nuclear pleomorphism. Different areas of the tumor may show variation in the cytologic appearance. Admixed small lymphocytes and histiocytes are readily seen. However, eosinophils or plasma cells are less common than in CHL. MGZL should be distinguished from tumor cell-rich forms of CHL, NS (grade 2)

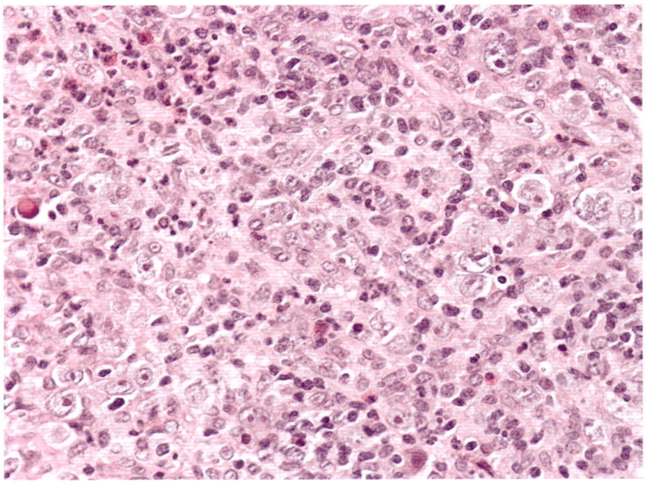

FIGURE 86.1 This example of mediastinal gray zone lymphoma was diagnosed in a 22-year-old woman with a large mediastinal mass. The growth pattern is diffuse and tumor cell rich but with an inflammatory background of histiocytes, small lymphocytes, and few granulocytes. Many large pleomorphic cells are present, with some of them resembling Hodgkin/Reed Sternberg cells. However, they show a spectrum in cell size, and many intermediate forms are present as well. Fine fibrosis can be seen in the background.

based on cytological and architectural features, as well as immunophenotype.

Sequential occurrences of CHL, NS, and PMBL are a related biological phenomenon to MGZL and in selected cases studied have shown evidence of clonal identity. It is somewhat more common for the disease to present as CHL and relapse as PMBL, but both situations have been reported. Cases with thymic involvement may show cystic changes within the gland, attesting to the likely thymic origin of the tumor.

Immunophenotype

Most cases of MGZL show upregulation of the B-cell program with expression of CD19, CD20, and CD79a, usually in the majority of tumor cells (Figure 86.2).[1,3] As CD20 can be focally and variably expressed in many cases of CHL, expression of at least two B-cell markers is desirable.[4] The transcription factors OCT2 and BOB.1 are usually positive as well. Some authors have applied less stringent criteria, accepting a diagnosis of MGZL in cases that would otherwise fulfill histological criteria for CHL, NS based on staining for CD20 in a subset of, or the majority of, tumor cells.[5] CD30 is nearly always positive in the majority of the tumor cells, but CD15 is either negative or positive in a small subset of tumor cells. MUM1 is strongly expressed. PD-L1 is often positive, with comparable alterations at the genetic level, leading to effective therapy with checkpoint inhibitors in some studies.[6,7]

The above-mentioned description applies to most cases of MGZL. However, a small subset of cases show a histologic appearance on hematoxylin and eosin that resembles PMBL but display a phenotype characteristic

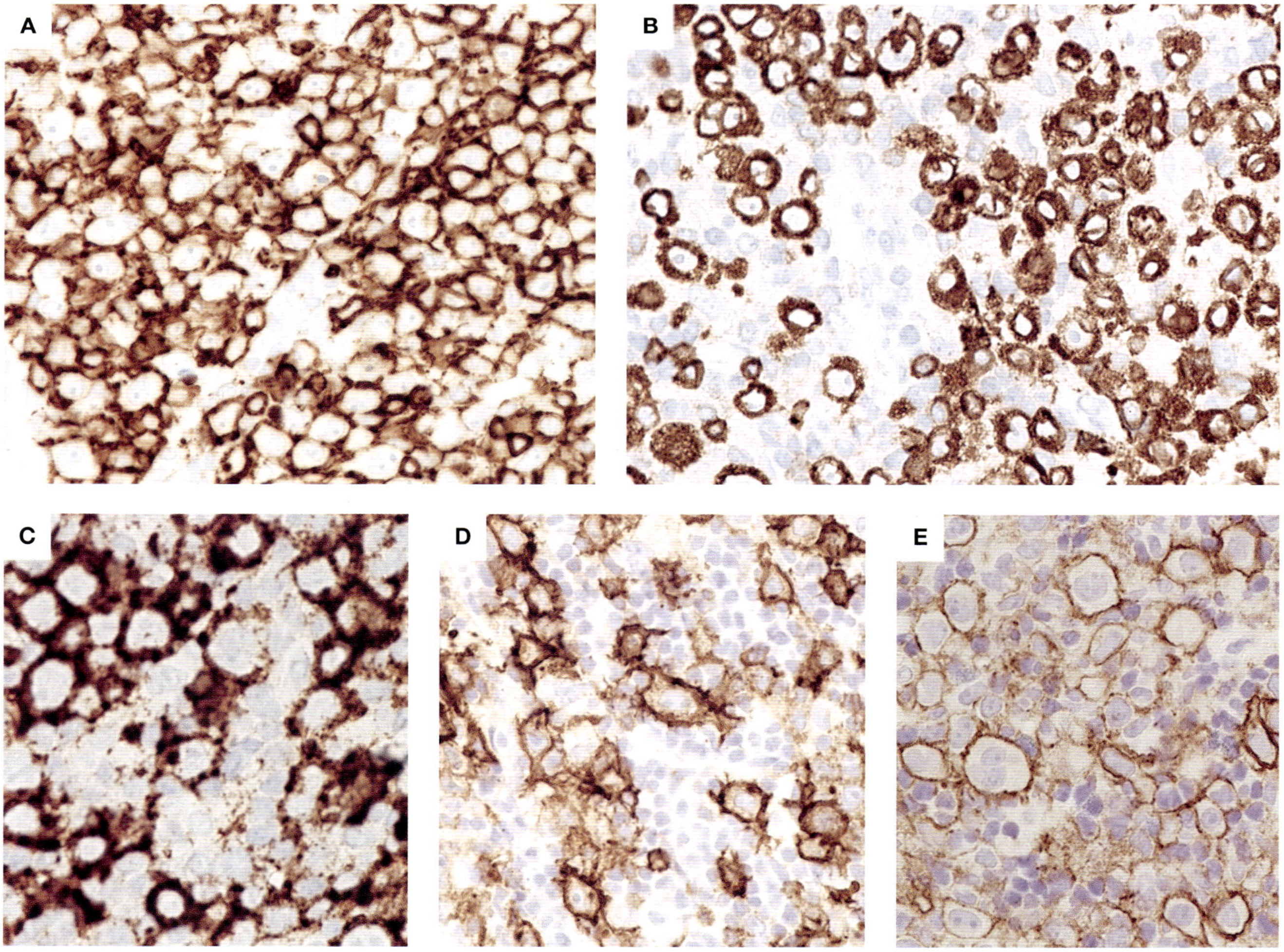

FIGURE 86.2 Immunohistochemical findings in mediastinal gray zone lymphoma. **A:** The tumor cells are strongly and uniformly positive for CD20. **B:** They are also strongly positive for CD79a, and CD30 **(C)**. **D:** A subset of tumor cells are positive for CD23, as might be seen in primary mediastinal large B-cell lymphoma. **E:** The tumor cells are positive for PD-L1, a finding that is associated with amplification of the PD-L1/L2 locus.

of CHL, with negative staining for B-cell markers and expression of both CD30 and CD15[3] (Figure 86.3).

Epstein-Barr virus (EBV) assessed by EBER in situ hybridization is typically negative, although rare cases of true MGZL can be EBV positive. EBV positivity should prompt consideration for a diagnosis of EBV-positive DLBCL, NOS, which can show partial loss of B-cell antigens and often express CD30.

Genetics

Fluorescence in situ hybridization studies have provided evidence for the close relationship of MGZL to both CHL, NS and PMBL. Common findings include amplifications in 2p16.1 (*REL/BCL11A* locus), alterations affecting the *JAK2/PDL2* locus at 9p24.1, and rearrangement of the *CIITA* locus at 16p13.13.[3] By next-generation sequencing, mutations in *SOCS1, B2M, TNFAIP3, GNA13, LRRN3,* and *NFKBIA* have been reported.[8] The involvement of JAK-STAT and NF-κB pathways is similar to that seen in CHL. Notably, the usual alterations most commonly seen in sporadic DLBCL are absent, eg, genes related to germinal center–derived DLBCL (*KMT2D, CREBBP,* and *BCL2*), with an absence of translocations involving *BCL2, BCL6,* and *MYC*.[8]

Studies employing methylation and gene expression profiling have confirmed a close relationship between MGZL and both PMBL and CHL.[9,10] Expression signatures related to germinal center B cells and IRF4 are low, while T-cell and macrophage signatures more closely resemble CHL rather than PMBL.

Prognosis and Clinical Comment

MGZL has a more aggressive clinical course than either PMBL or CHL. The most commonly used treatment regimen has been dose-adjusted etoposide phosphate (E), prednisone (P), vincristine sulfate (Oncovin), cyclophosphamide (C), and doxorubicin hydrochloride (H) (hydroxydaunorubicin), and rituximab (R), with the addition of radiation therapy in patients with locally resistant disease.[2] Both doxorubicin hydrochloride (Adriamycin), bleomycin

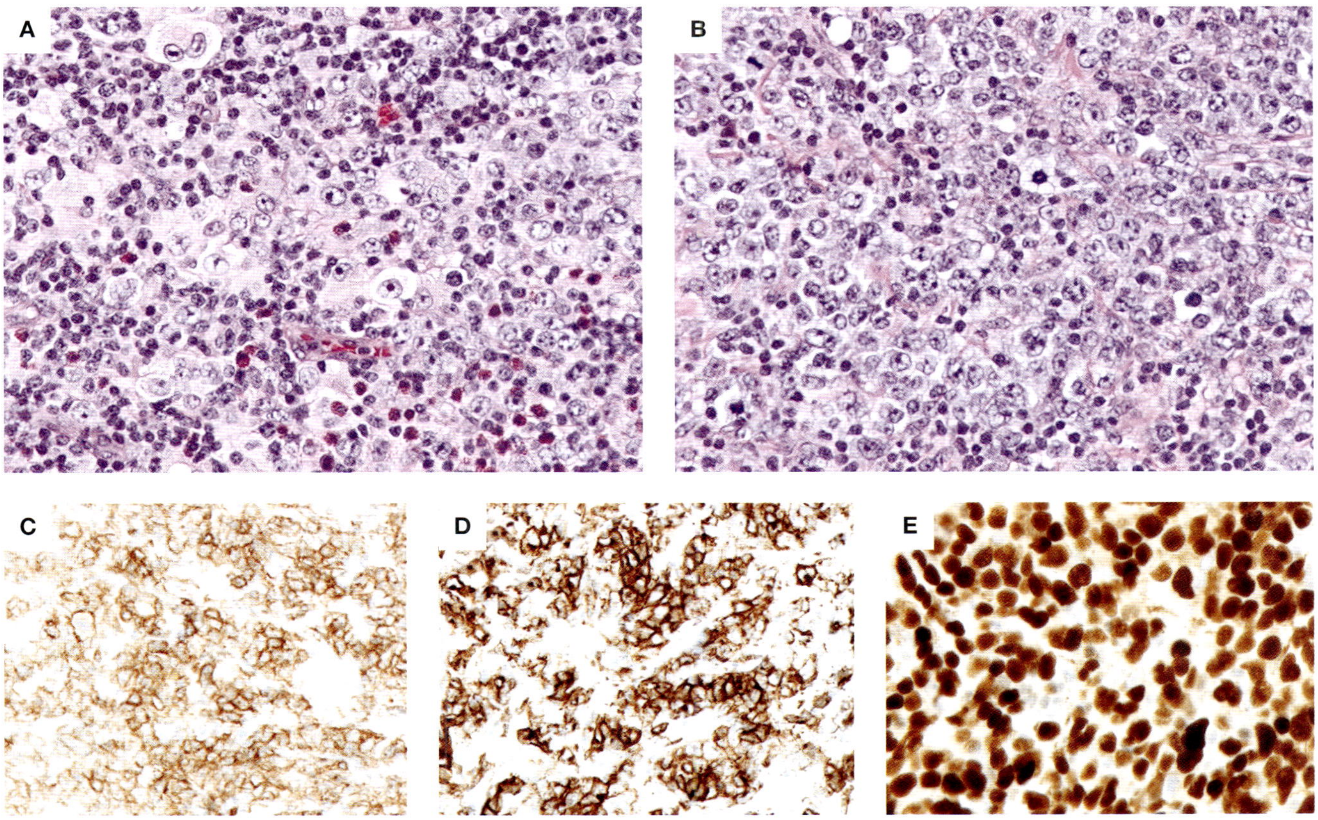

FIGURE 86.3 Variant histological patterns in mediastinal gray zone lymphoma. **A:** This area of the lesion closely resembles classic Hodgkin lymphoma with lacunar-type cells and admixed eosinophils. **B:** This portion of the same biopsy resembles primary mediastinal large B-cell lymphoma. By immunohistochemistry, tumor cells are positive for CD30 **(C)**, CD15 **(D)**, and OCT2 **(E)**.

sulfate, vinblastine sulfate, and dacarbazine and rituximab, cyclophosphamide, doxorubicin hydrochloride (hydroxydaunomycin), and vincristine sulfate (Oncovin), and prednisone have been less effective than other high-dose regimens such as escalated bleomycin sulfate, etoposide phosphate, doxorubicin hydrochloride (adriamycin), cyclophosphamide, vincristine sulfate (oncovin), procarbazine hydrochloride, prednisone.[11] In multivariate prognostic analysis, Eastern Cooperative Oncology Group-performance scale and anemia were the strongest factors associated with a shorter event-free survival and overall survival, respectively. For patients with nonlocalized relapsed/refractory disease, there is no standard approach but strategies such as immune checkpoint inhibition are rational and effective in albeit limited series.[6,7]

References

1. Traverse-Glehen A, Pittaluga S, Gaulard P, et al. Mediastinal gray zone lymphoma: the missing link between classic Hodgkin's lymphoma and mediastinal large B-cell lymphoma. *Am J Surg Pathol.* 2005;29(11):1411-1421.
2. Wilson WH, Pittaluga S, Nicolae A, et al. A prospective study of mediastinal gray-zone lymphoma. *Blood.* 2014;124(10):1563-1569.
3. Eberle FC, Salaverria I, Steidl C, et al. Gray zone lymphoma: chromosomal aberrations with immunophenotypic and clinical correlations. *Mod Pathol.* 2011;24(12):1586-1597.
4. Campo E, Jaffe ES, Cook JR, et al. The international consensus classification of mature lymphoid neoplasms: a report from the clinical advisory committee. *Blood.* 2022;140(11):1229-1253.
5. Sarkozy C, Copie-Bergman C, Damotte D, et al. Gray-zone lymphoma between cHL and large B-cell lymphoma: a histopathologic series from the LYSA. *Am J Surg Pathol.* 2019;43(3):341-351.
6. Melani C, Major A, Schowinsky J, et al. PD-1 blockade in mediastinal gray-zone lymphoma. *N Engl J Med.* 2017;377(1):89-91.
7. Santoro A, Moskowitz AJ, Ferrari S, et al. Nivolumab combined with brentuximab vedotin for relapsed/refractory mediastinal gray zone lymphoma. *Blood.* 2023;141(22):2780-2783.
8. Sarkozy C, Hung SS, Chavez EA, et al. Mutational landscape of gray zone lymphoma. *Blood.* 2021;137(13):1765-1776.
9. Eberle FC, Rodriguez-Canales J, Wei L, et al. Methylation profiling of mediastinal gray zone lymphoma reveals a distinctive signature with elements shared by classical Hodgkin's lymphoma and primary mediastinal large B-cell lymphoma. *Haematologica.* 2011;96(4):558-566.
10. Pittaluga S, Nicolae A, Wright GW, et al. Gene expression profiling of mediastinal gray zone lymphoma and its relationship to primary mediastinal B-cell lymphoma and classical Hodgkin lymphoma. *Blood Cancer Discov.* 2020;1(2):155-161.
11. Sarkozy C, Molina T, Ghesquieres H, et al. Mediastinal gray zone lymphoma: clinico-pathological characteristics and outcomes of 99 patients from the Lymphoma Study Association. *Haematologica.* 2017;102(1):150-159.

Chapter 87
Classic Hodgkin Lymphoma

Pierre Brousset, Steve M. Ansell, Ann LaCasce, Lauren B. Smith, Charlotte Syrykh, Thomas A. Tousseyn, and Girish Venkataraman

Definition

Classic Hodgkin lymphoma (CHL) is a monoclonal lymphoid neoplasm derived from germinal center B cells with an incomplete B-cell program,[1] characterized by the presence of scattered Hodgkin/Reed-Sternberg (HRS) cells, with a predominant tumor microenvironment (TME) made of nonneoplastic stromal and immune cells. There are four main subtypes: nodular sclerosis classic Hodgkin lymphoma (NSCHL), lymphocyte-rich classic Hodgkin lymphoma (LRCHL), mixed-cellularity classic Hodgkin lymphoma (MCCHL), and lymphocyte depleted classic Hodgkin lymphoma (LDCHL).

Synonyms

None

Epidemiology

The average annual age-adjusted incidence of CHL in the United States and Europe is 2 to 3 cases per 100,000 individuals. There is no significant increase over the last 2 decades compared to non-Hodgkin lymphomas.[2,3] Among noncutaneous lymphomas, CHL represents 14% of all cases.[4] The highest incidence is in patients with high socioeconomic index[5] with equal distribution by sex except for NSCHL subtype where there is a slight male predominance (1.5:1). CHL is rare in children (<18 years of age) with an increase in incidence peaking first in young adults between 25 and 35 years and peaking again after 55 years in Europe, Asia, and the United States. This bimodal distribution is not observed in Black or Hispanic populations.[5] There is a slight increase of CHL incidence in individuals with a first-degree relative affected with CHL.[6] In this regard, some genetic susceptibilities have been identified, with HLA-A*01:01 and B*37:01 being associated with an increased risk of Epstein-Barr virus (EBV)-positive CHL, whereas DRB1*15:01 and DPB1*01:01 are associated with a decreased risk.[7,8] For EBV-negative CHL, the class II SNP rs6903608 remained the strongest predictor of disease risk after adjusting for the effects of common HLA alleles.[8] Genome-wide association studies in populations of European ancestry have identified 18 genetic risk variants primarily in immune-related genes.[9,10] Several conditions illustrating some deficiency of immune response against EBV (infectious mononucleosis, HIV/AIDS, organ transplantations, or immunosuppressive drugs) increase the risk of developing CHL.[11] EBV itself is considered a risk factor, in particular in MCCHL cases and cases occurring in younger individuals from developing countries.[7,11] Latent EBV infection is present in 40% of the cases (75% in MCCHL and LDCHL, 15% in LRCHL, 10% in NSCHL).[8,12] The role of EBV is illustrated by a higher incidence of CHL after infectious mononucleosis (sometimes 10-15 years after)[10] and the frequency of EBV-positive cases in patients from developing countries.[11] Immune senescence might be associated with both the second peak of incidence of CHL after 55 years and the frequent presence of EBV in the tumor cells. EBV-positive CHL is more common in individuals with acquired immunodeficiency or those with organ transplantation.

General Clinical Features

CHL may involve various sites in the body with a predilection for lymph nodes: primary extranodal involvement is rare. Most patients present with asymptomatic lymphadenopathy. B symptoms are relatively uncommon in early-stage disease (20% of cases) but more frequently encountered in patients with advanced stage disease (60%). Two-thirds of early-stage CHL patients present with cervical, supraclavicular, or mediastinal involvement (Figure 87.1). Isolated abdominopelvic lymphadenopathy or presentation with splenic masses is rare, and more frequently encountered in the elderly. Involvement of extranodal sites such as the spleen, lung, liver, and bone marrow can be seen and is more likely in the setting of HIV. Paraneoplastic syndromes such as itching (pruritus), nephrotic syndrome, hemolytic anemia, and idiopathic thrombocytopenic purpura

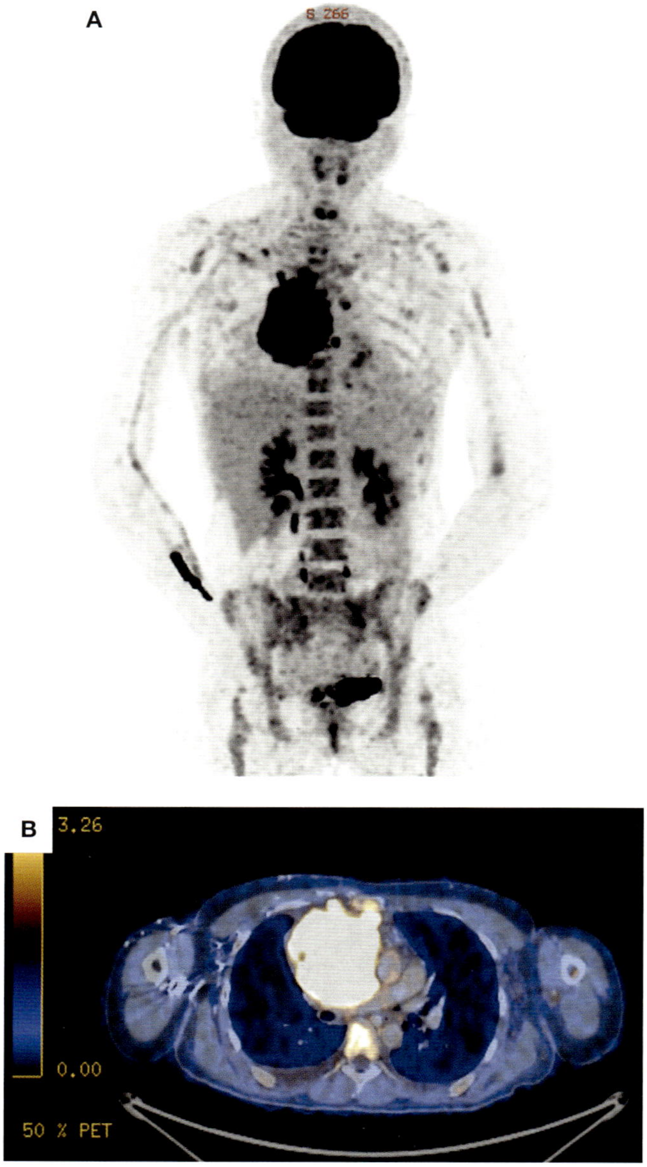

FIGURE 87.1 Radiological aspect of classic Hodgkin lymphoma involving the mediastinum. FDG-PET MIP **(A)** and axial fused PET/CT **(B)** showing increased FDG uptake in the mediastinum.

are rarely reported.[13] Laboratory findings often include microcytic anemia (often mimicking iron deficiency), leukocytosis with neutrophilia or eosinophilia, lymphopenia, and increased levels of inflammatory markers.

Different patterns of presentation and related symptoms are associated with different subtypes. NSCHL often presents with stage II disease and is associated with mediastinal involvement in 80% of the cases. In one-half of these patients, mediastinal involvement is characterized by bulky masses, which may cause respiratory symptoms and sometimes superior vena cava syndrome, although this is more common in primary mediastinal large B-cell lymphoma. B symptoms are seen in 30% to 40% of patients. MCCHL more frequently involves extranodal sites (stage IV disease) and patients more frequently suffer B symptoms. In LDCHL, widespread involvement of many lymph node areas and extranodal sites is often observed with frequent involvement of retroperitoneal lymph nodes and the bone marrow. B symptoms are common. There is no site predilection in LRCHL. Patients present with stage I or II disease and only rarely have B symptoms.

CHL very rarely involves the skin, Waldeyer ring, or the central nervous system and should be diagnosed with extreme caution in these sites where it is typically seen in the setting of advanced disease.

Morphology

Involved lymph nodes are significantly enlarged, and the macroscopic findings vary with the histological subtypes. Sclerotic hyaline fibrosis is characteristic of the NSCHL subtype. Necrosis may be apparent, and splenic involvement displays nodules of variable size.

Tumor cells characteristic of CHL are mononuclear Hodgkin cells and bi- or multinucleated Reed-Sternberg (RS) cells within a mixed inflammatory background corresponding to the TME. In some cases, the tumor cells are difficult to see as they may account for fewer than 1% to 10% of the number of cells in the infiltrate. It is possible to find typical RS cells in almost all cases, but they are usually not as numerous as mononucleated Hodgkin cells. RS cells display variable morphologic features and are generally very large (>30-40 μm) compared to mature lymphocytes (8-10 μm). They have large nuclei with prominent eosinophilic nucleoli. The characteristic RS cell has at least two nuclei, sometimes mirrored, with large eosinophilic nucleoli surrounded by a perinuclear halo (Figure 87.2A). Hodgkin cells are mononuclear cells with a round nucleus and a prominent nucleolus (Figure 87.2B).

Lacunar cells are characteristic of NSCHL. They correspond to large HRS cells with a single, large, central eosinophilic nucleolus. They have abundant cytoplasm and a characteristic "lacunar" or "empty space" with wisps of cytoplasm, resulting from formalin fixation–induced retraction of the cell cytoplasm producing a large space between the nucleus and surrounding TME (Figure 87.2C). Apoptotic cells, known as "mummified" cells, are frequently observed (Figure 87.2D). In some cases, mononuclear cells with morphologic features of

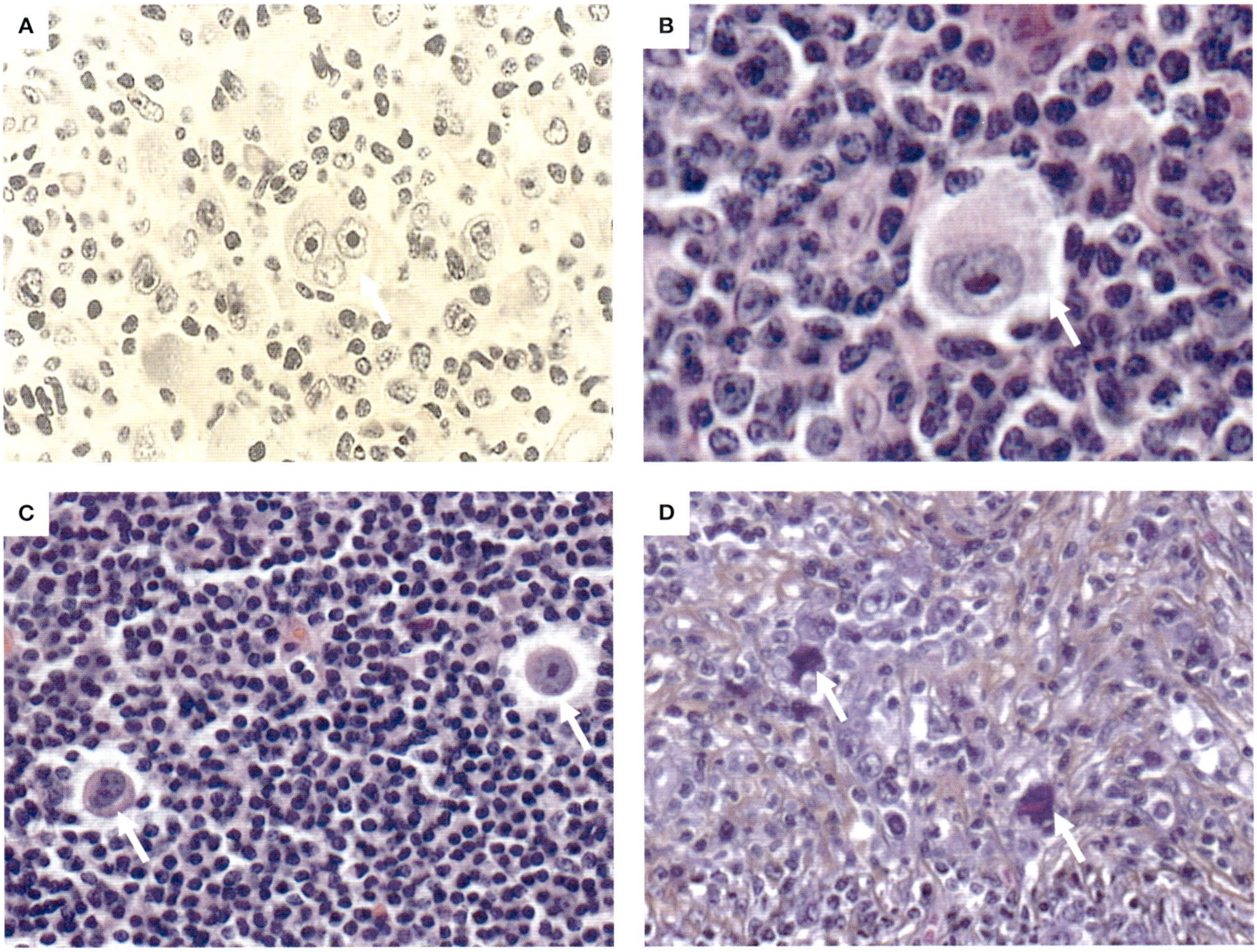

FIGURE 87.2 Cytologic features of classic Hodgkin lymphoma cell types. **A:** Reed-Sternberg cells (arrow) showing bilobated to multilobated nucleus, prominent eosinophilic nucleoli, and amphophilic cytoplasm. **B:** Hodgkin cell (arrow) showing a single round nucleus with prominent eosinophilic nucleolus. **C:** Lacunar cells (arrows) with pale retracted cytoplasm. **D:** Mummified cells (arrows) characterized by condensed hyperchromatic nuclei.

anaplastic cells predominate. They are homogeneous in size with crownlike or horseshoe-shaped nuclei. Mitoses are generally rare although the cells are in cycle (Ki-67$^+$).

The TME consists of T and B lymphocytes, plasma cells, histiocytes/macrophages (M1 and M2), neutrophils, eosinophils, mast cells, mesenchymal stromal cells, and endothelial cells. T cells predominate, and it is not clear whether or not the TME is skewed toward a TH2 cell-mediated immune response.[6] In some cases, T follicular helper (TFH) cells can be abundant and obscure the diagnosis, especially on core needle biopsies (see below). The lymphocyte-rich subtype may include abundant reactive B cells of mantle zone type within a dense follicular dendritic cell (FDC) network.

Subtypes

Four subtypes of CHL are recognized (NSCHL, MCCHL, LRCHL, and LDCHL), but the most important information for optimal therapeutic management is to distinguish CHL from other entities in the differential diagnosis.

NSCHL is the most frequent subtype, accounting for 70% of all CHL cases. The affected lymph node typically shows a characteristic pattern of nodules or discrete cellular areas, separated by bands of fibrous tissue ("compartmentalizing" sclerosis) associated with capsular thickening (Figure 87.3). This nodular appearance is a hallmark of NSCHL. Although classical HRS cells can be observed, lacunar cells predominate (Figure 87.4). The neoplastic HRS cells are embedded in an abundant polymorphous inflammatory TME composed of histiocytes,

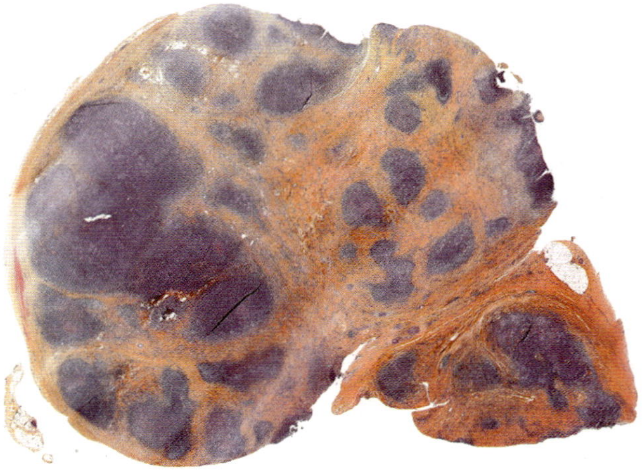

FIGURE 87.3 Nodular sclerosis classic Hodgkin lymphoma. Cellular nodules are separated by bands of collagen.

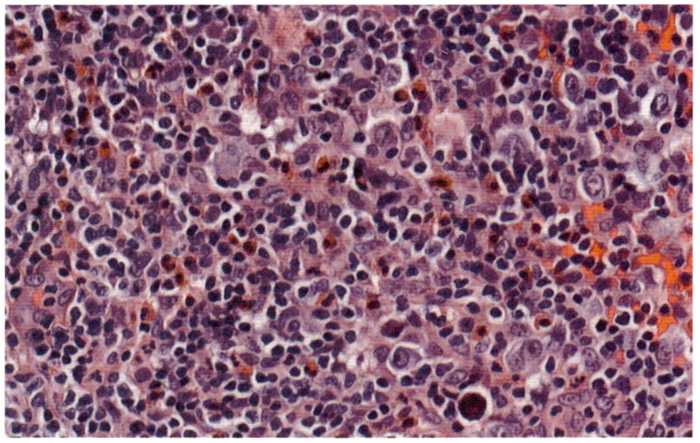

FIGURE 87.5 Nodular sclerosis classic Hodgkin lymphoma. Lymphoma cells are intermingled with a polymorphous inflammatory tumor microenvironment composed of histiocytes, eosinophils, few neutrophils, small lymphocytes, and plasma cells.

eosinophils, neutrophils, small lymphocytes, and variable numbers of plasma cells (Figure 87.5). The extent of obliteration of normal nodal architecture is variable. It is worth noting that the number of tumor cells may vary from case to case, but the grading system (grade 1/grade 2) proposed by the British National Lymphoma Investigation is no longer recommended.[14] Necrotic areas are frequently observed in tumor cell–rich cases.

MCCHL accounts for 20% to 25% of CHL cases. The lymph node architecture is frequently obliterated, but an interfollicular growth pattern can be observed. Necrosis and rarely bands of reticulin fibrosis may be present, but there is no capsular thickening or nodular pattern. Classical HRS and mononuclear variants are embedded in a TME-rich milieu consisting of small lymphocytes and histiocytes (sometimes epithelioid), with variable numbers of eosinophils and plasma cells (Figure 87.6). In rare instances, numerous epithelioid granulomata may obscure the diagnosis of CHL.

LRCHL is uncommon (5% of CHL cases) and is characterized by a predominantly nodular architecture ("nodular variant") (Figure 87.7) with frequent preservation of residual follicular architecture, although rare cases exhibit a diffuse pattern ("diffuse variant").[15] In contrast to NSCHL and MCCHL, the background is predominated by abundant small lymphocytes with a distinct paucity of other inflammatory cells (Figure 87.8).[14] Epithelioid histiocytes and other histiocytes, when present, are seen outside the nodules. The nodules are follicles composed of small mature B lymphocytes often surrounding regressed germinal centers containing attenuated FDC networks. In addition, the T zone is frequently attenuated. CD30-positive HRS cells are often seen within the mantle zones but not typically in the germinal centers (Figures 87.9-87.11). Rosettes of T cells (better appreciated using CD3 or PD1) can be seen around HRS cells (Figure 87.12). This, coupled with the

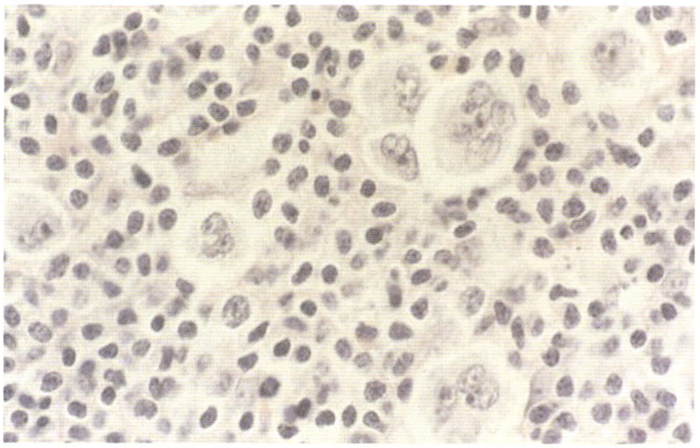

FIGURE 87.4 Nodular sclerosis classic Hodgkin lymphoma. Cellular nodule shows numerous lacunar cells with clear cytoplasm.

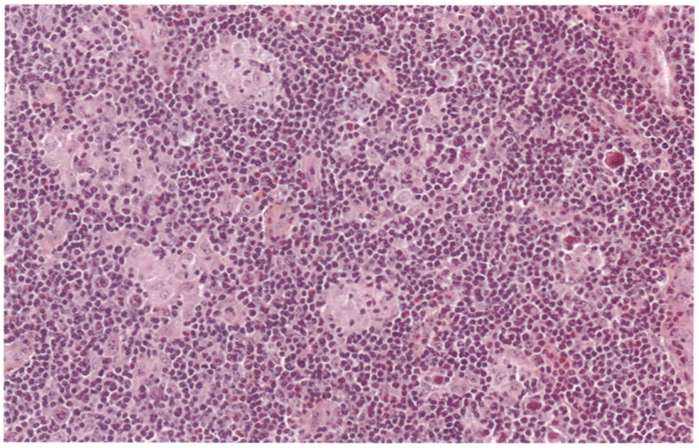

FIGURE 87.6 Mixed cellularity classic Hodgkin lymphoma. The infiltrate contains a mixed population of small lymphocytes, eosinophils, plasma cells, and histiocytes with epithelioid features associated with Hodgkin/Reed-Sternberg cells and variants.

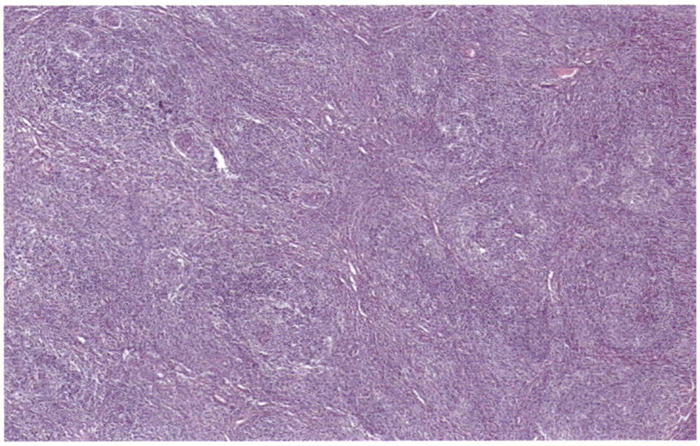

FIGURE 87.7 Lymphocyte-rich classic Hodgkin lymphoma, nodular variant. Cellular nodules are composed of small lymphocytes, frequently with atrophic germinal centers.

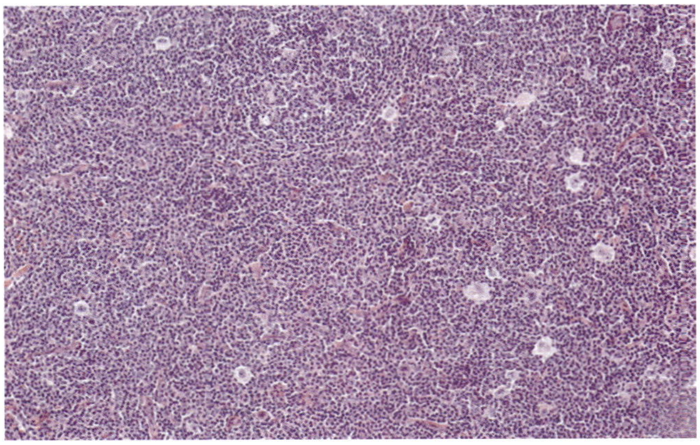

FIGURE 87.8 Lymphocyte-rich classic Hodgkin lymphoma. The tumor cells are located in expanded mantle zones and surrounded by a monotonous infiltrate made of small lymphocytes without eosinophils, neutrophils, or plasma cells.

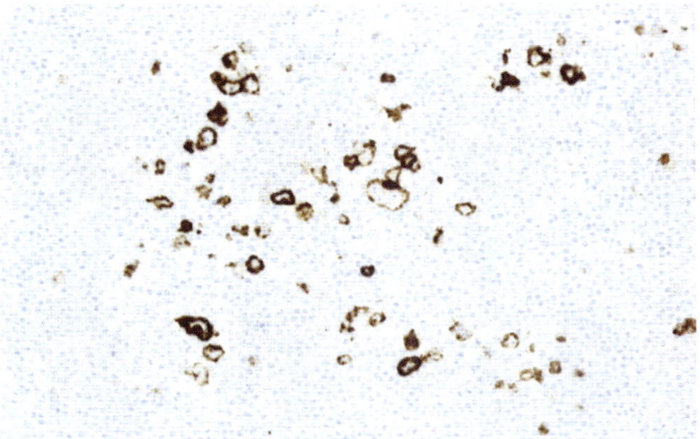

FIGURE 87.9 Lymphocyte-rich classic Hodgkin lymphoma. CD30 immunostain highlights the Hodgkin/Reed-Sternberg cells in a background of small lymphocytes.

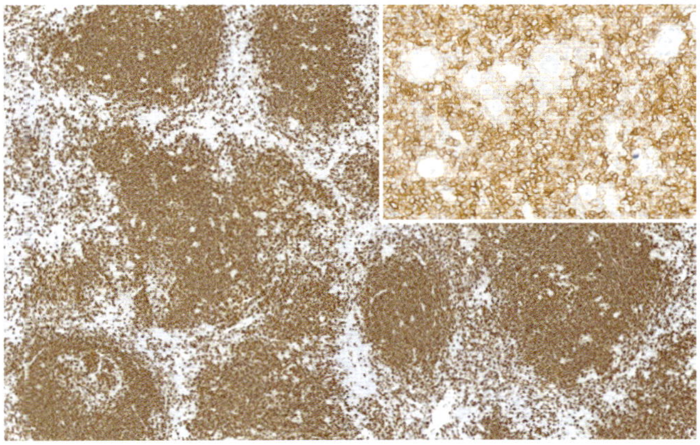

FIGURE 87.10 Lymphocyte-rich classic Hodgkin lymphoma. HRS cells are CD20 negative and located in a nodular small B cell–rich background.

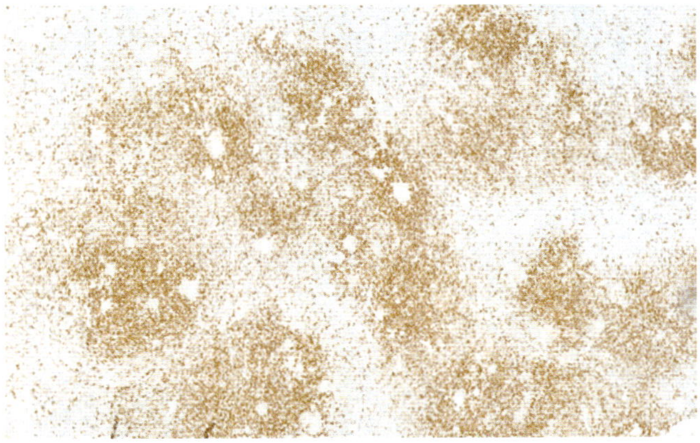

FIGURE 87.11 Lymphocyte-rich classic Hodgkin lymphoma. IgD immunostain reveals that the nodules consist with naïve B cells of normal mantle zones.

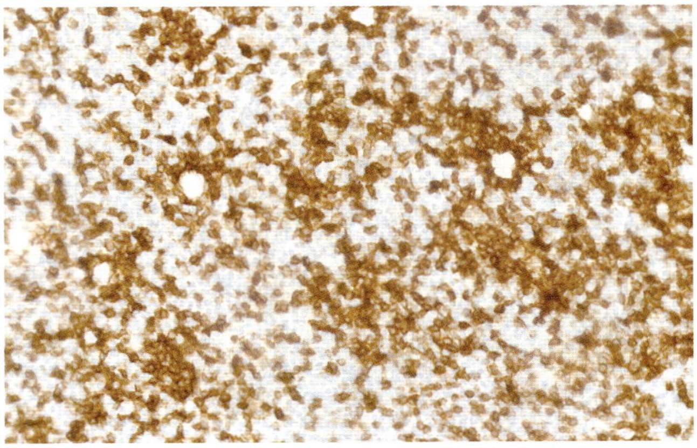

FIGURE 87.12 Lymphocyte-rich classic Hodgkin lymphoma. CD3 immunostain shows T cells forming rosettes around Hodgkin/Reed-Sternberg cells. The rosetting cells often express PD1.

fact that some of the constituent HRS cells may resemble lymphocyte-predominant (LP) cells, can lead to confusion with nodular lymphocyte-predominant B-cell lymphoma (NLPBL) (formerly nodular LP Hodgkin lymphoma). In the diffuse variant, the nodular architecture is dissolved with attenuated FDC networks. The background small lymphocytes may be admixed with histiocytes, with or without epithelioid features. The immunophenotype however is typical for classic HRS cells, although CD20 is more frequently positive in this subtype but never as strong and uniform as in NLPBL.

LDCHL is rare (≤1% of CHLs) and displays a diffuse growth pattern with abundant pleomorphic HRS cells (frequently EBV+). In LDCHL, the characteristic feature is the scarcity of normal lymphocytes, eosinophils, and plasma cells within the affected lymph node tissue, whereas histiocytes might be abundant. Fibrosis is generally absent.[16] Two patterns are classically described, one rich in neoplastic cells with pleomorphic and anaplastic features ("reticular") (Figure 87.13) and the other with abundant histiocytic infiltration and diffuse prominent fibroblastic proliferation without broad fibrous bands ("diffuse fibrosis") (Figure 87.14).

The differential diagnosis of CHL is summarized in Tables 87.1 and 87.2 and includes entities that either morphologically resemble CHL or have an overlapping immunophenotype.[17-21]

Immunophenotype

HRS cells strongly express CD30 in almost all cases (Figure 87.15).[22] CD15 is expressed in about 80% of cases (Figure 87.16).[23] The staining pattern of both antigens is quite similar, localized to the cell membrane with dot-like positivity corresponding to the Golgi apparatus. In

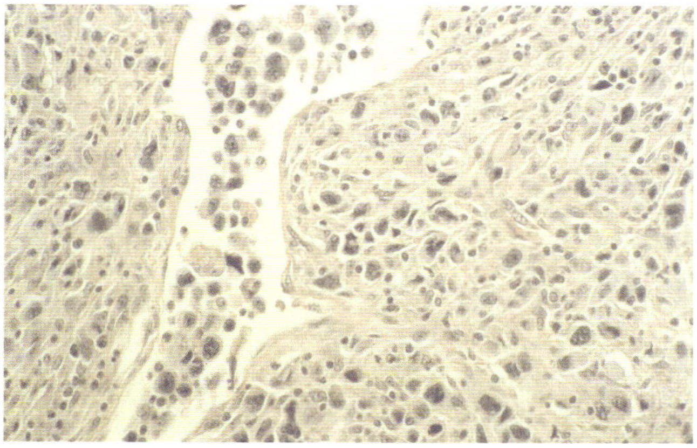

FIGURE 87.13 Lymphocyte-depleted classic Hodgkin lymphoma, rich in neoplastic cells pattern. Proliferation of large anaplastic and pleomorphic tumor cells with relatively few admixed inflammatory cells.

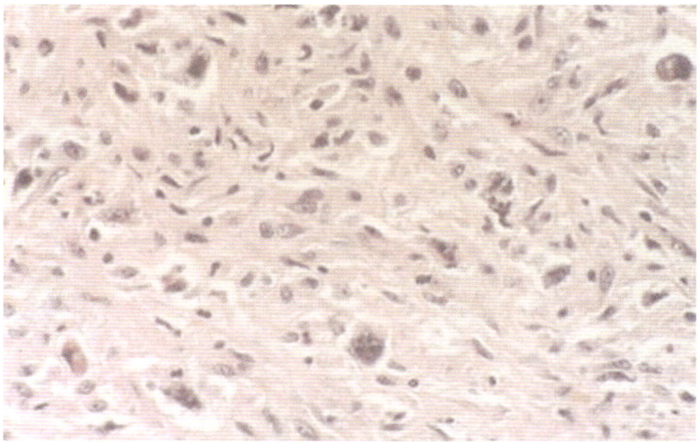

FIGURE 87.14 Lymphocyte-depleted classic Hodgkin lymphoma, diffuse fibrosis pattern. Hodgkin/Reed-Sternberg cells located in an hypocellular background composed of fibroblasts and histiocytes.

some cases, CD15 staining can be faint and restricted to cytoplasmic granules (usually in the Golgi area) (Figure 87.17). The leukocyte common antigen (CD45) should not be expressed. HRS cells correspond to germinal center cells with an incomplete B-cell program[1] with a frequent absence of B-cell markers, in particular the complete lack of immunoglobulin heavy and light chain gene expression. The B-cell lineage of HRS cells is demonstrated by PAX5 expression in almost all cases (Figure 87.18). PAX5 expression appears weaker than that of reactive surrounding B cells. CD20 may be detectable in 30% of cases with variable staining intensity, with strong expression being seen in only a small fraction of HRS cells, while others are completely negative (Figure 87.19). Other B-cell markers such as CD19, CD22, and CD79b are rarely observed although CD79a can be expressed in 5% to 10% of cases.[24] A clear homogenous expression of at least two B-cell markers should prompt consideration of gray zone lymphoma in mediastinal cases, or EBV-positive diffuse large B-cell lymphoma (DLBCL) in EBV+ cases. B-cell transcription factors such as OCT2, BOB.1, and PU.1 are downregulated or negative in most cases. BOB.1 and OCT2 expression can be either completely negative or mutually exclusive ($OCT2^+$/$BOB.1^-$ or $OCT2^-$/$BOB.1^+$),[25] although rare cases may have both. The transcription factor IRF4 (MUM1) is consistently and strongly expressed in HRS cells but is not lineage specific. MUM1 is useful in identifying rare HRS cells embedded in fibrotic posttherapy biopsies.

EBV infection can be documented in 70% to 75% of patients with MCCHL and LDCHL, whereas in NSCHL and LRCHL, EBV is detected in only around 10% of cases. EBV infection of HRS cells is highlighted by in situ hybridization techniques against EBV-encoded RNAs (Figure 87.20) or immunohistochemistry

TABLE 87.1 Main differential diagnoses of CHL with non-Hodgkin lymphomas

B-cell lymphomas	
Mediastinal Gray Zone Lymphoma	B-cell program maintained with a strong and homogeneous expression of at least two pan–B-cell markers (CD19, CD20, CD22, CD79a,b) Transcription factors OCT2, BOB.1$^+$ PAX5 (strong) CD30 heterogeneous, CD15$^-$, EBV–
Nodular lymphocyte-predominant B-cell lymphoma	Nodular architecture without frequent bandlike sclerosis Exceptional HRS cells Lymphocyte-predominant (LP) cells with full B-cell program (pan-B$^+$) in a background of mature naïve small B cells Follicular dendritic cell network hyperplastic (CD21$^+$) BOB.1, OCT2, PAX5 strongly positive OCT2 staining helpful in highlighting LP cells Rosettes of T cells (PD1$^+$) Variable expression of EMA and IgD Lack of CD30, CD15, and EBV (EBER$^-$, LMP1$^-$)
T-cell/histiocyte-rich large B-cell lymphoma	Aggressive clinical presentation (disseminated) Diffuse histological pattern Full B-cell program in the lymphoma cells No background of small B cells Lack of FDC network (CD21$^-$) CD30$^-$, CD15$^-$, EBV (EBER, LMP1)– EMA positive in half of the cases
T-cell lymphomas	
Angioimmunoblastic T-cell lymphoma	Aggressive lymphoma with polyadenopathy, hepatosplenomegaly, inflammatory syndrome, cutaneous rashes HRS-like cells similar to CHL but with frequent well-preserved B-cell program with variable EBV Predominance of malignant TFH cells (reactive TFH cells sometimes abundant in CHL may be challenging on needle core biopsies) Staining of neoplastic TFH cells: CD10$^+$, PD1$^+$, ICOS$^+$, IDH2R172$^+$ (10% of cases) High mitotic index Ki-67 >50% T-cell clone and/or mutated *RHOA*, *IDH2* genes
Peripheral T-cell lymphoma with HRS cells	Atypical malignant T cells with high mitotic rate Heterogeneous CD30 expression in malignant and HRS cells
Anaplastic large cell lymphoma (ALK–)	HRS-like cells, hallmark cells, cells with horseshoe-shaped nuclei Expression of pan–T-cell markers (CD3$^\pm$, CD2$^+$ with frequent cytotoxic markers, TIA1, granzyme B, and perforin); PAX5 is negative; homogeneous CD30 expression but CD15 frequently negative Absence of EBV infection Predominant T-cell clone, rearrangement of *DUSP22/IRF4*, *TP63* and/or *JAK1*, *STAT3* mutations

ALK, anaplastic lymphoma kinase; CHL, classic Hodgkin lymphoma; EBV, Epstein-Barr virus; EBER, EBV-encoded RNA; FDC, follicular dendritic cell; HRS, Hodgkin/Reed-Sternberg; TFH, T follicular helper.

TABLE 87.2 Differential diagnosis of CHL with other EBV-positive B-cell lymphoproliferative processes

Infectious mononucleosis with HRS-like cells	Teen age, young adults Cervical lymph nodes, tonsils, and adenoids involved, splenomegaly Admixture of large EBV+ immunoblasts (±HRS-like) with large reactive cytotoxic CD8$^+$ T cells seen in circulation Latency 3 (EBNA2$^+$, LMP1$^+$) IgM anti-EBV proteins in the serum
Infectious mononucleosis-like hyperplasia	Context of immune deficiency Localized in the Waldeyer ring (tonsils, adenoids) Pattern of nondestructive follicular hyperplasia with scattered EBV+ HRS cells
Lymphomatoid granulomatosis	Pulmonary involvement required for the diagnosis Angiocentric, angiodestructive EBV+ LPD Latency 2 or 3 (LMP1$^+$, EBNA2$^{-/+}$) B-cell program maintained; numerous perivascular T cells
Polymorphic lymphoproliferative disorders associated with immune deficiency (posttransplant, iatrogenic)	Mainly in extranodal sites Large polymorphism of B cells from small to HRS-like cells B-cell program frequently preserved Latency 2 (iatrogenic) or latency 3 (posttransplantation)
EBV-positive mucocutaneous ulcer	Almost exclusive to mucosal (gastrointestinal) and cutaneous sites; frequently isolated, self-limited Pleomorphic EBV+ B cells (some with HRS-like features) Full B-cell program in most cases EBV latency 2 or 3
EBV-positive diffuse large B-cell lymphoma	No obvious background of immune deficiency (except immune senescence)Mainly in extranodal sites Polymorphic or monomorphic with HRS-like cells B-cell program maintained

CHL, classic Hodgkin lymphoma; EBV, Epstein-Barr virus; HRS, Hodgkin/Reed-Sternberg; LPD, lymphoproliferative disease.

against the viral latent membrane protein 1 (LMP1) (Figure 87.21). Epstein-Barr nuclear antigen 1 (EBNA1) is expressed, whereas EBNA2 is never detected in EBV+ CHL. Altogether, HRS cells display a strict and constant latency 2 pattern.

Immunohistochemical detection of T-cell markers has been reported in rare cases (~5%).[26,27] The staining may look either spurious in the form of cytoplasmic dots with anti-CD3 antibodies or more specifically restricted to the cell membrane (CD3, CD2, CD4) often in a thick, crayon-like staining pattern. Similar to CD45 staining, there might be some false-positive staining due to reactive background T cells, including rosettes. In such cases, where some T-cell markers are expressed, caution should be taken and the B-cell

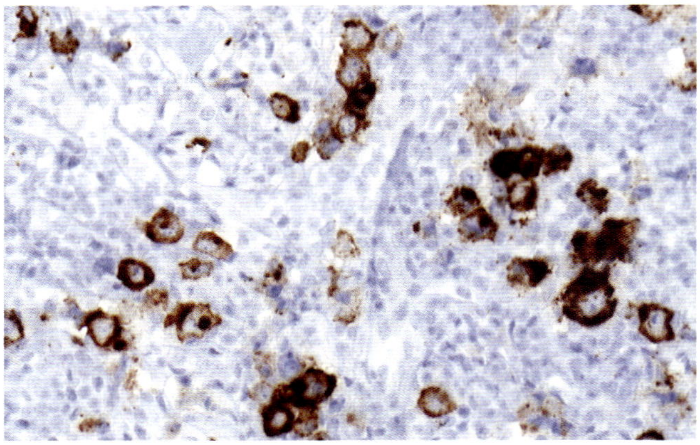

FIGURE 87.15 Immunophenotype of classical Hodgkin lymphoma. Strong expression of CD30 in Hodgkin/Reed-Sternberg cells and variants.

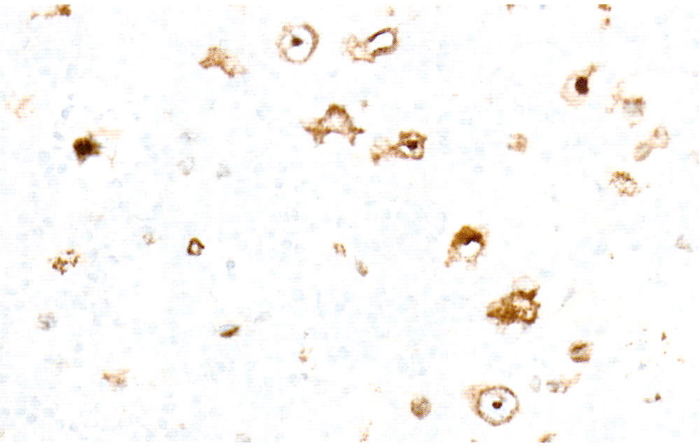

FIGURE 87.16 Immunophenotype of classic Hodgkin lymphoma. Expression of CD15 by neoplastic cells. Note the strong positivity of neutrophils, which serve as internal controls.

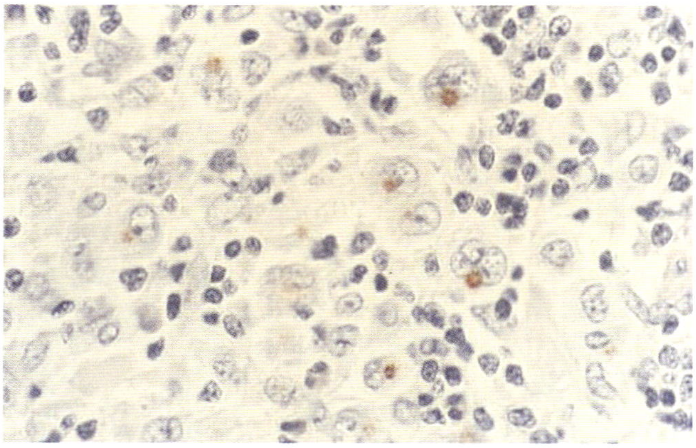

FIGURE 87.17 Immunophenotype of classic Hodgkin lymphoma. Expression of CD15 by neoplastic cells. Note the dotlike perinuclear staining pattern corresponding to the Golgi apparatus.

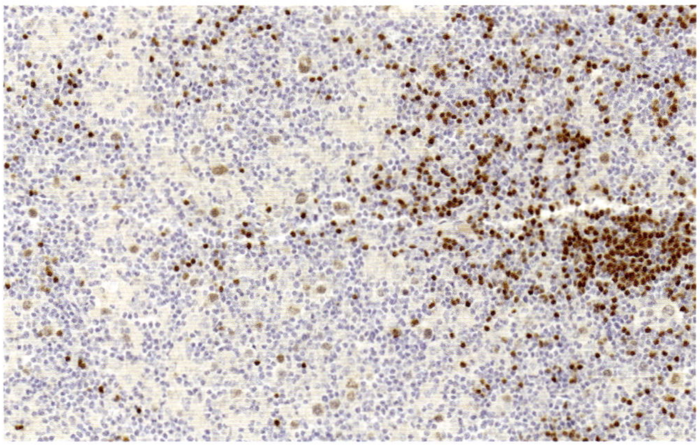

FIGURE 87.18 Immunophenotype of classic Hodgkin lymphoma. The nuclei of neoplastic cells are weakly stained by PAX5 compared to adjacent B cells with moderate PAX5 expression.

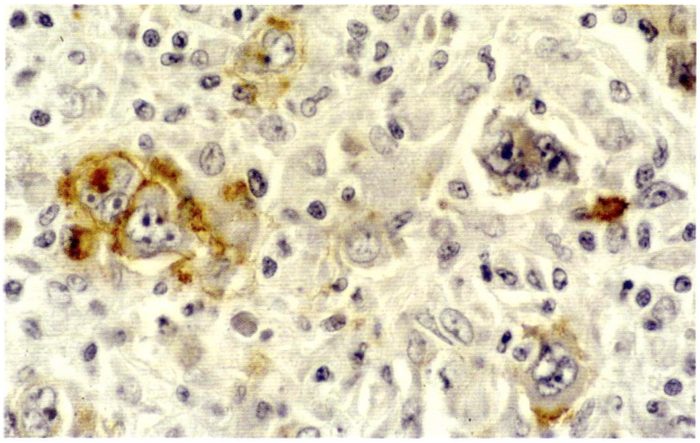

FIGURE 87.19 Immunophenotype of classic Hodgkin lymphoma. CD20 expression in HRS cells with variable and incomplete membranous pattern.

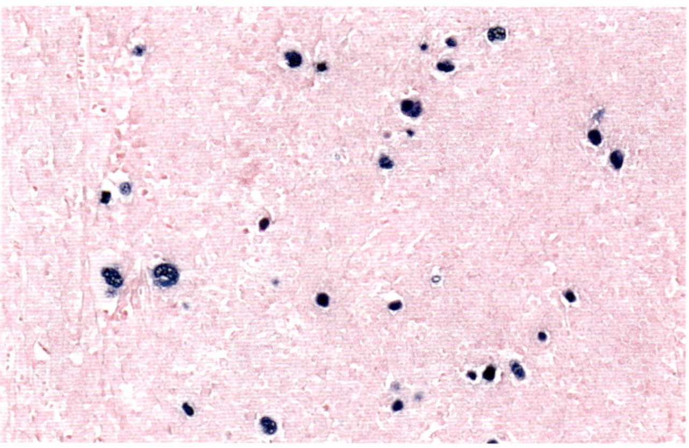

FIGURE 87.20 Epstein-Barr virus (EBV)-positive classic Hodgkin lymphoma. EBV-infected tumoral cells show strong nuclear expression of EBV-encoded small RNA by in situ hybridization.

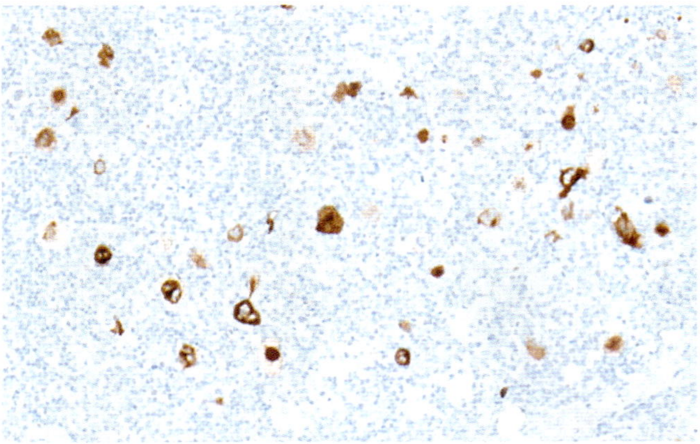

FIGURE 87.21 Epstein-Barr virus (EBV)-positive classic Hodgkin lymphoma. Expression of the EBV-encoded latent membrane protein 1 by Hodgkin/Reed-Sternberg cells.

nature of HRS neoplastic cells confirmed by PAX5 positivity and/or detection of immunoglobulin gene rearrangement. In rare instances, cytotoxic proteins (TIA1, perforin, granzyme A, granzyme B) may also been seen in HRS cells. Positive staining for transcription factors GATA3 and T-bet does not discriminate between CHL and T-cell lymphoma. GATA3 may help in distinguishing CHL from NLPBL.[28] PD-L1, STAT6, and pSTAT6 immunohistochemistry are helpful diagnostic tools to distinguish CHL (frequently positive) from PTCL with HRS-like cells (rarely positive).[29,30] HRS cells also often express PDL2, NOTCH1, CAMPATH1 antigen (CD52), and histone deacetylase 6 (HDAC6), which represent potential targets for therapy.[6] In cases with eosinophilia in the TME and the blood, HRS cells strongly express interleukin 5.[31]

Genetics

The paucity of HRS cells within the TME raises major challenges in the study of malignant cell molecular biology. Nonetheless, high-throughput molecular techniques, in particular genome-wide analyses, including sequencing of microdissected HRS cells and circulating tumor DNA (ctDNA), have led to a more refined molecular characterization of HRS cells and provides us with valuable tools for CHL diagnosis in the setting of atypical histological or clinical features.[32]

HRS cells are clonal B cells of germinal center derivation with an incomplete B-cell program. They harbor unproductive clonal immunoglobulin gene rearrangements with somatic hypermutations in the variable region.[1] However, immunoglobulin gene rearrangements are only detected in a minority of cases using whole section PCR in routine clinical diagnosis due to the low frequency of malignant HRS cells. Cases of CHL with clonal rearrangements of T-cell receptor genes have been historically reported.[33,34] However, it is likely that many of these represent unrecognized/misdiagnosed T-cell lymphomas (TFH T-cell lymphoma with HRS cells or anaplastic lymphoma kinase-negative anaplastic large cell lymphoma with a nodular sclerosis pattern). Furthermore, reactive T-cell lymphoproliferation in the TME is also conceivable, as reported in various infectious and immune dysregulation states. Indeed, a recent study based on ctDNA showed the presence of T-cell clones arising from the TME.[35] The mechanisms involved in downregulation of the B-cell program in HRS cells are not fully understood but include reduced expression of B-cell transcription factors (eg, *OCT2, BOB.1, PU.1*), upregulation of master regulators that inhibit B-cell gene expression (eg, *ID2, NOTCH1*),[36] and epigenetic mechanisms. In EBV+ CHL, viral proteins (eg, LMP1) also contribute to the downregulation of the B-cell program.[36]

CHL is characterized by a highly altered genomic landscape with considerable aneuploidy, recurrent chromosomal imbalances, and somatic mutations leading to constitutive activation of the oncogenic NF-kB and JAK/STAT signaling pathways and to enhanced immune evasion. However, no specific genetic lesions have been identified and almost all genes frequently altered in HRS cells have also been found involved in other B-cell malignancies. Comparative genomic hybridization documents copy number alterations in approximately 20% of cases, including gains in chromosome 2p (*REL*), 9p24.1 (*PD-L1, PD-L2, JAK2*), 12q13 (*STAT2, STAT6*), as well as losses of 1p36 (*TNFRSF14*), 6q (*TNFAIP3*), and 6p21 (*MHCI* and *MHCII*).[37-43] Translocations involving the MHC class II transactivator gene, *CIITA*, have also been detected in about 15% of CHL cases,[42,43] while breakpoints in the immunoglobulin loci were found in a minority (17%). The role of this latter alteration remains unclear since the immunoglobulin loci are silenced in HRS cells.

Besides cytogenetic alterations, several recurrent somatic mutations also affect components of the NF-kB pathway (*TNFAIP3, NFKBIA, NFKBIE, IKBKB*), the JAK/STAT pathway (*SOCS1, STAT6, PTPN1, CSF2RB*), and immune escape (*B2M, CIITA, HLA-B*).[42,44-50] Along with the key role of the NF-kB, JAK/STAT, and immune escape pathways in CHL pathogenesis, the PI3K/AKT and NOTCH1 pathways are also found constitutively activated in HRS cells.[51] Additional genes recurrently mutated in HRS cells include *ARID1A, XPO1* (mostly affected by the activating p.E571K mutation in codon

TABLE 87.3 Main recurrent genetic alterations in classic Hodgkin lymphoma

Gene	Type of genetic alteration	Approximate frequency (%)
NF-kB pathway		
REL	CNAs (2p16 gain)	30-60
TNFAIP3	SNVs, deletions	30-50
NFKBIA	SNVs, indels	10-20
NFKBIE	SNVs, indels	5-30
IKBKB	SNVs	10-15
JAK/STAT pathway		
SOCS1	SNVs, indels	35-70
JAK2 (9p24)	CNAs (9p24 gain)	10-60
STAT6	SNVs, gains	20-50
CSF2RB	SNVs	15-30
PTPN1	SNVs, indels	10-20
Immune escape		
B2M	SNVs, indels	20-70
PD-L1, PD-L2	CNAs (9p24 gain)	30-55
MHCI/MHCII	CNAs (6p21 loss)	40-50
TNFRSF14	CNAs (1p36 loss)	20-40
CIITA	Translocations, SNVs	5-15
HLA-B	SNVs, indels	15
PI3K/AKT pathway		
ITPKB	SNVs	15-40
GNA13	SNVs	15-30
NOTCH signaling		
SPEN	SNVs	10
FBXW7	SNVs	10
Others		
XPO1	SNVs (codon 571), gains	10-30
ARID1A	SNVs, indels	10-25
IGLL5	SNVs	10-25
TP53	SNVs	5-20

CNAs, copy number alterations; SNVs, single nucleotide variants; indels, insertions/deletions.

571), *IGLL5*, and *TP53* (Table 87.3).[42,44-50] Sequencing and gene expression studies suggest that the genotype of HRS cells influences cellular crosstalk within the TME, which is a critical determinant of CHL initiation and progression.[35] Thus, several genetic alterations are found to differ substantially in frequency between the histological CHL subtypes[35] and according to the EBV tumor status.[44,45,52] A recent study showed that molecular abnormalities of RS cells could be detected in ctDNA in parallel with single-cell transcriptional profile of CHL tumor tissues.[34] This approach revealed two distinct CHL genomic subtypes with characteristic clinical and prognostic correlates, as well as distinct transcriptional and immunological profiles.[34] In addition, the authors reported a novel class of truncating *IL4R* mutations depending on IL-13 signaling and potentially targetable with IL-4Rα–blocking antibodies.[34]

Prognosis and Clinical Comments

Staging is carried out according to the Lugano classification based on the Cotswold's modification to the original Ann Arbor staging system for Hodgkin lymphoma.[53,54] Standard staging consists of medical history,

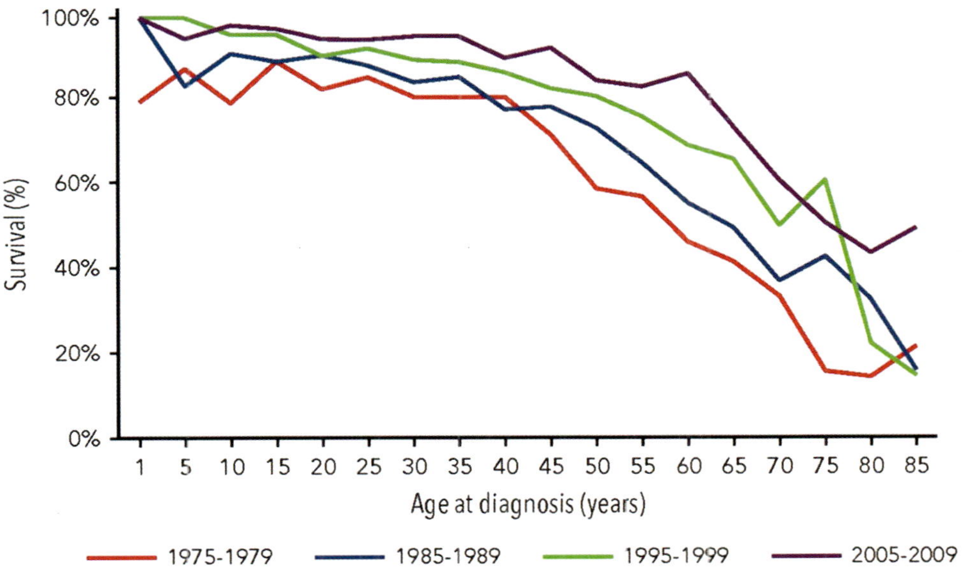

FIGURE 87.22 Survival curves for Hodgkin lymphoma from the Surveillance, Epidemiology, and End Results (SEER) database throughout decades of treatment. (From Flerlage JE, Metzger ML, Bhakta N. The management of Hodgkin lymphoma in adolescents and young adults: burden of disease or burden of choice? *Blood.* 2018;132(4):376-384.)

physical examination (with special attention to lymph node enlargement and abdominal organomegaly), and PET-CT scan, which should be repeated after completion of treatment for assessment of response. When PET scanning is unavailable, staging should rely on CT scanning, and bone marrow biopsy should be added to complete staging.

More than 80% of CHL patients can be cured with conventional polychemotherapy with or without radiotherapy. Principal multidrug regimens are ABVD (adriamycin, bleomycin, vinblastine, and dacarbazine) or BEACOPP (bleomycin, etoposide, doxorubicin, cyclophosphamide, vincristine, procarbazine, and prednisone). The antibody-drug conjugate brentuximab vedotin and PD-1 inhibitors are increasingly incorporated in initial therapy in combination with chemotherapy. Radiation therapy includes external beam radiation delivered with a linear accelerator with treatment fields designed using CT-guided simulation and 3D treatment planning.

Cure rates are 90% to 95% for nonbulky stage IA or stage IIA disease and 70% to 80% for advanced-stage disease.[55-57] Overall, up to 90% of patients in the age range 16 to 70 years can be cured with either standard chemotherapeutic regimens or with effective secondary interventions. With the advances in treatment regimens, survival across all age groups has increased over time but has always remained above 80% for pediatric and young adult patients before declining after 40 years of age (Figure 87.22).[58]

References

1. Kanzler H, Küppers R, Hansmann ML, Rajewsky K. Hodgkin and Reed-Sternberg cells in Hodgkin's disease represent the outgrowth of a dominant tumor clone derived from (crippled) germinal center B cells. *J Exp Med.* 1996;184(4):1495-1505.
2. SEER National Cancer Institute Surveillance Epidemiology and End Results Program. Cancer Stat Facts: Hodgkin Lymphoma. SEER; 2019. https://seer.cancer.gov/statfacts/html/hodg.html
3. Ebied A, Thanh Huan V, Makram OM, et al. The role of primary lymph node sites in survival and mortality prediction in Hodgkin lymphoma: a SEER population-based retrospective study. *Cancer Med.* 2018;7(4):953-965.
4. Laurent C, Baron M, Amara N, et al. Impact of expert pathologic review of lymphoma diagnosis: study of patients from the French lymphopath network. *J Clin Oncol.* 2017;35(18):2008-2017.
5. Evens AM, Antillón M, Aschebrook-Kilfoy B, Chiu BC. Racial disparities in Hodgkin's lymphoma: a comprehensive population-based analysis. *Ann Oncol.* 2012;23(8):2128-2137.
6. Connors JM, Cozen W, Steidl C, et al. Hodgkin lymphoma. *Nat Rev Dis Primers.* 2020;6(1):61.
7. Johnson PCD, McAulay KA, Montgomery D, et al. Modeling HLA associations with EBV-positive and -negative Hodgkin lymphoma suggests distinct mechanisms in disease pathogenesis. *Int J Cancer.* 2015;137(5):1066-1075.
8. Glaser SL, Lin RJ, Stewart SL, et al. Epstein-Barr virus-associated Hodgkin's disease: epidemiologic characteristics in international data. *Int J Cancer.* 1997;70(4):375-382.

9. Cozen W, Timofeeva MN, Li D, et al. A meta-analysis of Hodgkin lymphoma reveals 19p13.3 TCF3 as a novel susceptibility locus. *Nat Commun.* 2014;5:3856. doi:10.1038/ncomms4856
10. Sud A, Thomsen H, Orlando G, et al. Genome-wide association study implicates immune dysfunction in the development of Hodgkin lymphoma. *Blood.* 2018;132(19):2040-2052.
11. Latour S, Winter S. Inherited immunodeficiencies with high predisposition to Epstein-Barr virus-driven lymphoproliferative diseases. *Front Immunol.* 2018;9:1103. doi:10.3389/fimmu.2018.01103. eCollection 2018
12. Hjalgrim H, Askling J, Rostgaard K, et al. Characteristics of Hodgkin's lymphoma after infectious mononucleosis. *N Engl J Med.* 2003;349(14):1324-1332.
13. Cavalli F. Rare syndromes in Hodgkin's disease. *Ann Oncol.* 1998;9:S109-S113.
14. Haybittle JL, Hayhoe FG, Easterling MJ, et al. Review of British National Lymphoma Investigation studies of Hodgkin's disease and development of prognostic index. *Lancet.* 1985;1(8435):967-972.
15. Nam-Cha SH, Montes-Moreno S, Salcedo MT, Sanjuan J, Garcia JF, Piris MA. Lymphocyte-rich classical Hodgkin's lymphoma: distinctive tumor and microenvironment markers. *Mod Pathol.* 2009;22(8):1006-1015.
16. Slack GW, Ferry JA, Hasserjian RP, et al. Lymphocyte depleted Hodgkin lymphoma: an evaluation with immunophenotyping and genetic analysis. *Leuk Lymphoma.* 2009;50(6):937-943.
17. Campo E, Jaffe ES, Cook JR, et al. The international consensus classification of mature lymphoid neoplasms: a report from the clinical advisory committee. *Blood.* 2022;140(11):1229-1253.
18. Tousseyn TA, King RL, Fend F, Feldman AL, Brousset P, Jaffe ES. Evolution in the definition and diagnosis of the Hodgkin lymphomas and related entities. *Virchows Arch.* 2023;482(1):207-226.
19. Sarkozy C, Copie-Bergman C, Damotte D, et al. Gray-zone lymphoma between cHL and large B-cell lymphoma: a histopathologic series from the LYSA. *Am J Surg Pathol.* 2019;43(3):341-351.
20. Bosch-Schips J, Granai M, Quintanilla-Martinez L, Fend F. The Grey zones of classic Hodgkin lymphoma. *Cancers.* 2022;14(3):742.
21. Eladl AE, Satou A, Elsayed AA, et al. Clinicopathological study of 30 cases of peripheral T-cell lymphoma with Hodgkin and Reed-Sternberg-like B-cells from Japan. *Am J Surg Pathol.* 2017;41(4):506-516.
22. Stein H, Mason DY, Gerdes J, et al. The expression of the Hodgkin's disease associated antigen Ki-1 in reactive and neoplastic lymphoid tissue: evidence that Reed-Sternberg cells and histiocytic malignancies are derived from activated lymphoid cells. *Blood.* 1985;66(4):848-858.
23. Hall PA, D'Ardenne AJ. Value of CD15 immunostaining in diagnosing Hodgkin's disease: a review of published literature. *J Clin Pathol.* 1987;40(11):1298-1304.
24. Schmid C, Pan L, Diss T, Isaacson PG. Expression of B-cell antigens by Hodgkin's and Reed-Sternberg cells. *Am J Pathol.* 1991;139(4):701-707.
25. O'Malley DP, Fedoriw Y, Weiss LM. Distinguishing classical Hodgkin lymphoma, gray zone lymphoma, and large B-cell lymphoma: a proposed scoring system. *Appl Immunohistochem Mol Morphol.* 2016;24(8):535-540.
26. Venkataraman G, Song JY, Tzankov A, et al. Aberrant T-cell antigen expression in classical Hodgkin lymphoma is associated with decreased event-free survival and overall survival. *Blood.* 2013;121(10):1795-1804.
27. Tzankov A, Bourgau C, Kaiser A, et al. Rare expression of T-cell markers in classical Hodgkin's lymphoma. *Mod Pathol.* 2005;18(12):1542-1549.
28. Kezlarian B, Alhyari M, Venkataraman G, Karner K, Inamdar KV, Menon MP. GATA3 immunohistochemical staining in Hodgkin lymphoma: diagnostic utility in differentiating classic Hodgkin lymphoma from nodular lymphocyte predominant Hodgkin lymphoma and other mimicking entities. *Appl Immunohistochem Mol Morphol.* 2019;27(3):180-184.
29. Satou AT, Takahara T, Yamashita D, et al. Diagnostic utility of STAT6 and pSTAT6 immunohistochemistry for distinguishing classic Hodgkin lymphoma and peripheral T-cell lymphoma with Hodgkin and Reed-Sternberg–like cells. *Am J Surg Pathol.* 2023;47(8):897-906.
30. Van Slambrouck C, Huh J, Suh C, et al. Diagnostic utility of STAT6^{YE361} expression in classical Hodgkin lymphoma and related entities. *Mod Pathol.* 2020;33(5):834-845.
31. Samoszuk M, Nansen L. Detection of interleukin-5 messenger RNA in Reed-Sternberg cells of Hodgkin's disease with eosinophilia. *Blood.* 1990;75(1):13-16.
32. de Leval L, Alizadeh AA, Bergsagel PL, et al. Genomic profiling for clinical decision making in lymphoid neoplasms. *Blood.* 2022;140(21):2193-2227.
33. Seitz V, Hummel M, Marafioti T, Anagnostopoulos I, Assaf C, Stein H. Detection of clonal T-cell receptor gamma-chain gene rearrangements in Reed-Sternberg cells of classic Hodgkin disease. *Blood.* 2000;95(10):3020-3024.
34. Alig SK, Shahrokh Esfahani M, Garofalo A, et al. Distinct Hodgkin lymphoma subtypes defined by noninvasive genomic profiling. *Nature.* 2024;625(7996):778-787.
35. van Bladel DAG, Stevens WBC, van den Brand M, et al. Novel approaches in molecular characterization of classical Hodgkin lymphoma. *Cancers.* 2022;14(13):3222.
36. Küppers R, Engert A, Hansmann ML. Hodgkin lymphoma. *J Clin Invest.* 2012;122(10):3439-3447.
37. Joos S, Menz CK, Wrobel G, et al. Classical Hodgkin lymphoma is characterized by recurrent copy number gains of the short arm of chromosome 2. *Blood.* 2002;99(4):1381-1387.

38. Martín-Subero JI, Gesk S, Harder L, et al. Recurrent involvement of the REL and BCL11A loci in classical Hodgkin lymphoma. *Blood*. 2002;99(4):1474-1477.
39. Hartmann S, Martin-Subero JI, Gesk S, et al. Detection of genomic imbalances in microdissected Hodgkin and Reed-Sternberg cells of classical Hodgkin's lymphoma by array-based comparative genomic hybridization. *Haematologica*. 2008;93(9):1318-1326.
40. Green MR, Monti S, Rodig SJ, et al. Integrative analysis reveals selective 9p24.1 amplification, increased PD-1 ligand expression, and further induction via JAK2 in nodular sclerosing Hodgkin lymphoma and primary mediastinal large B-cell lymphoma. *Blood*. 2010;116(17):3268-3277.
41. Roemer MG, Advani RH, Ligon AH, et al. PD-L1 and PD-L2 genetic alterations define classical Hodgkin lymphoma and predict outcome. *J Clin Oncol*. 2016;34(23):2690-2697.N.
42. Wienand K, Chapuy B, Stewart C, et al. Genomic analyses of flow-sorted Hodgkin Reed-Sternberg cells reveal complementary mechanisms of immune evasion. *Blood Adv*. 2019;3(23):4065-4080.
43. Steidl C, Shah SP, Woolcock BW, et al. MHC class II transactivator CIITA is a recurrent gene fusion partner in lymphoid cancers. *Nature*. 2011;471(7338):377-381.
44. Reichel J, Chadburn A, Rubinstein PG, et al. Flow sorting and exome sequencing reveal the oncogenome of primary Hodgkin and Reed-Sternberg cells. *Blood*. 2015;125(7):1061-1072.
45. Spina V, Bruscaggin A, Cuccaro A, et al. Circulating tumor DNA reveals genetics, clonal evolution, and residual disease in classical Hodgkin lymphoma. *Blood*. 2018;131(22):2413-2425.
46. Tiacci E, Ladewig E, Schiavoni G, et al. Pervasive mutations of JAK-STAT pathway genes in classical Hodgkin lymphoma. *Blood*. 2018;131(22):2454-2465.
47. Sobesky S, Mammadova L, Cirillo M, et al. In-depth cell-free DNA sequencing reveals genomic landscape of Hodgkin's lymphoma and facilitates ultrasensitive residual disease detection. *Med*. 2021;2(10):1171-1193.e11.
48. Desch AK, Hartung K, Botzen A, et al. Genotyping circulating tumor DNA of pediatric Hodgkin lymphoma. *Leukemia*. 2020;34(1):151-166.
49. Camus V, Viennot M, Lequesne J, et al. Targeted genotyping of circulating tumor DNA for classical Hodgkin lymphoma monitoring: a prospective study. *Haematologica*. 2021;106(1):154-162.
50. Weniger MA, Küppers R. Molecular biology of Hodgkin lymphoma. *Leukemia*. 2021;35(4):968-981.
51. Jundt F, Anagnostopoulos I, Förster R, Mathas S, Stein H, Dörken B. Activated Notch1 signaling promotes tumor cell proliferation and survival in Hodgkin and anaplastic large cell lymphoma. *Blood*. 2002;99(9):3398-3403.
52. Lamaison C, Ferrant J, Gravelle P, et al. Histological subtypes drive distinct prognostic immune signatures in classical Hodgkin lymphoma. *Cancers*. 2022;14(19):4893.
53. Lister TA, Crowther D, Sutcliffe SB, et al. Report of a committee convened to discuss the evaluation and staging of patients with Hodgkin's disease: Cotswolds meeting. *J Clin Oncol*. 1989;7(11):1630-1636.
54. Cheson BD, Fisher RI, Barrington SF, et al. Recommendations for initial evaluation, staging, and response assessment of Hodgkin and non-Hodgkin lymphoma: the Lugano classification. *J Clin Oncol*. 2014;32(27):3059-3068.
55. Villa D, Sehn LH, Aquino-Parsons C, et al. Interim PET-directed therapy in limited stage Hodgkin lymphoma initially treated with ABVD. *Haematologica*. 2018;103(12):e590-e593.
56. Straus DJ, Jung SH, Pitcher B, et al. CALGB 50604: risk-adapted treatment of nonbulky early-stage Hodgkin lymphoma based on interim PET. *Blood*. 2018;132(10):1013-1021.
57. Meyer RM, Gospodarowicz MK, Connors JM, et al. ABVD alone versus radiation-based therapy in limited-stage Hodgkin's lymphoma. *N Engl J Med*. 2012;366(5):399-408.
58. Flerlage JE, Metzger ML, Bhakta N. The management of Hodgkin lymphoma in adolescents and young adults: burden of disease or burden of choice? *Blood*. 2018;132(4):376-384.

SECTION 12

Mature T- and NK-Cell Neoplasms

Chapter 88

T-Cell Prolymphocytic Leukemia

Claire Dearden, Emmanuel Bachy, Cristina López, and Sa A. Wang

Definition

T-cell prolymphocytic leukemia (T-PLL) is a rare postthymic T-cell malignancy with an aggressive clinical course and a poor prognosis, characterized by the proliferation of small to medium-sized lymphocytes, involving peripheral blood, bone marrow, lymph nodes, liver, spleen, and skin.[1] In 2019, the T-PLL International Study Group (TPLL-ISG) established criteria for the diagnosis, staging, and assessment of response to treatment of T-PLL with the goal of harmonizing research efforts and supporting clinical decision making.[2] The diagnostic criteria are adopted by the International Consensus Classification (Table 88.1).

Synonyms

Prolymphocytic leukemia, T-cell type; T-prolymphocytic leukemia; T-chronic lymphocytic leukemia (T-CLL) (not recommended).

Epidemiology

T-PLL is rare, with an incidence of only 2 per million per year in Western countries, accounting for about 2% of mature leukemias. This is a disease of older adults (median age: 65 years) and occurs more frequently in males (M:F = 2:1).[1]

Ataxia telangiectasia, an autosomal recessive condition caused by mutated *ATM*, has been reported to confer a 100-fold high risk than the general population of T-PLL. Furthermore, in these cases, presenting age is younger (median age 30 years), with some in adolescence. Nijmegen breakage syndrome has also been reported to be a risk factor. There are no other familial or geographical predisposing features.

General Clinical Features

Patients typically present with B symptoms, splenomegaly, edema, and serous effusions.[2] Periorbital or conjunctival edema is frequent in T-PLL. Almost half

TABLE 88.1 Clinical and biological features of T-PLL showing the major and minor diagnostic criteria defined by TPLL-ISG[2]

Characteristic	Description	Diagnostic criteria
Clinical presentation	Median age 65 years M:F 2:1 Splenomegaly, lymphadenopathy, skin rash, edema, and pleuroperitoneal effusions Very high WBC	Involvement of T-PLL specific site (eg, splenomegaly or pleural effusions) (**Minor**)
Morphology	Small to medium-sized lymphocytes with cytoplasmic blebs, basophilic cytoplasm, and single nucleolus. Small cell (20%) and cerebriform (5%) variants	
Immunophenotype	$CD2^+$, $CD3^+$, $CD5^+$, $CD7^{++}$, CD4/CD8 variable, TCL1+ (80%-90%), CD26 (60%-70%) CD1a−, TdT−, $CD25^{-/+}$ Clonal TRBC1	$>5 \times 10^9$/L cells of T-PLL phenotype in peripheral blood or bone marrow (**Major 1**)
Conventional karyotype	t(14;14)(q11;q32); inv(14)(q11q32);t(X;14)(q28;q11) Alterations of chromosome 8; complex	Complex karyotype (**Minor**) Abnormalities of chromosome 8 [idic(8)(p11); t(8;8), or trisomy 8(q)], chromosome 5, 12, 13, or 22 (**Minor**)
Molecular genetics	Rearrangement of *TCL-1, MTCP-1,* mutation or deletion of *ATM,* frequent mutations of JAK-STAT pathway genes (*IL2RG, JAK1, JAK3, and STAT5B*) (70%)	T-cell clonality (**Major 2**) Abnormalities of 14q32 or expression of *TCL1A/B* or *MTCP1* (**Major 3**) Abnormalities of chromosome 11 (11q22.3, *ATM*) (**Minor**)

T-PLL, T-cell prolymphocytic leukemia; TPLL-ISG, T-PLL International Study Group; WBC, white blood count.

the patients have hepatomegaly and/or lymphadenopathy, although these are rarely bulky. Skin involvement is seen in about 20% to 25% of patients and central nervous system involvement in rare cases. The white blood cell count is often high (≥100,000 × 10^9/l), with greater than 90% of the circulating cells being T-PLL cells, and tends to rise rapidly. Anemia and thrombocytopenia are seen in half the cases.

Lactate dehydrogenase levels are usually elevated, but hypercalcemia, common in human T-lymphotropic virus type 1 (HTLV-1)-related adult T-cell/leukemia lymphoma (ATLL), is not a feature of T-PLL. Serology and/or DNA analysis for HTLV-1 and -2 are consistently negative, and these retroviruses are not implicated in the pathogenesis of the disease.

A minority of patients, about 15%, may be asymptomatic, with a lower T-PLL count, at diagnosis and this "indolent" phase can persist for a variable length of time, which may extend to several years.[3] However, progression is inevitable and may be very rapid when it occurs.

Morphology

Diagnosis is based on the characteristic morphology, immunophenotype, and genetics of circulating T-PLL cells in the peripheral blood.[1,2] These cells are small to medium sized with a high nuclear-cytoplasmic ratio. In the majority of cases, the cells have a round to oval nucleus, a single prominent nucleolus, and basophilic agranular cytoplasm with cytoplasmic protrusions or blebs (Figure 88.1A). Two variants, small cell and cerebriform, are seen in approximately 20% to 25% and 5% of cases, respectively. The small cell variant contains small lymphocytes with condensed chromatin, scant cytoplasm, and often no visible nucleoli (Figure 88.1B), while the cerebriform variant shows marked nuclear irregularity, often with convolutions (Figure 88.1C), mimicking Sézary or ATLL cells. Both these morphologic variants have immunophenotypic, cytogenetic, and clinical features similar to typical T-PLL. Infiltration of the bone marrow is usually diffuse and interstitial (Figure 88.1D-F), and reticulin fibrosis is almost always present. Spleen histology shows a marked expansion of the red pulp, capsular and vascular infiltration, and atrophy of the white pulp. Infiltration of the lymph nodes is usually diffuse and predominates the paracortical areas. Liver involvement is characterized by varying degrees of periportal infiltrates and portal tract expansion. The skin histology shows a dermal infiltration, characterized by small to medium-sized lymphocytes with predominant perivascular distribution, absent epidermotropism, and inconspicuous cytological atypia. This is distinct from Sézary syndrome but may overlap with other T-cell neoplasms. It must be noted that, compared with peripheral blood, morphology of other tissues, eg, bone marrow and lymph nodes, is less informative and may not clearly discriminate between T-PLL and other mature T-cell malignancies.

Immunophenotype

Immunophenotyping by flow cytometry demonstrates the postthymic T-cell nature (TdT neg, CD1a neg, CD5 pos, CD2 pos, CD7 pos) of the prolymphocytes. The most common phenotype is expression of CD4 without CD8 (60% of cases) (Figure 88.2A and B), but coexpression of CD4/CD8 is seen in 25% of cases and a minority express CD8 alone.[2] Some cases may contain several immunophenotypic subsets reflecting intratumor heterogeneity (Figure 88.2C and D). T-PLL cells express CD7 with strong intensity in contrast to other mature T-cell leukemias, where this marker is often weakly positive or negative. Aberrant loss of the pan-T-cell markers CD2 and CD5 is not common. CD26 is positive in about two-thirds of cases. The majority of cases express surface CD3 and TCRαß with TRBC1 restriction, while occasional cases are negative for surface CD3 and TCR (null type). Commercially available TRBC1 antibody for flow cytometry can be used to confirm clonal TCR expression. Loss of CD45 can be occasionally observed. CD52 is expressed at high density in untreated patients and is of obvious therapeutic relevance. Cell surface antigens linked to T-cell activation such as CD25, CD38, and class II HLA-DR may be variably expressed, but markers of cytotoxic T cells such as CD56, CD16, CD94, granzyme B, and TIA-1 are negative, even in cases with a $CD8^+$ phenotype. Intracytoplasmic TCL1A (see Genetics section) protein expression assessment is a sensitive diagnostic test that can be performed by flow cytometry after cell permeabilization and by immunohistochemistry. TCL1 is positive in 80% to 90% T-PLL,[4] often associated with *TCL1* rearrangement, and negative in *MTCP*-rearranged cases, and TCL1-family negative T-PLL.

Genetics

The hallmark aberration of T-PLL, present in around 80% of the patients, is an inv(14)(q11q32) or t(14;14)(q11;q32) (10% of cases) involving TRA/TRD at 14q11 and the oncogene *TCL1* in 14q32[2] (Figure 88.3). Both rearrangements are generated via V(D)J recombination

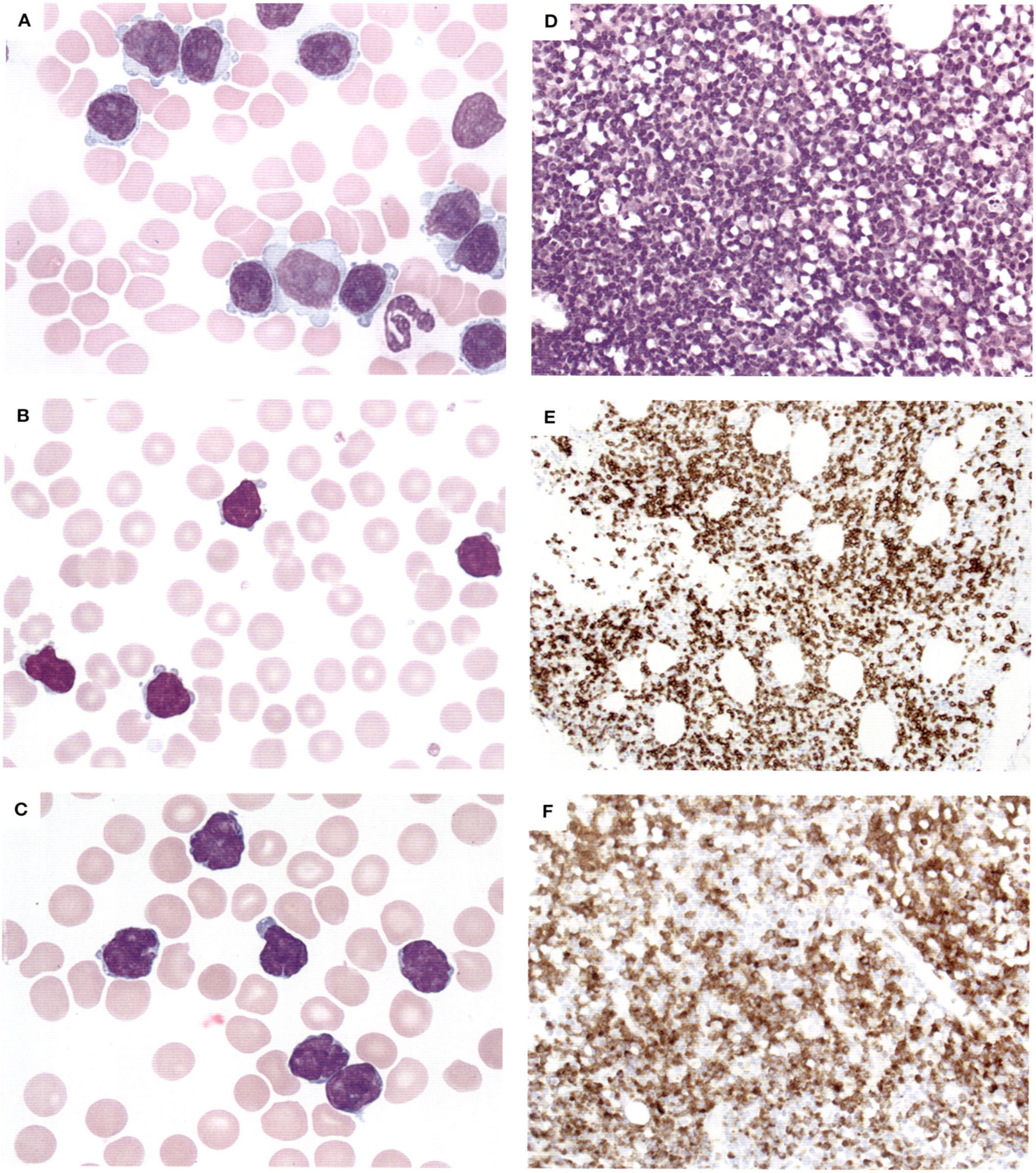

FIGURE 88.1 Morphological features of T-cell prolymphocytic leukemia (T-PLL). Typical T-PLL in peripheral blood (PB) shows small to medium-sized lymphocytes with round to oval nuclei, prominent nucleoli, and basophilic agranular cytoplasm with cytoplasmic protrusions or blebs **(A)**. Small cell variant T-PLL (PB) shows small lymphocytes with condensed chromatin, scant cytoplasm, and often no visible nucleoli **(B)**. Cerebriform variant T-PLL (PB) shows small lymphocytes with marked nuclear irregularity/convolutions **(C)**. Bone marrow typically shows an interstitial infiltrate by small to medium-sized lymphocytes **(D)**; and the infiltrating pattern is well illustrated by CD3 immunohistochemistry **(E)**. TCL1 is positive in 80% to 90% T-PLL **(F)**.

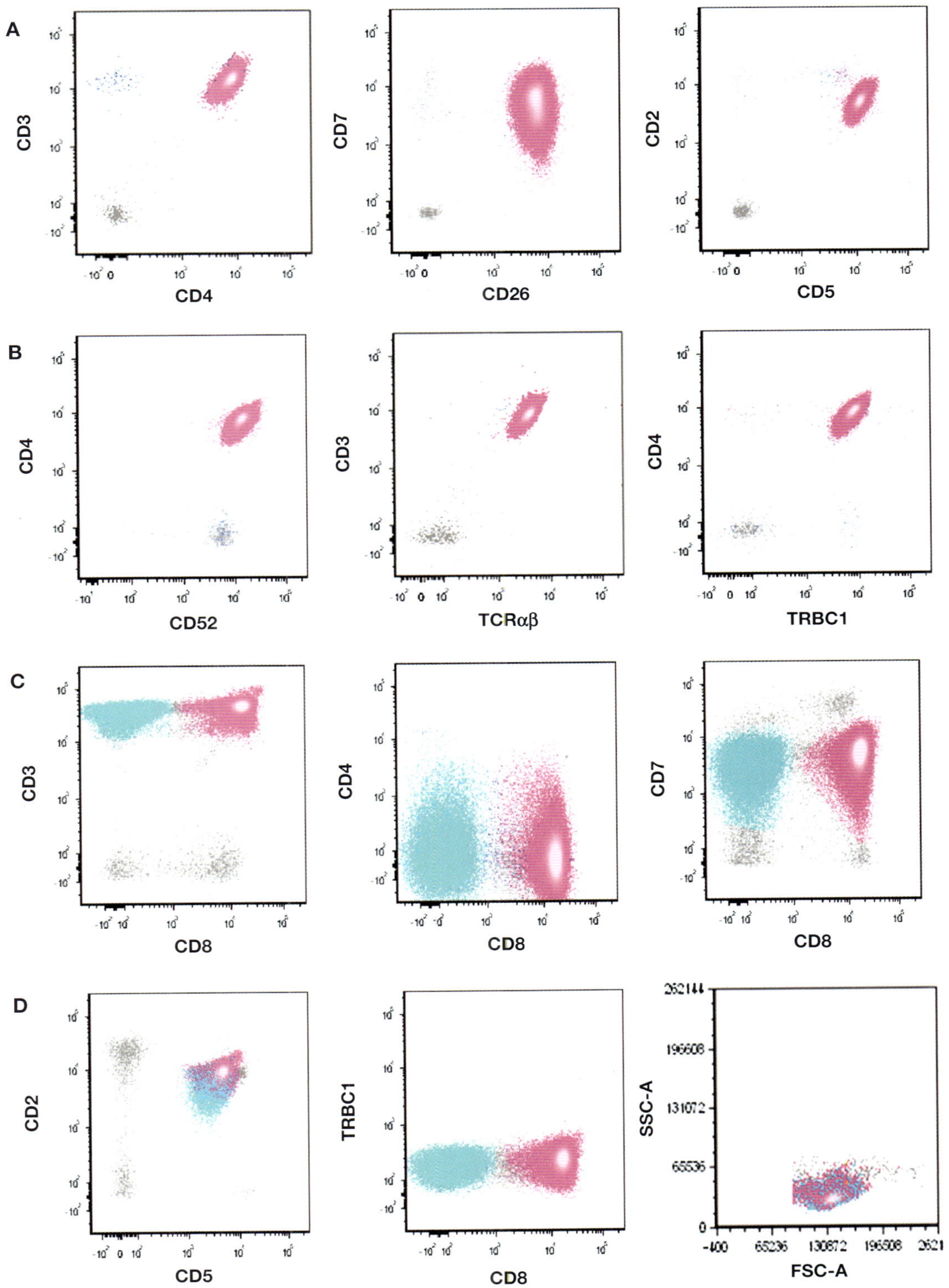

FIGURE 88.2 Flow cytometry immunophenotyping of T-cell prolymphocytic leukemia (T-PLL). Rows **A** and **B** illustrate a typical case of CD4$^+$ T-PLL, CD3$^+$, CD7bright+, CD26uniformly+, with no loss of CD2 and CD5, and CD52$^+$ (target for alemtuzumab). The T-PLL cells are TCRαβ+ and TRBC1+ (clonal pattern). Rows **C** and **D** show a case of T-PLL with immunophenotypic heterogeneity, the pink subset is CD8$^+$, and the turquoise subset is CD8 negative. Both populations show a minimal CD4 expression but are uniformly positive for CD7 (also CD26 and TCRαβ+, not shown), with no loss of CD2 and CD5. Both subsets are TRBC1 negative (clonal pattern) and small on forward scatter (FSC).

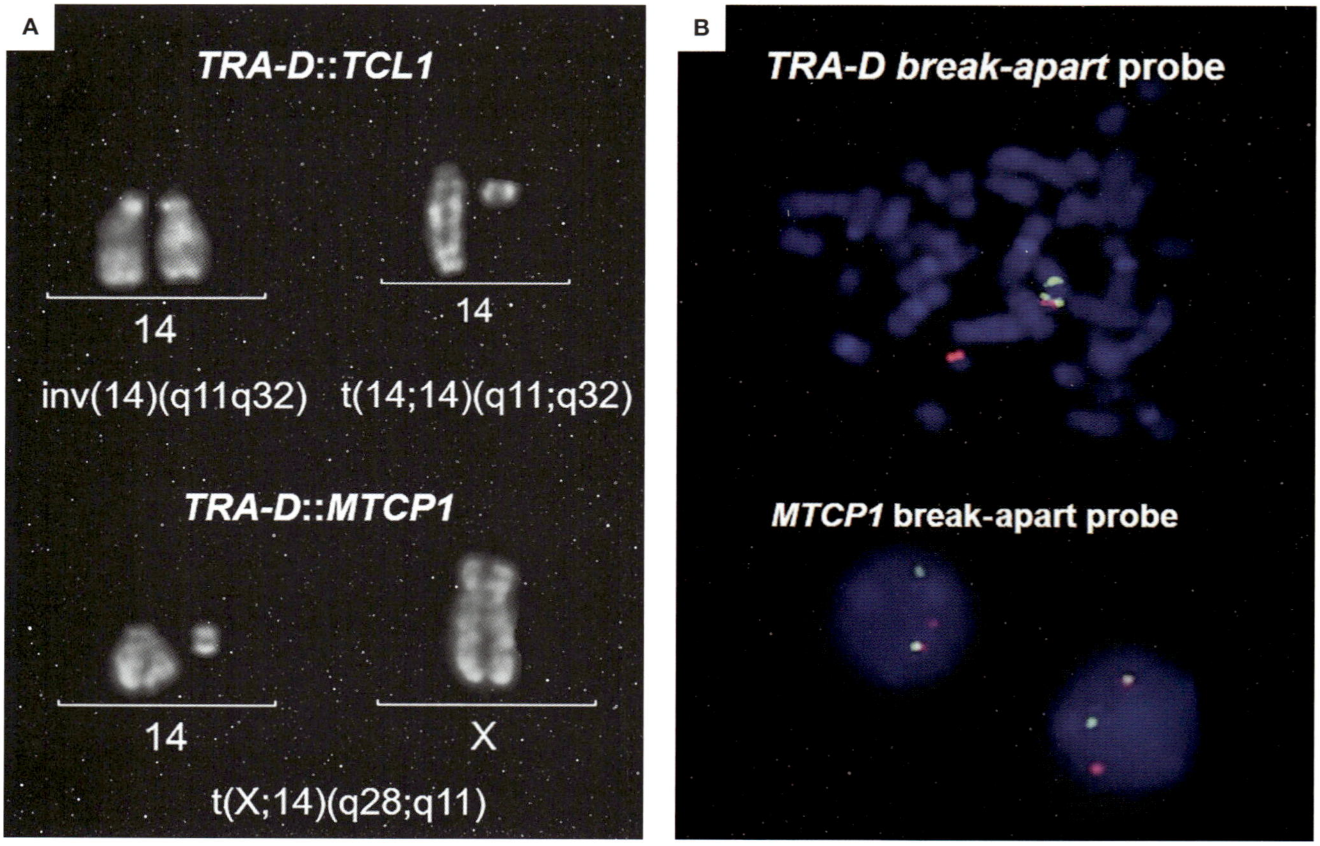

FIGURE 88.3 Cytogenetics in T-cell prolymphocytic leukemia (T-PLL). Panel **A** displays the hallmark structural aberrations in T-PLL: inv(14)(q11q32), t(14;14)(q11;q32), or t(X;14)(q28;q11) detected by conventional cytogenetics analysis, leading to upregulation of *TCL1* or its homologous gen *MTCP1*. The TRA-D rearrangement involved in the inv(14)(q11q32) or t(14;14)(q11;q32) could be analyzed using the fluorescence in situ hybridization (FISH) approach by *TRA-D* break-apart FISH probe, displayed in the upper part of panel **B**. The figure shows the *TRA-D* rearranged allele, corresponding to a green and red split signals, and the yellow signal indicating the unrearranged *TRA-D* allele. The lower part of panel **B** illustrates the FISH pattern detected in an exemplary case with *MCTP1* rearrangement. The yellow signal shows the unrearranged *MTCP1* allele, and the green and red signals show the rearranged allele.

and result in activation and overexpression of the proto-oncogene *TCL-1*.[4,5] Other translocations, t(X;14)(q28;q11) and t(X;7)(q28;q34), seen in around 10% of patients, involve rearrangement of the TRA/TRD with the *MTCP1* gene (belonging to the *TCL-1* gene family). A complex karyotype is a common finding. Alterations of chromosome 8, including idic(8p11),t(8;8)(p11-12;q12) among other unbalanced rearrangements of chromosome 8 are frequently detected. The *MYC* gene localized at 8q24 is not rearranged in these cases, but the encoded protein may be overexpressed. Loss-of-function mutations and/or deletion of *ATM*/11q22.3 (some can be cryptic, requiring fluorescence in situ hybridization study) resulting in somatic inactivation of *ATM* are common. In patients with ataxia telangiectasia with germline *ATM* mutation, a second *ATM* mutation is detected in patients who developed T-PLL. *TP53* mutation and/or deletion can reach up to one-third of cases.

There are several other recurrent chromosomal abnormalities, such as loss at 22q, 13q, 6q, 9p, 12p, and 17p and gains at 22q and 6p. Molecular genomic studies have revealed frequent somatic mutations involving the JAK-STAT pathway, such as activating mutations in *IL2RG, JAK1, JAK3,* and *STAT5B* (70%-80%) that are usually mutually exclusive. Studies have also found somatic mutations in epigenetic regulators and DNA repair genes, such as *EZH2, TET2, SMAHD1,* and *BCOR*. The role of the T-cell receptor, its downstream kinases, and JAK/STAT signaling in the pathogenesis of T-PLL has yet to be fully elucidated but may have therapeutic implications.

T-PLL pathogenesis is commonly driven by TCL1 overexpression and *ATM* loss, as well as genetic alterations that are incorporated into the TPLL-ISG diagnostic criteria. The co-operation between *TCL1* family members and *ATM* is unique to T-PLL across the spectrum of T-cell neoplasms.[6,7]

Notably, in around 10% of T-PLL cases, *TCL1 or MTCP* rearrangement or TCL1 overexpression is absent,[8] but such cases show characteristic clinicopathological features of T-PLL, harbor a complex karyotype, or chromosome 8, 12, 13, 22 abnormalities, with a high frequency of *ATM* inactivation, fulfilling the TPLL-ISG diagnostic criteria for T-PLL.[2,4] These cases, referred to as TCL1-family negative T-PLL, frequently start with a relatively indolent phase but progress to aggressive disease in a median interval less than 1 year.[9]

Prognosis and Clinical Comment

The median overall survival from the time of diagnosis remains less than 3 years. Risk factors associated with a poorer outcome include a high white blood cell count, short lymphocyte doubling time, older age, low hemoglobin, low platelets, and abnormal cytogenetics.[8] The most important predictor of outcome is response to alemtuzumab therapy, and this may be less favorable in patients with extramedullary disease.

In the few patients who present with indolent disease, it is reasonable to monitor them initially, but it is important to keep these patients under close surveillance due to the speed of progression when it occurs.

Alemtuzumab is still the recommended first-line treatment of choice (if available), given intravenously three times a week. It is associated with an overall response rate of over 80%.[10] There is no evidence that adding chemotherapy to alemtuzumab leads to a significant improvement in outcome. Despite encouraging response rates, relapse is inevitable, and so in those suitable, a stem cell transplant should be considered in first remission. Median progression-free survival post allogeneic stem cell transplant is about 18 to 24 months, with a high nonrelapse mortality. There is a plateau in the survival curves post allograft, suggesting that up to a third of patients will achieve a long-term response.[10] Autologous stem cell transplants have also been reported with some prolonged responses and could be considered if there is concern regarding fitness for allogeneic stem cell transplant or lack of a suitable donor.

With current treatment options, very few patients will have a successful outcome after relapse and most patients with T-PLL will still die from their disease. Future therapy will depend on the introduction of novel targeted agents, which as yet have not induced durable responses as single agents but may be more successful when used in combination strategies.

References

1. Swerdlow SH, Campo E, Pileri SA, et al. The 2016 revision of the World Health Organization classification of lymphoid neoplasms. *Blood*. 2016;127(20):2375-2390.
2. Staber PB, Herling M, Bellido M, et al. Consensus criteria for diagnosis, staging, and treatment response assessment of T-cell prolymphocytic leukemia. *Blood*. 2019;134(14):1132-1143.
3. Garand R, Goasguen J, Brizard A, et al. Indolent course as a relatively frequent presentation in T-prolymphocytic leukaemia. Groupe Français d'Hématologie Cellulaire. *Br J Haematol*. 1998;103(2):488-494.
4. Sun Y, Tang G, Hu Z, et al. Comparison of karyotyping, TCL1 fluorescence in situ hybridisation and TCL1 immunohistochemistry in T cell prolymphocytic leukaemia. *J Clin Pathol*. 2018;71(4):309-315.
5. Patil P, Cieslak A, Bernhart SH, et al. Reconstruction of rearranged T-cell receptor loci by whole genome and transcriptome sequencing gives insights into the initial steps of T-cell prolymphocytic leukemia. *Genes Chromosomes Cancer*. 2020;59(4):261-267.
6. Oberbeck S, Schrader A, Warner K, et al. Noncanonical effector functions of the T-memory-like T-PLL cell are shaped by cooperative TCL1A and TCR signaling. *Blood*. 2020;136(24):2786-2802.
7. Schrader A, Crispatzu G, Oberbeck S, et al. Actionable perturbations of damage responses by TCL1/ATM and epigenetic lesions form the basis of T-PLL. *Nat Commun*. 2018;9(1):697.
8. Fang H, Beird HC, Wang SA, et al. T-prolymphocytic leukemia: TCL1 or MTCP1 rearrangement is not mandatory to establish diagnosis. *Leukemia*. 2023;37(9):1919-1921.
9. Rose A, Zhang L, Jain AG, et al. Delineation of clinical course, outcomes, and prognostic factors in patients with T-cell prolymphocytic leukemia. *Am J Hematol*. 2023;98(6):913-921.
10. Dearden CE, Matutes E, Cazin B, et al. High remission rate in T-cell prolymphocytic leukemia with CAMPATH-1H. *Blood*. 2001;98:1721-1726.

Chapter 89

T-Cell Large Granular Lymphocytic Leukemia

Eric D. Hsi, Jarek P. Maciejewski, Min Shi, and Sa A. Wang

Definition

T-cell large granular lymphocytic leukemia (T-LGLL) is an indolent clonal proliferation of cytotoxic T cells resulting in cytopenias, usually along with lymphocytosis. Initially described in 1985, two general forms of large granular lymphocytic (LGL) neoplasias are recognized with approximately 90% being derived from T cells (T-LGLL) and 10% being derived from natural killer (NK) cells (chronic lymphoproliferative disorder of NK cells [CLPDNK], described in Chapter 90). T-LGLL may be diagnosed in the setting of a persistent increase in LGLs (preferably $>2.0 \times 10^9$/L) that are monoclonal. Lower numbers (0.5-2.0×10^9/L) of clonal LGLs may be acceptable for diagnosis in an appropriate clinical setting (persistent cytopenias and/or presence of an autoimmune disease) and in the presence of a bone marrow LGL infiltrate.[1-5]

Synonyms

T-gamma lymphocytosis (obsolete), T-cell large granular lymphocytosis, T-large granular lymphocytic leukemia (all not recommended).

Epidemiology

T-LGLL is a rare disorder with an estimated incidence of 0.2 to 0.72/million. It accounts for 2% to 5% of chronic lymphoproliferative disorders in North America and Europe, and up to 5% to 6% in Asia.[1]

General Clinical Features

T-LGLL is a disease of older adults, with a median age at diagnosis between 59 and 65 years and only 20% of patients being diagnosed before age 50. The M:F ratio is 1.0. There is an association with autoimmune diseases, most notably rheumatoid arthritis (RA). Felty syndrome (RA, splenomegaly, neutropenia) may be seen in 1% to 3% of RA patients, and RA is present in approximately 20% of T-LGLL patients, leading to the notion that they represent the spectrum of the same disease process. Other autoimmune diseases such as celiac disease, inflammatory bowel disease, pure red cell aplasia, and polymyalgia rheumatica, among others, may also occur and usually predate the diagnosis of T-LGLL. Cytopenias such as neutropenia, thrombocytopenia, and anemia are reported in 41% to 61%, 19% to 26%, and 24% to 41% of patients, respectively. Severe anemia (transfusion-dependent) or thrombocytopenia ($<50 \times 10^9$/L) are uncommon but severe neutropenia ($<0.5 \times 10^9$/L) is reported in 17% to 26% of patients.

Aphthous ulcers and recurrent infections may be presenting findings, a result of severe neutropenia. Splenomegaly is present in 25% to 30% of patients and hepatomegaly in 10%. Approximately one-third of patients may be asymptomatic and discovered due to cytopenias found on routine examination or during management of their autoimmune disorder.[4,5]

There is also an association of clonal T-LGL proliferations/leukemia with monoclonal gammopathy of undetermined significance, multiple myeloma, B-cell malignancies, and monoclonal B-cell lymphocytosis. Clonal T-LGL proliferations/LGL leukemia may occur concurrently with, or after treatment for, a hematologic disorder, or post-stem cell transplant. Many of these cases, particularly those after stem cell transplant, appear quite indolent.[6-9]

The LGL count is elevated (median 0.94-1.7×10^9/L) and approximately 60% of patients have an LGL count of $>1.0 \times 10^9$/L, while around 15% may have LGL counts of over 4.0×10^9/L.[4,5,7]

Morphology

The peripheral blood smear demonstrates increased numbers of large granular lymphocytes. Usually, the LGL cells are 15 to 18 μm in diameter and have moderate to abundant amounts of cytoplasm that contain fine to coarse azurophilic granules, round to slightly indented (reniform) nuclei, and mature chromatin. They may be morphologically indistinguishable from nonneoplastic activated cytotoxic lymphocytes (Figure 89.1A). However, some cases may exhibit abnormal features, such as irregular nuclear contours, reduced amount of cytoplasm, or reduced granules (Figure 89.1B). Bone marrow biopsy is not performed in all patients because a diagnosis of T-LGLL can sometimes be confidently made from peripheral blood studies in conjunction with clinical features. However, in cases with a low LGL count ($<2.0 \times 10^9$/L), bone marrow biopsy is highly recommended to demonstrate an LGL infiltrate to confirm the diagnosis. Bone marrow aspirate smears often show variable numbers of LGLs, similar to that in peripheral blood (Figure 89.1C). On bone marrow trephine biopsy, the LGL infiltrate can be difficult to see on hematoxylin and eosin staining (Figure 89.1D) and is best identified by immunohistochemistry using CD3, CD8, and cytotoxic markers TIA1 and granzyme B (Figure 89.1E and F). The infiltrate is often in an interstitial and/or a linear sinusoidal pattern and the latter is more characteristic of a neoplastic LGL infiltrate. Reactive lymphoid aggregates are frequently present, likely due to underlying autoimmune disorders.

Immunophenotype

Flow cytometry studies on the peripheral blood are critical for diagnosis. The majority of T-LGLL cells are $CD3^+CD8^+TCR\alpha\beta$ (80%-85%), expressing CD2, dim CD5, dim CD16, CD45RA, dim CD94, and CD57. Most will show restricted TCR Vβ family expression (Figure 89.2A). The use of the JOVI.1 antibody recognizing T-cell receptor β constant region 1 (TRBC1) has been shown to be useful in assessing T-cell clonality by flow cytometry with proposed cutoffs of <15%, >85%, or homogenous dim TRBC1 expression as evidence of clonality (Figure 89.2B).[10] Loss of pan-T-cell markers such as CD7, or rarely CD2 or CD5, may be seen. Increased CD16, CD94, and CD57 and decreased CD8 expression intensity as compared to normal/reactive LGL cells are frequently observed.[11] The $TCR\gamma\delta^+$ subtype comprises approximately 5% to 15% of T-LGLL. $TCR\gamma\delta^+$ T-LGLL cases are $CD3^+$, either $CD4^-/CD8^-$ or $CD8^+$, often $CD16^+$, $CD57^+$, and $CD56^-$/subset$^+$. While TRBC1 is not applicable to $TCR\gamma\delta^+$ T-LGLL, approximately 40% of TCRγδ T-LGLL cases demonstrate a single killer cell immunoglobulin-like receptor restriction, making it a potentially useful tool for assessing T-cell clonality (Figure 89.2C). While $TCR\gamma\delta^+$ T-LGLL shares morphological similarities with $TCR\alpha\beta^+$ T-LGLL, it tends to present with a higher frequency of cytopenias and exhibits a shorter overall survival.[12] Rare cases of LGL leukemia are $CD4^+/TCR\alpha\beta^+$ (2%-4%), which often coexpress dim/partial CD8, and are frequently positive

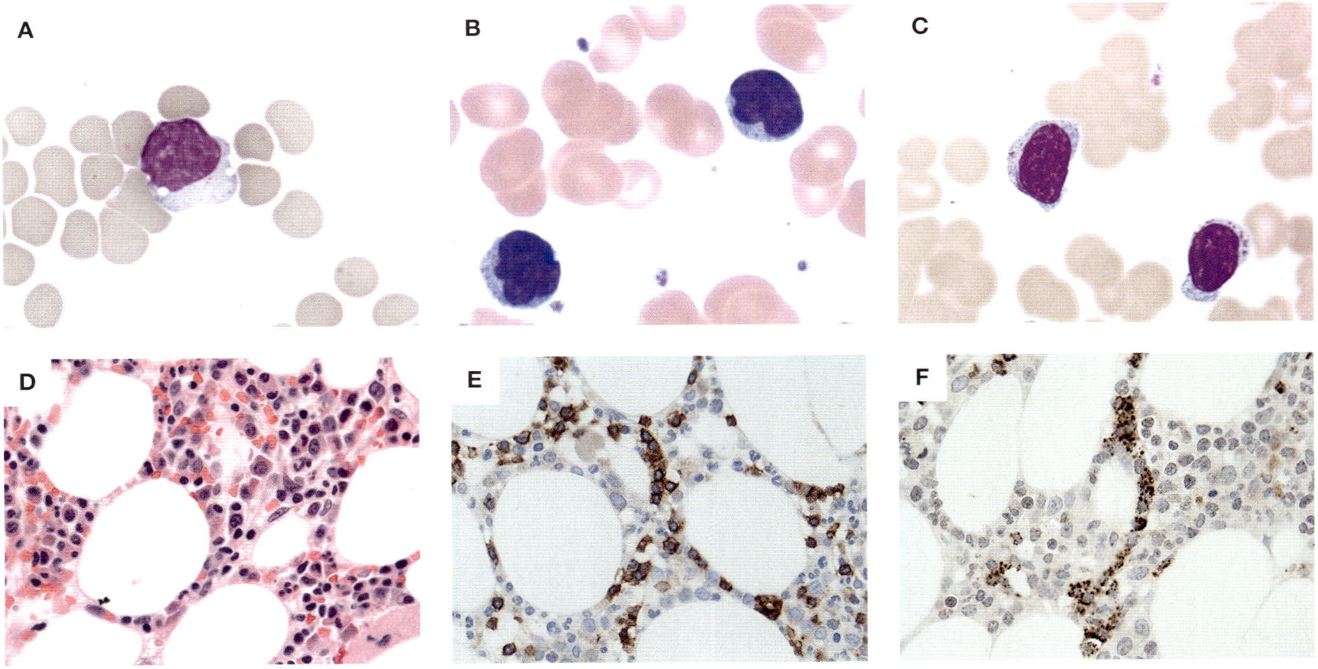

FIGURE 89.1 Morphology of T-cell large granular lymphocytic leukemia (T-LGLL) in peripheral blood (PB) and bone marrow (BM). **A:** Typical large granular lymphocytic (LGL) cells in PB have round or oval nuclei and abundant cytoplasm with azurophilic granules, indistinguishable from normal LGL cells. **B:** In some cases of T-LGLL, the cells in PB may demonstrate atypical features, such as small size, irregular nuclear contours, and reduced cytoplasm. **C:** LGL cells on BM aspirate smears are often similar to those on PB, in this case, with reduced cytoplasm and reduced granules. **D:** In the BM, the LGL infiltrate is difficult to visualize on hematoxylin and eosin staining. **E:** CD3 highlights small T cells, predominantly interstitial and focally sinusoidal. **F:** The sinusoidal infiltrate (highlighted by granzyme B) of T-LGLL is in a thin linear pattern, contrasting hepatosplenic T-cell lymphoma that expands the sinuses.

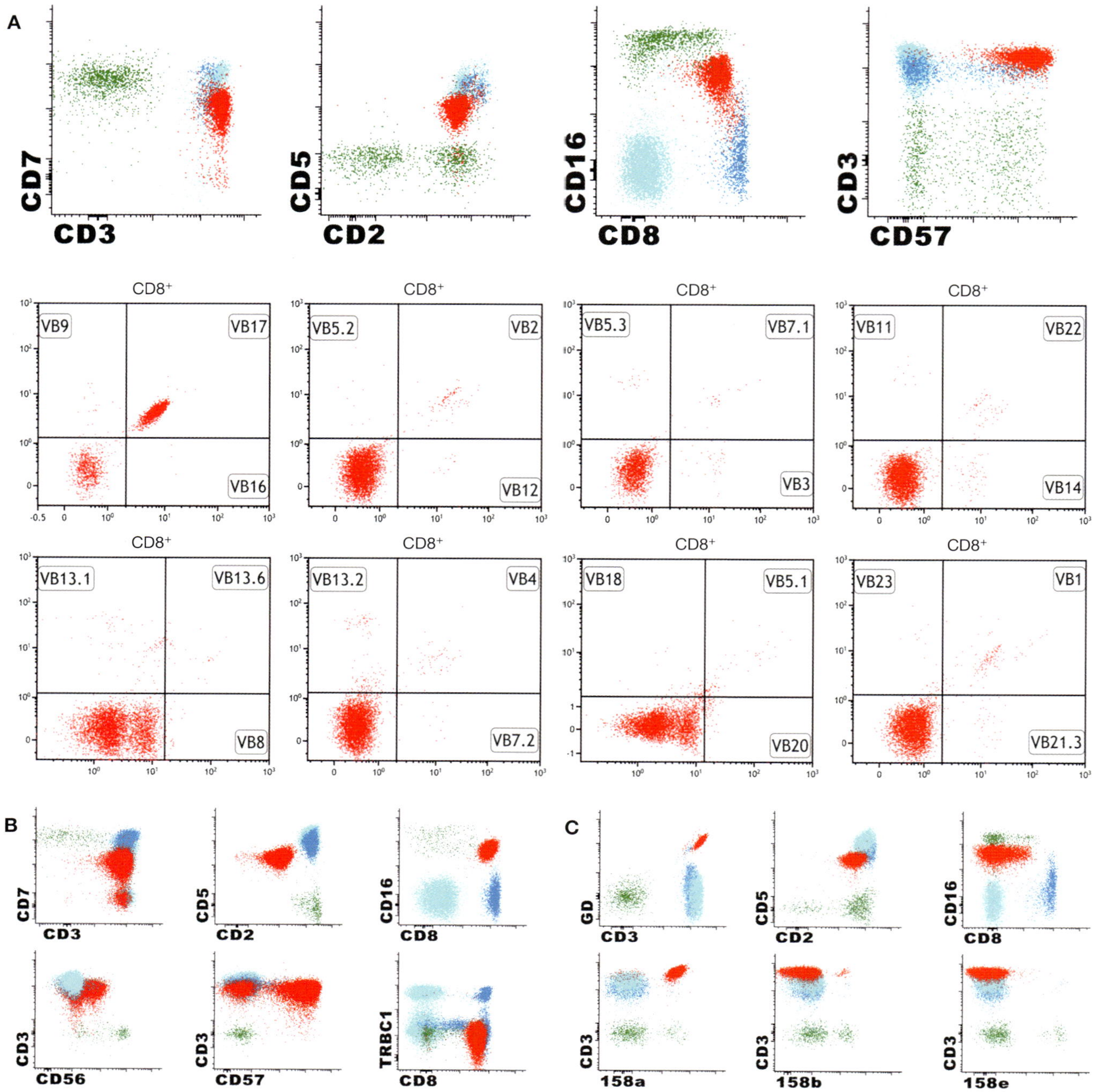

FIGURE 89.2 Flow cytometric immunophenotypes of T-cell large granular lymphocytic leukemia (T-LGLL) cases. **A:** In a CD3$^+$CD16$^+$CD57$^+$TCRαβ T-LGLL case (cells of interest colored in red), there is diminished expression of CD7, CD2, CD5, and CD8. The restricted V beta 17 expression on neoplastic cells confirms T-cell clonality. **B:** A CD3$^+$CD8$^+$CD16$^+$TCRαβ T-LGLL case reveals dim expression of CD7, CD2, CD5, CD56, and partial CD57 expression. The neoplastic cells uniformly lack TRBC1 expression, demonstrating T-cell clonality. **C:** A CD3$^+$CD16$^+$ TCRγδ T-LGLL case dimly expresses CD2 and CD5, which also shows restricted expression of the killer cell immunoglobulin-like receptor molecule CD158a, consistent with a clonal T-cell population.

for CD56 and CD57. Patients with CD4$^+$ LGL leukemia are less likely to present with cytopenia(s) or an autoimmune disease; instead, they more frequently associate with a primary malignancy than CD8$^+$ T-LGLL.[13,14]

Recommended markers for immunohistochemistry are CD3, CD8, and cytotoxic markers such as TIA1 and granzyme B. CD57 can be weak or partial, and often does not highlight all LGL cells. Granzyme B can be partially or completely lost in 30% to 40% T-LGLL. An algorithmic approach for diagnosis of T-LGLL and CLPDNK is illustrated in Figure 89.3.

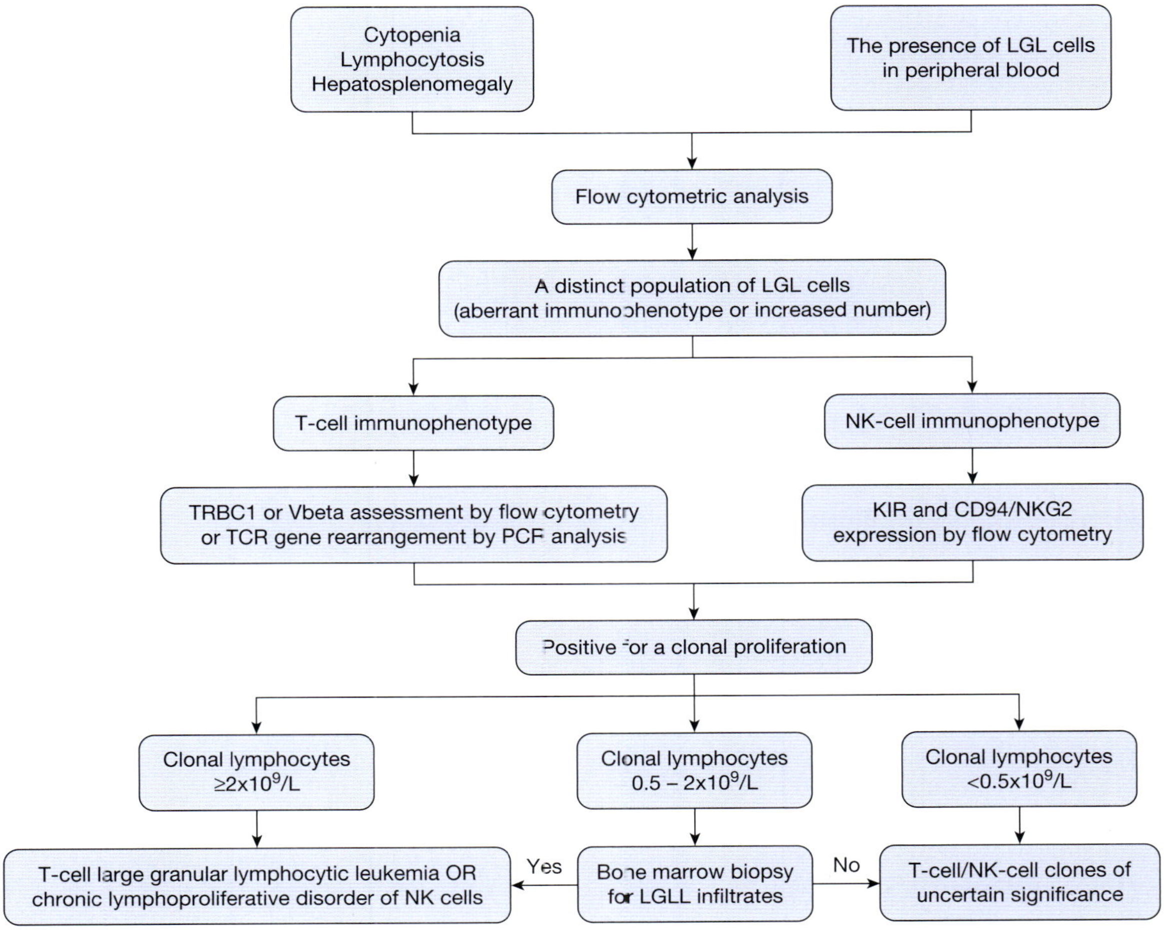

FIGURE 89.3 An algorithmic approach to large granular lymphocytic leukemia (LGLL) diagnosis. KIR, killer cell immunoglobulin-like receptor; LGL, large granular lymphocytic; NK, natural killer; PCR, polymerase chain reaction.

Genetics

By definition, T-cell receptor gene rearrangement studies show monoclonal results. Whole exome and transcriptome studies have shown putative driver mutations in *ARHGAP25, ABCC9, PCDHA11, SULF1, SLC6A15, DDX59, DNMT3A, FAS, KDM6A, KMT2D, PIK3R1, STAT3, STAT5B, TET2* and *TNFAIP3*. Among these, TCRγδ and TCRαβ cases shared *STAT3, KMT2D, PIK3R1,* and *SULF1* mutations.[15] Activating *STAT3* mutations are most common, seen in 30% to 50% of cases of T-LGLL and have been associated with a low neutrophil count ($<0.5 \times 10^9$/L), anemia (Hgb < 9.0 g/dL), need for treatment, and a shorter overall survival. *STAT3*-mutated cases show increased prevalence of comutations in the chromatin-modifying genes *KMT2D* and *SETD1B* as well as *TET2*. *DNMT3A* mutations are found in *STAT3* wild-type cases.[7,15,16] *STAT5B* mutations are found in few T-LGLL cases (2%) but appear to be enriched in CD4$^+$ T-LGLL (55%).[13]

Prognosis and Clinical Comment

A significant proportion of T-LGLL patients (30%-50%) are asymptomatic and only a minority show a proliferative from of this disease with a significant lymphocytosis. Because of its nonprogressive nature, expectant monitoring is warranted in many patients. The decision to initiate treatment is dictated by the presence/evolution of symptomatic cytopenias. Traditional chemotherapy is ineffective and chronic administration of immunosuppressive agents such as oral methotrexate, cyclosporine A and/or cyclophosphamide is commonly used when treatment is required. Refractory cases may require more potent immunosuppression that includes antithymocyte globulin and alemtuzumab.[7] The clinical context may be important in refractory cases. For example, patients may have coexisting hypogammaglobulinemia, plasma cell and B-cell dyscrasia, autoimmune hemolytic anemia, myelodysplastic syndrome or clonal cytopenia of undetermined significance, or organ transplant, which may suggest potential alternate therapeutic targets.[17-20] Overall survival (OS) is favorable (5-year OS of approximately 90% in some series) and prognosis is most dependent on comorbidities and severity and persistence of neutropenia.[4,7] To date, no widely accepted prognostic biomarkers have been found, including *STAT3* mutations which at best have only marginal impact.[7,21] Rare cases of T-LGLL have been reported to transform to a clonally related peripheral T-cell lymphoma.[22] Table 89.1 summarizes the features of T-LGLL.

T-Cell Clones of Uncertain Significance

The term T-cell clones of uncertain significance (T-CUS) is emerging. It may be used for cases in which small T-cell clones are found by sensitive flow cytometry or molecular analysis with minimal or no increase in LGLs ($<0.5 \times 10^9$/L) in the absence of clinical or laboratory features of a T-cell malignancy. T-CUS may occur in the setting of an immunodominant oligoclonal reactive expansion of cytotoxic T cells. T-CUS shows no significant bone marrow LGL infiltrate and thus also lacks sinusoidal infiltrates. Evaluation for somatic mutations such as in *STAT3* should be interpreted with caution since mutations have been reported in aplastic anemia, myelodysplasia, pure red cell aplasia, and carriers of HTLV1 and 2.[10,23-25]

TABLE 89.1 Summary of clinical and pathologic features of T-cell large granular lymphocytic leukemia (T-LGLL)

Clinical features
Median age of 60 years
Equal M:F ratio
Persistent T-LGLL–related symptoms (60%-70%)
Infections and fatigue
Splenomegaly
Hepatomegaly
Autoimmune disorders or other hematologic disorders (20%-30%)
Pathologic features
Large granular lymphocytes in the peripheral blood
Immunophenotypically distinct T cells (dim CD5, dim CD7, CD16, CD57)
Clonal T cells by flow cytometry or molecular studies
Intrasinusoidal distribution of cytotoxic T cells in the bone marrow
Somatic mutations in T cells (*STAT3* most commonly)

References

1. Lamy T, Moignet A, Loughran TP Jr. LGL leukemia: from pathogenesis to treatment. *Blood.* 2017;129(9):1082-1094. doi:10.1182/blood-2016-08-692590
2. Moosic KB, Ananth K, Andrade F, Feith DJ, Darrah E, Loughran , TP Jr. Intersection between large granular lymphocyte leukemia and rheumatoid arthritis. *Front Oncol.* 2022;12:869205. doi:10.3389/fonc.2022.869205
3. Park SH, Lee YJ, Kim Y, Kim HK, Lim JH, Jo JC. T-large granular lymphocytic leukemia. *Blood Res.* 2023;58(S1):S52-S57. doi:10.5045/br.2023.2023037
4. Bareau B, Rey J, Hamidou M, et al. Analysis of a French cohort of patients with large granular lymphocyte leukemia: a report on 229 cases. *Haematologica.* 2010;95(9):1534-1541. doi:10.3324/haematol.2009.018481
5. Dong N, Castillo Tokumori F, Isenalumhe L, et al. Large granular lymphocytic leukemia - a retrospective study of 319 cases. *Am J Hematol.* 2021;96(7):772-780. doi:10.1002/ajh.26183
6. Gill H, Ip AH, Leung R, et al. Indolent T-cell large granular lymphocyte leukaemia after haematopoietic SCT: a clinicopathologic and molecular analysis. *Bone Marrow Transplant.* 2012;47(7):952-956. doi:10.1038/bmt.2011.212
7. Sanikommu SR, Clemente MJ, Chomczynski P, et al. Clinical features and treatment outcomes in large granular lymphocytic leukemia (LGLL). *Leuk Lymphoma.* 2018;59(2):416-422. doi:10.1080/10428194.2017.1339880
8. Sidiqi MH, Aljama MA, Viswanatha DS, Dingli D. T-cell large granular lymphocytic leukemia and plasma cell disorders. *Haematologica.* 2019;104(3):e108-e110. doi:10.3324/haematol.2018.204099
9. Goyal T, Thakral B, Wang SA, et al. T-cell large granular lymphocytic leukemia and coexisting B-cell lymphomas: a study from the bone marrow Pathology Group. *Am J Clin Pathol.* 2018;149(2):164-171. doi:10.1093/ajcp/aqx146
10. Shi M, Olteanu H, Jevremovic D, et al. T-cell clones of uncertain significance are highly prevalent and show close resemblance to T-cell large granular lymphocytic leukemia. Implications for laboratory diagnostics. *Mod Pathol.* 2020;33(10):2046-2057. doi:10.1038/s41379-020-0568-2
11. Ohgami RS, Ohgami JK, Pereira IT, Gitana G, Zehnder JL, Arber DA. Refining the diagnosis of T-cell large granular lymphocytic leukemia by combining distinct patterns of antigen expression with T-cell clonality studies. *Leukemia.* 2011;25(9):1439-1443. doi:10.1038/leu.2011.107
12. Barila G, Grassi A, Cheon H, et al. Tγδ LGLL identifies a subset with more symptomatic disease: analysis of an international cohort of 137 patients. *Blood.* 2023;141(9):1036-1046. doi:10.1182/blood.2021013489

13. Bhattacharya D, Teramo A, Gasparini VR, et al. Identification of novel STAT5B mutations and characterization of TCRβ signatures in CD4+ T-cell large granular lymphocyte leukemia. *Blood Cancer J*. 2022;12(2):31. doi:10.1038/s41408-022-00630-8
14. Lima M, Almeida J, Dos Anjos Teixeira M, et al. TCRalphabeta+/CD4+ large granular lymphocytosis: a new clonal T-cell lymphoproliferative disorder. *Am J Pathol*. 2003;163(2):763-771. doi:10.1016/s0002-9440(10)63703-0
15. Cheon H, Xing JC, Moosic KB, et al. Genomic landscape of TCRαβ and TCRγδ T-large granular lymphocyte leukemia. *Blood*. 2022;139(20):3058-3072. doi:10.1182/blood.2021013164
16. Barila G, Teramo A, Calabretto G, et al. Stat3 mutations impact on overall survival in large granular lymphocyte leukemia: a single-center experience of 205 patients. *Leukemia*. 2020;34(4):1116-1124. doi:10.1038/s41375-019-0644-0
17. Awada H, Mahfouz RZ, Durrani J, et al. Large granular lymphocytic leukaemia after solid organ and haematopoietic stem cell transplantation. *Br J Haematol*. 2020;189(2):318-322. doi:10.1111/bjh.16336
18. Durrani J, Awada H, Kishtagari A, et al. Large granular lymphocytic leukemia coexists with myeloid clones and myelodysplastic syndrome. *Leukemia*. 2020;34(3):957-962. doi:10.1038/s41375-019-0601-y
19. Gurnari C, Durrani J, Pagliuca S, et al. Novel invariant features of Good syndrome. *Leukemia*. 2021;35(6):1792-1796. doi:10.1038/s41375-020-01114-z
20. Ogbue OD, Kewan T, Bahaj WS, Gurnari C, Visconte V, Maciejewski JP. New approaches to idiopathic neutropenia in the era of clonal hematopoiesis. *Exp Hematol Oncol*. 2023;12(1):42. doi:10.1186/s40164-023-00403-4
21. Munoz-Garcia N, Jara-Acevedo M, Caldas C, et al. STAT3 and STAT5B mutations in T/NK-cell chronic lymphoproliferative disorders of large granular lymphocytes (LGL): association with disease features. *Cancers*. 2020;12(12):3508. doi:10.3390/cancers12123508
22. Pastoret C, Llamas-Gutierrez F, Fouchard M, et al. Molecular mechanisms underlying transformation of large granular lymphocytic leukemia to high-grade T-cell lymphoma. *Leukemia*. 2023;37(7):1567-1571. doi:10.1038/s41375-023-01922-z
23. Semenzato G, Teramo A, Calabretto G, Gasparini VR, Zambello R. All that glitters is not LGL Leukemia. *Leukemia*. 2022;36(11):2551-2557. doi:10.1038/s41375-022-01695-x
24. Kim D, Myllymaki M, Kankainen M, et al. Somatic STAT3 mutations in CD8(+) T cells of healthy blood donors carrying human T-cell leukemia virus type 2. *Haematologica*. 2022;107(2):550-554. doi:10.3324/haematol.2021.279140
25. Yamagishi M, Kubokawa M, Kuze Y, et al. Chronological genome and single-cell transcriptome integration characterizes the evolutionary process of adult T cell leukemia-lymphoma. *Nat Commun*. 2021;12(1):4821. doi:10.1038/s41467-021-25101-9

Chapter 90

Chronic Lymphoproliferative Disorder of Natural Killer Cells

Eric D. Hsi, Jarek P. Maciejewski, Min Shi, and Sa A. Wang

Definition

Chronic lymphoproliferative disorder of natural killer cells (CLPD-NK) is an indolent proliferation characterized by a persistent increase in peripheral blood large granular lymphocytes of natural killer (NK) cell type (preferably greater than 2.0×10^9/L) without an identifiable reactive cause. Monoclonality may be demonstrated by molecular or flow cytometric methods.

Synonyms

NK-large granular lymphocytic leukemia, chronic NK lymphocytosis, NK-cell large granular lymphocytosis, indolent large granular NK-cell lymphoproliferative disorder, indolent leukemia of NK cells (not recommended).

Epidemiology

CLPD-NK is uncommon, comprising 5% to 10% of large granular lymphocytic (LGL) proliferations in series reporting both T-LGL leukemia (T-LGLL), and CLPD-NK. It occurs in adults with a median age in the late fifth and early sixth decade of life and slight male predominance (M:F = 1.4). There does not appear to be a geographic or ethnic predilection.[1,2]

General Clinical Features

Approximately 50% of patients are asymptomatic. The presenting symptoms include fatigue, splenomegaly, hepatomegaly, and recurrent infections. Similar to T-LGLL, patients with CLPD-NK often have a history of autoimmune disease.[1,3] Some patients have a history of hematologic malignancy such as lymphoma, MGUS/myeloma, or myeloid neoplasms (together about 10% of patients) or solid tumor (10%-15% of patients). Mild lymphocytosis with an absolute lymphocyte count of $>4.0 \times 10^9$/L is seen in approximately half of the patients. The median LGL count is 2.1×10^9/L, and around 30% have LGL counts $<1.0 \times 10^9$/L. Neutropenia is present in approximately 30% of patients, thrombocytopenia in 20% of patients, and Hgb < 11 g/dL in 20% of patients.[1,4] Hemolytic anemia appears to be more common in the context of CLPD-NK than T-LGLL.[5] In rare patients both forms of LGL proliferations can coexist.[3]

Morphology

The peripheral blood smear shows increased mature large granular lymphocytes. These cells may be smaller than usual LGL cells with relatively scant cytoplasm; some may show irregular nuclei but commonly show abundant pale blue cytoplasm with variable numbers of azurophilic granules (Figure 90.1A and B). Although bone marrow biopsy is not done in every case, it often shows an increase in interstitial cytotoxic lymphocytes, which is subtle on hematoxylin and eosin–stained slides and best seen by immunohistochemical stains (Figure 90.1C). Most cases will show at least a focal sinusoidal infiltrate in addition to an interstitial infiltrate but dense and diffuse involvement is not typically seen (Figure 90.1D and E).[6]

Immunophenotype

Immunophenotyping is critical for making a diagnosis of CLPD-NK. Normal NK cells lack surface CD3 and CD5 but express CD2, CD7, CD16, CD94, and CD56, with a small subset being positive for CD8 and CD57. In CLPD-NK, abnormal NK cells may partially or completely lose expression of CD7 or CD56 but only rarely lose CD2 (Figure 90.1F). Other immunophenotypic aberrations in CLPD-NK include uniform CD57 expression (in approximately 60% of cases), either complete loss or conversely uniform expression of CD8, and CD5 expression in rare cases. Similar to normal NK cells, the neoplastic cells in CLPD-NK express cytotoxic granules such as TIA1, granzyme B, and perforin, but granzyme B can be lost in a subset of cases.

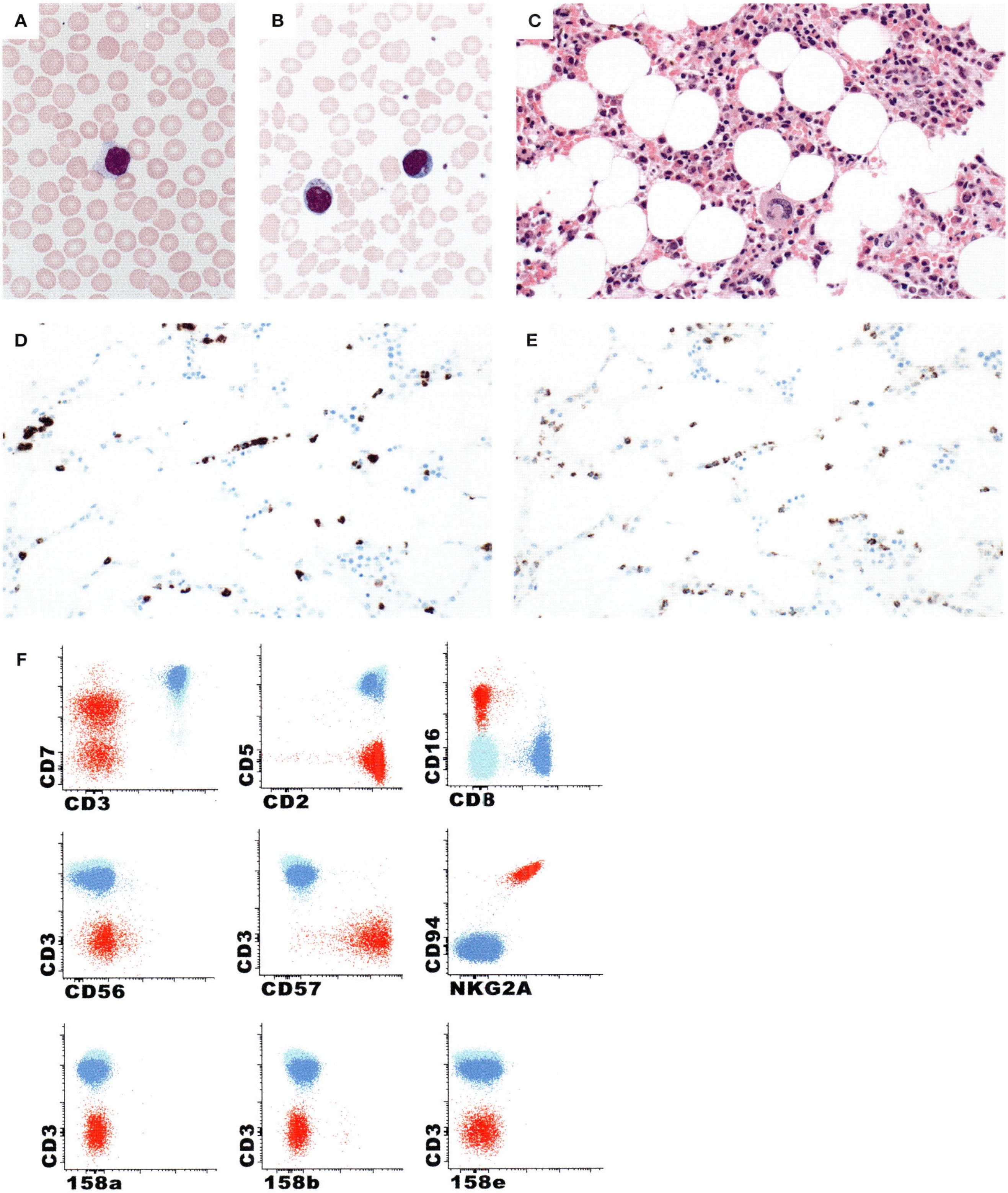

FIGURE 90.1 Morphologic and immunophenotypic characteristics of chronic lymphoproliferative disorder of natural killer cells (CLPD-NK). **A:** CLPD-NK cells typically display ample cytoplasm with variable granules. **B:** Sometimes CLPD-NK cells have less abundant cytoplasm and irregular nuclear contours. **C:** Patients with CLPD-NK often exhibit increased marrow cellularity without evident lymphocytic infiltrates on hematoxylin and eosin–stained slides. Immunohistochemical stains for granzyme B **(D)** and TIA-1 **(E)** reveal a linear arrangement of cytotoxic lymphocytes inside the sinuses. **F:** Flow cytometry analysis demonstrates that the CLPD-NK case is negative for CD3 and CD5, positive for CD2 and partially positive for CD7 with coexpression of CD16 and CD57; it lacks CD56 expression. The complete absence of CD158a, CD158b, and CD158e, along with uniform expression of CD94/NKG2A, suggests NK-cell clonality.

Recent studies have attempted to compare the phenotype of CLPD-NK with normal NK-cell subsets based on expression of CD16, CD56, and CD57. $CD16^{dim}/CD56^{bright}$ NK cells are found in tissues such as lymph node, tonsils, and gut, while $CD16^{+}/CD56^{dim/neg}$ NK cells are preferentially found in blood, bone marrow, spleen, and lung. $CD16^{dim}/CD56^{bright}$ NK cells secrete cytokines and chemokines facilitating communication with immune cells and the microenvironment, while $CD16^{+}/CD56^{dim/neg}$ cells are cytotoxic effectors that can further differentiate to a terminally differentiated $CD57^{+}$ adaptive ("memory") subset, seen preferentially in blood. Some studies suggest the $CD16^{+}/CD56^{dim/neg}/CD57^{neg}$ phenotype correlates with *STAT3* mutation and more symptomatic disease.[7,8]

Restricted expression or absence of killer cell immunoglobulin-like receptors such as CD158a, CD158b, and CD158e or homogeneous expression of CD94/NKG2A and CD94/NKG2C complexes can be used as surrogates of clonality in NK-cell populations (Figure 90.1F).[9] However, this is not widely available and requires experience in interpretation with the caveat that, as with other LGL proliferations, transiently restricted populations might be found in occasional reactive settings, so-called NK-cell clones of uncertain significance.[6,9,10]

Genetics

Recurrent somatic mutations have been reported in CLPD-NK (Table 90.1). Detailed studies of the commonly mutated genes such as *STAT3, TET2*, and *CCL22* show that these somatic mutations are indeed present in NK cells. Of interest, *TET2* mutations were often shared by both myeloid and NK cells, suggesting *TET2* alterations occur in hematopoietic stem cells. This might explain the association between CLPD-NK and myeloid malignancy in some patients.[4,11-13]

CCL22 and *STAT3* mutations seem to be mutually exclusive. *STAT3* mutations in CLPD-NK have been associated with a $CD16^{bright}/CD56^{dim}$ phenotype and lower hemoglobin and neutrophil counts.[4,7,12] *TET2* mutations may preferentially be associated with a $CD16^{dim}$ phenotype, a lower platelet count, the presence of other hematologic malignancy, and resistance to immunosuppressive agents.[4,11] *CCL22* mutations are associated with a $CD16^{dim}/CD56^{bright}$ immunophenotype. Demonstration of somatic mutations in NK cells such as *STAT3* mutation indicates NK clonality. It is a robust marker to help distinguish reactive and neoplastic NK-cell populations; however, caution is advised in using somatic mutation data in isolation for diagnosis of NK and T-LGLL since *STAT3* mutations have been found in asymptomatic carriers of HTLV 1 and 2.[14,15]

To differentiate CLPD-NK from reactive NK lymphocytosis, the practical diagnostic algorithm may follow that illustrated in Chapter 89.

Prognosis and Clinical Comment

Overall, the survival of CLPD-NK is similar to that of T-LGLL. Owing to the rarity of CLPD-NK, little treatment data are available. Methotrexate and cyclophosphamide seem to have similar response rates, but less

TABLE 90.1 Recurrent mutations reported in CLPD-NK[4,11,12]

Gene	Frequency	Pathway
STAT3	31%	JAK/STAT
CCL22	21%	CCL22
TET2	20%	Epigenetic
PIK3CA/PIK3AP1	10%	PI3K/AKT
TNFAIP3	10%	NF-κB
ATM	7%	DNA damage repair
DNMT3A	7%	Epigenetic
ASXL1	5%	Epigemetic
PPM1D	5%	TP53
KRAS	5%	RAS
STAT5B	5%	JAK/STAT

Pastoret C, Desmots F, Drillet G, et al. Linking the KIR phenotype with STAT3 and TET2 mutations to identify chronic lymphoproliferative disorders of NK cells. Blood. 2021;137(23):3237-3250; Olson TL, Cheon H, Xing JC, et al. Frequent somatic TET2 mutations in chronic NK-LGL leukemia with distinct patterns of cytopenias. Blood. 2021;138(8):662-673; and Baer C, Kimura S, Rana MS, et al. CCL22 mutations drive natural killer cell lymphoproliferative disease by deregulating microenvironmental crosstalk. *Nat Genet.* 2022;54(5):637-648.

experience exists with cyclosporine A, tacrolimus, and sirolimus. Improvement has been observed with splenectomy in a few reported patients.[2] In patients with cytopenia and clonal hematopoiesis it can be difficult to distinguish between symptomatic CLPD-NK with coincidental clonal hematopoiesis of indeterminate potential (CHIP) versus clonal cytopenia of undetermined significance (CCUS) with asymptomatic CLPD-NK.

References

1. Poullot E, Zambello R, Leblanc F, et al. Chronic natural killer lymphoproliferative disorders: characteristics of an international cohort of 70 patients. *Ann Oncol.* 2014;25(10):2030-2035. doi:10.1093/annonc/mdu369
2. Sanikommu SR, Clemente MJ, Chomczynski P, et al. Clinical features and treatment outcomes in large granular lymphocytic leukemia (LGLL). *Leuk Lymphoma.* 2018;59(2):416-422. doi:10.1080/10428194.2017.1339380
3. Jerez A, Clemente MJ, Makishima H, et al. STAT3 mutations unify the pathogenesis of chronic lymphoproliferative disorders of NK cells and T-cell large granular lymphocyte leukemia. *Blood.* 2012;120(15):3048-3057. doi:10.1182/blood-2012-06-435297
4. Pastoret C, Desmots F, Drillet G, et al. Linking the KIR phenotype with STAT3 and TET2 mutations to identify chronic lymphoproliferative disorders of NK cells. *Blood.* 2021;137(23):3237-3250. doi:10.1182/blood.2020006721
5. Ogbue OU S, Bravo-Perez C, Williams ND, et al. Insights into large granular lymphocytic leukemia-associated hemolytic anemia: clinical associations, therapeutic responses, and optimal management strategies from a large institutional study. Poster presented at American Society of Hematology Annual Meeting; 12/11/2023. 2023; San Diego, CA.
6. Morice WG, Jevremovic D, Olteanu H, et al. Chronic lymphoproliferative disorder of natural killer cells: a distinct entity with subtypes correlating with normal natural killer cell subsets. *Leukemia.* 2010;24(4):881-884. doi:10.1038/leu.2009.304
7. Barila G, Teramo A, Calabretto G, et al. Dominant cytotoxic NK cell subset within CLPD-NK patients identifies a more aggressive NK cell proliferation. *Blood Cancer J.* 2018;8(6):51. doi:10.1038/s41408-018-0088-1
8. Dogra P, Rancan C, Ma W, et al. Tissue determinants of human NK cell development, function, and residence. *Cell.* 2020;180(4):749-763 e13. doi:10.1016/j.cell.2020.01.022
9. Seheult JN, Otteson GE, Jevremovic D, et al. Establishing NK-cell receptor restriction by flow cytometry and detecting potential NK-cell clones of uncertain significance. *Mod Pathol.* 2023;36(8):100255. doi:10.1016/j.modpat.2023.100255
10. Bravo-Perez C, Carrillo-Tornel S, Garcia-Torralba E, Jerez A. Persistent large granular lymphocyte clonal expansions: "the root of many evils"-and of some goodness. *Cancers.* 2022;14(5):1340. doi:10.3390/cancers14051340
11. Olson TL, Cheon H, Xing JC, et al. Frequent somatic TET2 mutations in chronic NK-LGL leukemia with distinct patterns of cytopenias. *Blood.* 2021;138(8):662-673. doi:10.1182/blood.2020005831
12. Baer C, Kimura S, Rana MS, et al. CCL22 mutations drive natural killer cell lymphoproliferative disease by deregulating microenvironmental crosstalk. *Nat Genet.* 2022;54(5):637-648. doi:10.1038/s41588-022-01059-2
13. Jerez A, Clemente MJ, Makishima H, et al. STAT3 mutations indicate the presence of subclinical T-cell clones in a subset of aplastic anemia and myelodysplastic syndrome patients. *Blood.* 2013;122(14):2453-2459. doi:10.1182/blood-2013-04-494930
14. Yamagishi M, Kubokawa M, Kuze Y, et al. Chronological genome and single-cell transcriptome integration characterizes the evolutionary process of adult T cell leukemia-lymphoma. *Nat Commun.* 2021;12(1):4821. doi:10.1038/s41467-021-25101-9
15. Kim D, Myllymaki M, Kankainen M, et al. Somatic STAT3 mutations in CD8(+) T cells of healthy blood donors carrying human T-cell leukemia virus type 2. *Haematologica.* 2022;107(2):550-554. doi:10.3324/haematol.2021.279140

Chapter 91
Adult T-Cell Leukemia/Lymphoma

Koichi Ohshima, Philippe Gaulard, Steven M. Horwitz, and Shigeo Nakamura

Definition

Adult T-cell leukemia/lymphoma (ATLL) is a peripheral T-cell neoplasm, which is caused by the human T-lymphotropic virus 1 (HTLV-1). Most ATLL patients present with widespread lymph node involvement as well as involvement of peripheral blood. The histology shows remarkable pleomorphism. The leukemic cells show the multilobed appearance of so-called flower cells. Neoplastic cells show monoclonal integration of HTLV-1 and express T-cell–associated antigens (CD2, CD3, CD5), but usually lack CD7. Most cases are CD4-positive.

Synonyms

Adult T-cell leukemia/lymphoma (HTLV-1–positive) (acceptable); adult T-cell lymphoma; adult T-cell leukemia (not recommended).

Epidemiology

ATLL is endemic in several regions of the world, in particular south-western Japan, the Caribbean basin, and parts of central Africa. The distribution of the disease is closely linked to the prevalence of HTLV-1 in the population. The disease has a long latency, and affected individuals are usually exposed to the virus very early in life. The virus may be transmitted in breast milk, as well as through exposure to peripheral blood and blood products. The cumulative incidence of ATLL is estimated to be 2.5% among HTLV-1 carriers in Japan.[1] Sporadic cases have been described, but the affected patients often derive from an endemic region of the world. ATLL occurs only in adults, and the patient age at onset ranges from the third to the ninth decade of life, with an average age at diagnosis of 58 years. The male to female ratio is 1.5-1.2:1.[1,2]

HTLV-1 is causally linked to ATLL, resulting in neoplastic transformation of infected cells with accumulation of genetic alterations. HTLV-1 enters cells mainly through cell-to-cell contact. Three molecules are involved in HTLV-1 binding and entry: (1) heparan sulfate proteoglycan,[3] (2) neuropilin 1,[4] and (3) glucose transporter 1.[5]

Neuropilin 1 appears to function as the viral receptor. The p40 tax viral protein leads to transcriptional activation of many genes in HTLV-1–infected lymphocytes.[6] In addition, the HTLV-1 basic leucine zipper factor (HBZ) is thought to be important for T-cell proliferation and oncogenesis.[7] However, additional genetic alternations acquired over time may result in the development of a malignancy. DNA hypermethylation is associated with disease progression.[8] HTLV-1 can also indirectly cause other diseases (Table 91.1), such as HTLV-1– associated myelopathy/tropical spastic paraparesis.[9]

General Clinical Features

Most patients present with widespread lymph node involvement and involvement of the peripheral blood (Figure 91.1). The number of circulating neoplastic cells does not correlate with the degree of bone marrow involvement. This suggests that circulating cells are recruited from other organs, such as the skin, which is the most common extralymphatic site of involvement (involved in >50% of cases). The distribution of the disease is usually systemic, involving the spleen and extranodal sites including the skin, lungs, liver, gastrointestinal tract, and central nervous system. There are epidemiologic differences in the patterns

TABLE 91.1 Clinical spectrum of HTLV-1–associated diseases

Neoplastic disorders
Adult T-cell leukemia/lymphoma
Smouldering
Chronic
Acute
Lymphomatous
Nonneoplastic disorders[1]
HTLV-1–associated myelopathy (tropical spastic paraparesis)
HTLV-1–associated infective dermatitis
Other HTLV-1 inflammatory disorders
Uveitis
Thyroiditis
Pneumonitis
Myositis

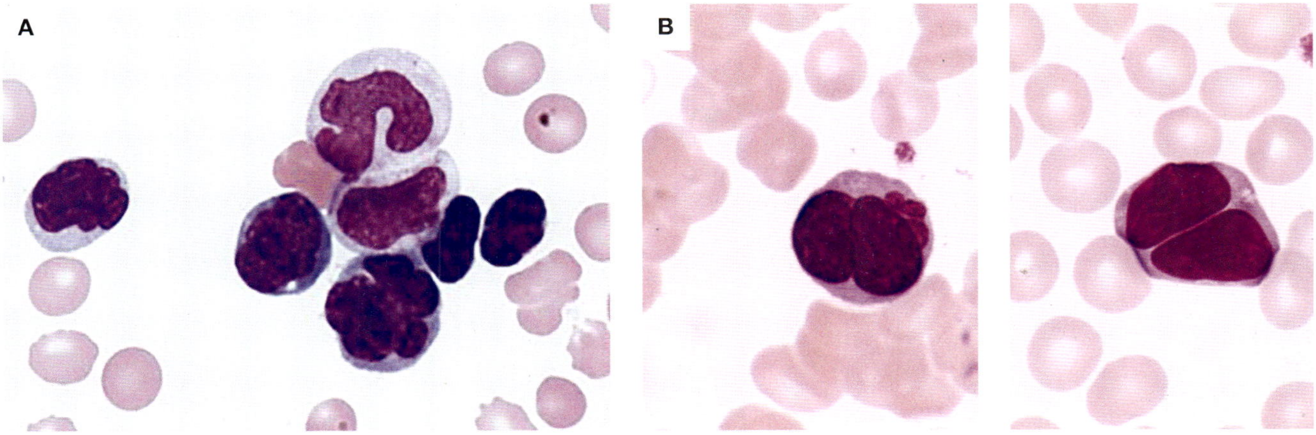

FIGURE 91.1 Adult T-cell leukemia/lymphoma (ATLL). Peripheral blood films. **A:** In the acute variant, the leukemic cells are medium-sized to large lymphoid cells with irregular nuclei and basophilic cytoplasm. The characteristic ATLL cells have been described as flower cells, with many nuclear convolutions and lobes. **B:** ATLL cells in the chronic variant are generally small, with slight nuclear abnormalities such as notching, indentation, and convolution.

of presentation. For example, a leukemic clinical presentation is much less common in patients from the Caribbean than in patients from Japan.[8]

Several clinical variants have been identified: acute, lymphomatous, chronic, and smoldering (Table 91.2).[10] The acute variant is most common and is characterized by a leukemic phase, often with a markedly elevated white blood cell count, skin rash, and generalized lymphadenopathy. Hypercalcemia, with or without lytic bone lesions, is a common feature. Patients with acute ATLL have systemic disease accompanied by hepatosplenomegaly, constitutional symptoms, and elevated lactate dehydrogenase. Many patients have an associated T-cell immunodeficiency, with frequent opportunistic infections such as *Pneumocystis jirovecii* pneumonia and strongyloidiasis. The lymphomatous variant is characterized by prominent lymphadenopathy but without peripheral blood involvement. Most patients present with advanced-stage disease similar to the acute form, although hypercalcemia is seen less often. Cutaneous lesions are common in both the acute and the lymphomatous forms of ATLL. They are clinically diverse and include erythematous rashes, papules, and nodules. Larger nodules may show ulceration. Rare cases show tumor-like lesions or erythroderma as seen in Sézary-like syndrome (Figure 91.2). The chronic variant is frequently associated with an exfoliative skin rash (Figures 91.2 and 91.3). An absolute lymphocytosis may be present, but atypical lymphocytes are not numerous in the peripheral blood. Hypercalcaemia is absent. In the smouldering variant, the white blood cell count is normal with >5% circulating neoplastic cells. ATLL cells are generally small, with a normal appearance (see Figure 91.1). Patients frequently have skin or pulmonary lesions, but there is no hypercalcaemia. Especially in patients with hypercalcemia, imaging studies may show lytic bone lesions

TABLE 91.2 Diagnostic criteria for clinical subtypes of adult T-cell leukemia/lymphoma

	Smouldering	Chronic	Lymphomatous	Acute
Lymphocytosis	No	Increased	No	Increased
Blood abnormal lymphocytes	>5%	Increased	<1%	Increased
Lactate dehydrogenase	Normal	Slightly increased	Variable	Increased
Calcium levels	Normal	Normal	Variable	Variable
Skin involvement	Erythema, papules	Variable	Variable	Variable
Lymphadenopathy	No	Mild	Yes	Variable
Hepatosplenomegaly	No	Mild	Variable	Variable
Bone marrow infiltration	No	No	Variable	Variable

Modified from Shimoyama M (1991). Diagnostic criteria and classification of clinical subtypes of adult T-cell leukaemia-lymphoma. A report from the Lymphoma Study Group (1984-87). *Br J Haematol.* 79:428-437.

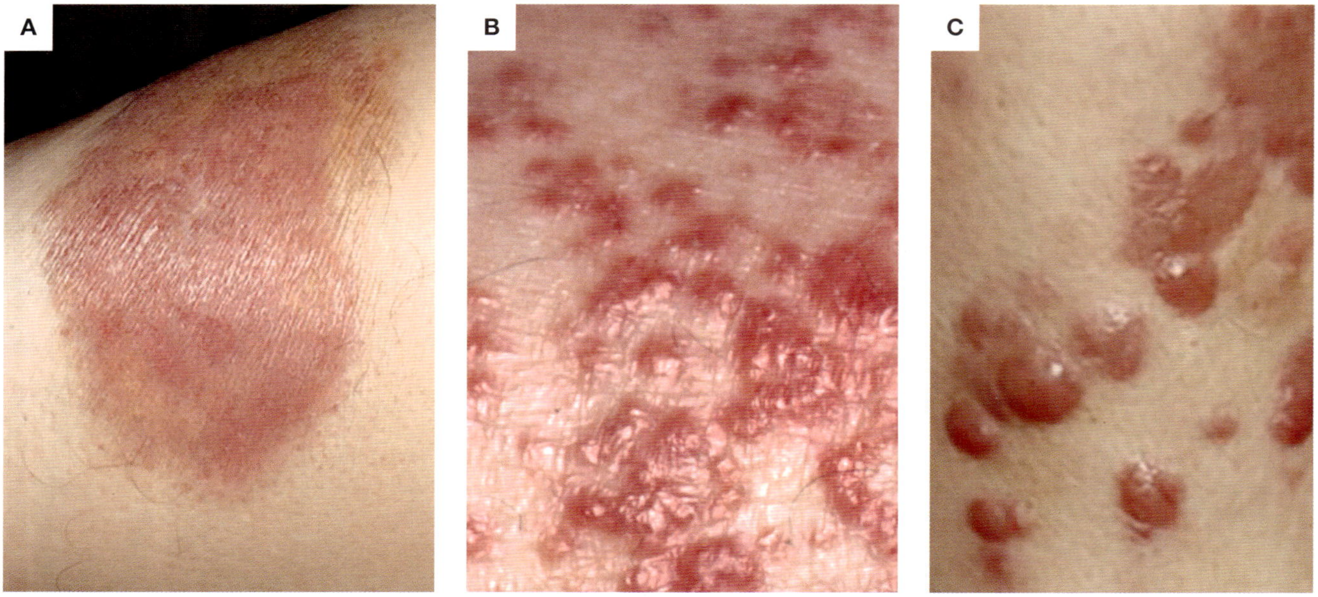

FIGURE 91.2 Adult T-cell leukemia/lymphoma. Cutaneous lesions classified as (A) erythema, (B) papules, and (C) nodules.

(Figures 91.4 and 91.5). Radiologically, FDG-PET/CT is usually positive in sites of disease activity.[11]

Morphology

Several morphologic variants have been described, reflecting this varied cytology and referred to as pleomorphic small, medium, and large cell types, anaplastic, and a rare form resembling angioimmunoblastic T-cell lymphoma[12] (Figures 91.6 and 91.7). The use of these variants is optional but they call attention to the spectrum of morphologic appearances. The inflammatory background is usually sparse, although eosinophilia may be present. The neoplastic lymphoid cells are typically medium-sized to large, often with pronounced nuclear pleomorphism. The nuclear chromatin is coarsely clumped with distinct, sometimes prominent, nucleoli. Blast-like cells with transformed nuclei and dispersed chromatin are present in variable proportions.[10] Giant cells with convoluted or multilobed nuclear contours are sometimes present. Rare cases are composed predominantly of small lymphocytes, with irregular nuclear contours. Cell size does not correlate with the clinical prognosis,[12] with the exception of the

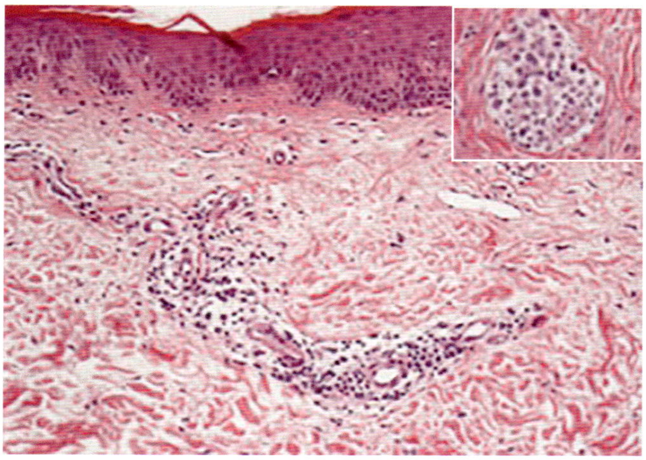

FIGURE 91.3 Adult T-cell leukemia/lymphoma, smoldering variant. A sparse infiltrate in perivascular lesion of the skin is seen with minimal cytologic atypia (inset).

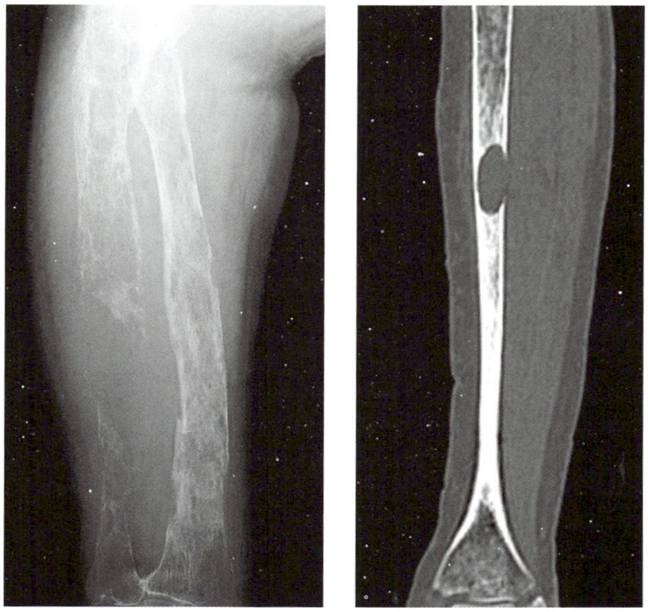

FIGURE 91.4 Adult T-cell leukemia/lymphoma. A radiograph shows extensive lytic bone lesions (left) and punched out lesion (right).

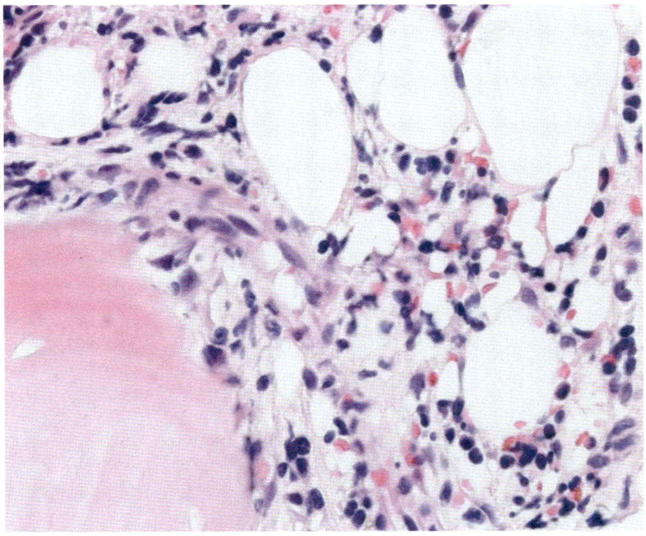

FIGURE 91.5 Adult T-cell leukemia/lymphoma. Bone marrow infiltrate is sparse. Osteoclastic activity along the trabeculae is prominent.

chronic and smoldering forms, in which the lymphocytes have a more normal appearance. Lymph nodes in some patients in an early phase of adult T-cell lymphoma/leukemia may exhibit a Hodgkin lymphoma–like histology[13] (Figure 91.8). The lymph nodes have expanded paracortical areas containing a diffuse infiltrate of small- to medium-sized lymphocytes with mild nuclear irregularities, indistinct nucleoli, and scant cytoplasm. EBV-positive B lymphocytes with Hodgkin-like features are interspersed in this background. The expansion of EBV-positive B cells is thought to be secondary to the underlying immunodeficiency seen in patients with ATLL. In the peripheral blood, the multilobed appearance of the neoplastic cells has led to the term flower cells. These cells have deeply basophilic cytoplasm, most readily observed with Giemsa staining of air-dried smears (see Figure 91.1). Marrow infiltrates are usually patchy, ranging from sparse to moderate. Osteoclastic activity may be prominent, even in the absence of bone marrow infiltration by neoplastic cells (Figure 91.5). Skin lesions are seen in >50% of patients with ATLL. Epidermal infiltration with Pautrier-like microabscesses is common (Figures 91.9 and 91.10). Dermal infiltration is mainly perivascular (see Figure 91.13), but larger tumor nodules may be observed. Diffuse infiltration of many organs is indicative of the systemic nature of the disease.

Immunophenotype

Tumor cells express T-cell–associated antigens (CD2, CD3, CD5), but usually lack CD7. Most cases are CD4-positive and CD8-negative, but a few are CD4-negative and CD8-positive or double positive for CD4 and CD8. CD25 is strongly expressed in nearly all cases. The large transformed cells may be positive for CD30, but are negative for ALK and cytotoxic molecules. Tumor cells frequently express the chemokine receptor CCR4. FOXP3, a feature of T regulatory (Treg) cells, is expressed in a subset of cases.[14] The postulated normal counterpart is a peripheral $CD4^+$ T cell. It has been hypothesized that the $CD4^+$, $CD25^+$, FOXP3+ Treg cells are the closest normal counterparts,[14] which would be consistent with the disease's characteristic association with immunodeficiency (Figure 91.11).

Genetics

Neoplastic cells show monoclonal integration of HTLV-1 (Figure 91.12). Clonal integration is not present in healthy carriers.[15] Tax, encoded by the HTLV-1 pX region, is a critical nonstructural protein that plays a key role in leukemogenesis and activates a variety

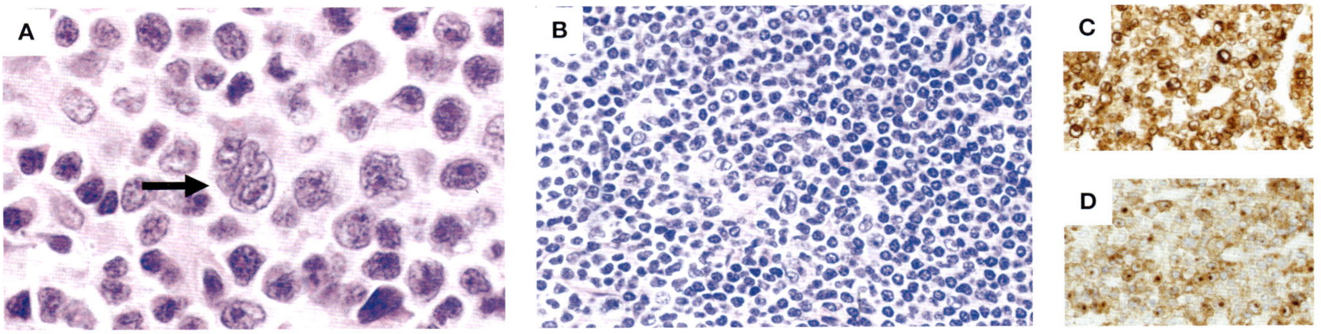

FIGURE 91.6 Adult T-cell leukemia/lymphoma. **A:** The pleomorphic (medium-sized and large cell) type shows a diffuse proliferation of atypical medium-sized to large lymphoid cells with irregular nuclei, intermingled with cerebriform giant cells (arrow). **B:** The lymph nodes in the pleomorphic small-cell type show a diffuse proliferation of atypical medium-sized to small lymphoid cells. The lymphoma cells usually express CD3 (**C**) and CCR4 (**D**).

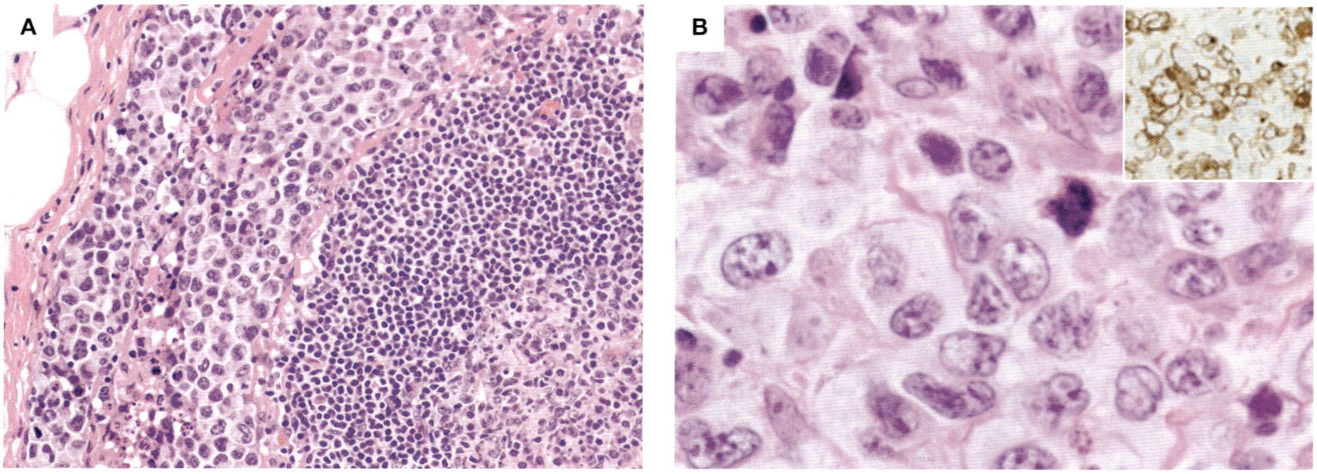

FIGURE 91.7 Adult T-cell leukemia/lymphoma. **A:** In this case, the lymphoma cells infiltrate the peripheral sinus of the lymph node. **B:** The morphology consists of large cells with anaplastic features. The cells are strongly CD30-positive (inset), raising the differential diagnosis with anaplastic large cell lymphoma.

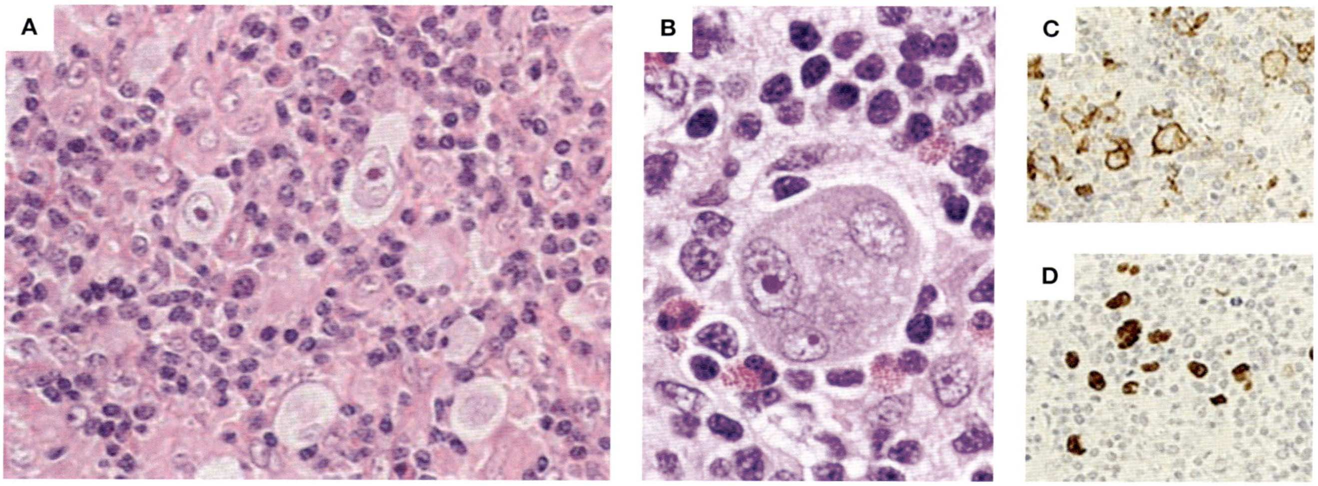

FIGURE 91.8 Adult T-cell leukemia/lymphoma (ATLL). **A:** The presence of pleomorphic tumor cells and background eosinophilia may simulate classic Hodgkin lymphoma. **B:** The lymph nodes in Hodgkin-like ATLL show Reed–Sternberg–like giant cells of B-cell (not T-cell) lineage, which react with CD30 antibody **(C)** and are EBV-positive (**D:** EBER1 in situ hybridization).

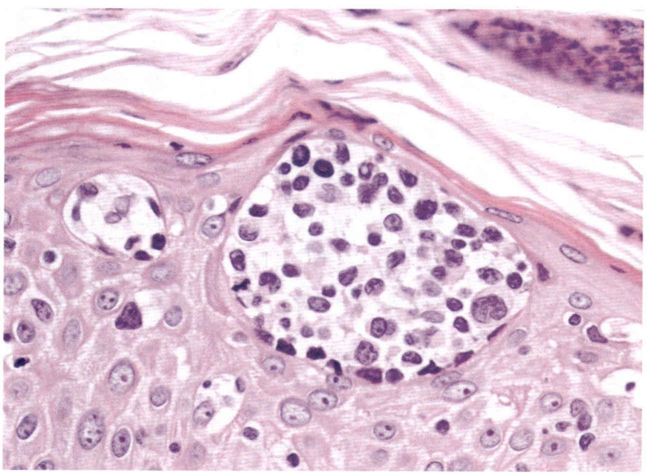

FIGURE 91.9 Adult T-cell leukemia/lymphoma. Neoplastic cells infiltrate the epidermis, producing Pautrier-like microabscesses.

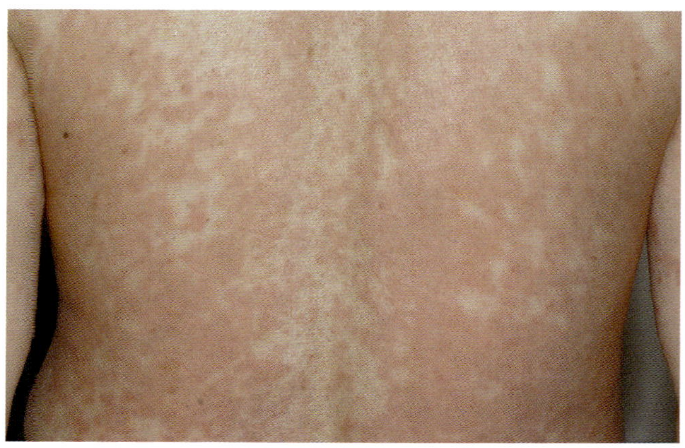

FIGURE 91.10 Adult T-cell leukemia/lymphoma, smoldering variant. Diffuse exfoliative skin rash.

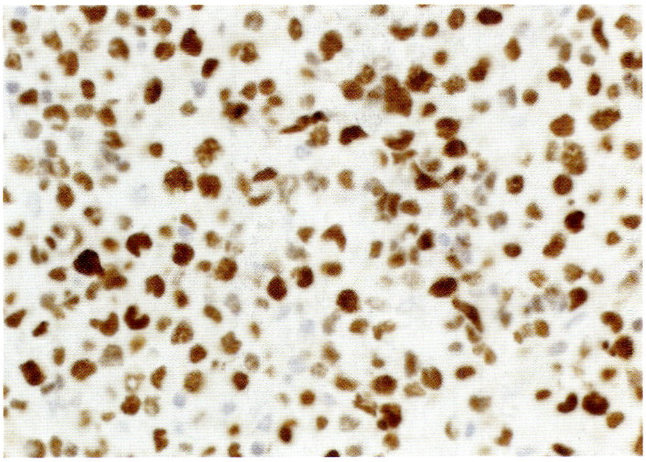

FIGURE 91.11 Adult T-cell leukemia/lymphoma cells frequently express FOXP3. The coexpression of FOXP3 and CD25 is characteristic of T regulatory (Treg) cells.

of cellular genes.[16] Enhancement of cAMP response element-binding (CREB) transcription factor phosphorylation by Tax appears to play a role in leukemogenesis and cell proliferation.[17] However, Tax is not critical to sustain tumor cell growth and is inactivated in a high proportion of cases of ATLL.[16] HBZ also appears to play a critical role in tumorigenesis.[18] HBZ is the only gene that is consistently expressed in all ATLL cases, which is contrasted with a temporary expression of Tax in a limited number of infected cells[19] (Figure 91.13). HBZ also drives cell proliferation, inhibits apoptosis, and induces the expression of TIGIT and CCR4 on cell surface, which is implicated in the proliferation and trafficking of malignant cells.[20]

A recent study provided an integrated genomic and transcriptomic analysis of >400 ATLL cases.[21] The authors identified a single viral integration site in most cases of ATLL, confirming the clonal nature of the disease. ATLL showed considerable genomic instability, with a high number of structural variations per case. A total of 50 genes were recurrently mutated. Among the most frequently mutated genes were *PLCG1, PRKCB, CCR4, CARD11, STAT3, TP53, VAV1, TBL1XR1, NOTCH1, GATA3, IRF4, FAS, CCR7 POT1*, some of which are involved in T-cell receptor signaling (Figure 91.14). This study also confirmed a high incidence of *CCR4* mutations and identified mutations in *CCR7* in some other cases. The additional mutations identified affect the NF-kappa B pathway and genes involved in T-cell signaling.

Recently, a clinicogenetic risk model for overall survival, m7-ATL-PI has been generated, which includes ATLL prognostic index (ATL-PI) and nonsilent mutations in seven genes. m7-ATL-PI was calculated by summing the following: high-risk ATL-PI category (+10), low-risk ATL-PI category (−4), and nonsilent mutations in *TP53* (+4), *IRF4* (+3), *RHOA* (+1), *PRKCB* (+1), *CARD11* (+0.5), *CCR7* (−2), and *GATA3* (−3).[22] Some genetic alterations are associated with immune escape mechanisms in ATLL. The genomic amplification of

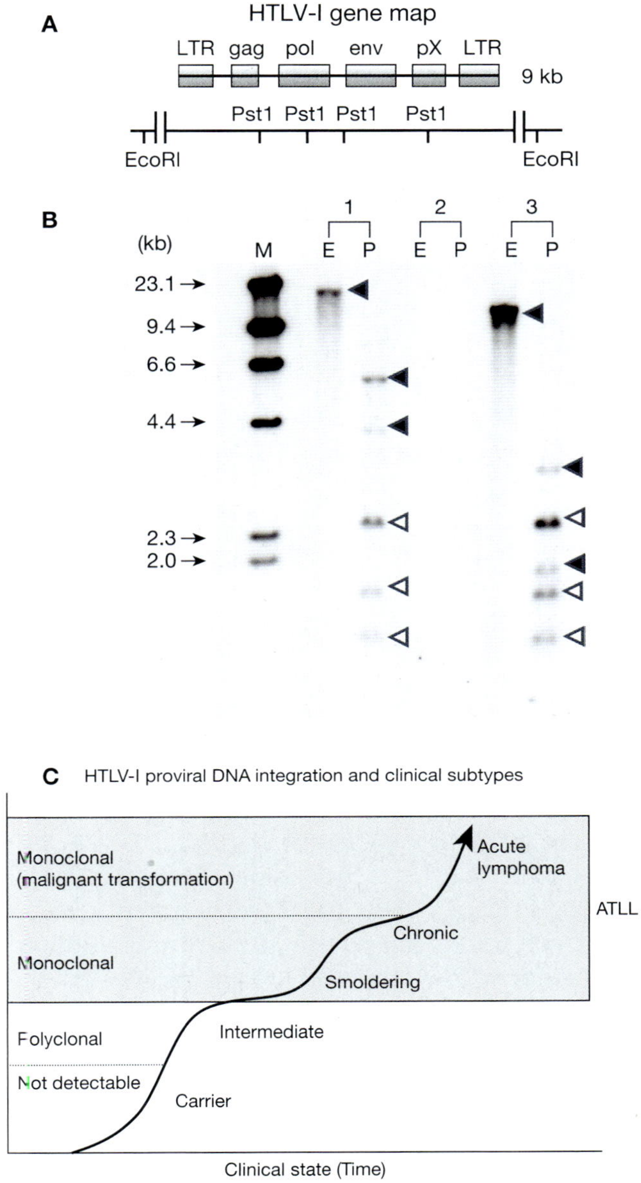

FIGURE 91.12 Adult T-cell leukamia/lymphoma (ATLL). **A:** HTLV-1 gene map. Restriction enzymes EcoRI (E) and PstI (P) recognition sites for each enzyme are shown. **B:** Southern blot analysis after DNA digestion with restriction enzymes EcoRI (E) and PstI (P). 1: positive control (adult T-cell leukemia/lymphoma [ATLL] cell line) 2: negative control. 3: ATLL case. M is size marker 1,3 display monoclonal proviral HTLV-1 DNA bands (▲) and internal bands (△). The difference in band sizes lane 1 and 3 for different cases is the result of the difference in integration sites. **C:** Adult T-cell leukemia/lymphoma. Status of HTLV-1 proviral DNA integration shown on the left is correlated to clinical status shown on the right.

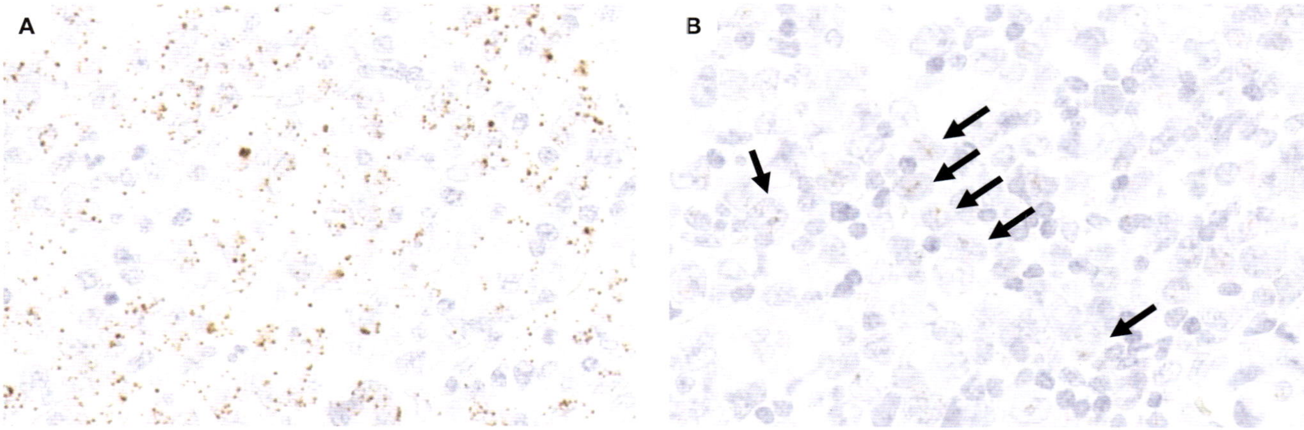

FIGURE 91.13 Adult T-cell leukemia/lymphoma (ATLL). **A:** In situ hybridization of HBZ mRNA. Target-specific signals showed dot-like pattern. The signals were expressed in a large number of ATLL cells. **B:** In situ hybridization of tax mRNA. At the most one or two signals were expressed per ATLL cell, and the intensity of many signals was weak. The signals (arrows) were expressed only in a small number of ATLL cells.

PD-L1, or disruption of the three prime untranslated regions (3′UTR) in *PD-L1* have been identified in 27% of ATLL cases. This disruption stabilizes the mRNA of *PD-L1* leading to overexpression, which allows ATLL cells to escape from the host immune response. Furthermore, deletions and mutations of genes related to major histocompatibility complex class I, including *HLA-A,-B* and *B2M*, have been identified in ATLL cases.[21] Young Japanese ATLL patients frequently have *CD28* fusions (*CTLA4::CD28, ICOS::CD28*), compared with unselected Japanese patients.[23,24] From a clinical perspective, *PD-L1* amplification is an independent negative prognostic factor among every subtype of ATLL case[21] (Figure 91.14).

Prognosis and Clinical Comments

Clinical subtype, patient age, performance status, and serum calcium and lactate dehydrogenase levels are major prognostic factors.[2] The survival time for the acute and lymphomatous variants ranges from 2 weeks to >1 year. Death is often caused by infectious complications, including *P. jirovecii* pneumonia, cryptococcal meningitis, disseminated herpes zoster, and hypercalcemia.[10] The chronic and smoldering forms have a more protracted clinical course and better survival, but can progress to an acute phase with an aggressive course in approximately 25% of patients[2] (Figure 91.15).

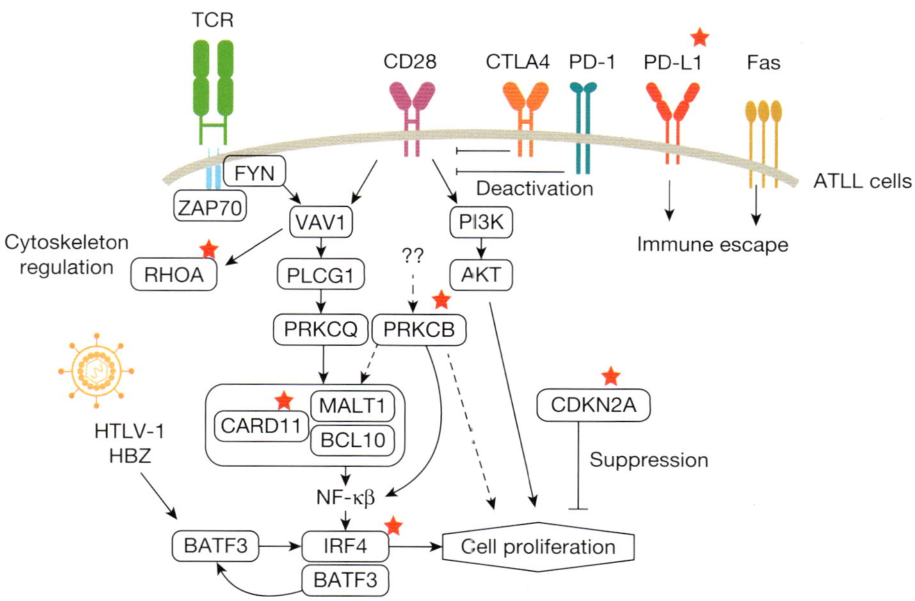

FIGURE 91.14 Adult T-cell leukemia/lymphoma (ATLL). Signaling pathways altered in ATLL are depicted. Red stars denote that the gene alterations related to prognosis in ATLL. (Modified from Yoshida N, Miyoshi H, Ohshima K. (2021) Clinical applications of genomic alterations in ATLL: predictive markers and therapeutic targets. *Cancers (Basel)*. 2021;13(8):1801. doi:10.3390/cancers13081801.)

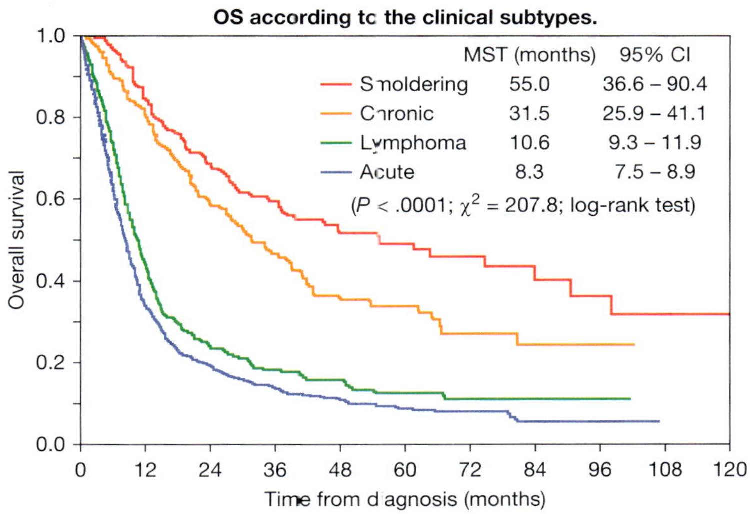

No. at risk

Smoldering	157	114	87	66	49	37	21	13	9	6	5
Chronic	187	121	80	49	33	24	15	9	3	0	0
Lymphoma	355	129	55	32	21	14	7	5	3	0	0
Acute	895	261	131	81	48	26	19	8	5	1	1

FIGURE 91.15 Adult T-cell leukemia/lymphoma. Overall survival of 1665 patients diagnosed between 2000 and 2009 in Japan. A total of 227 patients underwent allogeneic bone marrow transplantation; (OS) 25% of those patients had long survival. MST, median survival time. (Data from Katsuya H, Ishitsuka K, Utsunomiya A, et al. (2015). Treatment and survival among 1594 patients with ATL. *Blood.* 126:2570-2577.)

For aggressive ATLL, multiagent chemotherapy with or without allogeneic hematopoietic stem cell transplantation has been recommended, but for many patients the outcome remains poor. Recently, novel agents, including mogamulizumab, lenalidomide, brentuximab vedotin, tucidinostat and valemetostat, have been approved for those patients.[25]

References

1. Tajima K, Hinuma Y. Epidemiology of HTLV-I/II in Japan and the world. In: Takatsuki K, Hinuma Y, Yoshida M, eds. Advances in Adult T-Cell Leukemia and HTLV-I Research (Gann Monograph on Cancer Research). Japan Scientific Societies Press; 1992:129-149.
2. Katsuya H, Ishitsuka K, Utsunomiya A, et al. Treatment and survival among 1594 patients with ATL. *Blood*. 2015;126(24):2570-2577.
3. Jones KS, Petrow-Sadowski C, Bertolette DC, Huang Y, Ruscetti FW. Heparan sulfate proteoglycans mediate attachment and entry of human T-cell leukemia virus type 1 virions into CD4+ T cells. *J Virol*. 2005;79(20):12692-12702.
4. Ghez D, Lepelletier Y, Lambert S, et al. Neuropilin-1 is involved in human T-cell lymphotropic virus type 1 entry. *J Virol*. 2006;80(14):6844-6854.
5. Manel N, Kim FJ, Kinet S, Taylor N, Sitbon M, Battini JL. (2003) The ubiquitous glucose transporter GLUT-1 is a receptor for HTLV. , 115(4):449-459.
6. Franchini G. Molecular mechanisms of human T-cell leukemia/lymphotropic virus type I infection. *Blood*. 1995;86(10):3619-3639.
7. Satou Y, Yasunaga J, Yoshida M, Matsuoka M. HTLV-I basic leucine zipper factor gene mRNA supports proliferation of adult T cell leukemia cells. *Proc Natl Acad Sci U S A*. 2006;103(3):720-725.
8. Levine PH, Manns A, Jaffe ES, et al. The effect of ethnic differences on the pattern of HTLV-I-associated T-cell leukemia/lymphoma (HATL) in the United States. *Int J Cancer*. 1994;56(2):177-181.
9. Takatsuki K, Yamaguchi K, Watanabe T, et al. Adult T-cell leukemia and HTLV-1 related disease. *Gann Mono Can Res*. 1992;32:1-15.
10. Shimoyama M. Diagnostic criteria and classification of clinical subtypes of adult T-cell leukaemia-lymphoma. A report from the Lymphoma Study Group (1984-87). *Br J Haematol*. 1991;79(3):428-437.
11. Casulo C, Schöder H, Feeney J, et al. 18F-fluorodeoxyglucose positron emission tomography in the staging and prognosis of T cell lymphoma. *Leuk Lymphoma*. 2013;54(10):2163-2167.
12. Ohshima K. Pathological features of diseases associated with human T-cell leukemia virus type I. *Cancer Sci*. 2007;98(6):772-778.
13. Ohshima K, Suzumiya J, Kato A, Tashiro K, Kikuchi M. Clonal HTLV-I-infected CD4+ T-lymphocytes and non-clonal non-HTLV-I-infected giant cells in incipient ATLL with Hodgkin-like histologic features. *Int J Cancer*. 1997;72(4):592-598.

14. Karube K, Ohshima K, Tsuchiya T, et al. Expression of FoxP3, a key molecule in CD4CD25 regulatory T cells, in adult T-cell leukaemia/lymphoma cells. *Br J Haematol.* 2004;126(1):81-84.

15. Tsukasaki K, Tsushima H, Yamamura M, et al. Integration patterns of HTLV-I provirus in relation to the clinical course of ATL: frequent clonal change at crisis from indolent disease. *Blood.* 1997;89(3):948-956.

16. Peloponese JMJ., Kinjo T, Jeang KT. Human T-cell leukemia virus type 1 Tax and cellular transformation. *Int J Hematol.* 2007;86(2):101-106.

17. Kim YM, Ramírez JA, Mick JE, Giebler HA, Yan JP, Nyborg JK. Molecular characterization of the Tax-containing HTLV-1 enhancer complex reveals a prominent role for CREB phosphorylation in Tax transactivation. *J Biol Chem.* 2007;282(26):18750-18757.

18. Zhao T, Matsuoka M. HBZ and its roles in HTLV-1 oncogenesis. *Front Microbiol.* 2012;3:247.

19. Yamada K, Miyoshi H, Yoshida N, et al. Human T-cell lymphotropic virus HBZ and tax mRNA expression are associated with specific clinicopathological features in adult T-cell leukemia/lymphoma. *Mod Pathol.* 2021;34(2):314-326.

20. Bangham C.RM, Matsuoka M. Human T-cell leukaemia virus type 1: parasitism and pathogenesis. *Philos Trans R Soc Lond B Biol Sci.* 2017;372(1732):20160272.

21. Kataoka K, Nagata Y, Kitanaka A, et al. Integrated molecular analysis of adult T cell leukemia/lymphoma. *Nat Genet.* 2015;47(11):1304-1315.

22. Kameda T, Kataoka K, Kamiunten A, et al. Integrated genetic and clinical prognostic factors for aggressive adult T-cell leukemia/lymphoma. *Haematologica.* 2023;108(8):2178-2191.

23. Yoshida N, Shigemori K, Donaldson N, et al. Genomic landscape of young ATLL patients identifies frequent targetable CD28 fusions. *Blood.* 2020;135(17):1467-1471.

24. Yoshida N, Miyoshi H, Ohshima K. (2021) Clinical Applications of genomic alterations in ATLL: predictive markers and therapeutic targets. *Cancers.* 2021;13(8):1801. doi:10.3390/cancers13081801.

25. Makiyama J, Ishitsuka K, Munakata W, Maruyama D, Nagai H. An update on the developments in the treatment of adult T-cell leukemia-lymphoma: current knowledge and future perspective. *Jpn J Clin Oncol.* 2023;53(12):1104-1111. doi:10.1093/jjco/hyad108

Chapter 92

Epstein-Barr Virus-Positive T- and Natural Killer-Cell Lymphoproliferative Disorders of Childhood

Leticia Quintanilla-Martinez, Carlos Barrionuevo, Jeffrey I. Cohen, Young-Hyeh Ko, and Stefania Pittaluga

INTRODUCTION

Epstein-Barr virus (EBV)-associated T-cell and natural killer-cell lymphoproliferative disorders (LPDs) of childhood is a group of uncommon diseases that affects mainly pediatric population but can also occur in adults. This group of disorders has undergone a major revision in the 2022 International Consensus Classification (ICC) (Table 92.1).[1] In the 2017 WHO classification, two major groups were recognized: chronic active EBV (CAEBV) infection and systemic EBV-positive T-cell lymphoma of childhood.[2] The ICC now recognizes the following four major disorders: hydroa vacciniforme (HV) LPD, severe mosquito bite allergy, CAEBV disease, systemic, and systemic EBV-positive T-cell lymphoma of childhood. All occur with increased frequency in Asians and in Native Americans from Central and South America and Mexico.

The concept and definition of HV-LPD has changed considerably since this entity was first introduced in the 2008 WHO classification as HV-like lymphoma. The term HV-like LPD was introduced in the 2017 WHO classification.[2,3] Because recent studies have shown that classic HV, a photosensitivity dermatosis described in Western countries is also associated with EBV,[4,5] and therefore, belongs to the same disease spectrum as cases from Asia and Latin America, the term HV-LPD is introduced to the ICC. Two forms of HV-LPD are recognized, one indolent classic form, and one systemic form characterized by systemic symptoms during presentation and exacerbation of the skin lesions. The criteria and morphological features of severe mosquito bite allergy remain the same. CAEBV disease was previously referred as CAEBV infection[2]; however, because most adults are chronically, latently infected, and few acquire the disease, the term CAEBV disease is preferred and has been introduced in the ICC.[1,6] In previous classifications, CAEBV disease included cases with EBV-infected T, natural killer or B cells. Most patients with B-cell CAEBV disease have underlying primary immunodeficiency; therefore, these cases are now excluded and CAEBV disease should include only T- or natural killer-cell disease. Systemic EBV-positive T-cell lymphoma of childhood has a very fulminant course, usually associated with hemophagocytic lymphohistiocytosis (HLH). Cases presenting predominantly with lymphadenopathy are now recognized as part of the clinical spectrum of the disease.[7]

Hydroa Vacciniforme Lymphoproliferative Disorder

Definition

Hydroa vacciniforme lymphoproliferative disorder (HV-LPD) is a chronic EBV-positive LPD of childhood. HV-LPD is a primarily cutaneous disorder of polyclonal or monoclonal T cells or of natural killer cells, with a broad spectrum of clinical aggressiveness and usually a long clinical course. Two forms are recognized; the classic form, which is an indolent, self-limited photosensitivity dermatosis without systemic symptoms affecting mainly White populations, and the systemic form characterized by more severe and extensive skin lesions with systemic symptoms including fever, hepatosplenomegaly, and lymphadenopathy affecting mainly Asians and Latin America populations (Table 92.2).

Synonyms

Edematous, scarring vasculitic panniculitis, angiocentric cutaneous T-cell lymphoma of childhood, hydroa vacciniforme-like lymphoma, severe hydroa vacciniforme, and hydroa vacciniforme-like lymphoproliferative disorder (all not recommended).[2]

Epidemiology

This condition is seen mainly in children and adolescents with a median patient age at diagnosis of 8 years (range: 1-21 years), and a slightly male predominance

TABLE 92.1 Changes in the Epstein-Barr virus-positive T- and natural killer-cell lymphoproliferative disorders and lymphomas

2017 revised fourth WHO classification	2022 International consensus classification
EBV-positive T- and NK-cell LPD in childhood	**EBV-positive T- and NK-cell LPD in childhood**
Chronic active EBV infection • Cutaneous form - Hydroa vacciniforme-like LPD	Hydroa vacciniforme LPD - *Classic form:* indolent, self-limited - *Systemic form:* mild to severe disease, systemic symptoms, more common in Asia and Latin America
- Severe mosquito bite allergy	Severe mosquito bite allergy
• Chronic active EBV infection systemic form	Chronic active EBV disease, systemic form - Only of T- and NK-cell phenotype - B-cell type is excluded
Systemic EBV+ T-cell lymphoma of childhood	Systemic EBV+ T-cell lymphoma of childhood - A predominantly nodal form recognized
EBV-positive T- and NK cell lymphomas in adults	**EBV-positive T- and NK cell lymphomas in adults**
Extranodal NK/T-cell lymphoma, nasal type	Extranodal NK/T-cell lymphoma, nasal type
Aggressive NK-cell leukemia	Aggressive NK-cell leukemia - 10% of cases are EBV negative
Primary nodal EBV positive T/NK cell lymphoma, a variant of PTCL, NOS	Primary nodal EBV-positive T/NK cell lymphoma[a]

CAEBV, chronic active EBV; EBV, Epstein-Barr virus; LPD, lymphoproliferative disorder; NK, natural killer; PTCL, peripheral T-cell lymphoma; NOS, not otherwise specified.
[a]Recognized as a provisional entity.

TABLE 92.2 Hydroa vacciniforme lymphoproliferative disorder

	Classic HV-LPD	Systemic HV-LPD
Skin lesions	- Sun-exposed areas - Seasonal variation - Clearing after photoprotection	- Sun-exposed and nonexposed areas. - Protracted clinical course - Poor response to photoprotection
Systemic symptoms[a]	No	- Yes, during exacerbation of skin lesions. - Usually transitory, associated with the skin lesions
Morphology	- Epidermal reticular degeneration leading to intraepidermal spongiotic vesiculation. - The infiltrate is mainly around adnexa and blood vessels with angiocentricity	The same morphology as classic HV-LPD
EBV infected cells	- Usually T cells - Gamma-delta T cells predominate in Japanese population - <40% in Whites and Latin Americans	- Usually T cells - Alpha-beta T cells predominate - Rarely gamma-delta T cells and NK cells
Ethnicity	More common in White population	More common in Asian and Latin American populations
EBV DNA levels in blood	High but usually lower than in the systemic form	High
T-cell monoclonality	Approximately 30%	>80%
Prognosis and treatment	- In General good outcome with conservative treatment - Self-limited in adolescence - Some cases progress to the systemic form	- Risk to progress to an overt lymphoma - Initial response to immunomodulators - In severe cases HSCT is recommended

EBV, Epstein-Barr virus; HSCT, hematopoietic stem cell transplantation; HV, Hydroa vacciniforme; LPD, lymphoproliferative disorder.
[a]Systemic symptoms include fever >37.5, liver damage, and lymphadenopathy, excluding specific organ involvement. When the symptoms persist more than 3 months and organ damage is demonstrated, the diagnosis of CAEBV disease, systemic should be considered.

(2.3:1).[3,8-10] It is rare in adults.[11] The classic form affects mainly Whites,[4] whereas the systemic form is seen in Asians and in Native Americans from Central and South America and Mexico.[3,8-10,12-14]

General clinical features

HV-LPD is characterized by a papulovesicular eruption that generally proceeds to ulceration and scarring (Figure 92.1). The severity of the skin lesions and the clinical presentation varies between patients with a broad spectrum.[2]

Classic form: This form is characterized by an indolent clinical course and localized papulovesicular eruption on sun-exposed skin and no systemic symptoms. There is a seasonal variation with increased recurrence in spring and summer. Spontaneous remission during adolescence and clearing after photoprotection often occurs. Rarely patients progress to a more aggressive (systemic) form of the disease.[4,15]

Systemic form: Skin lesions are present in sun-exposed and nonexposed areas. Severe facial, lip, and periorbital edema might develop.[12] During the presentation and exacerbation of the skin lesions, transitory systemic symptoms including fever, wasting, lymphadenopathy, and hepatosplenomegaly may be present. The disease follows a protracted clinical course with weeks up to years of disease-free intervals.[3] However, as the disease progresses, there are more extensive and more severe skin lesions and systemic symptoms.[8,9] Patients might respond initially to photoprotection or immunomodulating therapies. Severe mosquito bite allergy might rarely develop in association with HV-LPD and conveys a worse prognosis.[16]

Morphology

The skin shows epidermal reticular degeneration leading to intraepidermal spongiotic vesiculation (see Figure 92.1). The lymphoid infiltrate predominates in the dermis but may extend into the subcutaneous tissue. The infiltrate is mainly localized around the adnexa and blood vessels often with angiodestructive features (Figures 92.1 and 92.2). The infiltrating cells are usually small- to medium-sized and lack significant atypia. The intensity of the infiltrate varies. In severe cases, the overlying epidermis is ulcerated (see Figure 92.2).[3]

Immunophenotype

The infiltrating cells have a cytotoxic phenotype with expression of TIA-1, granzyme B, and perforin. The cells are mostly CD8+ with few cases being CD4+

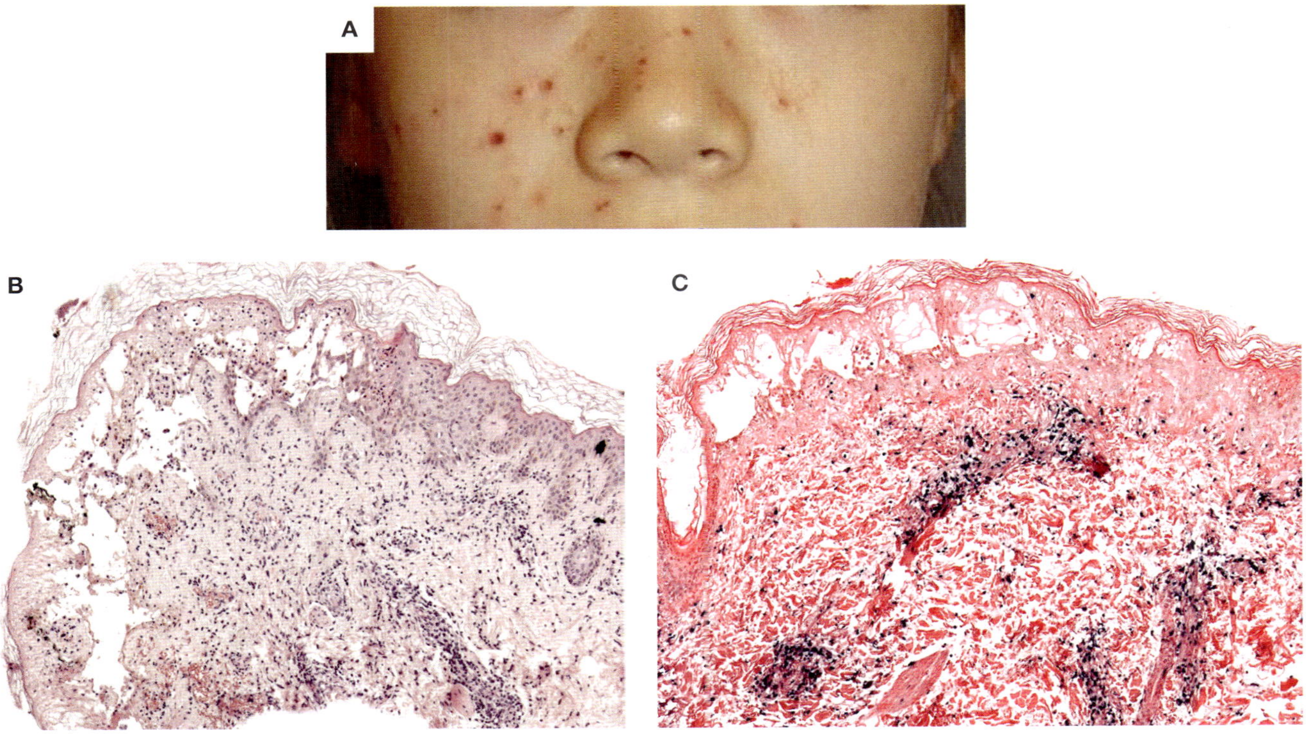

FIGURE 92.1 Hydroa-vacciniforme lymphoproliferative disorder. **A:** An 8-year-old girl with an Epstein-Barr virus (EBV) viral load of 6,069,512 copies/mL in peripheral blood. The skin exhibits papulovesicular eruptions. The lesions are ulcerated with a hemorrhagic crust. **B:** The skin biopsy shows reticular degeneration leading to intraepidermal spongiotic vesiculation. The lymphoid infiltrate predominates in the dermis surrounding adnexa and blood vessels. **C:** The lymphoid cells are positive for EBV, as demonstrated by in situ hybridization for EBV-encoded small RNA.

or even double positive for CD4 and CD8. Natural killer-cell phenotype with expression of CD56 is rare. Occasional cases have a mixture of T and natural killer cells. Cases with natural killer-cell phenotype tend to be more panniculitic and might mimic subcutaneous panniculitis-like T cell-lymphoma. Clonal expansion of gamma delta T cells has been documented in the peripheral blood of most cases of classic form in Japan, but less often in Whites and in Latin American populations (90% vs 40%),[4,13] and only in rare cases has been demonstrated in the infiltrating lymphocytes in the skin (see Figure 92.2).[3,4] Alpha beta T cells are more common in the systemic form. CD30 is often expressed. EBV-encoded RNA (EBER) in situ hybridization (ISH) is positive in a variable proportion of infiltrating cells. LMP1 is usually not detected.[3,8,13,17]

Genetics

The etiology is unknown; however, genetic predisposition might play a role as indicated by the increased risk of systemic disease in Asians and Native Americans. The systemic form has clonal rearrangements of the T-cell receptor (TCR) genes in most of the cases when compared to the classic form (80% vs 30%).[4] Monoclonal T-cell proliferation does not predict the clinical behavior of the disease.[4] EBV is monoclonal by terminal repeat analysis. Although LMP1 is negative by immunohistochemistry, it can be detected in most cases by PCR in peripheral blood, indicating type II EBV latency.[4,18] There are no data concerning the mutational landscape of the disease.

Prognosis and clinical outcome

The clinical course is variable and patients might have recurrent skin lesions for years with and without systemic symptoms. T-cell clonality, the number of EBV-positive infected cells, and the density of the infiltrate do not predict the clinical course.[3,4,19] The classic form is indolent with often complete resolution by adolescence. Conservative treatment with photoprotection and topical steroids are recommended.[4] In the systemic form, the clinical course is more aggressive. Studies have suggested that this form might be successfully treated with immunomodulators (thalidomide, antivirals, interferon);[3,20,21] however, hematopoietic stem cell transplantation (HSCT) is the only curative treatment.[4] Chemotherapy is not curative in the absence of HSCT. In the absence of HSCT patients often progress to liver failure, HLH or T- or natural killer-cell lymphoma.

Severe Mosquito Bite Allergy

Definition

Severe mosquito bite allergy (SMBA) is an EBV-positive natural killer-cell LPD characterized by high fever and intense local skin symptoms, including erythema, bullae, ulcers, skin necrosis, and deep scarring following mosquito bites. Patients have natural killer-cell lymphocytosis in the peripheral blood and an increased risk to develop hemophagocytic syndrome and natural killer/T-cell lymphoma or aggressive natural killer-cell leukemia in the longstanding clinical course.

Synonym

Hypersensitivity to mosquito bites (not recommended).

Epidemiology

SMBA is a very uncommon disease. Most cases have been reported in Japan,[19,22] with few cases from Taiwan, China, South Korea, Mexico, and South America. The patient's age at onset ranges from birth to 18 years (mean: 6.7 years). There is no sex predilection.[23]

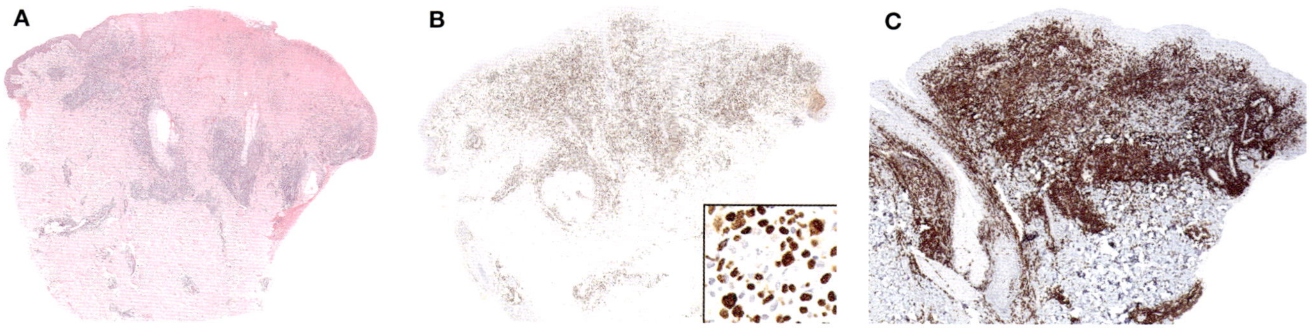

FIGURE 92.2 Hydroa vacciniforme lymphoproliferative disorder. Skin biopsy of a 10-year-old girl with papulovesicular skin lesions on the face scalp and neck who subsequently developed systemic symptoms. **A:** The skin is ulcerated and shows a lymphoid infiltrate concentrated in the superficial dermis surrounding blood vessels and adnexa. **B:** The lymphoid cells are positive for Epstein-Barr virus (EBV), as demonstrated by in situ hybridization for EBV-encoded small RNA (EBER). Inset: Higher magnification of the EBER-positive cells. **C:** The lymphoid infiltrate is positive for T-cell receptor delta. Peripheral blood showed also clonal gamma delta T cells.

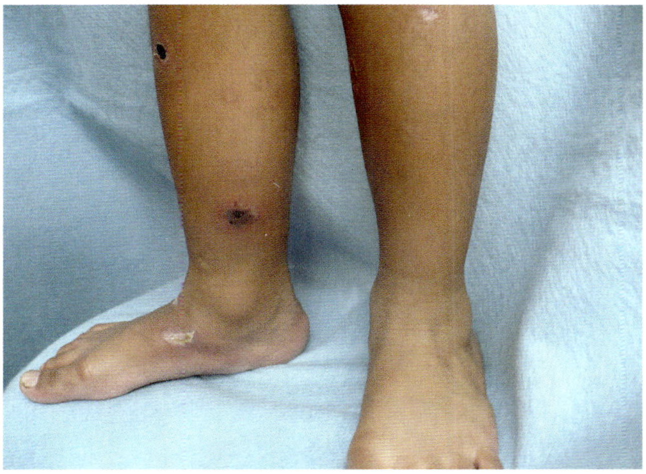

FIGURE 92.3 Severe mosquito bite allergy. The lower leg shows two recent lesions with necrosis, edema, and erythema in the sites of mosquito bite.

General clinical features

This disorder is characterized by transient intense skin reaction with skin ulceration and systemic symptoms including high fever and general malaise following mosquito bite (Figure 92.3). The distinguishing features are elevated serum IgE, high EBV DNA in peripheral blood, and natural killer-cell lymphocytosis.[22] Lymphadenopathy, hepatosplenomegaly, hepatic dysfunction, hematuria, and proteinuria are occasionally seen in the clinical course. After recovering, the patients are asymptomatic until the next mosquito bites.[15,19,24]

Morphology

The skin biopsy shows necrosis and ulceration or intraepidermal bullae at the bite site. The dermis shows edema and a dense lymphoid infiltration extending into the subcutaneous tissue. There is angioinvasion and angiodestruction. The infiltrate is polymorphic including small lymphocytes, large atypical cell, histiocytes, and abundant eosinophils (Figure 92.4). The morphological changes are similar to HV-LPD.[15,23]

Immunophenotype

The infiltrating cells show a natural killer-cell phenotype with expression of CD56, CD3, ε and cytotoxic molecules TIA1 and granzyme B. Reactive CD4 and CD8 positive cells are found at various intensities. CD30 is often positive. LMP1 is rarely positive.[15]

Genetics

Following a mosquito bite, $CD4^+$ cells react against the mosquito salivary gland secretions and induce reactivation of latently EBV-infected natural killer cells, which triggers a strong immunological reaction and infectious mononucleosis-like symptoms.[22] Natural killer cells are infected with monoclonal EBV as demonstrated by terminal repeat analysis indicating clonal expansion of the cells.[22] ISH for EBER shows that the majority of the infiltrating lymphoid cells are positive. TCR genes are polyclonal.

Prognosis and clinical outcome

Patients usually have a long clinical course. Symptoms usually resolve spontaneously at the beginning of the disease; however, these patients are at increased risk of developing hemophagocytic syndrome, systemic CAEBV disease, extranodal natural killer/T-cell lymphoma, nasal type, and aggressive natural killer-cell leukemia after 2 to 17 years.[15,19,23,24]

Chronic Active Epstein-Barr Virus Disease, Systemic

Definition

Chronic active EBV (CAEBV) disease of T-cell and natural killer-cell type is a systemic EBV-positive

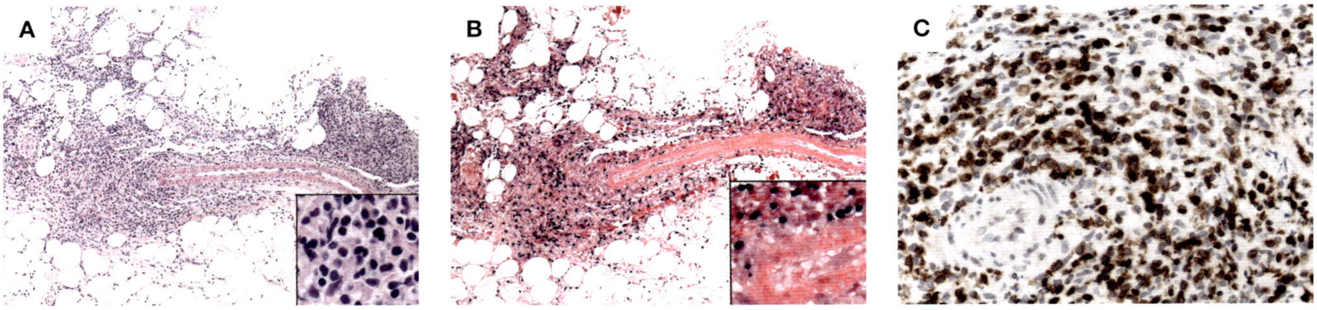

FIGURE 92.4 Severe mosquito bite allergy. **A:** The skin biopsy shows a dense infiltrate in the dermis and subcutaneous tissue with angiocentricity. Inset: At higher magnification, the infiltrate is polymorphic but mainly composed of medium-sized cells with bland nuclei and inconspicuous nucleoli. **B:** The infiltrating lymphocytes are positive for Epstein-Barr virus-encoded small RNA (EBER). Inset: EBER-positive cells surrounding the blood vessel. **C:** The infiltrating lymphocytes are CD56-positive.

polyclonal, oligoclonal, or monoclonal LPD characterized by infectious mononucleosis-like symptoms, which shows varying degrees of clinical severity depending on the host immune response and the EBV viral load. The revised diagnostic criteria include infectious mononucleosis-like symptoms persistent for >3 months, increased EBV DNA (>10,000 IU/mL) in peripheral blood, histological evidence of organ disease, and demonstration of EBV RNA or viral protein in T or natural killer cells of affected tissues in patients without known immunodeficiency, malignancy, or autoimmune disorders.[25]

Synonyms

Systemic chronic EBV infection of T-cell and natural killer-cell type (not recommended).

Epidemiology

CAEBV disease, systemic form has a strong racial predisposition with most cases reported from Asia[26-29] and Latin America and rarely in Western and African populations.[15] It occurs most often in children and adolescents. Adult-onset is rare and the disease seems to be more aggressive.[30] There is no sex predilection.

General clinical features

Approximately 50% of patients present with infectious mononucleosis-like symptoms including fever, hepatosplenomegaly, and lymphadenopathy.[6] Other frequent symptoms include SMBA (33%), skin rash (26%), HV-LPD eruptions (10%), diarrhea (6%), and uveitis (5%). Laboratory tests may show abnormal liver function tests, anemia, or thrombocytopenia. EBV DNA is increased in peripheral blood (>10,000 IU/mL). The clinical course varies but is usually protracted, with some individuals surviving for many years before disease progression. Patients with EBV-infected T cells have a shorter survival time than patients with natural killer-cell disease, more prominent systemic symptoms, and higher levels of EBV DNA in blood. Patients with natural killer-cell disease often have SMBA.[24,26] Some patients in South America present with periorbital and facial edema, high levels of EBV DNA in blood and systemic symptoms, and EBV in internal organs (Figure 92.5). These patients have an aggressive clinical course and lack the typical HV-LPD lesions.[1,31]

Morphology

The infiltrating lymphocytes in the different organs usually do not show changes suggestive of a neoplastic lymphoproliferation. The lymphoid cells are small without atypia; however, occasionally large atypical

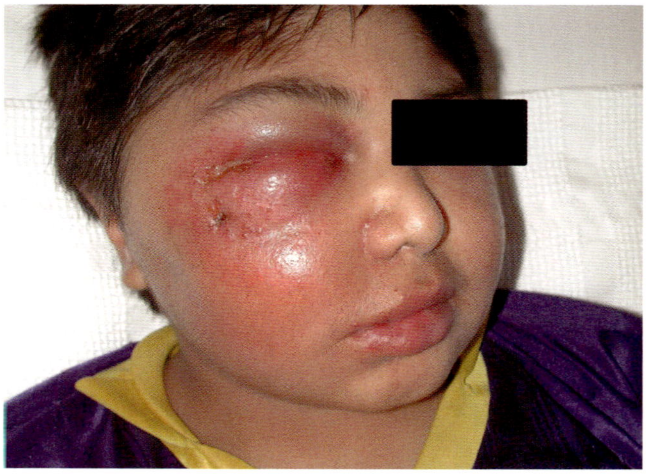

FIGURE 92.5 Chronic active Epstein-Barr virus disease, systemic. A young male patient presented with face edema accentuated in the periorbital region with lack of typical hydroa vacciniforme lesions.

cells often with natural killer or CD8 phenotype are observed (Figures 92.6 and 92.7). The liver shows sinusoidal and portal infiltration suggestive of viral hepatitis (see Figure 92.6). The spleen shows atrophy of the white pulp with congestion of the red pulp (Figure 92.7). The lymph nodes show reactive changes including paracortical and follicular hyperplasia, focal necrosis, and small granulomas (Figure 92.8). The bone marrow biopsies usually appear normal with a discrete interstitial lymphoid infiltrate. In cases complicated with hemophagocytic syndrome, sinus histiocytosis with erythrophagocytosis is present. In skin, a discrete lymphoid infiltrate without atypia in the dermis and surrounding blood vessels might be observed.[7,32]

Immunophenotype

In 59% of the cases, T cells are EBV infected and in 41% natural killer cells, and both T and natural killer cells in 4%. The infiltrating cells are predominantly CD4-positive and few cases show a cytotoxic CD8-positive phenotype. ISH for EBER is positive. The differential diagnosis of CAEBV disease includes other EBV-positive lymphoproliferative disorders (Table 92.3). The determination of the infected cells with double stainings for EBV and B, T, or natural killer cell markers is recommended. Cases with EBV-positive B-cell lymphoproliferative disease are excluded.

Genetics

The etiology is unknown; however, the strong racial predisposition suggests that genetic polymorphisms in genes related to the EBV immune response are responsible for the development of this disease.[15,33] HLA-A*26 is associated with increased frequency of

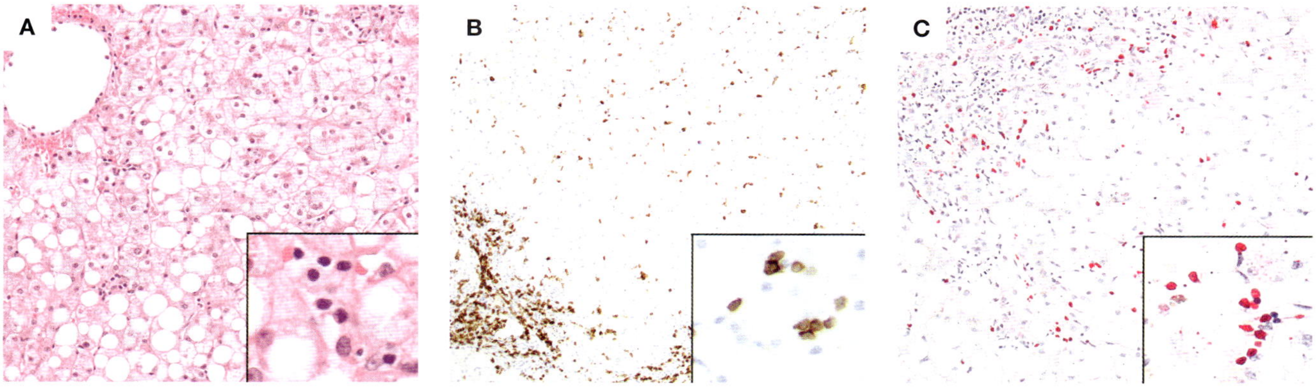

FIGURE 92.6 Chronic active Epstein-Barr virus disease, systemic. **A:** Liver biopsy shows a subtle lymphoid infiltrate both in the portal area and in the sinusoids. Inset: The lymphocytes do not show atypia. **B:** The lymphocytes are CD3 positive. Inset: Higher magnification to demonstrate the CD3-positive cells without atypia. **C:** EBER in situ hybridization shows that many of the infiltrating lymphocytes are EBV-encoded small RNA (EBER) positive (red). Inset: EBER-positive cells.

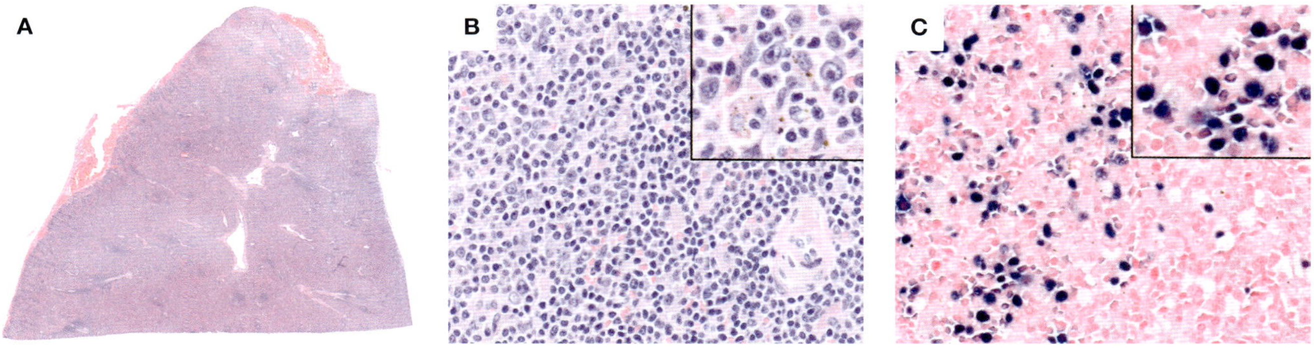

FIGURE 92.7 Chronic active Epstein-Barr virus disease, systemic. A young woman from Africa presented with spontaneous rupture of the spleen. **A:** Panoramic view of the spleen showing atrophic white pulp and expanded red pulp with two areas of subcapsular hemorrhage. **B:** At higher magnification, the atrophic white pulp is surrounded by a polymorphic infiltrate comprising large atypical cells, prominent nucleoli, and abundant cytoplasm. **C:** In situ hybridization for Epstein-Barr virus-encoded small RNA (EBER) shows many positive cells in the white pulp. The cells were positive for CD56 both by flow cytometric analysis and immunohistochemistry (data not shown).

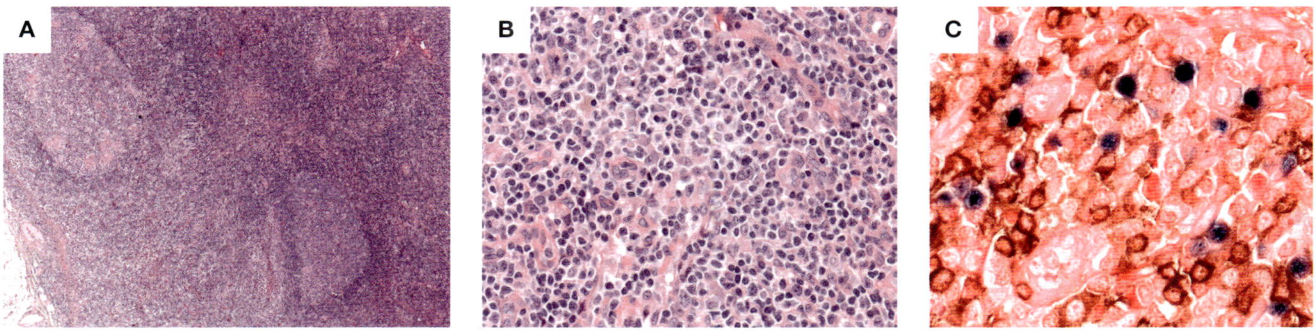

FIGURE 92.8 Chronic active Epstein-Barr virus disease, systemic. **A:** The lymph node shows follicular and paracortical hyperplasia with small epithelioid granulomas in the germinal center. **B:** At higher magnification, the interfollicular areas show a polymorphic infiltrate lacking cytological atypia. **C:** Double staining demonstrates that the Epstein-Barr virus-encoded small RNA positive cells (black) are CD4-positive (brown).

CAEBV in Japan and Taiwan.[34] TCR gene rearrangement may be monoclonal (84%), oligoclonal (11%), or polyclonal (5%).[27] Genetic studies suggest that some cases of CAEBV disease, especially natural killer-cell type, carry somatic mutations in *DDX3D* and *KMT2D* among other genes indicating that it is a premalignant condition. The EBV genome harbors frequent intragenic deletions not found in EBV-positive reactive disorders, suggesting a key role of these alterations in the development of CAEBV disease.[35]

TABLE 92.3 Differential diagnosis of systemic EBV-positive T- and natural killer-cell lymphoproliferative diseases

Disease	Age of presentation	Clinical features	Morphology	Immunophenotype	Lineage of EBV+ cells and molecular features
Nonfamilial EBV-associated HLH	Children/young adults	- Diagnostic criteria for HLH should be fulfilled (≥5 criteria)[a] - Systemic presentation - HLH always	- Hemophagocytosis in BM, spleen, or LNs - Bland cytology but a mild degree of atypia may be seen	- Predominantly cytotoxic $CD8^+$ T cells	- Relatively small numbers of EBV+ T cells, rarely NK cells - Monoclonal TR genes rearrangement in 50%-60% - Cytogenetic analysis normal
Chronic active EBV disease, Systemic (CAEBV)	Children/young adults Rarely adults	- Diagnostic criteria for CAEBV should be fulfilled[b] - Systemic presentation - HLH at progression	- No evidence of malignant lymphoproliferations - LN often with follicular hyperplasia and expanded paracortical areas - Bland cytology	T cell (60%) $CD4^+$>>$CD8^+$ NK cell: $CD56^+$ (40%)	- T or NK cells - Monoclonal TR genes rearrangement in 60% - Mutations in *DDX3X*, *KMT2D* in NK-cell phenotype
Systemic EBV+ T-cell lymphoma of childhood	Children/young adults	- Systemic presentation - Abnormal serology against EBV - Fulminant disease - HLH nearly always present	- Cytological atypia ranges from minimal to severe - LN subtle to complete infiltration by $CD8^+$ cells - Histiocytic hyperplasia and striking hemophagocytosis in BM, spleen, and liver	CD8>>>>CD4	- T cells - Monoclonal TR genes rearrangement (100%) - Not known mutational profile - Cytogenetic abnormalities (30%-35%)
Aggressive NK-cell leukemia (ANKL)	Young adults/adults	- Systemic, usually leukemic - High fever, general malaise, liver failure, hepatosplenomegaly, and pancytopenia. - HLH nearly always present	- Varying degrees of leukemic infiltrate in BM, liver, LN, and spleen. - LN with diffuse infiltration by neoplastic cells and striking hemophagocytosis - Broad cytological spectrum	NK-cell phenotype: $CD56^+$	- NK cells (100%) - 10% EBV negative - Polyclonal TR genes rearrangement - Mutations in JAK/STAT pathway, *TP53*, *DDX3X*, RAS/MAPK pathway
Primary nodal EBV+ T/NK-cell lymphoma	Adults, elderly patients	- Nodal (bulky) - No nasal involvement - Often associated to immunodeficiency, HIV+ - Aggressive disease - HLH uncommon	- LN involved by pleomorphic, large cells - Despite EBV+, necrosis and angiocentricity are uncommon	T cell $CD8^+$>>>>$CD4^+$ $CD56^+$ rare CD30 often expressed[c]	- T cells >>>>>NK cells - Monoclonal TR genes rearrangement in most of the cases - Mutations in *TET2*, *DNMT3A* and JAK/STAT pathway
Extranodal NK/T-cell lymphoma, nasal type	Adults	- 85% nasal region - 15% extranasal region (skin, gastrointestinal tract, lung, testis, CNS). - HLH uncommon	- Ulceration, angiocentricity, angiodestruction, and frequent coagulative necrosis with abundant apoptosis - Broad cytological spectrum	- Mostly NK-cell phenotype $CD56^+$ - Cytotoxic T-cell phenotype $CD8^+$>>>>$CD4^+$ (alpha-beta or gamma-delta)	- NK cells >>>>>T cells - Monoclonal TR genes rearrangement in a minority of the cases - Mutations in *DDX3X*, *BCOR*, *ARID1A*, *MSN*, *MAG*, and JAK/STAT pathway

BM, bone marrow; CNS, central nervous system; EBV, Epstein-Barr virus; HIV, human immunodeficiency virus; HLH, hemophagocytic lymphohistiocytosis; IM, infectious mononucleosis; LN, lymph node(s); NK: natural killer; TR, T-cell receptor.

[a](1) Fever >38.5 °C, (2) Splenomegaly, (3) Cytopenias, (4) Hypertriglyceridemia, (5) Hemophagocytosis, (6) Low/absent NK cell activity, (7) Elevated ferritin (8) Elevated CD25.

[b]Criteria for diagnosis of CAEBV. All criteria need to be fulfilled: (1) IM-like symptoms persistent for more than 3 months, (2) detection of >10,000 IU/mL EBV DNA in Blood, (3) detection of EBV in tissue, (4) no other chronic disease. IM-like symptoms include: fever, lymphadenopathy, hepatosplenomegaly, anemia, skin rash, diarrhea, and uveitis. Rare manifestations: myocarditis, coronary aneurism, interstitial pneumonia, digestive tract ulcer/perforation, CNS involvement.

[c]Differential diagnosis with anaplastic large cell lymphoma, ALK negative should be considered.

Prognosis and clinical outcome

The prognosis is variable with some patients following an indolent clinical course and others showing a rapidly progressive disease. The 5-year survival rates associated to T-cell type and natural killer-cell type are 59% and 87%, respectively.[24] The presence of a monoclonal T-cell proliferation does not correlate with increase in mortality or progression to a full-blown lymphoma.[27] HSCT is the only curative therapy and it is important to initiate transplantation before the disease progresses to an irreversible stage.[34] Relapses after transplantation is not uncommon.[36] Life-threatening complications include HLH (24%), coronary artery aneurysms (9%), liver failure (15%), interstitial pneumonia (5%), CNS involvement (7%), gastrointestinal perforation (11%) (Figure 92.9), myocarditis (4%), and progression to natural killer/T-cell lymphoma or aggressive natural killer leukemia (16%).[27,29,33]

Systemic Epstein-Barr Virus-Positive T-Cell Lymphoma of Childhood

Definition

Systemic EBV-positive T-cell lymphoma of childhood (SEBVTCL) is a life-threatening illness of children and young adults, characterized by a clonal proliferation of EBV-infected T cells with an activated cytotoxic phenotype. It usually occurs shortly after primary EBV infection or rarely in the setting of systemic CAEBV disease. It has a rapid progression, with multiorgan failure, sepsis, and death, usually within days to weeks. HLH is nearly always present. This entity has overlapping features with aggressive natural killer-cell leukemia.

Synonyms

Fulminant EBV-positive T-cell lymphoproliferative disorder of childhood,[37] sporadic fatal infectious mononucleosis, fulminant hemophagocytic syndrome in children in Taiwan, China, fatal EBV-associated hemophagocytic syndrome in Japan. Severe CAEBV with monoclonal EBV-positive T-cell proliferation represents part of the spectrum of systemic EBV-positive T-cell lymphoma of childhood.[38] All terms are not further recommended.

Epidemiology

The disorder is most prevalent in Asia, primarily in Japan and Taiwan and Southwest China.[26,39,40] It has been reported in Mexico and rarely in Western countries.[7,15,37,41] It occurs most often in children and young adults. However, it has been described in elderly individuals, mainly in Asia.[39,42] There is no sex predilection.

General clinical features

This is a systemic disease. The most commonly involved sites are the spleen and liver, followed by bone marrow, lymph nodes, skin, and lungs.[6,7,37,42] Previously healthy patients develop symptoms of infectious mononucleosis with fever, general malaise, and/or upper respiratory illness after primary EBV infection. Within a period of weeks, patients develop hepatosplenomegaly and liver failure, sometimes accompanied by lymphadenopathy and rash. Laboratory tests show pancytopenia, abnormal liver function tests, and often an abnormal EBV serology with low or absent anti-viral capsid antigen IgM antibodies, despite the acute EBV infection, which usually delays the diagnosis. The disease is usually complicated by HLH, coagulopathy, multiorgan failure, and sepsis.[7,37,41] Some cases occur in patients with a well-documented history of CAEBV disease.[37,41] A related disorder, presenting mainly with lymphadenopathy and high lactate dehydrogenase was reported originally in children from Peru.[43] These children have peripheral, mediastinal, and intra-abdominal lymphadenopathy with or without hepatosplenomegaly.[7,44] These cases should not be diagnosed as primary nodal EBV-positive T/natural killer-cell lymphoma, a disease of elderly patients, often associated with immunodeficiency.[6] The differential diagnosis includes other EBV-positive

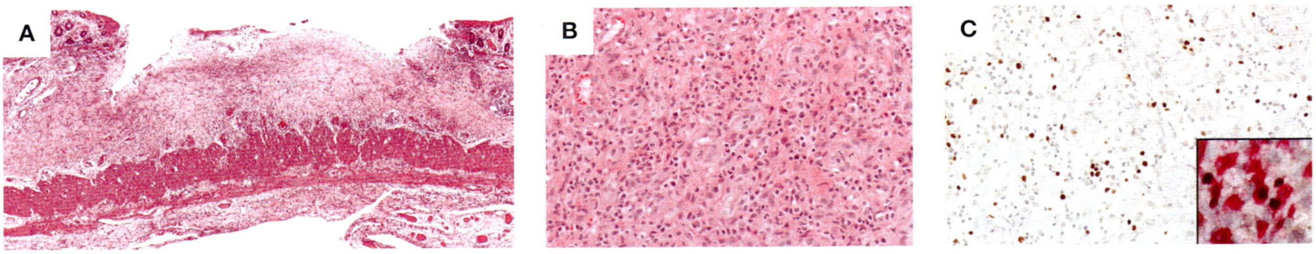

FIGURE 92.9 Chronic active Epstein-Barr virus disease, systemic. A 4-year-old girl with recurrent bowel perforation, natural killer lymphocytosis and history of severe mosquito bite allergy. **A:** Colon resection with ulceration of the mucosa. **B:** The submucosa shows granulation tissue and a subtle lymphoid infiltrate without atypia. **C:** In situ hybridization for Epstein-Barr virus-encoded small RNA (EBER) shows scattered positive cells. Inset: Double staining shows that the EBER-positive cells (black) are CD3-positive (red). CD56 was also positive in these cells (not shown).

T- and natural killer-cell lymphoproliferative disorders such as CAEBV, systemic type,[6,7,38,45] aggressive natural killer-cell leukemia and EBV-associated HLH (see Table 92.3).[41,46] Because HLH is often associated with SEBVTCL, the distinction between nonfamilial HLH and SEBVTCL is often difficult. Severe hyperbilirubinemia, hyperferritinemia, younger age, higher levels of EBV DNA, and cytologic atypia with extensive architectural effacement are parameters that favor the diagnosis of SEBVTCL. The most useful parameter is cytogenetic abnormalities that favors the diagnosis of SEBVTCL but it is only present in 30% to 35% of the cases.[7,46]

Morphology

The infiltrating T cells are usually small and lack significant cytologic atypia. However, cases with pleomorphic medium- to large-sized lymphoid cells, irregular nuclei, and frequent mitoses have been described.[7,32,37,39] The liver and spleen show mild to marked sinusoidal infiltration with striking hemophagocytosis. The splenic white pulp is depleted. The liver has prominent portal and sinusoidal infiltration, cholestasis, steatosis, and necrosis. The lymph nodes usually show preserved architecture with open sinuses. The B-cell areas are depleted, whereas the paracortical areas might be expanded and show a subtle to dense infiltration and a broad cytologic spectrum ranging from small- to medium-sized lymphocytes to large atypical lymphocytes with hyperchromatic and irregular nuclei (Figure 92.10). The more advanced the disease is the more depleted the lymph nodes look. A variable degree of sinus histiocytosis with

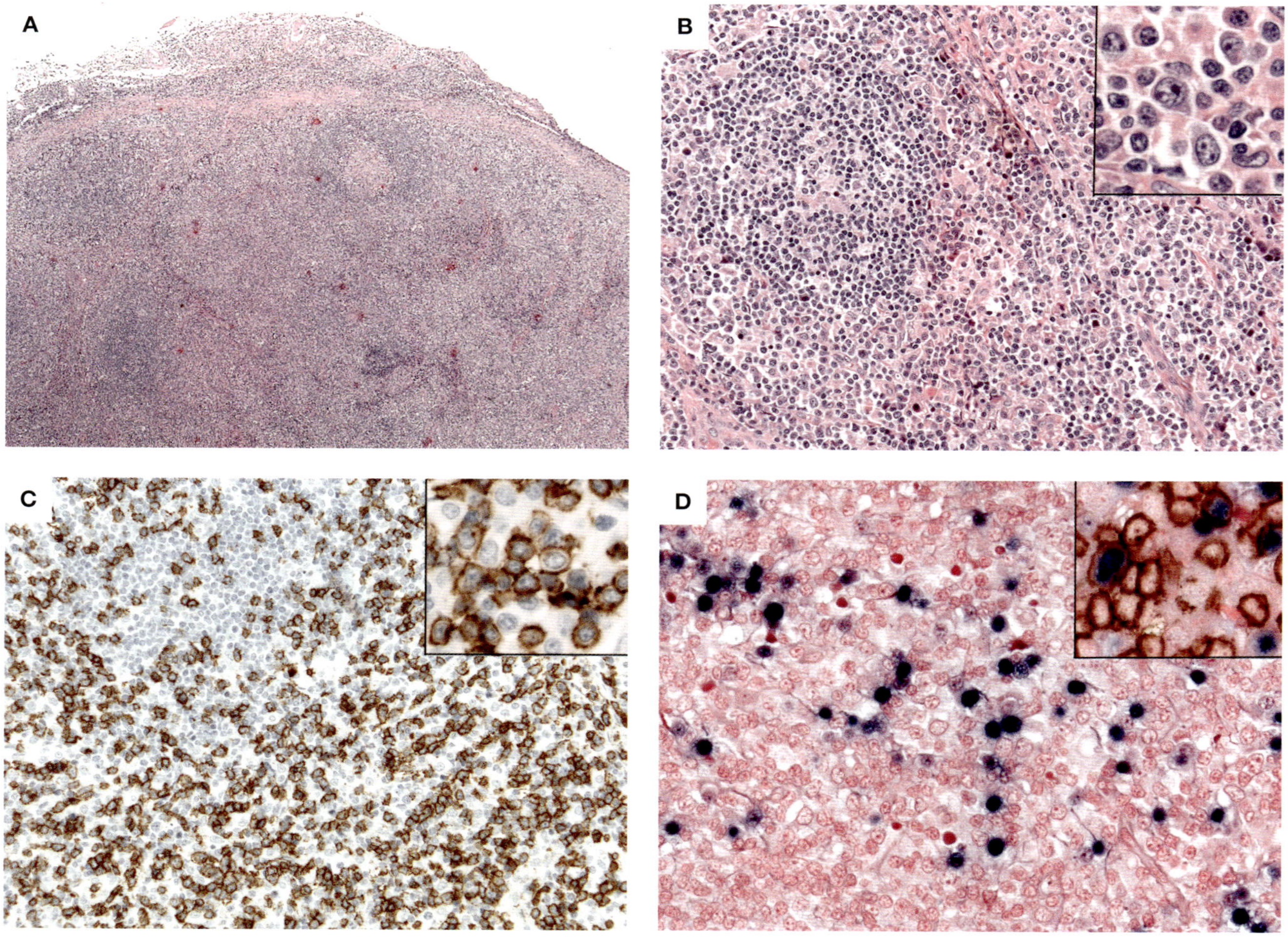

FIGURE 92.10 Systemic Epstein-Barr virus-positive T-cell lymphoma of childhood. **A:** The lymph node shows partial preservation of the architecture with residual regressive follicles and expanded interfollicular areas. **B:** Higher magnification of a regressive germinal center with expanded interfollicular area. Inset: The interfollicular infiltrate is polymorphic with some relatively large cells with irregular nuclei and prominent nucleoli with abundant cytoplasm. **C:** The infiltrate in the interfollicular region is predominantly CD8-positive. Inset: The atypical cells are CD8-positive. **D:** Many cells are positive for Epstein-Barr virus-encoded small RNA (EBER). Inset: Double staining demonstrates that the EBER-positive cells (black) are positive for CD8 (brown).

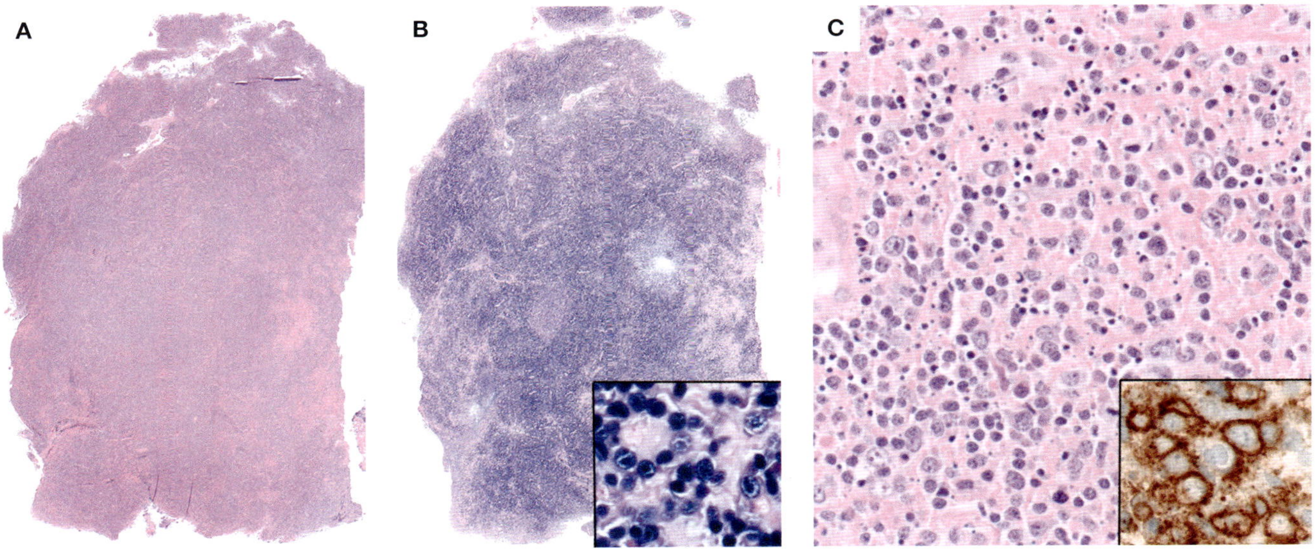

FIGURE 92.11 Systemic Epstein-Barr virus-positive T-cell lymphoma of childhood. An 18-year-old boy developed lymphadenopathy after infectious mononucleosis. **A:** Lymph node with effacement of the normal architecture by a diffuse lymphoid infiltrate. **B:** In situ hybridization for Epstein-Barr virus-encoded small RNA (EBER) shows that every single atypical cell is positive. Inset: Higher magnification demonstrates that not only the large atypical cells are positive but also the small lymphocytes. **C:** Higher magnification shows that the atypical infiltrate is composed of medium and large cells with irregular nuclei and prominent nucleoli. Note the increase apoptosis. Inset: The neoplastic cells are CD8-positive.

erythrophagocytosis is present. In cases presenting predominantly with lymphadenopathy, the lymph node shows partial or total replacement by a diffuse infiltrate of medium to large neoplastic atypical T cells (Figure 92.11).[7,43,44] Bone marrow biopsies show histiocytic hyperplasia with prominent erythrophagocytosis and a subtle infiltrate usually composed of medium to large lymphocytes (Figure 92.12).

Immunophenotype

The most typical immunophenotype of the neoplastic cells is $CD2^+$ $CD3^+$ $CD56^-$, and TIA1+. Most cases secondary to acute primary EBV infection are $CD8^+$,[15,32,37,39,41] whereas cases in the setting of CAEBV disease are $CD4^+$.[37,41] Rare cases show both $CD4^+$ and $CD8^+$ EBV-infected T cells.[37,41] EBER is positive.

Genetics

Although the etiology is unknown, its association with primary EBV infection, and the racial predisposition, strongly suggests a genetic defect in the host immune response to EBV.[7,15,37,41] The cells have monoclonal TR genes rearrangement. All cases harbor EBV in a clonal episomal form.[26,37,40] All cases analyzed carry type A EBV, either with wild-type or the 30 bp deleted product of *LMP1* gene.[40,47] ISH for EBER shows that the majority of the infiltrating lymphoid cells are positive. No consistent chromosomal aberrations or mutations have been identified.[32,41,46]

Prognosis and clinical outcome

Most cases have a fulminant clinical course resulting in death, usually from days to weeks of diagnosis. The disease is usually complicated by HLH. The rapidly progressive clinical course is similar to that of aggressive natural killer-cell leukemia. The optimal therapeutic approach for this disease is not standardized; however, the initial treatment should be directed to control the HLH. Recent data suggest that the HLH-94 protocol has advantages over HLH-2004 protocol.[34] The goal is to stop the hyperinflammatory process characteristic of HLH and continue with the therapy to prepare the patient for HSCT, which is the only definitive curative therapy for this disease.[48]

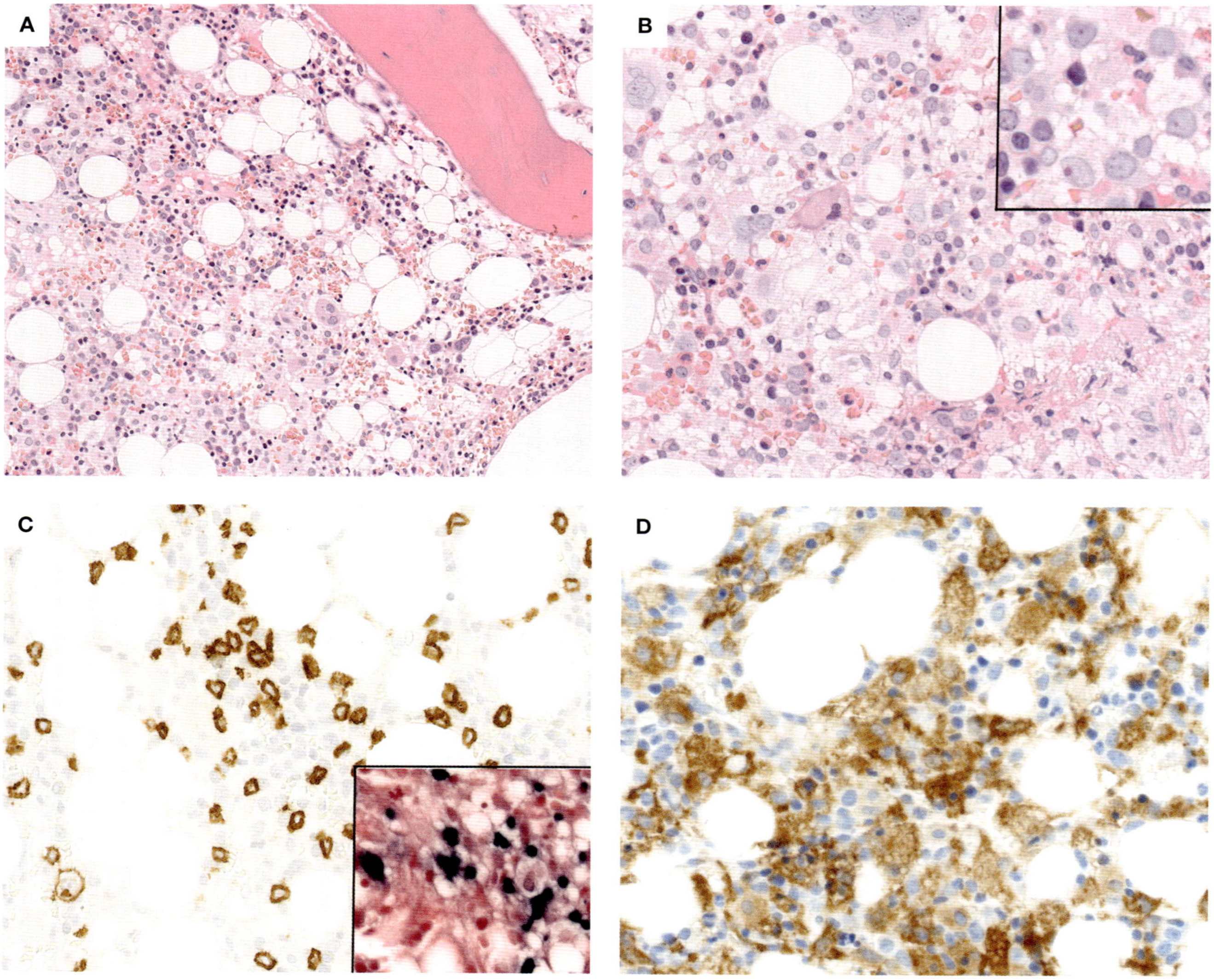

FIGURE 92.12 Systemic Epstein-Barr virus-positive T-cell lymphoma of childhood. **A:** The bone marrow is hypocellular and shows edema of the stroma. **B:** At higher magnification, there is histiocytic hyperplasia with erythrophagocytosis with a lymphoid infiltrate composed of relatively large cells. Inset: The large cells show inconspicuous nucleolus **C:** CD8 is positive in the large cells. Insert: In situ hybridization for Epstein-Barr virus-encoded small RNA shows that the lymphoid cells are positive. **D:** CD163 highlights the abundant histiocytes with erythrophagocytosis.

References

1. Campo E, Jaffe ES, Cook JR, et al. The international consensus classification of mature lymphoid neoplasms: a report from the clinical advisory committee. *Blood.* 2022;140(11):1229-1253.
2. Quintanilla-Martinez L, Ko YH, Kimura H, Jaffe ES. EBV-positive T-cell and NK-cell lymphoproliferative diseases of childhood. In: Swerdlow SH, Campo E, Harris NL, et al, eds. WHO Classification of Tumours of Haematopoetic and Lymphoid Tissues. IARC; 2017:355-363.
3. Quintanilla-Martinez L, Ridaura C, Nagl F, et al. Hydroa vacciniforme-like lymphoma: a chronic EBV+ lymphoproliferative disorder with risk to develop a systemic lymphoma. *Blood.* 2013;122(18):3101-3110.
4. Cohen JI, Manoli I, Dowdell K, et al. Hydroa vacciniforme-like lymphoproliferative disorder: an EBV disease with a low risk of systemic illness in whites. *Blood.* 2019;133(26):2753-2764.
5. Quintanilla-Martinez L, Fend F. Deciphering hydroa vacciniforme. *Blood.* 2019;133(26):2735-2737.
6. Quintanilla-Martinez L, Swerdlow SH, Tousseyn T, Barrionuevo C, Nakamura S, Jaffe ES. New concepts in EBV-associated B, T, and NK cell lymphoproliferative disorders. *Virchows Arch.* 2023;482(1):227-244.
7. Dojcinov SD, Quintanilla-Martinez L. How I diagnose EBV-positive B- and T-cell lymphoproliferative disorders. *Am J Clin Pathol.* 2023;159(1):14-33.
8. Sangueza M, Plaza JA. Hydroa vacciniforme-like cutaneous T-cell lymphoma: clinicopathologic and

immunohistochemical study of 12 cases. *J Am Acad Dermatol.* 2013;69(1):112-119.
9. Barrionuevo C, Anderson VM, Zevallos-Giampietri E, et al. Hydroa-like cutaneous T-cell lymphoma: a clinicopathologic and molecular genetic study of 16 pediatric cases from Peru. *Appl Immunohistochem Mol Morphol.* 2002;10(1):7-14.
10. Xu W, Tan J, Cai C, et al. Hydroa vacciniforme-like lymphoproliferative disorder: a retrospective study on clinicopathological characteristics of 32 cases. *Pediatr Dermatol.* 2022;39(3):372-375.
11. Liu Y, Ma C, Wang G, Wang L. Hydroa vacciniforme-like lymphoproliferative disorder: clinicopathologic study of 41 cases. *J Am Acad Dermatol.* 2019;81(2):534-540.
12. Magana M, Massone C, Magana P, Cerroni L. Clinicopathologic features of hydroa vacciniforme-like lymphoma: a series of 9 patients. *Am J Dermatopathol.* 2016;38(1):20-25.
13. Iwatsuki K, Miyake T, Hirai Y, Yamamoto T. Hydroa vacciniforme: a distinctive form of Epstein-Barr virus-associated T-cell lymphoproliferative disorders. *Eur J Dermatol.* 2019;29(1):21-28.
14. Oh SJ, Lee J, Park JH, et al. Hydroa vacciniforme-like lymphoproliferative disorder in Korea: prognostic implication of clinical signs and whole blood Epstein-Barr virus DNA. *Ann Dermatol.* 2021;33(3):222-227.
15. Cohen JI, Iwatsuki K, Ko YH, et al. Epstein-Barr virus NK and T cell lymphoproliferative disease: report of a 2018 international meeting. *Leuk Lymphoma.* 2020;61(4):808-819.
16. Hirai Y, Yamamoto T, Kimura H, et al. Hydroa vacciniforme is associated with increased numbers of Epstein-Barr virus-infected γδT cells. *J Invest Dermatol.* 2012;132(5):1401-1408.
17. Guo N, Chen Y, Wang Y, et al. Clinicopathological categorization of hydroa vacciniforme-like lymphoproliferative disorder: an analysis of prognostic implications and treatment based on 19 cases. *Diagn Pathol.* 2019;14(1):82.
18. Iwata S, Wada K, Tobita S, et al. Quantitative analysis of Epstein-Barr virus (EBV)-related gene expression in patients with chronic active EBV infection. *J Gen Virol.* 2010;91(pt 1):42-50.
19. Miyake T, Yamamoto T, Hirai Y, et al. Survival rates and prognostic factors of Epstein-Barr virus-associated hydroa vacciniforme and hypersensitivity to mosquito bites. *Br J Dermatol.* 2015;172(1):56-63.
20. Beltran BE, Maza I, Moises-Alfaro CB, et al. Thalidomide for the treatment of hydroa vacciniforme-like lymphoma: report of four pediatric cases from Peru. *Am J Hematol.* 2014;89(12):1160-1161.
21. Ruan Y, Shen X, Shi R, Zhao X, Zheng J. Hydroa vacciniforme-like lymphoproliferative disorder treated with intravenous immunoglobulin: long-term remission without haematopoietic stem cell transplantation or Chemotherapy. *Acta Derm Venereol.* 2020;100(13):adv00192.
22. Yamada M, Ishikawa Y, Imadome KI. Hypersensitivity to mosquito bites: a versatile Epstein-Barr virus disease with allergy, inflammation, and malignancy. *Allergol Int.* 2021;70(4):430-438.
23. Tokura Y, Ishihara S, Tagawa S, Seo N, Ohshima K, Takigawa M. Hypersensitivity to mosquito bites as the primary clinical manifestation of a juvenile type of Epstein-Barr virus-associated natural killer cell leukemia/lymphoma. *J Am Acad Dermatol.* 2001;45(4):569-578.
24. Kimura H, Hoshino Y, Hara S, et al. Differences between T cell-type and natural killer cell-type chronic active Epstein-Barr virus infection. *J Infect Dis.* 2005;191(4):531-539.
25. Kawada JI, Ito Y, Ohshima K, et al. Updated guidelines for chronic active Epstein-Barr virus disease. *Int J Hematol.* 2023;118(5):568-576.
26. Kimura H, Hoshino Y, Kanegane H, et al. Clinical and virologic characteristics of chronic active Epstein-Barr virus infection. *Blood.* 2001;98(2):280-286.
27. Kimura H, Ito Y, Kawabe S, et al. EBV-associated T/NK-cell lymphoproliferative diseases in nonimmunocompromised hosts: prospective analysis of 108 cases. *Blood.* 2012;119(3):673-686.
28. Ai J, Xie Z. Epstein-barr virus-positive T/NK-cell lymphoproliferative diseases in Chinese mainland. *Front Pediatr.* 2018;6:289.
29. Hong M, Ko YH, Yoo KH, et al. EBV-positive T/NK-cell lymphoproliferative disease of childhood. *Korean J Pathol.* 2013;47(2):137-147.
30. Arai A, Imadome KI, Watanabe Y, et al. Clinical features of adult-onset chronic active Epstein-Barr virus infection: a retrospective analysis. *Int J Hematol.* 2011;93(5):602-609.
31. Plaza JA, Sangueza M. Hydroa vacciniforme-like lymphoma with primarily periorbital swelling: 7 cases of an atypical clinical manifestation of this rare cutaneous T-cell lymphoma. *Am J Dermatopathol.* 2015;37(1):20-25.
32. Dojcinov SD, Fend F, Quintanilla-Martinez L. EBV-positive lymphoproliferations of B- T- and NK-cell derivation in non-immunocompromised hosts. *Pathogens.* 2018;7(1):28.
33. Cohen JI, Kimura H, Nakamura S, Ko YH, Jaffe ES. Epstein-Barr virus-associated lymphoproliferative disease in non-immunocompromised hosts: a status report and summary of an international meeting, 8-9 September 2008. *Ann Oncol.* 2009;20(9):1472-1482.
34. Bollard CM, Cohen JI. How I treat T-cell chronic active Epstein-Barr virus disease. *Blood.* 2018;131(26):2899-2905.
35. Okuno Y, Murata T, Sato Y, et al. Defective Epstein-Barr virus in chronic active infection and haematological malignancy. *Nat Microbiol.* 2019;4(3):404-413.
36. Davila Saldana BJ, John T, Bonifant C, et al. High risk of relapsed disease in patients with NK/T-cell chronic active Epstein-Barr virus disease outside of Asia. *Blood Adv.* 2022;6(2):452-459.

37. Quintanilla-Martinez L, Kumar S, Fend F, et al. Fulminant EBV(+) T-cell lymphoproliferative disorder following acute/chronic EBV infection: a distinct clinicopathologic syndrome. *Blood*. 2000;96(2):443-451.

38. Ohshima K, Kimura H, Yoshino T, et al. Proposed categorization of pathological states of EBV-associated T/natural killer-cell lymphoproliferative disorder (LPD) in children and young adults: overlap with chronic active EBV infection and infantile fulminant EBV T-LPD. *Pathol Int*. 2008;58(4):209-217.

39. Chen Z, Wang M, Guan P, et al. Comparison of systemic EBV-positive T-cell and NK-cell lymphoproliferative diseases of childhood based on classification evolution: new classification, old problems. *Am J Surg Pathol*. 2020;44(8):1061-1072.

40. Suzuki K, Ohshima K, Karube K, et al. Clinicopathological states of Epstein-Barr virus-associated T/NK-cell lymphoproliferative disorders (severe chronic active EBV infection) of children and young adults. *Int J Oncol*. 2004;24(5):1165-1174.

41. Coffey AM, Lewis A, Marcogliese AN, et al. A clinicopathologic study of the spectrum of systemic forms of EBV-associated T-cell lymphoproliferative disorders of childhood: a single tertiary care pediatric institution experience in North America. *Pediatr Blood Cancer*. 2019;66(8):e27798.

42. Wang Z, Kimura S, Iwasaki H, et al. Clinicopathological findings of systemic Epstein-Barr virus-positive T-lymphoproliferative diseases in younger and older adults. *Diagn Pathol*. 2021;16(1):48.

43. Rodriguez-Pinilla SM, Barrionuevo C, Garcia J, et al. Epstein-Barr virus-positive systemic NK/T-cell lymphomas in children: report of six cases. *Histopathology*. 2011;59(6):1183-1193.

44. Climent F, Nicolae A, de Leval L, et al. Cytotoxic peripheral T-cell lymphomas and EBV-positive T/NK-cell lymphoproliferative diseases: emerging concepts, recent advances, and the putative role of clonal hematopoiesis. A report of the 2022 EA4HP/SH lymphoma workshop. *Virchows Arch*. 2023;483(3):333-348.

45. Yonese I, Sakashita C, Imadome KI, et al. Nationwide survey of systemic chronic active EBV infection in Japan in accordance with the new WHO classification. *Blood Adv*. 2020;4(13):2918-2926.

46. Smith MC, Cohen DN, Greig B, et al. The ambiguous boundary between EBV-related hemophagocytic lymphohistiocytosis and systemic EBV-driven T cell lymphoproliferative disorder. *Int J Clin Exp Pathol*. 2014;7(9):5738-5749.

47. Kasahara Y, Yachie A, Takei K, et al. Differential cellular targets of Epstein-Barr virus (EBV) infection between acute EBV-associated hemophagocytic lymphohistiocytosis and chronic active EBV infection. *Blood*. 2001;98(6):1882-1888.

48. Bergsten E, Horne A, Hed Myrberg I, et al. Stem cell transplantation for children with hemophagocytic lymphohistiocytosis: results from the HLH-2004 study. *Blood Adv*. 2020;4(15):3754-3766.

Chapter 93

Extranodal Natural Killer/T-Cell Lymphoma, Nasal Type

Wing C. Chan, Won Seog Kim, Young-Hyeh Ko, and Stefania Pittaluga

Definition

Extranodal NK/T-cell lymphoma, nasal type (ENKTCL) is an aggressive lymphoma involving predominantly extranodal sites, which is derived from mature NK or T cells. The lymphoma is consistently associated with Epstein-Barr virus (EBV) infection and characterized by angiocentric and angiodestructive lesions associated with prominent necrosis. The tumor cells have a cytotoxic phenotype regardless of cell lineage derivation. The prototypical site of involvement is the nasal and paranasal regions including the palate (Figure 93.1) and therefore, similar tumors apparently originating in other extranodal sites are also designated as ENKTCL-NT. Similar tumors presenting with lymphadenopathy and lacking nasal involvement are now designated as primary nodal EBV$^+$ T-cell/NK-cell lymphoma and represent a distinct entity.

Synonyms

Malignant midline reticulosis, lethal midline granuloma, polymorphic reticulosis, angiocentric T-cell lymphoma, extranodal NK/T-cell lymphoma (all not recommended).

Epidemiology

ENKTCL has a much higher prevalence in eastern Asians and in the native populations in the Americas. It is rare outside of these regions. It occurs mostly in adults with a male predominance.[1-4]

General Clinical Features

Characteristically, the patients present with nasal involvement with nasal obstructive symptoms and/or bleeding. More advanced cases may present with destructive lesions of the nose and surrounding structures in the upper aerodigestive tract (Figure 93.1). The disease may disseminate to other extranodal sites, parenchymal organs, and lymph nodes. Systemic symptoms may be present and some patients may develop a hemophagocytic syndrome. Bone marrow staging biopsies are usually negative. Some patients present with extranasal disease, most commonly skin or gastrointestinal tract, and multiple sites may be involved. These patients generally have a more aggressive clinical disease with poor prognosis.

Patients with EBV-positive T-cell lymphoproliferative disorders (chronic active EBV disease, hydroa vacciniforme of systemic type) may develop a progressive systemic lymphoma resembling extranasal ENKTCL and a diagnosis of progression to ENKTCL may be made. ENKTCL has also been reported in patients with immunosuppression including in a posttransplant setting.[5,6] Table 92.3 summarizes the differential diagnosis of ENKTCL with other EBV-positive T- and NK-cell neoplasms.

Morphology

As the tumor is extranodal and frequently nasal/paranasal, the overlying epithelium is typically ulcerated but pseudoepitheliomatous hyperplasia has been described.[7] A key feature of the tumor is the presence of angiocentric and angiodestructive lesions with areas of necrosis and prominent single cell apoptosis.[8] Although the cell death may be related to vascular damage, proinflammatory/cytotoxic cytokines, Fas/FasL and TRAIL/TRAILR interaction, and cytotoxic proteins release may also contribute.[8-11] The infiltrate is diffuse and the cytomorphology is variable. Tumors most often comprise small- to medium-sized cells mixed with varying numbers of large cells, but tumors with mostly small or large cells are occasionally seen. Tumor nuclei tend to be round or oval with granular chromatin and some irregular folding. Nucleoli are generally not prominent even in large cells, but mitosis is often quite brisk irrespective of the morphology (Figure 93.2). Imprints

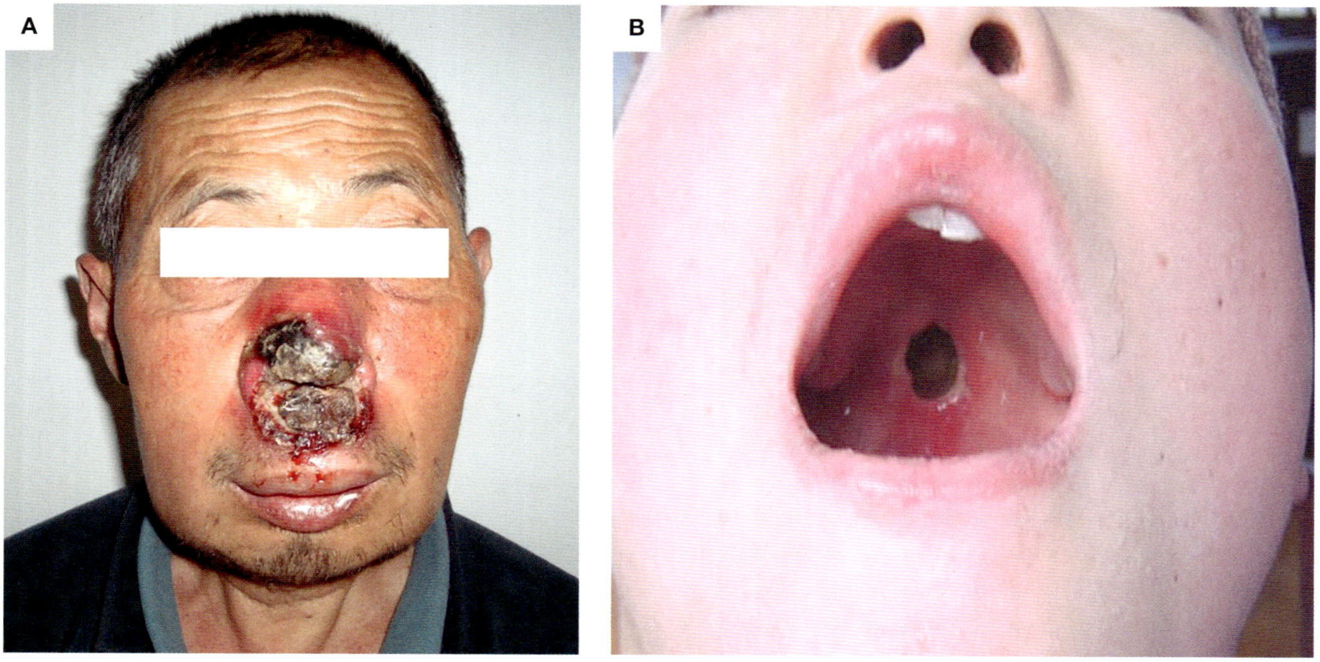

FIGURE 93.1 Images of patients with extranodal NK/T-cell lymphoma, nasal type (ENKTCL). **A:** ENKTCL presenting as a necrotizing lesion destroying much of the nose. **B:** Presentation of ENKTCL as a lesion in the hard palate with perforation. (Photographs Courtesy of Professor Wei-ping Liu, Department of Pathology, West-China Hospital, Sichuan University.)

show lymphoid cells with a moderate amount of cytoplasm containing azurophilic granules. Although most tumors are quite monomorphic, some tumors have a more prominent polymorphic background composed of variable amounts of small reactive lymphocytes, histiocytes, plasma cells, and eosinophils.[2] When the reactive component is prominent, it might be misinterpreted as an inflammatory lesion especially in small biopsies with predominantly small tumor cells.

An intravascular lymphoma of NK/T-cells has been described characterized by the unique intravascular distribution of the neoplastic cells often involving the skin or brain and not producing ulcers or mass lesions (Figure 93.3).[12] This may be considered a variant of ENKTCL.

Immunophenotype

The presence of EBV, as usually demonstrated by positive in-situ hybridization for EBV-encoded small RNAs (EBERs), is an essential diagnostic criterion (Figures 93.3C and 93.4A). Typically, most cells show a positive hybridization signal. In the absence of EBV infection, another NK-cell or T-cell lymphoproliferative disorder or lymphoma should be considered. False negative results for EBER in-situ hybridization may occur in cases with extensive RNA degradation. LMP1 is frequently negative by immunostaining and is not a reliable assay for EBV infection. Most cases express CD2, cCD3 (CD3ε), CD7, and CD56, but CD8, CD16 and CD57 are generally negative (Figures 93.3 and

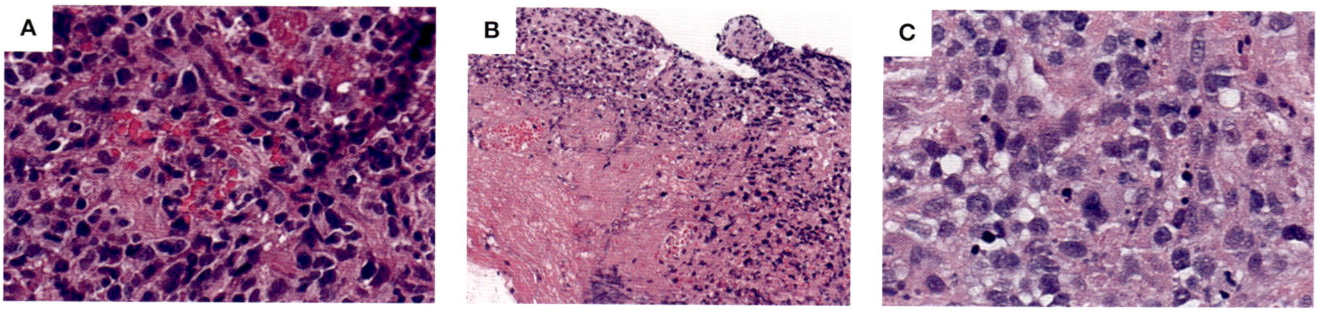

FIGURE 93.2 Morphologic features of extranodal NK/T-cell lymphoma, nasal type (ENKTCL). **A:** Tumor showing an angiocentric lesion. Tumor cells are mostly medium-sized cells with scattered large cells. **B:** Large area of necrosis. Remnants of blood vessels can be seen. **C:** Tumor consisting of mostly large cells. Apoptotic bodies are quite prominent.

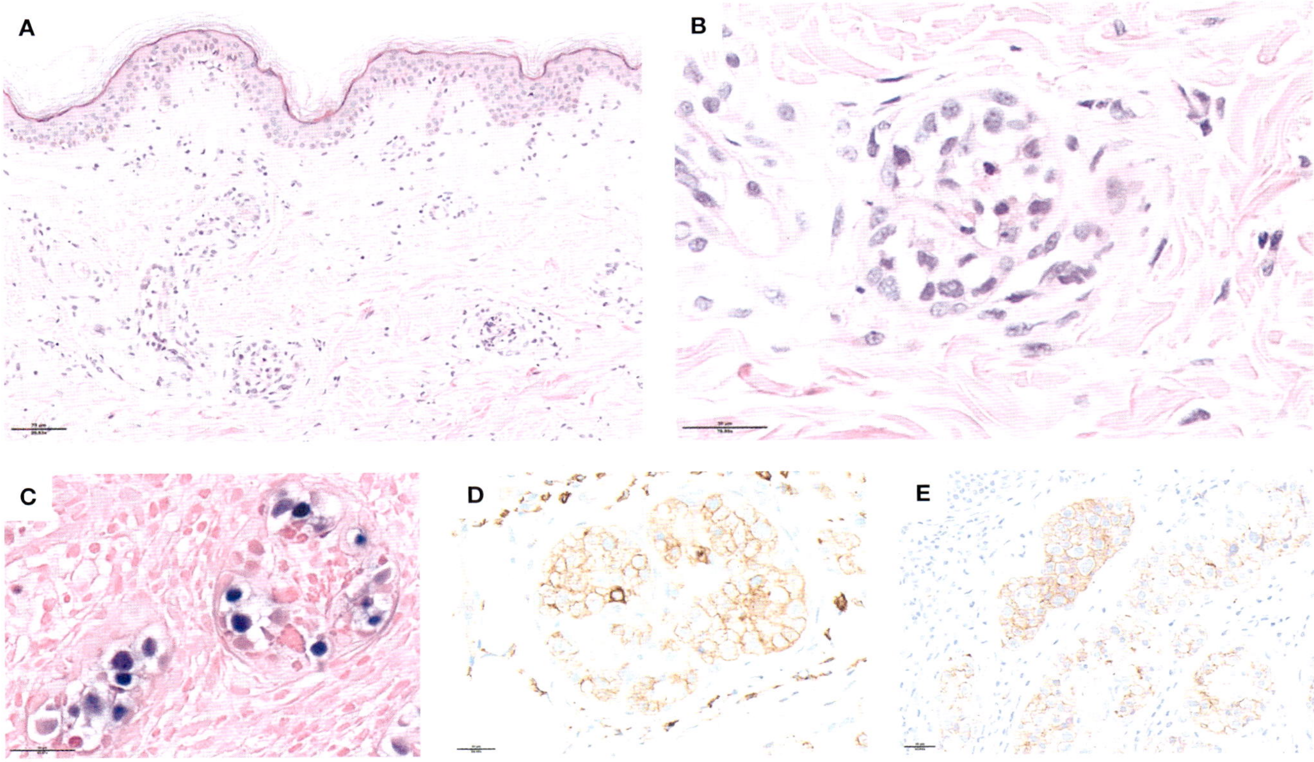

FIGURE 93.3 Intravascular variant of extranodal NK/T-cell lymphoma, nasal type (ENKTCL). **A:** Low-power view of a skin biopsy showing slightly distended microvessels. **B:** At high power, the vascular lumens are filled with atypical medium-sized lymphoid cells. **C:** The intravascular lymphoid cells show a positive hybridization signal for EBER probes. **D** and **E:** On immunostaining, the atypical cells are positive for CD7 (**D**) and CD56 (**E**).

93.4). Although CD56 is frequently expressed and is very useful for the diagnosis in both NK- and T-lineage tumors, about 10% to 20% of the cases may be negative.[13] Both lineages express cytotoxic molecules such as TIA1, granzyme B, and perforin 8 (Figure 93.4), but one or even two of these may be absent (eg, granzyme B may be negative in ~12% of cases). The expression of CD5 and the demonstration of TCRαβ or TCRγδ or cell surface CD3 support the T-cell derivation of the tumor.[13,14] However, failure to detect TCR/CD3 by immunohistochemistry does not definitively exclude a T-cell origin, and clonal rearrangement of the TRB or TRG genes is the most definitive criteria to distinguish between T- and NK-cell lineage. Nonetheless, determination of T- versus NK-cell lineage currently has no clinical implications on treatment and is not mandatory in routine diagnosis. Ki67 expression could be high even in cases without a high content of large cells (Figure 93.4F). CD30 expression can be prominent in some cases but is not strong and uniform as seen in anaplastic large cell lymphoma (Figure 93.4G). Some other markers have been reported to be commonly expressed ENKTCL including CD25, CD95 (FAS), CD178 (FASL), HLA-DR and megakaryocyte-associated tyrosine kinase (MATK)[9,13,14] but they are not generally used in routine clinical practice. PD-L1 is frequently expressed in the tumor cells as well as in the macrophages and assaying for its expression could be of interest in cases considered for immune checkpoint therapy.[15,16]

Genetics

Epstein-Barr virus

The consistent association of this disease with EBV and the clonal nature of the virus[17] in the tumor suggest that EBV infection is an important factor in its pathogenesis. EBV can be detected in the plasma of the majority of patients at diagnosis, and EBV load can be used as a prognostic marker as well as a marker for monitoring treatment response.[18] The tumor generally shows a type II latency profile (EBNA1$^+$, EBERs$^+$, LMP1$^+$, and LMP2$^+$). The majority of cases carry type A (type 1) EBV with a 30 bp deletion in the *LMP1* gene in a subset of the cases,[3] a finding which has not been clearly associated with a more aggressive disease in ENKTCL. More recently, sequencing of the EBV genome found a more complex picture.[19] Widespread single nucleotide variants, indels, and larger deletions compared with the

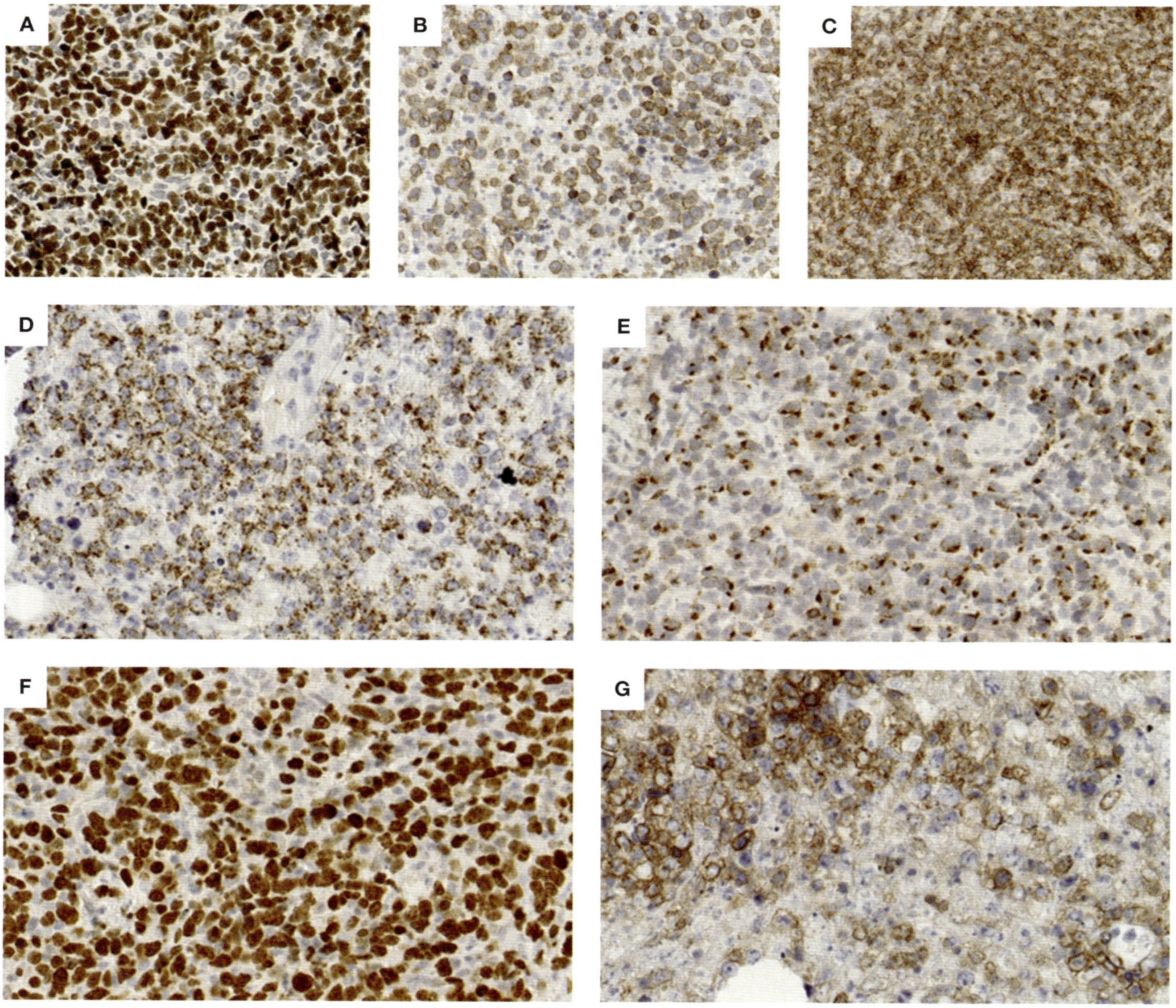

FIGURE 93.4 Representative immunostainings and EBER in-situ hybridization in extranodal NK/T-cell lymphoma, nasal type (ENKTCL). **A-E:** Typical staining pattern with tumor cells showing positivity for EBER **(A)**, expression of cCD3 **(B)** and CD56 **(C)**, and strong TIA1 **(D)** and Granzyme B **(E)** positivity in all tumor cells. **F:** Very high Ki67^{+} percentage is observed in this case showing mostly medium-sized cells. **G:** CD30 may be expressed in a substantial percentage of tumor cells, but it is not uniformly strongly positive as in anaplastic large cell lymphoma.

reference EBV genome were reported for the EBV in ENKTCL. Small insertions of EBV sequence into the host genome are also detected.[17] Additional investigations are needed to more fully define these changes and to determine the biological effects of these variants.

T-cell receptor rearrangement

A clonal T-cell receptor (TCR) gene rearrangement is the most definitive evidence of T-cell lineage derivation of the lymphoma. However, this has not been uniformly or systematically assessed. Of the larger series (reviewed in reference 20) with such information, about 75% of the cases lack TCR rearrangement and are presumed to be of NK-cell origin. Caution is required in interpreting small clonal T-cell populations as it could represent reactive T cells present. The size of the clonal population should be commensurate with the abundance of tumor cells present.

Gene expression profiling

Gene expression profiling studies showed that ENKTCL highly expressed a large group of genes associated with normal or activated NK cells regardless of lineage derivation.[20] A number of pathways were enriched including vascular endothelial growth factor-regulated genes, hypoxia signaling, genotoxic stress/TP53 pathway, Notch1 signaling, WNT3A signaling, and TGFβ signaling. Several important activated signaling molecules were also frequently detected including pSTAT3, pAKT, pPDGFRα, RELA, and cREL.[20,21] The data may suggest potential targets for therapy. ENKTCL cases share a unique gene expression signature that could be useful in diagnosis, particularly when combined with EBERs expression.[22]

Genetic and epigenetic studies

The unique geographic distribution of ENKTCL and its strong association with EBV infection suggest unique genetic susceptibility in its development. A genome-wide association study found significant association for 51 single nucleotide polymorphisms at the major histocompatibility complex class II region with rs9277378 showing the strongest association.[23] A later study found two loci at *IL18RAP* and *HLA-DRB1*.[24] These associations suggest that antigen presentation and immune regulation play important roles in the pathogenesis of ENKTCL (see Figure 93.5).

With the advent of next generation sequencing, multiple mutation analyses have been reported. Most of these are small series with different technical and analytical approaches. Although several common mutations have been reported, others have been reported at spuriously high or low levels. More recently, three large genetic studies[25-27] have been published with many shared frequent mutations, although still with substantial differences. The more consistently reported mutations with relatively high frequencies are briefly described in the following.

JAK/STAT pathway genes mutation, including *STAT3* (mostly missense mutations affecting the Src homology 2 (SH2) domain, in ~21% of patients), *JAK1/2/3* (~7%), *PTPRD*, *STAT5B*, *PTPN6*, and *IL7R* (1%-4%) are the most frequent oncogenic mutations.[25] Mutations that may affect the NOTCH and RAS/MAPK pathway are moderately common. Mutations of genes directly affecting the NF-κB pathway seem uncommon.

Mutations in tumor suppressor genes (TSGs) are found in almost half of the patients, with the most frequent in *DDX3X* and *TP53* in 19% and 12% of the patients, respectively. Interestingly, these mutations are mutually exclusive and reportedly associated with worse prognosis.[26] Loss-of-function mutation of *MGA* (8%) that regulates MYC activation[28] and other less-frequent mutations in TSGs or presumed TSGs (<5%) including *ZFHX3/ATBF1*, *PRDM1*, *SAMD9*,[29] and multiple members of protein tyrosine phosphatase families (*PTPN* and *PTPR*)[29-31] were identified. *PRDM1* is actually deficient in a much higher percentage of cases due to 6q21 copy number loss and promoter hypermethylation.[32,33] The death receptor pathway may be interrupted by *FAS* mutations.

Mutations in epigenetic modifiers collectively identified in 40% to 50% of patients, affect chromatin modifiers such as histone lysine N-methyltransferases or demethylases *KMT2D*, *KMT2C*, and *SETD2*; *KDM2B* and *KDM6A* & *B*; histone deacetylases, *BCOR*, *BCORL1*, and *NCOR1/2*; histone acetyltransferases *EP300* and *CREBBP*; the SWI/SNF family members *ARID1A* and *SMARCA4*; and the DNA demethylase, *TET2*.

Because ENKTCL is an EBV-associated lymphoma, escape from host immune surveillance is critical. Mutations affecting *B2M*, *HLA-A* and *B*, and *CIITA* or *CD58* are relatively infrequent. Frequent high PD-L1 expression in ENKTCL has been reported[34] and may be related to its upregulation by pSTAT3, IFNG, and HIF1α, all of which are often expressed.[35-37] Furthermore, genetic alterations leading to 3′ UTR disruption of *PD-L1* mRNA resulting in increased transcript persistence are often found in ENKTCL.[15,38] Thus, PDL1 overexpression may be an important mechanism of immune escape.

In addition to mutations, many frequent chromosomal copy number abnormalities were found (gains in 1q, 2q,7q, 17q, and 19q and losses in 6q, 7p, 10p, 11q, 13q, and 17p). Some of the frequent gains and losses harbor oncogenes or TSG, respectively, and may thus contribute to oncogene activity or TSG inactivation.[25]

Two large studies[25,27] attempted to find genetic subgroups that are prognostically significant. Weaknesses of these studies include the retrospective nature and nonuniformity of treatment, the small sizes of the subgroups and the lack of a large well-defined independent validation cohort. Whether these reported genetic subgroups are indeed prognostic awaits further confirmation.

ENKTCL exhibits a CpG island DNA hypermethylator phenotype (CIMP) similar to some other EBV-associated malignancies.[39] This is associated with the frequent methylation of the promoter of many TSGs.[40] Thus, in ENKTCL, a TSG could be inactivated by multiple mechanisms including mutation, promoter methylation, and copy number loss, and the relative contribution of these mechanisms on a TSG inactivation varies.

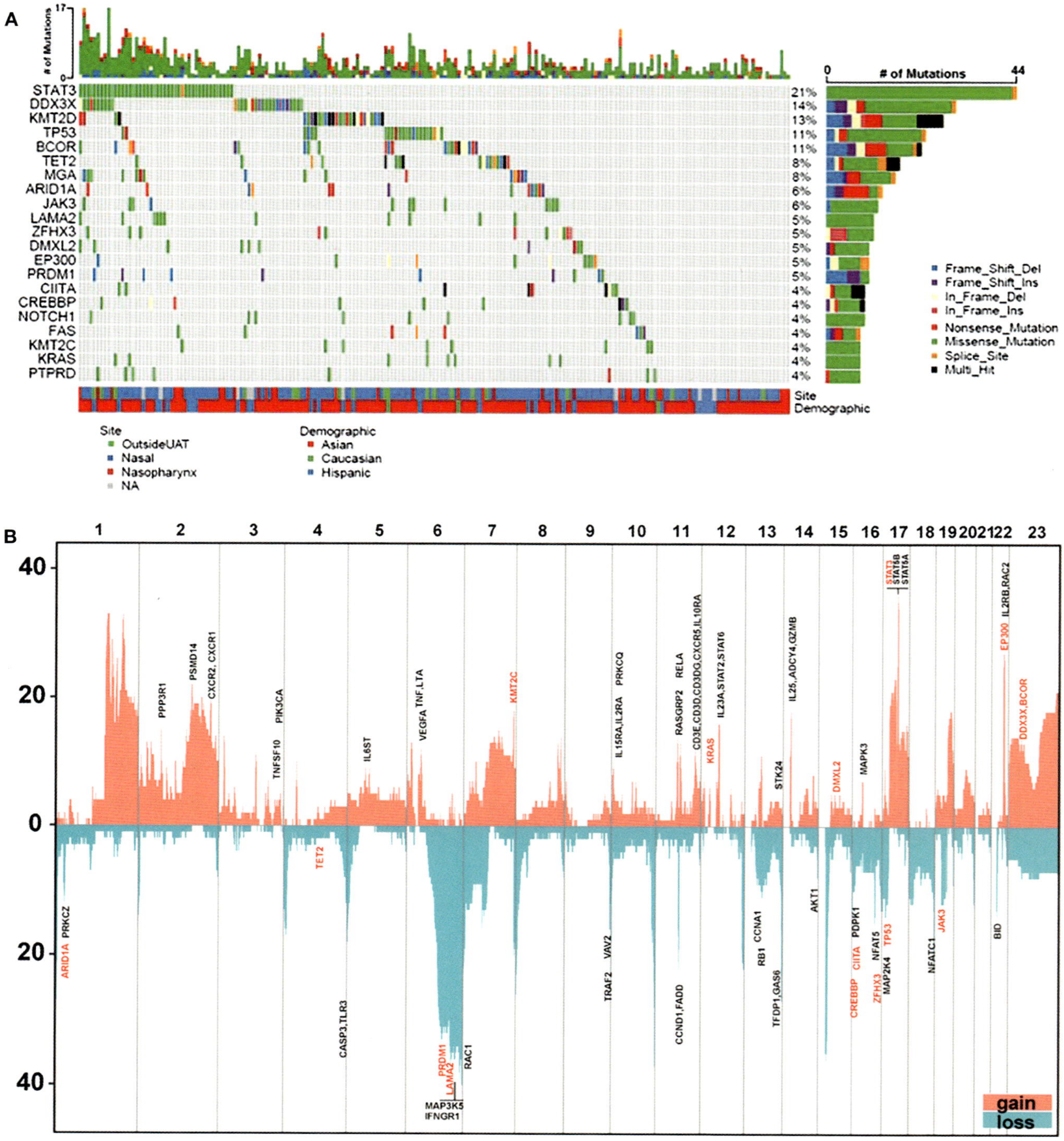

FIGURE 93.5 Representative genetic abnormalities in extranodal NK/T-cell lymphoma, nasal type (ENKTCL). **A:** The more frequent mutations detected in ENKTCL are represented; these mutations are detected in other studies although the frequency may vary. **B:** Copy number abnormalities detected in ENKTCL. Genes potentially significant in ENKTCL development are shown. Genes in red were found to be mutated in at least 4% of cases. (Modified from Dong G, Liu X, Wang L, et al Genomic profiling identifies distinct genetic subtypes in extra-nodal natural killer/T-cell lymphoma. *Leukemia*. 2022;36(8):2064-2075.)

Prognosis and Clinical Comment

The prognostic value of grading using cytologic features is not significant by multivariate analysis. In the international PTCL project, tumors with Ki 67 staining of >50% or transformed cells >40% were associated with worse outcome in nasal but not extranasal cases.[1]

Clinically, the Prognostic Index for Natural Killer Lymphoma and Prognostic Index for Natural Killer Lymphoma-E (adding EBV-DNA score) are now widely used prognostic models that can be employed to develop risk-adapted treatment approaches in the contemporary era.[41] It is possible that combining molecular parameters such as genetic subgroups may further improve the clinical prognostic models.[25,27] Plasma EBV DNA and/or PET/CT scan are highly useful in monitoring response to treatment and clinical decision making. In early-stage nasal disease, radiation therapy is the mainstay of treatment but the combination with chemotherapy provides better disease control and the combinatorial approach is now the standard of care. For advanced-stage disease or extranasal disease, intensive, asparaginase-containing chemotherapeutic regimen such as SMILE (methylprednisolone, methotrexate, ifosfamide, l-asparaginase, and etoposide) is superior to CHOP-based chemotherapy but has substantial toxicity. Alternative regimens with less toxicity have been proposed. The outcomes of patients treated with more current approaches are: 54% 5-year overall survival in patients with nasal disease and 34% in patients with extranasal disease.[42] Despite recent advances, relapsed and particularly primary refractory disease have very poor outcome even with salvage therapy using allogeneic HSC transplantation. Other approaches have been attempted and there are reports of impressive responses in these patients to PD1/PDL1 immune checkpoint blockade.[43] There are potential targets for novel therapeutic approaches from recent genomics and epigenomic studies that could be tested preclinically and promising ones confirmed through clinical trials.

References

1. Au WY, Weisenburger DD, Intragumtornchai T; International Peripheral T-Cell Lymphoma Project, et al. Clinical differences between nasal and extranasal natural killer/T-cell lymphoma: a study of 136 cases from the International Peripheral T-Cell Lymphoma Project. *Blood*. 2009;113(17):3931-3937.
2. Chan JK, Quintanilla-Martinez L, Ferry JA. Extranodal NK/T-cell lymphoma, nasal type. In: Swerdlow SH, ed. WHO Classification of Tumours of Haematopoietic and Lymphoid Tissues. 4th ed. 2017:368-371.
3. Montes-Mojarro IA, Fend F, Quintanilla-Martinez L. EBV and the pathogenesis of NK/T cell lymphoma. *Cancers*. 2021;13(6):1414.
4. Yoon SE, Song Y, Kim SJ, et al. Comprehensive analysis of peripheral T-cell and natural killer/T-cell lymphoma in Asian patients: a multinational, multicenter, prospective registry study in Asia. *Lancet Reg Health West Pac*. 2021;10:100126.
5. Hoshida Y, Li T, Dong Z, et al. Lymphoproliferative disorders in renal transplant patients in Japan. *Int J Cancer*. 2001;91(6):869-875.
6. Stadlmann S, Fend F, Moser P, Obrist P, Greil R, Dirnhofer S. Epstein-Barr virus-associated extranodal NK/T-cell lymphoma, nasal type of the hypopharynx, in a renal allograft recipient: case report and review of literature. *Hum Pathol*. 2001;32(11):1264-1268.
7. Ling YH, Zhu CM, Wen SH, et al. Pseudoepitheliomatous hyperplasia mimicking invasive squamous cell carcinoma in extranodal natural killer/T-cell lymphoma: a report of 34 cases. *Histopathology*. 2015;67(3):404-409.
8. Ng CS, Lo ST, Chan JK, Chan WC. CD56+ putative natural killer cell lymphomas: production of cytolytic effectors and related proteins mediating tumor cell apoptosis? *Hum Pathol*. 1997;28(11):1276-1282.
9. Ohshima K, Suzumiya J, Shimazaki K, et al. Nasal T/NK cell lymphomas commonly express perforin and Fas ligand: important mediators of tissue damage. *Histopathology*. 1997;31(5):444-450.
10. Sarhan D, D'Arcy P, Wennerberg E, et al Activated monocytes augment TRAIL-mediated cytotoxicity by human NK cells through release of IFN-gamma. *Eur J Immunol*. 2013;43(1):249-257.
11. Teruya-Feldstein J, Jaffe ES, Burd PR, et al. The role of Mig, the monokine induced by interferon-gamma, and IP-10, the interferon-gamma-inducible protein-10, in tissue necrosis and vascular damage associated with Epstein-Barr virus-positive lymphoproliferative disease. *Blood*. 1997;90(10):4099-4105.
12. Zanelli M, Parente P, Sanguedolce F, et al. Intravascular NK/T-Cell lymphoma: what we know about this diagnostically challenging, aggressive disease. *Cancers*. 2022;14(21):5458. doi:10.3390/cancers14215458
13. Ng SB, Lai KW, Murugaya S, et al. Nasal-type extranodal natural killer/T-cell lymphomas: a clinicopathologic and genotypic study of 42 cases in Singapore. *Mod Pathol*. 2004;17(9):1097-1107.
14. Pongpruttipan T, Sukpanichnant S, Assanasen T, et al. Extranodal NK/T-cell lymphoma, nasal type, includes cases of natural killer cell and αβ, γδ, and αβ/γδ T-cell origin: a comprehensive clinicopathologic and phenotypic study. *Am J Surg Pathol*. 2012;36(4):481-499.
15. Lim JQ, Huang D, Tang T, et al. Whole-genome sequencing identifies responders to Pembrolizumab in relapse/refractory natural-killer/T-cell lymphoma. *Leukemia*. 2020;34(12):3413-3419.
16. Nagato T, Ohkuri T, Ohara K, et al. Programmed death-ligand 1 and its soluble form are highly expressed in nasal natural killer/T-cell lymphoma: a potential rationale for immunotherapy. *Cancer Immunol Immunother*. 2017;66(7):877-890.
17. Peng RJ, Han BW, Cai QQ, et al. Genomic and transcriptomic landscapes of Epstein-Barr virus in extranodal natural killer T-cell lymphoma. *Leukemia*. 2019;33(6):1451-1462.
18. Yan Z, Yao Z, Wang H, et al. Plasma EBV-DNA and peripheral blood mononuclear cell EBV-DNA have disparate clinical relevance in patients with extranodal NK/T-cell lymphoma. *J Clin Virol*. 2022;157:105320.

19. Zanella L, Riquelme I, Buchegger K, Abanto M, Ili C, Brebi P. A reliable Epstein-Barr Virus classification based on phylogenomic and population analyses. *Sci Rep*. 2019;9(1):9829.
20. Iqbal J, Weisenburger DD, Chowdhury A; International Peripheral T-cell Lymphoma Project, et al. Natural killer cell lymphoma shares strikingly similar molecular features with a group of non-hepatosplenic γδ T-cell lymphoma and is highly sensitive to a novel aurora kinase A inhibitor in vitro. *Leukemia*. 2011;25(2):348-358.
21. Huang Y, de Reynies A, de Leval L, et al. Gene expression profiling identifies emerging oncogenic pathways operating in extranodal NK/T-cell lymphoma, nasal type. *Blood*. 2010;115(6):1226-1237.
22. Amador C, Bouska A, Wright G, et al. Gene expression signatures for the accurate diagnosis of peripheral T-cell lymphoma entities in the routine clinical practice. *J Clin Oncol*. 2022;40(36):4261-4275.
23. Li Z, Xia Y, Feng LN, et al. Genetic risk of extranodal natural killer T-cell lymphoma: a genome-wide association study. *Lancet Oncol*. 2016;17(9):1240-1247.
24. Lin GW, Xu C, Chen K; International NKTCL Working Group, et al. Genetic risk of extranodal natural killer T-cell lymphoma: a genome-wide association study in multiple populations. *Lancet Oncol*. 2020;21(2):306-316.
25. Dong G, Liu X, Wang L, et al. Genomic profiling identifies distinct genetic subtypes in extra-nodal natural killer/T-cell lymphoma. *Leukemia*. 2022;36(8):2064-2075.
26. Jiang L, Gu ZH, Yan ZX, et al. Exome sequencing identifies somatic mutations of DDX3X in natural killer/T-cell lymphoma. *Nat Genet*. 2015;47(9):1061-1066.
27. Xiong J, Cui BW, Wang N, et al. Genomic and transcriptomic characterization of natural killer T cell lymphoma. *Cancer Cell*. March 16, 2020;37(3):403-419.e6.
28. Hurlin PJ, Steingrìmsson E, Copeland NG, Jenkins NA, Eisenman RNJTE. Mga, a dual-specificity transcription factor that interacts with Max and contains a T-domain DNA-binding motif. *EMBO J*. 1999;18(24):7019-7028.
29. Davidsson J, Puschmann A, Tedgard U, Bryder D, Nilsson L, Cammenga J. SAMD9 and SAMD9L in inherited predisposition to ataxia, pancytopenia, and myeloid malignancies. *Leukemia*. 2018;32(5):1106-1115.
30. Jiang Y, Janku F, Subbiah V, et al. Germline PTPRD mutations in Ewing sarcoma: biologic and clinical implications. *Oncotarget*. 2013;4(6):884-889.
31. Kim M, Morales LD, Jang IS, Cho YY, Kim DJ. Protein tyrosine phosphatases as potential regulators of STAT3 signaling. *Int J Mol Sci*. 2018;19(9).
32. Iqbal J, Kucuk C, Deleeuw RJ, et al. Genomic analyses reveal global functional alterations that promote tumor growth and novel tumor suppressor genes in natural killer-cell malignancies. *Leukemia*. 2009;23(6):1139-1151.
33. Kucuk C, Iqbal J, Hu X, et al. PRDM1 is a tumor suppressor gene in natural killer cell malignancies. *Proc Natl Acad Sci U S A*. 2011;108(50):20119-20124.
34. Chen BJ, Chapuy B, Ouyang J, et al. PD-L1 expression is characteristic of a subset of aggressive B-cell lymphomas and virus-associated malignancies. *Clin Cancer Res*. 2013;19(13):3462-3473.
35. Bi XW, Wang H, Zhang WW, et al. PD-L1 is upregulated by EBV-driven LMP1 through NF-κB pathway and correlates with poor prognosis in natural killer/T-cell lymphoma. *J Hematol Oncol*. 2016;9(1):109.
36. Garcia-Diaz A, Shin DS, Moreno BH, et al. Interferon receptor signaling pathways regulating PD-L1 and PD-L2 expression. *Cell Rep*. 2017;19(6):1189-1201.
37. Sun C, Mezzadra R, Schumacher TN. Regulation and function of the PD-L1 checkpoint. *Immunity*. 2018;48(3):434-452.
38. Kataoka K, Shiraishi Y, Takeda Y, et al. Aberrant PD-L1 expression through 3'-UTR disruption in multiple cancers. *Nature*. 2016;534(7607):402-406.
39. Kang GH, Lee S, Kim WH, et al. Epstein-Barr virus-positive gastric carcinoma demonstrates frequent aberrant methylation of multiple genes and constitutes CpG island methylator phenotype-positive gastric carcinoma. *Am J Pathol*. 2002;160(3):787-794.
40. Kucuk C, Hu X, Jiang B, et al. Global promoter methylation analysis reveals novel candidate tumor suppressor genes in natural killer cell lymphoma. *Clin Cancer Res*. 2015;21(7):1699-1711.
41. Kim SJ, Yoon DH, Jaccard A, et al. A prognostic index for natural killer cell lymphoma after non-anthracycline-based treatment: a multicentre, retrospective analysis. *Lancet Oncol*. 2016;17(3):389-400.
42. Fox CP, Civallero M, Ko YH, et al. Survival outcomes of patients with extranodal natural-killer T-cell lymphoma: a prospective cohort study from the international T-cell Project. *Lancet Haematol*. 2020;7(4):e284-e294.
43. Tse E, Zhao WL, Xiong J, Kwong YL. How we treat NK/T-cell lymphomas. *J Hematol Oncol*. 2022;15(1):74.

Chapter 94
Aggressive Natural Killer-Cell Leukemia

Wing C. Chan, Won Seog Kim, Young-Hyeh Ko, and Stefania Pittaluga

Definition

Aggressive natural killer-cell leukemia (ANKL) is a natural killer-cell malignancy with systemic and leukemic manifestations at presentation. The tumor cells are Epstein-Barr virus (EBV)-positive in most cases and the clinical course is typically fulminant with very poor survival. It includes de novo cases as well as cases arising from a previous chronic natural killer-cell lymphoproliferative disorder (LPD), ie, chronic LPD of natural killer cells, chronic active EBV disease of natural killer cell type, severe mosquito bite allergy, or rarely hydroa vacciniforme LPD.

Synonyms

None.

Epidemiology

Most of the reported ANKL cases were from Asia with sporadic reports from other geographic regions including patients from other racial groups. There seems to be a higher representation of Caucasian and African patients compared with extranodal natural killer/T cell lymphoma, nasal type (ENKTCL). There is no gender predominance, and the majority of patients are adults with a median age of ~40 but adolescent and young adult cases are common (close to 40%), whereas childhood cases are rare.[1-3] Some of the younger patients represent cases arising from an EBV-positive natural killer-cell LPD of childhood.[1,4]

General Clinical Features

The disease is typically fulminant and manifests with high fever, night sweats, weight loss, hepatosplenomegaly, coagulopathy, and high LDH.[5] Peripheral blood often shows cytopenia with variable percentages of abnormal granulated lymphocytes on the smears. Hemophagocytic syndrome often develops during the clinical course and may be associated with coagulopathy, liver, and multiorgan failure.

Advanced stage ENKTCL of natural killer cell lineage with multiorgan involvement may simulate ANKL, particularly in patients with extranasal disease, but a secondary diagnosis of ANKL is not indicated in these cases. The diagnosis of ANKL should be reserved for cases with primary blood and bone marrow involvement, hepatosplenomegaly, and with the appropriate clinical features (see Table 92.3 for differential diagnosis of ANKL with ENKTCL and other EBV+ NK/T-cell neoplasms).

The intravascular variant of ENKTCL (see Chapter 93 Extranodal Natural Killer/T-Cell Lymphoma, Nasal Type)[6] may show clinicopathologic overlap with ANKL, but intravascular ENKTCL tends to have more frequent skin and central nervous system involvement that is largely confined to the intravascular compartment, rather than prominent hepatosplenomegaly. The clinical course, although aggressive, is less fulminant compared to ANKL and does not have the high incidence of hemophagocytic syndrome.

Morphology

The neoplastic cells may resemble the large granular lymphocytes seen in chronic LPD of natural killer cells but in most cases, they show more pleomorphism including many cells with larger, more irregular nuclei that may contain small nucleoli. Cases may contain highly pleomorphic or blastic cells and rare cases with agranular lymphocytes have been described[2,7] (Figure 94.1A-E). The peripheral blood often shows pancytopenia. Although neoplastic cells can often be identified, obvious leukemic manifestation with lymphocytosis is uncommon. Similarly, bone marrow involvement[3] ranges from 5% to 90% and the pattern of neoplastic infiltration is more often patchy or interstitial and better revealed by immunohistochemistry, rather than being massive (Figure 94.1F-I). A sinusoidal pattern of involvement has been described in some cases.[8] Mild dyserythropoiesis is often present and marrow stromal damage, such as edema, serous fat atrophy, and reticulin fibrosis has been described.[3] As hemophagocytic syndrome is a frequent complication, an increase in macrophages with hemophagocytosis may be

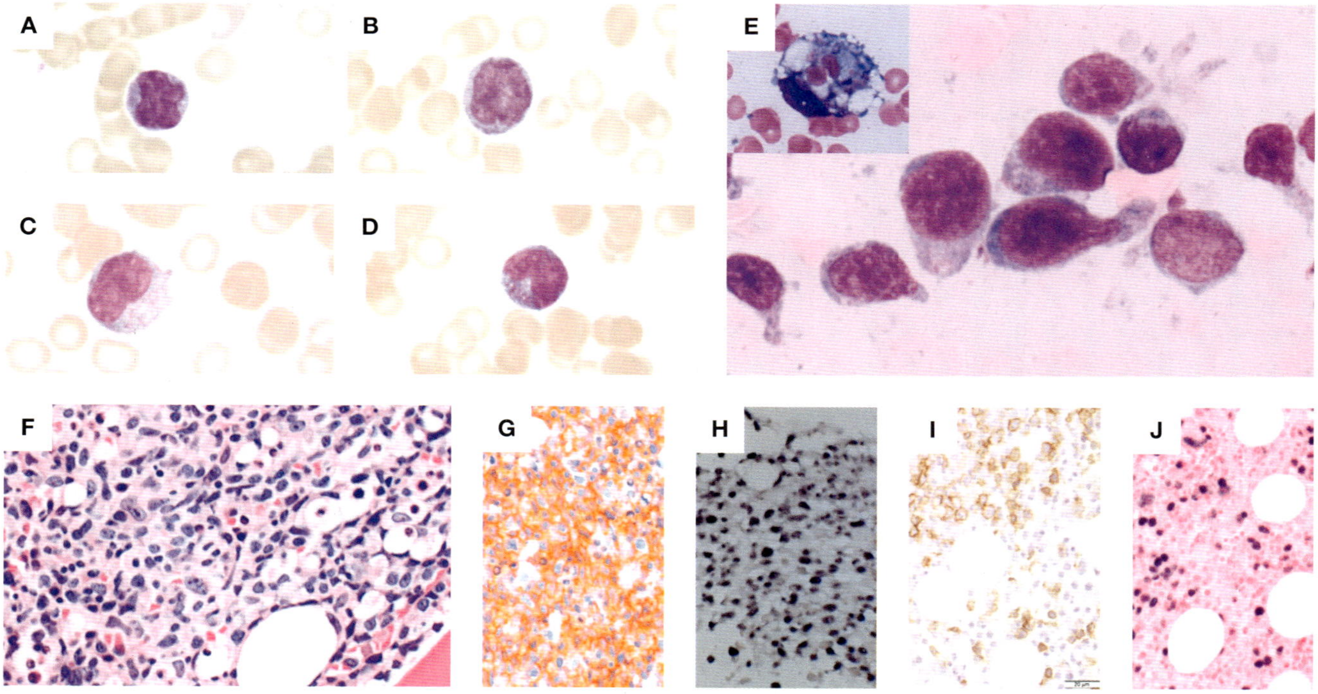

FIGURE 94.1 Blood and bone marrow involvement in aggressive natural killer-cell leukemia (ANKL). **A-D:** Blood leukemic cells with variable morphology (Wright Giemsa stain). **E:** A group of leukemic cells in the bone marrow. Inset, macrophage showing hemophagocytosis (Wright Giemsa stain). **F-H:** Bone marrow biopsy showing extensive infiltration by leukemic cells. **G:** CD56 staining (immunoperoxidase). **H:** EBERs in situ hybridization (ISH) highlighting the leukemic cells. **I** and **J:** Bone marrow biopsy showing interstitial infiltrate of leukemic cells that is underscored by immunostaining for CD56 and ISH for EBV-encoded small RNAs (EBER).

conspicuous in these cases (Figure 94.1E). Multiple parenchymal and secondary lymphoid organs are often involved, particularly the liver and spleen. The liver infiltrates may show a portal and sinusoidal pattern (Figures 94.2 and 94.3) and splenic red pulp is predominantly and often extensively involved. Apoptotic bodies are readily observed and there may be varying degrees of necrosis.

Immunophenotype

Flow cytometric analysis of blood or bone marrow has been frequently used for immunophenotyping. The tumor cells express many natural killer-cell associated markers (see Figures 94.2 and 94.3) including CD2, CD56, cytotoxic molecules, and CD94. Cytoplasmic CD3ε, CD11b, and HLA-DR are also often expressed. CD16, which is not usually expressed in ENKTCL, is reported frequently positive in some studies,[8-10] but not in others.[3,11] CD57 is generally negative and CD7 is inconsistently expressed, whereas CD8 is absent in most cases. T-cell markers such as surface CD3, T-cell antigen receptors, and CD5 are negative. EBV infection can be demonstrated by EBER in situ hybridization (ISH) in most of the cases (see Figures 94.2 and 94.3). LMP1 staining is usually negative.[3]

ANKL includes a minority of EBV-negative cases (10%-20% of cases) and this group seems to be enriched in non-Asian and older patients, compared with EBV+ ANKL.[7,12] The lack of Epstein-Barr virus (EBV) infection may raise concerns in the diagnosis. A case with the appropriate clinical features and pathologic findings similar to an EBV+ ANKL should be classified as ANKL, but specified as to its EBV status.

ANKL that has prominent sinusoidal involvement of the marrow, liver, and spleen could be confused with hepatosplenic T-cell lymphoma, which may not express CD4, CD5 or CD8 and may be TIA1- and CD56-positive. HSTCL is, however, of T-cell lineage with clonal TRG gene rearrangement and often shows TCRγδ/sCD3 expression; the tumor cells usually do not express granzyme B and perforin and CD94 tends to be absent or dim (see Table 99.1).

Genetics

ANKL is, by definition, derived from natural killer cells and the T-cell receptor genes are in the germline configuration.

Because of the rarity of the disease, genetic information is still quite limited. Cases with cytogenetic data

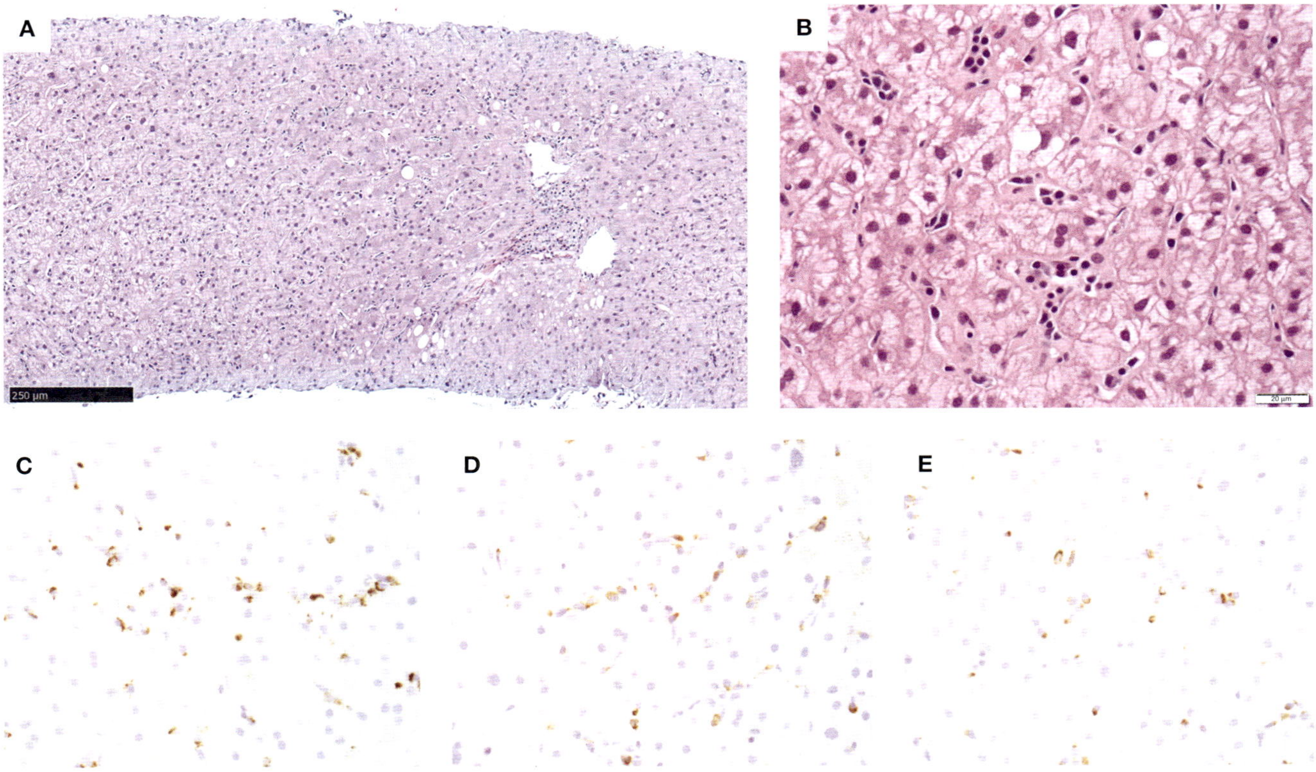

FIGURE 94.2 Liver involvement in aggressive natural killer-cell leukemia (ANKL). **A** and **B:** Liver biopsy showing a mild sinusoidal infiltration by rather small lymphoid cells. (H&E) **C-E:** immunostainings for TIA1, granzyme B, and perforin highlight the intrasinusoidal lymphocytes.

generally show complex chromosomal changes[3,8,13] with frequent chromosome 7 abnormalities and recurrent del(6q) and del(11q). Comparative genomic hybridization studies identified recurrent gains in multiple regions of 1q, Xq25-q28, 9p24, and 17q21 and losses in 1p36, 3q21.3, 6q21-q25, 7p22.1, 7q22.1, and 17p13.1.[14,15] Next-generation sequencing has identified frequent mutations that prominently affect the JAK/STAT pathway. *JAK3* and *STAT3* mutations are consistently reported but mutations in other genes of the pathway are reported in single studies.[16-18] Mutations in the RAS/MAPK pathway (*BRAF, KRAS,*

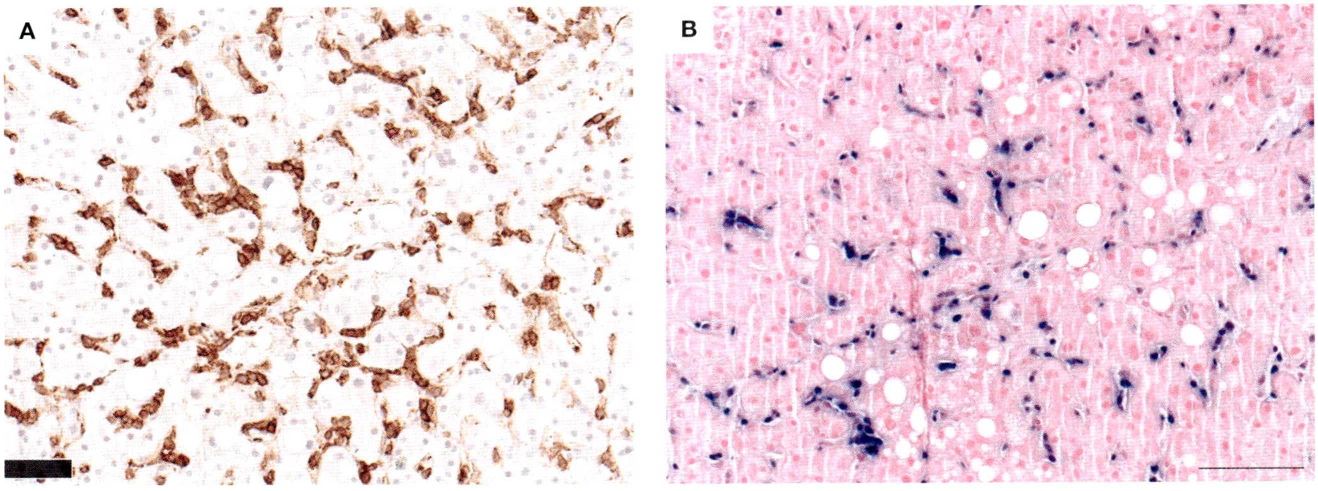

FIGURE 94.3 Liver involvement by aggressive natural killer-cell leukemia (ANKL). **A:** This case is characterized by an extensive sinusoidal infiltration by lymphocytes positive for CD56. **B:** The lymphoid cells are positive for EBV-encoded small RNAs (EBERs) by in situ hybridization.

NRAS, MAPK10) and in phosphotyrosine phosphatases are also quite frequent. Mutations in genes regulating or modifying the epigenome including *TET2, CREBBP, KMT2D, SETD2, ARID1A, ARID2, ASXL1-3, NCOR2*, and *BCOR* were also reported. The tumor suppressor genes *TP53* and *DDX3X* are often mutated at least in one of the reports. The genetic information available is still very limited but in general, most of the reported mutations are also represented in ENKTCL but with varying frequencies. Nevertheless, the similarity in the set of mutated genes with ENKTCL suggests shared oncogenic pathways. Information on EBV-negative cases is even more limited. In one report, 2/2 patients sequenced had *STAT3* missense mutations[7] whereas in two other patients[12], no JAK/STAT pathway mutations were found, although a number of mutations noted in EBV+ ANKL were detected.

The complex genetic abnormalities found in the neoplastic clone suggest the presence of these abnormal cells long before the onset of the disease. What induces the acute fulminant onset is unclear, but the possibility of cytokines as triggers has been raised.[18]

Prognosis and Clinical Comment

The prognosis of patients with ANKL is extremely poor with short survival. Aside from the widespread organ infiltrations by the neoplastic cells, many of the clinical manifestations could be related to the accompanying cytokine storm. The rapid expansion of activated natural killer cells leads directly or indirectly to the production of many cytotoxic or inflammatory factors,[19-21] including cytokines that induce the hemophagocytic syndrome and other adverse consequences. FasL is elevated in the plasma[21] and can induce apoptosis of Fas-expressing cells such as hepatocytes.

A minority of patients achieves complete remission on chemotherapy, but the disease often relapses. Allogeneic stem cell transplantation can produce lasting remission in a subset of patients, particularly in those who achieve complete remission on chemotherapy.[22,23] Genetic alterations that may enhance the expression of PD-L1 are frequent in ANKL, as observed in ENKTCL[24] but efficacy of immune checkpoint blockade has not been reported yet. Targeted agents against JAK and BCL2 may be helpful and have been preliminarily explored in in vitro studies.[17]

References

1. Ishida F. Aggressive NK-cell leukemia. *Front Pediatr*. 2018;6:292. doi:10.3389/fped.2018.00292
2. Ruskova A, Thula R, Chan G. Aggressive Natural Killer-Cell Leukemia: report of five cases and review of the literature. *Leuk Lymphoma*. 2004;45(12):2427-2438. doi:10.1080/10428190400004513
3. Ryder J, Wang X, Bao L, Gross SA, Hua F, Irons RD. Aggressive natural killer cell leukemia: report of a Chinese series and review of the literature. *Int J Hematol*. 2007;85(1):18-25. doi:10.1532/IJH97.A10612
4. Kimura H, Ito Y, Kawabe S, et al. EBV-associated T/NK-cell lymphoproliferative diseases in nonimmunocompromised hosts: prospective analysis of 108 cases. *Blood*. 2012;119(3):673-686. doi:10.1182/blood-2011-10-381921
5. Zhang H, Meng Q, Yin W, Xu L, Lie L. Adult aggressive natural killer cell leukemia. *Am J Med Sci*. 2013;346(1):56-63. doi:10.1097/MAJ.0b013e3182764b59
6. Zanelli M, Parente P, Sanguedolce F, et al. Intravascular NK/T-Cell lymphoma: what we know about this diagnostically challenging, aggressive disease. *Cancers*. 2022;14(21):5458. doi:10.3390/cancers14215458
7. Nicolae A, Ganapathi KA, Pham TH, et al. EBV-Negative aggressive NK-cell leukemia/lymphoma: clinical, pathologic, and genetic features. *Am J Surg Pathol*. 2017;41(1):67-74. doi:10.1097/PAS.0000000000000735
8. El Hussein S, Medeiros LJ, Khoury JD. Aggressive NK cell leukemia: current state of the art. *Cancers*. 2020;12(10):2900. doi:10.3390/cancers12102900
9. Imamura N, Kusunoki Y, Oda K, et al. Aggressive natural killer cell leukemia/lymphoma—possible existence of a new clinical entity originating from the third lineage of lymphoid cells. *Rinsho Ketsueki*. 1989;30(2):193-201. Japanese.
10. Suzuki R, Suzumiya J, Nakamura S; NK-Cell Tumor Study Group, et al. Aggressive natural killer-cell leukemia revisited: large granular lymphocyte leukemia of cytotoxic NK cells. *Leukemia*. 2004;18(4):763-770. doi:10.1038/sj.leu.2403262
11. Li Y, Wei J, Mao X, et al. Flow cytometric immunophenotyping is sensitive for the early diagnosis of de novo aggressive natural killer cell leukemia (ANKL): a multicenter retrospective analysis. *PLoS One*. 2016;11(8):e0158827. doi:10.1371/journal.pone.0158827
12. Gao J, Behdad A, Ji P, Wolniak KL, Frankfurt O, Chen YH. EBV-negative aggressive NK-cell leukemia/lymphoma: a clinical and pathological study from a single institution. *Mod Pathol*. 2017;30(8):1100-1115. doi:10.1038/modpathol.2017.37
13. Yang CF, Hsu CY, Ho DM. Aggressive natural killer (NK)-cell leukaemia and extranodal NK/T-cell lymphoma are two distinct diseases that differ in their clinical presentation and cytogenetic findings. *Histopathology*. 2018;72(6):955-964. doi:10.1111/his.13463

14. Nakashima Y, Tagawa H, Suzuki R, et al. Genome-wide array-based comparative genomic hybridization of natural killer cell lymphoma/leukemia: different genomic alteration patterns of aggressive NK-cell leukemia and extranodal Nk/T-cell lymphoma, nasal type. *Genes Chromosomes Cancer*. 2005;44(3):247-255. doi:10.1002/gcc.20245
15. Ohshima K, Haraokaa S, Ishihara S, et al. Analysis of chromosome 6q deletion in EBV-associated NK cell leukaemia/lymphoma. *Leuk Lymphoma*. 2002;43(2):293-300. doi:10.1080/10428190290006062
16. El Hussein S, Patel KP, Fang H, et al. Genomic and immunophenotypic landscape of aggressive NK-cell leukemia. *Am J Surg Pathol*. 2020;44(9):1235-1243. doi:10.1097/PAS.0000000000001518
17. Dufva O, Kankainen M, Kelkka T, et al. Aggressive natural killer-cell leukemia mutational landscape and drug profiling highlight JAK-STAT signaling as therapeutic target. *Nat Commun*. 2018;9(1):1567. doi:10.1038/s41467-018-03987-2
18. Huang L, Liu D, Wang N, et al. Integrated genomic analysis identifies deregulated JAK/STAT-MYC-biosynthesis axis in aggressive NK-cell leukemia. *Cell Res*. 2018;28(2):172-186. doi:10.1038/cr.2017.146
19. Henter JI, Elinder G, Söder O, Hansson M, Andersson B, Andersson U. Hypercytokinemia in familial hemophagocytic lymphohistiocytosis. *Blood*. 1991;78(11):2918-2922.
20. Teruya-Feldstein J, Setsuda J, Yao X, et al. MIP-1alpha expression in tissues from patients with hemophagocytic syndrome. *Lab Invest*. 1999;79(12):1583-1590.
21. Nakashima Y, Tagawa H, Suzuki R, et al. Genome-wide array-based comparative genomic hybridization of natural killer cell lymphoma/leukemia: different genomic alteration patterns of aggressive NK-cell leukemia and extranodal Nk/T-cell lymphoma, nasal type. *Genes Chromosomes Cancer*. 2005;44(3):247-255. doi:10.1002/gcc.20245
22. Hamadani M, Kanate AS, DiGilio A, et al. Allogeneic hematopoietic cell transplantation for aggressive NK cell leukemia. A center for international blood and marrow transplant research analysis. *Biol Blood Marrow Transplant*. 2017;23(5):853-856. doi:10.1016/j.bbmt.2017.01.082
23. Jung KS, Cho SH, Kim SJ, Ko YH, Kang ES, Kim WS. L-asparaginase-based regimens followed by allogeneic hematopoietic stem cell transplantation improve outcomes in aggressive natural killer cell leukemia. *J Hematol Oncol*. 2016;9:41. doi:10.1186/s13045-016-0271-4
24. Kataoka K, Miyoshi H, Sakata S, et al. Frequent structural variations involving programmed death ligands in Epstein-Barr virus-associated lymphomas. *Leukemia*. 2019;33(7):1687-1699. doi:10.1038/s41375-019-0380-5

Chapter 95

Primary Nodal Epstein-Barr Virus-positive T-Cell/NK-Cell Lymphoma

Shigeo Nakamura, Carlos Barrionuevo, Fina Climent, and Won seog Kim

Definition

Primary nodal Epstein-Barr virus (EBV)-positive T- or NK-cell lymphoma (EBV+ nTNKL) is an aggressive lymphoma of cytotoxic T-cell or more rarely NK-cell phenotype, characterized by lymphadenopathy and systemic symptoms at presentation and association with EBV.

By definition, it is a systemic disease without nasal involvement. This disease was introduced in the 2017 World Health Organization classification as a variant of peripheral T-cell lymphoma (PTCL), not otherwise specified (NOS). New findings have led to include this lymphoma as a new provisional entity in the 2022 International Consensus Classification.

Synonyms

Nodal PTCL, NOS, EBV+ (not recommended).

Epidemiology

This overall very rare disease has been largely documented in East Asia (Table 95.1).[1-9] Recent data emphasize the differences of those cases both from extranodal EBV-positive NK-/T-cell lymphomas (ENKTL) and from nodal EBV-negative cytotoxic T-cell lymphomas. Patients are older adults with a median age of 62 to 64 years often in the setting of immunosuppression (HIV, post transplant), immunosenescence or in association with autoimmune diseases.

TABLE 95.1 Summary of the clinicopathologic features of primary nodal EBV+ T/NK-cell lymphoma

Geographical cohorts	Japan	Singapore	Korea
Median age (y)	62	61	64
Clinical stage III/IV	86%	88%	87%
IPI high-intermediate/high	64%	NA	87%
Thrombocytopenia	55%	NA	53%
Extranodal involvement >1 site	15%	NA	29%
Median overall survival (mo)	8.0	2.5	3.5
Immunophenotype			
CD3	95%	NA	100%
CD4	19%	NA	20%
CD5	29%	NA	NA
CD8	63%	67%	67%
CD56	12%	22%	7%
TCRβ	43%	47%	64%
TCRγ and/or δ	12%	0%	0%
T-cell origin[a]	80%	84%	92%

NA, not available.

Modified from Kato S, Yamashita D, Nakamura S. Nodal EBV+ cytotoxic T-cell lymphoma: a literature review based on the 2017 WHO classification. *J Clin Exp Hematopathol.* 2020;60(2):30-36.

[a]T-cell origin based on TCR protein expression and/or clonal rearrangement of TR genes.

General Clinical Features

EBV+ nTNKL presents with lymphadenopathy with or without extranodal involvement. EBV+ nTNKL can involve the Waldeyer ring and should be distinguished from ENKTL with nodal disease. This distinction requires a thorough assessment of clinical, histopathological, and molecular features.[10] Some cases exhibit hepatic involvement (32%-60%) or bone marrow involvement (24%-29%), but there is no nasal involvement.

Clinical information, such as staging and history of lymphoma at nonnodal sites and any context of immunosuppression, is important in the diagnosis of this disease. Patients typically show aggressive clinical features, ie, advanced clinical-stage disease (86%-88%), B symptoms (72%-80%), high or high/intermediate International Prognostic Index (IPI) (64%-87%), and thrombocytopenia (53%-62%).[7]

ENKTL rarely involves lymph nodes and must be excluded clinically. The differential diagnosis also includes systemic chronic active EBV disease (CAEBV) of T-cell or NK-cell phenotype or systemic EBV positive T-cell lymphoma of childhood (Table 92.3). EBV+ nTNKL may arise in patients with a history CAEBV.[7]

Morphology

This disease diffusely affects the lymph node architecture with a monomorphic infiltrative pattern of medium- to large-sized cells (Figure 95.1) and lacks the angiocentric pattern and necrosis seen in ENKTL. Prototypic cases (about half) have a centroblastoid appearance morphologically raising a differential diagnosis with diffuse large B-cell lymphoma and distinct from the pleomorphic and elongated nuclei seen in ENKTL.[1]

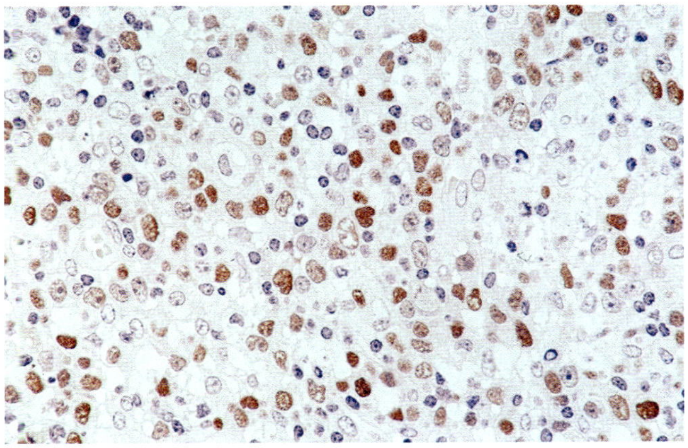

FIGURE 95.2 Primary nodal EBV-positive T/NK-cell lymphoma. Most tumor cells are positive for EBER.

Immunophenotype

EBV studies are essential to make the diagnosis. EBV-encoded small RNA (EBER) by in situ hybridization is positive in the majority of neoplastic cells (Figure 95.2) with latency type I or II but not III. Tumors express cytotoxic markers and more often are of T-cell rather than NK-cell origin, prototypically evidenced by a CD8^{+}/CD56^{-} phenotype and clonal TR gene rearrangements.[3,7,8] EBV+ nTNKL shows CD3 positivity in 95% to 100% of the cases, expression of cytotoxic molecules (TIA1, granzyme B, and/or perforin) in 100% (Figure 95.3), CD8 in 63% to 72% (Figure 95.4), and less frequently CD56 in 0% to 22%.[7] Positivity for CD30 (37%-39%), combined with the morphology

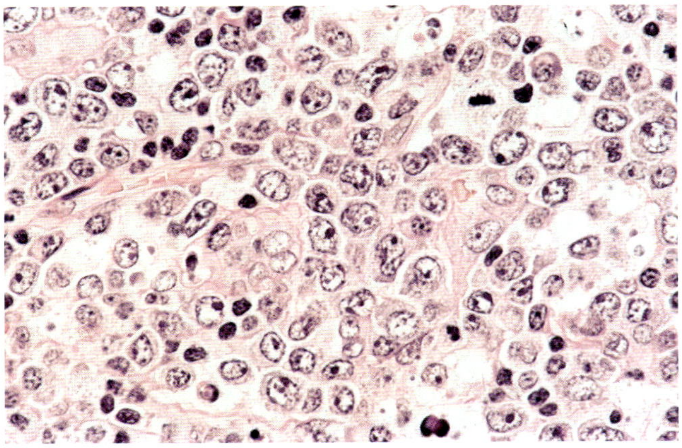

FIGURE 95.1 Primary nodal EBV-positive T/NK-cell lymphoma. The tumor cells prototypically show a centroblastoid appearance.

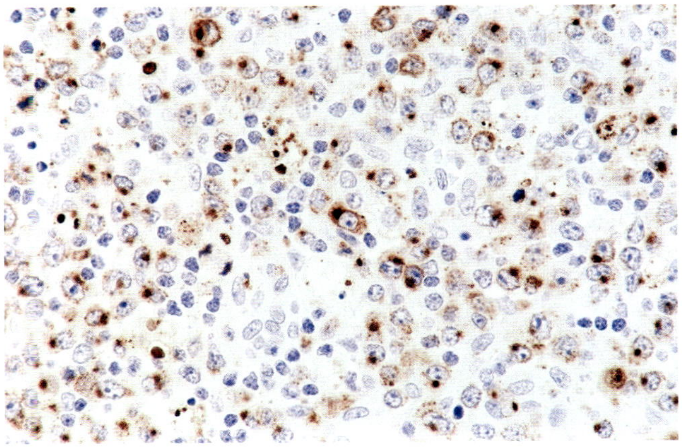

FIGURE 95.3 Primary nodal EBV-positive T/NK-cell lymphoma. The tumor cells express granzyme B.

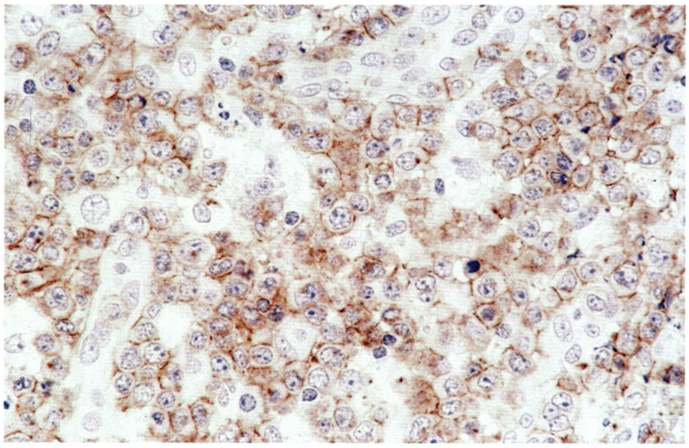

FIGURE 95.4 Primary nodal EBV-positive T/NK-cell lymphoma. The tumor cells are positive for CD8.

and cytotoxic phenotype, sometimes raises a differential diagnosis with anaplastic large cel lymphoma, requiring assessment of EBV status. Approximately 80% to 92% of cases show clonal TR rearrangements and/or expression of TCR proteins (TCR beta 43% to 64%, TCR gamma or TCR delta 0% to 12%; see Table 95.1). These findings support the assertion that they are of T-cell lineage contrasted with a minority (<20%) of NK-cell lineage lacking both of them.

PD-L1 protein is overexpressed in both tumor and nontumor cells (Figure 95-5).[5,6,9]

Genetics

EBV+ nTNKL has lower genomic instability than ENKTL and its expression signature is characterized by the upregulation of T-cell-related genes and downregulation of CD56, different from ENKTL. Its genomic landscape comprises frequent mutations of

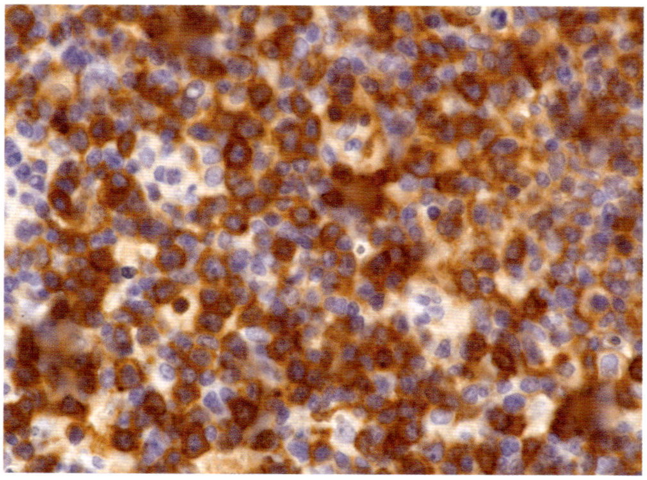

FIGURE 95.5 Primary nodal EBV-positive T/NK-cell lymphoma. PD-L1 expression is detected on neoplastic cells.

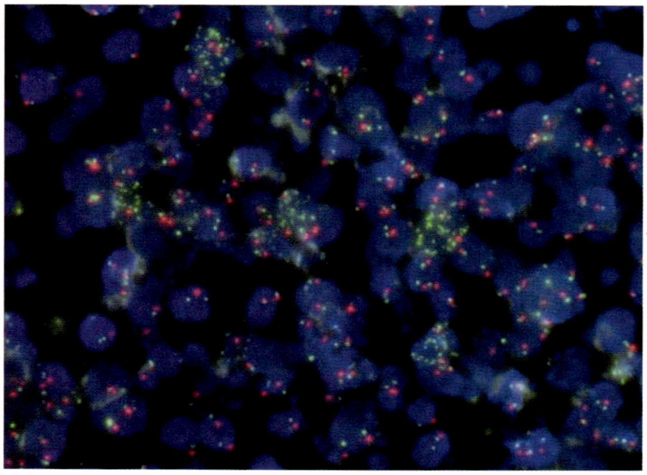

FIGURE 95.6 Fluorescence in situ hybridization analysis showing *PD-L1* gene amplification in a primary nodal EBV+ T-cell/NK-cell lymphoma using a SPEC CD274/PD-L1 (green signal), PDCD1LG2/CEN9 (red signal) Dual Color Probe.

TET2 (64%), *PIK3CD* (33%), *DDX3* (20%), and *STAT3* (19%), partially overlapping with ENKTL.[5,9,10,11] In addition, the presence of frequent mutations of epigenetic modifier genes is consistent with that observed in EBV-negative nodal cytotoxic PTCL[12] and might suggest a putative role of clonal hematopoiesis.[11] Compared to ENKTCL, EBV+ nTNKL shows upregulation of JAK/STAT signaling and immune-related pathways including PD-L1 (CD274) expression (Figure 95.6), and downregulation of EBV miRNAs.[10] Copy number analysis also showed recurrent losses of 3q26.1, 22q11.23, and 14q11.2.

Prognosis and Clinical Comment

Primary nodal EBV+ T/NK-cell lymphoma is an aggressive lymphoma with a high risk of disease progression and relapse, and has a median overall survival of 2.5 to 8.0 months.[7] There is no standard treatment approach. It remains uncertain if these patients will show a similar favorable response to L-asparaginase-based regimens as observed in patients with advanced ENKTL.[13] The use of immune checkpoint inhibitors targeting the PD1/PD-L1 axis has not yet been documented.

References

1. Kagami Y, Suzuki R, Taji H, et al. Nodal cytotoxic lymphoma spectrum: a clinicopathologic study of 66 patients. *Am J Surg Pathol.* 1999;23(10):1184-1200. doi:10.1097/00000478-199910000-00003
2. Kato S, Takahashi E, Asano N, et al. Nodal cytotoxic molecule (CM)-positive Epstein-Barr virus (EBV)-associated

peripheral T cell lymphoma (PTCL): a clinicopathological study of 26 cases. *Histopathology*. 2012;61(2):186-199. doi:10.1111/j.1365-2559.2012.04199.x

3. Kato S, Asano N, Miyata-Takata T, et al. T-cell receptor (TCR) phenotype of nodal Epstein-Barr virus (EBV)-positive cytotoxic T-cell lymphoma (CTL): a clinicopathologic study of 39 cases. *Am J Surg Pathol.* 2015;39(4):462-471. doi:10.1097/PAS.0000000000000323
4. Jeon YK, Kim JH, Sung JY, Han JH, Ko YH; Hematopathology Study Group of the Korean Society of Pathologists. Epstein-Barr virus-positive nodal T/NK-cell lymphoma: an analysis of 15 cases with distinct clinicopathological features. *Hum Pathol.* 2015;46(7):981-990. doi:10.1016/j.humpath.2015.03.002
5. Ng SB, Chung TH, Kato S, et al. Epstein-Barr virus-associated primary nodal T/NK-cell lymphoma shows a distinct molecular signature and copy number changes. *Haematologica.* 2018;103(2):278-287. doi:10.3324/haematol.2017.180430
6. Yamashita D, Shimada K, Kohno K, et al. PD-L1 expression on tumor or stromal cells of nodal cytotoxic T-cell lymphoma: a clinicopathological study of 50 cases. *Pathol Int.* 2020;70(8):513-522. doi:10.1111/pin.12950
7. Kato S, Yamashita D, Nakamura S. Nodal EBV+ cytotoxic T-cell lymphoma: a literature review based on the 2017 WHO classification. *J Clin Exp Hematop.* 2020;60(2):30-36. doi:10.3960/jslrt.20001
8. Feldman AL, Laurent C, Narbaitz M, et al. Classification and diagnostic evaluation of nodal T- and NK-cell lymphomas. *Virchows Arch.* 2023;482(1):265-279. doi:10.1007/s00428-022-03412-6
9. Climent F, Nicolae A, de Leval L, et al. Cytotoxic peripheral T-cell lymphomas and EBV-positive T/NK-cell lymphoproliferative diseases: emerging concepts, recent advances, and the putative role of clonal hematopoiesis. A report of the 2022 EA4HP/SH lymphoma workshop. *Virchows Arch.* 2023;483(3):333-348. doi:10.1007/s00428-023-03616-4
10. Wai CMM, Chen S, Phyu T, et al. Immune pathway upregulation and lower genomic instability distinguish EBV-positive nodal T/NK-cell lymphoma from ENKTL and PTCL-NOS. *Haematologica.* 2022;107(8):1864-1879. doi:10.3324/haematol.2021.280003
11. Kato S, Hamada M, Okamoto A, et al. EBV+ nodal T/NK-cell lymphoma associated with clonal hematopoiesis and structural variations of the viral genome. Blood Adv. 2024;8(9):2138-2147. doi:10.1182/bloodadvances.2023012019
12. Nicolae A, Bouilly J, Lara D, et al. Nodal cytotoxic peripheral T-cell lymphoma occurs frequently in the clinical setting of immunodysregulation and is associated with recurrent epigenetic alterations. *Mod Pathol.* 2022;35(8):1126-1136. doi:10.1038/s41379-022-01022-w
13. Yamaguchi M, Suzuki R, Oguchi M. Advances in the treatment of extranodal NK/T-cell lymphoma, nasal type. *Blood.* 2018;131(23):2528-2540. doi:10.1182/blood-2017-12-791418

Chapter 96

Type II Refractory Celiac Disease and Enteropathy-Associated T-Cell Lymphoma

Laurence de Leval, Julie Bruneau, Francesco d'Amore, and Ahmet Dogan

TYPE II REFRACTORY CELIAC DISEASE

Definition

Celiac disease (CD) is an immune-mediated enteropathy occurring in genetically susceptible individuals carrying HLA-DQ2 or HLA-DQ8, which is triggered and sustained by ingestion of gluten.[1] Refractory celiac disease (RCD) is defined as persistent gastrointestinal symptoms and villous atrophy despite a strict gluten-free diet for at least 6 to 12 months in patients diagnosed with celiac disease, after other etiologies for nonresponsiveness and malignancies have been excluded.[2] Type II RCD (RCD-II) is characterized by a clonal expansion of intraepithelial lymphocytes (IELs) showing an abnormal immunophenotype.[1] RCD-II is a severe complication of celiac disease associated with a poor prognosis and a 30% to 50% risk for transformation to overt enteropathy-associated T-cell lymphoma (EATL) within 5 years.[3]

An overview of T-cell and natural killer-cell neoplasms involving the gastrointestinal tract is presented in Table 96.1.

Synonyms

Intraepithelial T-cell lymphoma; cryptic intraepithelial T-cell lymphoma; low-grade intraepithelial lymphoma; in situ enteropathy-associated T-cell lymphoma (all not recommended).

Epidemiology

RCD-II is estimated to affect less than 1% of individuals with celiac disease.

General Clinical Features

Patients with RCD-II often present with severe malnutrition, more pronounced than in RCD-I (which is associated with polyclonal and phenotypically normal IELs) or CD, due to chronic diarrhea, hypoalbuminemia, or ulcerative jejunitis, sometimes complicated by strictures or perforations.[3,4]

Aberrant T lymphocytes in RCD-II are not strictly confined to the intestinal epithelium but may involve the lamina propria, other parts of the gastrointestinal tract, or extragastrointestinal locations, including the blood, bone marrow, and skin.[5,6]

Morphology

Small intestinal lesions in RCD-II show villous atrophy with expanded IELs (>25 lymphocytes per 100 enterocytes), which are small with no or limited cytologic atypia (Figure 96.1). The histologic features are similar to those of active CD or RCD-I, but mucosal ulceration is more frequent.

Immunophenotype

The abnormal IELs in RCD-II have innate lymphoid cell-like features with dual T- and natural killer-cell traits and are stimulated to expand by interleukin-15 (IL-15) overexpressed by the enterocytes in patients with CD.[7] They are $CD2^+$, $CD5^-CD7^+$, $CD30^-$, $CD56^-$, and express αE integrin (CD103) and cytotoxic molecules (TIA, granzyme B and/or perforin).[8] They do not express surface CD3 (sCD3) but retain intracellular CD3 expression (cCD3), and usually lack surface expression of CD8 and T-cell receptor (TCR) molecules. Flow cytometric analysis of isolated small intestinal IELs is the reference method for subtyping RCD (into types I and II) and a cut-off of 20% or more aberrant IELs is used to diagnose RCD-II (Figure 96.2A).[6] By immunohistochemistry (IHC) (Figure 96.1), a threshold of >50% $cCD3^+$ IELs showing loss of CD8 or TCRαβ expression is used to indicate an aberrant immunophenotype.[9] Rare cases of RCD-II develop from. $TCR\gamma\delta^+$ IELs or from $TCR\alpha\beta^+$ IELs expressing CD8.[2,8] IELs in RCD-II also express the natural killer receptor NKp46, and one study found that detection of

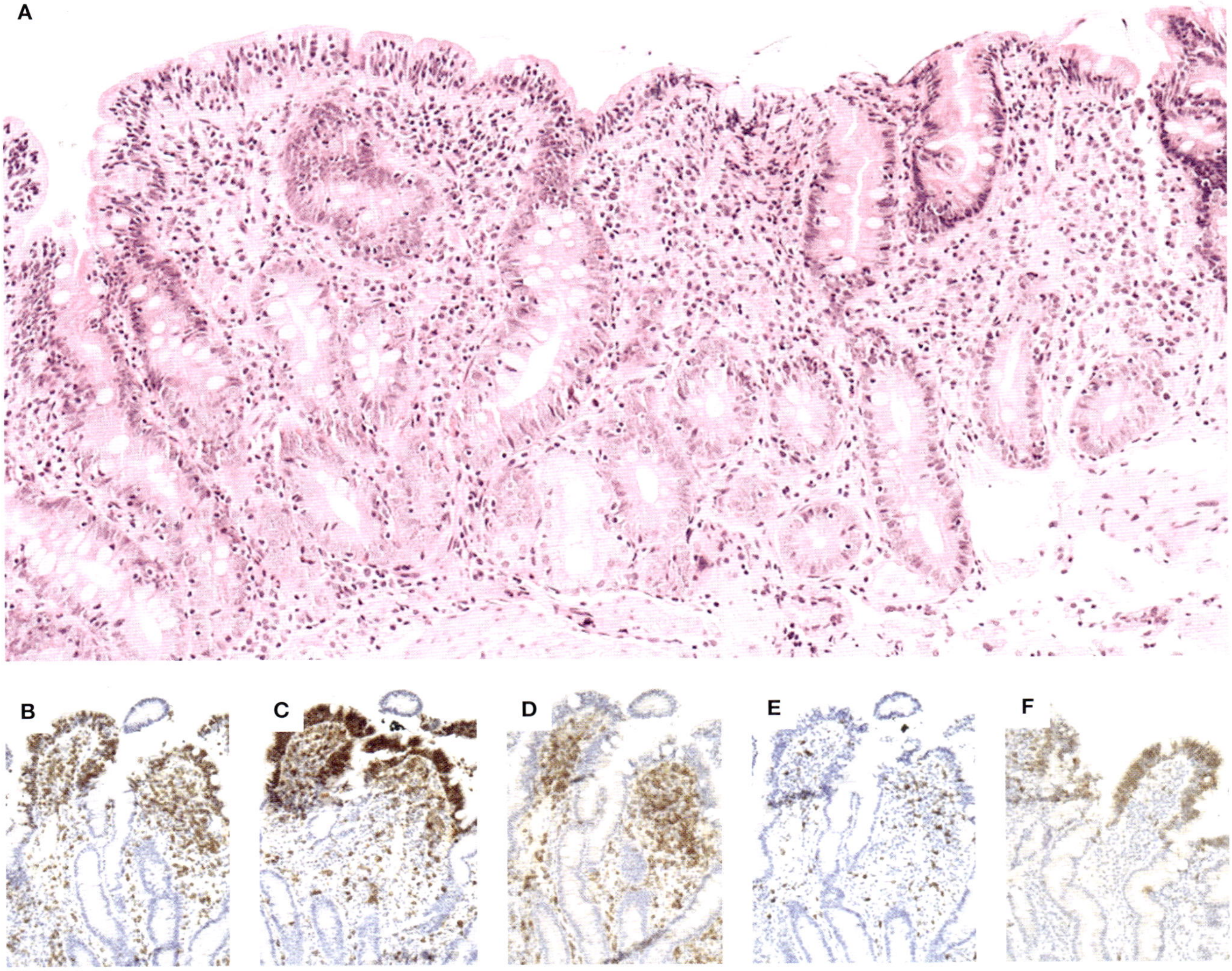

FIGURE 96.1 Refractory celiac disease type II. **A:** A duodenal biopsy shows a severe and total villous blunting (Marsh 3c) with a moderate increase of intraepithelial lymphocytes (IELs). **B:** Anti-CD3 and **C:** anti-CD103 highlight IELs and scattered lymphocytes in the lamina propria. **D:** The IELs are CD4-negative. **E:** The IELs are mostly negative (>50%) for CD8. **F:** NKp46 stains the IELs and scattered cells in the lamina propria.

>25 NKp46+ IELs per 100 epithelial cells discriminates RCD-II from CD and RCD-I.[10] The presence of atypical IELs with CD30 expression is rarely seen in RCD-II and is considered a sign of progression to EATL.[11]

Genetics

The abnormal IELs in RCD-II exhibit clonal TRG or TRB gene rearrangements (Figure 96.2B). Analysis of TCR clonality results may be difficult and, depending on the method used, a subset of RCD-II shows polyclonal patterns of TCR gene rearrangements.[12] The finding of reproducible peaks in independent samples is more specific. Combinatory TCR clonality and IHC testing is recommended if multiparametric flow cytometric analysis is not available.[13] Trisomy of 1q is the only known recurrent chromosome abnormality.[14] Recent sequencing studies[8,15] have identified genetic alterations in most cases, notably gain-of-function mutations in JAK-STAT pathway genes, including a *JAK1* p.G1097 hotspot mutations in about half of the cases and frequent *STAT3* mutations, which appear to be the main drivers of CD-associated lymphomagenesis and confer hyperresponsiveness to IL-15.[8] Other recurrent somatic events were observed in epigenetic regulators (*TET2, KMT2D, DDX3X*) and nuclear factor-κB (NFκB) pathway genes (*TNFAIP3, TNIP3*).

Prognosis and Clinical Comment

RCD-II is regarded as a precursor lesion to EATL or a cryptic intraepithelial T-cell lymphoma, associated with a 30% to 50% risk for transformation to overt

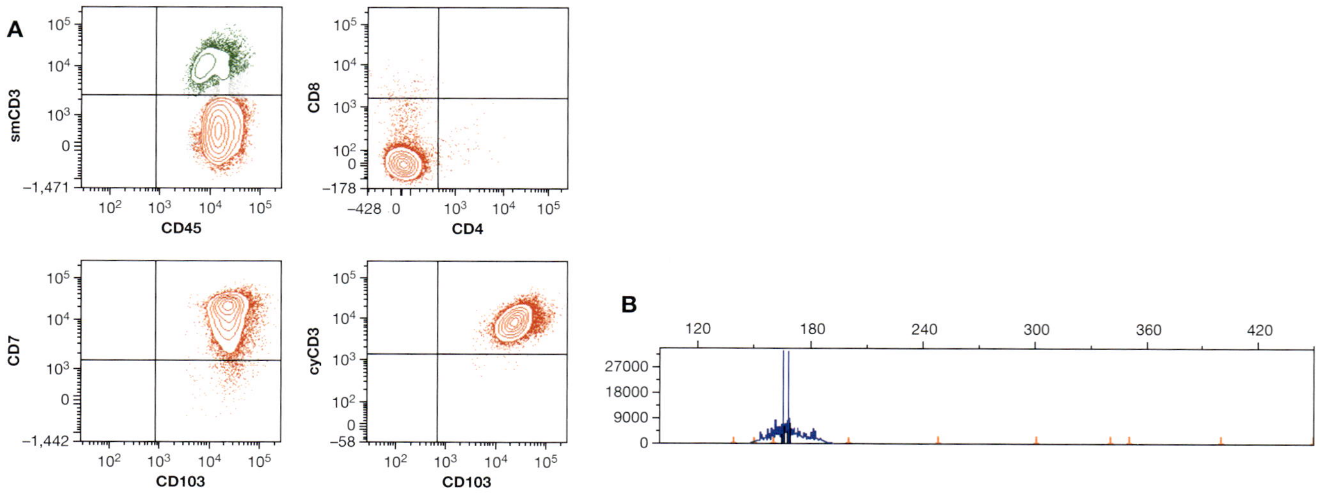

FIGURE 96.2 Refractory celiac disease type II. **A:** Flow cytometry after duodenal biopsy dissection of surface epithelium from lamina propria and IEL isolation: the green population illustrates the residual normal IELs with the expression of surface CD3 (sCD3), whereas the red population highlights the aberrant IEL population, $sCD3^- CD7^+ CD103^+ CD4^- CD8^-$, with high levels expression of the intracytoplasmic (cy)$CD3^+$. **B:** Representation of a monoclonal rearrangement of the TRG gene on a polyclonal background.

EATL within 5 years.[3] Homozygosity for HLA-DQ2 and genetic polymorphisms at the 7p14.3 locus or in the *MYO9B* gene appear to increase the likelihood to progress from CD to RCD-II and EATL.[3]

According to clinical practice guidelines of the American Gastroenterology Association,[16] for patients with persistently symptomatic and nontreatment responsive CD, if exposure to gluten-containing diet can be excluded, the patient should be referred to an esophagogastroduodenoscopy with multiple small bowel biopsies.[16] If villous atrophy persists, and other causes of villous atrophy can be excluded, IHC, flow cytometry, TCR clonality analysis, and if available mutation analysis should be performed to distinguish between type I and type II RCD based on the absence (type I) or presence (type II) of clonal IELs.[16] If clonal IELs are identified, small bowel imaging with capsule endoscopy and a positron emission tomograph (PET)–CT, possibly supplemented by magnetic resonance enterography, should be carried out under suspicion of EATL. Tissue biopsies should be submitted to an experienced hematopathologist to evaluate the presence of lesions suggestive of EATL (including CD30 expression).[16] If EATL is diagnosed, specific management for this entity should be initiated (see Chapter 96). If not, regular checks for EATL (eg, positron emission tomograph–CT, endoscopic biopsies at 6- to 12-month intervals) should be performed in a multidisciplinary team context (pathologist, hematologist, gastroenterologist, dietician). Corticosteroids, most commonly open-capsule budesonide or, if unavailable, prednisolone, are the medication of choice and should be used as first-line therapy regardless of whether the patient has a type I or type II RCD.

ENTEROPATHY-ASSOCIATED T-CELL LYMPHOMA

Definition

Enteropthy-assocaited T-cell lymphoma (EATL) is a lymphoma of intestinal intraepithelial T cells that occurs in individuals with celiac disease (CD) and shows cellular pleomorphism and a prominent inflammatory component.

Synonyms

Enteropathy-type T-cell lymphoma; enteropathy-associated T-cell lymphoma, type I (not recommended).

Epidemiology

EATL represents less than 5% of peripheral T-cell lymphomas and overall the main type of primary intestinal T-cell lymphoma worldwide.[17] The disease is most prevalent in Europe, followed by North American populations, where the genetic background of CD is more common. EATL was previously reported to be almost absent in Asians, but a recent epidemiological study conducted in South Korea, China, and other Asian countries indicates a prevalence close to that of monomorphic epitheliotropic intestinal T-cell lymphoma.[18]

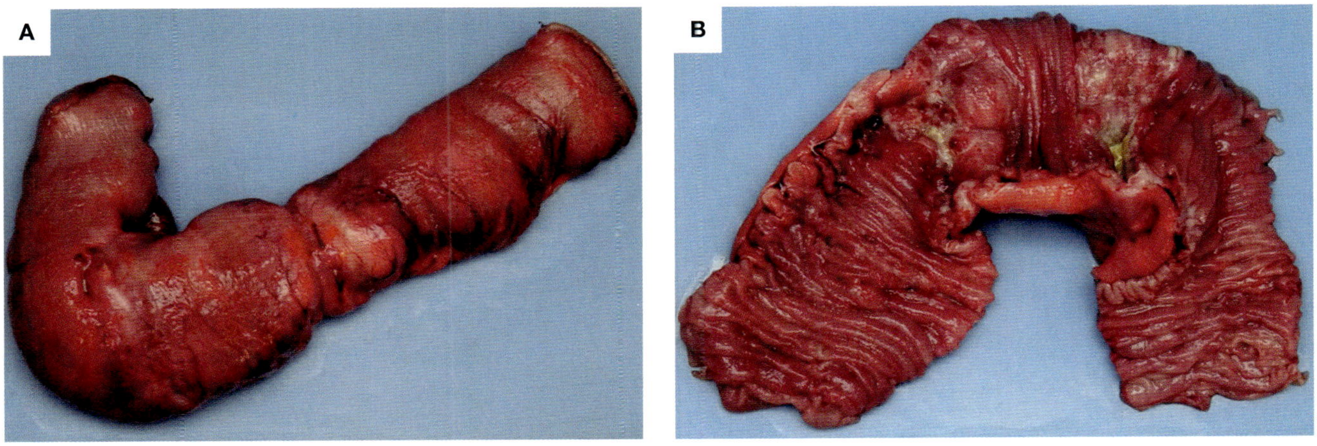

FIGURE 96.3 Macroscopic presentation of enteropathy-associated T-cell lymphoma. **A:** 71-year-old man known for celiac disease reported intermittent gastrointestinal discomfort, occasional blood in stool, recent weight loss, and presented with increased abdominal pain, due to jejunal intussusception with an obstructive syndrome. **A:** A segmental jejunal resection showed bowel dilatation above a stricture and peritonitis. **B:** The luminal side showed a large ulcerated tumor.

General Clinical Features

The median age at presentation is more than 60 years and most reports indicate a male predominance (whereas CD is more prevalent in females). EATL typically occurs in patients with a previous diagnosis of CD or refractory CD (RCD), but up to half of the patients have no previous history.[19] Homozygosity for HLA-DQ2 alleles and older age are risk factors.[20]

EATL most commonly affects the jejunum, less commonly other segments of the small bowel and rarely the large intestine or stomach; lesions are frequently multifocal. Occasionally, EATL may present outside the gastrointestinal tract (eg, skin, spleen, or CNS), especially cases evolving from RCD-II.[2,21] Abdominal pain, diarrhea, and weight loss are commonly reported, often culminating in an acute abdominal emergency due to intestinal perforation and peritonitis, or obstruction. The disease disseminates to abdominal lymph nodes, or extra-abdominal organs, including bone marrow, lung, or liver, and a large subset of the patients have stage IV disease at the time of diagnosis.[20]

Morphology

EATL manifests as ulcerative lesions with or without strictures, or tumor masses (Figure 96.3). Mesenteric infiltration and lymph node involvement is common (Figure 96.4).[19,20] The tumor can be monomorphic or pleomorphic, with a morphological spectrum ranging from medium to large cells with prominent nucleoli, to anaplastic-type or bizarre multinucleated cells (Figures 96.5-96.7).[20] Angiocentricity and angioinvasion, resulting in extensive necrosis, and a high mitotic rate are common. A polymorphic inflammatory infiltrate rich in eosinophils, plasma cells, and histiocytes is frequent, sometimes obscuring the lymphoma cells. Tumor cells may disseminate to distant intestinal epithelium or mucosa (Figure 96.8). Histopathologic features of CD may be seen distant from the tumor infiltration, but not always in the intestinal mucosa outside the tumor. Establishing a diagnosis of EATL in patients with no history of CD may be difficult if enteropathic features are not seen outside of the tumor. If the pathologic features are suggestive or consistent with EATL, especially if supported by CD30 and CD103 expression,[22] the diagnosis should be suggested, and serologic testing and HLA genotyping performed.

Immunophenotype

By IHC EATL cells are usually $CD2^+$, $CD3^+$, $CD4^-$, $CD5^-$, $CD7^+$, $CD8^-$, $CD30^+$, and $CD56^-$, and express cytotoxic markers (TIA1, garnzyme B and/or perforin) (Figures 96.8 and 96.9).[23] Up to 50% EATL presenting de novo with no prior diagnosis of celiac disease have been reported to express CD8.[20] Tumors displaying large cell morphology can resemble anaplastic large cell lymphoma.[23,24] EATL is negative for ALK and EBV. Most cases express CD103[22] and are negative for TCR expression (TCR-silent); approximately 25% are $TCR\alpha\beta^+$ or express cytoplasmic TCRβ chains, and TCRγ chain expression has been rarely described.[20,25-27] Overexpression of p53 is seen in many cases.

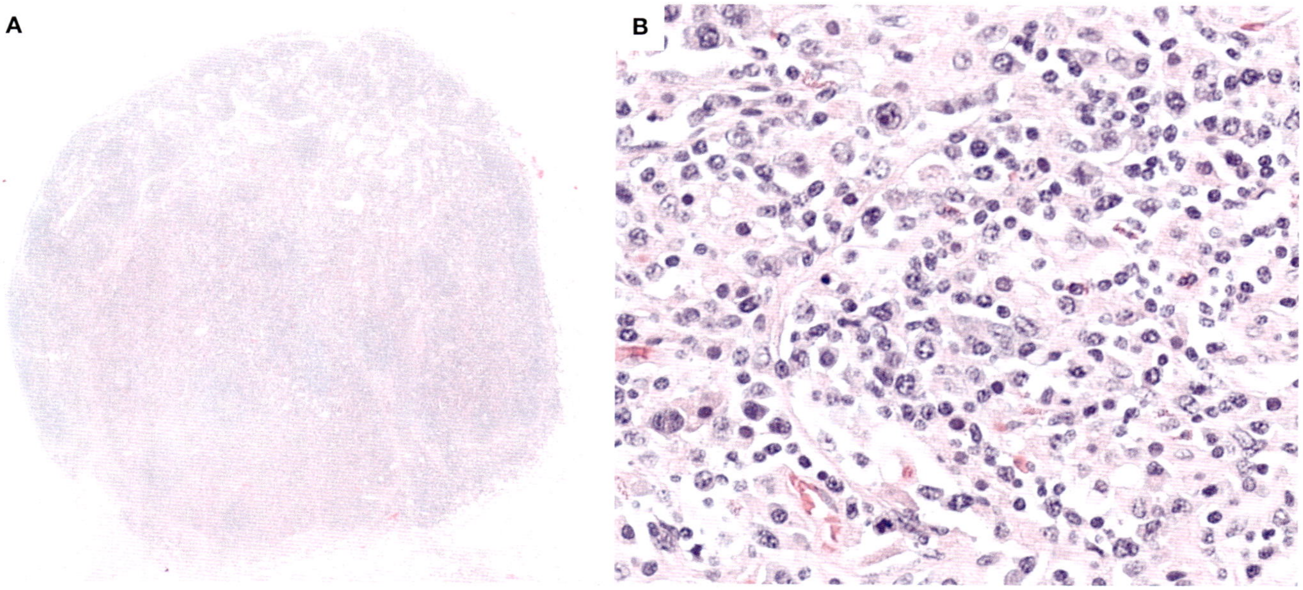

FIGURE 96.4 Lymph node involvement by enteropathy-associated T-cell lymphoma. **A:** This enlarged mesenteric lymph node shows partial involvement by enteropathy-associated T-cell lymphoma expanding the interfollicular and paracortical areas. **B:** The lymphoma infiltrate comprises pleomorphic neoplastic cells admixed with histiocytes, plasma cells, and small lymphocytes.

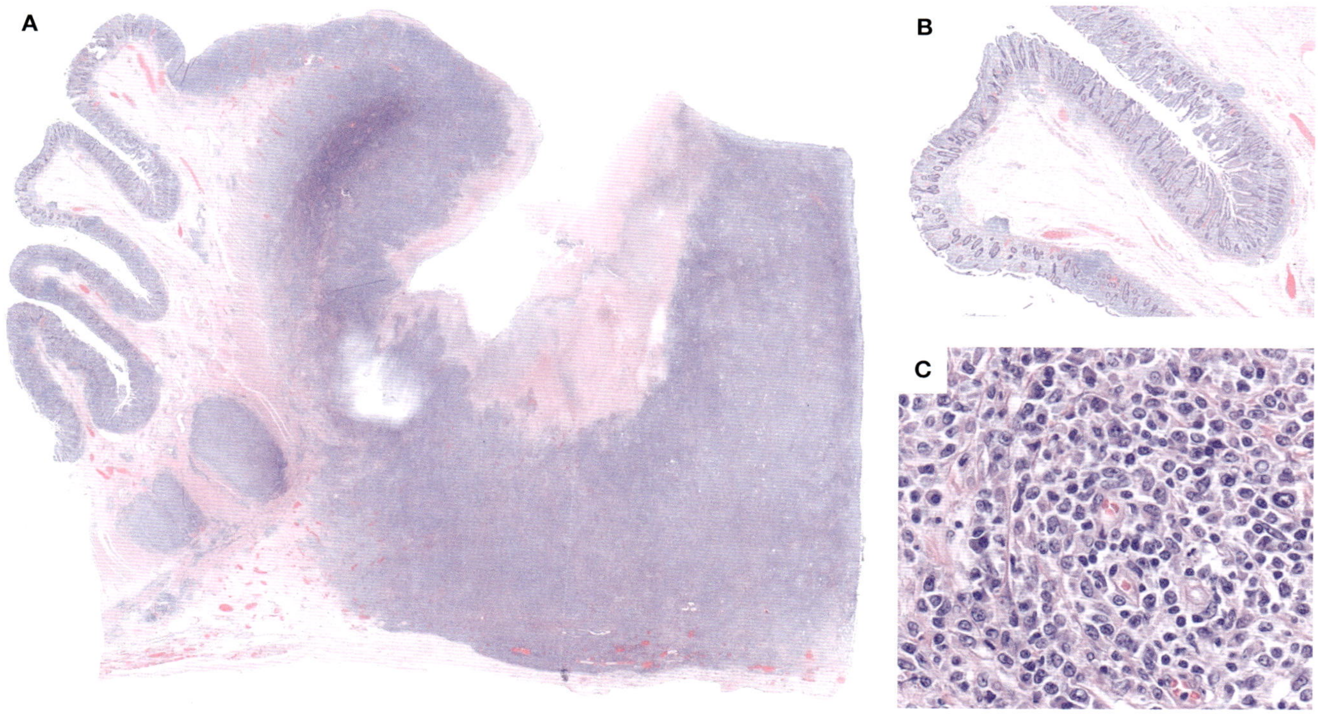

FIGURE 96.5 Histologic features of enteropathy-associated T-cell lymphoma. **A:** Low-power view showing an ulcerated transmural jejunal tumor, **(B)** arising in a background of flat mucosa. **C:** This tumor was composed of sheets of large atypical lymphoid cells.

Genetics

Clonal TCR gene rearrangements are detected in most cases. EATL demonstrates multiple chromosomal imbalances: 9q gains and nearly mutually exclusive losses at 16q12.1; gains of chromosome 7, 1q, and 5q; and losses involving 8p22 to 23.2, 16q21.1, 11q14.1-q14.2, and 9p21.2-p21.3.[28,29] The mutational landscape of EATL overlaps that of RCD-II and appears to be similar in cases developed from RCD-II and those occurring de novo.[15] Hence, EATL is characterized by highly recurrent activating

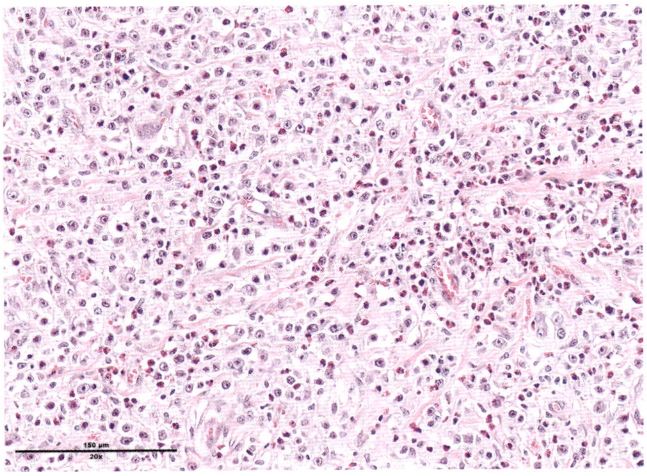

FIGURE 96.6 Histologic features of enteropathy-associated T-cell lymphoma. This tumor comprises pleomorphic medium to large atypical lymphoid cells admixed with inflammatory cells including many eosinophils.

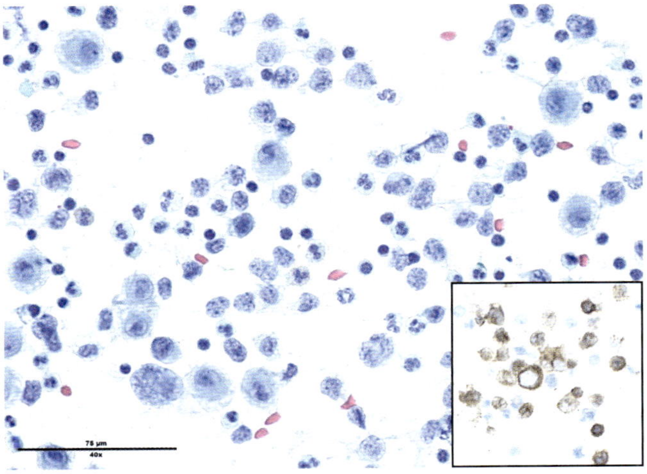

FIGURE 96.7 Cytology of enteropathy-associated T-cell lymphoma. This pericardial effusion represents relapsing enteropathy-associated T-cell lymphoma in a patient who initially presented with an intestinal mass. The smear (Papanicolaou staining) shows pleomorphic large atypical lymphoid cells with irregular nuclear contours, and scattered large cells. These cells are positive for CD3 (inset).

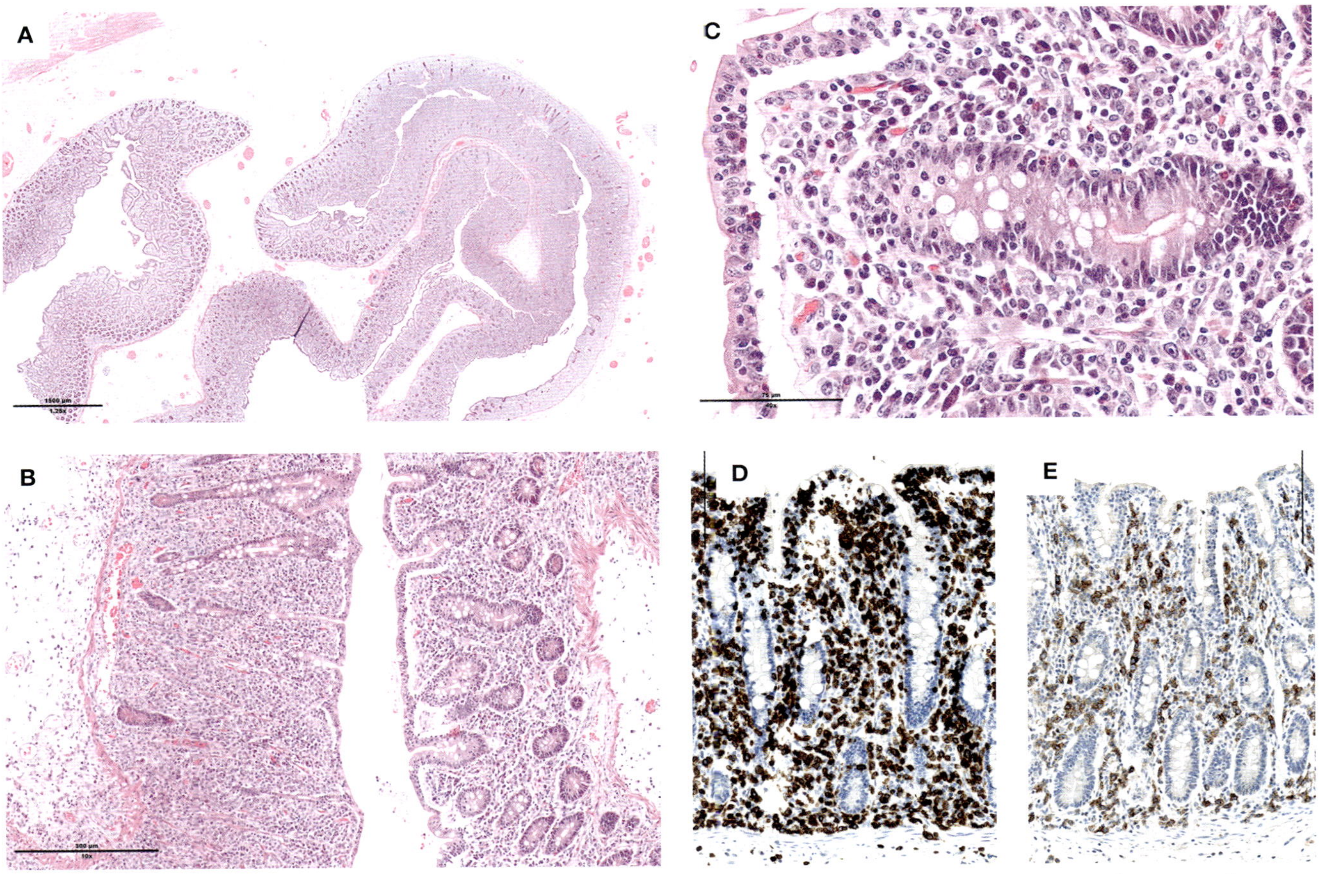

FIGURE 96.8 Intramucosal enteropathy-associated T-cell lymphoma. **A:** Low-power view of the jejunum at distance from a grossly invasive enteropathy-associated T-cell lymphoma, showing villous atrophy and variably increased mucosal cellularity. **B:** There is massive (left) or more subtle (right) infiltration of the lamina propria by large atypical lymphoid cells. **C:** Higher-power view demonstrating the atypical features of the lymphoid cells in the lamina propria. **D:** Intramucosal cells are positive for CD3. **E:** CD30 stains a subset of the cells in the lamina propria.

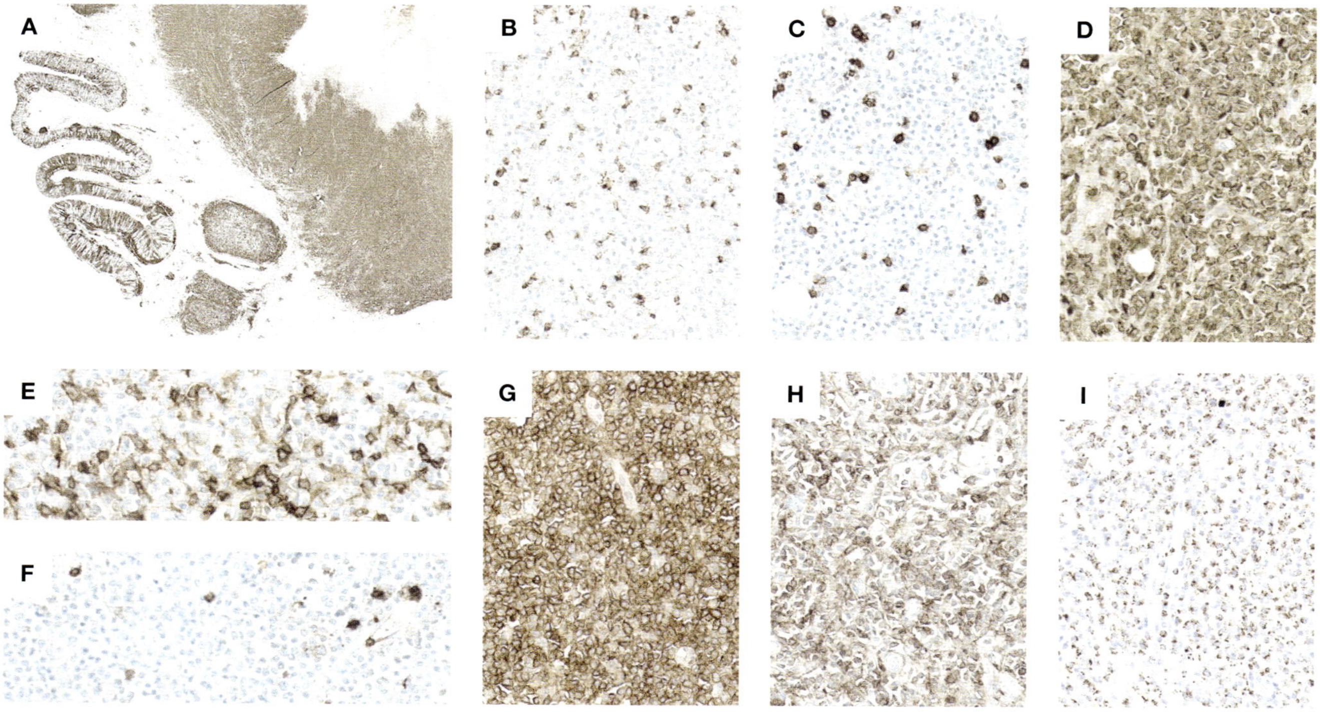

FIGURE 96.9 Immunophenotype of enteropathy-associated T-cell lymphoma. **A:** CD3 stains the infiltrating tumor and highlights increased intraepithelial lymphocytes in the adjacent atrophic mucosa. The neoplastic cells are **(B)** negative for CD2, **(C)** negative for CD5, **(D)** positive for CD7, **(E and F)** negative for CD4 and CD8, **(G)** positive for CD103, **(H)** positive for CD30, and **(I)** positive for TIA-1.

mutations in the JAK/STAT pathway, most commonly in *JAK1* (at the p.c1097 hotspot) and *STAT3,* and rarely in *JAK3, STAT5B, TYK2,* or *SOCS1*. Other mutations occur in NFκB genes (*TNFAIP3*), genes involved in epigenetic regulation, and gene expression (*KMT2D, BCOR, DDX3X*), mitogen-activated protein kinase pathway genes (*KRAS, NRAS, BRAF*), and *TP53*.[15,27-31]

Prognosis and Clinical Comment

The prognosis is poor, with a median survival of 7 months.[32] Patients presenting with de novo EATL have better outcomes than those with preceding RCD-II (50% vs 0%-8% 5-year overall survival).[20] A clinical prognostic model developed for EATL (EATL prognostic index [EPI]) stratifies the patients into three risk groups according to the presence of B symptoms and the international prognostic index.[33] The high mortality rate in patients with EATL probably reflects a combination of risk factors such as disease aggressivity, malnutrition deteriorating host performance and treatment tolerance, and a high risk of developing surgery-requiring complications, ultimately eroding the possibility of delivering an optimal treatment schedule.

Presently, CHOEP/CHOP-like chemotherapy with or without the addition of high-dose methotrexate and consolidated with autologous stem-cell transplantation (ASCT), is still considered the preferred treatment strategy. This approach has resulted in 5-year progression-free (PFS) and overall survival of 40% to 50% and 50% to 60%, respectively.[34,35] However, due to frequent patient frailty, these aggressive treatments are only feasible in approximately half of EATL patients. This may explain the real-world 5-year overall survival rates of 15% to 20% observed in unselected, population-based EATL cohorts.[36]

Encouraging preliminary results from the EATL-001 phase II study evaluating the use of brentuximab vedotin in combination with cyclophosphamide–doxorubicin–prednisolone (BV-CHP) in 14 patients with >10% CD30-positive tumor cells, followed by consolidative high-dose therapy (HDT)–autologous stem-cell transplantation in responding patients, have recently been presented.[37] BV-CHP was well tolerated, allowing most patients to undergo high-dose therapy–auto-hematopoietic stem cell transplantation translating into 2-year progression-free and overall survival rates of 63% and 68%, respectively.

TABLE 96.1 Comparative features and differential diagnosis of NK/T-cell neoplasms involving the gastrointestinal tract

	Refractory celiac disease type I (RCD-I)	Refractory celiac disease type II (RCD-II)	Enteropathy-associated T-cell lymphoma (EATL)	Monomorphic epitheliotropic intestinal T-cell lymphoma (MEITL)	Intestinal T-cell lymphoma, NOS (ITCL, NOS)	Indolent clonal T-cell LPD of the GI tract (iT-LPD-GI)	Indolent NK-cell LPD of the GI tract (iNK-LPD-GI)	Intestinal extranodal NK/T-cell lymphoma, nasal type (ENKTCL)
Clinical presenting features	Persistence or recurrence of diarrhea and villous atrophy in patients with CD under gluten-free diet	Same as RCD-I, but usually more severe	Abdominal symptoms, diarrhea Intestinal obstruction or perforation in patients with CD or RCD, or revealing CD	Intestinal obstruction or perforation	Abdominal symptoms or complication of a tumor mass	Abdominal symptoms	Incidental discovery or abdominal symptoms	Intestinal bleeding or perforation
Localization in the GI tract	Small intestine	Small intestine	Small intestine > colon, stomach, often multifocal	Small intestine > colon	Colon and small intestine > stomach	Small intestine and colon > upper GI tract	Stomach (lymphomatoid gastropathy) > small intestine and colon	Small intestine or colon
Macroscopy/ endoscopy	Mucosal atrophy	Mucosal atrophy and/or ulcerative lesions (ulcerative jejunitis)	Ulcerations, tumoral ulcer, or tumor mass	Tumor mass	Tumor mass	Mucosal ulcers or polyps, or normal-appearing mucosa	Erosions, ulcerations or normal-appearing mucosa	Tumor mass or tumoral ulcer, necrosis common
Histology	Villous atrophy, increased IEL	Villous atrophy, increased IEL, ulceration	Pleomorphic medium- to large-sized cells, angiocentrism, and angioinvasion common, inflammatory cells	Monomorphic, small- to medium-sized cells, or more atypical (40%), epitheliotropism	Pleomorphic mediujm-sized to large cells	Nondestructive infiltrate, small lymphocytes without significant atypia	Usually nondestructive infiltrate, medium to large atypical cells, no necrosis or IEL	Usually pleomorphic morphology, frequent angiocentrism, angioinvasion, and necrosis
Immunophenotype	$sCD3^{+}$ $cCD3^{+}$ $CD4^{-}$ $CD5^{-}$ $CD7^{+}$ $CD8^{+}$ $CD103^{+}$ $CD30^{-}$ CD56-	$sCD3^{-}$ $cCD3^{+}$ $CD4^{-}$ $CD5^{-}$ $CD7^{+}$ $CD8^{-}$ $CD103^{+}$ $CD30^{-}$ $CD56^{-}$	$cCD3^{+}$ $CD4^{-}$ $CD5^{-}$ $CD7^{+}$ $CD8^{-}$ $CD103^{+}$ $CD30^{+}$ CD56	$cCD3^{+}$ $CD4^{-}$ $CD5^{-}$ $CD7^{+}$ CD8 $CD103^{+}$ $CD30^{-}$ $CD56^{+}$	$cCD3^{+}$ $CD4^{\pm}$ $CD8^{-/+}$ $CD30^{-/+}$ $CD56^{-/+}$	cCD3+ $CD4^{+/-}$ $CD5^{+/-}$ $CD7^{+/-}$ $CD8^{-/+}$ $CD30^{-}$ $CD56^{-}$	$cCD3^{+}$ $CD4^{-}$ $CD5^{-}$ $CD7^{+}$ $CD8^{-}$ $CD30^{-}$ $CD56^{+}$	$cCD3^{+}$ $CD4^{-}$ $CD5^{-}$ $CD7^{+}$ $CD8^{-}$ $CD30^{\pm}$ $CD56^{+}$
TCR expression	positive, mostly TCR $\alpha\beta$	negative	negative > TCR$\alpha\beta$ > TCR$\gamma\delta$	TCR$\gamma\delta$ > TCR$\alpha\beta$ or TCR-negative > double positive	TCR-negative or TCR$\alpha\beta$ or TCR$\gamma\delta$	TCR$\alpha\beta$	TCR-negative	TCR-negative > TCR$\alpha\beta$ or TCR$\gamma\delta$

(Continued)

TABLE 96.1 *(Continued)*

	Refractory celiac disease type I (RCD-I)	Refractory celiac disease type II (RCD-II)	Enteropathy-associated T-cell lymphoma (EATL)	Monomorphic epitheliotropic intestinal T-cell lymphoma (MEITL)	Intestinal T-cell lymphoma, NOS (ITCL, NOS)	Indolent clonal T-cell LPD of the GI tract (iT-LPD-GI)	Indolent NK-cell LPD of the GI tract (iNK-LPD-GI)	Intestinal extranodal NK/T-cell lymphoma, nasal type (ENKTCL)
TCR gene rearrangement	polyclonal	monoclonal	monoclonal	monoclonal	monoclonal	monoclonal	polyclonal	Polyclonal or, less commonly, monoclonal
Cytotoxic markers	positive	positive	positive	positive	variable	variable	positive	positive
EBV	negative	negative	negative	negative	negative	negative	negative	positive
Genes altered	None	*JAK1*, *STAT3*, *TNFAIP3*, *KMT2D*, *TET2*	*JAK1 STAT3*, *TNFAIP3*, *KMT2D*, *TET2*	*SETD2*, *STAT5B*, *JAK3*, *GNAI2*, *TP53*, *MYC*	*JAK1*, *JAK3*, *SETD2*, *STAT5B*, *TET2*	JAK/STAT pathway genes, *STAT5::JAK2* fusion	*JAK3*, other miscellaneous genes	*BCOR*, *DDX3X*, *TP53*, *STAT3*
Differential diagnosis	CD and RCD-II	RCD-I and EATL	MEITL, ITCL,NOS, ALCL	EATL, ENKTCL, iNK-LPD-GI	MEITL, EATL, ATLL	Inflammatory bowel disease, EATL, ITCL, NOS	ENKTCL, MEITL	iNK-LPD-GI, MEITL, ITCL, NOS

ALCL, anaplastic large cell lymphoma; GI, gastrointestinal; LPD, lymphoproliferative disorder.

References

1. Rubio-Tapia A, Hill ID, Semrad C, et al. American College of Gastroenterology guidelines update: diagnosis and management of celiac disease. *Am J Gastroenterol.* 2023;118(1):59-76. doi:10.14309/ajg.0000000000002075
2. Malamut G, Cording S, Cerf-Bensussan N. Recent advances in celiac disease and refractory celiac disease. *F1000Res.* 2019;8doi:10.12688/f1000research.18701.1
3. Hujoel IA, Murray JA. Refractory celiac disease. *Curr Gastroenterol Rep.* 2020;22(4):18. doi:10.1007/s11894-020-0756-8
4. Malamut G, Afchain P, Verkarre V, et al. Presentation and long-term follow-up of refractory celiac disease: comparison of type I with type II. *Gastroenterology.* 2009;136(1):81-90. doi:10.1053/j.gastro.2008.09.069
5. Bisig B, Cairoli A, Gaide O, et al. Cutaneous presentation of enteropathy-associated T-cell lymphoma masquerading as a DUSP22-rearranged CD30+ lymphoproliferation. *Virchows Arch.* 2022;481(4):653-657. doi:10.1007/s00428-022-03309-4
6. Verbeek WH, Goerres MS, von Blomberg BM, et al. Flow cytometric determination of aberrant intra-epithelial lymphocytes predicts T-cell lymphoma development more accurately than T-cell clonality analysis in Refractory Celiac Disease. *Clin Immunol.* 2008;126(1):48-56.
7. Ettersperger J, Montcuquet N, Malamut G, et al. Interleukin-15-Dependent T-cell-like innate intraepithelial lymphocytes develop in the intestine and transform into lymphomas in celiac disease. *Immunity.* 2016;45(3):610-625. doi:10.1016/j.immuni.2016.07.018
8. Soderquist CR, Lewis SK, Gru AA, et al. Immunophenotypic spectrum and genomic landscape of refractory celiac disease type II. *Am J Surg Pathol.* 2021;45(7):905-916. doi:10.1097/PAS.0000000000001658
9. WHO Classification of Tumours of the Haematopoietic and Lymphoid Tissues Revised 4th ed. IARC; 2017.
10. Cheminant M, Bruneau J, Malamut G, et al. NKp46 is a diagnostic biomarker and may be a therapeutic target in gastrointestinal T-cell lymphoproliferative diseases: a CELAC study. *Gut.* 2019;68(8):1396-1405. doi:10.1136/gutjnl-2018-317371
11. Montes-Moreno S, King RL, Oschlies I, et al. Update on lymphoproliferative disorders of the gastrointestinal tract: disease spectrum from indolent lymphoproliferations to aggressive lymphomas. *Virchows Arch.* 2020;476(5):667-681. doi:10.1007/s00428-019-02704-8
12. Hussein S, Gindin T, Lagana SM, et al. Clonal T cell receptor gene rearrangements in coeliac disease: implications for diagnosing refractory coeliac disease. *J Clin Pathol.* 2018;71(9):825-831. doi:10.1136/jclinpath-2018-205023
13. Elli L, Leffler D, Cellier C, et al. Guidelines for best practices in monitoring established coeliac disease in adult patients. *Nat Rev Gastroenterol Hepatol.* 2024;21(3):198-215. doi:10.1038/s41575-023-00872-2
14. Verkarre V, Romana SP, Cellier C, et al. Recurrent partial trisomy 1q22-q44 in clonal intraepithelial lymphocytes in refractory celiac sprue. *Gastroenterology.* 2003;125(1):40-46.
15. Cording S, Lhermitte L, Malamut G, et al. Oncogenetic landscape of lymphomagenesis in coeliac disease. *Gut.* 2022;71(3):497-508. doi:10.1136/gutjnl-2020-322935
16. Green PHR, Paski S, Ko CW, Rubio-Tapia A. AGA clinical practice update on management of refractory celiac disease: expert review. *Gastroenterology.* 2022;163(5):1461-1469.
17. Delabie J, Holte H, Vose JM, et al Enteropathy-associated T-cell lymphoma: clinical and histological findings from the international peripheral T-cell lymphoma project. *Blood.* 2011;118(1):148-155. doi:10.1182/blood-2011-02-335216
18. Yoon SE, Song Y, Kim SJ, et al. Comprehensive analysis of peripheral T-cell and natural killer/T-cell lymphoma in Asian patients: a multinational, multicenter, prospective registry study in Asia. *Lancet Reg Health West Pac.* 2021;10:100126. doi:10.1016/j.lanwpc.2021.100126
19. Gale J, Simmonds PD, Mead GM, Sweetenham JW, Wright DH. Enteropathy-type intestinal T-cell lymphoma: clinical features and treatment of 31 patients in a single center. *J Clin Oncol.* 2000;18(4):795-803.
20. Malamut G, Chandesris O, Verkarre V, et al. Enteropathy associated T cell lymphoma in celiac disease: a large retrospective study. *Dig Liver Dis.* 2013;45(5):377-384. doi:10.1016/j.dld.2012.12.001
21. Verkarre V, Asnafi V, Lecomte T, et al. Refractory coeliac sprue is a diffuse gastrointestinal disease. *Gut.* 2003;52(2):205-211.
22. Morgan EA, Pihan GA, Said JW, et al. Profile of CD103 expression in T-cell neoplasms: immunoreactivity is not restricted to enteropathy-associated T-cell lymphoma. *Am J Surg Pathol.* 2014;38(11):1557-1570. doi:10.1097/PAS.0000000000000296
23. Sabattini E, Pizzi M, Tabanelli V, et al. CD30 expression in peripheral T-cell lymphomas. *Haematologica.* 2013;98(8):e81-e82. doi:10.3324/haematol.2013.084913
24. Bossard C, Dobay MP, Parrens M, et al. Immunohistochemistry as a valuable tool to assess CD30 expression in peripheral T-cell lymphomas: high correlation with mRNA levels. *Blood.* 2014;124(19):2983-2986. doi:10.1182/blood-2014-07-584953
25. Chott A, Haedicke W, Mosberger I, et al. Most CD56+ intestinal lymphomas are CD8+CD5-T-cell lymphomas of monomorphic small to medium size histology. *Am J Pathol.* 1998;153(5):1483-1490.
26. Murray A, Cuevas EC, Jones DB, Wright DH. Study of the immunohistochemistry and T cell clonality of enteropathy-associated T cell lymphoma. *Am J Pathol.* 1995;146(2):509-519.
27. Mutzbauer G, Maurus K, Buszello C, et al. SYK expression in monomorphic epitheliotropic intestinal T-cell lymphoma. *Mod Pathol.* 2018;31(3):505-516. doi:10.1038/modpathol.2017.145

28. Deleeuw RJ, Zettl A, Klinker E, et al. Whole-genome analysis and HLA genotyping of enteropathy-type T-cell lymphoma reveals 2 distinct lymphoma subtypes. *Gastroenterology*. 2007;132(5):1902-1911.
29. Moffitt AB, Ondrejka SL, McKinney M, et al. Enteropathy-associated T cell lymphoma subtypes are characterized by loss of function of SETD2. *J Exp Med*. 2017;214(5):1371-1386. doi:10.1084/jem.20160894
30. Nicolae A, Xi L, Pham TH, et al. Mutations in the JAK/STAT and RAS signaling pathways are common in intestinal T-cell lymphomas. *Leukemia*. 2016;30(11):2245-2247. doi:10.1038/leu.2016.178
31. Roberti A, Dobay MP, Bisig B, et al. Type II enteropathy-associated T-cell lymphoma features a unique genomic profile with highly recurrent SETD2 alterations. *Nat Commun*. 2016;7:12602. doi:10.1038/ncomms12602
32. Nijeboer P, de Baaij LR, Visser O, et al. Treatment response in enteropathy associated T-cell lymphoma; survival in a large multicenter cohort. *Am J Hematol*. 2015;90(6):493-498. doi:10.1002/ajh.23992
33. de Baaij LR, Berkhof J, van de Water JM, et al. A new and validated clinical prognostic model (EPI) for enteropathy-associated T-cell lymphoma. *Clin Cancer Res*. 2015;21(13):3013-3019. doi:10.1158/1078-0432.CCR-14-2195
34. Sieniawski M, Angamuthu N, Boyd K, et al. Evaluation of enteropathy-associated T-cell lymphoma comparing standard therapies with a novel regimen including autologous stem cell transplantation. *Blood*. 2010;115(18):3664-3670. doi:10.1182/blood-2009-07-231324
35. d'Amore F, Relander T, Lauritzsen GF, et al. Up-front autologous stem-cell transplantation in peripheral T-cell lymphoma: NLG-T-01. Clinical trial, phase II multicenter study research support, non-U.S. Gov't. *J Clin Oncol*. 2012;30(25):3093-3099. doi:10.1200/JCO.2011.40.2719
36. Awad AK, Awan RU, Awad AK, Nabeel A, Dar S, Abegunde AT. Patients with enteropathy-associated T-cell lymphoma in the United States from 2000 to 2018: SEER data-base analysis. *Cancer Treat Res Commun*. 2023;36:100745. doi:10.1016/j.ctarc.2023.100745
37. Sibon D, Khater S, Bruneau J, et al. The Eatl-001 trial: results of a phase 2 study of brentuximab vedotin and CHP followed by consolidation with high-dose therapy—autologous stem-cell transplantation (HDT-ASCT) in the frontline treatment of patients with enteropathy-associated T-cell lymphoma. *Blood*. 2021;138. doi:10.1182/blood-2021-153709

Chapter 97

Monomorphic Epitheliotropic Intestinal T-Cell Lymphoma

Luis Veloza, Laurence de Leval, Won Seog Kim, and Tadashi Yoshino

Definition

Monomorphic epitheliotropic intestinal T-cell lymphoma (MEITL) is a rare and aggressive primary intestinal T-cell lymphoma derived from intraepithelial T lymphocytes (IELs), typically characterized by a monomorphic cytomorphology (medium-sized cells with round nuclei and a rim of pale cytoplasm), prominent epitheliotropism, and no association with celiac disease (CD). The distinctive features from other gastrointestinal T- and NK-cell neoplasms is shown in Table 96.1.

Synonyms

Type II enteropathy-associated T-cell lymphoma (EATL), not recommended.

Epidemiology

MEITL occurs worldwide and is the most frequent primary intestinal T-cell lymphoma in Asia.[1-3] MEITL affects older adults with a median age in the sixth decade and has a male predominance in most series (M:F ratio being 2:1).[1,2,4-10]

General Clinical Features

In contrast to EATL, MEITL is not associated with CD. Most patients present with abdominal pain, gastrointestinal bleeding, weight loss, intestinal perforation, and/or obstruction, which is associated with an infiltrative tumor mass. MEITL usually develops in the small intestine, with rare concurrent colon and/or gastric disease. Regional lymph node involvement is occasionally seen (15%-44%), and dissemination to distant organs, mainly lung, liver, brain, and skin, occurs not uncommonly.[2,5-7,9,11] Bone marrow infiltration is rare.[2,5,7,9,10]

Morphology

MEITL presents as an ulcerated tumor mass with transmural invasion and frequent perforation (Figure 97.1). The typical histology, seen in the majority of cases consists of a monotonous proliferation of small to medium-sized tumor cells, with round nuclei, dispersed chromatin, inconspicuous nucleoli, ample pale cytoplasm, and absence of necrosis (Figure 97.2). Less commonly, the neoplastic cells may be larger or even pleomorphic, with vesicular chromatin or prominent nucleoli, or the tumors may present high-grade morphological features, such as starry-sky appearance, prominent apoptosis, angiotropism/angioinvasion, and necrosis away from the ulcerated surface[6,10] (Figure 97.2). In contrast to EATL, a prominent inflammatory component is not usually observed.[6] In the peripheral zone, tumor cells extend superficially to the adjacent mucosa, often showing prominent epitheliotropism and resulting in distortion, destruction, or expansion of villi[6,9] (Figure 97.2). The non-involved intestinal mucosa features normal architecture without villous atrophy but may present an increased number of morphologically bland IELs.[9]

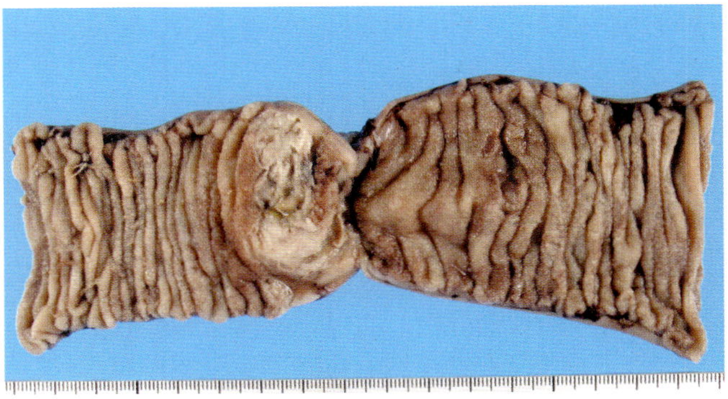

FIGURE 97.1 Monomorphic epitheliotropic intestinal T-cell lymphoma. Small intestinal resection specimen showing an ulcerated tumor mass involving the whole circumference of the intestinal wall.

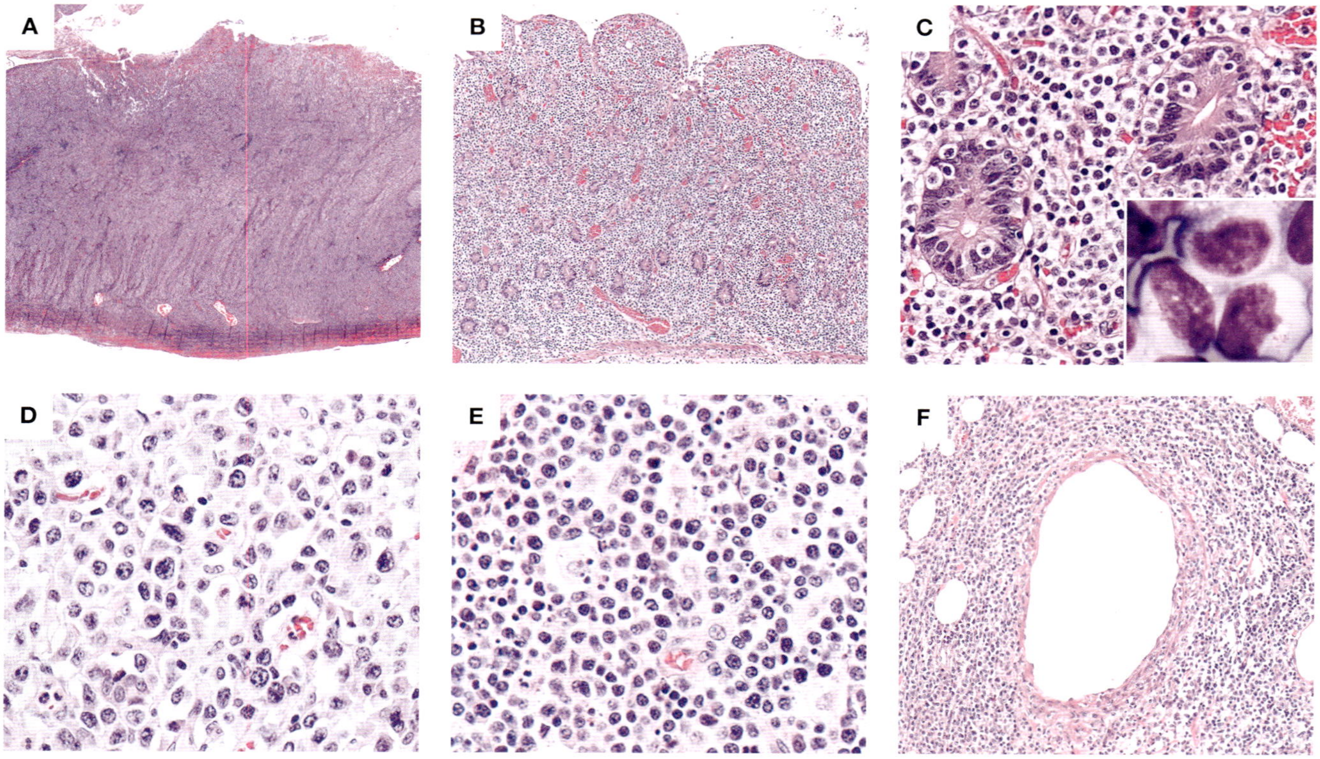

FIGURE 97.2 Monomorphic epitheliotropic intestinal T-cell lymphoma. The lymphoma shows transmural infiltration of the small intestinal wall with superficial ulceration (**A**). Lateral tumor spread (peripheral zone) is associated with shortening and widening of the villi (**B**). Tumor cells are monomorphic medium-sized with round nuclei, dispersed chromatin, inconspicuous nucleoli, and ample pale cytoplasm showing prominent epitheliotropism into the basal membrane side of the intestinal crypt epithelium. Inset is a cytology smear showing medium-sized lymphocytes with mild pleomorphism, inconspicuous nucleoli, and ample pale cytoplasm containing azurophilic granules (Giemsa) (**C**). In this case, medium-sized cells with irregular nuclei and open chromatin with inconspicuous nucleoli are intermingled with occasional large cells with vesicular chromatin and distinct nucleoli (**D**). This case is composed of small to medium-sized pleomorphic atypical cells with frequent apoptotic bodies some of which are phagocytized by histiocytes imparting a starry-sky appearance (**E**). Angiotropism and angioinvasion are evident in this case (**F**).

Immunophenotype

MEITL cells usually express CD3 and CD7 with double positivity for CD8 (56%-90%) and CD56 (73%-94%) in most cases, variably express CD2, and are negative for CD5, CD4, and CD30 (Figures 97.3 and 97.4). Most cases show an activated cytotoxic immunophenotype, with almost constant TIA1 expression and more variable positivity for granzyme B and perforin[1,2,4-11] (Figure 97.4). Aberrant expression of B-cell markers (CD20 or less commonly CD79a) has been reported in up to one-fourth of the cases (11%-24%)[6,7,9] (Figure 97.3). TCR is usually expressed, more commonly TCRγδ (23%-77%) than TCRαβ (10%-57%), while fewer cases are TCR silent (5%-40%) or more rarely coexpress both TCR isoforms (3%-16%)[5-11] (Figure 97.4). In contrast to EATL, MEITL expresses MATK and SYK.[7,11] MYC is variably expressed, in around one-third of the cases, partly reflecting *MYC* gene locus alterations.[6] Epstein-Barr virus is consistently absent in the neoplastic cells.[6,7,9]

Genetics

There is a clonal TCR gene rearrangement in most cases, even in the TCR-silent cases.[2,7] Apart from *MYC* alterations (gains and rarely translocations) reported in about 20% to 70% of the cases,[4,6-8,12] MEITL also shows gains at 9q34.3, 1q32.3, 4p15.1, 5q34, 7q34, 8p11.23, 9q22.31, 9q33.2, and 12p13.31 and losses of 7p14.1 and 16q12.1. Unlike in EATL, gains at 1q32.2-q41 and 5q34-q35.5 are uncommon.[4,8,13] The vast majority of MEITL (>90%) harbor disruptive mutations and/or deletions of the *SETD2* gene, which result in reduced or absent trimethylation of H3K36me3[5,6,10,12] (Figure 97.5). Many cases also present mutations in the JAK-STAT pathway genes, most commonly gain-of-function mutations in *STAT5B*

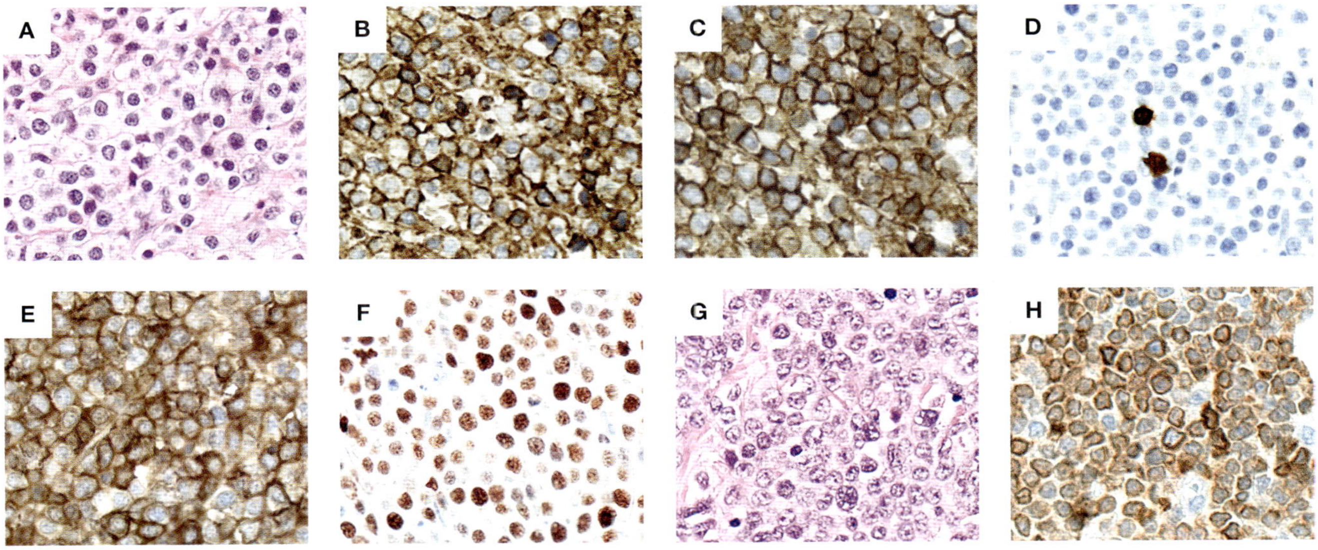

FIGURE 97.3 Monomorphic epitheliotropic intestinal T-cell lymphoma. **A-F:** This case showing typical morphology **(A)** is positive for CD8 **(B)** and CD56 **(C)** and is negative for CD5 **(D)**. CD103 is strongly expressed **(E)**, and intense nuclear positivity for p53 **(F)** is associated with the presence of a *TP53* mutation. In another case with atypical morphology including dispersed large cells with vesicular chromatin and distinct nucleoli **(G)** a B-cell marker, CD79a, is coexpressed **(H)**.

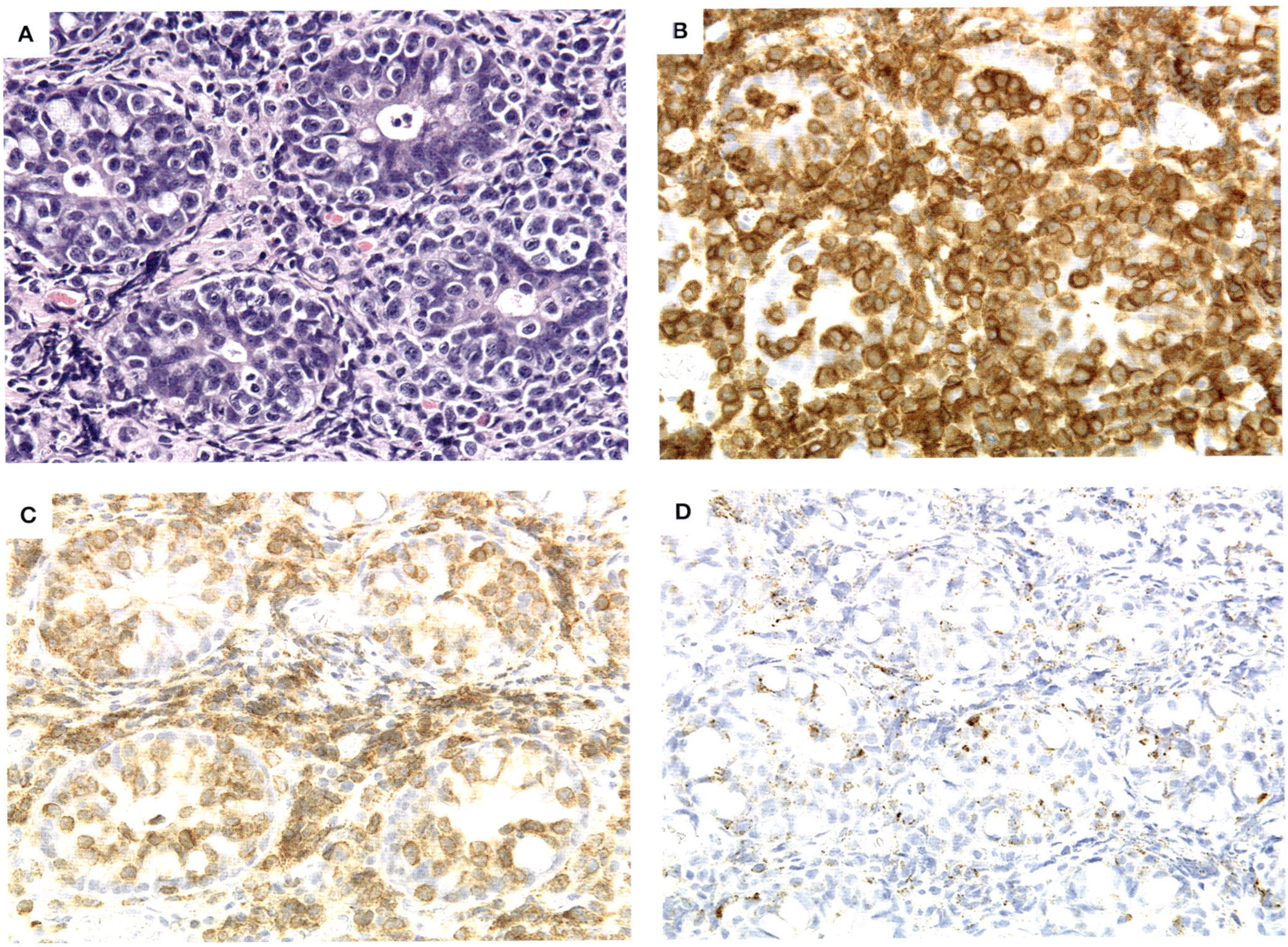

FIGURE 97.4 Monomorphic epitheliotropic intestinal T-cell lymphoma. Epitheliotropism into colonic crypt epithelium **(A)** is highlighted by immunostainings for CD3 **(B)**, TCRγ **(C)**, and TIA1 **(D)**.

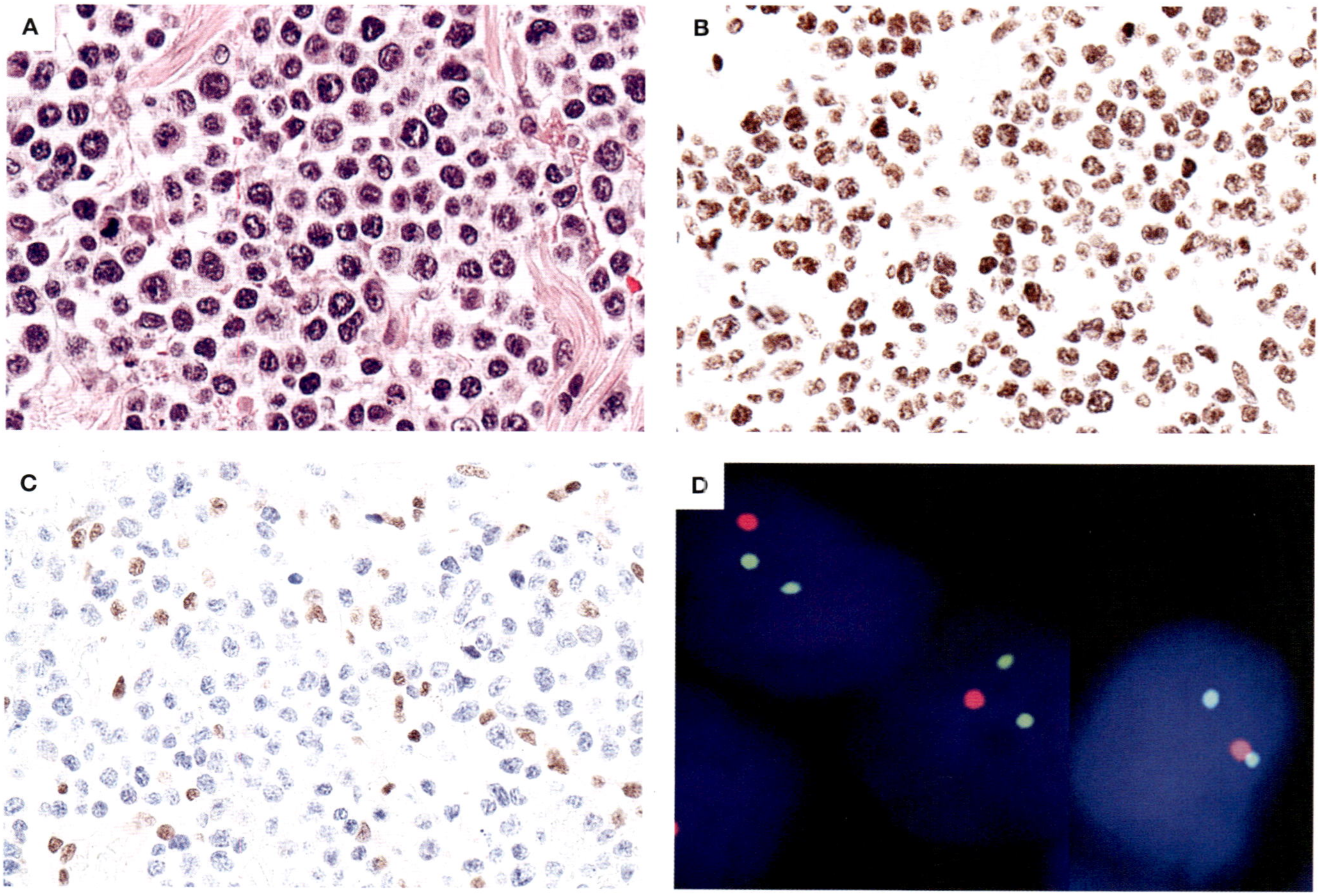

FIGURE 97.5 Monomorphic epitheliotropic intestinal T-cell lymphoma. In this case with typical morphology (**A**), lymphoma cells show strong nuclear positivity for H3K36me2 (**B**) and negativity for H3K36me3 (internal controls being positive) (**C**). Fluorescence in situ hybridization analysis with *SETD2* probes shows 1 single red (*SETD2*) and two green (control) signals per nucleus, demonstrating the deletion of one *SETD2* allele (**D**).

(>60%) and/or *JAK3* (35%-50%).[6,10,12,13] Mutually exclusive alterations of MAPK pathway genes (*BRAF, KRAS, NRAS*) are identified in about 30% to 46% of tumors.[10,12] *TP53* mutations are detected in one-third of the cases. Mutations of *GNAI2* have been reported in 9% to 24% of the tumors.[6,10,12,13] Mutations in epigenetic regulators other than *SETD2* (*CREBBP* histone acetyltransferase, *EP300*, *EZH2*, and *ARID1*) are infrequent.[6,12]

Prognosis and Clinical Comment

Prognosis is dismal with a median overall survival of 7 to 11 months.[2,5-7,10] In a large series of MEITL from Western Europe, MYC expression, mutations in *TP53* or *STAT5B*, and poor performance status correlated with shorter survival, while aberrant B-cell marker expression was associated with better outcome at multivariate analysis.[6]

References

1. Delabie J, Holte H, Vose JM, et al. Enteropathy-associated T-cell lymphoma: clinical and histological findings from the international peripheral T-cell lymphoma project. *Blood.* 2011;118(1):148-155.
2. Tse E, Gill H, Loong F, et al. Type II enteropathy-associated T-cell lymphoma: a multicenter analysis from the Asia lymphoma study Group. *Am J Hematol.* 2012;87(7):663-668.
3. Yoon SE, Song Y, Kim SJ, et al. Comprehensive analysis of peripheral T-cell and natural killer/T-cell lymphoma in Asian patients: a multinational, multicenter, prospective registry study in Asia. *Lancet Reg Health West Pac.* 2021;10:100126.
4. Deleeuw RJ, Zettl A, Klinker E, et al. Whole-genome analysis and HLA genotyping of enteropathy-type T-cell lymphoma reveals 2 distinct lymphoma subtypes. *Gastroenterology.* 2007;132(5):1902-1911.

5. Moffitt AB, Ondrejka SL, McKinney M, et al. Enteropathy-associated T cell lymphoma subtypes are characterized by loss of function of SETD2. *J Exp Med.* 2017;214(5):1371-1386.
6. Veloza L, Cavalieri D, Missiaglia E, et al. Monomorphic epitheliotropic intestinal T-cell lymphoma comprises morphologic and genomic heterogeneity impacting outcome. *Haematologica.* 2023;108(1):181-195.
7. Tan SY, Chuang SS, Tang T, et al. Type II EATL (epitheliotropic intestinal T-cell lymphoma): a neoplasm of intra-epithelial T-cells with predominant CD8αα phenotype. *Leukemia.* 2013;27(8):1688-1696.
8. Tomita S, Kikuti YY, Carreras J, et al. Genomic and immunohistochemical profiles of enteropathy-associated T-cell lymphoma in Japan. *Mod Pathol.* 2015;28(10): 1286-1296.
9. Chan JK, Chan AC, Cheuk W, et al. Type II enteropathy-associated T-cell lymphoma: a distinct aggressive lymphoma with frequent γδ T-cell receptor expression. *Am J Surg Pathol.* 2011;35(10):1557-1569.
10. Hang JF, Yuan CT, Chang KC, et al. Targeted next-generation sequencing reveals a wide morphologic and immunophenotypic spectrum of monomorphic epitheliotropic intestinal T-cell lymphoma. *Am J Surg Pathol.* 2022;46(9):1207-1218.
11. Mutzbauer G, Maurus K, Buszello C, et al. SYK expression in monomorphic epitheliotropic intestinal T-cell lymphoma. *Mod Pathol.* 2018;31(3):505-516.
12. Roberti A, Dobay MP, Bisig B, et al. Type II enteropathy-associated T-cell lymphoma features a unique genomic profile with highly recurrent SETD2 alterations. *Nat Commun.* 2016;7:12602.
13. Nairismägi ML, Tan J, Lim JQ, et al. JAK-STAT and G-protein-coupled receptor signaling pathways are frequently altered in epitheliotropic intestinal T-cell lymphoma. *Leukemia.* 2016;30(6):1311-1319.

Chapter 98

Intestinal T-Cell Lymphoma, Not Otherwise Specified and Indolent Lymphoproliferative Disorders of the Gastrointestinal Tract

Laurence de Leval, Anamarija M. Perry, Luis Veloza, Andrew L. Feldman, Steven M. Horwitz, Won Seog Kim, and Tadashi Yoshino

INTESTINAL T-CELL LYMPHOMA, NOT OTHERWISE SPECIFIED

Definition

Intestinal T-cell lymphoma, not otherwise specified (ITCL, NOS) is a diagnosis of exclusion reserved for aggressive primary gastrointestinal lymphomas that are not classified as either enteropathy-associated T-cell lymphoma (EATL) or monomorphic epitheliotropic intestinal T-cell lymphoma (MEITL) by the current criteria, after having excluded secondary intestinal involvement by other T/NK-cell lymphoma entities, such as extranodal NK/T-cell lymphoma, nasal type, anaplastic large cell lymphoma, and HTLV1-associated adult T-cell lymphoma/leukemia. This category can also be used for intestinal T-cell lymphomas that cannot be properly classified due to insufficient quality of the biopsy materials. The distinctive features from other gastrointestinal T- and NK-cell neoplasms are shown in Table 96.1.

Synonyms

None.

Epidemiology

Data on ITCL, NOS are scarce, because this disease entity was introduced for the first time in the 2017 revised fourth edition of the World Health Organization (WHO) classification. ITCL, NOS affects individuals worldwide and is overall much rarer than EATL and MEITL, accounting likely for 10% to 20% of all primary intestinal T-cell lymphomas.[1-3] ITCL, NOS occurs in older adults with a median age of 49 to 69 years and a male predominance (M:F ratio approximately 2:1).[1,2,4-9]

General Clinical Features

The small intestine and the colon are the most frequently involved organs, with common multifocal involvement.[1,4-6] Malabsorption has rarely been reported. Patients present frequently with B symptoms, fever, pain, or bleeding. Intestinal perforation and/or obstruction occur in less than 40% of patients, and about half present with stage III/IV disease.[1,4-6,8,9]

Morphology

ITCL, NOS usually presents as an ulcerated or exophytic luminal mass with transmural infiltration. Most cases are composed of pleomorphic medium-sized to large cells[4-6,9] (Figure 98.1). Few cases comprise monomorphic small to medium-sized cells resembling MEITL (Figure 98.1).[5,9] Epitheliotropism is not typically seen in cases involving the intestine[5,10] but has been described occasionally in gastric cases.[11] Enteropathy-related changes in the adjacent noninvolved mucosa are not described.[1,6,8]

Immunophenotype

ITCL, NOS is $CD3^+$, usually $CD7^+$, and variably positive for CD2 and CD5 (14%-56%), whereas CD20 is negative. Two-thirds of cases are $CD4^-/CD8^-$, and few are positive for either CD4 or CD8. A minority of cases are $CD56^+$. Most cases show an activated cytotoxic immunophenotype[1,4,5,8,9] and are TCR-silent or positive for TCR βF1 (20%-46%).[1,2,4,8,10] One-third of cases express CD30[1,4,8] (Figure 98.2). Although there have been occasional reports of EBV-positive ITCL, NOS, these cases should be better designed as EBV-positive NK/T-cell lymphoma nasal type.[8]

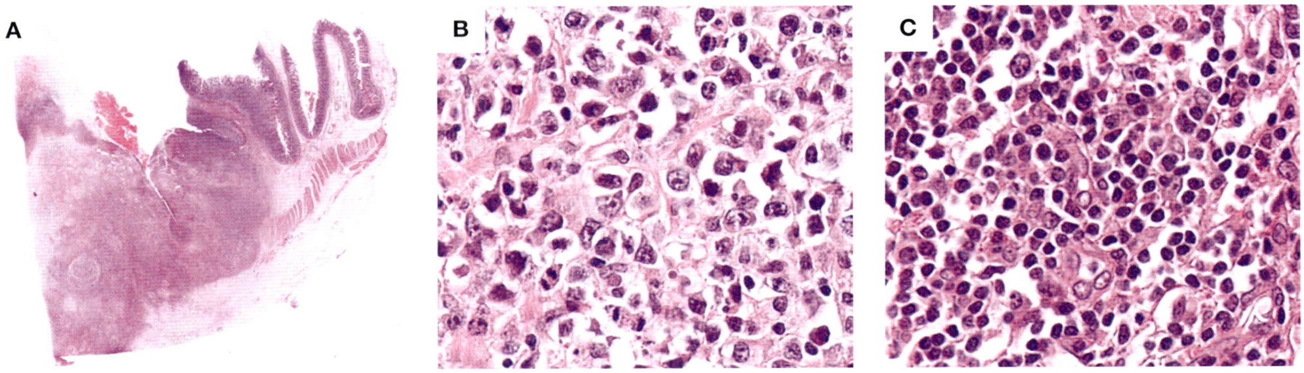

FIGURE 98.1 Intestinal T-cell lymphoma, not otherwise specified. Small intestinal resection specimen showing an ulcerated tumor mass with transmural infiltration and extensive necrosis (**A**). This case is composed of pleomorphic medium-sized and large cells with irregular nuclei, vesicular chromatin, prominent nucleoli, and frequent mitosis (**B**). Another case is composed predominantly of small monomorphic cells with scant amount of cytoplasm, intermingled with rare larger cells (**C**).

Genetics

Mutations in genes overlapping with those altered in MEITL and EATL have been reported in ITCL, NOS (*JAK3, JAK1, STAT5B, TET2, DNMT3A, SETD2* and *KRAS*).[2,4,7]

Prognosis and Clinical Comment

The median overall survival of patients with ITCL, NOS is 4 to 34 months.[1,5,6] Advanced clinical stage and large-cell morphology have been associated with worse outcome.[11]

INDOLENT CLONAL T-CELL LYMPHOPROLIFERATIVE DISORDER OF THE GASTROINTESTINAL TRACT

Definition

Indolent clonal T-cell lymphoproliferative disorder (LPD) of the gastrointestinal tract (GIT) is a T-cell LPD that involves the mucosa of the GIT, most commonly the small intestine and colon, and is characterized by a chronic, indolent, relapsing course, with a low risk of transformation to aggressive T-cell lymphoma. This disease was first included in the 2017 revision of the

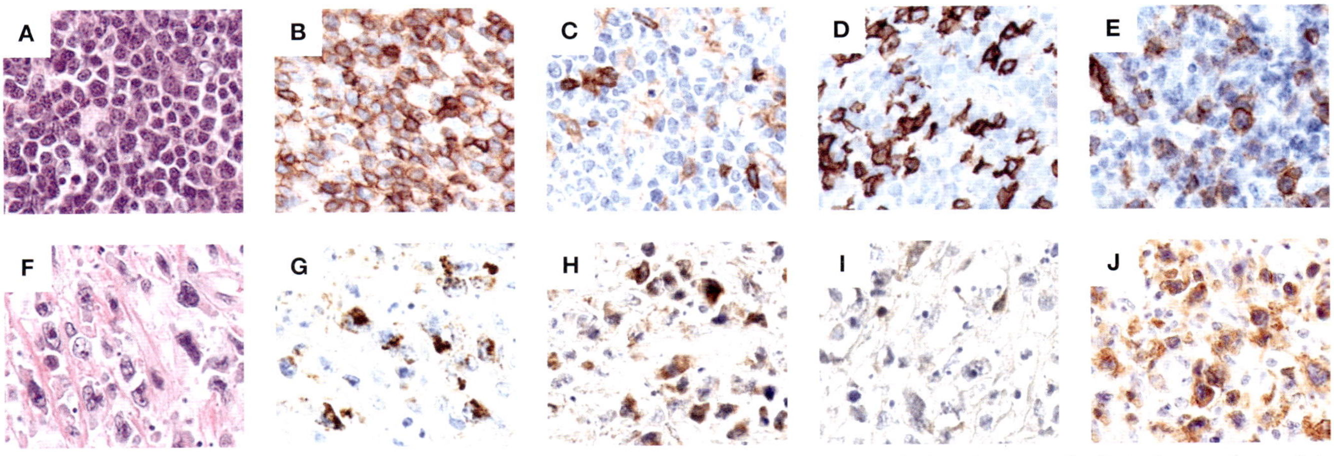

FIGURE 98.2 Intestinal T-cell lymphoma, not otherwise specified. This case (**A-E**) is composed of medium-sized cells with irregular nuclei, dispersed chromatin, and inconspicuous nucleoli, with occasional histiocytes and apoptotic bodies (**A**). Tumor cells are CD3$^+$ (**B**), CD4$^-$ (**C**), CD8$^-$ (**D**), and partially positive for CD5 (**E**). In the other case (**F-J**), tumor cells are large-sized, pleomorphic with open chromatin and prominent nucleoli (**F**). Lymphoma cells show a cytotoxic immunophenotype, with TIA1 expression (**G**). They are TCRβ$^+$ (**H**), TCRγ$^-$ (**I**), and CD30$^+$ (**J**).

WHO classification as a provisional entity and has been upgraded to a definitive entity in the current International Consensus Classification. The term "clonal" was added to the name to emphasize that documentation of clonality is essential to establish the diagnosis. The distinctive features from other gastrointestinal T- and NK-cell neoplasms are shown in Table 96.1.

Synonyms

Indolent T-cell lymphoproliferative disorder of the gastrointestinal tract, indolent T-cell lymphoma of the gastrointestinal tract (not recommended).

Epidemiology

The disease usually occurs in adults, with a median age of diagnosis in the fifth and sixth decades of life, and is very rarely reported in children. Men are more commonly affected than women, with a male-to-female ratio of 2 to 3:1.[12-14]

General Clinical Features

This disorder can occur in any site of the GIT; however, the most commonly involved sites are small intestine and colon. Involvement of multiple sites is frequently seen. The endoscopic appearance of the lesions is variable and includes polyps, mucosal nodularity, erosions, ulcers, and mucosal erythema or friability. Disease can spread beyond the GIT and involve lymph nodes (frequently mesenteric), bone marrow, and peripheral blood. The most common presenting symptoms are diarrhea, abdominal pain, bloating, and vomiting. Other symptoms and signs include rectal bleeding, weight loss, food intolerance, electrolyte imbalances, and malabsorption. Some patients have a previous history of inflammatory bowel disease, autoimmune disorder, or infection.[12,13,15]

Morphology

The lamina propria is involved by a diffuse, nondestructive infiltrate of small, monomorphic lymphocytes, which distorts and displaces the mucosal glands and occasionally involves the muscularis mucosae or submucosa (Figure 98.3A). Intestinal crypts are usually hyperplastic but typically without villous atrophy, and epitheliotropism is seen only occasionally. Thus, the features are clearly distinct from celiac disease. The lymphoid cells are round to slightly irregular with inconspicuous nucleoli (Figure 98.3B) and occasionally admixed with eosinophils. Rarely, scattered granulomas or lymphoid follicles can be seen. Vascular invasion and necrosis are absent.[12,13,15,16]

Immunophenotype

Indolent clonal T-LPD consists of mature TCRβF1$^+$ CD3$^+$ T cells (Figure 98.4). CD4$^+$ cases are slightly more common than CD8$^+$ ones, and rare cases are either double positive (CD4$^+$/CD8$^+$) or double negative (CD4$^-$/CD8$^-$). CD2 and CD5 are usually positive, while CD7 expression is variable, CD7 being the most frequently lost or downregulated marker. T-follicular helper markers are not expressed, and some cases show expression of t-bet and/or GATA-3. CD8$^+$ cases express TIA1, while granzyme B is usually negative. CD56 and in situ hybridization for EBV are negative. The proliferation index (Ki67) is very low (<10%).[12-14,16-18]

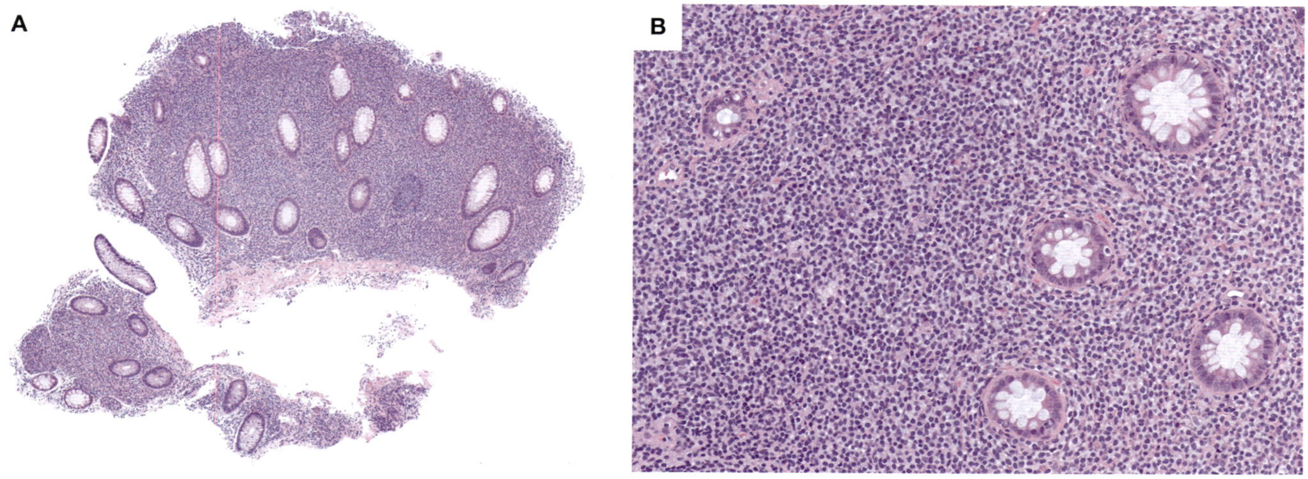

FIGURE 98.3 Indolent clonal T-cell lymphoproliferative disorder of the gastrointestinal tract. **A:** Colonic mucosa involved by diffuse, nondestructive lymphoid infiltrate that distorts and displaces the mucosal glands. **B:** The lymphoid infiltrate is monomorphic, composed of small lymphoid cells with round to slightly irregular nuclei and with inconspicuous nucleoli.

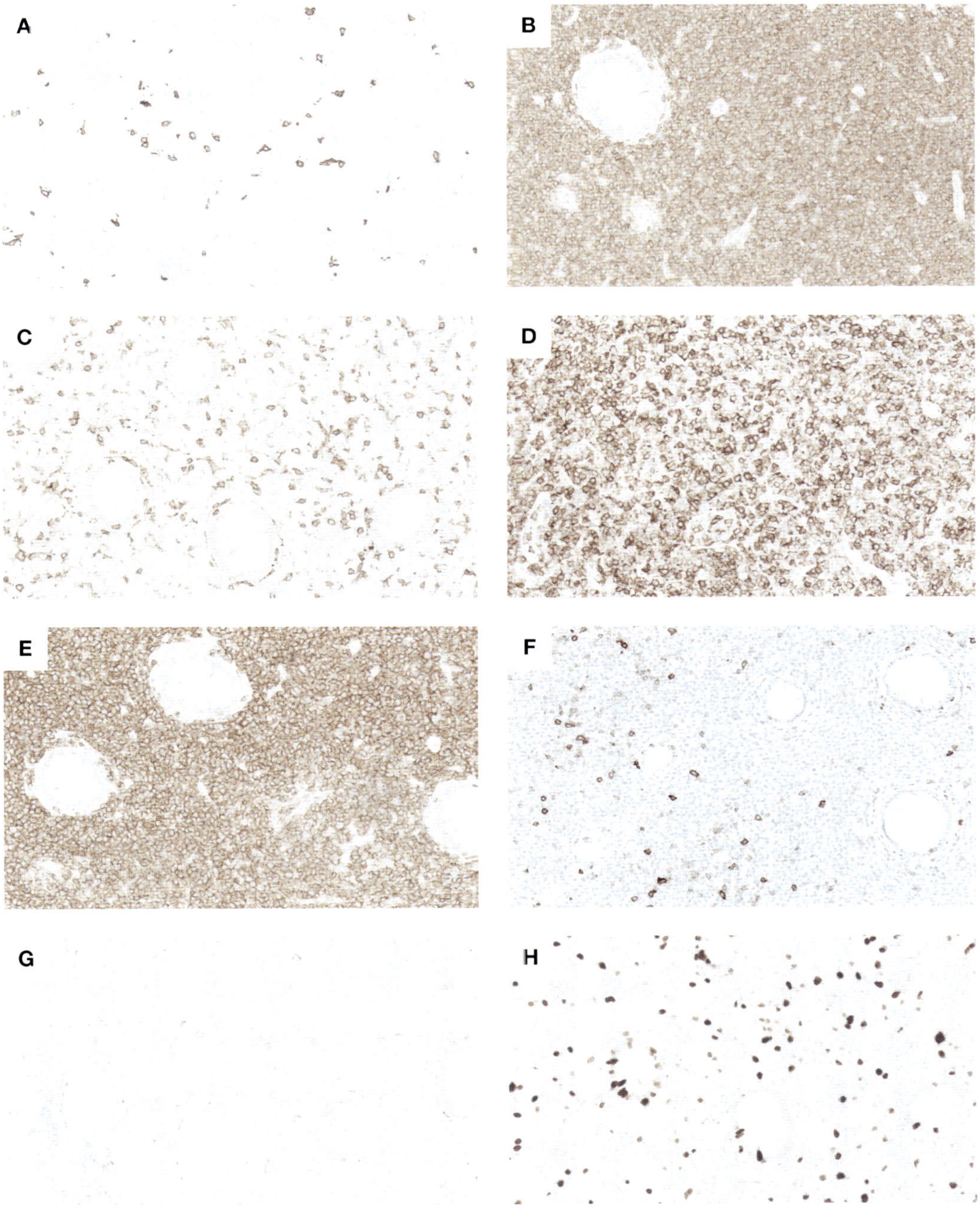

FIGURE 98.4 Immunophenotype of indolent clonal T-cell lymphoproliferative disorder of the gastrointestinal tract. The cells are positive for CD3 (**B**), CD8 (**D**), and CD5 (**E**) and are negative for CD4 (**C**), CD7 (**F**), and CD56 (**G**). CD20 (**A**) shows scattered small B cells in the background. Proliferative index (Ki67; **H**) is very low.

Genetics

All cases have clonal T-cell receptor gene rearrangements. Genetic data on this entity are relatively scarce and suggestive of a different pathogenesis between $CD4^+$ and $CD8^+$ cases. A subset of $CD4^+$ cases show a recurrent *STAT3::JAK2* fusion and phosphorylation of STAT5.[14,16,19] Furthermore, some CD4+ cases harbor other recurrent alterations of the JAK-STAT pathway, including *STAT3* mutations and *SOCS1* deletion, as well as concomitant mutations in epigenetic modifier genes (*TET2, DNMT3A, KMT2D*). In contrast, some $CD8^+$ cases harbor structural alterations in the *IL2* gene.[16,18]

Prognosis and Clinical Comment

Indolent clonal T-cell LPD of the GIT shows a protracted clinical course with frequent relapses. Reported patients who were treated with chemotherapy (various regimens) showed limited or no response, therefore chemotherapy is not recommended. There are anecdotal reports of responses to various mild and immunomodulatory agents.[20] However, the clinical course is chronic and many patients are alive with persistent disease more than 10 years after the initial diagnosis.[12,13,16,17] Occasional cases of dissemination outside of the GIT and progression/transformation to a more aggressive T-cell lymphoma have been reported, with median time to transformation of >10 years.[14-16,18,20]

INDOLENT NATURAL KILLER-CELL LYMPHOPROLIFERATIVE DISORDER OF THE GASTROINTESTINAL TRACT

Definition

Indolent NK-cell LPD of the GIT is a rare LPD of mature NK cells that involves the mucosa of the GIT, most commonly stomach and duodenum, and is not associated with EBV infection. This is a newly created entity in the International Consensus Classification, formerly described as "lymphomatoid gastropathy" or "NK-cell enteropathy." The terminology was chosen to mirror that of similar disorders of T-cell origin (indolent clonal T-cell LPD of the GIT see above). The distinctive features from other gastrointestinal T- and NK-cell neoplasms are shown in Table 96.1.

Synonyms

Lymphomatoid gastropathy; NK-cell enteropathy (not recommended).

Epidemiology

The disease usually occurs in adults with a median age of diagnosis in the sixth decade and shows a slight female predominance.[21-23] Rare cases have been reported in young adults and children.

General Clinical Features

The disease, initially described in Asia as "lymphomatoid gastropathy," often involves the upper GIT, in particular the stomach. It can also manifest as lesions in the small intestine (most commonly duodenum), or colon, and some patients show involvement of multiple sites including upper and lower GIT. Rarely, disease has been reported to involve the gallbladder, abdominal lymph nodes, the nasopharynx, or the lower genital tract.[24,25] Endoscopically, the lesions are solitary or often multiple and have variable appearance, including mucosal erythema, erosions, superficial ulcers, flat lesions, and occasionally polyps. Most patients are asymptomatic (particularly in cases of stomach involvement), and disease is discovered during elective endoscopy. The most common presenting symptom is abdominal pain or discomfort. Other, less frequent signs and symptoms include diarrhea, constipation, vomiting, bleeding, weight loss, and anemia.[21,22,24-27] Gastric lesions are frequently associated with concomitant *Helicobacter pylori* infection.[21,28]

Morphology

The lamina propria is expanded by a diffuse infiltrate of medium-sized to large cells with irregular nuclei, fine chromatin, inconspicuous nucleoli, and moderately abundant eosinophilic to pale cytoplasm (Figure 98.5A and B). Epitheliotropism is seen in some cases. Necrosis is usually absent but has been reported in occasional cases, and there is no angiocentricity or angiodestruction.[21,22,24,25]

Immunophenotype

The atypical cells show an NK-cell immunophenotype (Figure 98.5C-F), positive for cytoplasmic CD3, CD7, and CD56. CD2 is variably positive, CD4 and CD5 are negative, and occasional cases are CD8 positive. Cytotoxic markers (TIA-1, granzyme B, and/or perforin) are positive. In situ hybridization for EBV is negative. The proliferation index (Ki67) is variable, <50% in most cases, but >50% in a subset of cases.[21,22,24,25,28]

Genetics

Given the derivation from NK cells, indolent NK-cell LPD of the GIT is by definition negative for clonal T-cell receptor gene rearrangements. Genetic studies on this disease are very limited.[23,27] A recurrent somatic deletion in the autoinhibitory pseudokinase domain of *JAK3*, K563_C565del, has been detected in about 30% of cases investigated by high-throughput sequencing. A number of nonrecurrent mutations were reported involving *APOB*, *FOXO3*, *CREBBP*, *RP1L1*, *PTPRS*, *AURKB*, *AXL*, *CUL3*, *CHEK2*, *RUNX1T1*, *CIC*, *SMARCB1*, *ERBB4*, *IGF1R*, *PIK3CB,* and *SETD5*.[23,27]

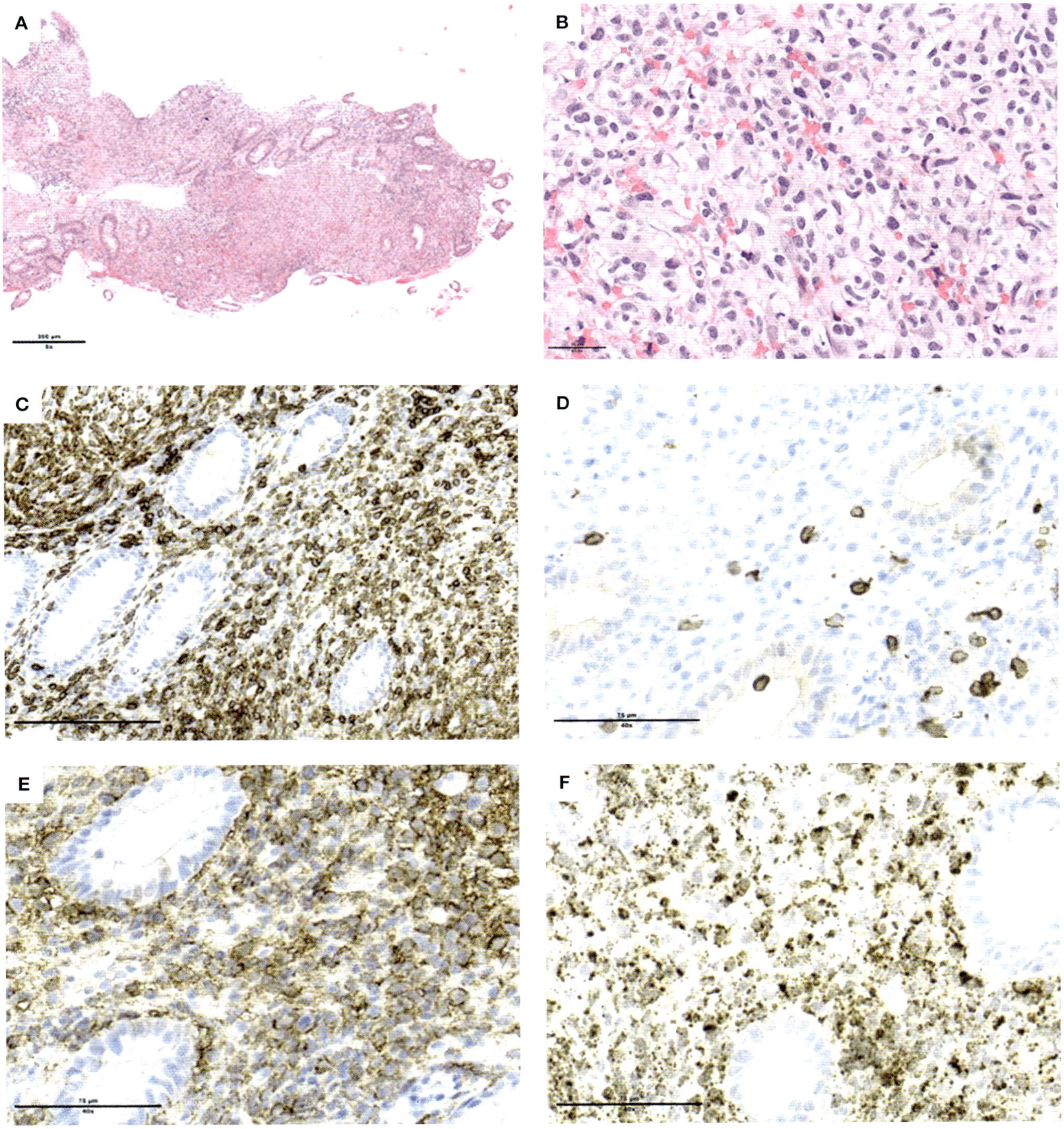

FIGURE 98.5 Indolent NK-cell lymphoproliferative disorder of the gastrointestinal tract. **A:** Low-power view of a colonic lesion discovered incidentally as a small ulcer during screening colonoscopy, showing a pale cellular infiltrate expanding the lamina propria and submucosa. **B:** The cells are medium-sized to large with elongated nuclei and abundant pale cytoplasm. By immunohistochemistry, they are **(C)** positive for CD3, **(D)** negative for CD5, **(E)** positive for CD56, and **(F)** positive for granzyme B. EBV was negative (not shown).

Prognosis and Clinical Comment

Indolent NK-cell LPD of the GIT may show spontaneous resolution or persist despite therapy. Patients who were treated with chemotherapy regimens showed limited to no response. In some cases of spontaneous resolution, disease may relapse at the same or different site in the GIT. There are no reports of progression/transformation to a more aggressive lymphoma.[21-23,25] Although the data in the literature are limited, it appears that watchful waiting is the preferred approach in this disease.[29]

References

1. Lucioni M, Fraticelli S, Santacroce G, et al. Clinical and histopathological features of an Italian monocentric series of primary small bowel T-cell lymphomas. *Cancers*. 2023;15(10):2743.
2. Nicolae A, Xi L, Pham TH, et al. Mutations in the JAK/STAT and RAS signaling pathways are common in intestinal T-cell lymphomas. *Leukemia*. 2016;30(11):2245-2247.
3. Yoon SE, Song Y, Kim SJ, et al. Comprehensive analysis of peripheral T-cell and natural killer/T-cell lymphoma in Asian patients: a multinational, multicenter, prospective registry study in Asia. *Lancet Reg Health West Pac*. 2021;10:100126.
4. Hang JF, Yuan CT, Chang KC, et al. Targeted next-generation sequencing reveals a wide morphologic and immunophenotypic spectrum of monomorphic epitheliotropic intestinal T-cell lymphoma. *Am J Surg Pathol*. 2022;46(9):1207-1218.
5. Kim EK, Jang M, Yang WI, Yoon SO. Primary gastrointestinal T/NK cell lymphoma. *Cancers*. 2021;13(11):2679.
6. Kim SJ, Choi CW, Mun YC, et al. Multicenter retrospective analysis of 581 patients with primary intestinal non-hodgkin lymphoma from the Consortium for Improving Survival of Lymphoma (CISL). *BMC Cancer*. 2011;11:321.
7. Lee G, Ryu HJ, Choi JW, et al. Characteristic gene alterations in primary gastrointestinal T- and NK-cell lymphomas. *Leukemia*. 2019;33(7):1797-1832.
8. Sun J, Lu Z, Yang D, Chen J. Primary intestinal T-cell and NK-cell lymphomas: a clinicopathological and molecular study from China focused on type II enteropathy-associated T-cell lymphoma and primary intestinal NK-cell lymphoma. *Mod Pathol*. 2011;24(7):983-992.
9. Wang RC, Chen BJ, Yuan CT, et al. The spectrum of intestinal mature T- and NK-cell neoplasms in a tertiary center in Taiwan with a high frequency of perforation. *Pathol Res Pract*. 2022;240:154184.
10. Attygalle AD, Cabeçadas J, Gaulard P, et al. Peripheral T-cell and NK-cell lymphomas and their mimics; taking a step forward - report on the lymphoma workshop of the XVIth meeting of the European Association for Haematopathology and the Society for Hematopathology. *Histopathology*. 2014;64(2):171-199.
11. Kawamoto K, Nakamura S, Iwashita A, et al. Clinicopathological characteristics of primary gastric T-cell lymphoma. *Histopathology*. 2009;55(6):641-653.
12. Perry AM, Warnke RA, Hu Q, et al. Indolent T-cell lymphoproliferative disease of the gastrointestinal tract. *Blood*. 2013;122(22):3599-3606. doi:10.1182/blood-2013-07-512830
13. Soderquist CR, Bhagat G. Gastrointestinal T- and NK-cell lymphomas and indolent lymphoproliferative disorders. *Semin Diagn Pathol*. 2020;37(1):11-23. doi:10.1053/j.semdp.2019.08.001
14. Sharma A, Oishi N, Boddicker RL, et al. Recurrent STAT3-JAK2 fusions in indolent T-cell lymphoproliferative disorder of the gastrointestinal tract. *Blood*. 2018;131(20):2262-2266. doi:10.1182/blood-2018-01-830968
15. de Leval L, Feldman AL, Pileri S, Nakamura S, Gaulard P. Extranodal T- and NK-cell lymphomas. *Virchows Arch*. 2023;482(1):245-264. doi:10.1007/s00428-022-03434-0
16. Soderquist CR, Patel N, Murty VV, et al. Genetic and phenotypic characterization of indolent T-cell lymphoproliferative disorders of the gastrointestinal tract. *Haematologica*. 2020;105(7):1895-1906. doi:10.3324/haematol.2019.230961
17. Malamut G, Meresse B, Kaltenbach S, et al. Small intestinal CD4+ T-cell lymphoma is a heterogenous entity with common pathology features. *Clin Gastroenterol Hepatol*. 2014;12(4):599-608 e1. doi:10.1016/j.cgh.2013.11.028
18. Fan W, Niu L, He H, et al. Indolent T-cell lymphoproliferative disorder of gastrointestinal tract with unusual clinical courses: report of 6 cases and literature review. *Virchows Arch*. 2023;482(4):729-743. doi:10.1007/s00428-022-03467-5
19. Montes-Moreno S, King RL, Oschlies I, et al. Update on lymphoproliferative disorders of the gastrointestinal tract: disease spectrum from indolent lymphoproliferations to aggressive lymphomas. *Virchows Arch*. 2020;476(5):667-681. doi:10.1007/s00428-019-02704-8
20. Stuver R, Epstein-Peterson ZD, Horwitz SM. Few and far between: clinical management of rare extranodal subtypes of mature T-cell and NK-cell lymphomas. *Haematologica*. 2023;108(12):3244-3260. doi:10.3324/haematol.2023.282717
21. Takeuchi K, Yokoyama M, Ishizawa S, et al. Lymphomatoid gastropathy: a distinct clinicopathologic entity of self-limited pseudomalignant NK-cell proliferation. *Blood*. 2010;116(25):5631-5637.
22. Xia D, Morgan EA, Berger D, Pinkus GS, Ferry JA, Zukerberg LR. NK-cell enteropathy and similar indolent lymphoproliferative disorders: a case series with literature review. *Am J Clin Pathol*. 2019;151(1):75-85.
23. Xiao W, Gupta GK, Yao J, et al. Recurrent somatic JAK3 mutations in NK-cell enteropathy. *Blood*. 2019;134(12):986-991.
24. Soderquist CR, Bhagat G. Gastrointestinal T- and NK-cell lymphomas and indolent lymphoproliferative disorders. *Semin Diagn Pathol*. 2020;37(1):11-23.
25. Mansoor A, Pittaluga S, Beck PL, Wilson WH, Ferry JA, Jaffe ES. NK-cell enteropathy: a benign NK-cell lymphoproliferative disease mimicking intestinal lymphoma—clinicopathologic features and follow-up in a unique case series. *Blood*. 2011;117(5):1447-1452.
26. Dargent JL, Tinton N, Trimech M, de Leval L. Lymph node involvement by enteropathy-like indolent NK-cell proliferation. *Virchows Arch*. 2021;478(6):1197-1202.
27. Yi H, Li A, Ouyang B, et al. Clinicopathological and molecular features of indolent natural killer-cell lymphoproliferative disorder of the gastrointestinal tract. *Histopathology*. 2023;82(4):567-575.
28. Takata K, Noujima-Harada M, Miyata-Takata T, et al. Clinicopathologic analysis of 6 lymphomatoid gastropathy cases: expanding the disease spectrum to CD4-CD8+ cases. *Am J Surg Pathol*. 2015;39(9):1259-1266.
29. Stuver R, Epstein-Peterson ZD, Horwitz SM. Few and far between: clinical management of rare extranodal subtypes of mature T-cell and NK-cell lymphomas. *Haematologica*. 2023;108(12):3244-3260.

Chapter 99
Hepatosplenic T-Cell Lymphoma

Philippe Gaulard, Carmen Barcena, Andrew L. Feldman, and Barbara Pro

Definition

Hepatosplenic T-cell lymphoma (HSTCL) is a rare aggressive extranodal lymphoma characterized by a hepatosplenic presentation without lymphadenopathy and a poor outcome. A background of immune dysregulation is frequent. The neoplasm results from a proliferation of γδ (or less commonly αβ) cytotoxic T cells likely belonging to the innate immune system, recirculating between spleen, bone marrow, and liver. HSTCL is usually composed of medium-sized lymphoid cells, demonstrating marked sinusoidal infiltration of spleen, liver, and bone marrow. Isochromosome 7q and alterations in members of the JAK/STAT pathway are common.

Synonyms

Hepatosplenic γδ T-cell lymphoma (not recommended).

Epidemiology

HSTCL is a rare form of lymphoma, reported in both Western and Asian countries. It represents 1% to 2% of all peripheral T-cell lymphomas.[1] Peak incidence occurs in adolescents and young adults, with a male predominance (median age around 35 years).[1-3] However, the elderly may be affected.

General Clinical Features

Up to 40% of patients show a context of chronic immune suppression, most commonly long-term immunosuppressive therapy for solid organ transplantation.[2] In this context, HSTCL is regarded as a late-onset posttransplant lymphoproliferative disorder of host origin. Cases occur also in patients with autoimmune disorders, most often Crohn's disease and less frequently rheumatoid arthritis, systemic lupus erythematosus, psoriasis, or autoimmune hepatitis. The simultaneous exposure to thiopurine immunomodulators (azathioprine, 6-mercaptopurine) or tumor necrosis factor alpha (TNFα) antagonists (eg, infliximab) likely account for a higher risk of HSTCL, especially in children treated for Crohn's disease. Occasional cases have been observed following acute myeloid leukemia or Epstein-Barr virus (EBV)–positive lymphoproliferative disorders, in patients with *Plasmodium falciparum* infection,[2] or during pregnancy.

Patients typically present with marked splenomegaly, usually with hepatomegaly, but with no lymphadenopathy, and with systemic symptoms. Cytopenias are common, related to hypersplenism, bone marrow involvement, cytokine release, or immune dysregulation. Thrombocytopenia is almost constant, often with anemia (~75%) and neutropenia (~50%). Although lymphocytosis is uncommon, a minor population of atypical lymphoid cells can be identified by careful examination of blood smears or by flow cytometry in approximately half of the patients.[2] An overt leukemic picture, rare at presentation, can be seen in advanced disease. Hemophagocytic syndrome may occur. Owing to the almost constant bone marrow involvement, most patients have Ann Arbor stage IV disease. They frequently present with two or three adverse risk factors of the age-adjusted International Prognostic Index, thus falling into the high-risk group.[2]

HSTCL is easily distinguishable from other γδ T-cell lymphomas, involving extranodal sites (skin and subcutaneous tissue, intestine, or the nasal region), but may be more difficult to differentiate clinically from some T-cell large granular lymphocytic leukemia (T-LGLL) with a γδ phenotype or from aggressive natural killer (NK)-cell leukemia.[3]

Morphology

The spleen is enlarged with diffuse involvement of the red pulp, without any gross lesions identifiable. Similarly, diffuse hepatic enlargement in the absence of focal lesions is seen. This is consistent with the diffuse uptake of spleen, liver, and bone marrow on FDG-PET/CT.

Histologically (Figure 99.1), the cells of HSTCL are monotonous, small- to medium-sized with a rim of pale cytoplasm. The nuclear chromatin is loosely

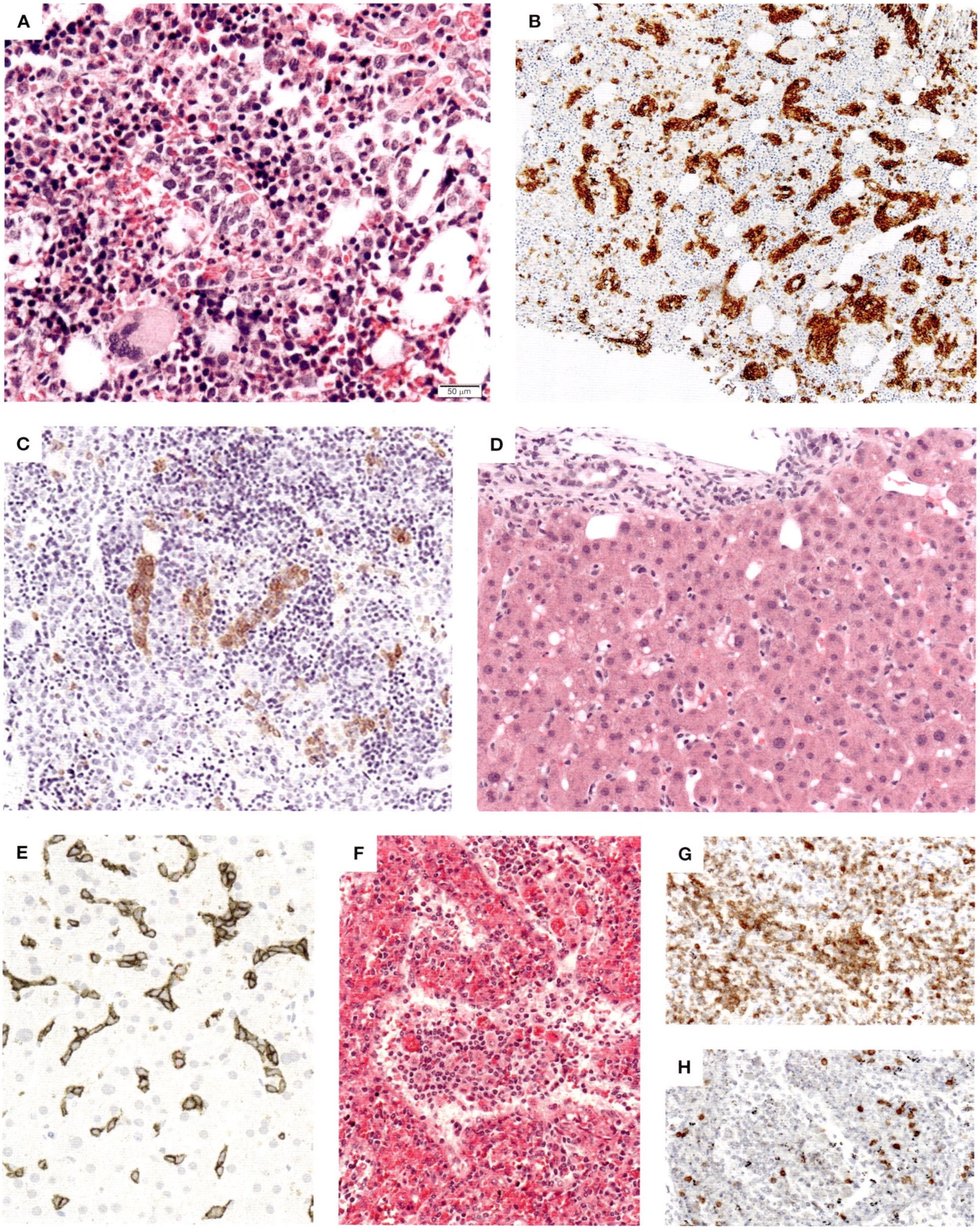

FIGURE 99.1 Hepatosplenic T-cell lymphoma (HSTCL). **A:** The bone marrow biopsy involved by HSTCL is highly cellular and shows intrasinusoidal infiltration by atypical medium-sized lymphoid cells highlighted by **(B)** CD2 and **(C)** T-cell receptor delta. **D:** The liver biopsy reveals a lymphoid infiltrate in the sinusoids and in the portal tracts; the cells are slightly atypical and are immunohistochemically positive for **(E)** T-cell receptor delta. **F:** Cords and sinusoids of the spleen are infiltrated by atypical lymphoid cells; by immunohistochemistry the cells express **(G)** CD3, but are negative for **(H)** CD5.

condensed with small inconspicuous nucleoli. Some pleomorphism may be occasionally seen.[3] The tumor cells involve the cords and sinuses—which may be dilated—of the splenic red pulp, with atrophy of the white pulp (Figure 99.1F). Histiocytes may be numerous, sometimes showing erythrophagocytosis. The liver shows a predominantly sinusoidal infiltration, which can lead to pseudopeliotic lesions (Figure 99.1D). Neoplastic cells are almost constantly present in the bone marrow, with an almost exclusive intrasinusoidal single file or aggregate-like distribution within variably distended bone marrow sinusoids (Figure 99.1A). This latter pattern, often subtle and difficult to recognize on morphology alone, is highlighted by CD3 immunostaining. It is highly characteristic and thus, an essential diagnostic criterion for HSTCL. In addition, at presentation, the bone marrow is usually hypercellular with trilineage hyperplasia. It may show mild dysmyelopoiesis, which can be mistaken as myelodysplastic syndrome in settings of peripheral cytopenias.[2,3] Although usually not enlarged, splenic hilar lymph nodes commonly manifest some degree of lymphomatous involvement confined to the sinuses or perisinusal areas, without destruction of the normal architecture.

With disease progression, cytologic atypia with pleomorphic large cell or blastic changes may be seen.[3] These cytologic variants show a similar tissue distribution in sites involved by HSTCL. However, in advanced disease, the bone marrow infiltration may extend beyond the sinuses resulting in an interstitial or diffuse pattern of involvement.

The diagnosis of HSTCL is based on histopathologic and immunophenotypic criteria. In the past, the diagnosis was often made on splenectomy. Currently, bone marrow biopsy is the recommended diagnostic procedure.[4] Although examination of the bone marrow aspirate allows for cytologic, flow cytometric, and cytogenetic analysis, this alone does not suffice for the diagnosis.[2,3] Although recommended by the National Comprehensive Cancer Network guidelines,[4] liver biopsy appears less useful in clinical practice given the overlapping morphological finding of HSTCL with other lymphomas or reactive conditions.

Immunophenotype

The neoplastic cells are $CD3^+$, $CD5^-$, $CD2^+$, $CD7^{+/-}$, and $CD4^-$, $CD8^-$, with rare cases $CD8^+$. Most cases are $CD56^+$ and $CD57^-$; some are $CD16^+$ (Figure 99.1). Neoplastic cells show granular cytoplasmic expression of T-cell intracellular antigen 1 (TIA-1) (Figure 99.1), but are usually negative for granzyme B and perforin, consistent with a nonactivated cytotoxic phenotype. Expression of killer immunoglobulin-like receptors, especially KIR3DL2, which is targetable, and to a lesser degree CD94/NKG2A, are common. HSTCL cells are negative for CD25 and CD30. Most cases (~80%) are $TCR\gamma\delta^+$ and $TCR\alpha\beta^-$ (Figure 99.1C and E).[5,6] Most γδ HSTCLs express the Vδ1 chain.[2] However, approximately 20% of cases express TCRαβ and <5% show a TCR-silent phenotype either at presentation or at relapse.[3,6,7] The αβ variant is classified together with the more common γδ form of the disease based on overlapping clinicopathologic, cytogenetic, and molecular features.[7] By in situ hybridization with EBV-encoded small RNA (EBER) probes, HSTCL is EBV-negative in almost all cases, with EBV being reported in exceptional cases with cytologic features of transformation (suggesting that EBV in such cases is a secondary event).[2]

Although determination of an αβ or γδ phenotype is nowadays possible in histologic sections, flow cytometric analysis of bone marrow aspirates is recommended, enabling not only complete immunophenotyping of neoplastic cells, but also cytogenetics and molecular studies.

Altogether (Table 99.1), the features of HSTCL contrast with those of T-cell large granular lymphocytic leukemia (T-LGLL), in which the cells have a more mature lymphocytic appearance, a $CD8^+$ and often $CD57^+$ phenotype with granzyme B expression, and a subtle, diffuse interstitial pattern in the marrow with minimal (not prominent) infiltration of sinuses.[3] HSTCL also differs from aggressive NK-cell leukemia, which has less-monotonous neoplastic cells with an interstitial pattern rather than a sinusoidal distribution in the bone marrow, shows an activated cytotoxic granzyme B+, perforin+ phenotype, lacks TCR expression, and above all discloses EBV by in situ hybridization (ISH; EBV-encoded small RNA probes) in most cases.

Genetics

The cells have rearranged TRG genes. Cases of γδ origin show a biallelic rearrangement of TRD genes. TRB genes are rearranged in αβ cases; however, unproductive rearrangement of TRB genes has been reported in some γδ cases. Isochromosome 7q (i[7][q10]) and trisomy 8 are detected in up to 80% and 50% of both γδ and αβ HSTCL cases, respectively.[7,8] With disease progression, a variety of FISH patterns equivalent to two to five

TABLE 99.1 Main clinical, pathologic, and genetic features of hepatosplenic T-cell lymphoma, T-cell large granular lymphocytic leukemia, and aggressive natural killer-cell leukemia

	Clinical features	Morphology (cytology, pattern)	Phenotype	Cytotoxic profile	Cell of origin	EBV (EBER; ISH)	Genetics	Bone marrow biopsy
HSTCL	B symptoms, splenomegaly, hepatomegaly, cytopenias, no lymphadenopathy	Monomorphic, medium-sized cells,sinusal/ sinusoidal pattern (spleen, liver, BM)	$CD3^+$, $CD5^-$, $CD4^-$, $CD8^-$, $CD56^+$, $CD57^-$	Nonactivated (TIA1+, GrB-, Perf-)	Tγδ >> Tαβ	Negative	iso7q, trisomy 8 Mutations: - epigenetics (*SETD2, INO1*), - JAK-STAT (*STAT5B*)	Almost exclusively sinusoidal involvement
T-LGLL	Neutropenia, lymphocytosis, mild splenomegaly, no lymphadenopathy, auto-immune manifestations, indolent presentation	Small to medium-sized cells with azurophilic granules,interstitial pattern (BM)	$CD3^+$, $CD5^{-/+}$, $CD4^-$, $CD8^+$, $CD56^-$, $CD57^+$	Activated (TIA1+, GrB+, Perf+)	Tαβ (>>Tγδ)	Negative	Mutations: - JAK-STAT (*STAT3, STAT5B*), - epigenetics (*TET2, DNMT3A*...)	Interstitial ± sinusoidal (often subtle) + nodules and nodular, myeloid maturation arrest
Aggressive NK-cell leukemia	B symptoms, cytopenias, variable (mild) leukemic spread, HPS, splenomegaly, +/– involvement of lymphadenopathy, other extranodal sites	Variable, small, medium-sized to alrge lymphoid cells interstitial + patchy pattern in involved organs	$CD3^+$, $CD5^{-/+}$, $CD4^-$, $CD8^-$, $CD56^+$, $CD57^-$	Activated (TIA1+, GrB+, Perf+)	NK	Positive (most cases)	Absence of TCR gene rearrangement;del 6q, del 11q, mutations *STAT3, DDX3X, TET2, TP53*...	Interstitial diffuse ± patchy involvement, hemophagocytosis

BM, bone marrow; EBER, EBV-encoded small RNA; EBV, Epstein-Barr virus; GrB, granzyme B; HPS, hemophagocytic syndrome; HSTCL, hepatosplenic T-cell lymphoma; ISH, in situ hybridization; iso7q, isochromosome 7q; NK, natural killer; Perf, perforin; TIA1, T-cell intracellular antigen; T-LGLL, T-cell large granular lymphocytic leukemia.

copies of i(7)(q10) or numerical and structural aberrations of the second chromosome 7 have been detected.[8] A ring chromosome leading to 7q amplification has also been reported, which may result from illegitimate somatic rearrangements of both TRG and TRB loci.[9] The common gained region, which has been mapped to 7q22, associates with increased expression of several genes including the multidrug resistance gene *ABCB1, RUNDC3, PPP1R9A, CHN2/β2-chimerin* genes, which may be responsible for the intrinsic drug resistance of the neoplastic cells and their growth advantage.[9] Loss of chromosomes Y, 21, 10p, and 11q14 and gain of chromosome 1q may also be present.[6,9] Although i(7)(q10) is a characteristic feature, it is not specific for HSTCL as it has also been reported in acute myeloid and lymphoblastic leukemias, myelodysplastic syndrome, rare cases of extranodal NK/T-cell lymphoma, nasal type, and anaplastic large cell lymphoma. Gene expression profiling studies have shown that HSTL discloses a distinct molecular signature unifying αβ and γδ cases. A high expression of sphingosine-1-phosphatase receptor 5 involved in cell trafficking has been reported, which might explain the peculiar sinusoidal pattern seen in HSTCLs.[7] Sequencing studies have shown that more than 60% of HSTCL disclose genetic changes in chromatin modifying genes such as *SETD2, INO80, TET3,* and *SMARCA2*.[5,6] In addition, *STAT5B* and more rarely *STAT3* missense mutations have been found in approximately 40% of HSTCL,[5] consistent with the significant enrichment in genes of the JAK-STAT pathway.[5-7] These alterations have been linked to HSTCL pathogenesis, but are not unique to HSTCL and occur in other mature, cytotoxic T/NK-cell lymphomas. Conversely, HSTCL lacks *RHOA* mutations and rarely exhibits *CD28* and *CCR4* gene alterations, which are commonly seen in other T-cell neoplasms.[6]

Prognosis and Clinical Comment

The course is aggressive. Patients may initially respond to chemotherapy, but relapses are seen in the vast majority of cases. Overall, HSTL is refractory to conventional anthracycline-based chemotherapy.[10] The median survival is <2 years.[2] Platinum-cytarabine and pentostatin have been shown to be active agents.[2,10] Early use of high-dose therapy followed by hematopoietic stem cell transplantation, especially allogeneic, may improve survival.

References

1. de Leval L, Feldman AL, Pileri S, Nakamura S, Gaulard P. Extranodal T- and NK-cell lymphomas. *Virchows Arch.* 2023;482(1):245-264.
2. Belhadj K, Reyes F, Farcet JP, et al. Hepatosplenic gammadelta T-cell lymphoma is a rare clinicopathologic entity with poor outcome: report on a series of 21 patients. *Blood.* 2003;102(13):4261-4269.
3. Attygalle AD, Cabeçadas J, Gaulard P, et al. Peripheral T-cell and NK-cell lymphomas and their mimics; taking a step forward—report on the lymphoma workshop of the XVIth meeting of the European Association for Haematopathology and the Society for Hematopathology. *Histopathology.* 2014;64(2):171-199.
4. Horwitz SM, Ansell S, Ai WZ, et al. NCCN guidelines insights: T-cell lymphomas, version 1.2021. *J Natl Compr Canc Netw.* 2020;18(11):1460-1467.
5. Nicolae A, Xi L, Pittaluga S, et al. Frequent STAT5B mutations in γδ hepatosplenic T-cell lymphomas. *Leukemia.* 2014;28(11):2244-2248.
6. McKinney M, Moffitt AB, Gaulard P, et al. The genetic basis of hepatosplenic T-cell lymphoma. *Cancer Discov.* 2017;7(4):369-379.
7. Travert M, Huang Y, de Leval L, et al. Molecular features of hepatosplenic T-cell lymphoma unravels potential novel therapeutic targets. *Blood.* 2012;119(24):5795-5806.
8. Wlodarska I, Martin-Garcia N, Achten R, et al. Fluorescence in situ hybridization study of chromosome 7 aberrations in hepatosplenic T-cell lymphoma: isochromosome 7q as a common abnormality accumulating in forms with features of cytologic progression. *Genes Chromosomes Cancer.* 2002;33(3):243-251.
9. Finalet Ferreiro J, Rouhigharabaei L, Urbankova H, et al. Integrative genomic and transcriptomic analysis identified candidate genes implicated in the pathogenesis of hepatosplenic T-cell lymphoma. *PLoS One.* 242014;9(7):e102977.
10. Pro B, Allen P, Behdad A. Hepatosplenic T-cell lymphoma: a rare but challenging entity. *Blood.* 2020;136(18):2018-2026.

Chapter 100
Mycosis Fungoides

Nneka I. Comfere, Eduardo Calonje, and Lorenzo Cerroni

Definition

Mycosis fungoides (MF) is a form of epidermotropic cutaneous T-cell lymphoma (CTCL) characterized by patches, plaques, and/or tumors with a chronic and indolent course. Folliculotropic mycosis fungoides (FMF), pagetoid reticulosis, and granulomatous slack skin disease are recognized variants of MF with unique clinicopathologic characteristics, clinical behavior, and prognosis. Cutaneous T-cell lymphoma (CTCL) is an imprecise and inconsistently applied label that has been used as a collective term for MF and Sezary syndrome, but is also employed as terminology to encompass all types of T-cell lymphoma arising primarily in skin. Whilst it is acceptable to use CTCL as a catch all for all types of primary cutaneous T-cell lymphoma, it's use as a surrogate for MF is to be avoided.

Synonyms

Alibert-Bazin disease (not recommended).

Epidemiology

The majority (75%-80%) of primary cutaneous lymphomas in the Western world are of T lineage, and MF is the most common type (60% of CTCL). Most cases are of classic type with FMF, pagetoid reticulosis, and granulomatous slack skin variants in the minority (10%, <1%, and <1% of all MF cases, respectively).[1,2] MF accounts for 62% of all CTCL with notable heterogeneity of frequencies characterized by geographical clustering, suggesting a role for environmental factors or industrial pollution in its pathogenesis.[3] Surveillance, Epidemiology, and End Results program–based analysis of incidence rates of cutaneous lymphoma by gender and race/ethnicity (2001-2005) demonstrates significantly higher rates in men than in women (14 vs 8.2/1,000,000 person years, respectively). Incidence rates are highest among blacks and non-Hispanic whites (both 15/1,000,000 person-years) and increase exponentially with age, peaking at 80 years in MF.[4] Notably, there appears to be a trend toward earlier MF disease stage presentations in non-whites including African American patient populations and in younger age groups (median age at diagnosis = 47 years) with a female predominance (1.4:1).[5]

General Clinical Features

MF is characterized by persistent and progressive well-circumscribed, erythematous patches that evolve over years to decades into plaques (plaque lesions) and in some cases ulcerated tumors (tumor lesions) (Figures 100.1A and 100.2-100.4). While patches, plaques, and tumors may be present at any given time, in some cases one or more lesion types will predominate. Lesions present on non–sun exposed (bathing trunk distribution) body sites predominantly and may be pruritic and bear secondary features of scale, atrophy, follicular prominence, poikiloderma, and/or hypopigmentation.[6] Some patients present with tumor stage lesions or erythroderma.[7] However, the vast majority of the former probably represent other, more aggressive forms of CTCL. Also, most patients presenting primarily with erythroderma usually display the full clinical picture of Sezary syndrome, erythrodermic MF more usually representing a late stage, of the disease. Early-stage lesions of MF may bear significant clinical resemblance to inflammatory dermatoses including eczematous dermatitis, psoriasis, drug reactions, and morphea, resulting in diagnostic delays (median delay, 36 months).[6] Recognized variants of MF have distinct clinical features that are described under the relevant headings (see also Table 100.1).

Morphology

Epitheliotropism with infiltration of the epidermis by neoplastic lymphocytes (epidermotropism) is the histological hallmark of MF, although hair follicle and sweat duct epithelium may also be involved (folliculotropism and syringotropism, respectively). The neoplastic lymphocytes possess highly irregular, hyperchromatic nuclei with convoluted outlines

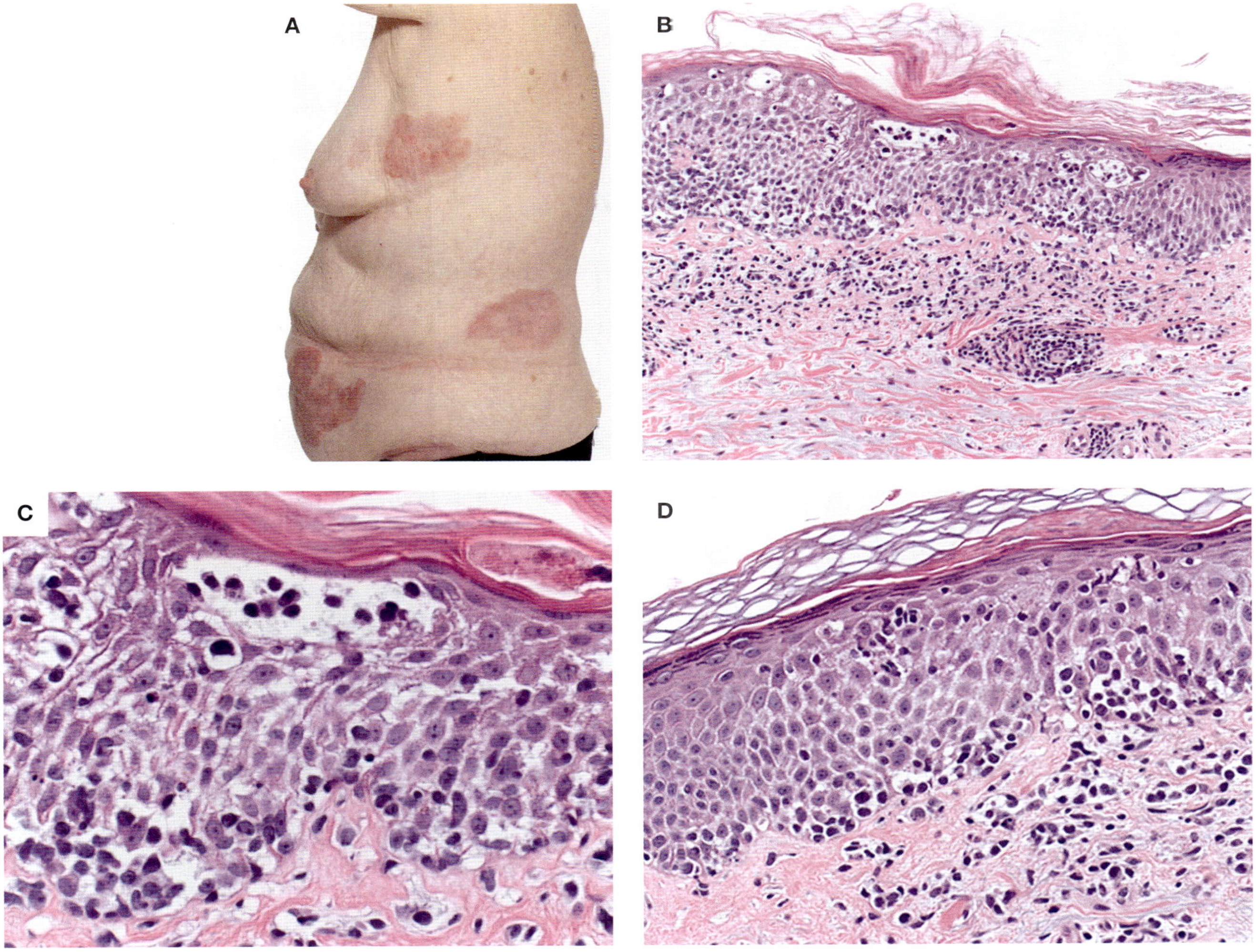

FIGURE 100.1 Patch stage mycosis fungoides (MF). **A:** Erythematous patches with minimal scale and slight central clearing in mycosis fungoides. **B:** Epidermotropism of atypical T lymphocytes (20× magnification; hematoxylin and eosin stain). **C:** Patch stage MF. Clusters of atypical T lymphocytes in the epidermis (Pautrier microabscesses); 40× magnification; hematoxylin and eosin stain **D:** Patch stage MF. Wiry papillary dermal collagen fibers, haloed lymphocytes, and lymphocyte tagging along the basement membrane zone; 20× magnification, hematoxylin and eosin stain.

(cerebriform nuclei). They can be of small to medium size in earlier stages of the disease but are more often of medium to large size in advanced stage. Different patterns of epidermotropism may be seen. Often there are long linear arrays of lymphocytes with halos situated along the dermal-epidermal junction ("lymphocyte tagging"). A pagetoid distribution of intraepidermal cerebriform cells may also be seen, as may discrete clusters of intraepidermal lymphoid cells (Pautrier microabscesses/Darier nests). In patch and early plaque stage of MF the changes can be subtle and inflammatory features such as psoriasiform hyperplasia, spongiosis, and interface dermatitis may be seen, along with a mixed reactive inflammatory cell infiltrate in the papillary dermis, including small lymphocytes, histiocytes, and sometimes eosinophils (Figure 100.1B-D). Distinction from benign dermatoses is often fraught and dependent on identifying intraepidermal medium-large cerebriform cells, lymphocyte tagging, Pautrier microabscesses, and a degree of epidermotropism in excess of that expected for any spongiosis that might be present. In established plaque and tumor stage lesions, the atypical infiltrate is denser and more diffuse with extension throughout the dermis and into the subcutaneous tissue. Tumor stage lesions may not demonstrate epitheliotropism.[8]

Large cell transformation of MF is associated with disease progression and very poor prognosis. It is defined by the presence of large neoplastic T cells, which account for 25% or more of the infiltrate or are seen forming distinct tumor nodules in a patient with established MF.

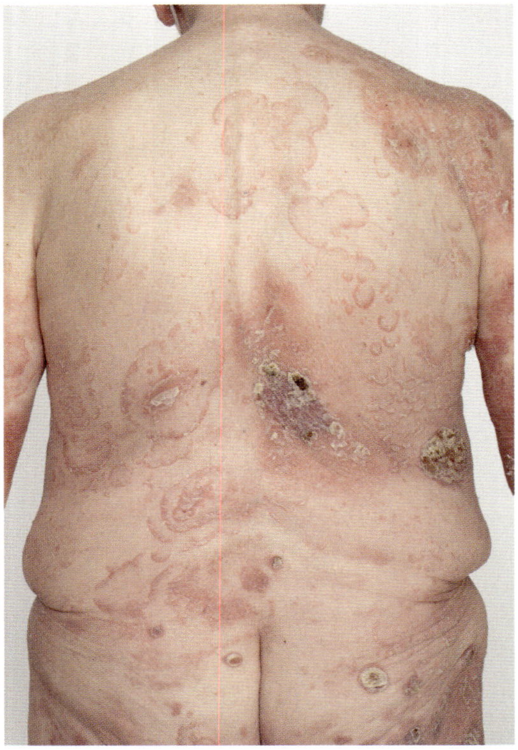

FIGURE 100.2 Mycosis fungoides. Erythematous scaly arciform/gyriform patches and hyperkeratotic infiltrated plaques on torso.

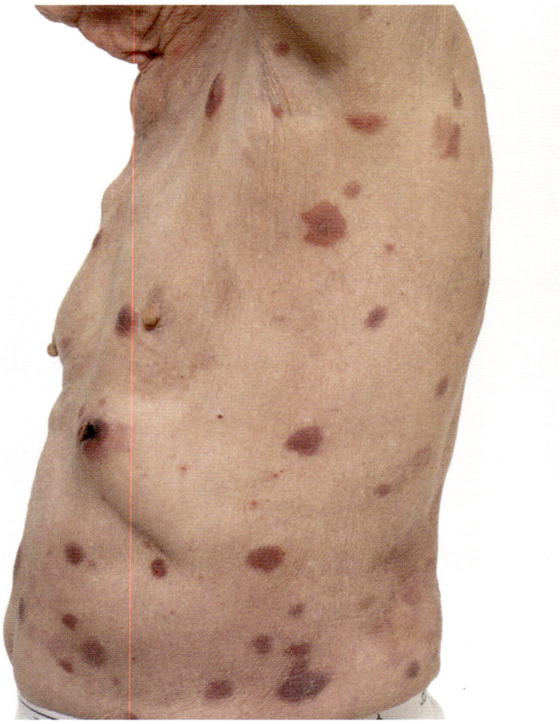

FIGURE 100.3 Mycosis fungoides. Erythematous to violaceous, infiltrated plaques, some with central hemorrhagic eschar on torso.

Immunophenotype

The neoplastic T lymphocytes are almost all of α/β-type (TCR-β F1 positive), CD3 and CD4 positive, and CD8 negative. In the earlier stages of the disease, the only phenotypic aberrancy may be loss of CD7, absence of CD2, and C5 usually only being seen later on in the course of the disease.[8,9] Partial loss of CD7 should be interpreted with caution as the antigen may also be focally absent in benign dermatoses. Complete loss of CD7 carries greater significance.[10] Strong expression of PD1, suggestive of immune exhaustion, is often seen, but other markers of follicular helper T cells such as CD10 and CXCL13 are typically absent. CD30 may be expressed by a minority of cells but is more frequently encountered and more extensively positive following large cell transformation. Rare, unusual phenotypes include CD8-positive and/or TCR-γδ-positive cases. For these to qualify as MF the clinical phenotype must be typical. CD8-positive MF is more often associated with pediatric patients, black and Asian populations, and hypopigmented skin lesions.

Variants of mycosis fungoides

Folliculotropic mycosis fungoides

In FMF, patients present with patches, plaques, or grouped papules with a predilection for the head and neck area (Figures 100.5-100.8). Acneiform lesions, pruritus, and alopecia are common. Histopathologic features include mild to dense perifollicular, superficial to mid-dermal cerebriform T-cell infiltrates with predominant folliculotropism, secondary follicular mucinous degeneration with follicular rupture, basaloid folliculolymphoid hyperplasia, dilated follicular infundibula, milia-like cysts, and comedones. Secondary features include angiocentric and angiodestructive atypical T-lymphoid infiltrates, rare interfollicular epidermotropism, syringotropism, and/or ulceration. Admixed eosinophils are a common finding in FMF, and other secondary inflammatory changes such as plasma cells and granulomas are frequent.

Pagetoid reticulosis

Pagetoid reticulosis manifests as a solitary, slowly growing lesion that evolves into a thick, often verruciform, plaque or localized group of plaques, on a distal extremity (Figure 100.9), on occasion reaching up to 30 cm in diameter. Histologically, there is epidermal hyperplasia and parakeratosis associated with an intraepidermal infiltrate of medium-large cerebriform T cells with abundant clear cytoplasm. Epidermotropism is striking

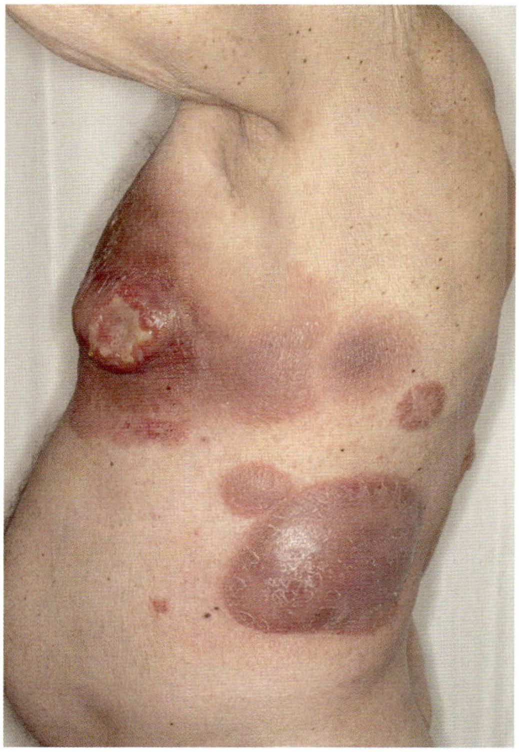

FIGURE 100.4 Mycosis fungoides. Erythematous to brawny appearing patches, infiltrated plaques, and ulcerated tumors on torso.

and neoplastic lymphocytes are almost exclusively present within the epidermis, often predominately colonizing the lower half with pagetoid distribution. Pautrier microabscesses may be seen. Papillary dermal lymphocytes are usually sparse and reactive in nature. The neoplastic T cells are of α/β type and frequently CD8⁺, although CD4⁻/CD8⁻ and CD4⁻/CD8⁺ phenotypes are occasionally observed. CD30 may be positive.

Granulomatous slack skin

Granulomatous slack skin is exceedingly rare. Patients are often young adults who present with red-purple papules and plaques that evolve into large pendulous skin folds, usually in the axillary or inguinal regions. Histopathologic features include a dense dermal infiltrate of atypical T lymphocytes, often of small to medium size and CD4⁺. These are admixed with prominent multinucleated giant cells, which may show elastophagocytosis and lymphophagocytosis. Elastolysis with loss and fragmentation of elastic tissue fibers is also seen.

Genetics

Clonal TCR gene rearrangements are present in MF but not always detectable, with a higher false-negative rate in patch compared with plaque and tumor stage lesions.[11] Moreover, clonal TCR rearrangements can be found in a variety of inflammatory dermatoses, meaning results of such studies should always be interpreted with caution. Demonstration of the same clone in two or more lesions from the same patient is most predictive of neoplasia. Emerging technical advances in array-based comparative genomic hybridization and next-generation sequencing has facilitated detailed analysis of genetic and transcriptional changes in MF, implicating several signaling pathways and epigenetic mechanisms in its pathogenesis, some of which are potentially amenable to therapeutic targeting. Examples include overactivation of JAK/STAT signaling secondary to reduced *SOCS1* expression, the latter as a consequence of deletions or unbalanced translocations, upregulation of miR-155 (which targets *SOCS1* mRNA), or DNA methylation of the *SOCS1* promoter.[12] *TET2, DNMT3A,* and *IDH2* mutations, resulting in DNA hypermethylation and oncometabolite (IDH2) production, have also been detected.[12,13]

Prognosis and Clinical Comment

Extent of disease, as determined by the International Society for Cutaneous Lymphomas (ISCL) and European Organization for Research and Treatment of Cancer (EORTC) staging system, is the most important predictor of outcome and, to an extent, dictates the therapeutic approach[14,15] (Table 100.2). Five-year

TABLE 100.1 Mycosis fungoides (MF) variants—clinical and histopathologic features

MF variant	Clinical features	Histopathologic features
Folliculotropic MF (Figures 100.5-100.8)	Follicular papules or plaques, acneiform lesions, comedones, milia, cysts; head and neck region with associated alopecia	Folliculocentric atypical lymphoid infiltrate with folliculotropism, follicular mucinosis and destruction, milia-like cysts
Pagetoid reticulosis (Figure 100.9)	Solitary or few erythematous patches or plaques on acral skin	Marked epidermotropism of atypical lymphocytes within hyperplastic epithelium
Granulomatous slack skin	Erythematous plaques that develop into bulky, pendulous skin within flexural skin such as the inguinal creases	Granulomatous infiltrate including multinucleated giant cells admixed with atypical lymphocytes

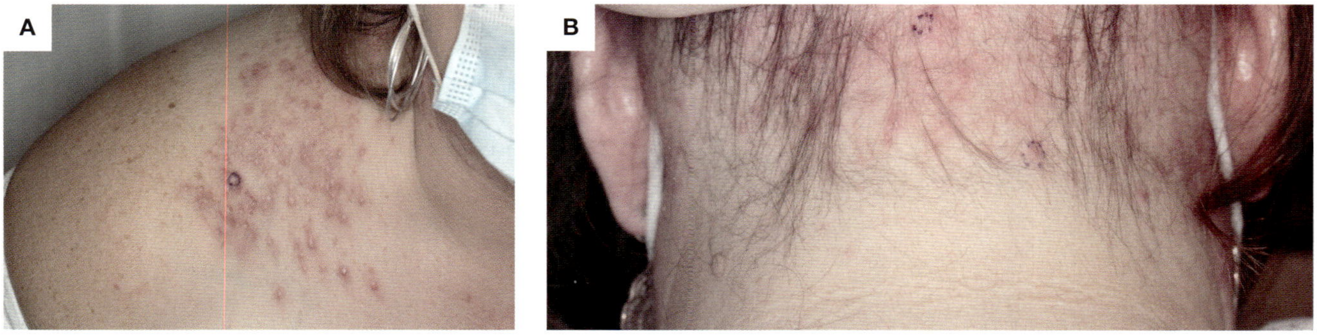

FIGURE 100.5 Folliculotropic mycosis fungoides. **A:** Acneiform papules and pustules on shoulder. **B:** Acneiform papules on nape of neck with background erythema and associated alopecia.

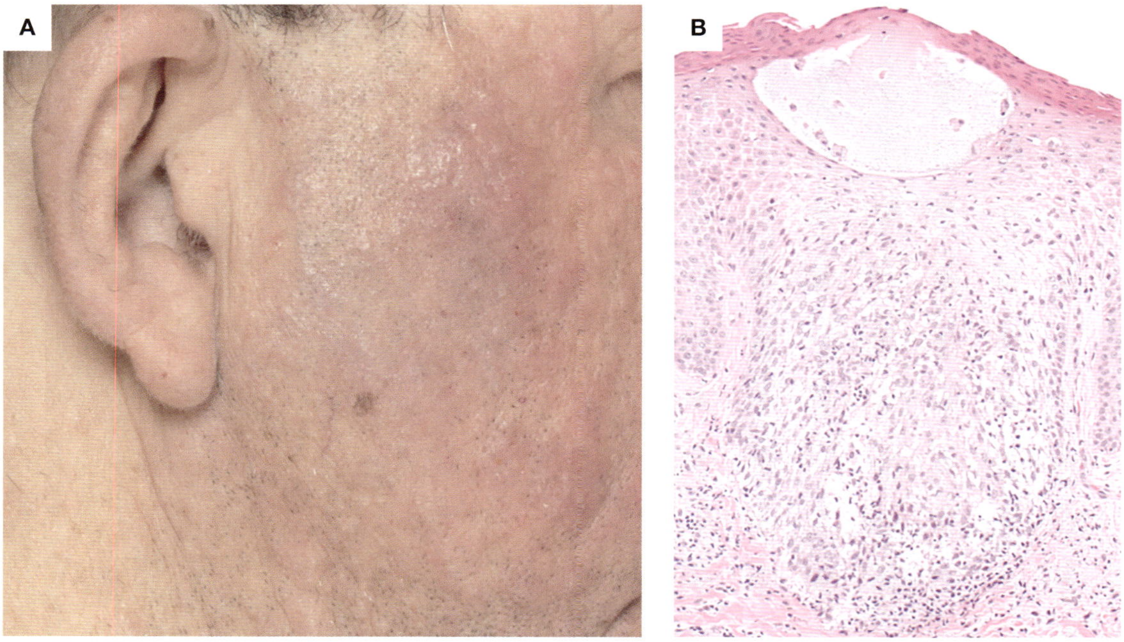

FIGURE 100.6 Folliculotropic mycosis fungoides. **A:** Erythematous plaques on face. **B:** Folliculotropic atypical lymphoid infiltrate with marked follicular mucinosis (20× magnification; hematoxylin and eosin stain).

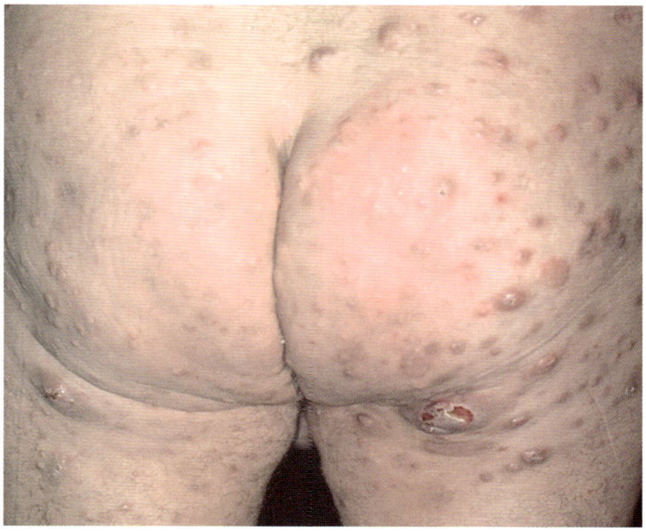

FIGURE 100.7 Folliculotropic mycosis fungoides. Papules, pustules, milia-like cysts, and nodules with secondary erosion on buttocks. (Image courtesy of Lorenzo Cerroni.)

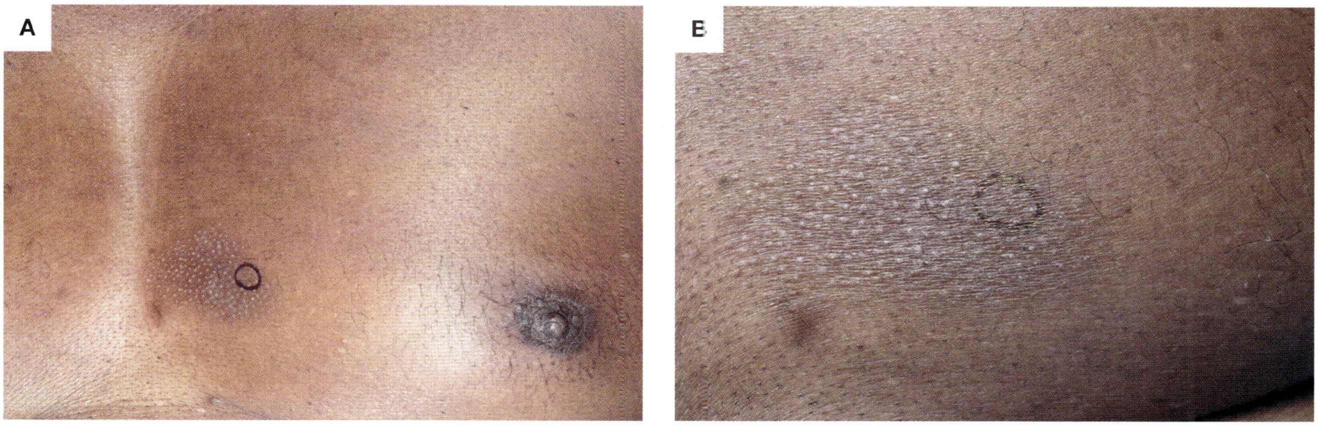

FIGURE 100.8 Folliculotropic mycosis fungoides. **A:** Hyperpigmented infiltrated plaques with follicular accentuation on the central chest. **B:** Inset: high magnification of hyperpigmented plaque with follicular prominence.

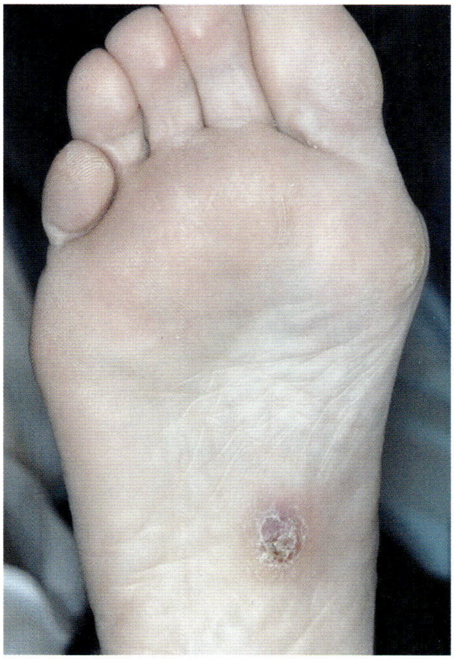

FIGURE 100.9 Pagetoid reticulosis. Localized hyperkeratotic plaque on plantar foot.

overall survival (OS) rates for MF and Sezary syndrome are 85.8% for stage IB and 62.2% for stage IIB and drop significantly in stage IVB disease, with OS rates of only 23.3%.[16] Multivariate analysis incorporating ISCL/EORTC staging criteria, including multiple clinicopathologic factors, confirms that advanced skin stage, presence of a peripheral blood clone in the absence of Sezary cells (B0b), increased lactate dehydrogenase, and folliculotropic MF were independent predictors of worse survival and elevated risk of disease progression; large cell transformation and tumor distribution were independent predictors of only elevated risk of disease progression; and NMB stages, age, male sex, and poikilodermatous MF were significant for survival.[16]

In FMF, two distinct prognostic subsets have been defined. Early presentation characterized by follicular papules, acneiform lesions, comedones, and cysts with a relatively mild atypical lymphoid infiltrate is associated with an indolent course similar to patch stage MF (5-yr OS 92%). Conversely, advanced presentation typified by thick plaques and a dense and deep perifollicular atypical lymphoid infiltrate has a prognosis similar to tumor stage MF (5-yr OS 55%).[17] Patients presenting with plaques fall between these two groups and are more heterogeneous; poor prognosis in these patients is associated with percentage of atypical cells, cell size, percentage of Ki-67+ cells, and coexistent interfollicular epidermotropism, while extensive follicular mucinosis is associated with more favorable outcome.[18] Prognosis for pagetoid reticulosis is generally excellent. Treatment of choice for this variant is excision or local radiotherapy.

TABLE 100.2 ISCL/EORTC staging classification of cutaneous T-cell lymphoma[15]

TNMB classification skin (T)	Findings
T1	Patches/plaques on ≤10% of skin surface
T2	Patches/plaques on >10% of skin surface
T3	Tumors (≥1 with diameter >1 cm)
T4	Erythroderma (>80% of skin surface)
Lymph node (N)	
N0	No clinically abnormal lymph nodes; pathology not required
N1[a]	Clinically abnormal lymph nodes; pathology Dutch grade 1 or NCI LN0-2
N2[a]	Clinically abnormal lymph nodes; pathology Dutch grade 2 or NCI LN3
N3	Clinically abnormal lymph nodes; pathology Dutch grade 3-4 or NCI LN4; clone positive or negative
NX	Clinically abnormal peripheral or central lymph nodes; no pathologic confirmation
Visceral (M)	
M0	No visceral involvement
M1	Visceral involvement present (pathologic confirmation required with exception of spleen and liver involvement, which may be determined by imaging)
Blood (B)	
B0[a]	No or less than 5% circulating atypical (Sezary) cells
B1[a]	Low blood tumor burden (>5% of lymphocytes are Sezary cells but not B2)
B2	High blood tumor burden (>1000 µL Sezary cells and positive T-cell clone)

Stage					
IA	T1, N0, M0, B0-1	IB	T2, N0, M0, B0-1		
II	T1-2, N1-2, M0, B0-1	IIB	T3, N0-2, M0, B0-1		
III	T4, N0-2, M0, B0-1	IIIA	T4, N0-2, M0, B0	IIIB	T4,N0-2, M0, B1
IVA1	T1-4, N0-2, M0, B2	IVA2	T1-4, N3, M0, B0-2	IVB	T1-4, N0-3, M1, B0-2

[a]N and B compartments subdivided into a and b representing clone-negative and clone-positive categories, respectively.

References

1. Willemze R, Cerroni L, Kempf W, et al. The 2018 update of the WHO-EORTC classification for primary cutaneous lymphomas. *Blood*. 2019;133(16):1703-1714.
2. Kempf W, Mitteldorf C. Cutaneous T-cell lymphomas – an update 2021. *Hematol Oncol*. 2021;39(suppl 1):46-51.
3. Dobos G, Pohrt A, Ram-Wolff C, et al. Epidemiology of cutaneous T-cell lymphomas: a systematic review and meta-analysis of 16,953 patients. *Cancers*. 2020;12(10):2921
4. Bradford PT, Devesa SS, Anderson WF, Toro JR. Cutaneous lymphoma incidence patterns in the United States: a population based study of 3884 cases. *Blood*. 2009;113(21):5064-5073.
5. Geller S, Lebowitz E, Pulitzer M, Myskowski PL. Understanding racial disparities in mycosis fungoides through international collaborative studies. *Br J Dermatol*. 2019;180(5):1263-1264.
6. Scarisbrick JJ, Quaglino P, Prince HM, et al. The PROCLIPI international registry of early-stage mycosis fungoides identifies substantial diagnostic delay in most patients. *Br J Dermatol*. 2019;181(2):350-357.
7. Jawed SI, Myskowski PL, Horwitz S, Moskowitz A, Querfeld C. Primary cutaneous T-cell lymphoma (mycosis fungoides and Sezary syndrome): Part 1. Diagnosis—clinical and histopathologic features and new molecular and biologic markers. *J Am Acad Dermatol*. 2014;70(2):204.e1-16.
8. Pimpinelli N, Olsen EA, Santucci M, et al. Defining early mycosis fungoides. *J Am Acad Dermatol*. 2005;53(6):1053-1063.
9. Ormsby A, Bergfeld WF, Tubbs RR, Hsi ED. Evaluation of a new paraffin-reactive CD7 T-cell deletion marker and a polymerase chain reaction-based T-cell receptor gene rearrangement assay: implications for diagnosis of mycosis fungoides in community clinical practice. *J Am Acad Dermatol*. 2001;45(3):405-413.

10. Murphy M, Fullen D, Carlson JA. Low CD7 expression in benign and malignant cutaneous lymphocytic infiltrates: experience with an antibody reactive with paraffin-embedded tissue. *Am J Dermatopathol.* 2002;24(1):6-16.
11. Ponti R, Quaglino P, Novelli M, et al. T-cell receptor γ gene rearrangement by multiplex polymerase chain reaction/heteroduplex analysis in patients with cutaneous T-cell lymphoma (mycosis fungoides/Sezary syndrome) and benign inflammatory disease: correlation with clinical, histological and immunophenotypical findings. *Br J Dermatol.* 2005;153(3):565-573.
12. Tensen CP, Quint KD, Vermeer MH. Genetic and epigenetic insights into cutaneous T-cell lymphoma. *Blood.* 2022;139(1):15-33.
13. Choi J, Goh G, Walradt T, et al. Genomic landscape of cutaneous T cell lymphoma. *Nat Genet.* 2015;47(9):1011-1019.
14. Mourad A, Gniadecki R. Overall survival in mycosis fungoides: a systematic review and meta-analysis. *J Invest Dermatol.* 2020;140(2):495-497.e5.
15. Olsen E, Vonderheid E, Pimpinelli N, et al. Revisions to the staging and classification of mycosis fungoides and Sezary syndrome: a proposal of the International Society for Cutaneous Lymphomas (ISCL) and the cutaneous lymphoma task force of the European Organization of Research and Treatment of Cancer (EORTC). *Blood.* 2007;110(6):1713-1722.
16. Aga NS, Wedgeworth E, Crichton S, et al. Survival outcomes and prognostic factors in mycosis fungoides/Sézary syndrome: validation of the revised International Society for Cutaneous Lymphomas/European Organisation for Research and Treatment of Cancer staging proposal. *J Clin Oncol.* 2010;28(31):4730-4739.
17. van Santen S, Roach REJ, van Doorn R, et al. Clinical staging and prognostic factors in folliculotropic mycosis fungoides. *JAMA Dermatol.* 2016;152(9):992-1000.
18. van Santen S, Jansen PM, Quint KD, Vermeer MH, Willemze R. Plaque stage folliculotropic mycosis fungoides: histopathologic features and prognostic factors in a series of 40 patients. *J Cutan Pathol.* 2020;47(3):241-250..

Chapter 101
Sézary Syndrome

Nneka I. Comfere, Eduardo Calonje, and Lorenzo Cerroni

Definition

Sézary syndrome is a rare, aggressive, leukemic form of cutaneous T-cell lymphoma (CTCL) that is characterized by the triad of (1) pruritic erythroderma (confluent erythema over >80% of body), (2) generalized lymphadenopathy, and (3) circulating clonally related malignant T lymphocytes with cerebriform nuclei (Sézary cells) in the peripheral blood, lymph nodes, and skin. However, Sézary cells may be seen in the peripheral blood of patients with benign dermatoses and the clinical and histological picture may not be specific. Confirmation of peripheral blood involvement is therefore a prerequisite for definitive diagnosis, and at least one of the following criteria must be fulfilled: (1) an absolute Sézary count of ≥1000/μL, and/or (2) a CD4:CD8 ratio of ≥10 due to an increase in circulating $CD4^+$ T-cells, and/or (3) an aberrant T-cell phenotype defined as $CD4^+/CD7^-$ T cells ≥40% or $CD4^+/CD26^-$ T cells ≥30%.[1,2] Although related to mycosis fungoides (MF), it is considered a separate entity due to differences in ontogeny and clinical behavior. Therefore, use of the imprecise and inconsistently applied term Cutaneous T-cell Lymphoma (CTCL) as a collective surrogate for both SS and MF should be discontinued. CTCL should only be employed as a generic term to encompass all types of cutaneous T-cell lymphoma as a whole.

Synonyms

None.

Epidemiology

Sézary syndrome is a disease of adults, most patients are aged >60 years at presentation, with a slight male predominance. While MF represents the most common form of CTCL, Sézary syndrome is rare. The relative incidence of Sézary syndrome globally remains stable at 3% with a slightly increased incidence noted in Europe[3]; but, in general, there are limited data on the incidence and disease prevalence.

General Clinical Features

Sézary syndrome develops de novo acutely or subacutely. Putative, rare cases preceded by classic MF are best considered erythrodermic variants of MF. It should also be noted that erythroderma is not specific for Sézary syndrome or advanced-stage MF; it may also be seen in association with other lymphomas that involve peripheral blood (eg, T-prolymphocytic leukemia, adult T-cell leukemia/lymphoma) as well as reactive dermatoses such as psoriasis, atopic and contact dermatitis, and drug reactions. Common clinical features of Sézary syndrome include variable degrees of erythema and, in severe presentations, generalized erythroderma with keratoderma and secondary fissures of the palmoplantar surfaces, alopecia, onychodystrophy, and blepharoconjunctivitis and ectropion[1] (Figures 101.1 and 101.2). Pruritus is a debilitating symptom that significantly impairs quality of life. Notably, erythroderma may not be the presenting sign of Sézary syndrome, resulting in a mean diagnostic delay of 5 years. Therefore, early disease should be considered as a differential diagnosis in nonerythrodermic dermatitis that fails to respond to standard therapy.[4]

Morphology

The histopathologic features are similar to those seen in MF with the exception that epidermotropism, Pautrier microabscesses/Darier nests, and haloed lymphocytes are less prominent features in Sézary syndrome (Figure 101.3) and up to a third of skin biopsies may demonstrate nonspecific findings.[5,6] Thus, distinction between MF and Sézary syndrome and between Sézary syndrome and erythroderma secondary to inflammatory dermatoses based on histopathologic features alone is challenging. Enlarged lymph nodes typically show features of dermatopathic lymphadenopathy. Involvement by Sézary syndrome ranges from small collections of Sézary cells to more extensive effacement of architecture by a relatively monotonous infiltrate of neoplastic T cells. Bone marrow may be involved, but

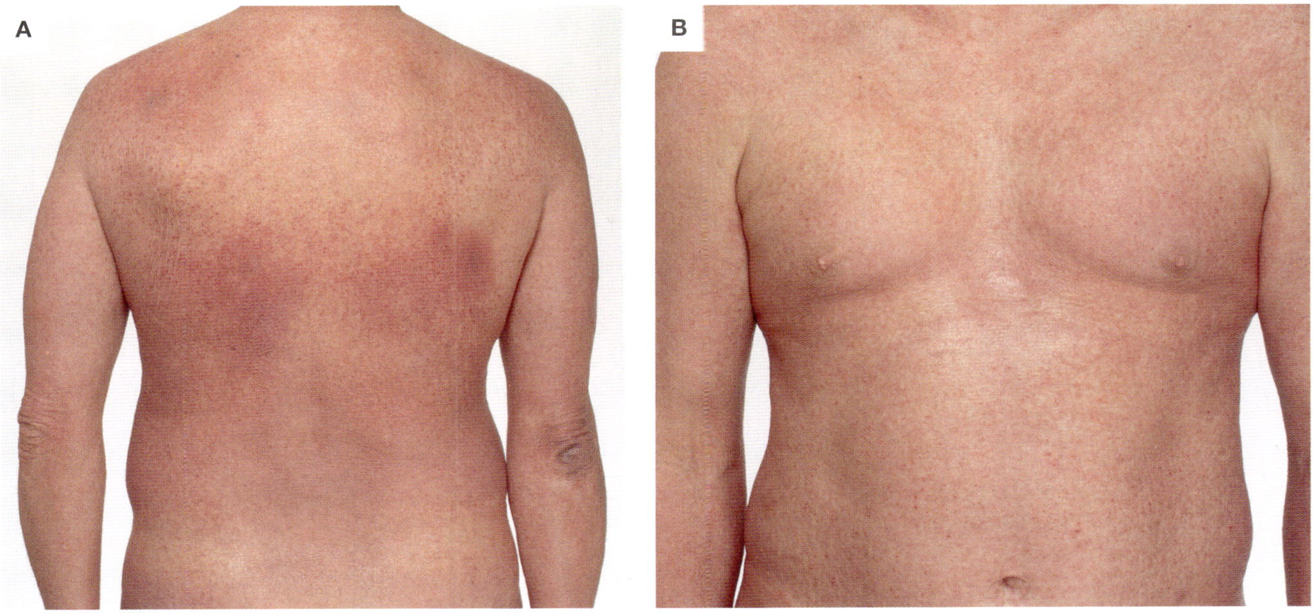

FIGURE 101.1 Sézary syndrome. Erythroderma (>80% body surface area involvement) of the **(A)** posterior and **(B)** anterior torso.

neoplastic cells are often sparse and usually distributed in an interstitial fashion.

Immunophenotype

Sézary syndrome cells are mature TCR-α/β helper T cells that demonstrate an immunophenotypic profile similar to that of MF. The clonal T cells are $CD3^+$, $CD4^+$, and $CD8^-$ with frequent aberrant loss of pan T-cell markers including CD2, CD3, CD4, CD5, CD7, and/or CD26 (Figure 101.4). CD7 and/or CD26 loss is most commonly observed.[7] Almost all cases express PD1 (see Figure 101.4), and there is frequent reactivity with antibodies to CD25, ICOS, and less commonly CXCL13. Sézary cells also express cutaneous lymphocyte antigen and the skin homing receptors CCR4 and CCR7.

Genetics

T-cell receptor genes are clonally rearranged. Complex numerical and structural changes similar to those found in MF are encountered. Detailed analysis of the genetic, epigenetic, and transcriptional changes in Sézary syndrome have demonstrated recurrent alterations in genes implicated in epigenetic remodeling, cell cycle regulation, DNA damage repair, JAK-STAT signaling, and NF-kappa B activation, generating insights into disease pathogenesis and uncovering new therapeutic targets.[8]

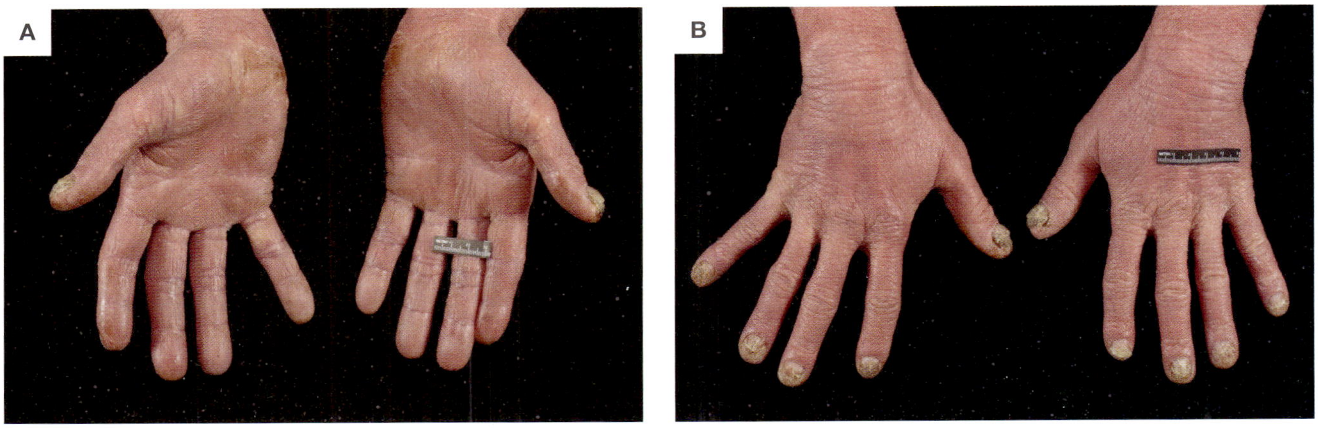

FIGURE 101.2 Sézary syndrome. **A:** Palmar keratoderma. **B:** Onychodystrophy of fingernails.

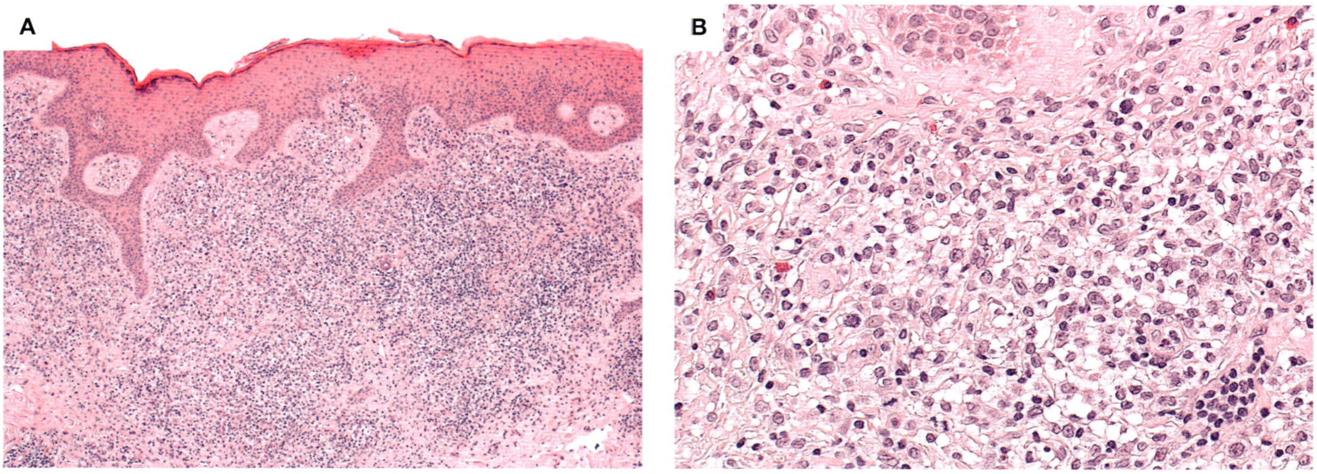

FIGURE 101.3 Sézary syndrome. **A:** Low-power view showing prominent dermal infiltrate with little or no epidermotropism. **B:** The infiltrate consists of a relatively uniform population of intermediate-size lymphocytes with irregular nuclear contours. (Images courtesy of Dr JR Goodlad.)

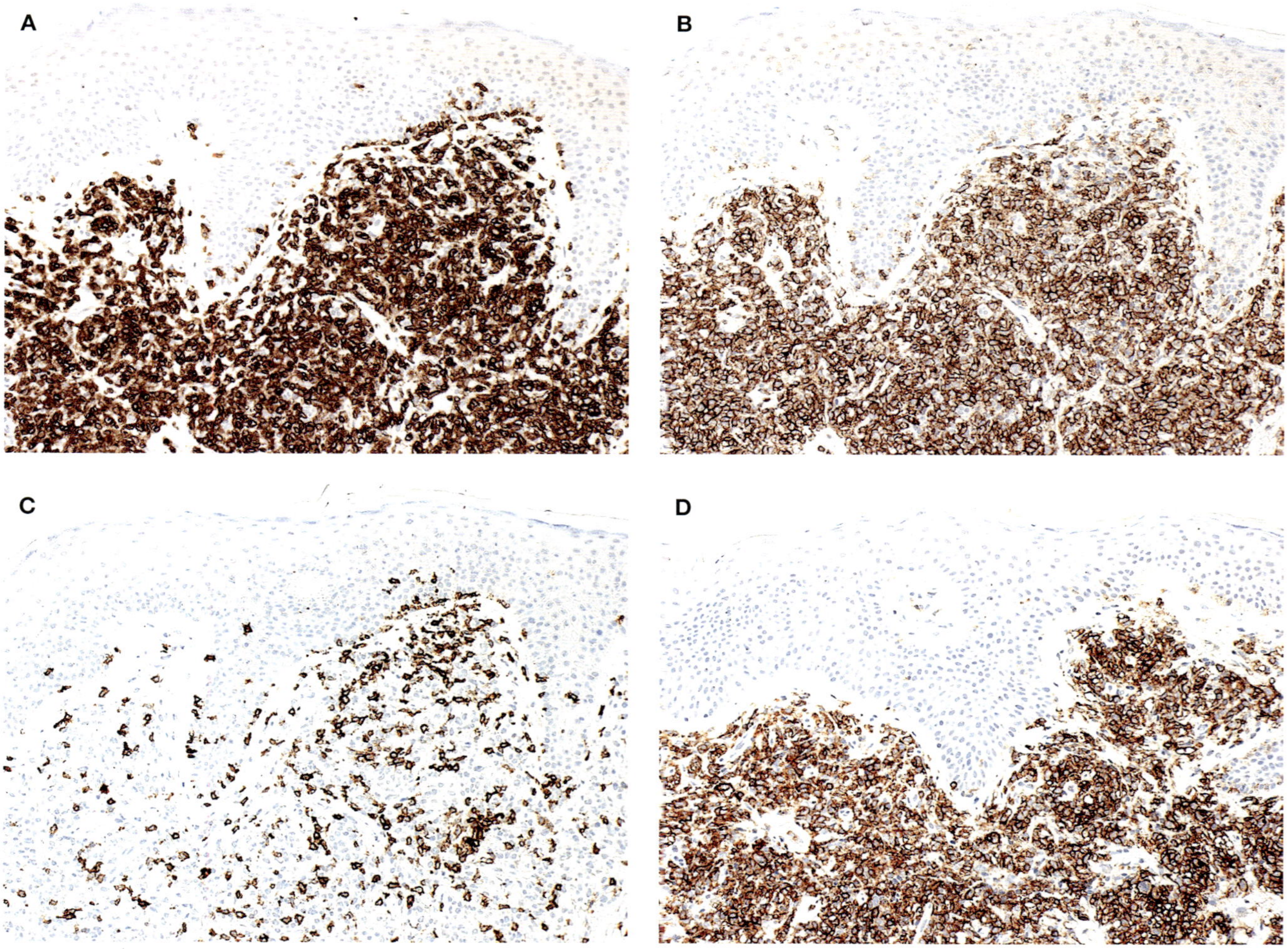

FIGURE 101.4 Sézary syndrome, immunophenotype. **A:** The neoplastic lymphoid cells express CD3. **B:** They are also positive for CD4. **C:** Loss of CD7, as in this case, is typical. **D:** Strong uniform expression of PD1 is also the norm and can be a clue to the diagnosis. (Images courtesy of Dr JR Goodlad.)

Prognosis and Clinical Comment

Sézary syndrome is an aggressive disease with a median survival of 32 months. Outcome is related to staging according to the same International Society for Cutaneous Lymphoma and European Organization for Research and Treatment of Cancer system as used for MF (see Table 100.2, Chapter 100, p. 678). Adverse prognostic factors for patients with late-stage disease include male gender, age >60 years, stage B1/B2 or N2/N3 disease, and visceral disease, with 10-year overall survival of 53.2% for low-risk patients and 15% for high-risk patients (three to five risk factors).[9] Health-related quality of life measures in CTCL are adversely affected especially in newly diagnosed women with MF or Sézary syndrome and in those with alopecia.[10]

References

1. Willemze R, Cerroni L, Kempf W, et al. The 2018 update of the WHO-EORTC classification for primary cutaneous lymphomas. *Blood*. 2019;133(16):1703-1714.
2. Vonderheid E, Bernengo MG, Burg G, et al. Update on erythrodermic cutaneous T-cell lymphoma: report of the International Society for cutaneous lymphomas. *J Am Acad Dermatol*. 2002;46(1):95-106.
3. Dobos G, Pohrt A, Ram-Wolff C, et al. Epidemiology of cutaneous T-cell lymphomas: a systematic review and meta-analysis of 16,953 patients. *Cancers*. 2020;12(10):2921.
4. Mangold A, Thompson A, Davis MD, et al. Early clinical manifestations of Sezary syndrome: a multicenter retrospective cohort study. *J Am Acad Dermatol*. 2017;77(4):719-727.
5. Trotter MF, Whitaker SJ, Orchard GE, Smith NP. Cutaneous histopathology of Sezary syndrome: a study of 41 cases with a proven circulating T-cell clone. *J Cutan Pathol*. 1997;24(5):286-291.
6. Burg G, Kempf W, Cozzio A, et al. WHO/EORTC classification of cutaneous lymphomas 2005: histological and molecular aspects. *J Cutan Pathol*. 2005;32(10):647-674.
7. Hristov A, Tejasvi T, Wilcox RA. Mycosis fungoides and Sézary syndrome: 2019 update on diagnosis, risk-stratification, and management. *Am J Hematol*. 2019;94(9):1027-1041. 1-27-1041.
8. Tensen CP, Quint KD, Vermeer MH. Genetic and epigenetic insights into cutaneous T-cell lymphoma. *Blood*. 2022;139(1):15-33.
9. Benton EC, Crichton S, Talpur R, et al. A cutaneous lymphoma international prognostic index (CLIPi) for mycosis fungoides and Sezary syndrome. *Eur J cancer*. 2013;49(13):2859-2868.
10. Molloy K, Jonak C, Woei-A-Jin FJSH, et al. Characteristics associated with significantly worse quality of life in mycosis fundgoides/Sezary syndrome from the Prospective Cutaneous Lymphoma International Prognostic Index (PROCLIPI) study. *Br J Dermatol*. 202(182):541-542.

Chapter 102
Primary Cutaneous CD30-Positive T-Cell Lymphoproliferative Disorders

Andrew L. Feldman and Lorenzo Cerroni

Primary cutaneous CD30-positive T-cell lymphoproliferative disorders (pcCD30^{+} T-LPDs) encompass a spectrum of neoplastic T-cell proliferations arising primarily in the skin. This spectrum includes lymphomatoid papulosis (LyP), primary cutaneous anaplastic large cell lymphoma (pcALCL), and borderline cases with intermediate features. There are diverse and sometimes overlapping histological and immunophenotypic findings, and correlation with the clinical presentation and course is essential for accurate diagnosis. Cases of mycosis fungoides (MF) expressing CD30, with or without histological transformation, are specifically excluded from this group. In addition, pcCD30^{+} T-LPDs must be distinguished from benign cutaneous infectious or inflammatory processes, as well as from secondary cutaneous involvement by systemic CD30-positive T-cell lymphomas, particularly ALCL.

LYMPHOMATOID PAPULOSIS

Definition

LyP is a chronic, indolent primary cutaneous T-LPD characterized by recurrent, self-healing skin lesions. It comprises at least six pathologic subtypes with varying pathological and genetic features.

Synonyms

None.

Epidemiology

LyP is predominantly a disease of adults, with a median age of 45 years, although pediatric cases have been reported.[1-4] The male:female ratio is 2 to 3:1. The cause of LyP is unknown. In some patients, LyP occurs before, during, or after another lymphoma such as ALCL, Hodgkin lymphoma, or particularly MF.[5,6]

General Clinical Features

Depending on subtype, LyP presents with crops of papular or papulonodular skin lesions, sometimes with necrosis (Figure 102.1).[1-3] The lesions may be few or numerous. Individual lesions typically show different stages of development and generally resolve several weeks to several months after appearing, sometimes with residual scarring. The lesions most often affect the trunk and extremities and occasionally involve the oral or genital mucosa in addition to the skin.

Morphology

The histologic features of LyP vary markedly by subtype (Table 102.1).[1,2] In addition, the appearance differs depending on the stage of development of the individual lesion.

Type A LyP is the most common subtype seen (>80%). There is typically a wedge-shaped dermal infiltrate containing scattered or occasionally clustered large atypical lymphoid cells in a background of small lymphocytes, histiocytes, and acute inflammatory cells (Figure 102.2). Eosinophils are commonly found. The large cells may be multinucleated or Reed-Sternberg-like. Occasionally, there may be epidermotropism. The lesions may resemble those of classic Hodgkin lymphoma.

Type B LyP is rare (<5%) and shows histological features resembling plaque-stage MF (Figure 102.3). Cerebriform cells are typically present, and there is epidermotropism. Large transformed cells are typically absent. The upper dermis is often involved by a band-like or perivascular dermal infiltrate. Reactive immune cells are typically sparse. Distinction from MF relies on the clinical presentation and course.

Type C LyP (about 10%) shows sheets or prominent clusters of atypical lymphoid cells in the dermis with relatively few admixed reactive cells (Figure 102.4). The tumor cells account for >50% of the infiltrate. They are medium-sized to large, and hallmark-like cells may

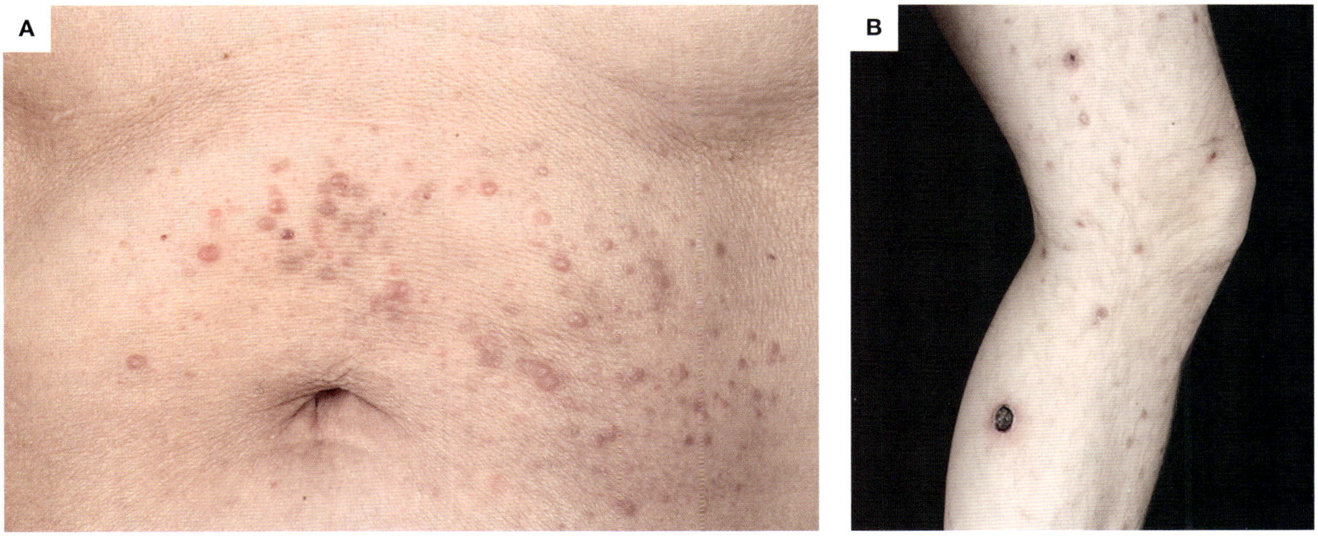

FIGURE 102.1 Clinical appearance of lymphomatoid papulosis. Examples from two patients are shown.

TABLE 102.1 Features of the subtypes of lymphomatoid papulosis

Subtype	Relative frequency	Histologic features	Phenotype	Differential diagnosis
LyP, type A	>80%	Wedge-shaped dermal infiltrate containing scattered large cells in a mixed inflammatory background	$CD4^+/CD8^-$; $CD30^+$; cytotox±	CHL, pcALCL, MF (tumor stage)
LyP, type B	<5%	Epidermotropic infiltrate of small to medium-sized lymphocytes with cerebriform nuclei	$CD4^+/CD8^-$; $CD30^{+a}$; cytotox−	MF (plaque stage)
LyP, type C	10%	Nodular dermal proliferation of large transformed cells	$CD4^+/CD8^-$; $CD30^+$; cytotox±	pcALCL, transformed MF
LyP, type D	<5%	Epidermotropic infiltrate of medium-sized lymphocytes with ulceration	$CD4^-/CD8^+$; $CD30^+$; cytotox+	CD8+ aggressive epidermotropic TCL, PLEVA
LyP, type E	<5%	Angiocentric infiltrate of pleomorphic lymphocytes with necrosis	$CD4^-/CD8^+$; $CD30^+$; cytotox±	Benign necroulcerative diseases (eg, vasculitides); angiocentric/angiodestructive lymphomas
LyP with *DUSP22*-R	<5%	Nodular dermal proliferation of large transformed cells with epidermotropic infiltrate of smaller lymphocytes	$CD4^-/CD8^+$ or $CD4^-/CD8^-$; $CD30^+$, biphasic; cytotox−	Transformed MF

CHL, classic Hodgkin lymphoma; cytotox, cytotoxic markers (TIA-1, granzyme B, and/or perforin); LyP, lymphomatoid papulosis; MF, mycosis fungoides; pcALCL, primary cutaneous anaplastic large cell lymphoma; PLEVA, pityriasis lichenoides et varioliformis acuta; R, rearrangement; TCL, T-cell lymphoma.

[a]Older reports considered LyP, type B, a CD30-negative variant; however, these cases are always positive with standard, modern immunohistochemical techniques, although the positivity may be weak.

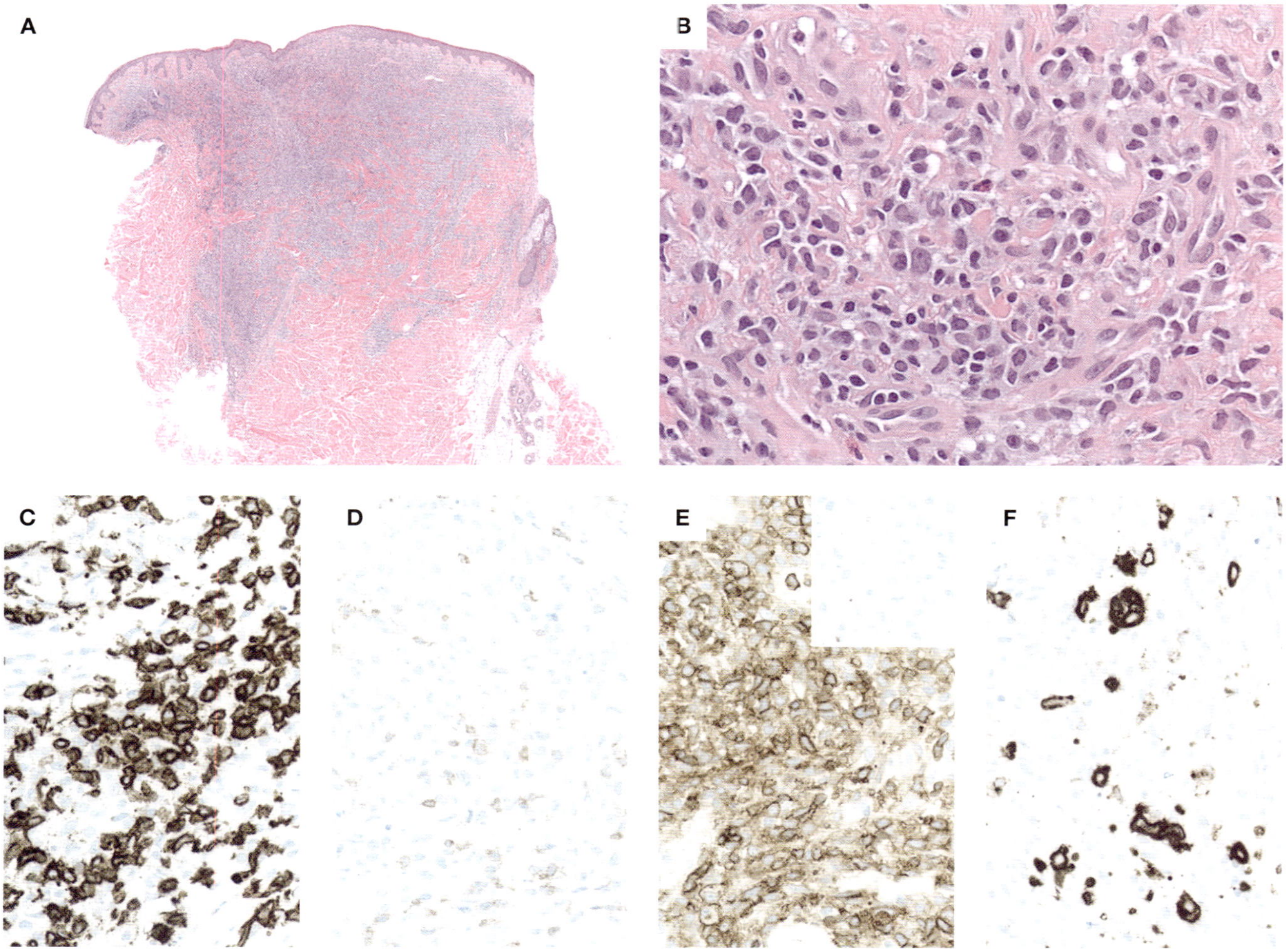

FIGURE 102.2 Type A lymphomatoid papulosis. **A:** Biopsy of a papule on the back shows a wedge-shaped dermal infiltrate. **B:** The infiltrate contains medium-sized to large atypical lymphocytes in a background of small lymphocytes, histiocytes, and occasional eosinophils. **C:** The tumor cells are positive for CD3. **D:** They show loss of CD7 expression. **E:** CD4 stains the tumor cells and background histiocytes. The tumor cells are negative for CD8 (inset). **F:** CD30 highlights a subset of the atypical cells.

be seen. Epidermotropism may be present but is not the dominant feature. The lesion may show ulceration. Distinction from pcALCL relies on the clinical presentation and course.

Type D LyP is rare (<5%). The neoplastic cells show marked epidermotropism and are typically medium in size, slightly larger than those seen in most cases of type B LyP (Figure 102.5). Large transformed cells are typically absent. There is often epidermal hyperplasia with a pagetoid appearance. There is a varying degree of dermal involvement. The features may mimic $CD8^+$ aggressive epidermotropic T-cell lymphoma.[7]

Type E LyP is also rare (<5%) and shows an angiocentric or angioinvasive dermal infiltrate of pleomorphic lymphocytes, which may be associated with angiodestruction, necrosis, hemorrhage, and/or overlying ulceration (Figure 102.6).[8] Acute inflammatory cells are typically admixed. There may be epidermotropism and/or extension into the subcutaneous fat. Lesions typically progress from papulonodular to papulonecrotic and may coalesce to form larger areas of ulceration with eschar formation.

LyP with *DUSP22* rearrangement (R) also is rare (<5%). It tends to occur in an older age group than the other subtypes, mostly in males.[9] It typically presents with only a single site of involvement, showing papulonodular lesions without ulceration. Histologically, it shows a characteristic biphasic pattern (Figure 102.7), with a sheet-like or nodular infiltrate of medium-sized to large transformed lymphocytes in the dermis and an epidermotropic component of small to medium-sized lymphocytes, sometimes including Pautrier-like microabscesses. These features can mimic transformed MF or pcALCL.

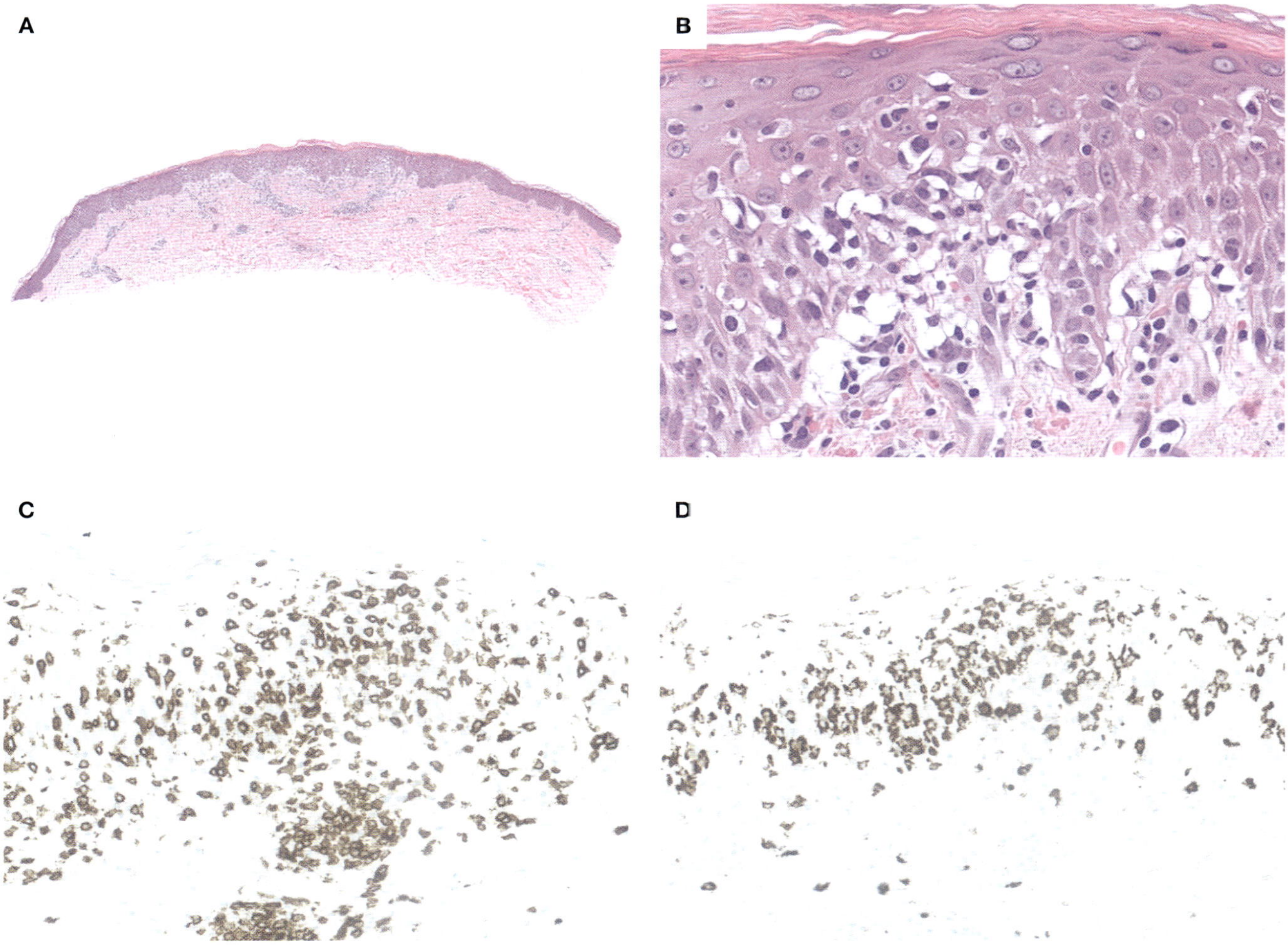

FIGURE 102.3 Type B lymphomatoid papulosis. **A:** Biopsy of a papule on the wrist shows an infiltrate in the upper dermis. **B:** There is epidermotropism of small atypical lymphocytes. The epidermotropic infiltrate is positive for CD3 **(C)** and CD30 **(D)**. The epidermotropic T cells also expressed CD4, CD5, and TCR-β (not shown).

Immunophenotype

The neoplastic cells in most LyP subtypes consistently express CD30, with the exception that CD30 expression in type B may be weaker. Types A, B, and C are typically $CD4^+$ T-LPDs (Figures 102.2-102.4), while types D and E are typically $CD8^+$ and express cytotoxic markers (Figures 102.5 and 102.6). LyP with *DUSP22*-R tends to be $CD8^+$ or double negative for CD4/CD8. These cases often show a biphasic pattern of CD30 expression, with strong expression in the dermal tumor component and weak expression in the epidermotropic component (Figure 102.7). The phenotype of types A and C LyP is similar to that of pcALCL and systemic ALK-negative ALCL. LyP typically either expresses T-cell receptor (TCR)-β or is TCR silent, but cases with a γδ phenotype have been reported (Figure 102.8).[10]

Genetics

The T-cell receptor genes are clonally rearranged in most cases and may show the same rearrangement as other T-cell lymphomas occurring in the same patient (eg, MF or pcALCL).[11] Mutations have been reported in epigenetic modifying genes, including *SETD2*, *KMT2A*, *KMT2D*, and *CREBBP*.[12] Gene fusions involving *TYK2* or *JAK2* and mutations of *STAT5A*, *DNMT3A*, and *PLCG1* have been identified in both LyP and MF lesions occurring in the same patient.[13]

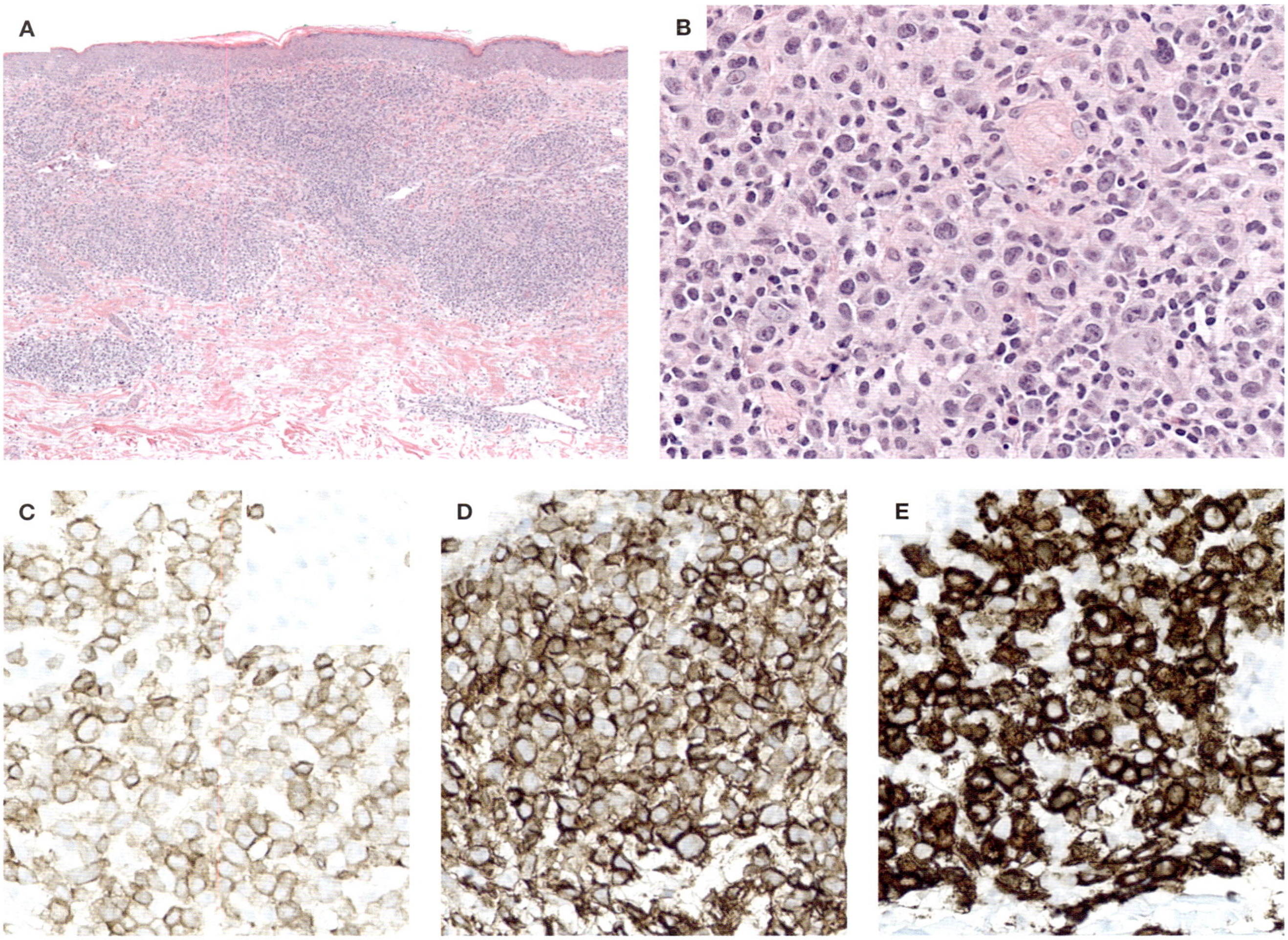

FIGURE 102.4 Type C lymphomatoid papulosis. **A:** Biopsy of a lesion on the arm shows a nodular infiltrate in the mid- to upper dermis without epidermotropism. **B:** The infiltrate contains sheets of medium-sized to large atypical lymphocytes. **C:** The atypical cells show weak expression of CD5 and aberrant loss of CD3 (inset). They are strongly and uniformly positive for CD4 **D:** and CD30 (**E**).

In addition, different genetic alterations have been observed in distinct lesions from a patient with clonally related LyP and ALCL, suggesting divergent evolution of a common precursor.[14] Rearrangements of the *TYK2* tyrosine kinase gene have been reported in a subset of patients with LyP occurring in isolation.[15] By definition, LyP with *DUSP22*-R shows rearrangement of the *DUSP22* locus on 6p25.5[9]; this alteration is not specific for LyP and is also seen in 20% to 30% of pcALCL (see later discussion) and systemic ALK-negative ALCL.

Prognosis and Clinical Comment

The lesions of LyP regress spontaneously and the prognosis is excellent, regardless of pathological subtype.[3,5] Rare deaths have been reported attributable to associated lymphomas, and long-term follow-up is recommended.[6] Local treatment may alleviate symptoms but systemic therapy is not typically required.

PRIMARY CUTANEOUS ANAPLASTIC LARGE CELL LYMPHOMA

Definition

pcALCL is a primary cutaneous T-cell lymphoma with pathological features resembling systemic ALK-negative ALCL but with initial presentation in the skin. CD30 is expressed in >75% of the neoplastic cells. Cases corresponding to transformed MF with extensive CD30 expression are excluded.

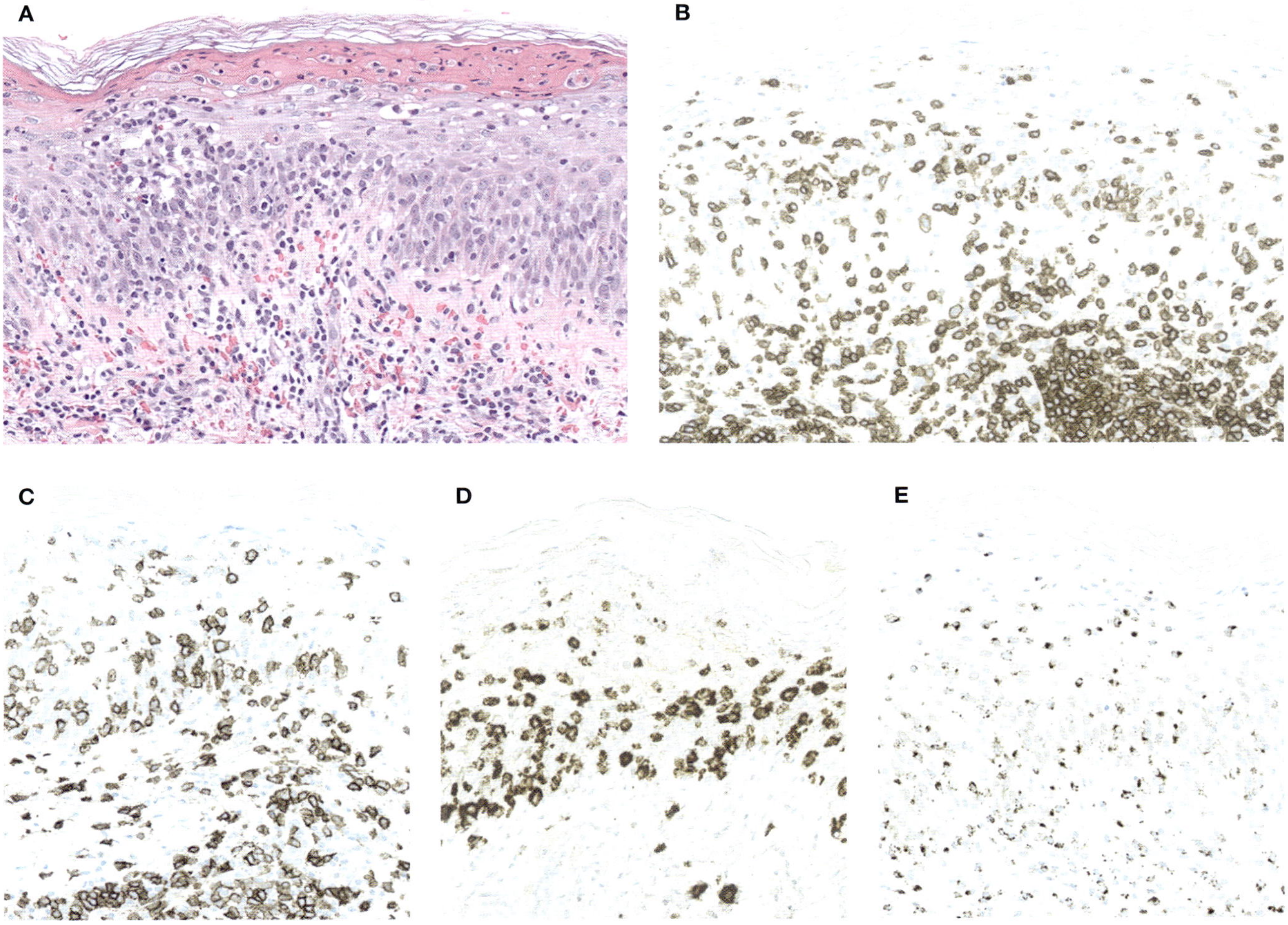

FIGURE 102.5 Type D lymphomatoid papulosis. **A:** Biopsy of a papule on the thigh shows a superficial dermal infiltrate with epidermotropism. The epidermis is hyperplastic. **B:** Antibodies to CD3 highlight the epidermotropism. The tumor cells are positive for CD8 **(C)**, CD30 **(D)**, and the cytotoxic marker TIA1 **(E)**. The tumor cells also expressed TCR-β and showed diminished expression of CD7 (not shown).

Synonyms

None.

Epidemiology

pcALCL is predominantly a tumor of adults, with a median age of 60 years.[3,5] The male:female ratio is 2 to 3:1. It is the third most common pcCD30$^+$ T-LPD (after MF and LyP). Patients may have coexistent pcALCL and LyP. While it has been suggested that pcALCL should not be diagnosed when there is clinical evidence or a history of MF, other data suggest that MF and pcALCL may coexist in some patients.[16] The cause of pcALCL is unknown.

General Clinical Features

Patients typically present with solitary or clustered localized skin nodules, frequently with ulceration (Figure 102.9).[2,3,5,17] The most common sites are the trunk, face, and extremities. About 20% of patients present with multifocal lesions. Locoregional lymph node involvement is seen in about 10% of patients, but widespread dissemination is very rare. Although spontaneous complete regression may be seen, this finding is more characteristic of LyP. Partial regression, however, is not rare.

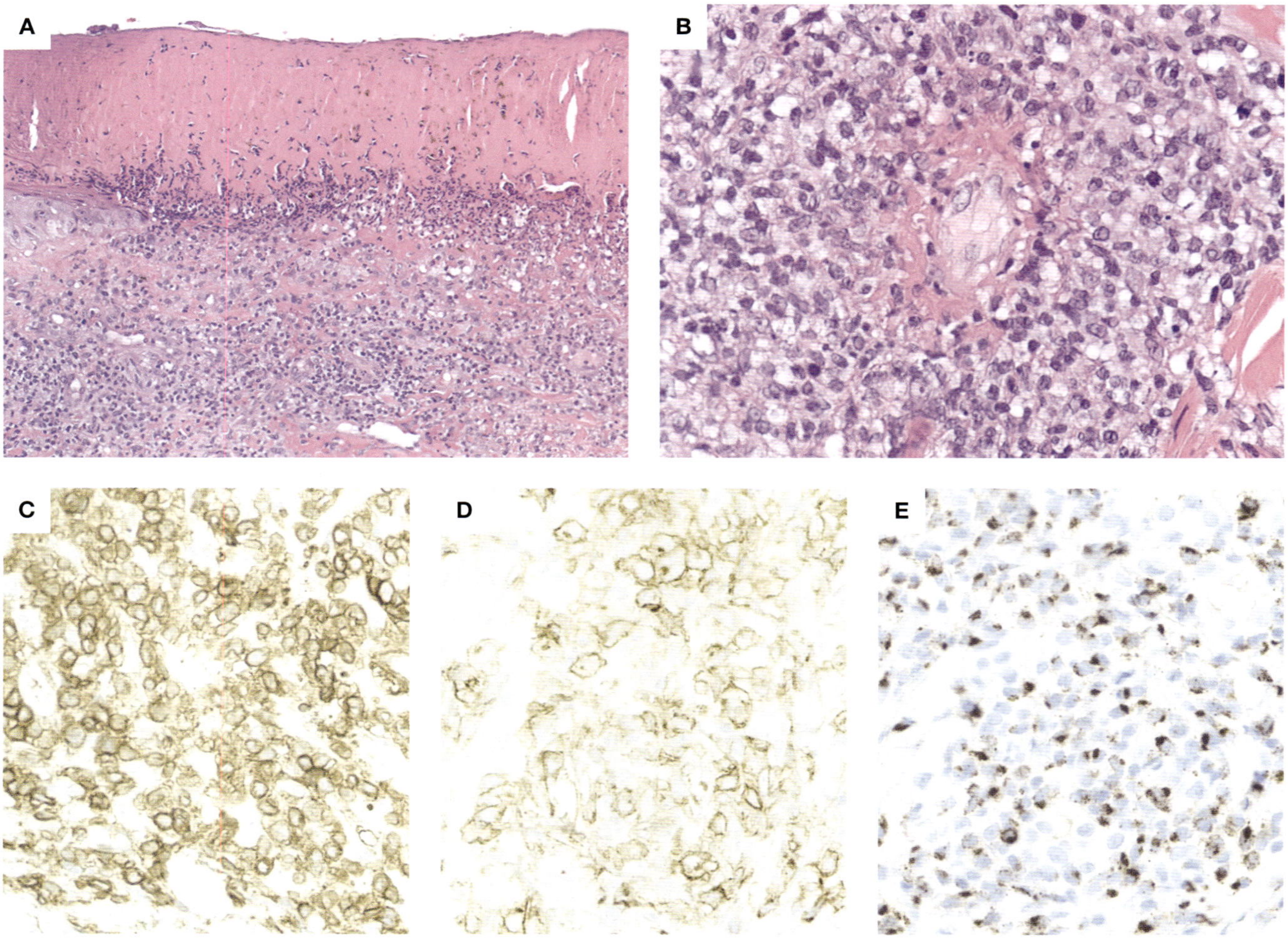

FIGURE 102.6 Type E lymphomatoid papulosis. **A:** Biopsy of a nodule on the leg shows a dermal infiltrate with epidermal necrosis. **B:** The infiltrate consists of medium-sized, atypical lymphocytes with accompanying angiodestruction. The tumor cells are positive for CD3 **(C)**, CD30 **(D)**, and the cytotoxic marker granzyme B **(E)**. The tumor cells showed loss of CD7 expression and diminished expression of CD2 (not shown).

Morphology

Tumors are composed of medium-sized to large cells with nuclear pleomorphism, including hallmark cells (Figure 102.10).[17] Most commonly, these diffusely infiltrate the dermis with varying admixed numbers of reactive inflammatory cells, including small lymphocytes, histiocytes, and/or acute inflammatory cells, particularly eosinophils. Intralymphatic involvement is common.[18] There may be extension into the subcutaneous fat. Overlying ulceration is common, and cases with a prominent inflammatory component often show epidermal hyperplasia. An epidermotropic component also may be seen, particularly in cases with *DUSP22*-R (Figure 102.11; see also later discussion).

Immunophenotype

By definition, all cases express CD30 in >75%of tumor cells (see Figure 102.10).[3,5,17] They should lack expression of ALK, although cases with otherwise similar clinical and pathological features but expressing ALK have been reported.[19,20] Because these rare cases remain incompletely understood, careful clinical correlation is recommended for the management of ALK-positive pcCD30$^+$ T-LPDs.[2] pcALCL has an immunophenotype similar to systemic ALCL, including a predominance of CD4 expression over CD8 expression; variable loss of pan-T-cell antigens such as CD2, CD3, CD5, and CD7; and frequent expression of cytotoxic markers such as TIA1, granzyme B, and perforin. Cases with *DUSP22*-R (see later discussion) typically express the

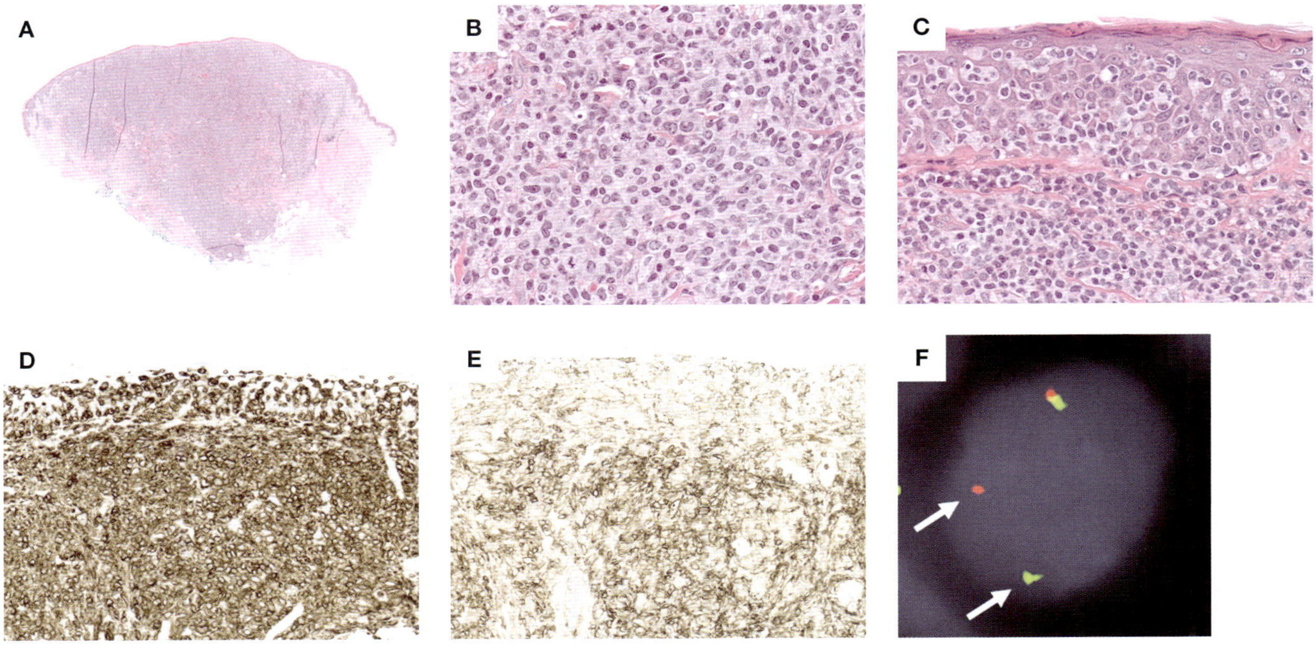

FIGURE 102.7 Lymphomatoid papulosis with *DUSP22* (6p25.3) rearrangement. **A:** Biopsy of a papular lesion from the antecubital fossa shows a wedge-shaped dermal infiltrate. **B:** The dermis contains a population of medium-sized to large transformed lymphoid cells. **C:** There is marked epidermotropism by a population of smaller lymphocytes. **D:** Antibodies to CD3 highlight the marked epidermotropism. **E:** CD30 is positive and shows a biphasic staining pattern, with stronger expression in the dermis and weaker expression in the epidermis. **F:** Fluorescence in situ hybridization shows a *DUSP22* rearrangement, characterized by separation of the red and green probes flanking the *DUSP22/IRF4* locus on 6p25.3 (arrows). The tumor cells also expressed CD2 and TCR-β and were negative for CD4, CD5, CD7, CD8, and ALK (not shown).

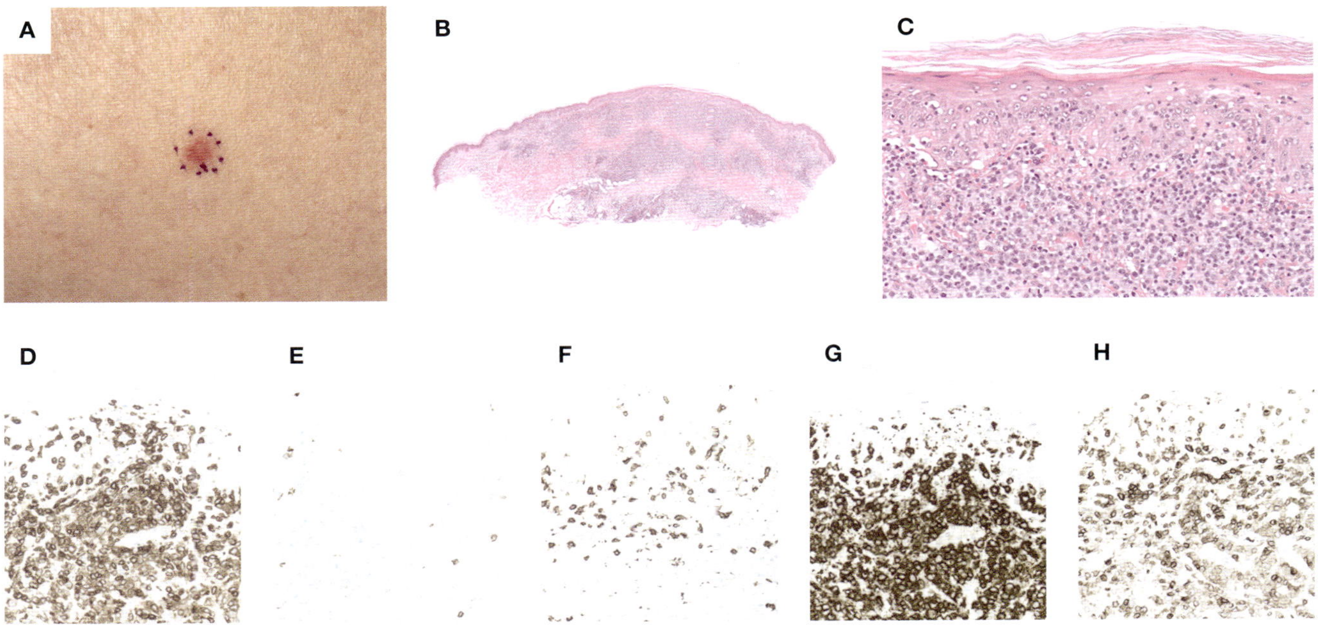

FIGURE 102.8 Lymphomatoid papulosis with a γδ phenotype. **A:** Papular lesion on the thigh. **B:** The dermis contains a nodular lymphoid infiltrate. **C:** The tumor cells are small to medium in size and show epidermotropism. **D:** Antibodies to CD3 highlight the epidermotropism. (**E:** CD5 is negative. **F:** Anti-CD8 stains rare cells. **G:** The tumor cells show strong and uniform expression of CD30. **H:** TCR-δ is positive. The tumor cells were negative for CD2, CD5, CD7, and TCR-β (not shown). This case had a *DUSP22* rearrangement.

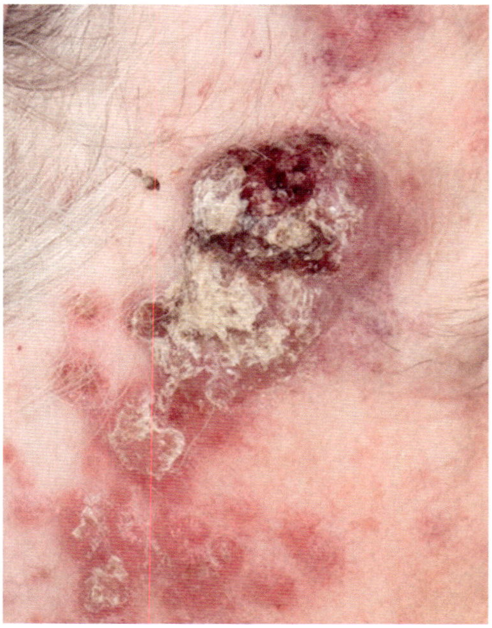

FIGURE 102.9 Clinical appearance of primary cutaneous anaplastic large cell lymphoma. There is an ulcerated tumor mass on the right temple with multiple small satellite lesions.

T-cell transcription factor LEF1 and lack cytotoxic marker expression (Figure 102.11).[21]

Genetics

The TCR genes are clonally rearranged in most cases.[3,17] Recurrent mutations in pcALCL involve the epigenetic modifying genes mutated in LyP (see earlier discussion), as well as mutations in *STAT3*.[12,22] *DUSP22*-R is seen in up to 30% of pcALCL, similar to systemic ALK-negative ALCL; this finding presently has no known clinical significance in pcALCL. Occasional rearrangements of *TP63* or *TYK2* have been reported.[15,23] Although experience is limited, pcALCL with *TP63*-R may behave aggressively. As discussed earlier, *ALK*-R may be seen in cases with clinicopathologic features of pcALCL but should be kept separate until more data are available. Deletions of *PRDM1* and *TNFRSF14* and gains of *EZH2* and *TNFRSF8* (encoding CD30) also have been reported.[24]

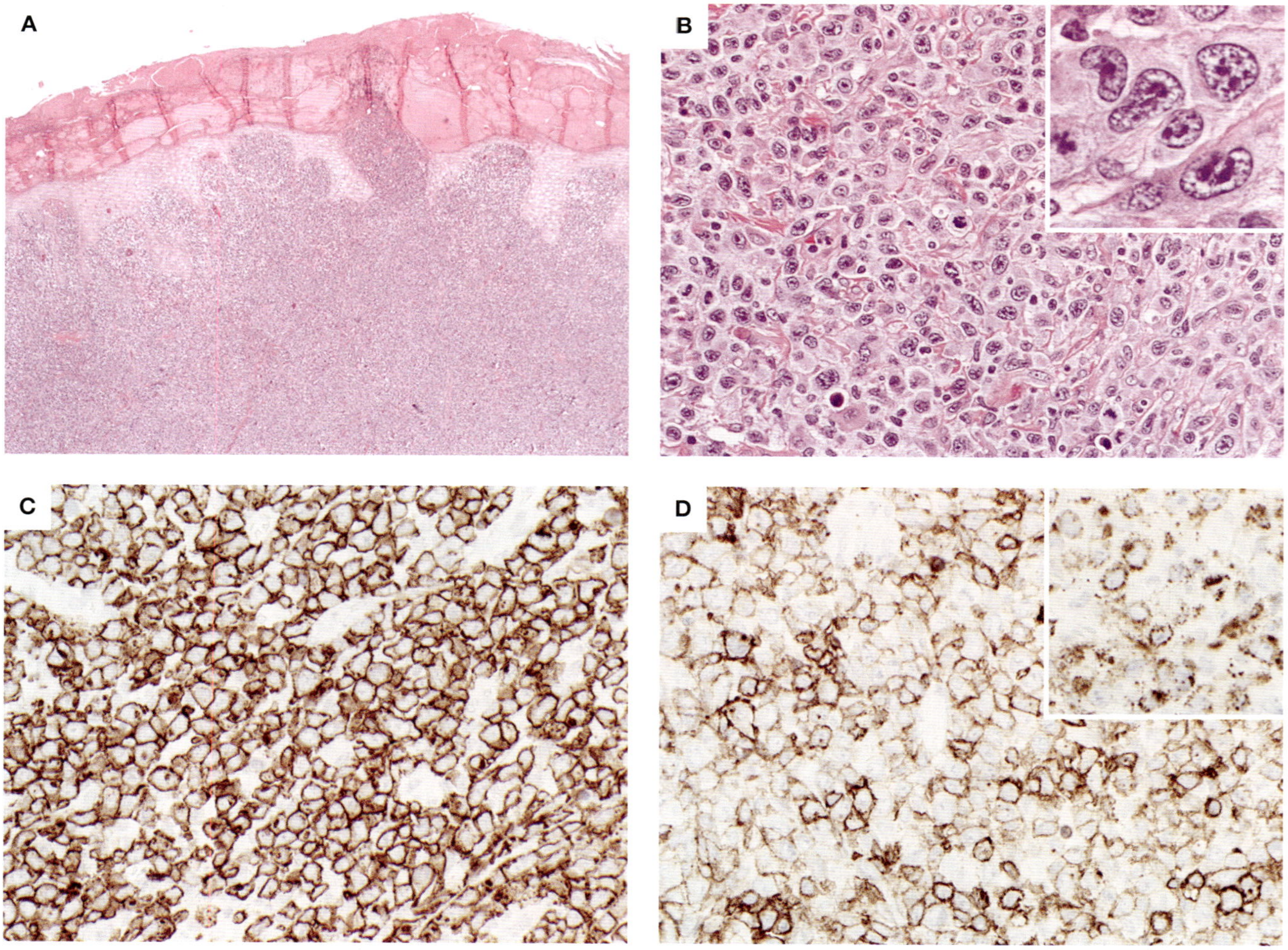

FIGURE 102.10 Primary cutaneous anaplastic large cell lymphoma. **A:** Biopsy of a thigh lesion shows the dermis to be extensively involved by sheets of tumor cells. The epidermis shows hyperkeratosis. **B:** The tumor cells are large and include hallmark cells (inset). **C:** The tumor cells are strongly and uniformly positive for CD30. **D:** They express CD2 (variable intensity) and the cytotoxic marker TIA1 (inset). They also expressed CD4 and granzyme B and were negative for CD3, CD5, CD8, and ALK (not shown).

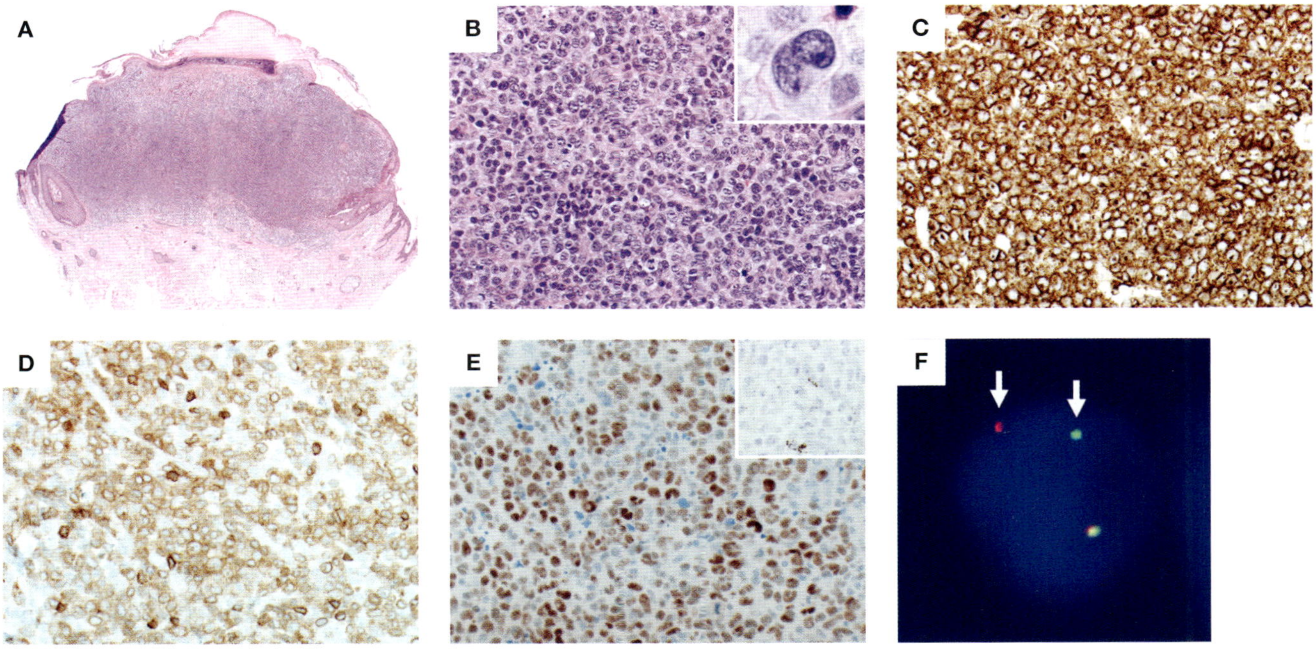

FIGURE 102.11 Primary cutaneous ALCL with *DUSP22* rearrangement. **A:** Biopsy of a forehead lesion shows a nodular growth pattern with hyperkeratosis and a diffuse dermal infiltrate. **B:** The infiltrate consists of sheets of medium-sized to large cells, including hallmark cells (inset). **C:** The tumor cells show strong and uniform expression of CD30. **D:** They are weakly positive for CD3 (compared with strong expression in background small reactive T cells). **E:** The tumor cells are positive for the transcription factor LEF1 and negative for the cytotoxic marker TIA1 (inset). **F:** Fluorescence in situ hybridization shows a *DUSP22* rearrangement, characterized by separation of the red and green probes flanking the *DUSP22/IRF4* locus on 6p25.3 (arrows). The tumor cells were also positive for CD2, CD45, and TCR-β and negative for CD4, CD5, CD7, CD8, granzyme B, and ALK (not shown).

Prognosis and Clinical Comment

The prognosis of pcALCL is generally good, with a 5-year disease-specific survival rate of 86% to 96%.[3,5,25] Patients with locoregional lymph node involvement have outcomes similar to those with disease limited to the skin. A variant with extensive involvement of the lower limbs has a worse prognosis. Treatment typically consists of local therapy, including resection and/or radiation. Some patients may benefit from systemic therapy such as brentuximab vedotin and/or anthracycline-based chemotherapy.[5,25,26] Skin recurrences are common, but most do not herald more aggressive clinical behavior or widespread dissemination. The 5-year cumulative risk of developing systemic lymphoma/extracutaneous disease is 9% to 14%.[5,25]

References

1. Goodlad JR. The many faces of lymphomatoid papulosis. *Diagn Histopathol.* 2014;20(7):263-270.
2. Willemze R, Cerroni L, Kempf W, et al. The 2018 update of the WHO-EORTC classification for primary cutaneous lymphomas. *Blood.* 2019;133(16):1703-1714.
3. Goodlad JR, Cerroni L, Swerdlow SH. Recent advances in cutaneous lymphoma-implications for current and future classifications. *Virchows Arch.* 2023;482(1):281-298.
4. Wieser I, Wohlmuth C, Nunez CA, Duvic M. Lymphomatoid papulosis in children and adolescents: a systematic review. *Am J Clin Dermatol.* 2016;17(4):319-327.
5. Bekkenk MW, Geelen FA, van Voorst Vader PC, et al. Primary and secondary cutaneous CD30(+) lymphoproliferative disorders: a report from the Dutch Cutaneous Lymphoma Group on the long-term follow-up data of 219 patients and guidelines for diagnosis and treatment. *Blood.* 2000;95(12):3653-3661.
6. Melchers RC, Willemze R, Bekkenk MW, et al. Frequency and prognosis of associated malignancies in 504 patients with lymphomatoid papulosis. *J Eur Acad Dermatol Venereol.* 2020;34(2):260-266.
7. Saggini A, Gulia A, Argenyi Z, et al. A variant of lymphomatoid papulosis simulating primary cutaneous aggressive epidermotropic CD8+ cytotoxic T-cell lymphoma. Description of 9 cases. *Am J Surg Pathol.* 2010;34(8):1168-1175.
8. Kempf W, Kazakov DV, Scharer L, et al. Angioinvasive lymphomatoid papulosis: a new variant simulating aggressive lymphomas. *Am J Surg Pathol.* 2013;37(1):1-13.

9. Karai LJ, Kadin ME, Hsi ED, et al. Chromosomal rearrangements of 6p25.3 define a new subtype of lymphomatoid papulosis. *Am J Surg Pathol.* 2013;37(8):1173-1181.
10. Torres-Cabala CA, Huen A, Iyer SP, Miranda RN. Gamma/delta phenotype in primary cutaneous T-cell lymphomas and lymphoid proliferations: challenges for diagnosis and classification. *Surg Pathol Clin.* 2021;14(2):177-194.
11. de la Garza Bravo MM, Patel KP, Loghavi S, et al. Shared clonality in distinctive lesions of lymphomatoid papulosis and mycosis fungoides occurring in the same patients suggests a common origin. *Hum Pathol.* 2015;46(4):558-569.
12. Abdulla FR, Zhang W, Wu X, et al. Genomic analysis of cutaneous CD30-positive lymphoproliferative disorders. *JID Innov.* 2022;2(1):100068.
13. Wobser M, Roth S, Appenzeller S, et al. Oncogenic mutations and gene fusions in CD30-positive lymphoproliferations and clonally related mycosis fungoides occurring in the same patients. *JID Innov.* 2021;1(3):100034.
14. Xerri L, Adelaide J, Avenin M, et al. Common origin of sequential cutaneous CD30+ lymphoproliferations with nodal involvement evidenced by genome-wide clonal evolution. *Histopathology.* 2019;74(4):654-662.
15. Velusamy T, Kiel MJ, Sahasrabuddhe AA, et al. A novel recurrent NPM1-TYK2 gene fusion in cutaneous CD30-positive lymphoproliferative disorders. *Blood.* 2014;124(25):3768-3771.
16. Gao C, McCormack CJ, van der Weyden C, et al. The importance of differentiating between Mycosis Fungoides with CD30 positive large cell transformation and mycosis fungoides with co-existent primary cutaneous anaplastic large cell lymphoma. *J Am Acad Dermatol.* 2021;84(1):185-187.
17. Xing X, Feldman AL. Anaplastic large cell lymphomas: ALK positive, ALK negative, and primary cutaneous. *Adv Anat Pathol.* 2015;22(1):29-49.
18. Ferrara G, Ena L, Cota C, Cerroni L. Intralymphatic spread is a common finding in cutaneous CD30+ lymphoproliferative disorders. *Am J Surg Pathol.* 2015;39(11):1511-1517.
19. Oschlies I, Lisfeld J, Lamant L, et al. ALK-positive anaplastic large cell lymphoma limited to the skin: clinical, histopathological and molecular analysis of 6 pediatric cases. A report from the ALCL99 study. *Haematologica.* 2013;98(1):50-56.
20. Melchers RC, Willemze R, van de Loo M, et al. Clinical, histologic, and molecular characteristics of anaplastic lymphoma kinase-positive primary cutaneous anaplastic large cell lymphoma. *Am J Surg Pathol.* 2020;44(6):776-781.
21. Feldman AL, Oishi N, Ketterling RP, Ansell SM, Shi M, Dasari S. Immunohistochemical approach to genetic subtyping of anaplastic large cell lymphoma. *Am J Surg Pathol.* 2022;46(11):1490-1499.
22. Crescenzo R, Abate F, Lasorsa E, et al. Convergent mutations and kinase fusions lead to oncogenic STAT3 activation in anaplastic large cell lymphoma. *Cancer Cell.* 2015;27(4):516-532.
23. Vasmatzis G, Johnson SH, Knudson RA, et al. Genome-wide analysis reveals recurrent structural abnormalities of TP63 and other p53-related genes in peripheral T-cell lymphomas. *Blood.* 2012;120(11):2280-2289.
24. Bastidas Torres AN, Melchers RC, Van Grieken L, et al. Whole-genome profiling of primary cutaneous anaplastic large cell lymphoma. *Haematologica.* 2022;107(7):1619-1632.
25. Hapgood G, Pickles T, Sehn LH, et al. Outcome of primary cutaneous anaplastic large cell lymphoma: a 20-year British Columbia Cancer Agency experience. *Br J Haematol.* 2017;176(2):234-240.
26. Horwitz SM, Scarisbrick JJ, Dummer R, et al. Randomized phase 3 ALCANZA study of brentuximab vedotin vs physician's choice in cutaneous T-cell lymphoma: final data. *Blood Adv.* 2021;5(23):5098-5106.

Chapter 103

Primary Cutaneous CD4-Positive Small/Medium T-Cell Lymphoproliferative Disorder

Socorro Maria Rodriguez-Pinilla and Lorenzo Cerroni

Definition

Primary cutaneous CD4-positive small/medium T-cell lymphoproliferative disorder (pcSMTLPD) is a clonal proliferation of CD4-positive T cells presenting as a solitary lesion in the absence of patches and plaques typical for mycosis fungoides. The clinical course is remarkably indolent, and there is considerable overlap with cases that previously would have been designated cutaneous T-cell pseudolymphoma. Cases of CD4-positive primary cutaneous lymphoma presenting with multiple, large, rapidly growing lesions, sheets of large cells, and/or a high proliferation index have a much more aggressive clinical course and are excluded from this entity. They are better regarded as peripheral T-cell lymphoma, not otherwise specified. pcSMTLPD is now regarded as a definite rather than provisional entity.[1]

Synonyms

None.

Epidemiology

pcSMTLPD is reportedly a rare disorder but may be underrecognized, many cases previously being labeled cutaneous T-cell pseudolymphoma.

General Clinical Features

pcSMTLPD usually presents as a solitary erythematous nodule/tumor in the head and neck area (70%) and less frequently as a plaque/papular lesion (Figure 103.1). Cases occurring on the trunk or upper limbs have been reported.[2] Most patients are middle aged, although pediatric cases have been described.[3] The clinical course is indolent with spontaneous remissions in up to 32% of the cases.[2]

Morphology

pcSMTLPD is characterized by a dermal infiltrate, usually with a nodular and/or diffuse growth (Figure 103.2), although a superficial band-like pattern is also described. Lesional cells are in the minority and can be scattered individually and often also form small clusters. They are typically of intermediate size with variable amounts of pale cytoplasm and nuclei with highly irregular contours (Figure 103.2) and can be seen rosetting around large immunoblast-like lymphoid cells. By definition, large lymphocytes do not exceed 30% of the total infiltrate. There is always an admixture of reactive small B cells (Figure 103.2); T cells, many of which express CD8; plasma cells; and histiocytes, the last occasionally forming microgranulomas. Neutrophils and eosinophils are less commonly present. Lymphoid follicles with reactive germinal centers are not a feature. Epidermotropism is never marked.

Immunophenotype

The neoplastic cells express CD3 and CD4 and show bright expression of PD1 (Figure 103.2). Other "follicular helper T-cell antigens" such as CXCL13, ICOS, and

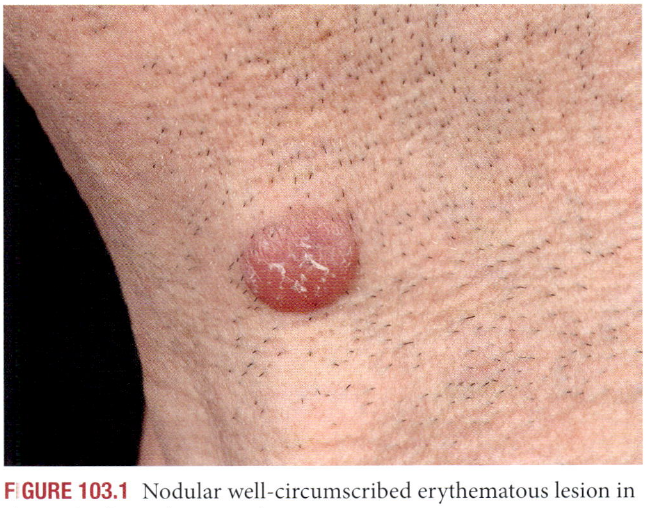

FIGURE 103.1 Nodular well-circumscribed erythematous lesion in the neck of a medium-aged man.

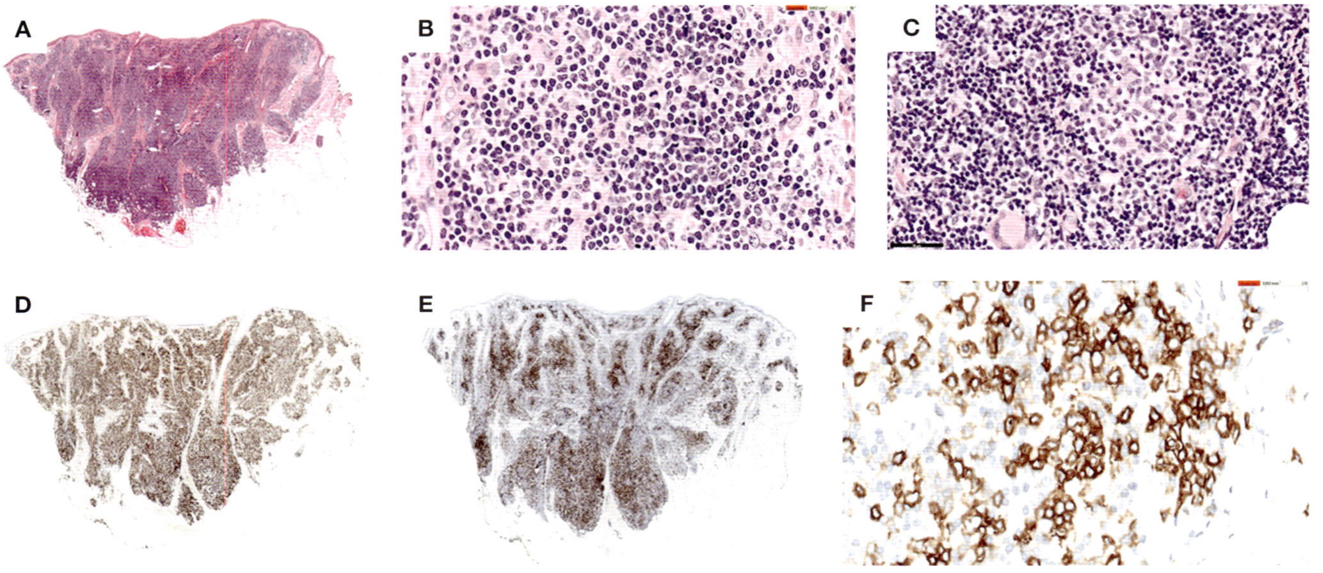

FIGURE 103.2 **A:** Panoramic view of primary cutaneous CD4-positive small/medium T-cell lymphoproliferative disorder showing a nodular growth pattern. **B:** Higher magnification highlighting the polymorphic infiltration with small to medium-sized atypical lymphocytes. **C:** Granulomatous aggregates present. **D:** Staining with anti-CD20 highlights numerous reactive B cells. **E:** Aggregates of PD1-positive cells. **F:** PD1-positive T lymphocytes surrounding a large B cell.

BCL6 may be demonstrated, but CD10 is usually negative.[4] Cyclin D1 is often positive. The Ki67 index is low and should not exceed 30%.[4] Many of the bystander T cells are CD8 positive. Occasionally, plasma cells with light chain restriction can be seen, but when germinal centers and/or light chain–restricted plasma cells are present a differential diagnosis of primary cutaneous marginal zone lymphoproliferative disorder should be considered.[5] Nevertheless, cases with overlapping features of pcSMTLPD and primary cutaneous marginal zone lymphoproliferative disorder are described and the distinction between these two entities cannot always be readily made.[5]

Genetics

Clonal TCR gene rearrangements are usually found. Little is known about the mutational profile of pcSMTLPD. Isolated somatic mutations in *DNMT3*, *ARID1A*, *EP300*, *SETD2*, *TP53*, *SH2B3*, and *NF1* have been described.[2,5]

Prognosis and Clinical Comment

Only locally directed therapy, either surgical excision or radiotherapy, is required. Cutaneous relapses are rare, and survival is 100%.

References

1. Willemze R, Kerl H, Sterry W, et al. EORTC classification for primary cutaneous lymphomas: a proposal from the cutaneous lymphoma study group of the European Organization for research and treatment of cancer. *Blood*. 1997;90(1):354-371.
2. Beltzung F, Ortonne N, Pelletier L, et al. Primary cutaneous CD4+ small/medium T-cell lymphoproliferative disorders: a clinical, pathologic, and molecular study of 60 cases presenting with a single lesion—a multicenter study of the French cutaneous lymphoma study group. *Am J Surg Pathol*. 2020;44(7):862-872.
3. Beltraminelli H, Leinweber B, Kerl H, Cerroni L. Primary cutaneous CD4+ small-/medium-sized pleomorphic T-cell lymphoma: a cutaneous nodular proliferation of pleomorphic T lymphocytes of undetermined significance? A study of 136 cases. *Am J Dermatopathol*. 2009;31(4):317-322.
4. Rodríguez Pinilla SM, Roncador G, Rodríguez-Peralto JL, et al. Primary cutaneous CD4+ small/medium-sized pleomorphic T-cell lymphoma expresses follicular T-cell markers. *Am J Surg Pathol*. 2009;33(1):81-90.
5. Obiorah IE, Karrs J, Brown L, et al. Overlapping features of primary cutaneous marginal zone lymphoproliferative disorder and primary cutaneous CD4+ small/medium T-cell lymphoproliferative disorder: a diagnostic challenge examined by genomic analysis. *Am J Surg Pathol*. 2023;47(3):344-353.

Chapter 104

Subcutaneous Panniculitis-Like T-Cell Lymphoma

Philippe Gaulard, John R. Goodlad, and Barbara Pro

Definition

Subcutaneous panniculitis-like T-cell lymphoma (SPTCL) is a lymphoma derived from cytotoxic alpha/beta (α/β) T cells composed of atypical lymphoid cells of varying size, typically with karyorrhexis and fat necrosis. The neoplastic cells preferentially infiltrate subcutaneous tissue and typically mimic panniculitis. Lymphomas infiltrating subcutaneous fat with a gamma-delta phenotype are specifically excluded from this category.

Synonyms

None.

Epidemiology

SPTCL is a rare panniculitis-like T-cell lymphoma subtype. Age distribution is broad (median age around 35 years),[1] but approximatively 20% are infants, children, or young adults under 20 years.[2] There is a slight female predominance. Up to 20% to 40% of patients with SPTCL have a prior history of autoimmune disease, most commonly systemic lupus erythematosus, less frequently rheumatoid arthritis or other conditions, and presence of autoantibodies, including antinuclear antibodies, has been reported in up to 65% of SPTCL.[1,3,4] In some patients an inflammatory panniculitis, particularly lupus erythematosus panniculitis (LEP), may precede SPTCL. In addition, SPTCL may have morphological features overlapping with LEP, and whether these lesions are related remains to be clarified. Individuals harboring biallelic, germline, loss-of-function mutations of *HAVCR2* (encoding TIM3) are highly susceptible to SPTCL, often with associated hemophagocytic lymphohistiocytosis (HLH). This phenomenon is associated with younger age and seems more prevalent in Asian populations.[3,5] It is worth noting that the *HVACR2* mutation has also been reported in idiopathic HLH.[6]

General Clinical Features

Patients typically present with multiple subcutaneous nodules or deep plaques, most frequently on the extremities or trunk, usually in the absence of other sites of disease (Figure 104.1). The nodules range in diameter from 0.5 to several centimeters,[1-4,7,8] and larger nodules may become necrotic but ulceration is typically

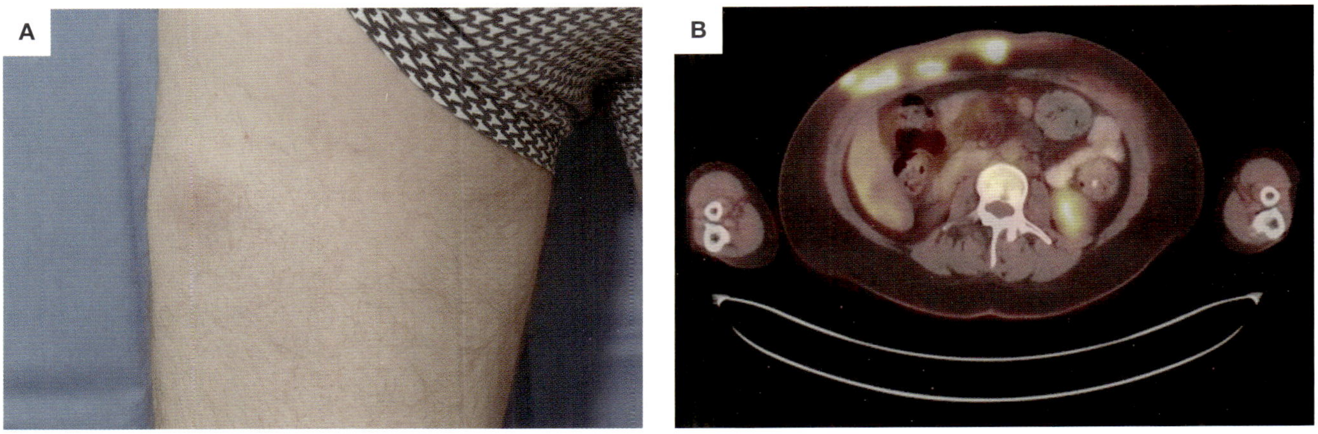

FIGURE 104.1 Subcutaneous panniculitis-like T-cell lymphoma (SPTCL). **A:** This patient presented with a dusky, erythematous nodule on the upper leg. **B:** Another patient with SPTCL. Positron emission tomography scan shows multiple lesions in abdominal fat.

not seen. Mesenteric or bone marrow involvement may rarely be present,[7] but other sites are generally spared. Lymphadenopathy and hepatosplenomegaly can occur but generally not due to lymphoma involvement. Systemic symptoms are seen in approximately 60% of patients. Cytopenias and abnormal liver function tests are common, and HLH is reported in 15% to 35% of cases.

Morphology

SPTCL shows a dense panniculitis-like infiltrate involving the subcutaneous fat lobules, usually sparing septa (Figure 104.2). There is an absence of superficial dermal and epidermal involvement, but minimal periadnexal extension into the reticular dermis is occasionally present. Most often, lymphoma cells are small or medium sized with irregular and hyperchromatic nuclei, often with a rim of pale-staining cytoplasm, typically associated with karyorrhexis (Figure 104.3). They infiltrate between adipocytes diffusely and in small aggregates, with a characteristic rimming of individual adipocytes, which constitutes a helpful diagnostic feature (see Figure 104.3). Lymphoma cells are often admixed with numerous histiocytes while other inflammatory cells, including plasma cells, are generally scarce. Vascular invasion is occasionally seen (Figure 104.4), and necrosis is frequent. Erythrophagocytic histiocytes may be seen in cases with an associated HLH.

Immunophenotype

The lymphoma cells have a mature CD3-positive, commonly CD8-positive, CD56-negative T-cell phenotype, with expression of cytotoxic molecules, including granzyme B, perforin, and T-cell intracellular antigen (TIA-1) (Figure 104.5). They are α/β T cells, expressing TCR-beta (βF1) or, when negative, not expressing the TCR gamma or TCR delta chains. Variable loss of pan-T antigens, particularly CD5, may be seen.[1,2] Neoplastic cells are negative for CD30, and EBV is absent.

The differential diagnosis with LEP may be challenging as both SPTCL and LEP demonstrate clinical and histopathologic overlap. The presence of atypical $CD8^+$ T cells with frequent Ki-67 positivity in clusters and/or rimming individual adipocytes (see Figure 104.5) is highly characteristic of SPTCL while predominance of CD4-positive T cells, dermal

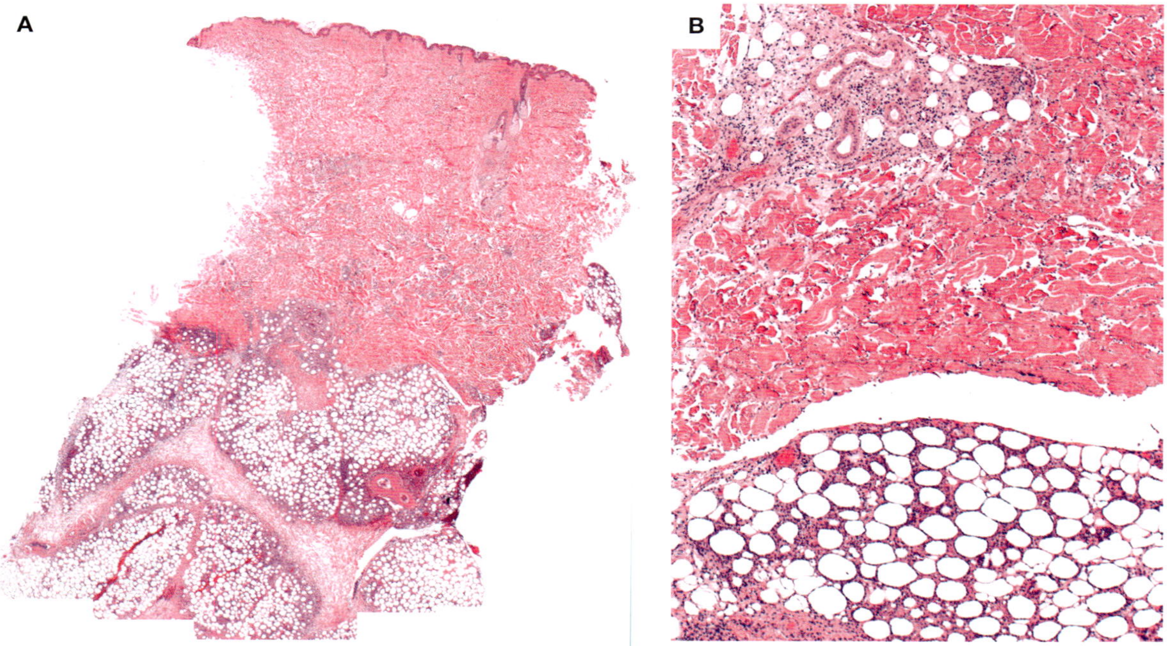

FIGURE 104.2 Subcutaneous panniculitis-like T-cell lymphoma. **A:** Low-power view showing infiltration of subcutaneous fat with periseptal accentuation. **B:** The superficial dermis and epidermis are typically spared, but there may be periadnexal infiltration within reticular dermis, as seen here.

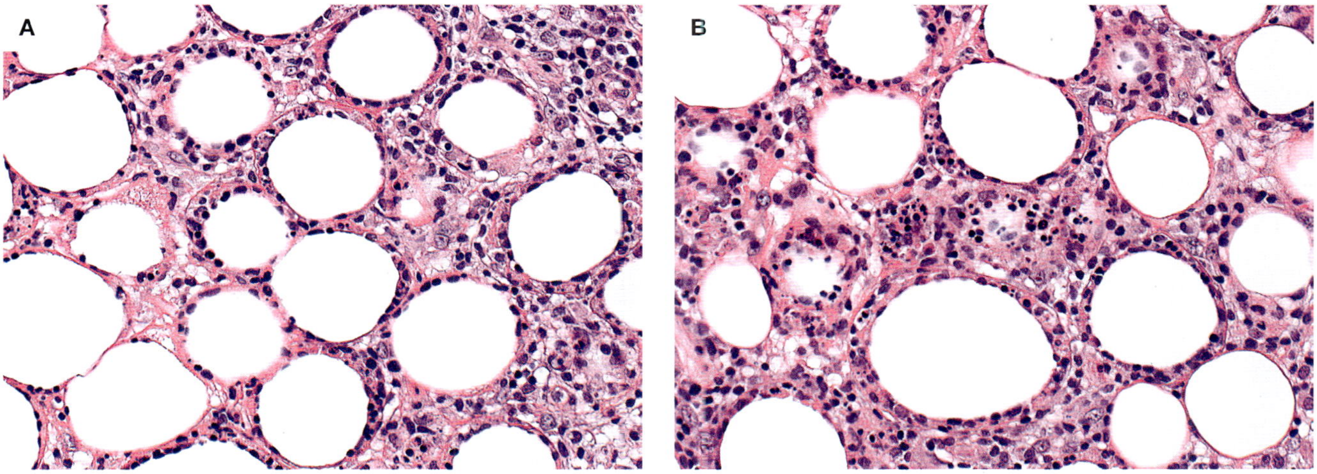

FIGURE 104.3 Subcutaneous panniculitis-like T-cell lymphoma. **A:** Medium-sized cells with hyperchromatic nuclei infiltrate between fat cells and encircle individual adipocytes. **B:** Nuclear karyorrhexis, present in several foci in this example, is often prominent.

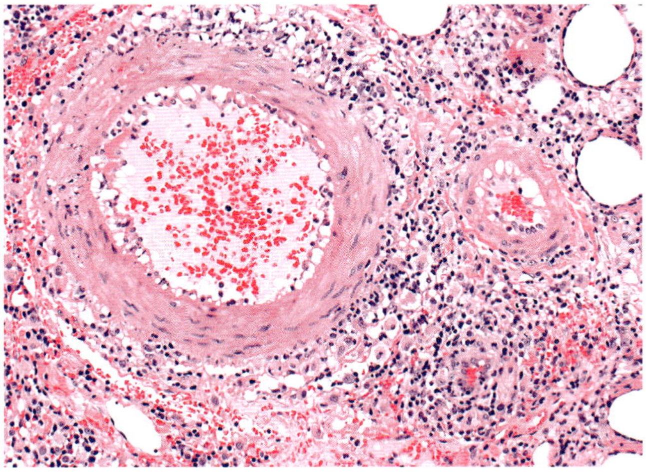

FIGURE 104.4 Subcutaneous panniculitis-like T-cell lymphoma. Varying degrees of vascular infiltration may occasionally be seen. This case shows focal infiltration of blood vessel walls by the neoplastic infiltrate.

CD20-predominant lymphoid aggregates or follicles, clusters of CD123-positive or IRF-8-positive plasmacytoid dendritic cells, numerous plasma cells, and hyaline fat necrosis favor LEP[8,9] (Table 104.1). Primary cutaneous gamma/delta T-cell lymphomas may show panniculitis-like features. In these cases, dermal and epidermal involvement, ulceration, a TCR gamma/delta phenotype, and CD56 expression exclude SPTCL[1] (see Table 104.1). The distinction from cutaneous gamma/delta T-cell lymphomas is important, because SPTCL has a much better prognosis.

Genetics

The neoplastic cells show clonal rearrangement of T-cell receptor genes. Besides the germline loss-of-function *HAVCR2* variant abrogating TIM-3 expression and leading to persistent immune activation and increased production of inflammatory cytokines in a subset of SPTCL (see earlier discussion), recurrent somatic mutations in genes associated with epigenetic regulation and PI3K/AKT/mTOR and JAK-STAT signal transduction pathways have been reported.[10,11]

Prognosis and Clinical Comment

The 5-year overall survival rate across all patients with SPTCL is around 80%.[1,4] However, the presence of HLH portends an adverse prognosis.[1] *HAVCR2* mutations have been associated with severe HLH.[3] Combination chemotherapy has traditionally been used, but more recent studies suggest that more conservative immunosuppressive regimens (prednisone, ciclosporin, low-dose methotrexate, chlorambucil, hydroxychloroquine) may be more effective in uncomplicated cases.[2] In general, initial therapy with corticosteroids and/or other immunomodulatory agents is currently recommended for patients without HLH. Patients with HLH may also benefit from immunosuppressive therapy and/or the *JAK1/2* inhibitor ruxolitinib.[2,6] However, those with more severe disease or inadequate response to immunosuppression require

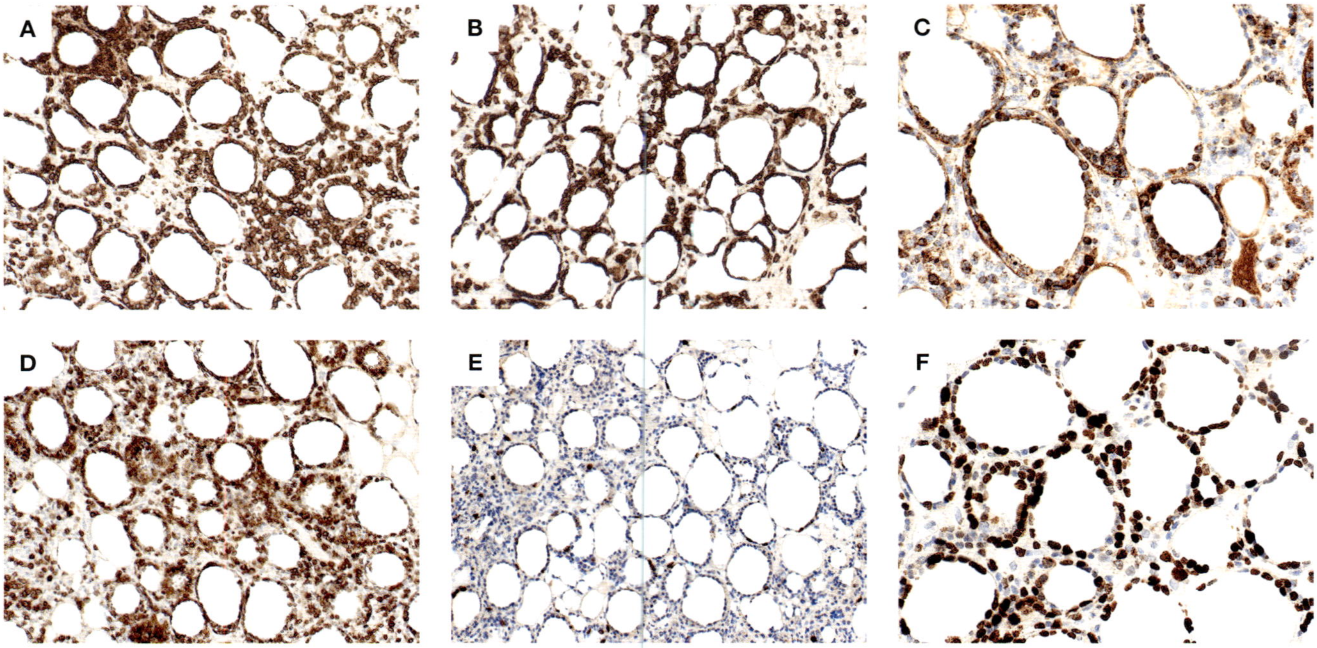

FIGURE 104.5 Subcutaneous panniculitis-like T-cell lymphoma, immunophenotype. **A:** Antibodies to CD3 confirm a T lineage in this example. The neoplastic lymphocytes have a cytotoxic phenotype. **B:** They express CD8. **C:** They also express granzyme B. **D:** Staining for TCR-βF1 is positive. **E:** The tumor cells are negative for TCR-δ. **F:** Antibodies to Ki-67 highlight the neoplastic lymphocytes rimming fat cells and can be useful in differentiating subcutaneous panniculitis-like T-cell lymphoma from reactive panniculitides such as lupus profundus.

TABLE 104.1 Comparison of main clinical, pathological, and genetic features between subcutaneous panniculitis-like T-cell lymphoma (SPTCL), lupus erythematous panniculitis (LEP), and primary cutaneous γ/δ T-cell lymphoma (PCGDTCL)

	SPTCL	LEP	PCGDTCL
Sites of involvement	Skin, rarely mesentery or bone marrow	Skin	Skin, extracutaneous involvement is rare
M/F ratio	1/3-4	1/3-4	1/2
Median age (range)	Wide range (any age but 20% <20 y of age at presentation)	40-50 y	50-60 y
Clinical context/setting	History of autoimmune disease (up to 40%), autoantibodies (up to 65%)	Frequent history of autoimmune disease and/or autoantibodies, often associated with DLE or SLE	Most cases have no association with autoimmune disease
Clinical features/symptoms	Multiple skin nodules or deep plaques, typically nonulcerated, in the trunk or (upper and lower) extremities. B symptoms (<70%), HLH (20%-50%)[b]	Multiple erythematous nodules or plaques in the trunk, face, or (upper) extremities. Absence of HLH	Disseminated plaques and ulceronecrotic nodules, preferentially affecting the extremities (lower > upper) and the trunk. B symptoms (~70%), HLH (up 45%)[b]
Morphology	Lymphocyte atypia (pleomorphism, irregular nuclei), adipocyte rimming, karyorrhexis. Infiltrate confined to subcutis and periadnexal fat	Small lymphocytes without atypia, often with hyalinization of fat. Lymphocytes surround adipocytes but without adipocyte rimming or karyorrhexis. Often associated interface changes in overlying epidermis	Panniculitis-like lesions, atypical medium- to large-sized pleomorphic T cells extension to the dermis, sometimes epidermis
Cell of origin	αβ T cell (activated cytotoxic profile)	N/A	γδ T cell (Vδ2 subset)(activated cytotoxic profile)

TABLE 104.1 *(Continued)*

	SPTCL	LEP	PCGDTCL
Phenotype	CD8+, TIA1+, CD56− TCRαβ (βF1)+, Ki-67+ atypical lymphocytes surrounding (disrupting) adipocytes. CD123+ clusters and CD20+ follicles almost absent within infiltrate	Absence of CD8+ Ki-67+ adipocyte rimming by atypical lymphocytes; CD4+ T cells predominant; CD20+ B-cell follicles, CD138+ plasma cell aggregates, CD123+ clusters, IRF8+ clusters within the dermis (50%)	CD3+, CD5−, CD4−/CD8−, CD56+, TCRγδ+, TIA1+, perforin+, granzyme B+
Genetic features	Clonal TCR gene rearrangement (~100%). *HVACR2* germline mutation (25%-60% reported)	Absent (rare) clonal TCR gene rearrangement	Clonal TCR gene rearrangement mutations in the JAK/STAT, MAPK, MYC, and chromatin modification pathways[a]
Prognosis, treatment	80%-85% 5-y survival, immunosuppressive drugs, polychemotherapy, ruxolitinib	Indolent but residual scarring possible, steroids or hydroxychloroquine as first line	Aggressive clinical course, <20% 5-y overall survival, polychemotherapy, allogeneic stem cell transplant in eligible patients

DLE, discoid lupus erythematosus; HLH hemophagocytic lymphohistiocytosis; SLE, systemic lupus erythematosus.
[a]Patients with HLH may have extracutaneous manifestations such as lymphadenopathy, splenomegaly, or hepatomegaly.
[b]According to Daniels J et al. Cellular origins and genetic landscape of cutaneous gamma delta T cell lymphomas. *Nat Commun.* 2020;11(1):806.

multiagent chemotherapy,[2] and consolidation with allogeneic stem cell transplantation should be considered in eligible patients.

References

1. Willemze R, Jansen PM, Cerroni L, et al. Subcutaneous panniculitis-like T-cell lymphoma: definition, classification, and prognostic factors—an EORTC Cutaneous Lymphoma Group Study of 83 cases. *Blood.* 2008;111(2):838-845. doi:10.1182/blood-2007-04-087288
2. Michonneau D, Petrella T, Ortonne N, et al. Subcutaneous panniculitis-like T-cell lymphoma: immunosuppressive drugs induce better response than polychemotherapy. *Acta Derm Venereol.* 2017;97(3):358-364. doi:10.2340/00015555-2543
3. Sonigo G, Battistella M, Beylot-Barry M, et al. HAVCR2 mutations are associated with severe hemophagocytic syndrome in subcutaneous panniculitis-like T-cell lymphoma. *Blood.* 2020;135(13):1058-1061. doi:10.1182/blood.2019003811
4. López-Lerma I, Peñate Y, Gallardo F, et al. Subcutaneous panniculitis-like T-cell lymphoma: clinical features, therapeutic approach, and outcome in a case series of 16 patients. *J Am Acad Dermatol.* 2018;79(5):892-898. doi:10.1016/j.jaad.2018.05.1243
5. Gayden T, Sepulveda FE, Khuong-Quang DA, et al. Germline HAVCR2 mutations altering TIM-3 characterize subcutaneous panniculitis-like T cell lymphomas with hemophagocytic lymphohistiocytic syndrome. *Nat Genet.* 2018;50(12):1650-1657. doi:10.1038/s41588-018-0251-4
6. Zhang Q, Zhou CJ, Li DH, et al. Efficacy of ruxolitinib for HAVCR2 mutation-associated hemophagocytic lymphohistiocytosis and panniculitis manifestations in children. *Br J Haematol.* 2023;202(1):135-146. doi:10.1111/bjh.18817
7. Attygalle AD, Cabeçadas J, Gaulard P, et al. Peripheral T-cell and NK-cell lymphomas and their mimics; taking a step forward—report on the lymphoma workshop of the XVIth meeting of the European Association for Haematopathology and the Society for Hematopathology. *Histopathology.* 2014;64(2):171-199. doi:10.1111/his.12251
8. LeBlanc RE, Tavallaee M, Kim YH, Kim J. Useful parameters for distinguishing subcutaneous panniculitis-like T-cell lymphoma from lupus erythematosus panniculitis. *Am J Surg Pathol.* 2016;40(6):745-754. doi:10.1097/PAS.0000000000000596
9. Wong J, Roy SF, McNiff JM, Xu ML. IRF8 in conjunction with CD123 and CD20 to distinguish lupus erythematosus panniculitis from subcutaneous panniculitis-like T-cell lymphoma. *Am J Surg Pathol.* 2023;47(12):1425-1431. doi:10.1097/PAS.0000000000002133
10. Li Z, Lu L, Zhou Z, et al. Recurrent mutations in epigenetic modifiers and the PI3K/AKT/mTOR pathway in subcutaneous panniculitis-like T-cell lymphoma. *Br J Haematol.* 2018;181(3):406-410. doi:10.1111/bjh.14611
11. Polprasert C, Takeuchi Y, Kakiuchi N, et al. Frequent germline mutations of HAVCR2 in sporadic subcutaneous panniculitis-like T-cell lymphoma. *Blood Adv.* 2019;3(4):588-595. doi:10.1182/bloodadvances.2018028340

Chapter 105
Primary Cutaneous Gamma-Delta T-Cell Lymphoma

Socorro Maria Rodriguez-Pinilla and Barbara Pro

Definition

Primary cutaneous γδ T-cell lymphoma (PCGDTCL) was initially recognized as a subtype of subcutaneous panniculitis T-cell lymphoma on account of inferior outcome when compared with counterparts with αβ-T-cell receptor expression (TCR-αβ).[1,2] The morphological spectrum of PCGDTCL has since broadened, and it is now defined as a clonal proliferation of mature activated cytotoxic T cells of γδ origin limited to skin with no extracutaneous manifestations at diagnosis. Currently, cases expressing γδ-TCR but otherwise displaying typical clinical features of mycosis fungoides or lymphomatoid papulosis are excluded.[3]

Synonyms

None.

Epidemiology

PCGDTCL is a rare form of primary cutaneous lymphoma accounting for <1% of all lymphomas. Consequently, very little epidemiological and clinical information is available. Most studies report a median age at presentation of >50 years with male predominance.

General Clinical Features

PCGDTCL usually presents with widespread skin lesions, most frequently multiple rapidly progressive deep plaques, although patches, superficial plaques, nodules, or tumors can also be the presenting features (Figure 105.1). Ulceration is frequent, reported in up to 50% of cases, and panniculitis-like presentation has been documented.[1,4] Extracutaneous dissemination, especially to mucosal and extranodal sites such as lung, thyroid, breast, liver, spleen, intestine, central nervous system, or testis is frequent but lymph nodes, spleen, and bone marrow are rarely involved. B-symptoms are common, and a hemophagocytic syndrome may be encountered. Staging employs the TNM system for cutaneous lymphomas other than MF and Sezary syndrome.[5]

Patients with cutaneous γ/δ T-cell lymphoma presenting with initially indolent disease have also been reported. The majority manifest as epidermotropic lymphomas characterized by slowly evolving patches and plaques typical of mycosis fungoides, with rare cases of indolent panniculitis-like γ/δ T-cell lymphoma also recorded.[6-9] While the former are currently labeled as mycosis fungoides, a significant proportion of these neoplasms, as well as cases of indolent panniculitis-like γ/δ T-cell lymphoma, ultimately progress and pursue an aggressive clinical course much more typical of the usual type PCGDTCL.[6-9] How best to identify and classify such cases requires further exploration.

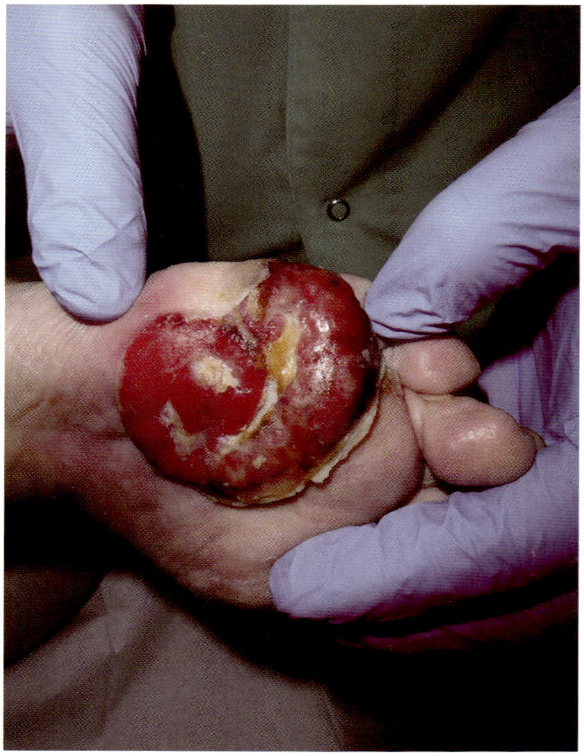

FIGURE 105.1 Primary cutaneous gamma delta T-cell lymphoma. This patient presented with a rapidly growing, well-delineated erythematous tumor on the sole of the foot.

Morphology

Tumor cells are usually of medium to large size with coarse chromatin (Figure 105.2), although small neoplastic lymphocytes may occasionally predominate. The pattern of infiltration is heterogeneous with intraepidermal, dermal, and subcutaneous variants seen (Figure 105.3). More than one pattern may be present in the same biopsy, and/or different patterns may be seen in separate biopsies from the same patient. Epidermotropism correlates with the presence of patches and plaques. It can be subtle or marked with a pagetoid reticulosis–like appearance.[10] Differentiation of such cases from mycosis fungoides and primary cutaneous CD8-positive aggressive epidermotropic cytotoxic T-cell lymphoma is dependent on phenotyping and clinical correlation. Involvement of dermis and subcutaneous fat more often correlates with tumor formation and angioinvasion, and necrosis may be seen. Subcutaneous infiltrates involve septae and lobules and may closely resemble subcutaneous panniculitis-like T-cell lymphoma with rimming of adipocytes, prominent apoptosis, and abundant karyorrhectic debris. In contrast to subcutaneous panniculitis-like T-cell lymphoma, involvement of fat is usually associated with concomitant dermal infiltration.[10]

Immunophenotype

The tumor cells express surface TCR-γ and TCR-δ and lack TCRβ (TCR-βF1). The morphological heterogeneity of PCGDTCL may be related to origin from different γ/δ T-cell subsets: expression of the Vδ1 isoform (physiologically associated with cutaneous and mucosal γδ T cells) correlates with an epidermal/dermal pattern of infiltration, whereas Vδ2 expression (normally present in circulating γδ T cells) associates with prominent

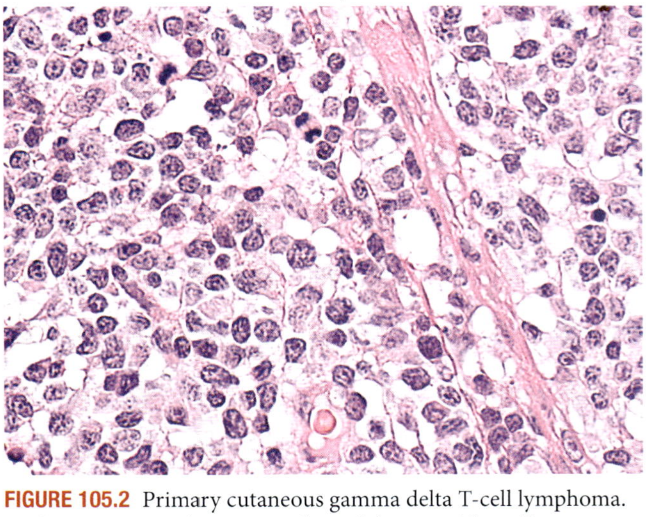

FIGURE 105.2 Primary cutaneous gamma delta T-cell lymphoma. High-power view showing cytological features. The cells are of intermediate to large size with coarsely clumped chromatin. (Image provided by Dr J.R. Goodlad.)

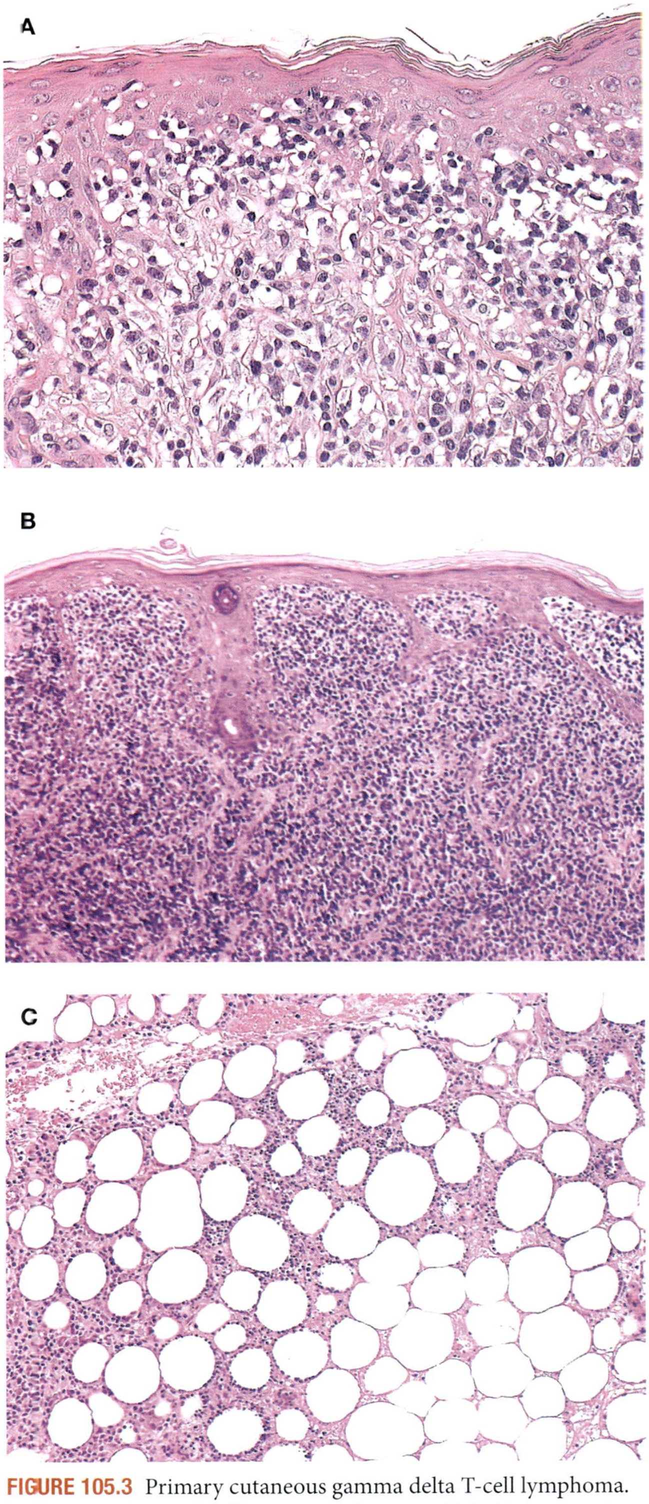

FIGURE 105.3 Primary cutaneous gamma delta T-cell lymphoma. Different patterns of infiltration can be seen. A) Epidermotropism. B) Diffuse infiltration of the dermis. C) Permeation of subcutaneous fat. (Image provided by Dr J.R. Goodlad.)

subcutaneous distribution.[7] Typically, there is expression of CD2 and CD3, with CD7 also often present, but CD5 is frequently lost. Most cases are double negative for CD4 and CD8 but express cytotoxic molecules such as TIA-1, granzyme B, and perforin[10] (Figure 105.4). Occasional CD8-positive cases are documented. CD56 is frequently positive (Figure 105.4), and CD30 is seen in a minority. By definition, EBV is negative, facilitating easy distinction for extranodal NK/T-cell lymphoma infiltrating skin.[10]

By definition, a γδ-TCR phenotype should be demonstrated; absence of TCRβ (βF1) expression is no longer considered adequate for the diagnosis of PCGDTCL. However, as a variety of other primary cutaneous T-cell lymphomas on occasion display a γδ-T cell phenotype, close clinical-pathological correlation is always required for correct diagnosis. In addition, cases of primary cutaneous T-cell lymphoma expressing TCR-γ and/or δ, as well as TCR-βF1 have been described. These display varied clinical presentations and include some which run an indolent course, and the significance of such a finding remains to be fully elucidated. Staging is also mandatory to exclude secondary skin involvement by extracutaneous TCRγδ-positive lymphomas, such as monomorphic epitheliotropic intestinal T-cell lymphoma and hepatosplenic T-cell lymphoma.

Genetics

TCR γ and δ genes are clonally rearranged. Recurrent mutations in the *JAK/STAT, MAPK, MYC,* and chromatin modifying pathways are frequent. While Vδ1 epidermal/dermal lymphomas are transcriptionally different from Vδ2 panniculitic lymphomas, no molecular differences have been found between these two groups.[7]

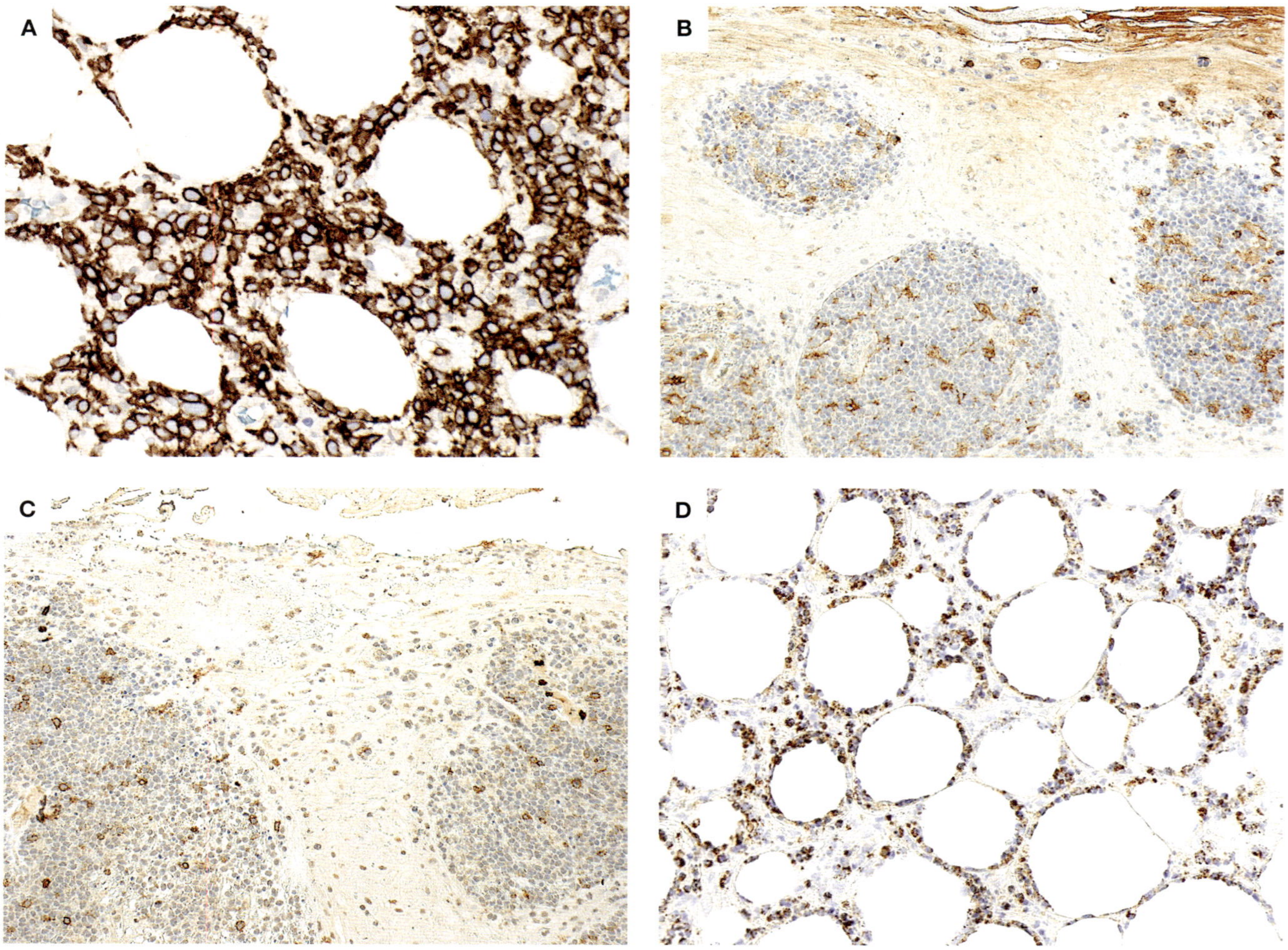

FIGURE 105.4 Primary cutaneous gamma delta T-cell lymphoma. **A:** TCRδ antibody highlights the neoplastic cells. Cases are typically negative for CD4 (B) and CD8 (C). **D:** CD56 is frequently expressed.

Prognosis and Clinical Comment

PCGDTCL is considered an aggressive disease. Response to systemic polychemotherapy is poor and the prognosis dismal. The median survival is 31 months, although allogeneic stem cell transplant may offer a better chance of longer-term remission.[4] Longer survival is observed for lesions centered on the epidermis compared with those involving the subcutaneous fat while the presence of a hemophagocytic syndrome and extracutaneous spread are associated with a more unfavorable outcome.[7,8]

References

1. Toro JR, Liewehr DJ, Pabby N, et al. Gamma-delta T-cell phenotype is associated with significantly decreased survival in cutaneous T-cell lymphoma. *Blood*. 2003;101(9):3407-3412.
2. Willemze R, Jansen PM, Cerroni L, et al. Subcutaneous panniculitis-like T-cell lymphoma: definition, classification, and prognostic factors—an EORTC Cutaneous Lymphoma Group Study of 83 cases. *Blood*. 2008;111(2):838-845.
3. Willemze R, Cerroni L, Kempf W, et al. The 2018 update of the WHO-EORTC classification for primary cutaneous lymphomas. *Blood*. 2019;133(16):1703-1714.
4. Guitart J, Weisenburger DD, Subtil A, et al. Cutaneous γδ T-cell lymphomas: a spectrum of presentations with overlap with other cytotoxic lymphomas. *Am J Surg Pathol*. 2012;36(11):1656-1665.
5. Kim YH, Willemze R, Pimpinelli N, et al. TNM classification system for primary cutaneous lymphomas other than mycosis fungoides and Sezary syndrome: a proposal of the International Society for Cutaneous Lymphomas (ISCL) and the cutaneous lymphoma task force of the European Organization of Research and Treatment of Cancer (EORTC). *Blood*. 2007;110(2):479-484.
6. Merrill ED, Agbay R, Miranda RN, et al. Primary cutaneous T-cell lymphomas showing gamma-delta (γδ) phenotype and predominantly epidermotropic pattern are clinicopathologically distinct from classic primary cutaneous γδ T-cell lymphomas. *Am J Surg Pathol*. 2017;41(2):204-215.
7. Daniels J, Doukas PG, Escala MEM, et al. Cellular origins and genetic landscape of cutaneous gamma delta T cell lymphomas. *Nat Commun*. 2020;11(1):1806.
8. von Dücker L, Fleischer M, Stutz N, et al. Primary cutaneous gamma-delta T-cell lymphoma with long-term indolent clinical course initially mimicking lupus erythematosus profundus. *Front Oncol*. 2020;10:133.
9. Hosler GA, Liégeois N, Anhalt GJ, Moresi JM. Transformation of cutaneous gamma/delta T-cell lymphoma following 15 years of indolent behavior. *J Cutan Pathol*. 2008;35(11):1063-1067.
10. Willemze R. Cutaneous lymphomas with a panniculitic presentation. *Semin Diagn Pathol*. 2017;34(1):36-43.

Chapter 106

Primary Cutaneous Acral CD8-Positive T-Cell Lymphoproliferative Disorder

Tony Petrella, John R. Goodlad, and Barbara Pro

Definition

Primary cutaneous acral CD8-positive T-cell lymphoproliferative disorder is characterized by a dermal-based infiltrate of clonal, medium-sized CD8-positive, cytotoxic lymphocytes. The tumor was initially described in ear localization[1] and then in other acral sites (nose, hand, and foot). It typically displays indolent behavior with an excellent prognosis, and is now classified as a lymphoproliferative disorder rather than an overt lymphoma.[2]

Synonyms

Indolent CD8 positive lymphoid proliferation of the ear (not recommended). Indolent CD8 positive lymphoid proliferations of acral sites (not recommended). Primary cutaneous acral CD8$^+$ T-cell lymphoma (not recommended).

Epidemiology

The disease affects adults with a male predominance (male/female ratio 3.2:1). The median age is around 56 years.[3]

General Clinical Features

Presentation is most often with a unique, nonulcerated, reddish nodule or papule of 0.5 to 2 cm in diameter. Sometimes, particularly on the feet, disease may manifest as an erythematous scaly plaque (up to 5 cm). Lesions grow slowly over several weeks or months with a median duration of 20 months before biopsy. A different diagnosis should be considered for fast-growing lesions, particularly when ulceration is present. Ear is the most frequent site affected (two-thirds of the cases), followed by nose and feet. Presentations on eyelids, hands, arms, or leg are also reported. Occasionally, lesions are multiple and particularly bilateral for ears[1,2] and for feet. Only one case with disseminated nodules (face, arm, trunk) has been reported.[4]

Morphology

Skin biopsy shows dense and diffuse dermal infiltration by monotonous medium-sized lymphoid cells with irregular and folded nuclei, and small nucleoli (Figures 106.1 and 106.2). Mitoses and apoptotic figures are absent or very rare. A single case with signet

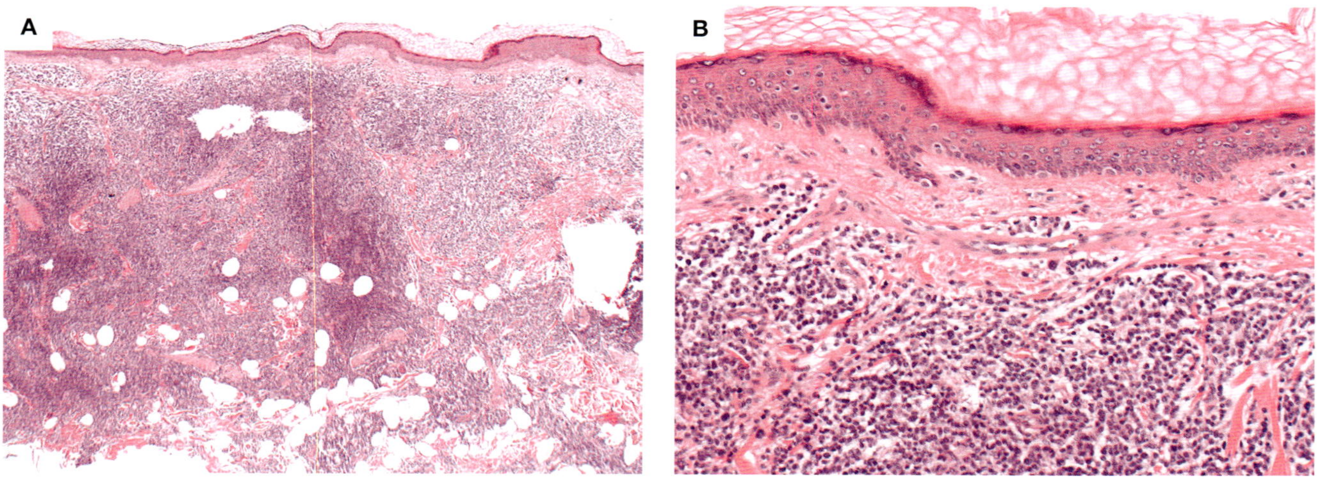

FIGURE 106.1 **A:** Primary cutaneous acral CD8-positive T-cell lymphoma showing characteristic diffuse infiltration of the dermis. In this case, there is also involvement of subcutaneous fat. **B:** The epidermis is typically spared.

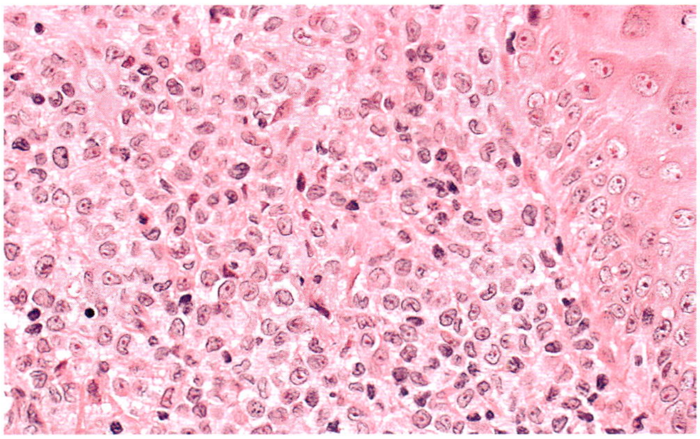

FIGURE 106.2 The neoplastic lymphocytes have irregular nuclear contours, finely dispersed chromatin, and small nucleoli.

ring cells has been reported. Reactive follicular B-cell aggregates may be seen in association with the infiltrate, but plasma cells, neutrophils, and eosinophils are absent or very rare. The epidermis is most often spared with a grenz zone, although infiltration of superficial dermis, with or without minimal epidermotropism, is occasional present, particularly in plaque lesions. Skin appendages are always spared. Angiotropism can be occasionally present but never angiodestruction and necrosis. The infiltrate frequently involves subcutaneous fat.

Immunophenotype

By definition, the tumor cells express CD8 (Figure 106.3), and they are always positive for CD3, TIA-1, and TCR-Beta-F1. TIA-1 staining shows a very characteristic Golgi dot-like pattern (Figure 106.4A). Other cytotoxic molecules, such as granzyme B and perforin, are

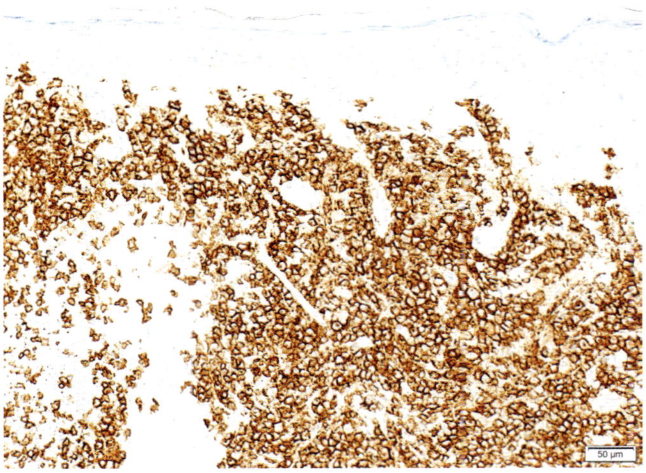

FIGURE 106.3 Staining for CD8. By definition the tumor cells are positive.

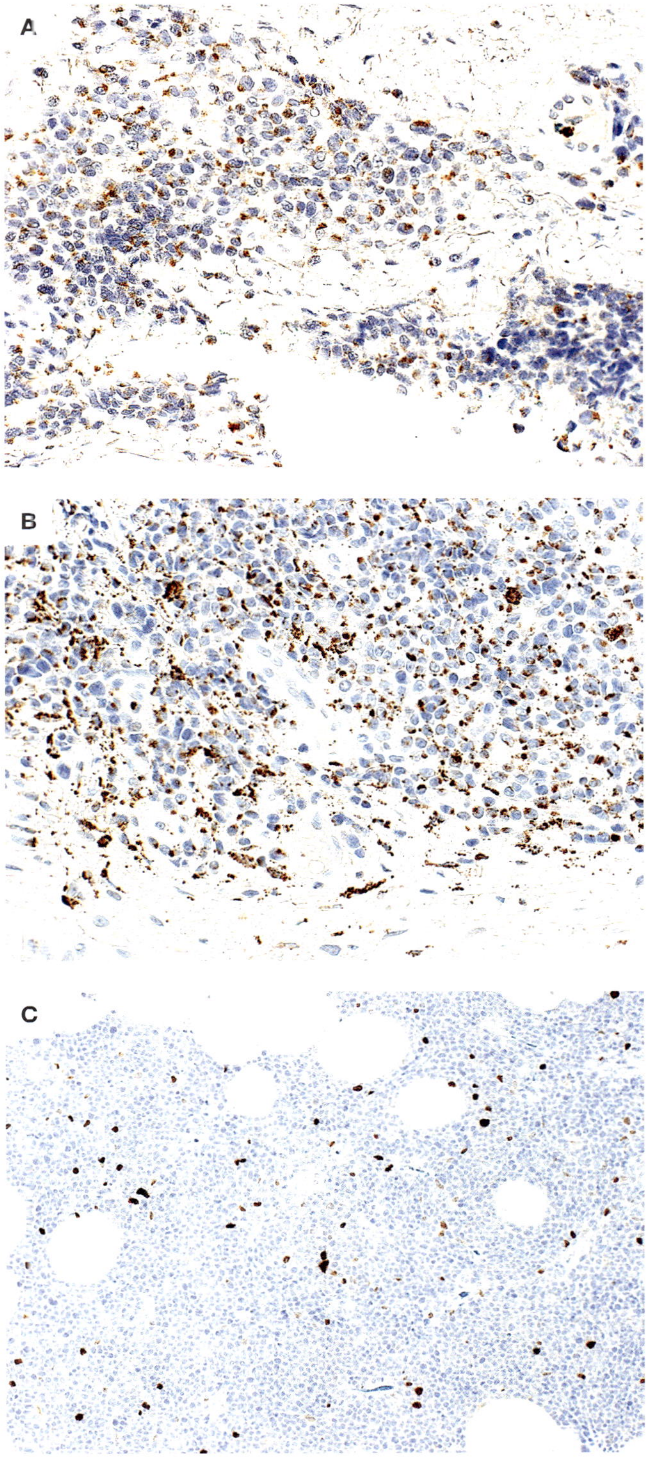

FIGURE 106.4 Primary cutaneous acral CD8-positive T-cell lymphoma typically shows positive Golgi dot-like staining for **(A)** TIA-1 and **(B)** CD68. **C:** A low Ki-67 index is also to be expected.

variably expressed. CD2, CD5, and CD7 are regularly positive, but one or more can be lost or only weakly expressed. CD99 is generally strongly positive, and a

Golgi dot-like pattern of staining is also seen for CD68 in the vast majority of cases (Figure 106.4B). Presence of the latter may aid discrimination from other types of T-cell lymphoma.[5] CD4, CD30, CD56, CD57, and TdT are always negative as are follicular T-helper markers (eg, CD10, BCL6, PD1, and CXCL13). The proliferative index demonstrated by Ki-67 staining is typically very low (<10%): the diagnosis should be questioned, and other CD8-positive cutaneous lymphomas carefully considered, when over 50% (Figure 106.4C). Staining for Epstein-Barr virus (LMP1 and EBER) is always negative.

Genetics

The neoplastic T cells show clonal T-cell receptor gene rearrangements. Specific genetic abnormalities have not yet been described. To date there is no published study focusing on gene mutational profile in this disease.

Prognosis and Clinical Comment

Treatment consists of surgical excision or local radiotherapy. No chemotherapy is required. Sometimes the lesion disappears spontaneously after biopsy. Most cases achieve long-lasting remission with only locally directed therapy, but recurrence/progression occurs in around 20% of the cases, more frequently in young people.[6] Except for one case with extracutaneous involvement, only cutaneous relapses have been described. In rare cases, recurrence may occur at other cutaneous sites.[6]

References

1. Petrella T, Maubec E, Cornillet-Lefebvre P, et al. Indolent CD8-positive lymphoid proliferation of the ear: a distinct primary cutaneous T-cell lymphoma? *Am J Surg Pathol.* 2007;31(12):1887-1892. doi:10.1097/PAS.0b013e318068b527
2. Greenblatt D, Ally M, Child F, et al. Indolent CD8(+) lymphoid proliferation of acral sites: a clinicopathologic study of six patients with some atypical features. *J Cutan Pathol.* 2013;40(2):248-258. doi:10.1111/cup.12045
3. Kluk J, Kai A, Koch D, et al. Indolent CD8-positive lymphoid proliferation of acral sites: three further cases of a rare entity and an update on a unique patient. *J Cutan Pathol.* 2016;43(2):125-136. doi:10.1111/cup.12633
4. Kempf W, Petrella T, Willemze R, et al. Clinical, histopathological and prognostic features of primary cutaneous acral CD8(+) T-cell lymphoma and other dermal CD8(+) cutaneous lymphoproliferations: results of an EORTC Cutaneous Lymphoma Group workshop. *Br J Dermatol.* 2022;186(5):887-897. doi:10.1111/bjd.20973
5. Wobser M, Roth S, Reinartz T, Rosenwald A, Goebeler M, Geissinger E. CD68 expression is a discriminative feature of indolent cutaneous CD8-positive lymphoid proliferation and distinguishes this lymphoma subtype from other CD8-positive cutaneous lymphomas. *Br J Dermatol.* 2015;172(6):1573-1580. doi:10.1111/bjd.13628
6. Maubec E, Marinho E, Laroche L, Mitchell A, Grange F, Petrella T. Primary cutaneous acral CD8(+) T-cell lymphomas relapse more frequently in younger patients. *Br J Haematol.* 2019;185(3):598-601. doi:10.1111/bjh.15572

Chapter 107

Primary Cutaneous CD8-Positive Aggressive Epidermotropic Cytotoxic T-Cell Lymphoma

John R. Goodlad, Lorenzo Cerroni, and Barbara Pro

Definition

Primary cutaneous CD8-positive aggressive epidermotropic cytotoxic T-cell lymphoma ($CD8^+$ AECTL) is a clinically aggressive epidermotropic lymphoma composed of cytotoxic T cells and confined to the skin at presentation. Listed as a provisional subtype of lymphoma in the World Health Organization revised fourth edition, it is now considered a definite entity. It is important to distinguish $CD8^+$ AECTL from other epidermotropic T-cell lymphomas with a $CD8^+$-positive cytotoxic phenotype and, while there are certain histological clues, this is largely achieved on the basis of distinctive clinical features.

Synonyms

Ketron-Goodman disease (not recommended)
Berti's lymphoma.

Epidemiology

This is a rare lymphoma of adults, accounting for <1% of all cutaneous lymphomas, with few published series of significant size.

General Clinical Features

Patients present with a short history of widespread rapidly evolving infiltrated plaques, papules, and tumors, which are frequently crusted and ulcerated (Figure 107.1). A hemorrhagic appearance is also common. Lesions present on trunk, arms, and legs. Mucosal membranes may also be involved. Importantly, a prodromal period characterized by slow-growing patches and plaques typical for mycosis fungoides is absent. The clinical course is characterized by early dissemination to visceral sites such as testes, lungs, spleen, and central nervous system but rarely to peripheral lymph nodes.[1-3]

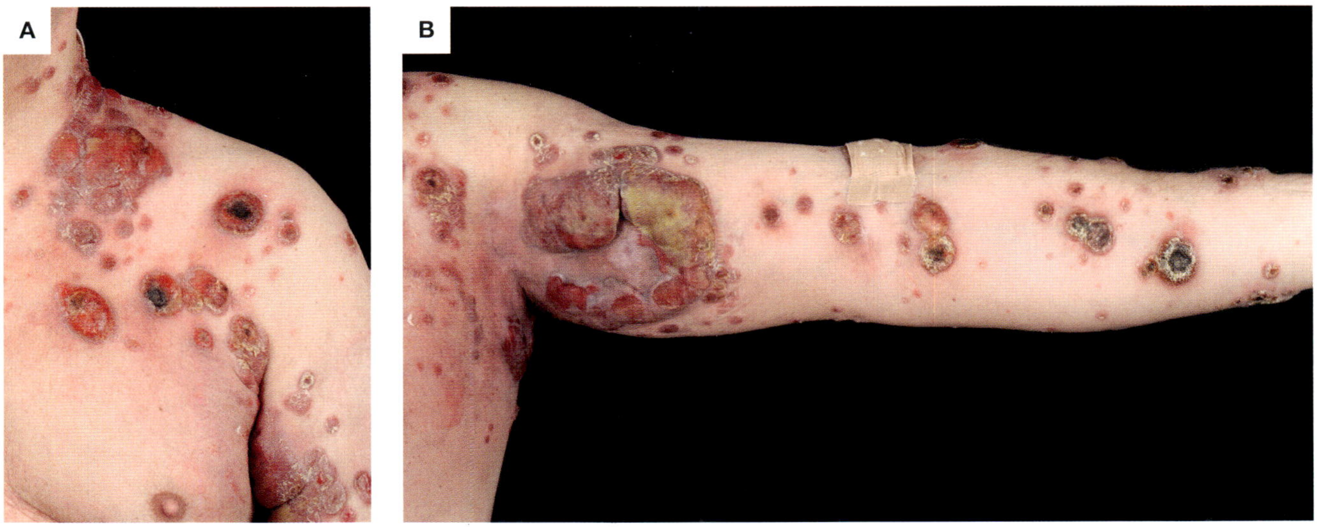

FIGURE 107.1 Primary cutaneous CD8-positive aggressive epidermotropic cytotoxic T-cell lymphoma. Patient presenting with multiple plaques and ulcerated tumors on the trunk (**A**) and limbs (**B**).

Morphology

The individual tumor cells in CD8+ AECTL are usually of intermediate to large size with enlarged hyperchromatic nuclei and coarse chromatin, without the cerebriform appearance typical of mycosis fungoides. Cells with an immunoblast-like appearance may also be seen. Epidermotropism is the hallmark of this disease. It is usually prominent, particularly in lesions clinically manifesting as plaques. It typically takes the form of epidermal replacement by single cells, imparting a pagetoid reticulosis–like appearance (Figure 107.2). Pautrier microabscesses are rarely seen, and basal cell tagging, typical of mycosis fungoides, is not a feature. There is often associated hyperkeratosis and/or acanthosis. Epidermal necrosis and ulceration are frequent (Figure 107.2). A variable dermal infiltrate can be present and is most pronounced in tumors. Dermal infiltration may be associated with angioinvasion ± angiodestruction and, less commonly, dermal necrosis. Infiltration of hair follicle epithelium is often also seen but without follicular mucinosis.[1,3,4]

Immunophenotype

The neoplastic lymphocytes are T cells of alpha-beta type (TCR-beta-F1 positive, TCR-delta negative) with a cytotoxic phenotype. They express CD8 together with TIA and/or granzyme B and lack CD4 (Figure 107.3). Most cases are positive for CD3 and a high proportion express CD7, but CD2 and CD5 are frequently lost. They are usually CD45RA positive, CD45RO negative. Staining for CD30 and CD56 is typically negative, as is in situ hybridization for Epstein-Barr virus.[1,3,4]

Genetics

Molecular analysis implicates abnormalities of genes involved in cell cycle regulation, chromatin regulation, and JAK-STAT pathway signaling in the pathogenesis of this neoplasm. Upregulation of *JAK2* signaling secondary to genomic alterations appears particularly important. Nearly all cases harbor rearrangements of *JAK2* with formation of oncogenic fusion genes. Deletions or loss-of-function mutations of *SH2B3* or *SOCS1* (negative regulators of the JAK-STAT pathway) and pathogenic activating mutations of JAK-STAT pathway genes such as *JAK3* or *STAT5B* are also common.[5]

Prognosis and Clinical Comment

CD8+ AECTL runs a very aggressive clinical course. There is no standardized treatment, but most cases are managed with systemic chemotherapy using cyclophosphamide, doxorubicin hydrochloride, vincristine and prednisone (CHOP), CHOP-like regimens or gemcitabine. Outlook is poor with a median survival of 12 months quoted in one recent series.[1] Novel therapies such as *JAK2* or histone deacetylase inhibitors may offer more hope in the future.

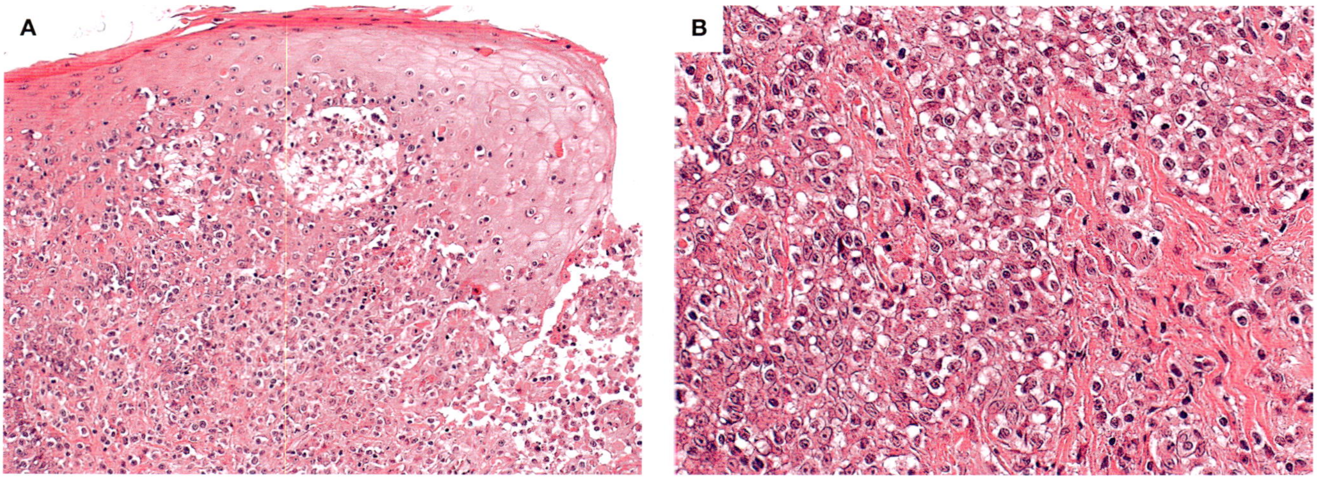

FIGURE 107.2 Primary cutaneous CD8-positive aggressive epidermotropic cytotoxic T-cell lymphoma. **A:** Low-power view showing epidermal infiltration adjacent to an area of epidermal necrosis and ulceration. **B:** Prominent epidermotropism by intermediate to large lymphoid cells.

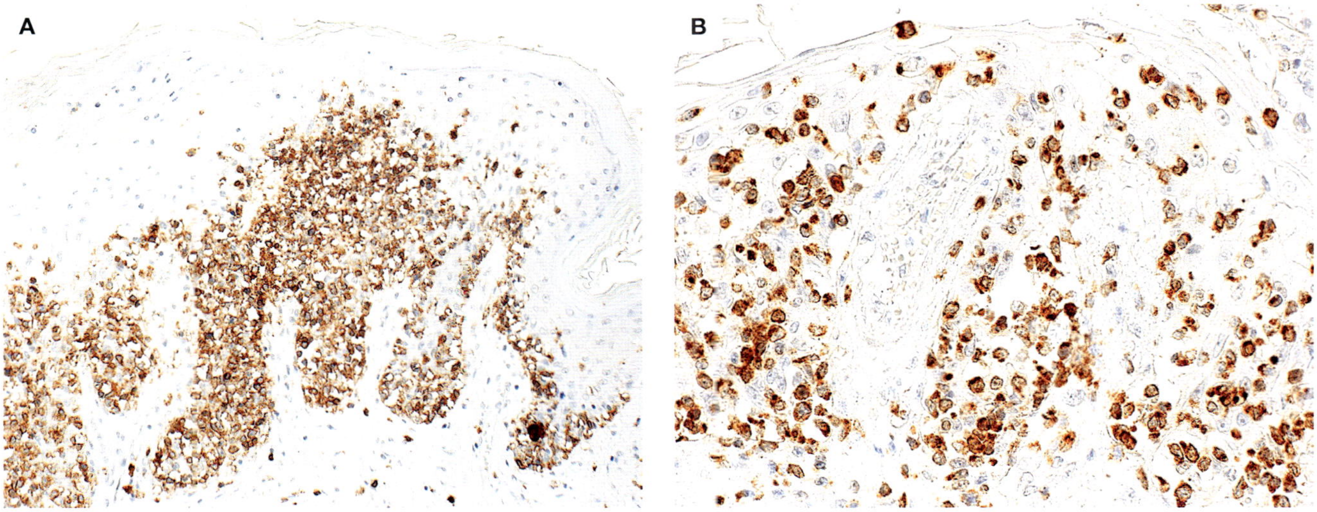

FIGURE 107.3 Primary cutaneous CD8-positive aggressive epidermotropic cytotoxic T-cell lymphoma. **A:** Antibodies to CD8 stain the neoplastic T-cells and emphasize the marked pagetoid epidermotropism. **B:** Staining for perforin is also positive.

References

1. Robson A, Assaf C, Bagot M, et al. Aggressive epidermotropic cutaneous CD8+ lymphoma: a cutaneous lymphoma with distinct clinical and pathological features. Report of an EORTC Cutaneous Lymphoma Task Force Workshop. *Histopathology*. 2015;67(4):425-441.
2. Agnarsson BA, Vonderheid EC, Kadin ME. Cutaneous T cell lymphoma with suppressor/cytotoxic (CD8) phenotype: identification of rapidly progressive and chronic subtypes. *J Am Acad Dermatol*. 1990;22(4):569-577.
3. Berti E, Tomasini D, Vermeer MH, Meijer CJ, Alessi E, Willemze R. Primary cutaneous CD8-positive epidermotropic cytotoxic T cell lymphomas. A distinct clinicopathological entity with an aggressive clinical behavior. *Am J Pathol*. 1999;155(2):483-492.
4. Goodlad JR, Cerroni L, Swerdlow SH. Recent advances in cutaneous lymphoma-implications for current and future classifications. *Virchows Arch*. 2023;482(1):281-298.
5. Bastidas Torres AN, Cats D, Out-Luiting JJ, et al. Deregulation of JAK2 signaling underlies primary cutaneous CD8(+) aggressive epidermotropic cytotoxic T-cell lymphoma. *Haematologica*. 2022;107(3):702-714.

Chapter 108

Peripheral T-Cell Lymphoma, Not Otherwise Specified

Philippe Gaulard, Wing C. Chan, Fina Climent, Laurence de Leval, Andrew L. Feldman, Miguel A. Piris, and Julie M. Vose

Definition

Peripheral T-cell lymphoma, not otherwise specified (PTCL, NOS) is a heterogeneous category including all mature (peripheral) T-cell lymphomas that do not correspond to any specified entity in the current classification. Excluded from this category are follicular helper T-cell (TFHL) lymphoma and primary nodal Epstein-Barr virus (EBV)-positive T/NK-cell lymphoma. PTCL, NOS likely does not constitute a single entity, and additional studies may identify further subgroups. It remains a diagnosis of exclusion, requiring a comprehensive integration of clinical, pathological, phenotypic, and, when necessary, molecular features to rule out a more specific entity.[1] Most cases are thought to derive from activated mature T cells, most commonly the CD4$^+$ central memory type of the adaptive immune system.

Synonyms

Peripheral T-cell lymphoma, unspecified; mature T-cell lymphoma, NOS (not recommended).

Epidemiology

In recent studies in North America, Europe, and Asia, PTCL, NOS is the second or third most common PTCL entity following angioimmunoblastic T-cell lymphoma/TFHL or extranodal NK/T-cell lymphoma, nasal-type in Asia, and accounts for around 20% to 25% of non-cutaneous T-cell lymphomas.[2-4] The higher prevalence of PTCL, NOS previously reported was likely due to incomplete phenotypic characterization, and particularly lack of systematic investigation for TFH markers. A context of immune dysfunction has been reported in some patients, especially those with cytotoxic molecule-positive PTCL, NOS. In particular, patients with chronic lymphocytic leukemia (CLL) may develop PTCL, NOS, often cytotoxic, usually after several years history of CLL.[5] PTCL, NOS in this setting has been linked to the accumulation of oligoclonal or monoclonal T-cell populations observed in patients with CLL. PTCL, NOS may also occur in patients with HIV infection and autoimmune disease and post transplantation.[1,6] Patients with the lymphocytic variant of hypereosinophilic syndrome may also develop PTCL, NOS.

General Clinical Features

Most patients are adults (median age around 60 years), with a male predominance in most series.[7] PTCL, NOS is very rare in children and young adults. Most patients present with peripheral lymph node involvement, but any site can be affected. Constitutional symptoms, poor performance status, and elevated lactate dehydrogenase levels are reported in 40% to 60% of the cases. Advanced-stage disease is common (about 70%), with involvement of the bone marrow, liver, spleen, and extranodal tissues.[8] The peripheral blood may be involved, but leukemic presentation is uncommon. Overall, 50% to 70% of the patients have an intermediate- to high-risk international prognostic index (IPI).[8] Primary extranodal presentation can occur in the skin, where it has been designated as "primary cutaneous PTCL, NOS"[9] and more rarely in the lungs or central nervous system. In this setting, the diagnosis of PTCL, NOS should be made only after more specific entities, especially spread of cutaneous T-cell lymphoma (mycosis fungoides or Sézary syndrome, in particular), or any extranodal lymphoma has been excluded. When EBV is present in most neoplastic cells, involvement by extranodal NK/T lymphoma, nasal-type or primary nodal EBV-positive T/NK cell lymphoma should be considered. Eosinophilia, pruritus, or hemophagocytic syndrome may be seen.

Morphology

PTCL, NOS encompasses a broad morphological spectrum. Besides the rare lymphoepithelioid variant, there are no specific morphological features. In the lymph nodes, these lymphomas usually grow diffusely and efface the normal architecture. When the involvement is interfollicular or paracortical, sparing residual follicles (a pattern formerly referred to as "T-zone variant"), and the infiltrate has a CD4+ phenotype, the case should be carefully investigated for TFHL-NOS. The cytological spectrum ranges from pleomorphic to monomorphic.[1,10] Most cases consist of medium-sized and/or large cells with irregular, pleomorphic nuclei; prominent nucleoli; and many mitotic figures (Figure 108.1). Clear cells and Reed-Sternberg (RS)-like cells can be seen. Rare cases have a predominance of small cells with atypical irregular nuclei (Figure 108.2). Hyperplastic high endothelial venules and open marginal sinuses characteristic of TFHL-AI (angioimmunoblastic T-cell lymphoma) are not usually seen. Follicular dendritic cell expansion is absent. An inflammatory background may be present, including small lymphocytes, eosinophils, plasma cells, large B cells, and clusters of epithelioid histiocytes. Abundance of epithelioid histiocytes is characteristic of the lymphoepithelioid variant.

In the skin, the lymphoma cells tend to infiltrate the dermis and subcutis, often producing nodules, which may undergo central necrosis. In the spleen, the pattern is variable, from solitary or multiple fleshy nodules to diffuse white pulp involvement with colonization of the periarteriolar sheaths or predominant infiltration of the red pulp. These cases must be distinguished from splenic involvement by T-cell leukemias or hepatosplenic T-cell lymphoma.

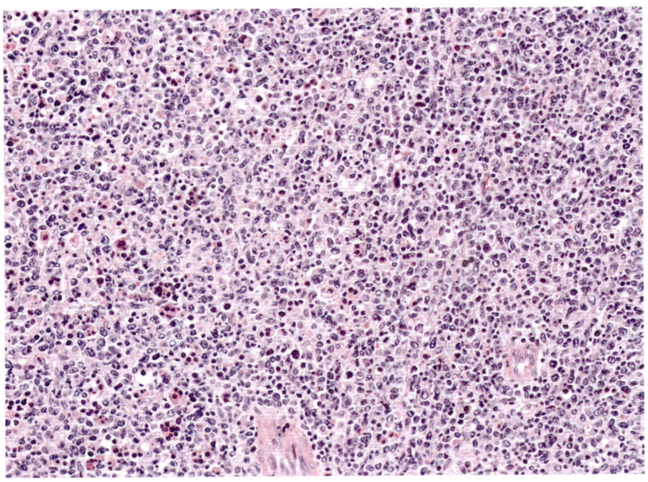

FIGURE 108.1 Example of a peripheral T-cell lymphoma, not otherwise specified consisting of a diffuse proliferation of medium-sized and large cells with pleomorphic often irregular nuclei, admixed with apoptotic figures, histiocytes, and small lymphocytes.

The lymphoepithelioid variant of PTCL, NOS, also known as Lennert lymphoma, usually has a diffuse growth pattern and consists predominantly of small cells with slightly irregular nuclear contours, numerous and sometimes confluent clusters of epithelioid histiocytes, and some larger, more atypical cells (Figure 108.3). There can be admixed inflammatory cells and scattered RS-like B cells (usually EBV-positive). High endothelial venules are not prominent. In most cases, the neoplastic cells are CD8-positive and have a cytotoxic profile (see Figure 108.3B).[10-12] This variant may have a better prognosis. Its cytotoxic profile is helpful in excluding epithelioid cell–rich TFHL.

Immunophenotype

Neoplastic cells in PTCL, NOS express T-cell antigens (CD3, CD2, CD5, CD7), but most cases show an aberrant T-cell phenotype with loss of one or more T-cell antigens, most commonly CD7 and/or CD5 (Figure 108.4).[1] Most cases are CD4-positive, more rarely CD8-positive, or uncommonly CD4/CD8 double positive or double negative. In such cases, especially when the neoplastic infiltrate is monotonous, negativity for TdT and other markers of immaturity are required to exclude T-lymphoblastic lymphoma. T-cell receptor (TCR) beta (βF1) is expressed (>85%), whereas a minority of cases are derived from γ/δ T cells (positive for TCR gamma and/or delta) or negative for both (TCR silent). CD30 is variably expressed from occasional tumor cells to >25% of tumor cells in half of cases.[13] Up to 20% of PTCL, NOS have been reported to contain >50% CD30-positive cells; in such cases, anaplastic large cell lymphoma (ALCL) should be considered and investigation for expression of ALK and cytotoxic molecules as well as *DUSP22* rearrangement should be performed. Recently, PTCL, NOS containing CD30-positive RS-like cells in a polymorphous background associated with *JAK2* rearrangements have been reported.[14] Such cases may express CD15, raising the differential diagnosis with classic Hodgkin lymphoma. CD25, another potential target for immunotherapy, is expressed at significant levels in around 40% of PTCL, NOS. Loss of BCL2 is observed in 45% to 60% of PTCL, NOS and may be used as an indicator of T-cell malignancy.[15] Occasional cases aberrantly express CD20 (or less frequently CD79a). A high Ki67 proliferation index is common.

A proportion of PTCL, NOS, even when $CD4^+$, express one or several cytotoxic granule-associated molecules (eg, TIA1, granzyme B, and/or perforin) (see Figure 108.4).[6,16] This subgroup frequently occurs

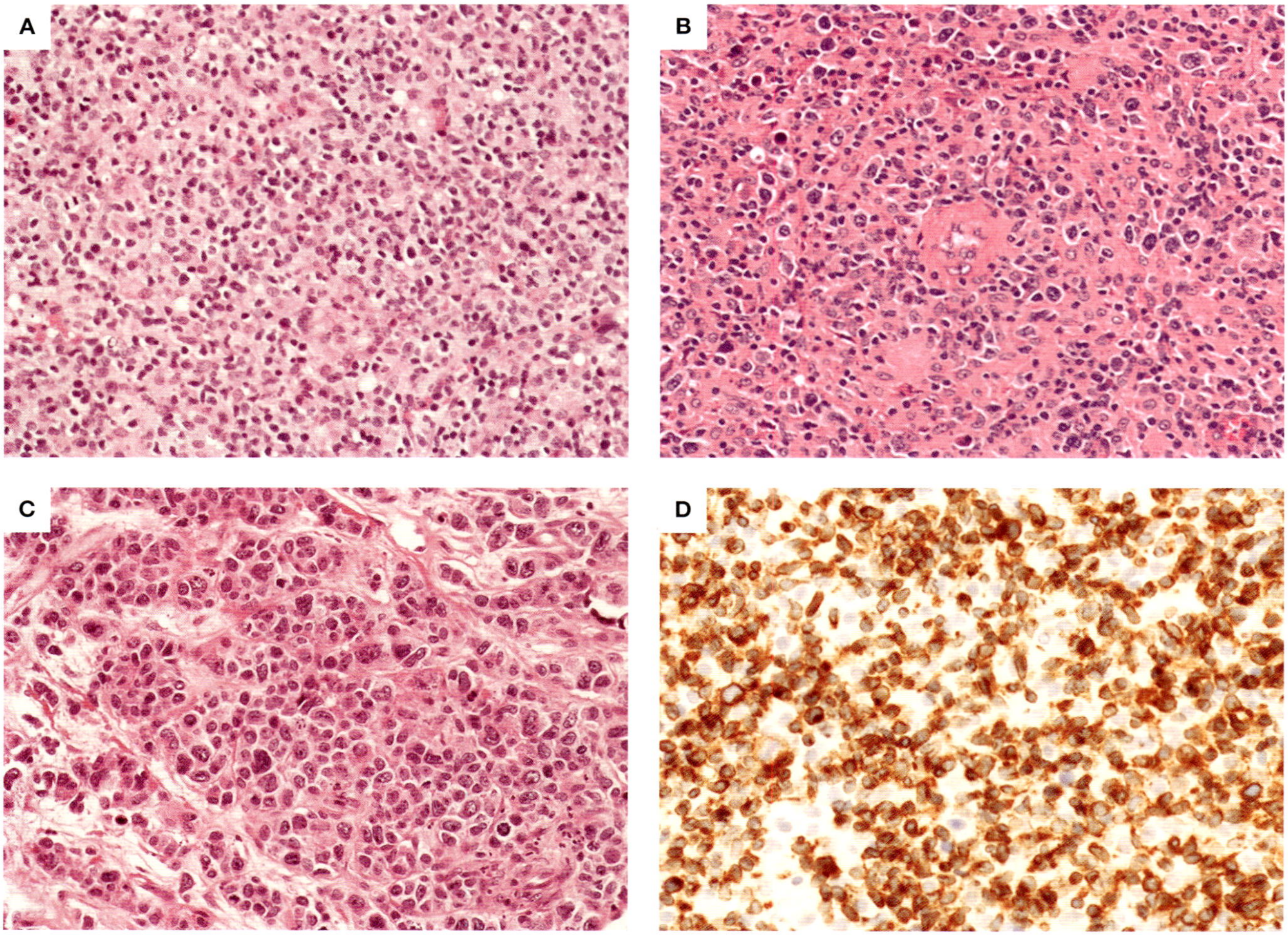

FIGURE 108.2 Other examples of peripheral T-cell lymphoma, not otherwise specified illustrating the spectrum of pathological aspects from cases mainly composed of small to medium-sized **(A)**; pleomorphic small, medium, to large neoplastic cells with irregular nuclei **(B)**; predominantly large neoplastic cells sometimes with anaplastic features **(C)**. Neoplastic cells are usually CD3-positive **(D)**.

in clinical settings of immune dysregulation.[6,16] It is commonly $CD8^+$ or $CD4^-/CD8^-$, and more rarely $CD4^+$, and often expresses TBX21 and/or CXCR3 (see Figure 108.4).

By definition, the neoplastic cells in PTCL, NOS should be EBV-negative, as the rare nodal PTCLs showing EBV in virtually all tumor cells (by EBER in situ hybridization) are now classified as primary nodal EBV-positive T/NK-cell lymphoma (see Chapter 95: Primary Nodal Epstein-Barr Virus+ T-Cell/NK-Cell Lymphoma).[1,16] The presence of scattered EBER-positive cells, likely representing bystander EBV-positive B cells, has been reported in up to 50% of PTCL, NOS, prior to the recognition of TFHL-NOS.[6,16]

Genetics

TCR genes are clonally rearranged in most cases.[17] Next-generation sequencing–based assays using primers sets targeting various regions of the TRB or TRG genes may overcome low sensitivity or false-negative results with polymerase chain reaction–based assays.[17]

By conventional cytogenetics, PTCL, NOS usually has complex karyotypes, which have been correlated with worse outcome. By array comparative genomic hybridization, genomic imbalances include recurrent gains affecting chromosomes 7q, 8q, 17q, and 22q and losses in chromosomes 4q, 5q, 6q, 9p, 10q, 12q, and 13q. Amplification at 7q22 targets cyclin-dependent kinase 6, while gains at 8q involve the *MYC* locus, losses at 9p21 are associated with reduced expression of cyclin-dependent kinases inhibitors, and gains at 7p22 correlate with increased levels of *CARMA1/CARD11*, an NF-kappaB activator.[18] *CDKN2A* deletions, found in around half of PTCL, NOS, may associate with *PTEN* deletions,[19] are preferentially observed in the GATA3 molecular subgroup and have been associated with shorter survival.[20] Chromosomal breaks involving the TCR gene loci (mostly the TRA/TRD locus at 14q11.2) are rare. Among them, the t(14;19)(q11;q13) translocation

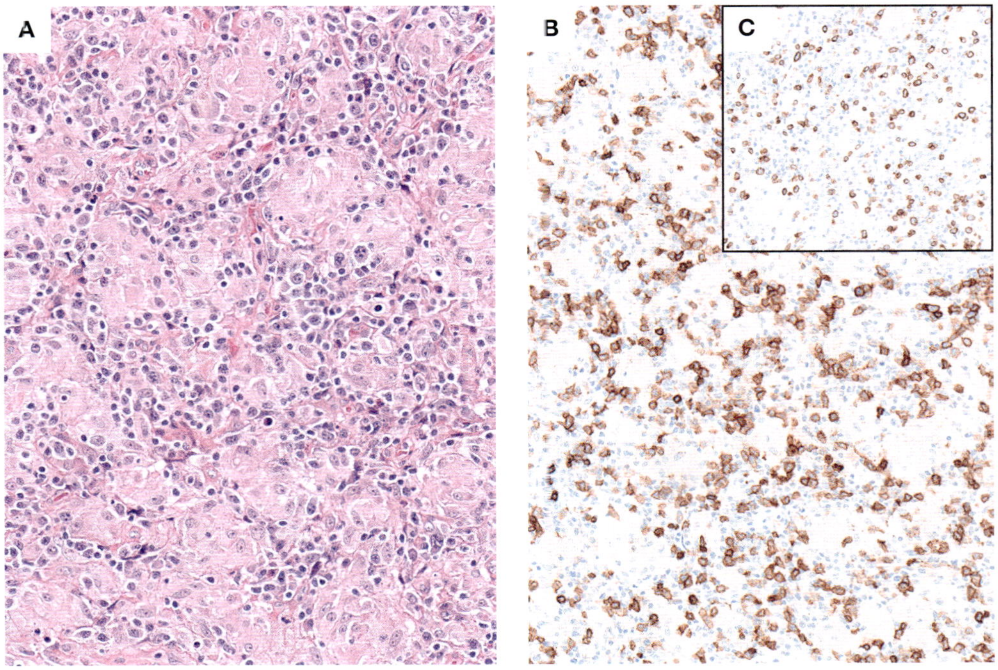

FIGURE 108.3 Lennert lymphoma variant: the architecture of the lymph node is effaced by a diffuse population of slightly atypical small to medium-sized lymphoid cells, admixed with numerous clusters of epithelioid histiocytes (**A**); atypical cells are highlighted by CD8 (**B**) and perforin (**C**) immunostaining.

involving *PVRL2* has been reported in single cases[21] and the t(6;14)(p25;q11.2) translocation involving *IRF4* may define a rare subset of aggressive cytotoxic PTCL, NOS involving the bone marrow and skin, or spleen.[22]

Several recurrent fusion transcripts have been reported with an overall low incidence.[21] These are not specific for PTCL, NOS, as they also occur in ALK-negative ALCL or TFHL.[17,21] *TP63* rearrangements with *TBL1XR1* or other partner genes, reported in about 5% of PTCL, NOS, are associated with poor outcome.[23] Fusions involving *VAV1* with different partners (*VAV1::MYOF1, VAV1::THAP4, VAV1::S100A7*) result in activation of the VAV1 effector pathway.[24] The *FYN::TRAF3IP2* fusion described in PTCL, NOS and TFHL activates the NF-kappaB pathway.[25] Fusions involving CD28 (*CD28::CTLA4* and *CD28::ICOS*) occur in PTCL, NOS.

Reflecting the heterogeneity of PTCL, NOS, there is no characteristic mutational pattern. PTCL, NOS harbors recurrent mutations in epigenetic modifiers, most often *TET2* or *DNMT3A*[26] and less commonly *SMARCA4* or *KMT2D*, and in genes related to the TCR signaling pathway, notably activating mutations in *PLCG1, CD28*, and *VAV1*.[6,17,27] Mutations in *RHOA* and *IDH2* are typically absent. *DNMT3A* mutations have been associated with poor outcome and a cytotoxic phenotype.[26] Alterations in *TP53* and/or *CDKN2A* may delineate a group of PTCL, NOS characterized by marked genomic instability and adverse outcome.[28]

PTCL, NOS with a cytotoxic granule-associated phenotype frequently harbors mutations in epigenetic modifiers, notably *TET2* and *DNMT3A*, and recurrent alterations in the TCR and JAK/STAT signaling pathways, including fusions involving *VAV1* and *CD28*.[6] PTCL-TBX21 and PTCL-GATA3 molecular subgroups are defined by distinct gene expression signatures at least partly reflecting genes regulated by the transcription factors TBX21 and GATA3, respectively.[10,20,29] A simplified NanoString transcriptomic assay applicable to routinely processed biopsies has been published for the molecular diagnosis of the PTCLs but is not commercially available.[29] An immunohistochemical algorithm using four antibodies may be used as a surrogate to gene expression profiling to identify these subgroups: expression of TBX21 or its target gene CXCR3 in >20% of tumor cells is associated with the TBX21 subgroup, and in cases negative for TBX21/CXCR3, expression of GATA3, or its target gene CCR4 in >50% neoplastic cells is indicative of the GATA3 subgroup (Figure 108.5).[10]

Histologically, PTCL-TBX21 tends to be polymorphous, with a background of reactive cells, and includes cases with a cytotoxic phenotype and Lennert lymphomas, while PTCL-GATA3 tends to consist of sheets of medium-sized or large tumor cells.[10] It is unclear from the literature to what extent the TBX21 subgroup overlaps with the group of PTCL, NOS expressing cytotoxic molecules. PTCL-TBX21 has fewer copy number

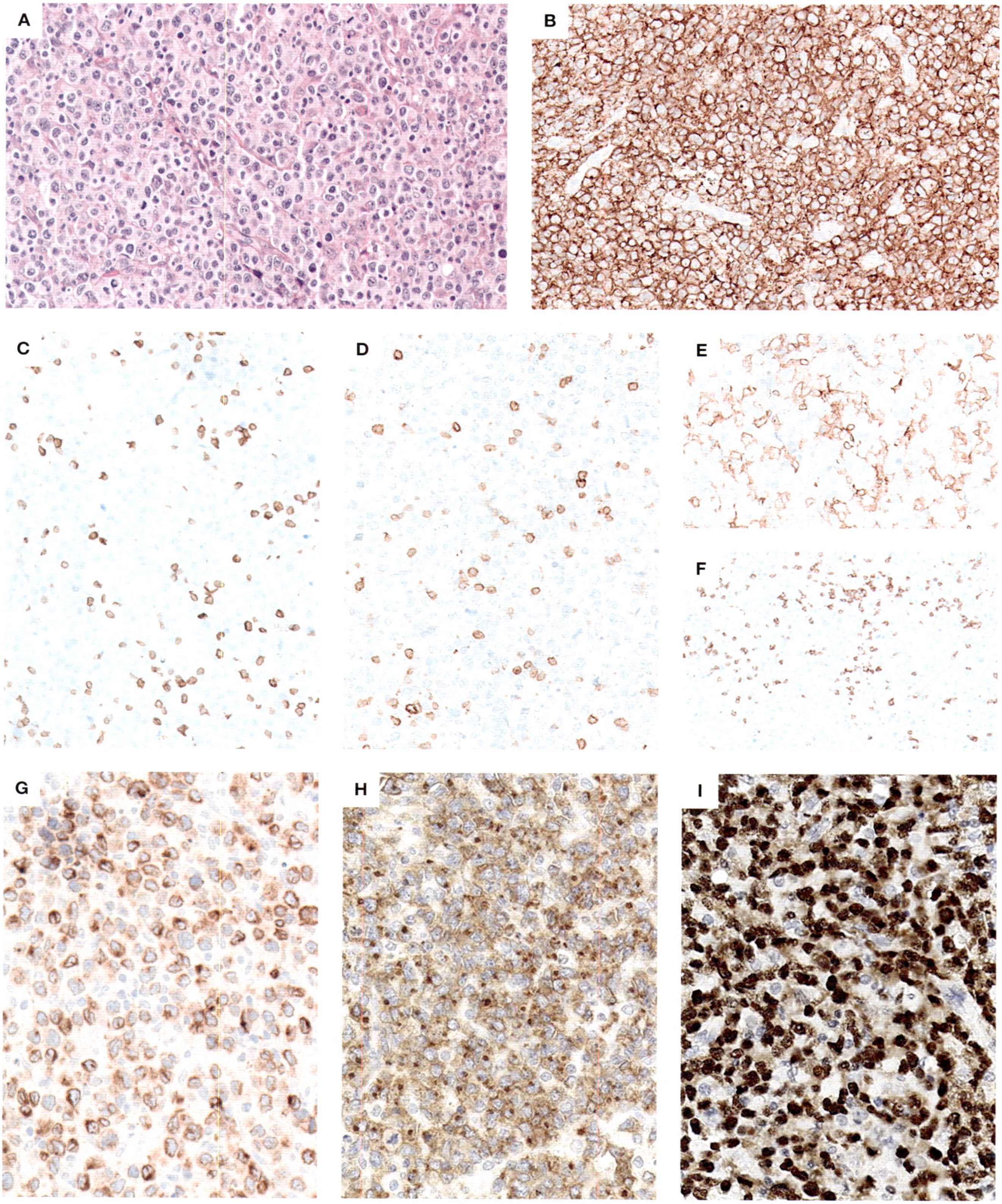

FIGURE 108.4 Cytotoxic molecule-positive PTCL, NOS in a lymph node: the architecture is replaced by a diffuse proliferation of atypical lymphoid cells with small to large nuclei surrounded by a abundant clear cytoplasm (**A**). By immunohistochemistry, neoplastic cells are strongly positive for CD2 (**B**) and negative for CD5 (**C**) and CD7 (**D**). They do not express CD4 (**E**) or CD8 (**F**) but are strongly positive for perforin (**G**). Almost all neoplastic cells are positive for CXCR3+ (**H**) and TBX21 (**I**). They were negative for GATA3 (not shown), and EBV by EBER in situ hybridization was absent (not shown).

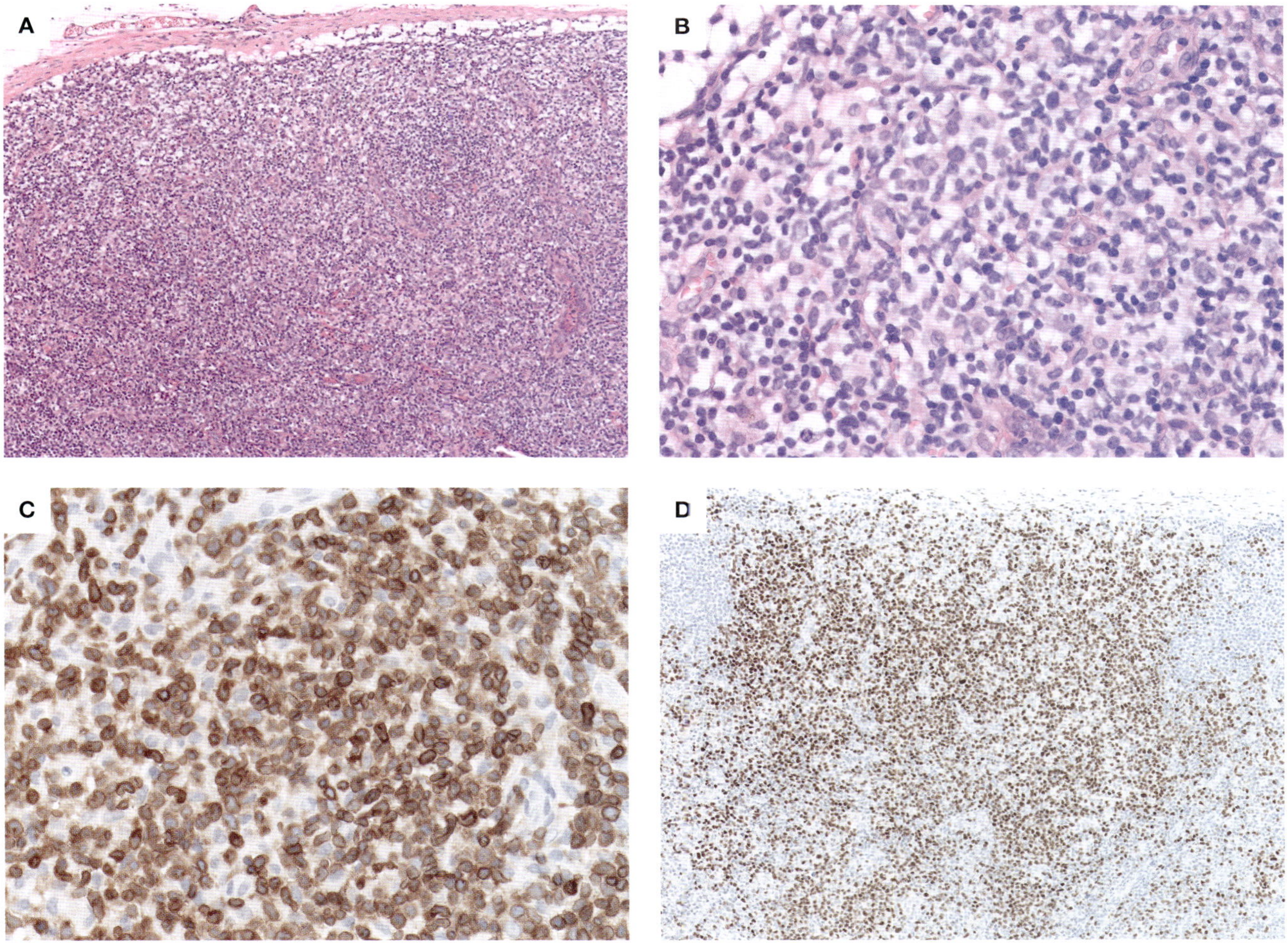

FIGURE 108.5 Peripheral T-cell lymphoma, not otherwise specified with GATA3 expression. The lymph node architecture is effaced by a diffuse proliferation of atypical small to large lymphocytes with irregular nuclei (**A** and **B**), which by immunohistochemistry are CD3 positive (**C**) and strongly and uniformly express GATA3 (**D**). They were negative for TBX21 and CXCR3 (not shown).

aberrations and more frequent mutations of epigenetic modifying genes, whereas PTCL-GATA3 has greater genomic complexity, frequent losses of *TP53, PTEN, RB1, CDKN2A/B*, and *PRDM1*, gains of *STAT3* and *MYC*, and mutations of *TP53* and *PRDM1*.[20] PTCL-GATA3 is reported to have the worst outcome. The identification of the TBX21 and GATA3 subgroups currently has no impact on frontline clinical management of the patients and is not required in standard diagnostic practice.

Overall, the diagnosis of PTCL, NOS is based on histopathologic and immunophenotypic criteria. Investigation for EBV is also critical. Molecular analysis, together with clinical features, can be helpful especially in difficult cases or to exclude another better-defined PTCL entity.[17]

Altogether, given its markedly variable features, PTCL, NOS encompasses broad differential diagnoses, which are sources of misdiagnoses. T-lymphoblastic lymphoma is usually easy to distinguish based on the immature, monotonous cellular appearance and TdT expression, whereas human T-lymphotropic virus 1 (HTLV1) serology and/or search for expression of CD25 by immunohistochemistry, HTLV1 by in situ hybridization or viral integration should be performed in PTCL, occurring in patients from endemic regions to exclude adult T-cell leukemia/lymphoma. When the lymphoma is composed of large cells with uniform expression of CD30, distinction from ALCL can be problematic; demonstration of ALK staining or *DUSP22* rearrangement by fluorescence in situ hybridization supports a diagnosis of ALK+ ALCL and *DUSP22*-rearranged ALK-ALCL, respectively. In addition, hallmark cells (with kidney- or horseshoe-shaped nuclei), sinusoidal involvement, expression of cytotoxic molecules and/or EMA, and strong and uniform expression of CD30 are characteristic of ALCL. Diagnosis of PTCL, NOS also requires exclusion of a TFHL-NOS. A diagnosis of TFHL should be considered in all cases of $CD4^+$ nodal PTCL. Expression of at least two TFH markers among CD10, PD1, ICOS, CXCL13, and BCL6 is required, and the presence of scattered EBV-infected cells (typically B cells) and expansion of follicular dendritic cells may be additional supporting features. In difficult cases, molecular studies showing a *RHOAG17V* mutation supports TFHL and rules out PTCL, NOS. Clinical features and history are also critical to exclude nodal involvement by a specific extranodal entity, such as mycosis fungoides or Sézary syndrome. EBV needs to be assessed in every suspected PTCL, NOS, especially CD4-negative, to evaluate for primary nodal EBV+ T-cell/NK-cell lymphoma. When $CD30^+$ RS-like cells are present, a pleomorphic background with cell atypia, negativity for PAX5, and the demonstration of a clonal T-cell population are helpful to distinguish PTCL, NOS with HRS-like cells from classic Hodgkin lymphoma, especially in those rare cases where RS cells express T-cell antigens.[30] Intact normal lymph node architecture, a predominant CD8+ phenotype of the T-cell population with no or mild cytologic atypia, and absence of a clonal T-cell population or somatic mutation help exclude PTCL, NOS in conditions associated with immune dysregulation, benign EBV+ lymphoproliferations, and other reactive conditions.

Prognosis and Clinical Comments

PTCL, NOS are aggressive lymphomas with a poor response to therapy, frequent relapses, and low 5-year overall and failure-free survival rates (20%-30%).[7,8] The factors consistently associated with prognosis are stage and IPI score. Other scoring systems have been developed. Bone marrow involvement and a Ki-67 proliferation index >70% have been proposed as adverse prognostic factors, as well as EBV positivity, NF-kappaB pathway deregulation, a high proliferation signature by gene expression, >70% transformed cells, a GATA3 or cytotoxic profile, and *TP53* mutations.[31]

Treatment of PTCL, NOS remains challenging. Current standards of care for frontline chemotherapy include combination chemotherapy with anthracycline containing regimens ± etoposide ± consolidation with high-dose chemotherapy and autologous stem cell transplantation. For those patients with PTCL, NOS expressing CD30, brentuximab vedotin may be added to the anthracycline and cyclophosphamide backbone. These treatments only produce long-term disease-free survival in approximately 20% to 30% of patients. Standard-of-care treatments at relapse include pralatrexate, belinostat, and gemcitabine-containing regimens. In younger patients, the use of allogeneic stem cell transplantation could also be considered. Many new agents are being tested for treatment of PTCL including PI3Kinase inhibitors, JAK-STAT inhibitors, and checkpoint inhibitors. Hopefully, collaborations on clinical research can improve the outcomes for patients with PTCL, NOS.

References

1. Feldman AL, Laurent C, Narbaitz M, et al. Classification and diagnostic evaluation of nodal T- and NK-cell lymphomas. *Virchows Arch.* 2023;482(1):265-279. doi:10.1007/s00428-022-03412-6
2. Hsi ED, Said J, Macon WR, et al. Diagnostic accuracy of a defined immunophenotypic and molecular genetic approach for peripheral T/NK-cell lymphomas. A North American PTCL study group project. *Am J Surg Pathol.* 2014;38(6):768-775. doi:10.1097/PAS.0000000000000188
3. Laurent C, Baron M, Amara N, et al. Impact of expert pathologic review of lymphoma diagnosis: study of patients from the French lymphopath network. *J Clin Oncol.* 2017;35(18):2008-2017. doi:10.1200/JCO.2016.71.2083
4. Yoon SE, Song Y, Kim SJ, et al. Comprehensive analysis of peripheral T-cell and natural killer/T-cell lymphoma in Asian patients: a multinational, multicenter, prospective registry study in Asia. *Lancet Reg Health West Pac.* 2021;10:100126. doi:10.1016/j.lanwpc.2021.100126
5. Chihara D, Dores GM, Flowers CR, Morton LM. The bidirectional increased risk of B-cell lymphoma and T-cell lymphoma. *Blood.* 2021;138(9):785-789. doi:10.1182/blood.2020010497
6. Nicolae A, Bouilly J, Lara D, et al. Nodal cytotoxic peripheral T-cell lymphoma occurs frequently in the clinical setting of immunodysregulation and is associated with recurrent epigenetic alterations. *Mod Pathol.* 2022;35(8):1126-1136. doi:10.1038/s41379-022-01022-w
7. Weiss J, Reneau J, Wilcox RA. PTCL, NOS: an update on classification, risk-stratification, and treatment. *Front Oncol.* 2023;13:1101441. doi:10.3389/fonc.2023.1101441
8. Weisenburger DD, Savage KJ, Harris NL, et al. Peripheral T-cell lymphoma, not otherwise specified: a report of 340 cases from the international peripheral T-cell lymphoma project. *Blood.* 2011;117(12):3402-3408. doi:10.1182/blood-2010-09-310342
9. Willemze R, Cerroni L, Kempf W, et al. The 2018 update of the WHO-EORTC classification for primary cutaneous lymphomas. *Blood.* 2019;133(16):1703-1714. doi:10.1182/blood-2018-11-881268

10. Amador C, Greiner TC, Heavican TB, et al. Reproducing the molecular subclassification of peripheral T-cell lymphoma-NOS by immunohistochemistry. *Blood.* 2019;134(24):2159-2170. doi:10.1182/blood.2019000779
11. Hartmann S, Agostinelli C, Klapper W, et al. Revising the historical collection of epithelioid cell-rich lymphomas of the Kiel Lymph Node Registry: what is Lennert's lymphoma nowadays? *Histopathology.* 2011;59(6):1173-1182. doi:10.1111/j.1365-2559.2011.04069.x
12. Geissinger E, Odenwald T, Lee SS, et al. Nodal peripheral T-cell lymphomas and, in particular, their lymphoepithelioid (Lennert's) variant are often derived from CD8(+) cytotoxic T-cells. *Virchows Arch.* 2004;445(4):334-343. doi:10.1007/s00428-004-1077-2
13. Bossard C, Dobay MP, Parrens M, et al. Immunohistochemistry as a valuable tool to assess CD30 expression in peripheral T-cell lymphomas: high correlation with mRNA levels. *Blood.* 2014;124(19):2983-2986. doi:10.1182/blood-2014-07-584953
14. Fitzpatrick MJ, Massoth LR, Marcus C, et al. JAK2 rearrangements are a recurrent alteration in CD30+ systemic T-cell lymphomas with anaplastic morphology. *Am J Surg Pathol.* 2021;45(7):895-904. doi:10.1097/PAS.0000000000001708
15. O'Malley DP, Chizhevsky V, Grimm KE, Hii A, Weiss LM. Utility of BCL2, PD1, and CD25 immunohistochemical expression in the diagnosis of T-cell lymphomas. *Appl Immunohistochem Mol Morphol.* 2014;22(2):99-104. doi:10.1097/PAI.0b013e31828ef1f7
16. Climent F, Nicolae A, de Leval L, et al. Cytotoxic peripheral T-cell lymphomas and EBV-positive T/NK-cell lymphoproliferative diseases: emerging concepts, recent advances, and the putative role of clonal hematopoiesis. A report of the 2022 EA4HP/SH lymphoma workshop. *Virchows Arch.* 2023;483(3):333-348. doi:10.1007/s00428-023-03616-4
17. de Leval L, Alizadeh AA, Bergsagel PL, et al. Genomic profiling for clinical decision making in lymphoid neoplasms. *Blood.* 2022;140(21):2193-2227. doi:10.1182/blood.2022015854
18. Fujiwara Si, Yamashita Y, Nakamura N, et al. High-resolution analysis of chromosome copy number alterations in angioimmunoblastic T-cell lymphoma and peripheral T-cell lymphoma, unspecified, with single nucleotide polymorphism-typing microarrays. *Leukemia.* 2008;22(10):1891-1898. doi:10.1038/leu.2008.191
19. Maura F, Dodero A, Carniti C, et al. CDKN2A deletion is a frequent event associated with poor outcome in patients with peripheral T-cell lymphoma not otherwise specified (PTCL-NOS). *Haematologica.* 2021;106(11):2918-2926. doi:10.3324/haematol.2020.262659
20. Heavican TB, Bouska A, Yu J, et al. Genetic drivers of oncogenic pathways in molecular subgroups of peripheral T-cell lymphoma. *Blood.* 2019;133(15):1664-1676. doi:10.1182/blood-2018-09-872549
21. Drieux F, Ruminy P, Sater V, et al. Detection of gene fusion transcripts in peripheral T-cell lymphoma using a multiplexed targeted sequencing assay. *J Mol Diagn.* 2021;23(8):929-940. doi:10.1016/j.jmoldx.2021.04.013
22. Feldman AL, Law M, Remstein ED, et al. Recurrent translocations involving the IRF4 oncogene locus in peripheral T-cell lymphomas. *Leukemia.* 2009;23(3):574-580. doi:10.1038/leu.2008.320
23. Vasmatzis G, Johnson SH, Knudson RA, et al. Genome-wide analysis reveals recurrent structural abnormalities of TP63 and other p53-related genes in peripheral T-cell lymphomas. *Blood.* 2012;120(11):2280-2289. doi:10.1182/blood-2012-03-419937
24. Cortes JR, Filip I, Albero R, et al. Oncogenic Vav1-Myo1f induces therapeutically targetable macrophage-rich tumor microenvironment in peripheral T cell lymphoma. *Cell Rep.* 2022;39(3):110695. doi:10.1016/j.celrep.2022.110695
25. Debackere K, Marcelis L, Demeyer S, et al. Fusion transcripts FYN-TRAF3IP2 and KHDRBS1-LCK hijack T cell receptor signaling in peripheral T-cell lymphoma, not otherwise specified. *Nat Commun.* 2021;12(1):3705. doi:10.1038/s41467-021-24037-4
26. Herek TA, Bouska A, Lone W, et al. DNMT3A mutations define a unique biological and prognostic subgroup associated with cytotoxic T cells in PTCL-NOS. *Blood.* 2022;140(11):1278-1290. doi:10.1182/blood.2021015019
27. Manso R, Rodríguez-Pinilla SM, González-Rincón J, et al. Recurrent presence of the PLCG1 S345F mutation in nodal peripheral T-cell lymphomas. *Haematologica.* 2015;100(1):e25-e27. doi:10.3324/haematol.2014.113696
28. Watatani Y, Sato Y, Miyoshi H, et al. Molecular heterogeneity in peripheral T-cell lymphoma, not otherwise specified revealed by comprehensive genetic profiling. *Leukemia.* 2019;33(12):2867-2883. doi:10.1038/s41375-019-0473-1
29. Amador C, Bouska A, Wright G, et al. Gene expression signatures for the accurate diagnosis of peripheral T-cell lymphoma entities in the routine clinical practice. *J Clin Oncol.* 2022;40(36):4261-4275. doi:10.1200/JCO.21.02707
30. Venkataraman G, Song JY, Tzankov A, et al. Aberrant T-cell antigen expression in classical Hodgkin lymphoma is associated with decreased event-free survival and overall survival. *Blood.* 2013;121(10):1795-1804. doi:10.1182/blood-2012-06-439455
31. Johnson WT, Ganesan N, Epstein-Peterson ZD, et al. TP53 mutations identify high-risk events for peripheral T-cell lymphoma treated with CHOP-based chemotherapy. *Blood Adv.* 2023;7(17):5172-5186. doi:10.1182/bloodadvances.2023009953

Chapter 109

Follicular Helper T-Cell Lymphoma

Ahmet Dogan, Philippe Gaulard, François Lemonnier, Sarah L. Ondrejka, and Pier Luigi Zinzani

Definition

Follicular helper T-cell lymphoma (TFHL) is a neoplasm of mature follicular helper T cells comprising three histological subtypes related by cell of origin, clinical behavior, and molecular pathogenesis (Table 109.1):

1. Follicular helper T-cell lymphoma, angioimmunoblastic type (TFHL-AI)
2. Follicular helper T-cell lymphoma, follicular type (TFHL-F)
3. Follicular helper T-cell lymphoma, not otherwise specified (TFHL-NOS)

Following the discovery that T follicular helper (TFH) cells represent the cell state of the neoplastic cells in angioimmunoblastic T-cell lymphoma (AITL), it was recognized that a subset of cases previously classified as peripheral T-cell lymphoma (PTCL), NOS, have a TFH-cell phenotype.[1,2] Additional studies supported that AITL and PTCL with TFH immunophenotype share clinical features, gene expression, and molecular genetic characteristics in addition to phenotype.[3-6] The 2016 World Health Organization (WHO) classification created an umbrella category of "nodal lymphomas of TFH origin" to encompass angioimmunoblastic T-cell lymphoma and peripheral T-cell lymphoma with TFH phenotype (follicular T-cell lymphoma and diffuse or T-zone pattern). The International Consensus Classification carries this notion forward by creating a single entity, TFHL, with three subtypes having in common clinical and molecular genetic features and requiring demonstration of TFH phenotype. These subtypes are distinguished by immune architecture and the tumor microenvironment.[7] This entity excludes specified subtypes of primary cutaneous T-cell lymphoma that may frequently

TABLE 109.1 Histological characteristics of follicular helper T-cell lymphoma subtypes

Subtype	Architecture	Follicles	Vasculature	B immunoblasts	Differential diagnosis
AI-Pattern 1	Preserved	Hyperplastic	Mild increase	Subtle	Reactive lymphoid hyperplasia (viral infections, drug reactions, autoimmune disease)
AI-Pattern 2	Partly preserved	Atretic	Moderate increase	Variable	Castleman disease
AI-Pattern 3	Effaced	Lost	Marked increase	Prominent	CHL Reactive lymphadenitis (viral infections such as HIV, drug reactions such as phenytoin)B-cell lymphomas CHL
F-FL	Nodular	Replaced by TFHL	Unremarkable	Subtle	Follicular lymphoma
F-PTGC	Nodular	Replaced by small B cells and TFHL cells	Unremarkable	Subtle	NLPBCL CHL PTGC
NOS	Paracortical or diffuse	Atretic or lost	Variable	Variable	PTCL, NOS Secondary lymph node involvement by cutaneous T-cell lymphoma

AI, angioimmunoblastic variant of TFHL; CHL, classic Hodgkin lymphoma; F-FL, follicular subtype of TFHL, follicular lymphoma-like; F-PTGC, follicular subtype of TFHL, PTGC-like; PTCL, peripheral T-cell lymphoma; NLPBCL, nodular lymphocyte predominant B-cell lymphoma; NOS, not otherwise specified; PTGC, progressive transformation of germinal centers; TFHL, follicular helper T-cell lymphoma.

express TFH markers (for example, mycosis fungoides and primary cutaneous small/medium CD4+ T-cell lymphoproliferative disorder).[8] Likewise, tumors with less convincing expression of TFH markers would be better categorized PTCL, NOS, and are best excluded from this category.

Synonyms

Angioimmunoblastic T-cell lymphoma (acceptable for TFHL-AI), nodal lymphomas of T follicular helper cell origin (not recommended).

Epidemiology

TFHL incidence data are mainly based on angioimmunoblastic T-cell lymphoma, which is the most common subtype accounting for 60% to 80% TFHL cases. TFHL-F is very rare. TFHL-NOS may account for up to 20% of nodal PTCLs, but the incidence is difficult to precisely estimate given variances in approach to diagnosis of T-cell lymphoma over the past few decades. Collectively, TFHL is one of the most common types of nodal, systemic PTCL, accounting for approximately 20% to 36% of noncutaneous T-cell lymphomas.[9-11] TFHL occurs in middle-aged to elderly individuals and has a slightly higher incidence in males than in females.[12]

The etiology of TFHL is unknown, but a strong association with underlying clonal hematopoiesis (CH) has emerged.[13] Up to 80% of patients with TFHL have underlying CH with *TET2* and/or *DNMT3A* mutations in the early progenitor cells (ie, hematopoietic stem cells), shared with the lymphoma which may predispose to myeloid neoplasms after TFHL-directed therapy.[14-16] There is a possible role for the Epstein-Barr virus in the etiology of TFHL, as it can drive associated B-cell proliferations especially in TFHL-AI. The precise mechanism is not known, although immunodeficiency and reactivation of EBV or TFH cell activation by EBV has been proposed.[17]

General Clinical Features

TFHL is a lymph node–based, systemic disease of older adults. Patients usually present with generalized lymphadenopathy and occasionally extranodal involvement (skin, tonsil, liver, spleen, and bone marrow) and B symptoms. A characteristic systemic presentation is known to occur especially in TFHL-AI, variably consisting of skin rash, pleural effusion, arthritis, and ascites. Accompanying laboratory abnormalities include cytopenia, polyclonal hypergammaglobulinemia (30%), circulating immune complexes, cold agglutinins with hemolytic anemia, warm autoimmune hemolytic anemia, absolute eosinophilia, positive rheumatoid factor, or other transiently induced autoimmune antibodies.[18,19] The median survival is less than 3 years, but a subset of patients experience long-term survival.[20]

Morphology

Histopathological features of TFHL are complex and require examination of lymph node architecture, microenvironment, and cytological features of the neoplastic cells. These features can be rarely comprehensively assessed in core biopsies, and in most cases a firm diagnosis can be only established by examination of excisional biopsies. The neoplastic T cells of TFHL are small to medium-sized lymphocytes with clear to pale cytoplasm and small irregular nuclei (Figures 109.1 to 109.4). Of the subtypes, TFHL-AI/angioimmunoblastic T-cell lymphoma is prototypic and best studied. TFHL-AI is associated with increased vascularity and clustering of the abnormal lymphocytes around arborizing high endothelial venules (HEVs). There is a polymorphous inflammatory microenvironment with eosinophils, plasma cells, histiocytes, and large immunoblastic cells, which may resemble Hodgkin/Reed-Sternberg (HRS) cells (see Figure 109.4). In some cases abnormal follicular dendritic cell (FDC) meshworks can be visualized. In excisional biopsy specimens, a perinodal lymphoma infiltrate often sparing of the peripheral cortical sinuses, can be seen[21,22] (see Figure 109.4). Three histological patterns are described (see Table 109.1): pattern I, with hyperplastic follicles (see Figure 109.1); pattern II, with regressive follicles (see Figure 109.2); and the most common pattern III with diffuse growth (see Figures 109.3 and 109.4). The patterns of FDC meshwork staining are helpful in consideration of histologic growth pattern. These are typically minimally or subtly expanded in pattern I, progressively expanded and disrupted in pattern II, and highly disrupted and proliferated with encircling of HEVs in pattern III[23] (see Figure 109.4). Rarely, patients with evidence of disseminated disease but low tumor burden in lymph nodes manifesting as clusters of abnormal TFH cells in the paracortex or surrounding follicles with regressively transformed germinal centers have been reported.[24]

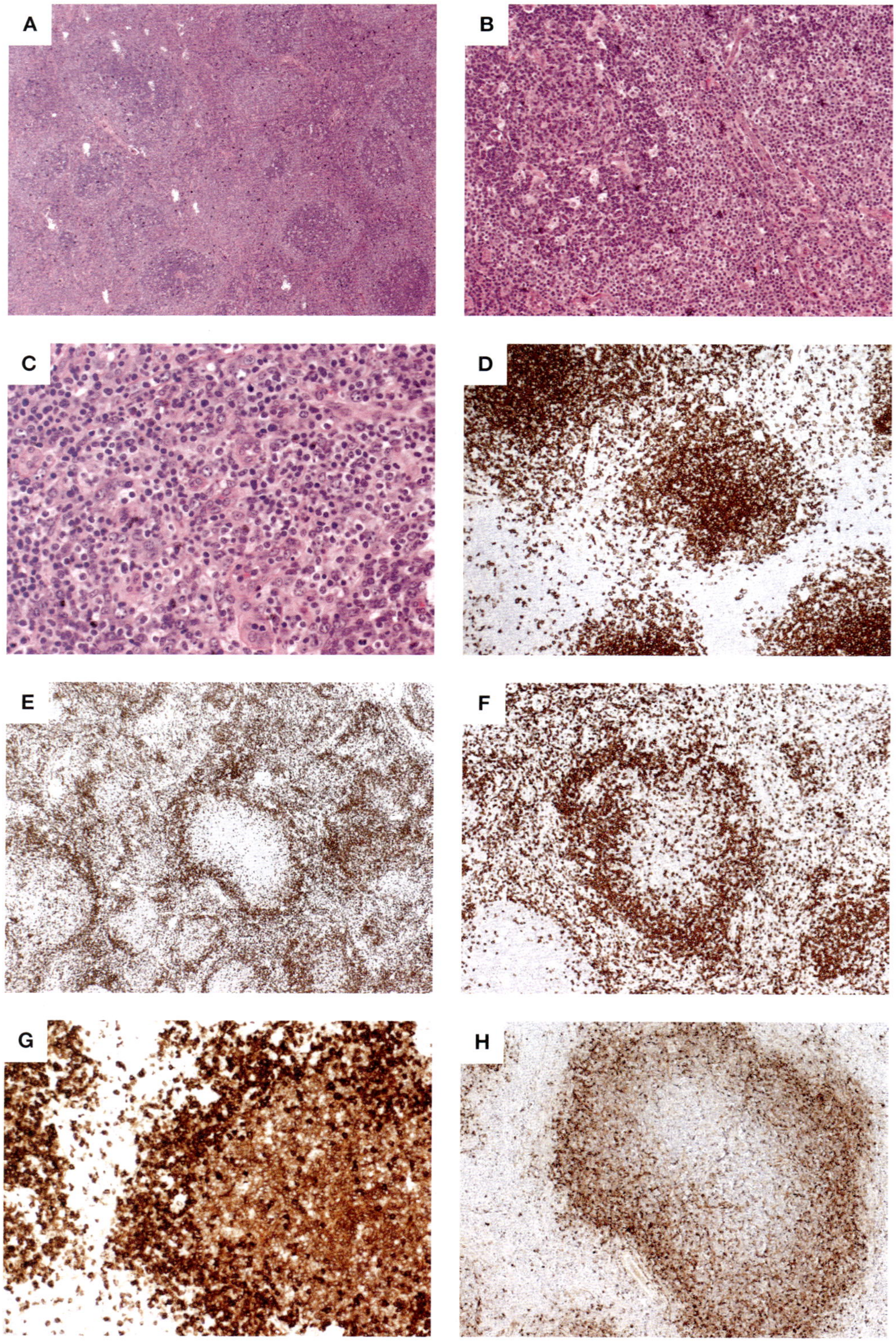

FIGURE 109.1 Histological and immunophenotypic features of follicular helper T-cell lymphoma, angioimmunoblastic-type, pattern I. Low- and medium-power views of the lymph node biopsy show hyperplastic germinal centers rimmed by a halo of intermediate-sized lymphocytes giving the impression of prominent marginal zones (**A** and **B**). Interfollicular areas show subtle expansion with prominent microvessels (**C**). Immunohistochemistry for CD20 highlights preserved germinal centers (**D**), which are surrounded by a rim of CD3-positive T cells (**E**). The neoplastic T cells express TCR beta chain (**F**), CD10 (**G**), and CXCL13 (**H**), confirming TFH phenotype. Note the difference in CD10 expression intensity between perifollicular neoplastic T cells (bright) compared with reactive germinal center B cells (dim) (**G**).

TFHL-F refers to a nodular or follicular proliferation of neoplastic TFHL cells that are intermediate sized and monotonous with less polymorphic background with lack of extrafollicular proliferation of FDCs and HEV as compared with TFHL-AI (Table 109.1). TFHL-F presents with two distinct growth patterns: either a follicular pattern, mimicking follicular lymphoma (FL-like) (Figure 109.5), or a pattern resembling progressive transformation of germinal centers (PTGC-like) (Figure 109.6).[25] HRS-like immunoblasts,

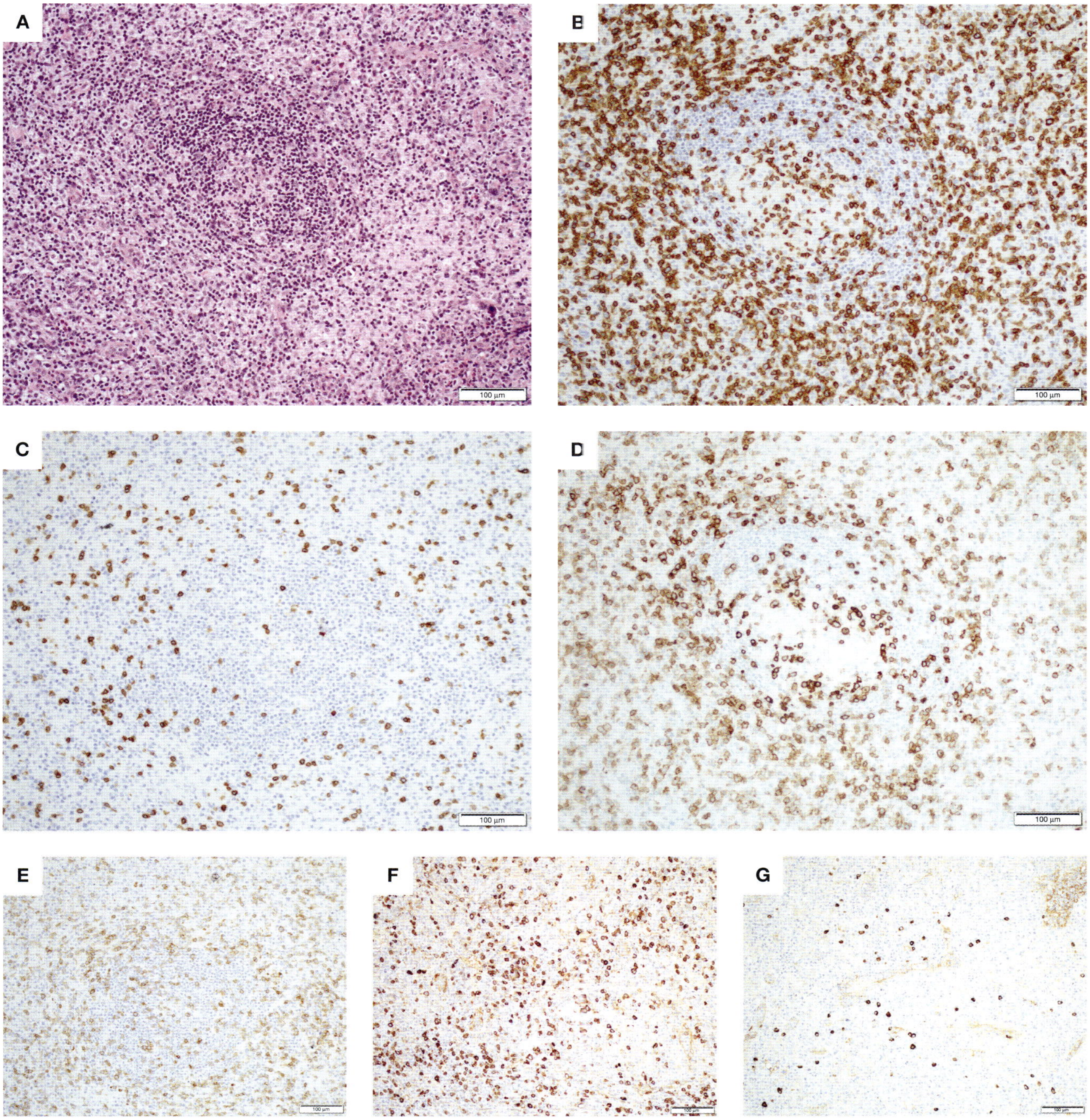

FIGURE 109.2 Histological and immunophenotypic features of follicular helper T-cell lymphoma, angioimmunoblastic-type, pattern II. Medium power view of the lymph node shows a small atrophic follicle center surrounded by small to intermediate lymphocytes and a prominent polymorphic expansion of paracortex (**A**). The T-cells rimming the atrophic follicle express TCR alpha chain (**B**) but lacks TRBC1 expression establishing a clonal T-cell proliferation (**C**). The neoplastic T-cells are positive for PD1 (**D**) and ICOS (**E**) confirming TFH cell-of origin. Immunoglobin kappa (**F**) and lambda (**G**) light chain staining highlights the presence of kappa light chain restricted plasma cells in the paracortex, a feature commonly seen in TFHLs. In this case the plasma cell proliferation was negative for EBV.

either EBV+ or EBV-, surrounded by neoplastic T cells are present in some cases. In FL-like TFHL-F, the neoplastic cells form intrafollicular aggregates sustained by a meshwork of FDC (see Figure 109.5). In PTGC-like TFHL-F, aggregates of medium-sized pale or clear neoplastic T cells are distributed within large nodules mainly composed of expanded mantle zones containing small IgD+ mantle zone B cells (see Figure 109.6).

TFHL-NOS may have some features of TFHL-AI, such as B-cell blasts or increased vascularity, but lacks the typical prominent inflammatory background, or FDC expansion (see Table 109.1). The growth pattern

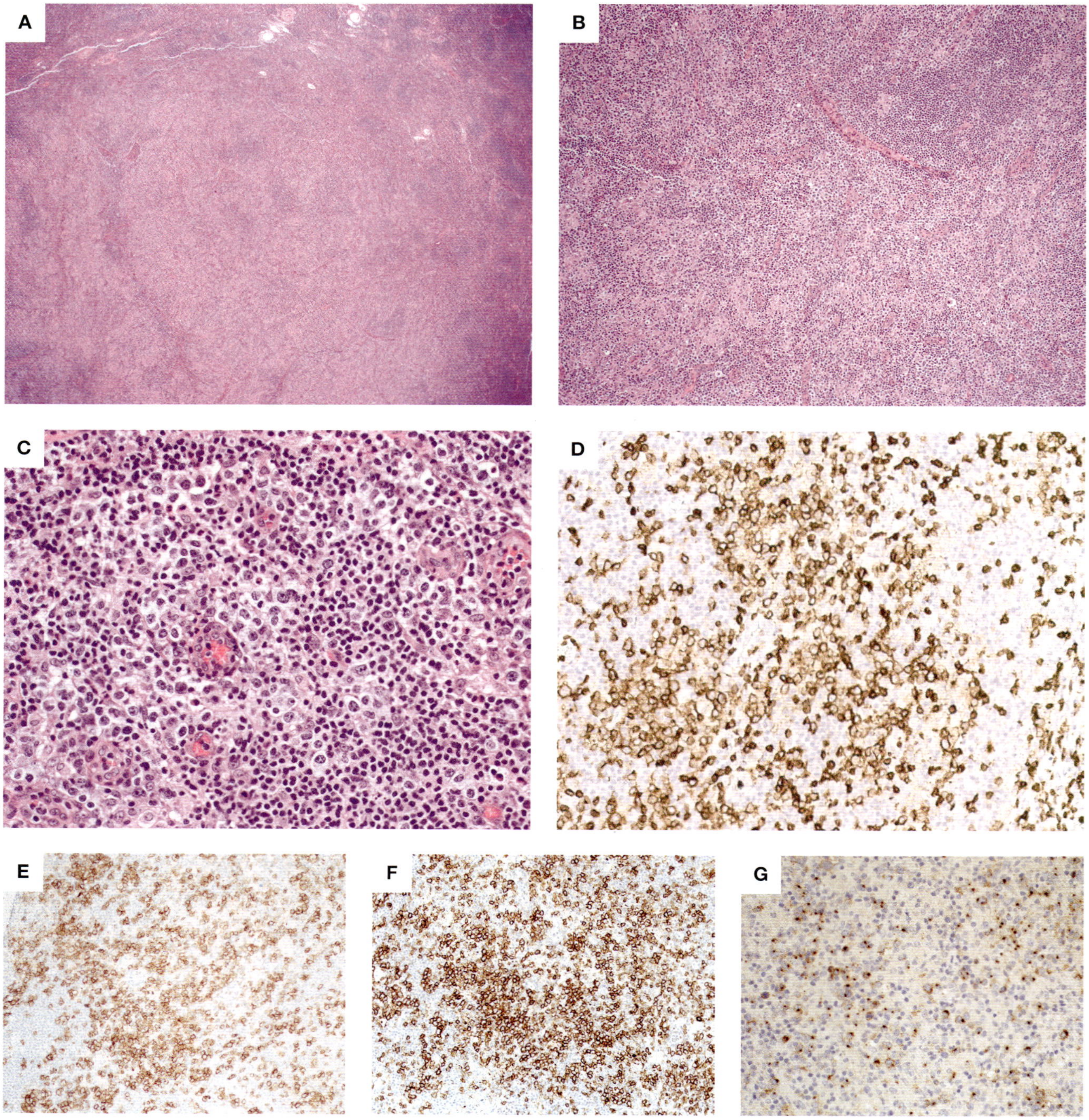

FIGURE 109.3 Histological and immunophenotypic features of follicular helper T-cell lymphoma, angioimmunoblastic-type, pattern III. Low and medium power views of the lymph node biopsy show complete effacement of the architecture by a polymorphic cellular infiltrate and marked microvascular proliferation (**A&B**). High power view highlights sheets of intermediate size neoplastic lymphocytes with clear cytoplasm (**C**). The neoplastic lymphocytes express CD3 (**D**), PD1 (**E**), ICOS (**F**) and CXCL13 (**G**) confirming TFH phenotype.

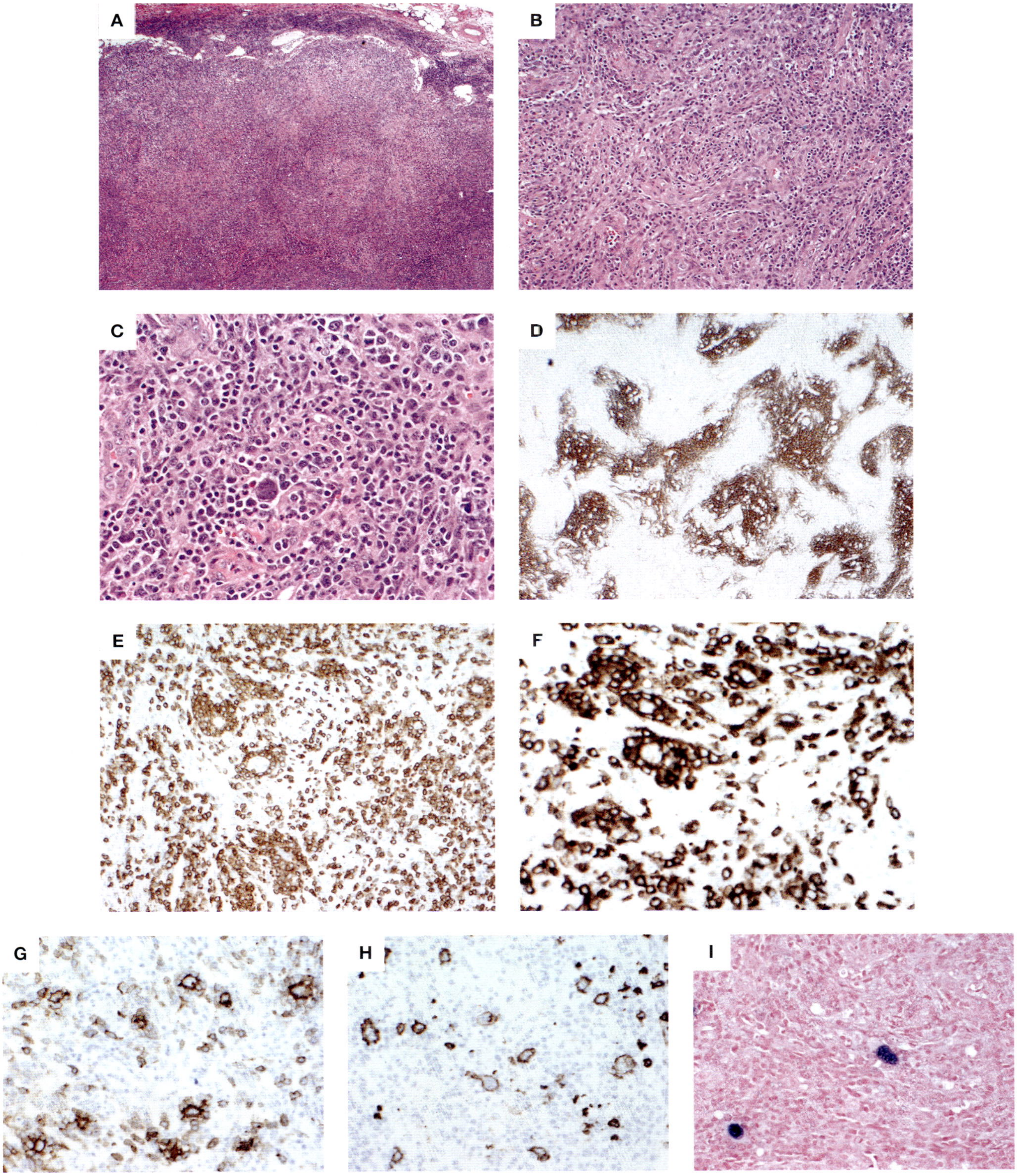

FIGURE 109.4 Histological and immunophenotypic features of follicular helper T-cell lymphoma, angioimmunoblastic-type, pattern III with Hodgkin/Reed-Sternberg (HRS)-like cells Low- and medium-power views of the lymph node biopsy show complete effacement of the architecture by a polymorphic cellular infiltrate and marked microvascular proliferation (**A** and **B**). Note preservation of peripheral sinus and involvement of perinodal tissues (**A**). High-power view highlights large HRS-like cells (**C**). Florid expansion follicular dendritic cell meshworks are seen with CD21 stain (**D**). The neoplastic TFH -cells resetting around HRS-like cells express CD3 (**E**) and TFH marker CD10 (**F**), whereas HRS-like cells express CD30 (**G**), CD15 (**H**) and are positive for EBV by EBER in situ hybridization (**I**).

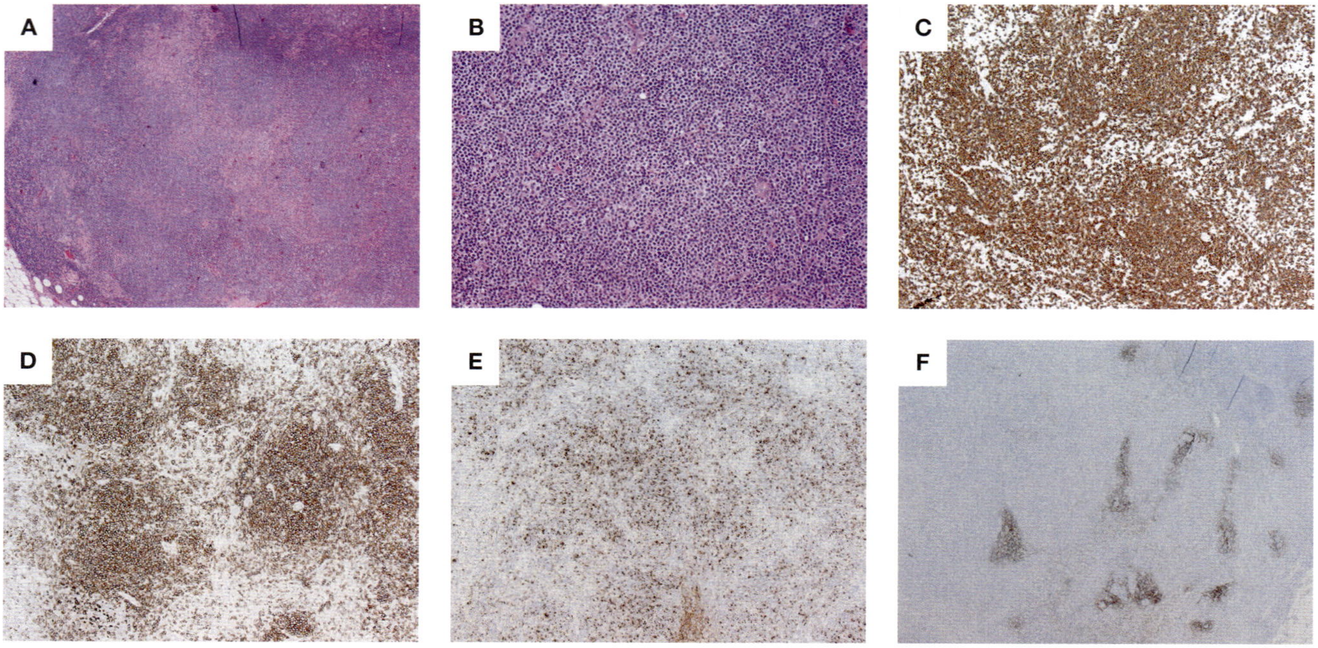

FIGURE 109.5 Histological and immunophenotypic features of follicular helper T-cell lymphoma, follicular type with follicular lymphoma–like growth pattern. Low-power view of the lymph node biopsy shows effacement of the architecture by a nodular proliferation of lymphocytes reminiscent of follicular lymphoma (**A**). At medium power, the nodular neoplastic infiltrate is composed of a monotonous population of intermediate-sized lymphocytes with moderate amount of clear cytoplasm (**B**). The neoplastic cells express CD3 (**C**), PD1 (**D**), and CXCL13 (**E**). CD21 staining shows that follicular dendritic cells are restricted to the follicles without expansion (**F**).

may be perifollicular mimicking marginal zone lymphoma, may be primarily interfollicular (T-zone variant), or may be diffuse. Cases with a diffuse pattern and less polymorphic inflammation may resemble a tumor cell–rich TFHL-AI, but in these cases a lack of FDC meshwork expansion favors TFHL-NOS.

Variable numbers of B cells are present in all subtypes of TFHL. The morphology of the B-cell component varies greatly. Some cases may contain significant numbers of physiological B cells with primary and secondary follicles that vary and range in size and degree of expansion (see Figure 109.1). In other cases, plasma cells may be prominent (see Figure 109.2), but in many cases, the most prominent B-cell component is a paracortical proliferation of polymorphic B cells including numerous immunoblasts, and occasionally, Reed-Sternberg-like cells (see Figure 109.4). The B-cell component may represent clonal expansion in up to 25% of the cases, often driven by EBV infection. The B-cell or plasma-cell component can at times obscure the underlying T-cell lymphoma. Well-documented cases of EBV-positive B immunoblastic proliferations progressing to an EBV-positive diffuse large B-cell lymphoma have been reported, either at diagnosis or at relapse.[26]

TFHLs are systemic disorders, and extranodal dissemination can be documented in most cases. The most common sites of extranodal involvement include bone marrow, skin, spleen, and mucosal tissues. At these sites, the neoplastic T cells frequently retain the morphological and phenotypic characteristics seen in the lymph node (Figure 109.7).

Immunophenotype

By immunohistochemistry, the neoplastic T cells express pan-T-cell antigens CD2, CD3, CD5, and TCR alpha/beta, with frequent loss of CD7 (see Figures 109.1-109.6). By flow cytometry, loss of surface CD3 expression with retention of cytoplasmic CD3 can be seen in some cases (Figure 109.8). If surface CD3 expression is retained, monoclonal TRBC1 restriction can be demonstrated[27] (see Figure 109.8). Inherent to the definition, the tumors must demonstrate a $CD4^+$ T helper cell phenotype, and in support of TFH-cell origin, ideally expression of three or more TFH markers (eg, PD1, CXCL13, BCL6, CD10, ICOS).[28,29] However, CD4 expression can be dim or sometimes absent in a small proportion of cases and assessment of TFH marker expression by immunohistochemistry

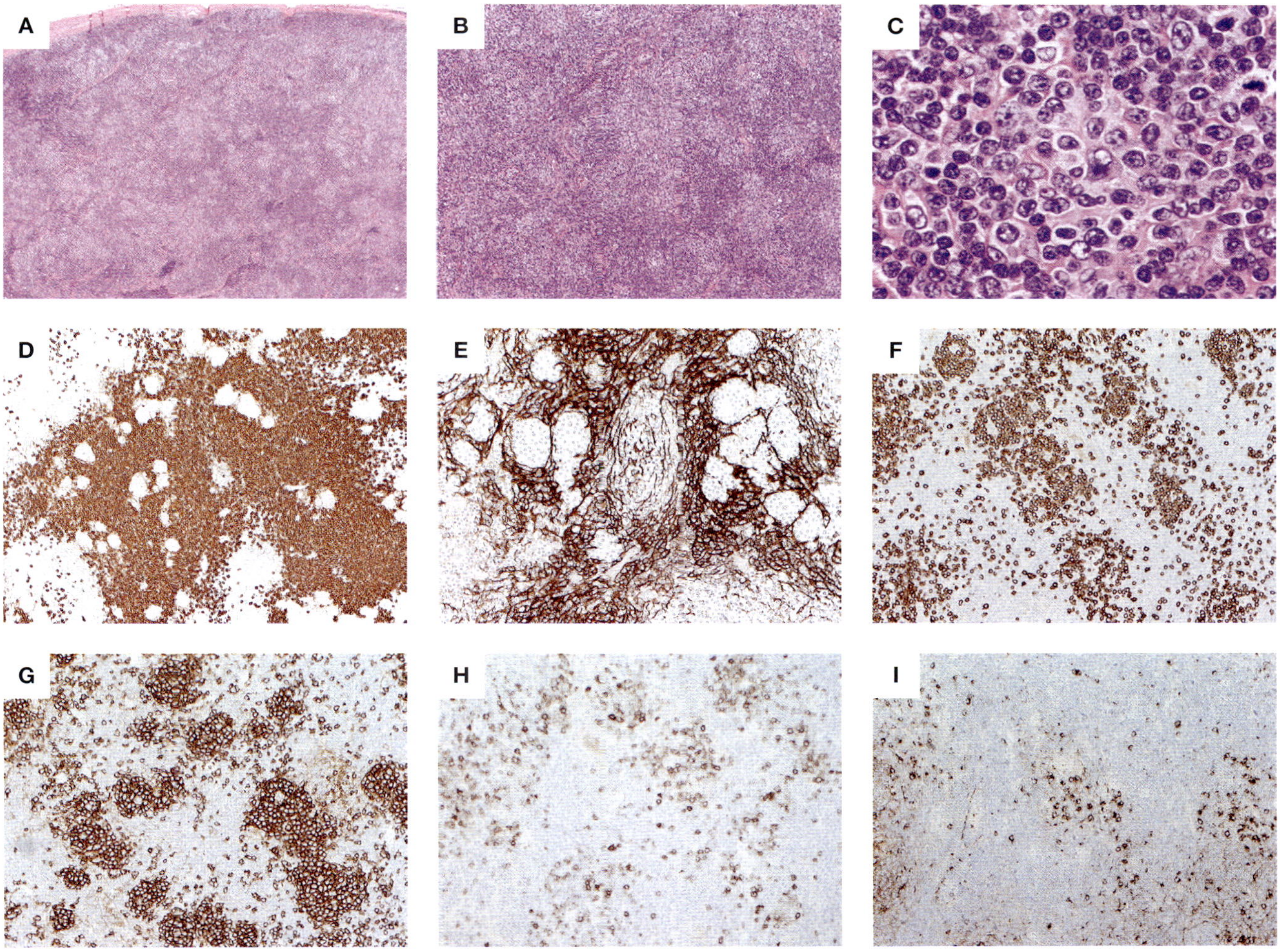

FIGURE 109.6 Histological and immunophenotypic features of follicular helper T-cell lymphoma, follicular type with PTGC-like growth pattern. Low- and medium-power views of the lymph node biopsy show effacement of the architecture by a nodular proliferation of lymphocytes reminiscent of PTGC with nests of intermediate-sized lymphoid cells with pale cytoplasm and sheets of smaller darker staining lymphoid cells with scanty cytoplasm consistent with residual mantle zone B cells (**A** and **B**). At high power, this dual cytology is better highlighted and the larger cells with more abundant cytoplasm show cytological atypia (**C**). The small lymphocytes within the nodules are mostly CD20 mantle zone B-cells (**D**) and follow the distribution of CD21-positive follicular dendritic cells underlying the nodules (**E**). CD3 labels nests of atypical intermediate-sized neoplastic T cells (**F**), which express CD4 (**G**), CD10 (**H**), and CXCL13 (**I**), consistent with the TFH phenotype.

may be challenging in biopsies with low tumor cell content. Of the TFH markers, CD10 and CXCL13 are more specific for the TFH phenotype, whereas PD-1 and ICOS are more sensitive. Both PD-1 and ICOS are physiologically expressed by T cells with exhausted/memory phenotype, albeit quite weakly. In TFHL, expression of PD-1 and ICOS is typically much brighter than reactive background memory/exhausted T cells allowing recognition of neoplastic TFHL cells (see Table 109.2).

Variable numbers of CD8-positive T cells may be present in the background, sometimes outnumbering the neoplastic TFHL cells. Florid disordered expansion of FDC meshworks is a hallmark of TFHL-AI and should be explored by FDC immunophenotypic markers such as CD21, CD23, and CD35 (see Figure 109.4). CD30 expression can be quite variable and can be detected on a subset of the neoplastic T cells and also frequently in B immunoblasts. B-cell lineage markers such as CD20, PAX5, and CD79a identify the heterogenous populations of B cells including immunoblasts and plasma cells. These may show evidence of clonality by flow cytometry and immunohistochemistry for immunoglobulin light chains (see Figure 109.2). EBV-positive B cells and plasma cells of varying numbers are present in 80% to 95% of the TFHL cases.

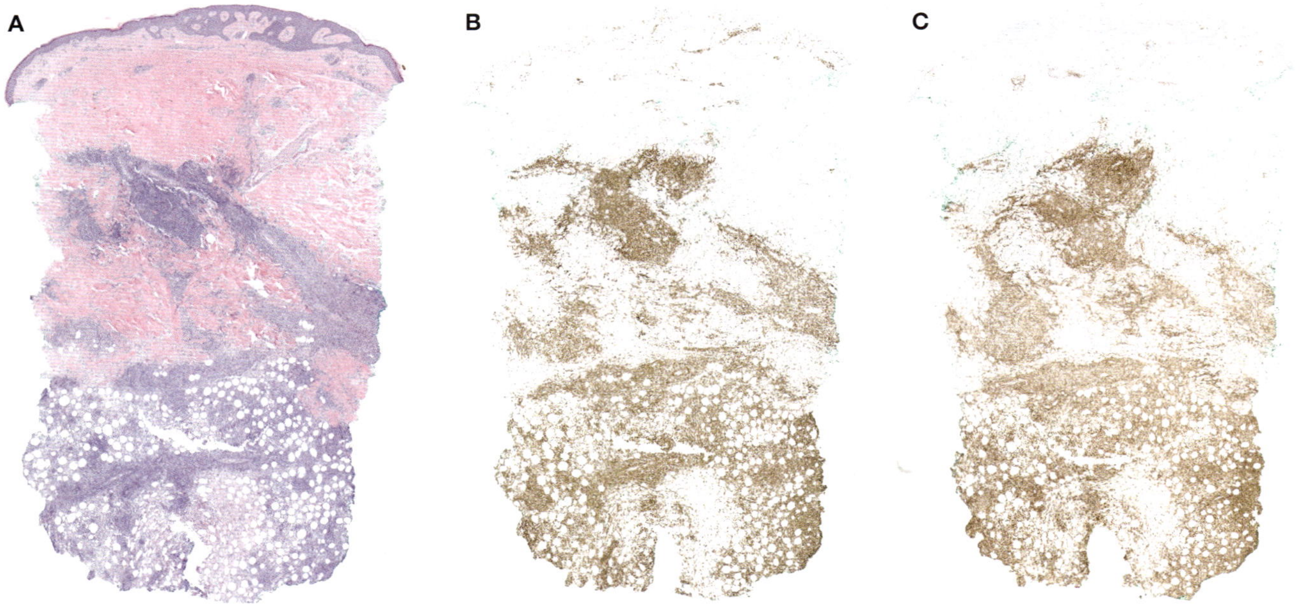

FIGURE 109.7 Histological and immunophenotypic features of skin involvement by follicular helper T-cell lymphoma, not otherwise specified (TFHL-NOS). Skin biopsy shows an extensive lymphoid infiltrate of lymphoid cells with a periadnexal and perivascular distribution in the dermis and a more interstitial pattern in the subcutaneous tissue **(A)**. The lymphoid cells are strongly positive for CD3 **(B)** and PD1 **(C)**. The patient had systemic disease and a lymph node biopsy was diagnosed as TFHL-NOS.

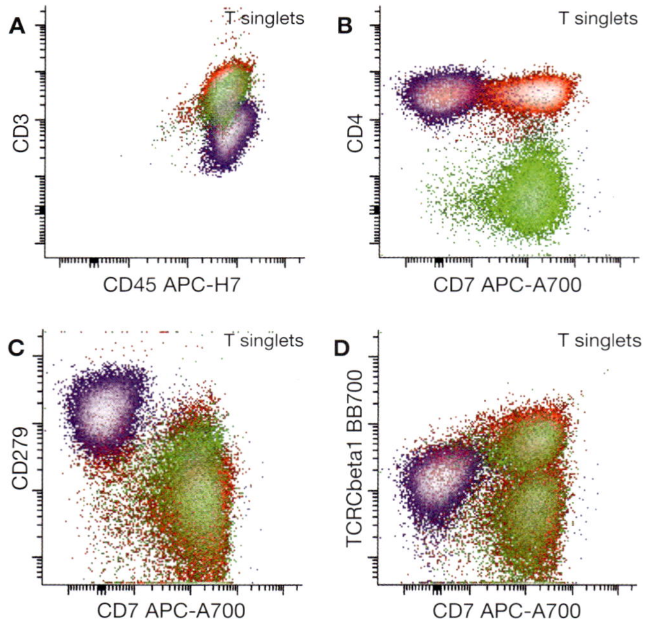

FIGURE 109.8 Flow cytometric immunophenotyping of a lymph node involved by follicular helper T-cell lymphoma, angioimmunoblastic type. In the flow histograms, the neoplastic T cells are shown in purple, reactive CD4-positive T cells in red, and reactive CD8-positive cells in green. The neoplastic T cells uniformly express CD45 but show dim expression of CD3 **(A)**. They are positive for CD4 but lack expression of CD7 **(B)**. CD7-negative abnormal T-cell population expresses bright CD279 (PD1) consistent with TFH phenotype **(C)**. The abnormal T-cell population shows dim but restricted TRBC1 expression confirming the clonal nature of the TFH proliferation. Note that reactive CD4- and CD8-positive T cells show a polytypic pattern by TRBC1 **(D)**.

Genetics

A clonal TCR gene rearrangement can be demonstrated in most cases of TFHL, and in combination with acquired somatic mutations, genetic evidence for a monoclonal T-cell population can be demonstrated in virtually all cases.[30] The genetics of TFHL is best characterized for TFHL-AI, less so for TFHL-F and TFHL-NOS. At the chromosomal level, the most frequent copy number alterations are gains of chromosome 5 and chromosome 21, and in smaller subset of cases, gains of chromosome 7, 11, 19, and 22.[31] Comprehensive genomic profiling has identified several characteristic recurrent mutations in TFHL. Most of the frequently identified fall into two broad biological processes that control cell differentiation (epigenetic) and cell proliferation/survival (T-cell receptor signaling). Up to 80% of TFHL carry loss-of-function mutation affecting epigenetic modifier gene *TET2* and up to 30% for *DNMT3A*.[32,33] These mutations have been detected not only in neoplastic T cells but also in myeloid precursor cells in the marrows of TFHL cases suggesting that TFHL may arise from a myeloid stem cell precursor by consequentially acquiring mutations allowing the tumor to develop in T-cell niche in the lymph nodes[15] (Figure 109.9). Secondary mutations that are seen exclusively in the neoplastic T cells but not in the myeloid precursors include activating mutations such as *RHOA* G17V in 50% to 70% of cases and *IDH2* R172* in around 30% of

TABLE 109.2 Immunophenotypic markers used in diagnosis of TFHL

Marker	Method of detection	Biology	Utility in TFHL	Pitfalls
CD2	IHC/Flow	Pan T	Expressed	
CD3	IHC/Flow	Pan T	Expressed in cytoplasm, may be lost on surface	
CD5	IHC/Flow	Pan T	Variable loss	
CD7	IHC/Flow	Pan T	Frequently lost or dim	
CD4	IHC/Flow	Helper T cells	Expressed	Level of expression can be low in some cases
CD8	IHC/Flow	Cytotoxic T cells	Negative	Background $CD8^+$ cytotoxic cells can be significantly increased
TCRαβ	IHC/Flow	T-cell subset	Expressed	Lost if CD3 surface expression is lost
TCRγδ	IHC/Flow		Negative	Increased reactive g/d T cell can be present
TRBC1	IHC/Flow	T-cell subset	Clonality	Only interpretable if surface CD3 is expressed
CD10	IHC/Flow	GC B cells Small subset of TFH	TFH phenotype	Often heterogeneous and limited to a subset of tumor cells. Specific for TFHL but not sensitive
CXCL13	IHC	TFH, FDC	TFH phenotype	Specific for TFHL (among lymphocytes) but not sensitive
PD1	IHC/Flow	TFH, exhausted T cells	TFH phenotype	Sensitive for TFHL but may be expressed in exhausted T cells
ICOS	IHC/Flow	TFH, exhausted T cells	TFH phenotype	Sensitive for TFHL but may be expressed in exhausted/activated T cells
BCL6	IHC	GC B cells,TFH	TFH phenotype	Ubiquitously expressed by other lineages
IDH2 R172*	IHC	Absent	Expressed in 30%	Only expressed in TFHL with the $IDH2^{R172*}$ mutation. Cytoplasmic, granular staining
CD21/CD23	IHC	FDC	Marked expansion	Castleman disease, follicular dendritic cell sarcoma
EBER	ISH	Rare EBV-infected cells	Increase in B cells	EBV-positive B-cell lymphoproliferative disorders, CHL

CHL, classic Hodgkin lymphoma; EBER, EBV-encoded RNAs; EBV, Epstein-Barr virus; FDC, follicular dendritic cell; Flow, flow cytometry; GC, germinal center; IHC, immunohistochemistry; ISH, in situ hybridization; TFH, T follicular helper cell; TFHL, follicular helper T-cell lymphoma.

cases.[34,35] The other genes frequently altered by gain-of-function mutations in the TCR signaling pathway include *PLCG1, CD28, FYN, PIK3* components, *CARD11*,[35,36] and rare fusions involving genes coding for costimulatory molecules such as *CD28, ICOS,* or *CTLA4*.[37]

Although most common mutations are seen across the histological spectrum of TFHL, several subtype-specific mutational patterns have emerged. For example, *IDH2* R172* mutations are restricted to TFHL-AITL, whereas rare *ITK::SYK* fusions have been almost exclusively reported in TFHL-F.

Prognosis and Clinical Comment

The prognosis of TFHL remains dismal with 32% to 44% patients surviving for 5 years based on large retrospective registry studies. The backbone of therapy

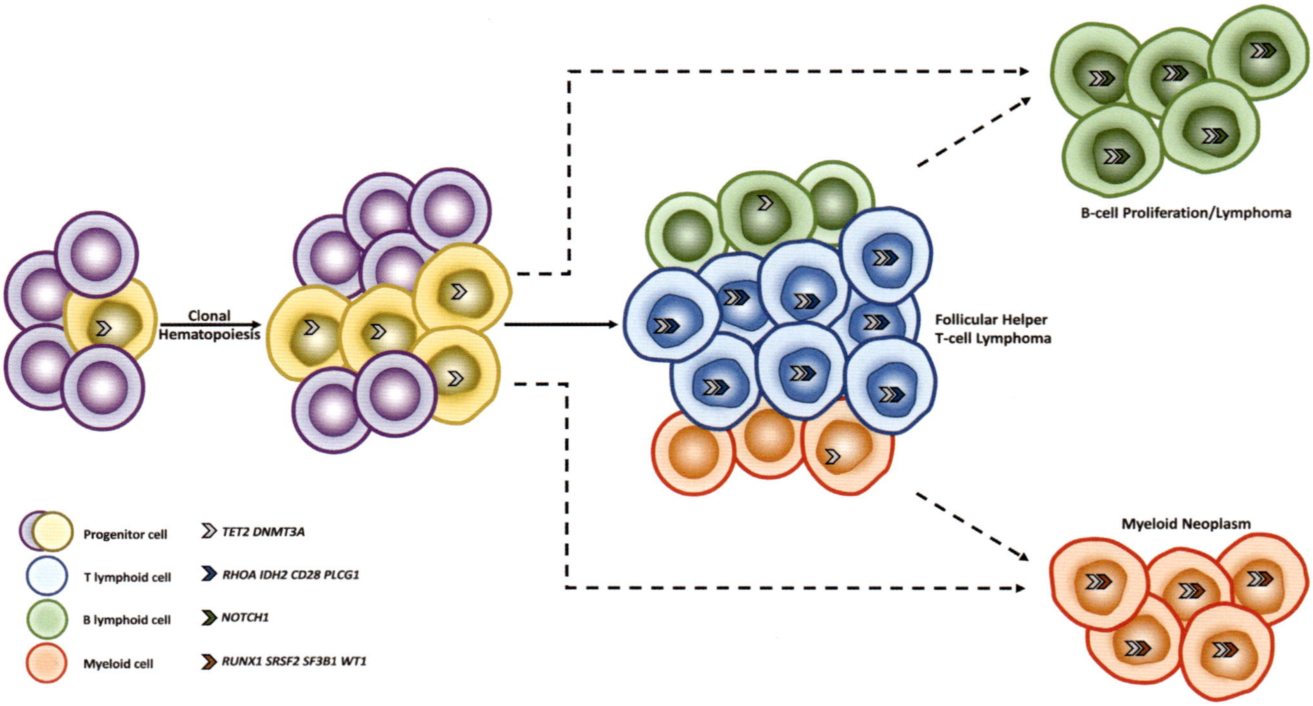

FIGURE 109.9 Schematic representation of clonal evolution of follicular helper T-cell lymphoma (TFHL). Most cases of TFHL arise from a background of myeloid clonal hematopoiesis often carrying mutation in *TET2* and/or *DNMT3A*. Development of TFHL from this background requires additional mutations frequently involving *RHOA* and *IDH2*. In a subset of the cases B-cell and/or myeloid neoplasms may arise from the same background clonal hematopoiesis through acquisition of mutations private for each lineage.

for TFHL remains CHOP (cyclophosphamide, doxorubicin, vincristine, prednisone)-based regimens.[38] Recently brentuximab vedotin–CHP (cyclophosphamide, doxorubicin, prednisone) combination has been approved by the US Food and Drug Administration for treatment of CD30-positive PTCL including TFHL in the United States, but its superiority to CHOP-based regimens remains debatable. As the chance of long-term disease control with CHOP-based regimens remains poor, consolidation with autologous transplantation is recommended in first remission. Beyond chemotherapy, there are efforts to develop "chemofree" approaches for management of TFHL.[39] These attempt to target biological vulnerabilities of TFHL such as the epigenetic machinery and TCR signaling pathway. Such approaches promise to alter the natural history of these tumors but may be limited by toxicity due to off-target effects.

References

1. de Leval L, Rickman DS, Thielen C, et al. The gene expression profile of nodal peripheral T-cell lymphoma demonstrates a molecular link between angioimmunoblastic T-cell lymphoma (AITL) and follicular helper T (TFH) cells. *Blood*. 2007;109(11):4952-4963.
2. Piccaluga PP, Agostinelli C, Califano A, et al. Gene expression analysis of angioimmunoblastic lymphoma indicates derivation from T follicular helper cells and vascular endothelial growth factor deregulation. *Cancer Res*. 2007;67(22):10703-10710.
3. Iqbal J, Wright G, Wang C, et al. Gene expression signatures delineate biological and prognostic subgroups in peripheral T-cell lymphoma. *Blood*. 2014;123(19):2915-2923.
4. Dobay MP, Lemonnier F, Missiaglia E, et al. Integrative clinicopathological and molecular analyses of angioimmunoblastic T-cell lymphoma and other nodal lymphomas of follicular helper T-cell origin. *Haematologica*. 2017;102(4):e148-e151.
5. Rodríguez-Pinilla SM, Atienza L, Murillo C, et al. Peripheral T-cell lymphoma with follicular T-cell markers. *Am J Surg Pathol*. 2008;32(12):1787-1799.
6. Grogg KL, Attygalle AD, Macon WR, Remstein ED, Kurtin PJ, Dogan A. Expression of CXCL13, a chemokine highly upregulated in germinal center T-helper cells, distinguishes angioimmunoblastic T-cell lymphoma from peripheral T-cell lymphoma, unspecified. *Mod Pathol*. 2006;19(8):1101-1107.
7. Campo E, Jaffe ES, Cook JR, et al. The international consensus classification of mature lymphoid neoplasms: a report from the clinical Advisory Committee. *Blood*. 2022;140(11):1229-1253.

8. Bosisio FM, Cerroni L. Expression of T-follicular helper markers in sequential biopsies of progressive mycosis fungoides and other primary cutaneous T-cell lymphomas. *Am J Dermatopathol.* 2015;37(2):115-121.
9. Abouyabis AN, Shenoy PJ, Lechowicz MJ, Flowers CR. Incidence and outcomes of the peripheral T-cell lymphoma subtypes in the United States. *Leuk Lymphoma.* 2008;49(11):2099-2107.
10. Vose J, Armitage J, Weisenburger D; International T-Cell Lymphoma Project. International peripheral T-cell and natural killer/T-cell lymphoma study: pathology findings and clinical outcomes. *J Clin Oncol.* 2008;26(25):4124-4130.
11. de Leval L, Parrens M, Le Bras F, et al. Angioimmunoblastic T-cell lymphoma is the most common T-cell lymphoma in two distinct French information data sets. *Haematologica.* 2015;100(9):e361-e364.
12. de Leval L, Gisselbrecht C, Gaulard P. Advances in the understanding and management of angioimmunoblastic T-cell lymphoma. *Br J Haematol.* 2010;148(5):673-689.
13. Tiacci E, Venanzi A, Ascani S, et al. High-risk clonal hematopoiesis as the origin of AITL and NPM1-mutated AML. *N Engl J Med.* 2018;379(10):981-984.
14. Couronné L, Bastard C, Bernard OA. TET2 and DNMT3A mutations in human T-cell lymphoma. *N Engl J Med.* 2012;366(1):95-96.
15. Lewis NE, Petrova-Drus K, Huet S, et al. Clonal hematopoiesis in angioimmunoblastic T-cell lymphoma with divergent evolution to myeloid neoplasms. *Blood Adv.* 2020;4(10):2261-2271.
16. Kommalapati A, Tella SH, Go RS, Bennani NN, Goyal G. A population-based analysis of second primary malignancies in T-cell neoplasms. *Br J Haematol.* 2019;185(2):338-342.
17. Chiba S, Sakata-Yanagimoto M. Advances in understanding of angioimmunoblastic T-cell lymphoma. *Leukemia.* 2020;34(10):2592-2606.
18. Lachenal F, Berger F, Ghesquières H, et al. Angioimmunoblastic T-cell lymphoma: clinical and laboratory features at diagnosis in 77 patients. *Medicine (Baltim).* 2007;86(5):282-292.
19. Mourad N, Mounier N, Brière J, et al. Clinical, biologic, and pathologic features in 157 patients with angioimmunoblastic T-cell lymphoma treated within the Groupe d'Etude des Lymphomes de l'Adulte (GELA) trials. *Blood.* 2008;111(9):4463-4470.
20. Federico M, Rudiger T, Bellei M, et al. Clinicopathologic characteristics of angioimmunoblastic T-cell lymphoma: analysis of the international peripheral T-cell lymphoma project. *J Clin Oncol.* 2013;31(2):240-246.
21. Yoon SE, Cho J, Kim YJ, et al. Comprehensive analysis of clinical, pathological, and genomic characteristics of follicular helper T-cell derived lymphomas. *Exp Hematol Oncol.* 2021;10(1):33.
22. Xie Y, Jaffe ES. How I diagnose angioimmunoblastic T-cell lymphoma. *Am J Clin Pathol.* 2021;156(1):1-14.
23. Attygalle AD, Kyriakou C, Dupuis J, et al. Histologic evolution of angioimmunoblastic T-cell lymphoma in consecutive biopsies: clinical correlation and insights into natural history and disease progression. *Am J Surg Pathol.* 2007;31(7):1077-1088.
24. Ondrejka SL, Amador C, Climent F, et al. Follicular helper T-cell lymphomas: disease spectrum, relationship with clonal hematopoiesis, and mimics. A report of the 2022 EA4HP/SH lymphoma workshop. *Virchows Arch.* 2023;483(3):349-365.
25. Huang Y, Moreau A, Dupuis J, et al. Peripheral T-cell lymphomas with a follicular growth pattern are derived from follicular helper T cells (TFH) and may show overlapping features with angioimmunoblastic T-cell lymphomas. *Am J Surg Pathol.* 2009;33(5):682-690.
26. Huppmann AR, Roullet MR, Raffeld M, Jaffe ES. Angioimmunoblastic T-cell lymphoma partially obscured by an Epstein-Barr virus-negative clonal plasma cell proliferation. *J Clin Oncol.* 2013;31(2):e28-e30.
27. Alikhan M, Song JY, Sohani AR, et al. Peripheral T-cell lymphomas of follicular helper T-cell type frequently display an aberrant CD3(-/dim)CD4(+) population by flow cytometry: an important clue to the diagnosis of a Hodgkin lymphoma mimic. *Mod Pathol.* 2016;29(10):1173-1182.
28. Basha BM, Bryant SC, Rech KL, et al. Application of a 5 marker panel to the routine diagnosis of peripheral T-cell lymphoma with T-follicular helper phenotype. *Am J Surg Pathol.* 2019;43(9):1282-1290.
29. Feldman AL, Laurent C, Narbaitz M, et al. Classification and diagnostic evaluation of nodal T- and NK-cell lymphomas. *Virchows Arch.* 2023;482(1):265-279.
30. Syrykh C, Gorez P, Péricart S, et al. Molecular diagnosis of T-cell lymphoma: a correlative study of PCR-based T-cell clonality assessment and targeted NGS. *Blood Adv.* 2021;5(22):4590-4593.
31. Heavican TB, Bouska A, Yu J, et al. Genetic drivers of oncogenic pathways in molecular subgroups of peripheral T-cell lymphoma. *Blood.* 2019;133(15):1664-1676.
32. Lemonnier F, Couronné L, Parrens M, et al. Recurrent TET2 mutations in peripheral T-cell lymphomas correlate with TFH-like features and adverse clinical parameters. *Blood.* 2012;120(7):1466-1469.
33. Sakata-Yanagimoto M, Enami T, Yoshida K, et al. Somatic RHOA mutation in angioimmunoblastic T cell lymphoma. *Nat Genet.* 2014;46(2):171-175.
34. Palomero T, Couronné L, Khiabanian H, et al. Recurrent mutations in epigenetic regulators, RHOA and FYN kinase in peripheral T cell lymphomas. *Nat Genet.* 2014;46(2):166-170.
35. Vallois D, Dobay MP, Morin RD, et al. Activating mutations in genes related to TCR signaling in angioimmunoblastic and other follicular helper T-cell-derived lymphomas. *Blood.* 2016;128(11):1490-1502.
36. Rohr J, Guo S, Huo J, et al. Recurrent activating mutations of CD28 in peripheral T-cell lymphomas. *Leukemia.* 2016;30(5):1062-1070.

37. Vallois D, Dupuy A, Lemonnier F, et al. RNA fusions involving CD28 are rare in peripheral T-cell lymphomas and concentrate mainly in those derived from follicular helper T cells. *Haematologica*. 2018;103(8):e360-e363.

38. Ngu HS, Savage KJ. Past, present and future therapeutic approaches in nodal peripheral T-cell lymphomas. *Haematologica*. 2023;108(12):3211-3226.

39. Stuver R, Lewis N, Dogan A, Horwitz SM. Moving towards biologically informed treatment strategies for T-cell lymphomas. *Int J Hematol*. 2023;117(4):492-503.

Chapter 110

Anaplastic Large Cell Lymphoma, ALK Positive

Andrew L. Feldman, Bettina Bisig, Steven M. Horwitz, Marina Narbaitz, and Kerry J. Savage

Definition

Anaplastic large cell lymphoma, ALK positive (ALK+ ALCL) is a systemic lymphoma of mature T-cell origin containing characteristic cells with pleomorphic nuclei and abundant cytoplasm that express CD30 and have gene fusions involving *ALK*.

Synonyms

None.

Epidemiology

ALK+ ALCL represents about 3% of all non-Hodgkin lymphomas.[1-4] Among peripheral (postthymic) T-cell lymphomas, its relative incidence varies geographically, from 3% in Asia to 6% in Europe and 16% in North America. ALK+ ALCL represents 10% to 15% of lymphomas in children and frequently presents in the first 3 decades of life, with a mean age of 22 years. It is more common in males, with a M:F ratio of about 1.5:1. The causes of ALK+ ALCL are unknown. Rare cases have been associated with insect bites,[5] but the biologic basis for this remains unclear.

General Clinical Features

ALK+ ALCL typically presents with lymphadenopathy, often with B symptoms, but may occur in virtually any anatomic site, including the mediastinum and spleen.[1,6] The most commonly involved extranodal sites are bone, lung, and skin. Rare ALCLs that express ALK but have isolated skin involvement have been reported to have a clinical course more similar to primary cutaneous ALCL[7]; the classification of these cases has not been established but they should be distinguished from patients with systemic disease and secondary skin involvement. Up to 70% of patients present with stage III or IV disease. Bone marrow involvement by ALK+ ALCL is present in 10% to 30% of patients at diagnosis. Peripheral blood involvement is rare, but can be seen, particularly in the small cell variant of ALK+ ALCL (see below). Rare central nervous system involvement at diagnosis or at relapse can occur.

Morphology

A characteristic cell type, called the hallmark cell, is seen in all cases of ALK+ ALCL.[3,8] Hallmark cells are typically large and have horseshoe- or kidney-shaped nuclei and abundant cytoplasm, with a prominent perinuclear eosinophilic area corresponding to the Golgi zone (Figure 110.1A). Depending on the plane of section, these cells may also appear to have round or oval nuclei, sometimes with a nuclear pseudoinclusion ("doughnut" cells). Aside from the shared feature of containing hallmark cells, ALK+ ALCLs have a wide spectrum of morphological appearances, some of which constitute recognized histologic patterns.

The common pattern is seen in about 60% of cases and shows sheets of tumor cells that are typically large (Figure 110.1B). Hallmark cells are generally abundant. Very large cells with marked nuclear pleomorphism, sometimes with a wreath-like pattern, may be present (Figure 110.1C). In lymph nodes, the tumor cells typically replace the paracortex but may spare residual follicles. Sinusoidal involvement is common, either as single cells or extensive sinusoidal expansion, and is helpful in recognizing the disease (Figure 110.1D). Sometimes, subtle sinusoidal involvement may be the only feature of involvement of a given lymph node.

The lymphohistiocytic pattern is seen in about 10% of cases. The tumor cells have cytological features similar to the common pattern but are distributed in a background of reactive cells including histiocytes and small lymphocytes (Figure 110.2). In some cases, the cells may be smaller and preferentially cluster around blood vessels (see small cell pattern, below). The histiocytes may exhibit erythrophagocytosis. Sometimes, they may be so abundant that the tumor cells are

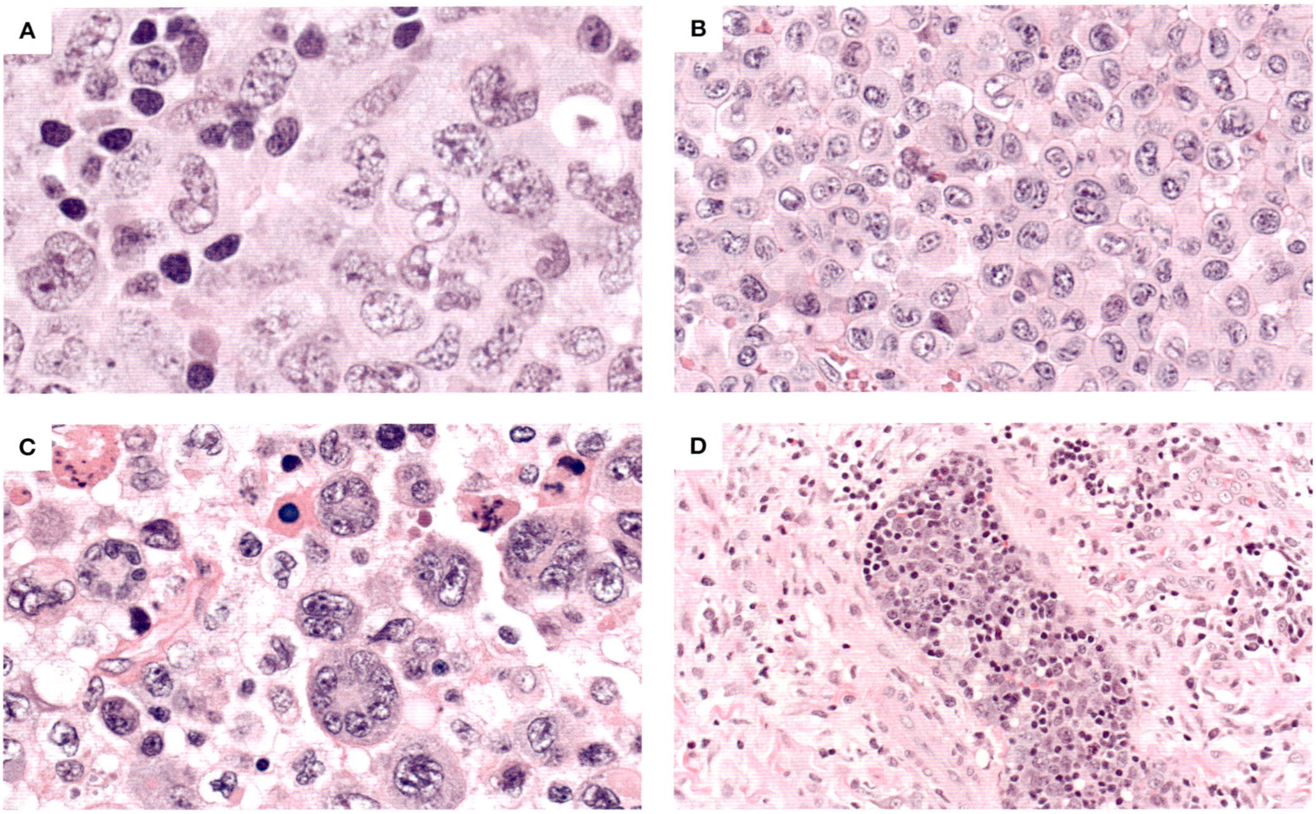

FIGURE 110.1 Anaplastic large cell lymphoma, ALK positive (ALK+ ALCL), common pattern. **A:** Hallmark cells in ALK+ ALCL. **B:** Common pattern of ALK+ ALCL, with sheets of large pleomorphic cells, including hallmark cells. **C:** Prominent wreath-like nuclei in ALK+ ALCL. **D:** Sinusoidal involvement by ALK+ ALCL.

difficult to identify, leading to misdiagnosis as a reactive condition.

The small cell pattern of ALK+ ALCL is seen in 5% to 10% of cases. Most of the cells in this pattern are small- or medium-sized, often showing a central round nucleus and clear cytoplasm ("fried egg" cells; Figure 110.3A and C). Nevertheless, hallmark cells are present, and often cluster around blood vessels (Figure 110.3D). Because the predominant tumor cell population lacks features of hallmark cells, this pattern can mistakenly be diagnosed as peripheral T-cell lymphoma, not otherwise specified. Therefore, a high index of suspicion with careful evaluation of morphology in perivascular tumor cells is necessary to prompt appropriate phenotypic studies (see below). Leukemic involvement by ALK+ ALCL is predominantly seen in cases with the small cell pattern. The tumor cells in the peripheral blood often are small and have folded nuclear contours, although large pleomorphic cells with cytoplasmic vacuoles also may be present.

A Hodgkin-like pattern has been described but is rare (<5%; Figure 110.4A and B).[9] These cases have some features resembling the nodular sclerosis variant of classic Hodgkin lymphoma, including a nodular growth pattern, bands of fibrosis, and sometimes cells reminiscent of lacunar variants of Reed-Sternberg cells. The tumor cells of ALK+ ALCL may also rarely have other cytologic appearances, at least in some areas of the tumor, including signet ring cells (Figure 110.4C), spindle cells ("sarcomatoid" pattern; Figure 110.4D), a predominance of markedly pleomorphic cells ("giant cell" pattern), and smaller cells in a myxoid/edematous background ("hypocellular" pattern). Multiple morphologic patterns may be seen in the same biopsy ("composite" pattern), in different biopsies at the same time point, and at different time points in the same patient.[8]

Immunophenotype

All cases express CD30.[3,8,10] Expression is typically strong and uniform, with a membranous and Golgi pattern of distribution (Figure 110.5A). Expression may be more variable in the small cell pattern, which may show strong CD30 expression in the perivascular hallmark cells but weak or even absent expression in the small cell

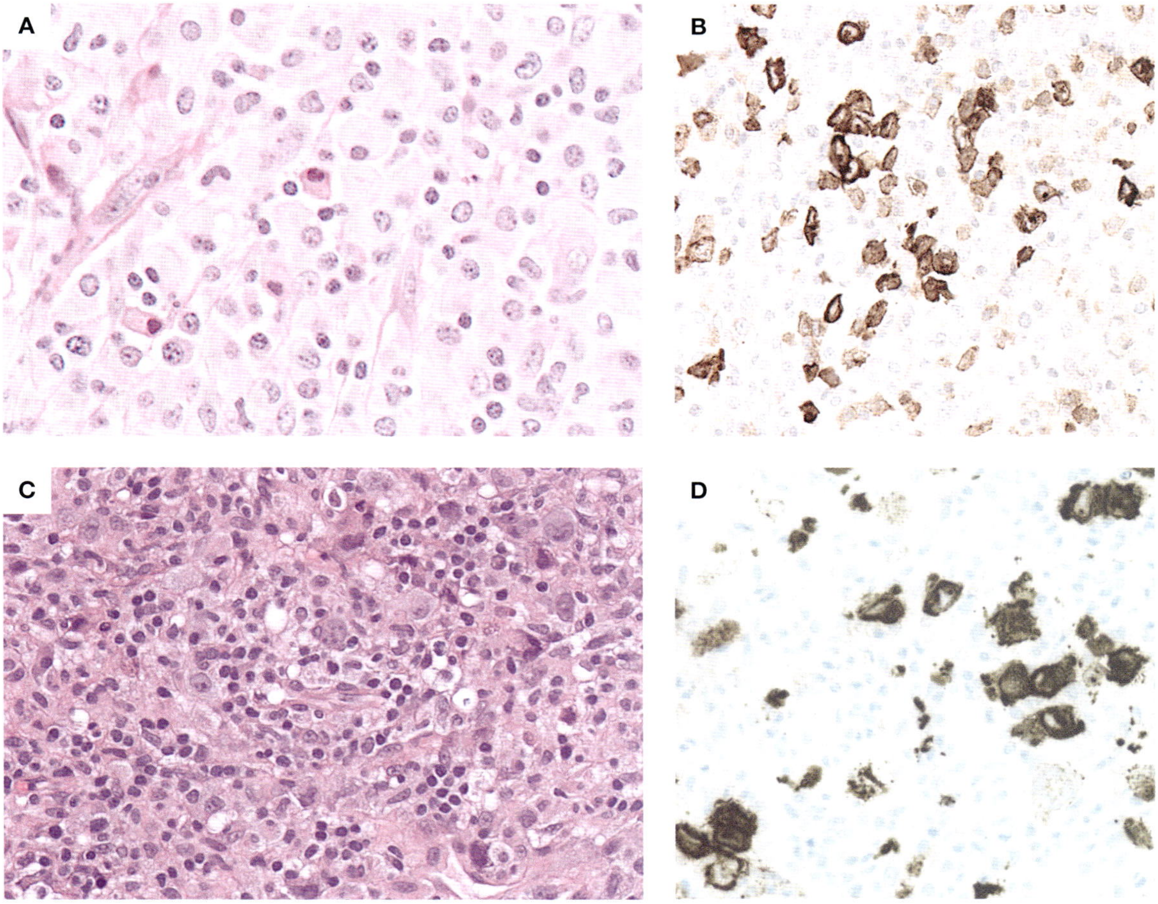

FIGURE 110.2 Anaplastic large cell lymphoma, ALK positive lymphohistiocytic pattern. **A:** The background in this case contains predominantly histiocytes. **B:** CD30 highlights the tumor cells. **C:** The background in this case contains predominantly small lymphocytes. **D:** CD30 highlights the tumor cells.

component (Figure 110.5B). Immunohistochemistry for ALK is positive and is a good surrogate for the presence of an *ALK* gene fusion. The pattern of staining depends on the fusion partner, with the most common fusion, *NPM1::ALK*, having a nuclear and cytoplasmic pattern[11] (Table 110.1; Figure 110.5C and D). Most cases show aberrant loss of T-cell antigens (Figure 110.6A-D). CD2 and CD4 are the T-cell antigens most commonly preserved. Occasional cases express CD8. Some cases lack any T-cell antigen expression (null cell phenotype). Cytotoxic markers (TIA1, granzyme B, and/or perforin) are frequently expressed, including cases lacking other T-cell antigens. MUM1 (IRF4) is typically positive (Figure 110.6E). CD56, EMA, and/or clusterin may be expressed. CD45 expression is variable (Figure 110.6F). Occasional cases aberrantly express PAX5, CD33, CD15, cytokeratins, or other non–T-cell markers.[3]

Genetics

The T-cell receptor genes are clonally rearranged in most but not all cases.[12] By definition, all cases have *ALK* fusions with various partners, the most common being *NPM1* encoding nucleophosmin, corresponding to the t(2;5)(p23;q35) translocation.[11] *ALK* fusions and their relative frequencies are shown in Table 110.1. Recurrently mutated genes include genes involved in T-cell receptor signaling and *NOTCH1*, which may represent a therapeutic target.[13] *TP53* mutations occur in approximately 10% of cases.[14] Acquisition of *ALK* mutations has been reported as a mechanism of resistance to ALK small molecule inhibitors.[15] ALK+ ALCL has a unique gene expression signature enriched for genes in the JAK-STAT3 pathway, which is activated by ALK fusion proteins.[16-18]

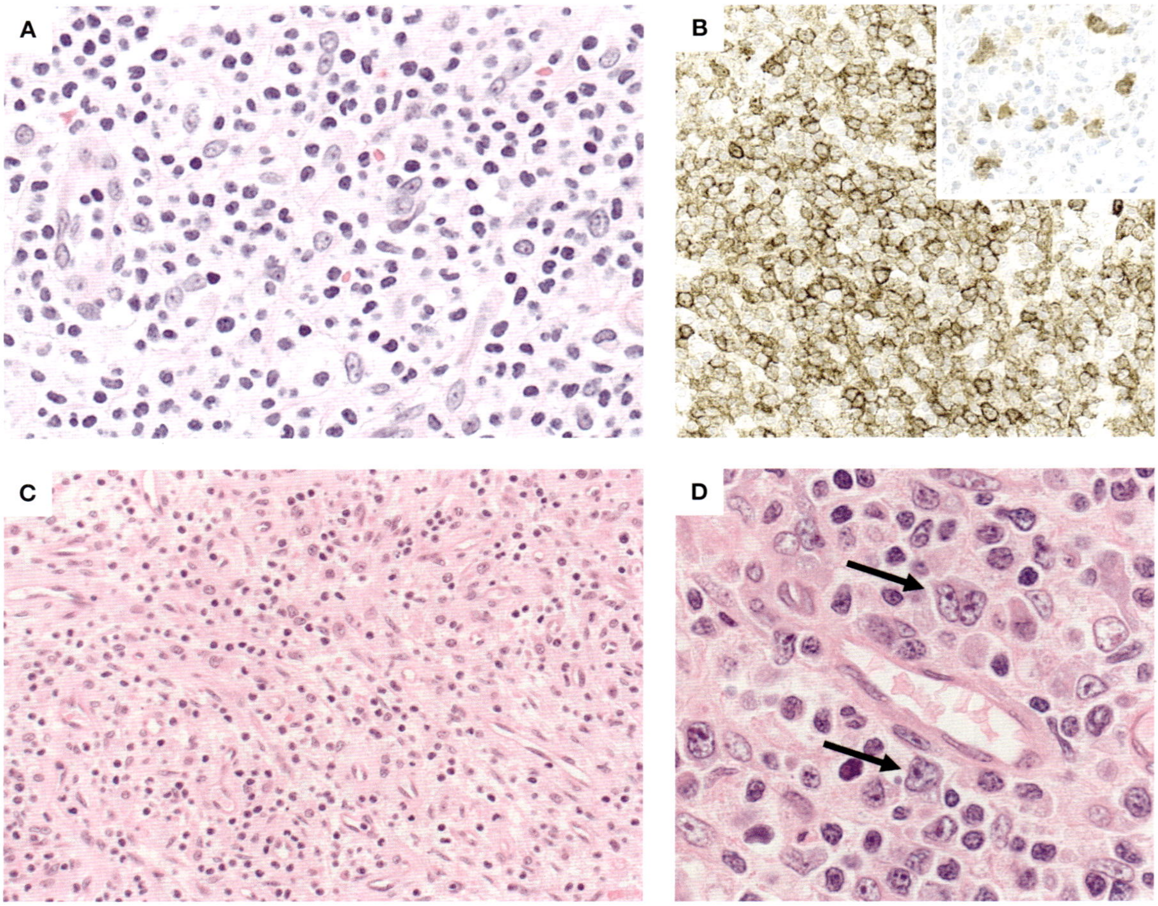

FIGURE 110.3 Anaplastic large cell lymphoma, ALK positive, small cell pattern. **A:** This tumor is composed predominantly of small cells with clear cytoplasm. **B:** The cells are positive for CD30, as well as ALK (inset). **C:** Another case showing the small cell pattern. **D:** Larger tumor cells are present around vessels (arrows).

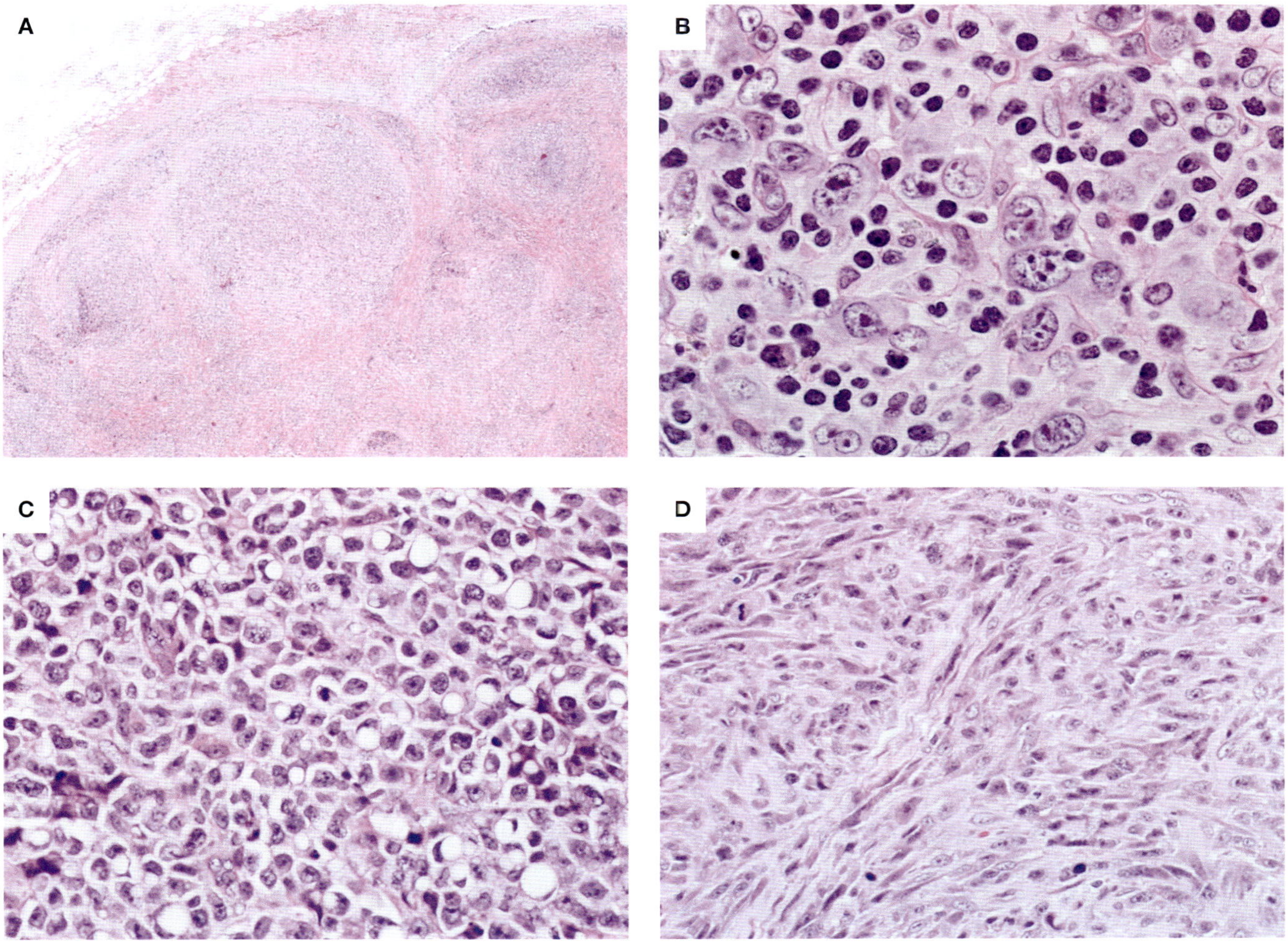

FIGURE 110.4 Anaplastic large cell lymphoma, ALK positive (ALK+ ALCL), rare histologic patterns. **A:** Hodgkin-like pattern, with nodules surrounded by bands of fibrosis, similar to nodular sclerosis classic Hodgkin lymphoma at low power. **B:** At high power, the tumor cells are scattered in a background of lymphocytes, histiocytes, and plasma cells, but do not have the typical cytological features of Reed-Sternberg cells. **C:** ALK+ ALCL with signet ring cells. **D:** ALK+ ALCL with spindled cells ("sarcomatoid" pattern).

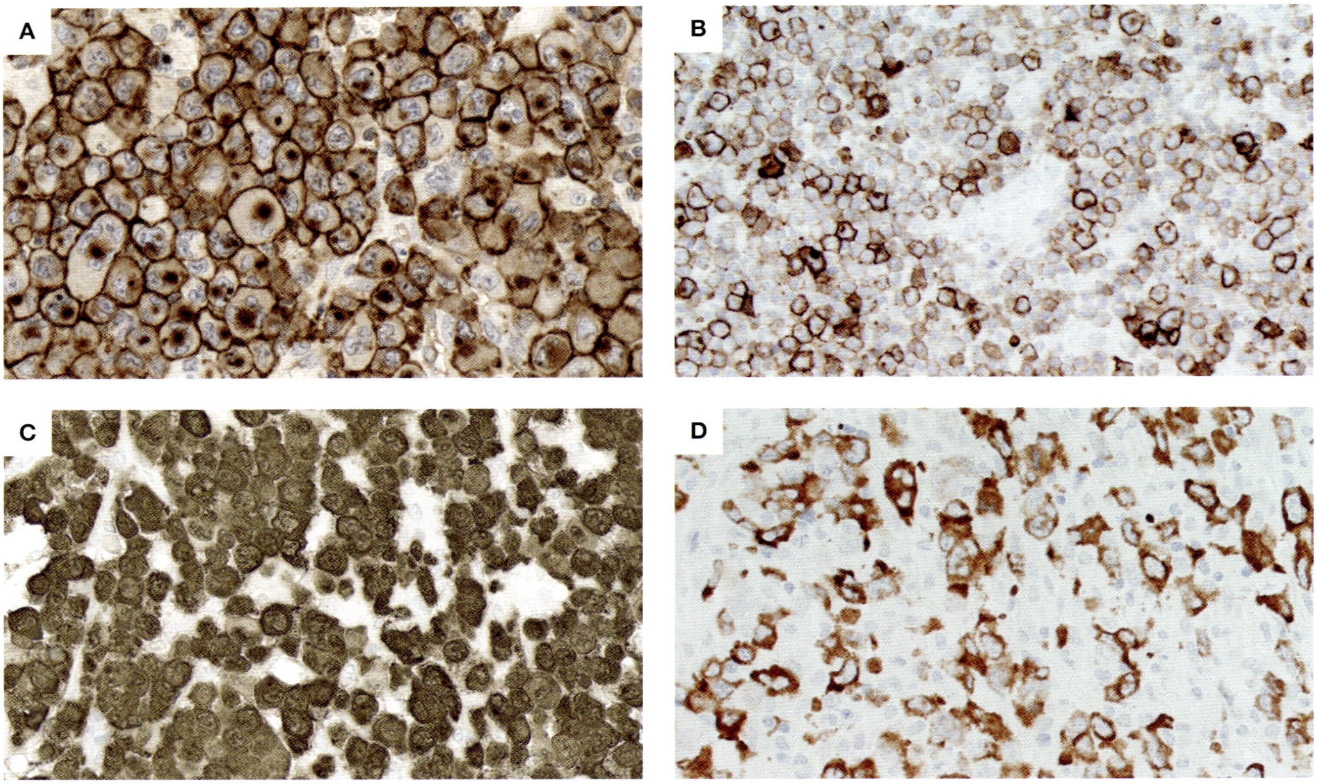

FIGURE 110.5 CD30 and ALK staining in anaplastic large cell lymphoma, ALK positive (ALK+ ALCL). **A:** Characteristic staining pattern for CD30 in ALK+ ALCL. The staining is strong and uniform, with a membranous and Golgi pattern of distribution. **B:** The intensity of CD30 staining is more variable in this case of ALK+ ALCL, small cell pattern. **C:** Characteristic nuclear and cytoplasmic pattern of ALK staining in ALK+ ALCL with *NPM1::ALK* fusion. **D:** Cytoplasmic staining only in ALK+ ALCL with *TRAF1::ALK* fusion (Table 110.1).

TABLE 110.1 Frequency and immunohistochemical staining patterns with different ALK fusions in anaplastic large cell lymphoma, ALK positive

Partner gene	Cytogenetic alteration	MW of fusion protein	ALK staining pattern	Frequency
NPM1	t(2;5)(p23;q35)	80 kD	Nuclear and diffuse cytoplasmic	84%
TPM3	t(1;2)(q25;p23)	104 kD	Diffuse cytoplasmic and membranous	13%
ATIC	inv(2)(p23;q35)	96 kD	Diffuse cytoplasmic	1%
CLTC	t(2;17)(p23;q23)	250 kD	Granular cytoplasmic	<1%
EEF1G	t(2;11)(p23;q12.3)	87 kD	Diffuse cytoplasmic	<1%
MSN	t(X;2)(q11;p23)	125 kD	Membranous	<1%
MYH9	t(2;22)(p23;q11)	220 kD	Diffuse cytoplasmic	<1%
PAPBC1	t(2;8)(p23;q22)	112 kD	Diffuse cytoplasmic	<1%
RNF213	t(2;17)(p23;q25)	unknown	Diffuse cytoplasmic	<1%
TFG	t(2;3)(p23;q21)	varies[a]	Diffuse cytoplasmic	<1%
TPM4	t(2;19)(p23;p13)	95 kD	Diffuse cytoplasmic	<1%
TRAF1	t(2;9)(p23;q33)	varies[b]	Diffuse cytoplasmic	<1%

ALK, anaplastic lymphoma kinase; kD, kilodalton; MW, molecular weight.

[a]The same portion of *ALK* may be fused to *TFG* fragments of different lengths, resulting in short (85 kD), long (97 kD), and extralong (113 kD) fusion proteins.

[b]Estimates of ~95 kD and slightly less than 75 kD have been reported.

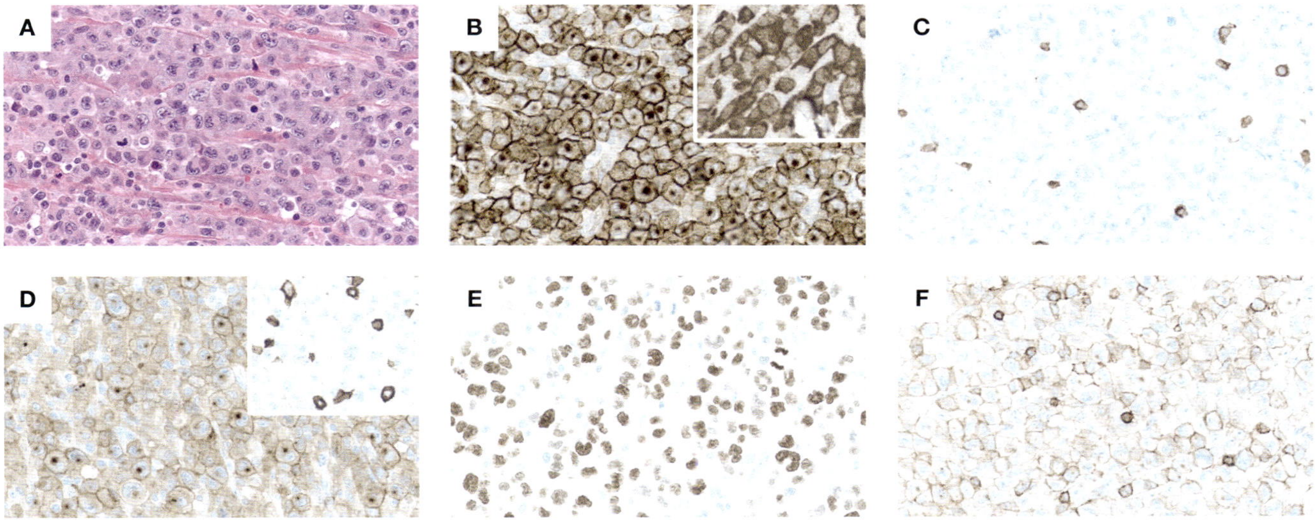

FIGURE 110.6 Anaplastic large cell lymphoma, ALK positive, additional immunophenotypic features. **A:** Hematoxylin and eosin staining demonstrates sheets of tumor cells (common pattern). **B:** The cells are strongly and uniformly positive for CD30, as well as ALK (inset). **C:** The tumor cells show aberrant loss of CD3. **D:** They are positive for CD4 and negative for CD8 (inset). **E:** The tumor cells show strong nuclear positivity for IRF4 (MUM1). **F:** CD45 expression is variable, with weaker intensity than in admixed small reactive lymphocytes.

Prognosis and Clinical Comment

The prognosis of ALK+ ALCL is generally favorable.[1,2] Outcomes are superior to those of ALCL, ALK negative, independent of patient age (Figure 110.7). Adverse prognostic factors include advanced age, advanced stage, peripheral blood and/or bone marrow involvement, CNS involvement, small cell or lymphohistiocytic histologic pattern, *TP53* mutation, and MYC expression.[1-3,14,20,21] The international prognostic index (IPI) can identify a high risk group with a poor outcome (IPI, 3-5; 5-year overall survival of ~30%).[4,22] Frontline treatment with brentuximab vedotin (BV)–cyclophosphamide, doxorubicin, and prednisone (CHP) is considered standard based on superiority over CHOP in those with IPI ≥2 as shown in the ECHELON-2 trial.[23] CHOEP has also been found to be associated with improved progression-free survival in retrospective studies, but has not been compared to BV-CHP.[6,24] BV alone may be used in relapsed/refractory ALK+ ALCL; small molecule ALK inhibitors may also have a role in this setting, though relapse after discontinuation remains an issue and these agents may be best utilized as a bridge to transplant.[25]

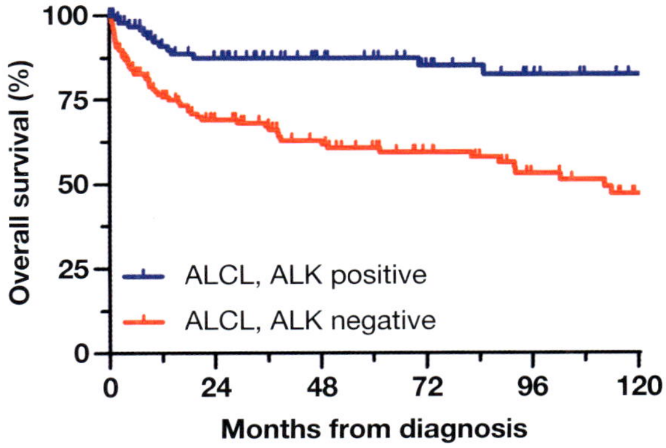

FIGURE 110.7 Outcomes of anaplastic large cell lymphoma, ALK positive and ALK negative. Five-year overall survival rates in a series of 257 systemic ALCLs were 87% and 61%, respectively ($P < .0001$, log-rank test) (Feldman AL, Dasari S, Rimsza LM, et al. Gene expression profiling reveals two overarching types of anaplastic large cell lymphoma with distinct targetable biology: an L.L.M.P.P. study. *Blood.* 2023;142(suppl 1):847-847.)

References

1. Ferreri AJ, Govi S, Pileri SA, Savage KJ. Anaplastic large cell lymphoma, ALK-positive. *Crit Rev Oncol Hematol.* 2012;83(2):293-302.

2. Vose J, Armitage J, Weisenburger D; International T-Cell Lymphoma Project. International peripheral T-cell and natural killer/T-cell lymphoma study: pathology findings and clinical outcomes. *J Clin Oncol.* 2008;26(25):4124-4130.
3. Xing X, Feldman AL. Anaplastic large cell lymphomas: ALK positive, ALK negative, and primary cutaneous. *Adv Anat Pathol.* 2015;22(1):29-49.
4. Falini B, Pileri S, Zinzani PL, et al. ALK+ lymphoma: clinico-pathological findings and outcome. *Blood.* 1999;93(8):2697-2706.
5. Lamant L, Pileri S, Sabattini E, Brugieres L, Jaffe ES, Delsol G. Cutaneous presentation of ALK-positive anaplastic large cell lymphoma following insect bites: evidence for an association in five cases. *Haematologica.* 2010;95(3):449-455.
6. Sibon D, Nguyen DP, Schmitz N, et al. ALK-positive anaplastic large-cell lymphoma in adults: an individual patient data pooled analysis of 263 patients. *Haematologica.* 2019;104(12):e562-e565.
7. Melchers RC, Willemze R, van de Loo M, et al. Clinical, histologic, and molecular characteristics of anaplastic lymphoma kinase-positive primary cutaneous anaplastic large cell lymphoma. *Am J Surg Pathol.* 2020;44(6):776-781.
8. Benharroch D, Meguerian-Bedoyan Z, Lamant L, et al. ALK-positive lymphoma: a single disease with a broad spectrum of morphology. *Blood.* 1998;91(6):2076-2084.
9. Vassallo J, Lamant L, Brugieres L, et al. ALK-positive anaplastic large cell lymphoma mimicking nodular sclerosis Hodgkin's lymphoma: report of 10 cases. *Am J Surg Pathol.* 2006;30(2):223-229.
10. Feldman AL, Laurent C, Narbaitz M, et al. Classification and diagnostic evaluation of nodal T- and NK-cell lymphomas. *Virchows Arch.* 2023;482(1):265-279.
11. Damm-Welk C, Klapper W, Oschlies I, et al. Distribution of *NPM1-ALK* and *X-ALK* fusion transcripts in paediatric anaplastic large cell lymphoma: a molecular-histological correlation. *Br J Haematol.* 2009;146(3):306-309.
12. Tan BT, Seo K, Warnke RA, Arber DA. The frequency of immunoglobulin heavy chain gene and T-cell receptor gamma-chain gene rearrangements and Epstein-Barr virus in ALK+ and ALK- anaplastic large cell lymphoma and other peripheral T-cell lymphomas. *J Mol Diagn.* 2008;10(6):502-512.
13. Larose H, Prokoph N, Matthews JD, et al. Whole exome sequencing reveals *NOTCH1* mutations in anaplastic large cell lymphoma and points to Notch both as a key pathway and a potential therapeutic target. *Haematologica.* 2021;106(6):1693-1704.
14. Lobello C, Tichy B, Bystry V, et al. *STAT3* and *TP53* mutations associate with poor prognosis in anaplastic large cell lymphoma. *Leukemia.* 2021;35(5):1500-1505.
15. Hare L, Burke GAA, Turner SD. Resistance to targeted agents used to treat paediatric ALK-positive ALCL. *Cancers.* 2021;13(23):6003.
16. Chiarle R, Simmons WJ, Cai H, et al. Stat3 is required for ALK-mediated lymphomagenesis and provides a possible therapeutic target. *Nat Med.* 2005;11(6):623-629.
17. Piva R, Agnelli L, Pellegrino E, et al. Gene expression profiling uncovers molecular classifiers for the recognition of anaplastic large-cell lymphoma within peripheral T-cell neoplasms. *J Clin Oncol.* 2010;28(9):1583-1590.
18. Luchtel RA, Dasari S, Oishi N, et al. Molecular profiling reveals immunogenic cues in anaplastic large cell lymphomas with *DUSP22* rearrangements. *Blood.* 2018;132(13):1386-1398.
19. Feldman AL, Dasari S, Rimsza LM, et al. Gene expression profiling reveals two overarching types of anaplastic large cell lymphoma with distinct targetable biology: an L.L.M.P.P. study. *Blood.* 2023;142(suppl 1):847.
20. Qiu L, Medeiros LJ, Tang G, et al. The leukemic phase of ALK-negative anaplastic large cell lymphoma is associated with CD7 positivity, complex karyotype, *TP53* deletion, and a poor prognosis. *Cancers.* 2021;13(24):6316.
21. Lyapichev KA, Tang G, Li S, et al. MYC expression is associated with older age, common morphology, increased MYC copy number, and poorer prognosis in patients with ALK+ anaplastic large cell lymphoma. *Hum Pathol.* 2021;108:22-31.
22. Savage KJ, Harris NL, Vose JM, et al. ALK- anaplastic large-cell lymphoma is clinically and immunophenotypically different from both ALK+ ALCL and peripheral T-cell lymphoma, not otherwise specified: report from the International Peripheral T-Cell Lymphoma Project. *Blood.* 2008;111(12):5496-5504.
23. Horwitz S, O'Connor OA, Pro B, et al. Brentuximab vedotin with chemotherapy for CD30-positive peripheral T-cell lymphoma (ECHELON-2): a global, double-blind, randomised, phase 3 trial. *Lancet.* 2019;393(10168):229-240.
24. Brink M, Meeuwes FO, van der Poel MWM, et al. Impact of etoposide and ASCT on survival among patients aged <65 years with stage II to IV PTCL: a population-based cohort study. *Blood.* 2022;140(9):1009-1019.
25. Brugieres L, Cozic N, Houot R, et al. Efficacy and safety of crizotinib in ALK-positive systemic anaplastic large-cell lymphoma in children, adolescents, and adult patients: results of the French AcSe-crizotinib trial. *Eur J Cancer.* 2023;191:112984.

Chapter 111

Anaplastic Large Cell Lymphoma, ALK Negative

Andrew L. Feldman, Bettina Bisig, Steven M. Horwitz, Marina Narbaitz, and Kerry J. Savage

Definition

Anaplastic large cell lymphoma, ALK negative (ALK− ALCL) is a systemic lymphoma of mature T-cell origin characterized by an infiltrate of cells with pleomorphic nuclei and abundant cytoplasm that express CD30 and lack gene fusions involving *ALK*. The histologic appearance should otherwise resemble ALCL, ALK positive (ALK+ ALCL). ALK− ALCL is a systemic disease that must be distinguished from localized forms of ALCL, including primary cutaneous (pc) ALCL and breast implant–associated ALCL.

Synonyms

None.

Epidemiology

ALK− ALCL represents about 2% to 3% of all non-Hodgkin lymphomas overall.[1-4] It constitutes 8% to 9% of peripheral (postthymic) T-cell lymphomas (PTCLs) in Europe and North America and 3% in Asia. In contrast to ALK+ ALCL, ALK− ALCL preferentially affects older adults. The median age is 58 years. It is more common in males, with a M:F ratio of about 1.5:1. The causes of ALK− ALCL are unknown.

General Clinical Features

Patients typically present with lymphadenopathy and often have B symptoms.[1,4] Peripheral lymph node involvement is most common, although mediastinal lymph nodes may be involved. While ALK− ALCL is predominantly a nodal form of PTCL, about 20% of cases involve extranodal sites, particularly skin, lung, liver, and the gastrointestinal tract. ALK− ALCL with secondary skin involvement must be distinguished from pcALCL, which is a form of pcCD30-positive lymphoproliferative disorder (see Chapter 102). In addition, pcALCL and breast implant–associated ALCL (Chapter 112) can secondarily involve locoregional lymph nodes.[2,5] About 60% of patients with ALK− ALCL present with stage III or IV disease. Bone marrow involvement by ALK− ALCL is relatively infrequent (<10%) and peripheral blood is rarely involved.

Morphology

Hallmark cells, as described in ALK+ ALCL (Chapter 110), are seen in all cases of ALK− ALCL (Figure 111.1A).[2,4] In general, the morphologic features of ALK− ALCL should resemble those of the common pattern of ALCL (Figure 111.1B), with cohesive sheets of tumor cells that in lymph nodes typically replace the paracortex but may spare residual follicles. Sinusoidal involvement is common, either as single cells or extensive sinusoidal expansion, and is a helpful clue both in recognizing the presence of neoplastic cells in subtle cases and in distinguishing ALK− ALCL from other PTCLs (Figure 111.1C).

Unlike ALK+ ALCL, distinct morphologic patterns are not recognized in ALK− ALCL. Although there is some variation in cell size, a small cell pattern is not acknowledged. Cases resembling the small cell pattern of ALK+ ALCL but lacking ALK expression should be diagnosed as PTCL, not otherwise specified (NOS). While a lymphohistiocytic variant is not recognized, a modest inflammatory background may be seen in some cases of ALK− ALCL. Similarly, while a Hodgkin-like pattern is not recognized, some cases have a predominance of very large, anaplastic cells with marked nuclear pleomorphism, sometimes with a wreath-like pattern and occasionally with Reed-Sternberg–like features (Figure 111.1D). These cases may be accompanied by a prominent mixed inflammatory background and occasionally show a nodular growth pattern with bands of fibrosis, reminiscent of classic Hodgkin lymphoma (CHL), nodular sclerosis type. Unless areas typical for ALK− ALCL are also present, most of these cases are better classified as PTCL, NOS once T-cell lineage is confirmed.[6]

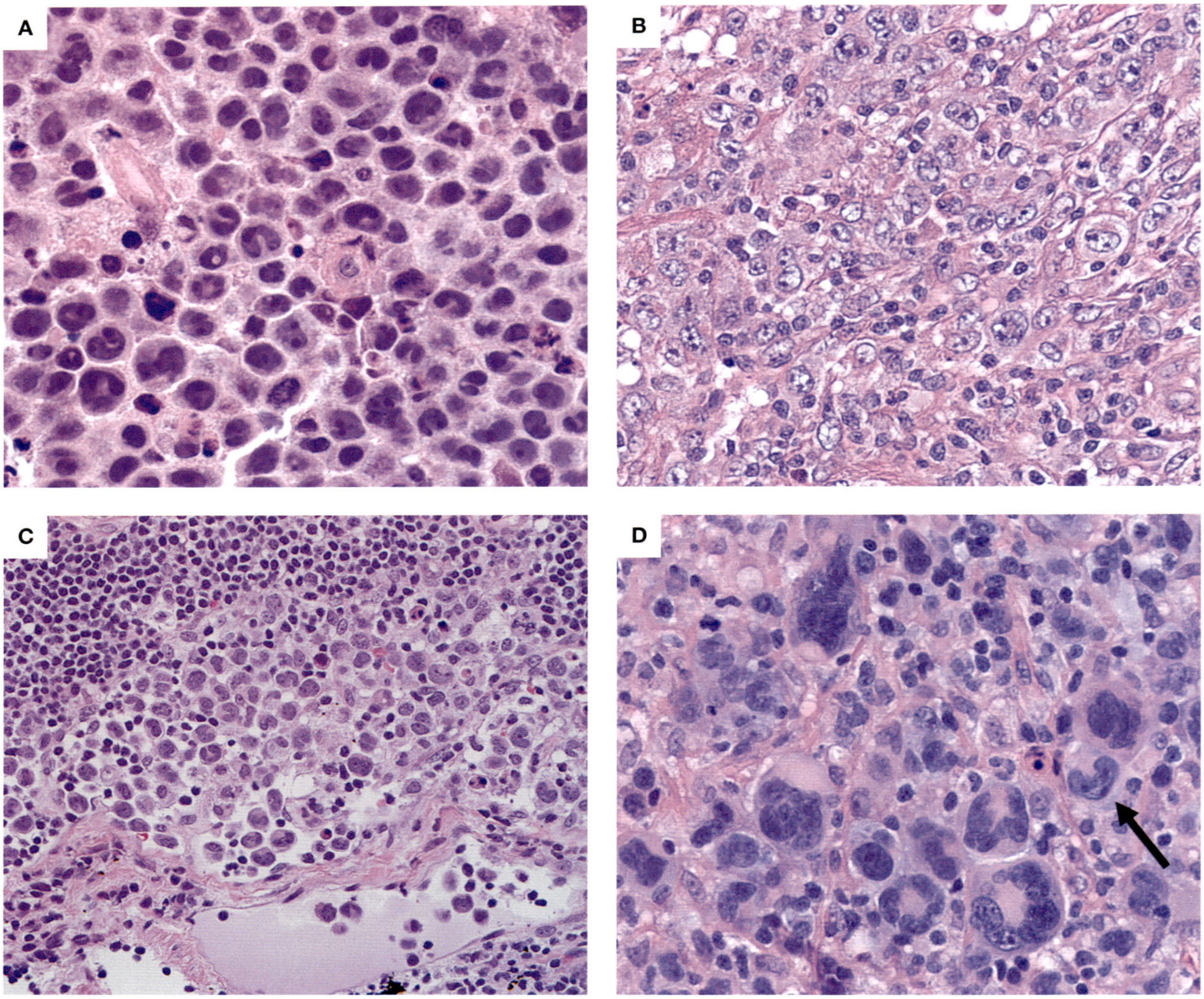

FIGURE 111.1 Morphological features of anaplastic large cell lymphoma, ALK negative (ALK− ALCL). **A:** Hallmark cells in ALK− ALCL. **B:** Typical sheetlike growth pattern of ALK− ALCL, resembling the common pattern seen in ALK+ ALCL. **C:** Sinusoidal involvement by ALK− ALCL. **D:** ALK− ALCL with pleomorphic giant cells, some with multinucleation or wreath-like nuclei. Typical hallmark cells also are present (arrow). There are scattered inflammatory cells in the background.

Immunophenotype

By definition, all cases express CD30 and lack expression of ALK.[1,2,4] CD30 expression should be strong and uniform, typically with a membranous and Golgi pattern of distribution (Figure 111.2A and B). The presence of variable CD30 expression should raise the possibility of another entity, such as PTCL, NOS (Figure 111.2C). CD30 expression may be diminished after treatment with the anti-CD30 antibody-drug conjugate brentuximab vedotin (BV).[7] Most cases show some loss of pan–T-cell antigen expression, including T-cell receptor proteins, and some lack all T-cell antigens (null cell phenotype). CD2 is the most commonly retained pan–T-cell antigen (Figure 111.2D and E). Occasional cases express CD8. MUM1 (IRF4) is typically positive. Cytotoxic markers (TIA1, granzyme B, and/or perforin) are often expressed. CD56, EMA, and/or clusterin may be expressed, but this is less common than in ALK+ ALCL. CD45 expression is variable. CD15 may be expressed in cases with or without CHL-like features (Figure 111.2F). EBV should be negative. Differentiating ALK− ALCL from CHL and PTCL, NOS requires integration of clinical data, morphology (see above), other phenotypic features, and sometimes molecular studies (see below).

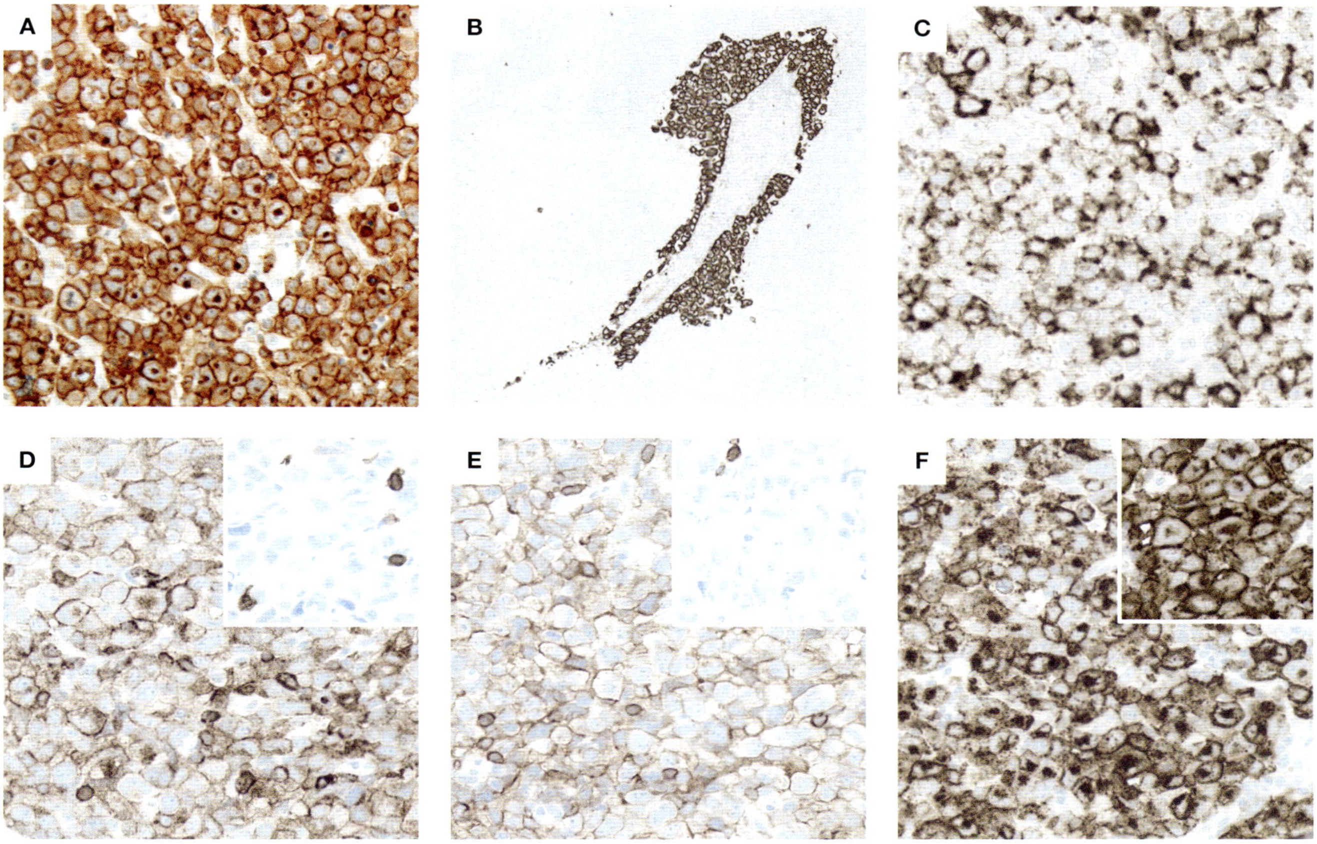

FIGURE 111.2 Immunophenotype of anaplastic large cell lymphoma, ALK negative (ALK− ALCL). **A:** CD30 staining in ALK− ALCL is strong and uniform, with a membranous and Golgi staining pattern. **B:** CD30 staining highlights sinusoidal involvement by ALK− ALCL in a lymph node biopsy. **C:** Peripheral T-cell lymphoma, not otherwise specified with partial CD30 expression. Although CD30 is strongly expressed in some of the cells, other cells are negative or only weakly positive. This staining pattern is not typical of ALK− ALCL. **D:** ALK− ALCL showing weak positivity for CD2 and loss of CD3 (inset). **E:** Same case as panel D. The tumor is weakly positive for CD4 and negative for CD8 (inset). **F:** Same case as panel D. This case was strongly positive for CD15. CD30 is shown in the inset.

Occasional ALK− ALCLs aberrantly express PAX5, CD33, keratins, or other non–T-cell markers (Figure 111.3).[2] Cases with *TP63* rearrangement (*TP63*-R; see below) are positive for p63 by immunohistochemistry, but this finding can also be seen in some cases lacking *TP63*-R.[8] Cases with *DUSP22*-R typically express LEF1 and lack expression of cytotoxic markers and phosphorylated STAT3.[9]

Genetics

The T-cell receptor genes are clonally rearranged in most but not all cases.[10] *ALK* fusions are absent. Chromosomal rearrangements of the *DUSP22* locus on 6p25.3, most commonly with a noncoding partner locus on 7q32.3, are seen in 19% to 45% of cases[11-15] (Figure 111.4). Fusions involving *TP63* with *TBL1XR1* or other partners are seen in 2% to 8% of cases (Figure 111.5),[16] including rare cases with concomitant *DUSP22*-R.[17] Cases lacking rearrangements of *ALK*, *DUSP22*, and *TP63* are designated “triple negative.”[12] A subset of cases has fusions involving non-*ALK* tyrosine kinase genes, including *ROS1*, *TYK2*, *FRK*, and *JAK2*.[18-20] *JAK2* rearrangements have been reported to occur in cases with markedly anaplastic morphologic features (Figure 111.6).[20] A subset of cases with aberrant *ERBB4* transcripts has also been described.[21] Recurrently mutated genes include *JAK1*, *JAK3*, *STAT3*, *MSC*, *TP53*, and *PRDM1*.[18,22,23] *MSC* mutations have been specifically associated with the presence of *DUSP22*-R (see below).[23] Copy number losses of *TP53* and *PRDM1* have been reported.[22] About two-thirds of ALK− ALCLs have a gene expression signature enriched for genes in the JAK-STAT3 pathway.[13,18] The remaining cases

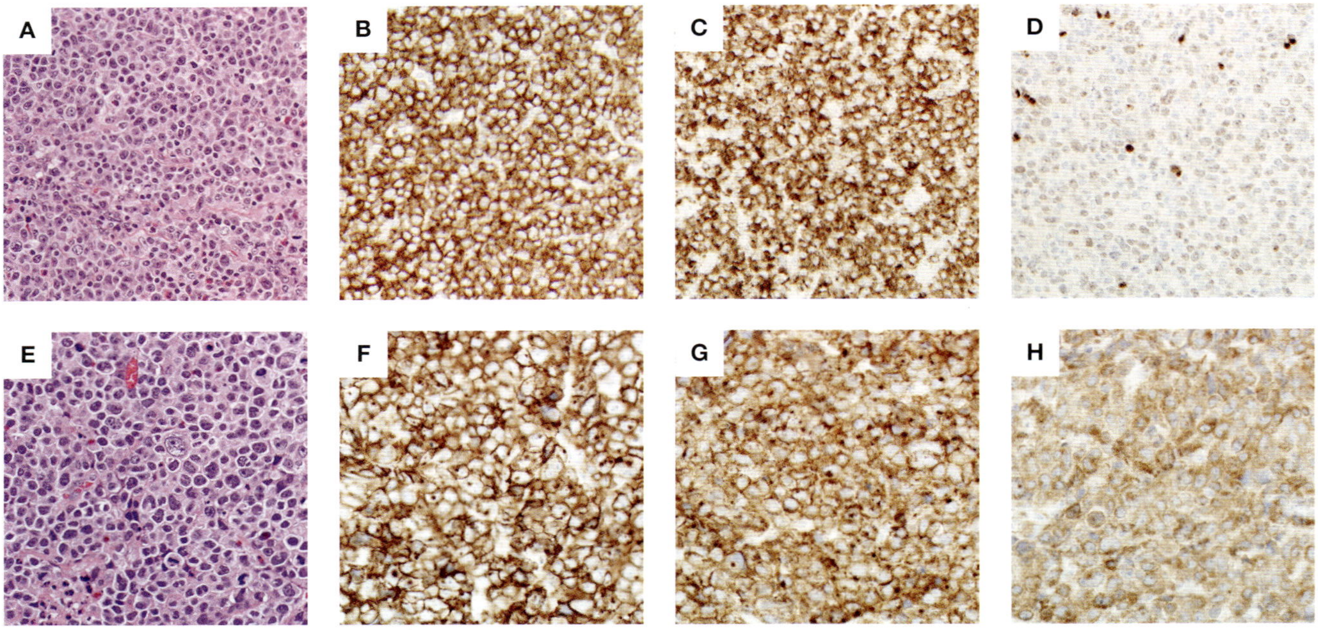

FIGURE 111.3 Aberrant antigen expression in anaplastic large cell lymphoma, ALK negative (ALK− ALCL). Case 1: Hematoxylin and eosin (H&E) staining **(A)** shows sheets of medium-sized to large tumor cells that are positive for CD30 **(B)** and CD2 **(C)**, and weakly positive for PAX5 **(D)**. Strong expression is seen in small reactive B cells. Case 2: H&E staining **(E)** shows sheets of large tumor cells that are positive for CD30 **(F)**, CD2 **(G)**, and OSCAR cytokeratin **(H)**. Clonal T-cell receptor gene rearrangements were detected by molecular studies in both cases (not shown).

lacking this signature are particularly enriched for *DUSP22*-R and may represent a distinct type of ALCL showing high expression of genes related to epigenetic pathways.[13,24]

Genetic subtype: ALK− ALCL with *DUSP22-R*

ALK− ALCL with *DUSP22*-R is recognized as a genetic subtype of ALK− ALCL based on a number of distinguishing features. Morphologically, cases tend to have sheetlike growth of cells that are somewhat smaller than in other ALK− ALCLs, with frequent doughnut cells.[25] Most cases express LEF1 and HLA class II and are negative for cytotoxic markers, phosphorylated STAT3, and PD-L1.[9,13] *MSC*[E116K] point mutations are seen in ~35% of ALK− ALCLs with *DUSP22*-R and are highly specific (>90%) for the presence of *DUSP22*-R among ALK− ALCLs.[23] ALK− ALCLs with *DUSP22*-R show global DNA hypomethylation and have a unique gene expression signature enriched for expression of cancer-testis antigen genes. Prognostic significance is discussed later. *DUSP22*-R is not specific for ALK− ALCL, and is seen with a similar frequency in pcALCL,[11] in a subset of lymphomatoid papulosis,[26] and rarely in other entities.[27]

Prognosis and Clinical Comment

The prognosis of ALK− ALCL is poorer than ALK+ ALCL, with 5-year overall survival (OS) rates of ~50%.[1,4,12] Frontline treatment consists of BV-CHP (BV, cyclophosphamide, doxorubicin, and prednisone) given improved outcomes compared with CHOP chemotherapy.[28] Autologous stem cell transplantation is typically recommended in first remission, which may still be of benefit following BV-CHP.[29] Despite frequent responses to first-line therapy, relapses are common and management of relapsed/refractory disease remains a significant clinical challenge. Data suggest the prognostic importance of genetic subgroups of ALK− ALCL. *DUSP22*-R has been associated with excellent prognosis, with 5-year OS up to 90% and similar to ALK+ ALCL in some studies, whereas other studies have reported the existence of high-risk cases and poorer OS rates, which may be impacted by clinical factors.[12,14,15,30,31] *TP63*-R is nearly always associated with aggressive disease and poor outcomes[12,30]; more data are needed to determine whether this should be considered a distinct genetic subtype. *STAT3* mutations and combined mutations and/or deletions involving *TP53* and *PRDM1* also are associated with adverse prognosis.[22,32]

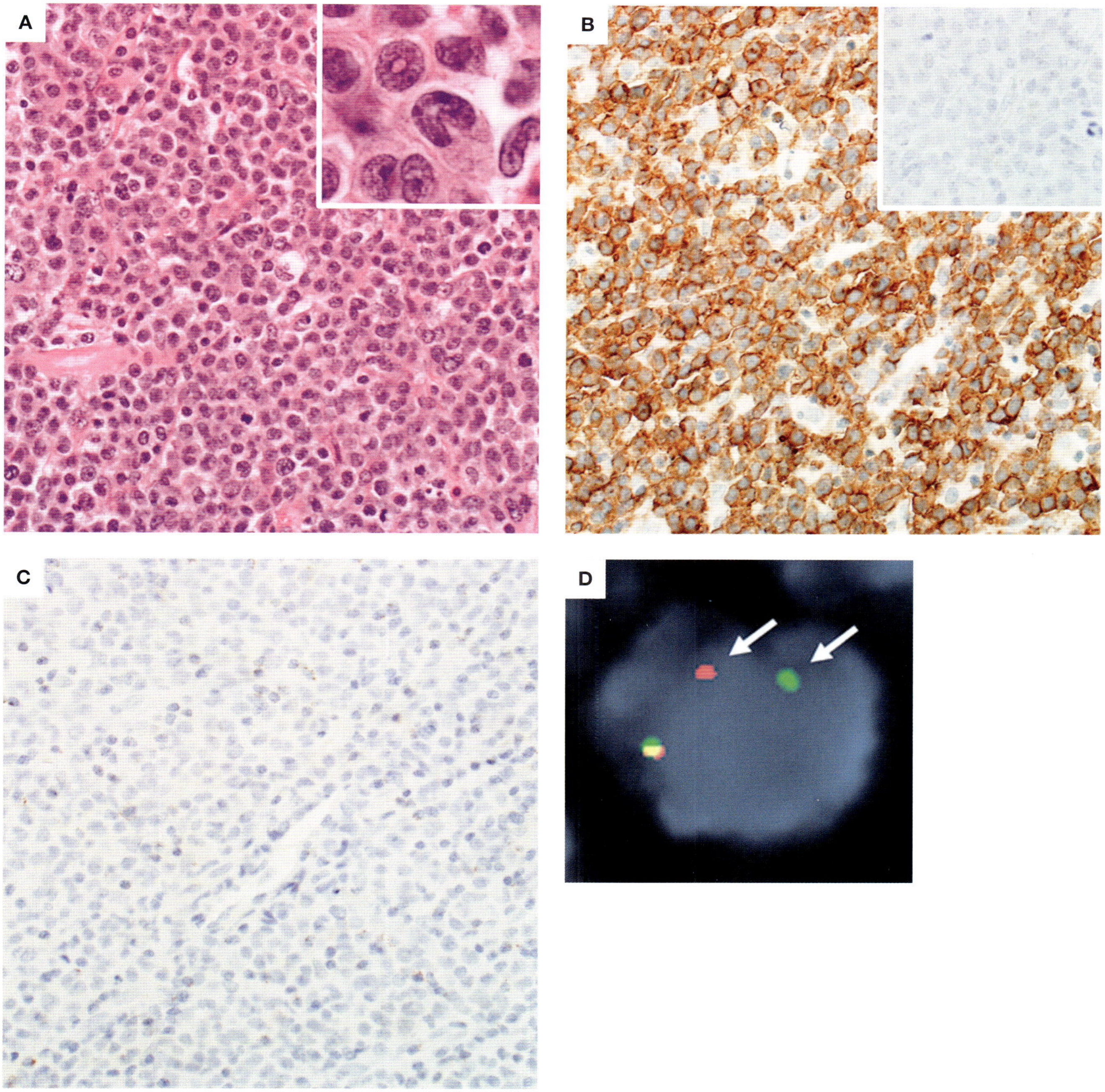

FIGURE 111.4 Anaplastic large cell lymphoma, ALK negative (ALK− ALCL) with *DUSP22* rearrangement. **A:** Hematoxylin and eosin staining shows sheets of medium-sized tumor cells, including hallmark and doughnut cells (inset). **B:** The tumor cells are strongly and uniformly positive for CD30 and negative for ALK (inset). **C:** They are negative for the cytotoxic marker TIA1, a characteristic finding in ALK− ALCL with *DUSP22* rearrangement. **D:** Fluorescence in situ hybridization using a breakapart probe to the *DUSP22* locus on 6p25.3 shows separation of the 5' (red) and 3' (green) signals (arrows), indicating the presence of a *DUSP22* rearrangement.

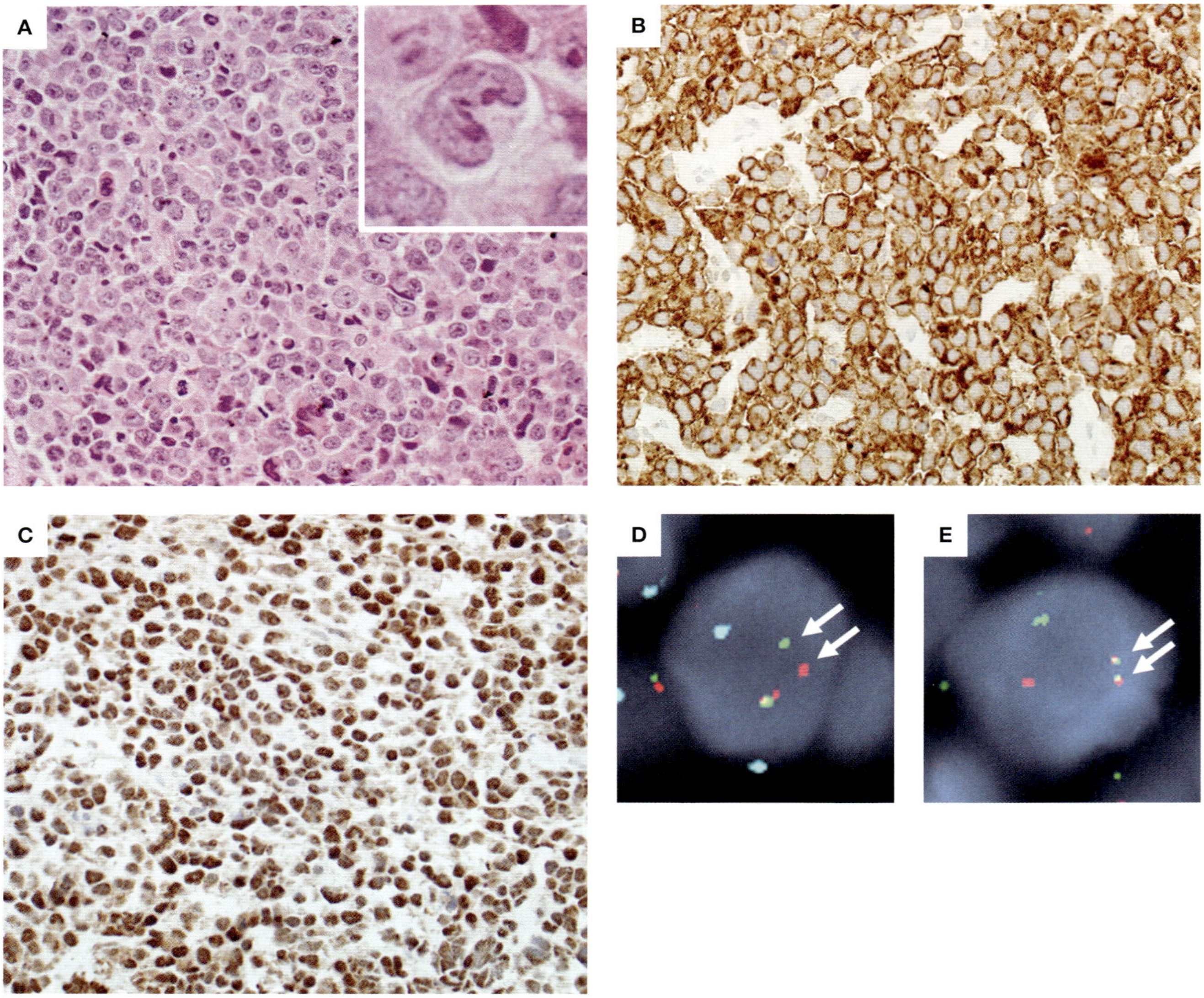

FIGURE 111.5 Anaplastic large cell lymphoma, ALK negative with *TP63* rearrangement. **A:** Hematoxylin and eosin staining shows sheets of large tumor cells, including hallmark cells (inset). The tumor cells are strongly and uniformly positive for both CD30 **(B)** and p63 **(C)**. **D:** Fluorescence in situ hybridization (FISH) using a breakapart probe to the *TP63* locus on 3q28 shows separation of the 5' (red) and 3' (green) signals (arrows). The cyan signals represent centromere 3. **E:** Dual-color, dual-fusion FISH shows two abnormal fusion signals (arrows), indicating the presence of *TBL1XR1::TP63*.

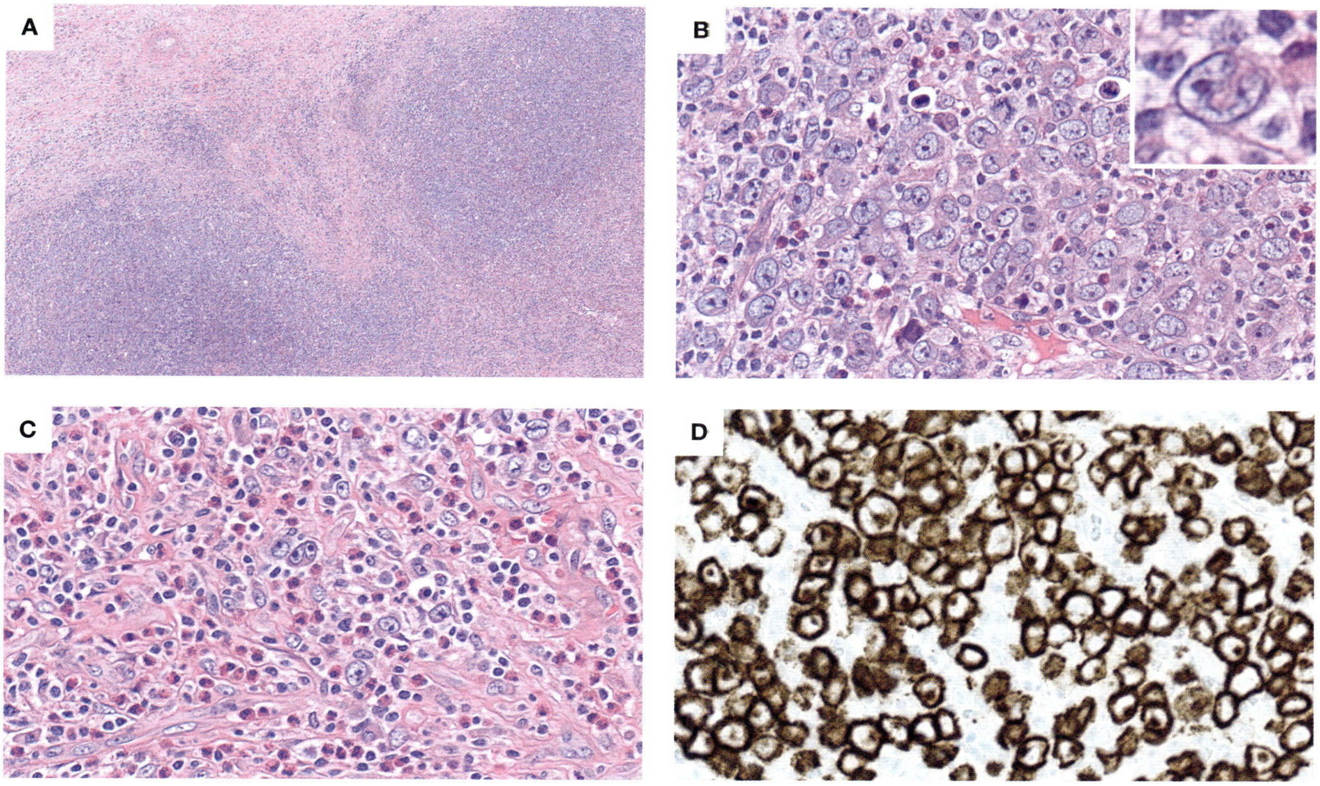

FIGURE 111.6 Anaplastic large cell lymphoma, ALK negative with *JAK2* rearrangement. **A:** At low power, the lymph node shows a macronodular architecture with capsular thickening and bands of fibrosis. **B:** Some areas show sheets of large tumor cells, including characteristic hallmark cells (inset). **C:** In other areas, the tumor cells are scattered in a mixed inflammatory background containing numerous eosinophils. **D:** CD30 shows strong and uniform staining, with a membranous and Golgi pattern. Fluorescence in situ hybridization demonstrated a *JAK2* rearrangement (not shown).

References

1. Ferreri AJ, Govi S, Pileri SA, Savage KJ. Anaplastic large cell lymphoma, ALK-negative. *Crit Rev Oncol Hematol.* 2013;85(2):206-215.
2. Xing X, Feldman AL. Anaplastic large cell lymphomas: ALK positive, ALK negative, and primary cutaneous. *Adv Anat Pathol.* 2015;22(1):29-49.
3. Vose J, Armitage J, Weisenburger D; International T-Cell Lymphoma Project. International peripheral T-cell and natural killer/T-cell lymphoma study: pathology findings and clinical outcomes. *J Clin Oncol.* 2008;26(25):4124-4130.
4. Savage KJ, Harris NL, Vose JM, et al. ALK- anaplastic large-cell lymphoma is clinically and immunophenotypically different from both ALK+ ALCL and peripheral T-cell lymphoma, not otherwise specified: report from the International Peripheral T-Cell Lymphoma Project. *Blood.* 2008;111(12):5496-5504.
5. Ferrufino-Schmidt MC, Medeiros LJ, Liu H, et al. Clinicopathologic features and prognostic impact of lymph node involvement in patients with breast implant-associated anaplastic large cell lymphoma. *Am J Surg Pathol.* 2018;42(3):293-305.
6. Attygalle AD, Cabecadas J, Gaulard P, et al. Peripheral T-cell and NK-cell lymphomas and their mimics; taking a step forward - report on the lymphoma workshop of the XVIth meeting of the European Association for Haematopathology and the Society for Hematopathology. *Histopathology.* 2014;64(2):171-199.
7. Al-Rohil RN, Torres-Cabala CA, Patel A, et al. Loss of CD30 expression after treatment with brentuximab vedotin in a patient with anaplastic large cell lymphoma: a novel finding. *J Cutan Pathol.* 2016;43(12):1161-1166.
8. Wang X, Boddicker RL, Dasari S, et al. Expression of p63 protein in anaplastic large cell lymphoma: implications for genetic subtyping. *Hum Pathol.* 2017;64:19-27.
9. Feldman AL, Oishi N, Ketterling RP, Ansell SM, Shi M, Dasari S. Immunohistochemical approach to genetic subtyping of anaplastic large cell lymphoma. *Am J Surg Pathol.* 2022;46(11):1490-1499.
10. Tan BT, Seo K, Warnke RA, Arber DA. The frequency of immunoglobulin heavy chain gene and T-cell receptor gamma-chain gene rearrangements and Epstein-Barr virus in ALK+ and ALK- anaplastic large cell lymphoma and other peripheral T-cell lymphomas. *J Mol Diagn.* 2008;10(6):502-512.

11. Feldman AL, Dogan A, Smith DI, et al. Discovery of recurrent t(6;7)(p25.3;q32.3) translocations in ALK-negative anaplastic large cell lymphomas by massively-parallel genomic sequencing. *Blood.* 2011;117(3):915-919.
12. Parrilla Castellar ER, Jaffe ES, Said JW, et al. ALK-negative anaplastic large cell lymphoma is a genetically heterogeneous disease with widely disparate clinical outcomes. *Blood.* 2014;124(9):1473-1480.
13. Luchtel RA, Dasari S, Oishi N, et al. Molecular profiling reveals immunogenic cues in anaplastic large cell lymphomas with *DUSP22* rearrangements. *Blood.* 2018;132(13):1386-1398.
14. Hapgood G, Ben-Neriah S, Mottok A, et al. Identification of high-risk *DUSP22*-rearranged ALK-negative anaplastic large cell lymphoma. *Br J Haematol.* 2019;186(3):e28-e31.
15. Sibon D, Bisig B, Bonnet C, et al. ALK-negative anaplastic large cell lymphoma with *DUSP22* rearrangement has distinctive disease characteristics with better progression-free survival: a LYSA study. *Haematologica.* 2023;108(6):1590-1603.
16. Vasmatzis G, Johnson SH, Knudson RA, et al. Genome-wide analysis reveals recurrent structural abnormalities of *TP63* and other p53-related genes in peripheral T-cell lymphomas. *Blood.* 2012;120(11):2280-2289.
17. Karube K, Feldman AL. "Double-hit" of *DUSP22* and *TP63* rearrangements in anaplastic large cell lymphoma, ALK-negative. *Blood.* 2020;135(9):700.
18. Crescenzo R, Abate F, Lasorsa E, et al. Convergent mutations and kinase fusions lead to oncogenic STAT3 activation in anaplastic large cell lymphoma. *Cancer Cell.* 2015;27(4):516-532.
19. Hu G, Dasari S, Asmann YW, et al. Targetable fusions of the *FRK* tyrosine kinase in ALK-negative anaplastic large cell lymphoma. *Leukemia.* 2018;32(2):565-569.
20. Fitzpatrick MJ, Massoth LR, Marcus C, et al. *JAK2* rearrangements are a recurrent alteration in CD30+ systemic T-cell lymphomas with anaplastic morphology. *Am J Surg Pathol.* 2021;45(7):895-904.
21. Scarfo I, Pellegrino E, Mereu E, et al. Identification of a new subclass of ALK-negative ALCL expressing aberrant levels of ERBB4 transcripts. *Blood.* 2016;127(2):221-232.
22. Boi M, Rinaldi A, Kwee I, et al. PRDM1/BLIMP1 is commonly inactivated in anaplastic large T-cell lymphoma. *Blood.* 2013;122(15):2683-2693.
23. Luchtel RA, Zimmermann MT, Hu G, et al. Recurrent *MSC* (E116K) mutations in ALK-negative anaplastic large cell lymphoma. *Blood.* 2019;133(26):2776-2789.
24. Feldman AL, Dasari S, Rimsza LM, et al. Gene expression profiling reveals two overarching types of anaplastic large cell lymphoma with distinct targetable biology: an L.L.M.P.P. study. *Blood.* 2023;142(suppl 1):847.
25. King RL, Dao L, McPhail E, et al. Morphology of ALK-negative anaplastic large cell lymphomas with *DUSP22* rearrangements. *Lab Invest.* 2015;95:355A.
26. Karai LJ, Kadin ME, Hsi ED, et al. Chromosomal rearrangements of 6p25.3 define a new subtype of lymphomatoid papulosis. *Am J Surg Pathol.* 2013;37(8):1173-1181.
27. Bisig B, Cairoli A, Gaide O, et al. Cutaneous presentation of enteropathy-associated T-cell lymphoma masquerading as a DUSP22-rearranged CD30+ lymphoproliferation. *Virchows Arch.* 2022;481(4):653-657.
28. Horwitz S, O'Connor OA, Pro B, et al. Brentuximab vedotin with chemotherapy for CD30-positive peripheral T-cell lymphoma (ECHELON-2): a global, double-blind, randomised, phase 3 trial. *Lancet.* 2019;393(10168):229-240.
29. Savage KJ, Horwitz SM, Advani R, et al. Role of stem cell transplant in CD30+ PTCL following frontline brentuximab vedotin plus CHP or CHOP in ECHELON-2. *Blood Adv.* 2022;6(19):5550-5555.
30. Pedersen MB, Hamilton-Dutoit SJ, Bendix K, et al. *DUSP22* and *TP63* rearrangements predict outcome of ALK-negative anaplastic large cell lymphoma: a Danish cohort study. *Blood.* 2017;130(4):554-557.
31. Qiu L, Tang G, Li S, et al. DUSP22 rearrangement is associated with a distinctive immunophenotype but not outcome in patients with systemic ALK-negative anaplastic large cell lymphoma. *Haematologica.* 2023;108(6):1604-1615.
32. Lobello C, Tichy B, Bystry V, et al. *STAT3* and *TP53* mutations associate with poor prognosis in anaplastic large cell lymphoma. *Leukemia.* 2021;35(5):1500-1505.

Chapter 112

Breast Implant–Associated Anaplastic Large Cell Lymphoma

Camille Laurent, Arianna Di Napoli, Andrew L. Feldman, and Steven M. Horwitz

Definition

Breast implant–associated anaplastic large cell lymphoma (BIA-ALCL) is rare form of ALCL arising primarily in association with a breast implant. BIA-ALCL is upgraded to a definite entity distinct from other ALCLs.

Synonyms

None.

Epidemiology

The risk of developing BIA-ALCL is very low, with an incidence ranging from 1/30,000 to 1/1000 women with breast implants.[1,2] Several studies have implicated high-texture implants and chronic inflammation due to implant debris and bacterial biofilm. Single reports suggest that patients with HLA-A*26 antigen or *BRCA1/2* mutations have an increased risk of BIA-ALCL.[1,3]

General Clinical Features

The mean patient age is 61 years with a median interval between last implant surgery and BIA-ALCL diagnosis of ~7 to 9 years.[4,5] Most patients present with a peri-implant seroma, while a minority have a palpable tumor mass, generally limited to the breast or associated with axillary lymphadenopathy.[4,5]

Morphology

The tumor cells can be identified by cytological examination of periprosthetic effusion fluid. Capsulectomy in patients with a seroma shows tumor cells that are typically large and pleomorphic. Scattered hallmark-like cells may be observed. The tumor cells are most commonly confined to the luminal surface of the capsule and/or encased within fibrinoid material (so-called in situ BIA-ALCL) (Figure 112.1A and B).[5] Some cases show early capsular invasion, while others present with a tumor mass in which malignant cells infiltrate deeper in the caspule (Figure 122.1C and D) and often the surrounding tissues (Figure 112.2). These tumors usually contain sheets of large anaplastic cells, sometimes resembling Hodgkin and Reed-Sternberg cells, within an inflammatory background often rich in eosinophils. Necrosis and/or sclerosis may also be observed.[5] Occasionally the lymphoma is first identified in regional nodes. In this case, the presence of CD30+ large cells in a lymph node may lead to a misdiagnosis of classic Hodgkin lymphoma, especially if the history of breast implants is unknown and the possibility of BIA-ALCL is not suspected.[5,6]

Immunophenotype

The phenotype is similar to that of ALK-negative ALCL, with strong and diffuse positivity for CD30 (see Figures 112.1 and 112.2). Incomplete expression of T-cell markers is common. The tumor cells are ALK and EBV negative. EMA, nuclear phospho-STAT3, and PD-L1 are frequently expressed.[5,6]

Genetics

T-cell receptor (TCR) genes are usually clonally rearranged. *ALK*, *DUSP22*, and *TP63* rearrangements are absent.[6] Copy number analyses show a complex karyotype; 20q13.13 loss appears to be a specific genomic feature of BIA-ALCLs that distinguishes them from other ALCLs.[7] Recurrent mutations in the JAK-STAT pathway genes, notably *STAT3* and *JAK1*, and in epigenetic modifier genes, including *KMT2C*, *KMT2D*, *CHD2*, and *CREBBP*, are commonly observed.[6,8] Both somatic and germline mutations in *TP53* have been found in BIA-ALCL. Like many other ALCLs, BIA-ALCLs show a gene expression profile enriched for JAK/STAT pathway genes with downregulation of TCR signaling genes.[9]

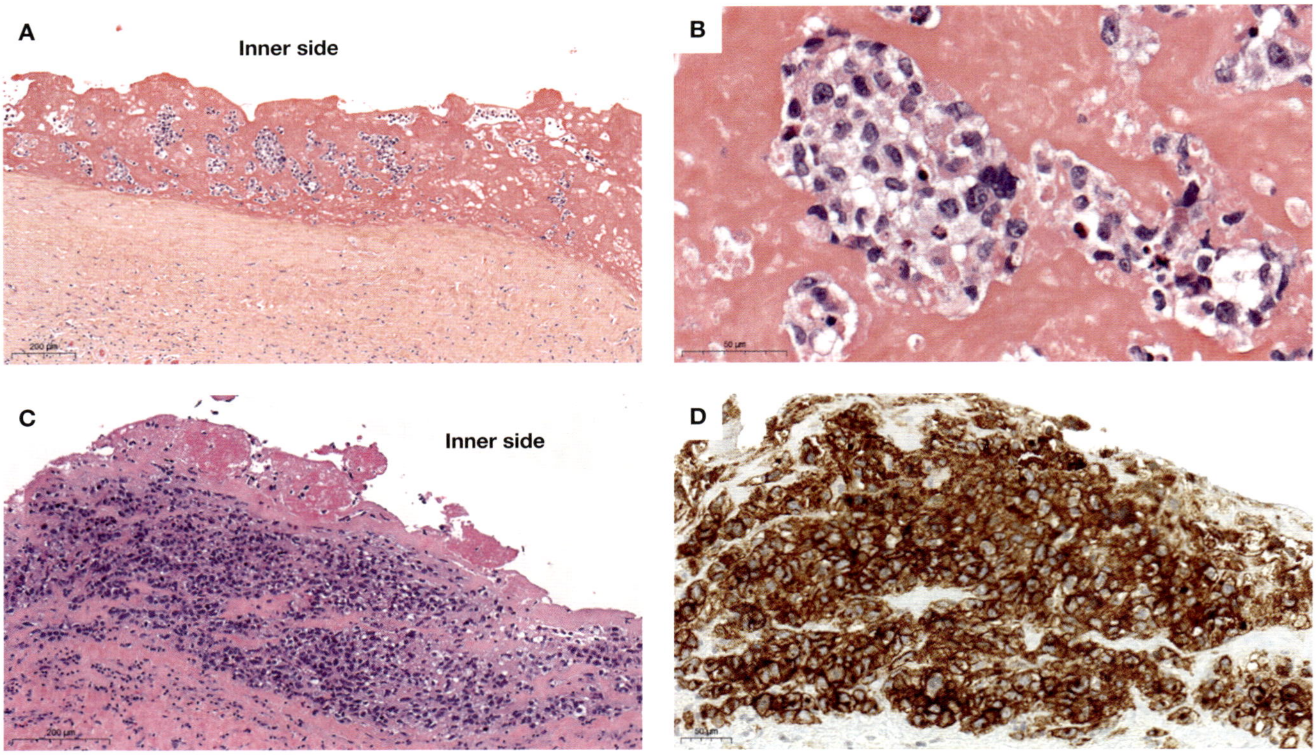

FIGURE 112.1 Breast implant–associated anaplastic large cell lymphoma (BIA-ALCL). **A:** pT1 BIA-ALCL (in situ) showing atypical cells in the fluid and exudate without capsule invasion. **B:** pT1 BIA-ALCL with atypical anaplastic cells encased within fibrinoid material. **C:** pT3 BIA-ALCL showing tumor cells aggregates or sheets within the capsule. **D:** Neoplastic cells strongly express CD30.

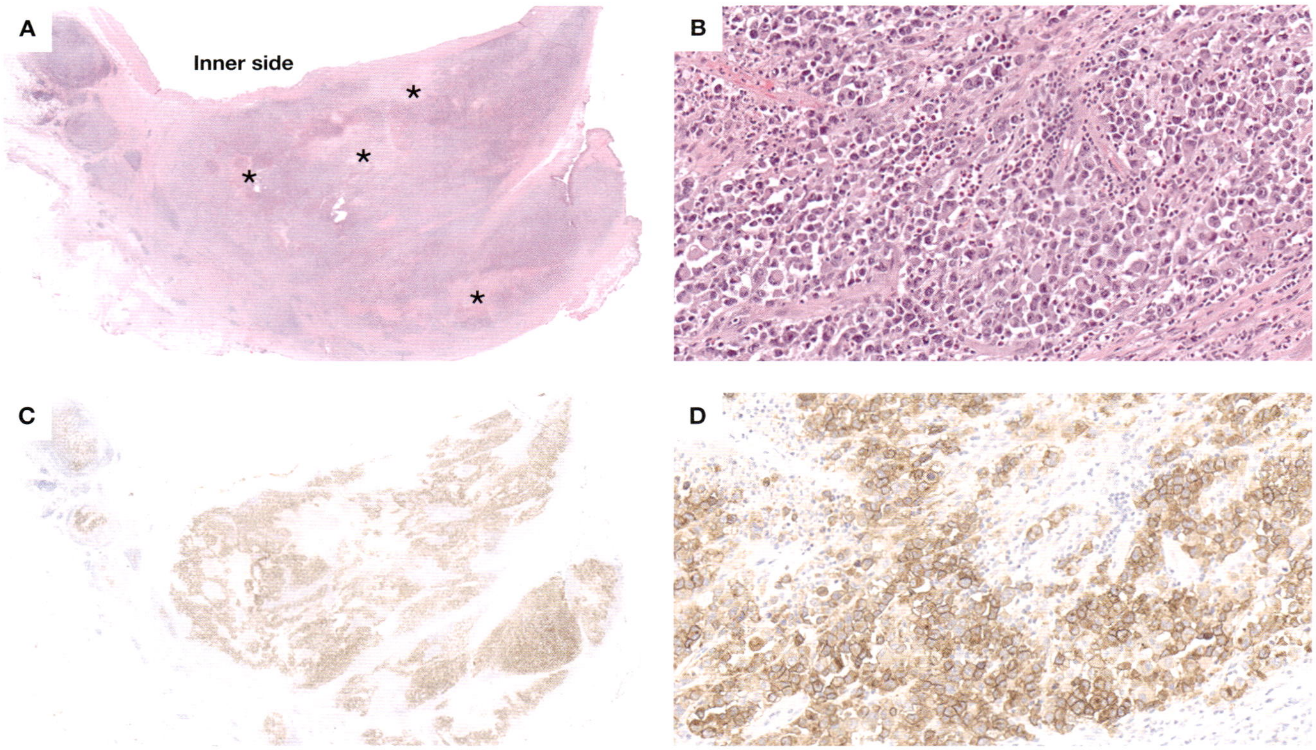

FIGURE 112.2 Breast implant–associated anaplastic large cell lymphoma (BIA-ALCL). **A:** pT4 BIA-ALCL tumor mass infiltrating the capsule and the soft tissue beyond (asterisk, necrotic areas). **B:** pT4 BIA-ALCL with large anaplastic tumor cells mixed with eosinophils. **C** and **D:** Tumor cells strongly express CD30.

They also are enriched for genes associated with regulatory T cells, hypoxia signaling, and the cytokine milieu.[9,10]

Prognosis and Clinical Comment

En bloc total capsulectomy with margin evaluation is the optimal treatment of most patients with BIA-ALCL. The use of the MD Anderson tumor-node-metastasis (TNM) staging (T1: in situ, tumor cells in seroma and/or on capsular luminal surface; T2: early capsule infiltration; T3: aggregates or sheets infiltrating capsule; T4: infiltration beyond capsule) is highly recommended.[11] Patients with stage I disease (T1-T3 N0 M0) who are treated with implant removal and total capsulectomy have excellent outcomes. In contrast, patients with II-IV stage disease (T4 N0 M0; T1-T4 N1-2 M0-1) have a more aggressive clinical course and are usually treated with systemic therapy consisting of an anthracycline-based regimen and/or brentuximab-vedotin akin to systemic ALCL. Radiation therapy is occasionally used for larger tumors within (T3) or extending through the capsule (T4).

References

1. Laurent C, Haioun C, Brousset P, Gaulard P. New insights into breast implant-associated anaplastic large cell lymphoma. *Curr Opin Oncol.* 2018;30(5):292-300.
2. Collett DJ, Rakhorst H, Lennox P, Magnusson M, Cooter R, Deva AK. Current risk estimate of breast implant-associated anaplastic large cell lymphoma in textured breast implants. *Plast Reconstr Surg.* 2019;143(3S A Review of Breast Implant-Associated Anaplastic Large Cell Lymphoma):30S-40S.
3. Carbonaro R, Accardo G, Mazzocconi L, et al. BIA-ALCL in patients with genetic predisposition for breast cancer: our experience and a review of the literature. *Eur J Cancer Prev.* 2023;32(4):370-376.
4. Miranda RN, Aladily TN, Prince HM, et al. Breast implant-associated anaplastic large-cell lymphoma: long-term follow-up of 60 patients. *J Clin Oncol.* 2014;32(2):114-120.
5. Laurent C, Delas A, Gaulard P, et al. Breast implant-associated anaplastic large cell lymphoma: two distinct clinicopathological variants with different outcomes. *Ann Oncol.* 2016;27(2):306-314.
6. Oishi N, Miranda RN, Feldman AL. Genetics of breast implant-associated anaplastic large cell lymphoma (BIA-ALCL). *Aesthetic Surg J.* 2019;39(suppl_1):S14-S20.
7. Los-de Vries GT, de Boer M, van Dijk E, et al. Chromosome 20 loss is characteristic of breast implant-associated anaplastic large cell lymphoma. *Blood.* 2020;136(25):2927-2932.
8. Laurent C, Nicolae A, Laurent C, et al. Gene alterations in epigenetic modifiers and JAK-STAT signaling are frequent in breast implant-associated ALCL. *Blood.* 2020;135(5):360-370.
9. Di Napoli A, De Cecco L, Piccaluga PP, et al. Transcriptional analysis distinguishes breast implant-associated anaplastic large cell lymphoma from other peripheral T-cell lymphomas. *Mod Pathol.* 2019;32(2):216-230.
10. Oishi N, Hundal T, Phillips JL, et al. Molecular profiling reveals a hypoxia signature in breast implant-associated anaplastic large cell lymphoma. *Haematologica.* 2021;106(6):1714-1724.
11. Clemens MW, Medeiros LJ, Butler CE, et al. Complete surgical excision is essential for the management of patients with breast implant-associated anaplastic large-cell lymphoma. *J Clin Oncol.* 2016;34(2):160-168.

SECTION 13

Immunodeficiency-Associated Lymphoproliferative Disorders

Chapter 113
Posttransplant Lymphoproliferative Disorders

Thomas A. Tousseyn, Genevieve M. Crane, Thomas M. Habermann, Elaine S. Jaffe, and Rebecca L. King

IATROGENIC IMMUNODEFICIENCY-ASSOCIATED LYMPHOPROLIFERATIVE DISORDERS

The group of iatrogenic immunodeficiency-related lymphoproliferative disorders (LPDs) includes two separately designated groups: posttransplant lymphoproliferative disorders (PTLDs) and other iatrogenic immunodeficiency-related lymphoproliferative disorders (OIIA-LPDs) that occur in patients undergoing immunosuppressive drug treatments, other than in the posttransplant setting. While certain histologic characteristics are commonly observed in Epstein-Barr virus (EBV)-associated B-cell LPDs across various clinical contexts, PTLD should be maintained as a distinct subgroup primarily due to differences in clinical management.[1,2] Despite the limited research on OIIA-LPDs, it is advisable to categorize them in a similar manner to PTLD and to broaden their scope to include cancer therapy–related LPDs.

Definition

PTLDs encompass a heterogeneous spectrum of lymphoid and plasmacytic proliferations that arise in recipients of solid organ or stem cell allograft. The majority (60%-80%) of PTLDs result from reactivation of EBV in B lymphocytes, occurring within the context of immunosuppression (IS) and diminished activity of EBV-specific cytotoxic T cells. Nonetheless, the PTLD diagnosis does not necessarily depend on an association with EBV, since there are lymphoid neoplasms arising late after transplantation that are EBV negative.[3]

The underlying principle of the 2022 International Consensus Classification (ICC) approach is that, when lymphoid or plasmacytic proliferations emerge in patients post solid organ (SOT) or stem cell transplantation (SCT), the initial focus lies in determining whether it constitutes a PTLD or if alternative explanations such as a particular infection, a nonspecific inflammatory reaction, or potential organ rejection are more applicable.[1] Clearly not all lymphoid hyperplasias observed after SOT or SCT should automatically be designated PTLD, and importantly the diagnosis cannot be established solely based on the existence of occasional EBV-positive cells in the biopsy sample.

After confirming the presence of a PTLD, the subsequent priority is to recognize reactive, overt malignant, or borderline histologic patterns. The 2022 ICC recognizes the major PTLD categories: nondestructive (ND), polymorphic (Poly), and monomorphic (Mono), for which the criteria remain largely unchanged from the World Health Organization (WHO) 4R (Table 113.1). Classic Hodgkin lymphoma (CHL) PTLD is integrated in the monomorphic category, as it is a lymphoid neoplasm, and EBV+ mucocutaneous ulcer (MCU) is assigned a separate entity (Table 113.1).[4] Association with EBV is generally required for ND- and Poly-PTLDs but not for all Mono-PTLDs.

Diagnosing cases as PTLD and subsequently identifying the specific subcategories remains crucial due to the significant implications for prognosis and treatment strategies. Individuals could potentially exhibit multiple PTLD types at either a single location or at distinct locations, and these types may or may not be clonally related. Hence, it is recommended to have access to excisional biopsies of the most concerning site, such as the one exhibiting the highest metabolic rate on positron emission tomography scan. Biopsies displaying intralesional heterogeneity should be categorized within the most elevated 'high grade" classification. However, one should be very careful in making the diagnosis of Mono-PTLD and restrict only to cases that would fulfill the criteria for lymphoma if occurring in an immunocompetent host. The presence of more densely populated areas of EBV+ B cells, even if sheeting out, in an otherwise Poly-PTLD, is not sufficient for the diagnosis of Mono-PTLD, and that is

TABLE 113.1 Categories of posttransplant lymphoproliferative disorder (PTLD) and other iatrogenic immunodeficiency-associated lymphoproliferative disorders (OIIA-LPD)[a]

PTLD	OIIA-LPD
Nondestructive PTLD (5%)	**Nondestructive OIIA-LPD (10%)**
• Plasmacytic hyperplasia	• Plasmacytic hyperplasia
• Infectious mononucleosis	• Infectious mononucleosis
• Follicular hyperplasia	• Follicular hyperplasia
EBV+ MCU	**EBV+ MCU**
Polymorphic PTLD (20%)	**Polymorphic OIIA-LPD (12%)**
Monomorphic PTLD (70%)	**Monomorphic OIIA-LPD (64%)**
B-cell neoplasms (69%)	B-cell neoplasms (57%)
• EBV+ DLBCL (48%)	• EBV+ DLBCL (28%)
• DLBCL NOS (EBV–) (20%)	• DLBCL NOS (EBV-) (27%)
• Burkitt lymphoma	• Burkitt lymphoma
• Plasmablastic lymphoma	• Plasmablastic lymphoma
• Multiple myeloma	• Multiple myeloma
• Plasmacytoma	• Plasmacytoma
• MALT lymphoma, EBV+	• MALT lymphoma, EBV+
Classic Hodgkin lymphoma (5%)	Classic Hodgkin lymphoma (14%)
T-cell neoplasms (1%)	T-cell neoplasms (7%)
• PTCL NOS	• PTCL NOS
• Hepatosplenic T-cell lymphoma	• Hepatosplenic T-cell lymphoma
• Other	• Other

DLBCL, diffuse large B-cell lymphoma; EBV, Epstein-Barr virus; MALT, mucosa-associated lymphoid tissue; MCU, mucocutaneous ulcer; NOS, not otherwise specified; PTCL, peripheral T-cell lymphoma.

[a]The two main changes, in comparison with the WHO fourth revised edition, are indicated in *italic*: CHL PTLD is merged into the Monomorphic category and EBV+ MCU should be categorized separately. EBV-negative small B-cell lymphomas are still excluded. OIIA-LPDs are categorized according to the PTLD scheme. (% indicates the relative frequency).

particularly true if occurring early after transplantation. Mono-PTLD represents not merely a progression along a single path but rather constitutes a distinct lesion characterized by genetic alterations that result in an autonomous entity resistant to regression upon IS withdrawal. Over time patients can present with different PTLD subtypes, leaving the question open to whether progression is possible from Poly- to Mono-PTLD. In small-size or low-quality biopsies one might not come further than making a diagnosis of PTLD, *not further classifiable*.

Synonyms

None.

Epidemiology

Recipients of a SOT are at increased risk of an LPD because of immune suppression. The risk of PTLD post SOT is influenced by a multitude of factors including the type of organ transplanted, the duration from the time of the transplant, the age of the patient, the EBV status of the donor/recipient, and the type and intensity of IS, as well as underlying and poorly understood characteristics of the recipient's immune system.[5] In the adult population, the incidence varies per organ: kidney transplants (0.8%-2.5%), pancreas transplants (0.5%-5.0%), liver transplants (1.0%-5.5%), heart transplants (3.0%-8.0%), lung transplants (3.0%-10.0%), and multiorgan transplants (up to 20%).[5] In allogeneic hematopoietic stem cell transplantation, the risk is highest (>20%) with selective T-cell depletion, 4% to 10% in unrelated donors, 4% to 5% with umbilical cord transplants, and 1% to 3% with matched related donors. Underestimation of the risk of PTLD is a potential pitfall if patients are not followed long term.[6] While the risk of PTLD is highest in the first year following transplantation, incidence continues to increase over time, even late post transplant. In a liver SOT experience, the incidence was 2.1% at 5 years but rose to 5.4% at 19.75 years. The incidence of PTLD is higher in children because of the risk of EBV mismatch, as well as underlying differences in immune function at varying ages, peaking with an intestinal transplant risk of 20%.[5]

Large transplant registries have reported standardized incidence ratios (SIRs) representing the observed number of lymphoma cases in the population of transplant recipients divided by the expected number of cases in the population of individuals who are not transplant recipients. In SOT recipients, the SIRs are approximately 10 for non-Hodgkin lymphoma and 4 for CHL.[7]

EBV seronegativity before transplantation in SOT recipients is a significant risk factor for PTLD, which develops primarily from the recipient's lymphocytes, leading to an increase in risk by a factor of 10 to 75 (vs the risk in seropositive patients). The risk is higher among children versus adults because primary EBV infection in EBV-negative organ recipients is the primary etiology in children.[8]

Calcineurin inhibition (CNI), tacrolimus, and belatacept are associated with increased risks of developing PTLD. Mycophenolate mofetil is associated with a higher risk of developing primary central nervous system (CNS) PTLD as compared with PTLD in non-CNS sites.[9] In a nonrandomized single-institution follow-up study in 2006 of 523 cardiac transplant patients who were switched over from CNI-based IS to sirolimus-based IS after 6 months, there was a significant decrease in PTLD.[10]

General Clinical Features

Relevant history includes the age of the patient, type of transplant, timing of transplant, and past and present immunosuppressive treatment. The clinical presentation ranges from incidental asymptomatic findings to fulminant organ failure, related to the direct expansion of EBV-infected B cells and profound decrease in performance status. Infectious mononucleosis (IM) PTLD occurs at a younger age than other PTLD types and is often present in children or adult SOT recipients who are EBV seronegative. They have a tendency to regress spontaneously upon reduction of IS; however, fulminant IM can be fatal. The clinical features of Mono-PTLD are overall similar to those of lymphoma in immunocompetent patients with the exception of more extranodal disease presentations.[11,12] Extranodal PTLD has been reported to involve the gastrointestinal tract (in 20%-30% of cases), SOT graft organs (in 10%-15% of cases), and the CNS (in 5%-20% of cases) in different series.[5,9] PTLD is defined as early onset or late onset, depending on whether the time interval between diagnosis and transplantation is less or more than 12 months, respectively. Early-onset cases are characterized by more frequent EBV positivity and SOT graft organ involvement and less often have monomorphic subtype and extranodal disease.[5]

Morphology

Ideally, the diagnosis is confirmed through the assessment of an excisional biopsy specimen, enabling the evaluation of the tissue architecture and providing sufficient tissue for comprehensive ancillary studies, including EBV-encoded RNA in situ hybridization (EBER ISH), to detect the presence of EBV. The major PTLD categories remain largely unaltered from the 2017 WHO 4R, and their diagnostic criteria and clinicopathologic characteristics are summarized in Tables 113.1 and 113.2.[1,2,4] EBV+ MCU is designated a separate PTLD category, and the Hodgkin PTLDs are placed under the monomorphic umbrella. A comprehensive framework to understand the spectrum of PTLD, indicating areas of histopathologic overlap, is provided in Figure 113.1. In particular, the PTLDs characterized by a polymorphic EBV+ B-cell component including Hodgkin/Reed-Sternberg (HRS)-like cells can cause differential diagnostic challenges, and some diagnostic clues are provided in Table 113.2. Certain individuals with nondestructive PTLDs might experience synchronous or metachronous instances of destructive PTLD subtypes in other locations. Hence, when clinically suspicious, multiple biopsies might be required.

Nondestructive PTLD

Nondestructive PTLD (ND-PTLD) refers to EBV-driven B-cell lymphoid hyperplasias within an intact tissue structure (Figure 113.2). It involves lymph nodes, tonsils, and adenoids more often than extranodal sites. Three growth patterns (florid follicular hyperplasia, IM-like hyperplasia, plasmacytic hyperplasia) are recognized, mimicking reactive lymphoid hyperplasias in the immunocompetent setting, and the lesions are only diagnosable as PTLD through identification of EBV positivity. However, very low or modest numbers of EBV+ cells without mass formation and/or architectural distortion do not fulfill criteria for PTLD and in these cases a descriptive diagnosis acknowledging focal EBV reactivation is suggested. Cases with features of more than one of these three patterns are not infrequent and can be diagnosed as such.

Florid follicular hyperplasia

Follicular hyperplasia PTLD (see Figure 113.2A and B) occurs most commonly in children and is characterized by the proliferation of B lymphocytes in a pattern that resembles reactive follicular hyperplasia. Histologically, lymphoid follicles are present with well-organized germinal centers containing a central light zone and a surrounding dark zone. The follicular dendritic cell network is intact, and the germinal center B cells in some of the follicles express EBER.

Infectious mononucleosis PTLD

This subtype is usually diagnosed in biopsies of tonsils, adenoids, and lymph nodes of children or in adult SOT recipients who have not had a prior EBV infection. The specimens display changes typical of IM as seen in immunocompetent individuals, characterized by an abundant proliferation of small lymphocytes, plasma cells, and often prominent transformed cells and immunoblasts (see Figure 113.2C-F). Not infrequently cells resembling HRS cells are observed, and immunophenotyping along with careful morphologic evaluation may be necessary to distinguish such cases from CHL. Although nodal sinuses may become less visible, the core structural integrity of the lymph node or tonsil

TABLE 113.2 Clinicopathologic features of the spectrum of the most frequently encountered posttransplant lymphoproliferative disorder (PTLD) subtypes[a]

	Nondestructive					Monomorphic			
Subtype	**FH**	**IM**	**PH**	**EBV+ MCU**	**Polymorphic**	**DLBCL, EBV+**	**DLBCL, EBV-**	**EBV+ MALT**	**CHL**
Age	Young	Young	Young	Variable	Variable	Variable	Elderly	Variable	Bimodal
Nodal	Possible	Cervical LN	Nodal	No	Less frequent	Nodal	cfr IC host	Rare	Nodal
Extranodal	Waldeyer	Often Waldeyer	EN/SOT graft	Solitary ulcer in skin/GI/ tonsil	Often EN (GI, lung, CNS)	Often EN/SOT graft	cfr IC host	Skin/GI	Rare
Ann Arbor	I	I-II	I	IE	I-II	III-IV	III-IV	IE	II-III
B symptoms	No	Possible	No	No	Possible	Yes	Yes	No	Yes
Time after transplant	<1 y	<1 y	<1 y	Variable	Variable	>1 y (rare <1 y!)	>1 y	>1 y	>1 y
Architecture	Preserved	Preserved	Preserved	Effaced	Effaced	Effaced	Effaced	Effaced	Effaced
Major histopathology findings	Prominent hyper-plastic follicles, (at least some) EBER+	Small/IM/ IBs; ± sheets of large IBs, possible HRS-like	EBER+ plasma cells	Well-circumscribed ulceration, bordered by rim of T cells; small/IM/IBs, incl HRS-like; no sheets; ± eos	Often necrosis; variation small/IM/ IBs, incl HRS-like cells and plasma cells; rich immune-inflammatory background, incl T, M2	cfr EBV+ DLBCL, NOS; sheets of large IBs or THRLBCL-like; often necrosis, angiodestruction, M2++	cfr IC host	cfr EBV-MZL	cfr IC host, mainly mixed cellularity subtype: HRS cells in mixed inflammatory back-ground + eos
Immuno-phenotype	No HHV8	Variably sized EBER+ cells	Polytypic light chains; no IgG4	Variably sized EBER+ cells; CD30$^+$	Variably-sized EBER+ B cells; CD30$^+$, CD15$^-$; B-cell markers present, but CD20 can be down; plc can be monotypic	CD30$^+$, CD20 +/–, non-GCB, PDL1+	cfr IC host	EBER+ B cells and monotypic plc	CD30$^+$, CD15$^+$, prominent loss of B-cell markers, except for weak PAX5
Association with EBV	100%	100%	100%	100%	100% (wide spectrum of cells)	100%	0%	100%	50% (HRS only)
EBV latency	3 or 2	3 or 2	3 or 2	3 or 2	3 or 2	3 or 2	-	?	2, not 3
Differential diagnosis	If no EBV, consider infection or HHV8+ GLPD	Consider Poly-PTLD in EBV sero+ patient	If no EBV, consider infection, IgG4-LPD or acute rejection (if in SOT graft)	Consider Poly/ Mono-PTLD if multiple lesions, lymphadenopathy, EBV cell free DNA	Consider CHL if only HRS cells, and not smaller cells are EBER+; diagnose EBV+ MCU in well-circumscribed solitary ulcer	Consider Poly-PTLD when <1 year post-Tx; perform extra panel of B-cell markers to confirm B-cell origin when CD20 is downregulated	cfr IC host	Poly-PTLD can have monotypic plc; EBV-negative MZL is not (yet) PTLD	Consider Poly-PTLD when extranodal, retained B-cell program, mixture of small to medium-sized EBV+ cells, latency 3

(Continued)

TABLE 113.2 (Continued)

	Nondestructive					Monomorphic			
Subtype	**FH**	**IM**	**PH**	**EBV+ MCU**	**Polymorphic**	**DLBCL, EBV+**	**DLBCL, EBV-**	**EBV+ MALT**	**CHL**
PCR poly/monoclonal	P	P/M	P	P	P/M	M	M	M	M/P
Cell-free EBV DNA	No	Yes	No	No	Yes	Yes	No	?	No
Genetic aberrations	No	No	No	No	Rare (*BCL6* SHM)	9p gain	*TP53* mutation	?	cfr IC host

CHL, classic Hodgkin lymphoma; CNS, central nervous system; DLBCL, diffuse large B-cell lymphoma; EBER, EBV encoded RNA in situ hybridization; EBV, Epstein-Barr virus; EN, extranodal; eos, eosinophils; FH, follicular hyperplasia; GCB, germinal center B-cell; GI, gastrointestinal; GLPD, germinotropic lymphoproliferative disorder; HHV8, human herpes virus 8; HRS, Hodgkin and Reed-Sternberg; IB, immunoblasts; IC, immunocompetent; IM, infectious mononucleosis; IM, intermediate; LN, lymph node; M, monoclonal; M2, M2 polarized macrophages; MALT, mucosa-associated lymphoid tissue lymphoma; MCU, mucocutaneous ulcer; Mono-PTLD, monomorphic posttransplant lymphoproliferative disorder; MZL, marginal zone lymphoma; P, polyclonal; PCR, polymerase chain reaction; PH, plasma cell hyperplasia; plc, plasma cell; Poly-PTLD, polymorphic posttransplant lymphoproliferative disorder; SHM, somatic hypermutation; SOT, solid organ transplant; T, T cell; THRLBCL, T-cell/histiocyte-rich large B-cell lymphoma; Tx, transplant.)

[a]Monomorphic PTLD subtypes that do not show significant differences from the immunocompetent hosts (like Burkitt, plasmablastic lymphoma, or PTCL) were not included.

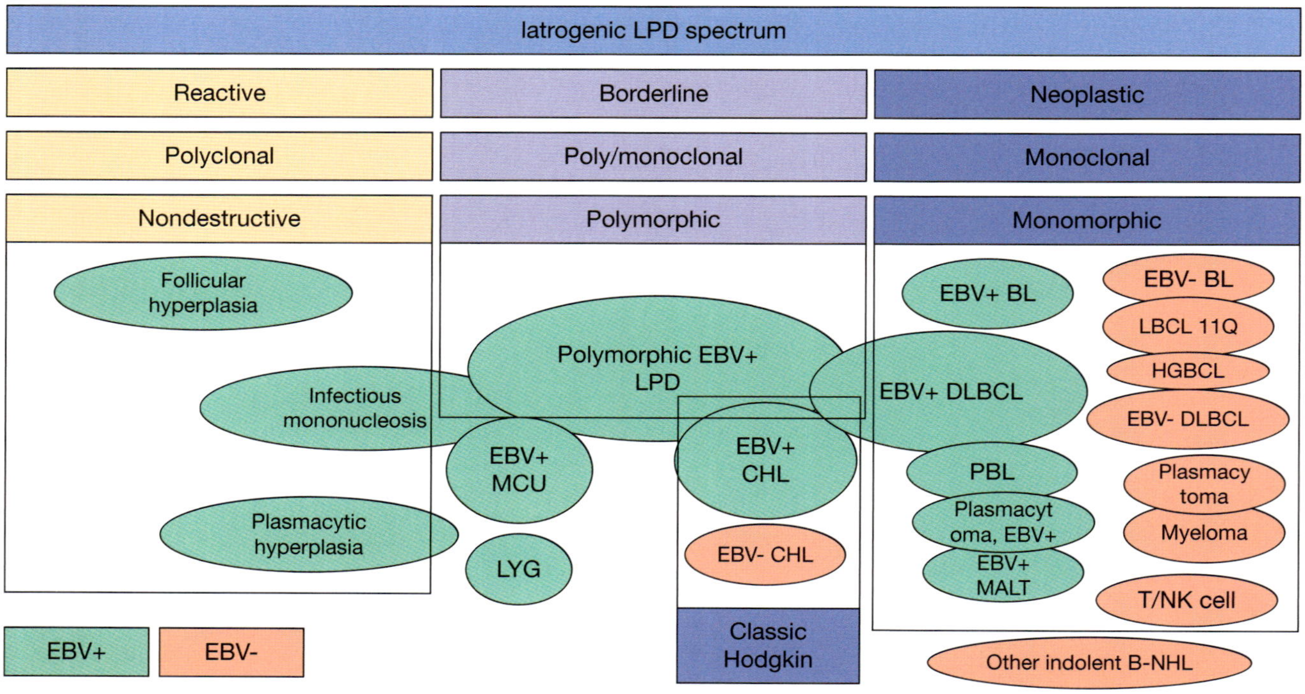

FIGURE 113.1 Framework for categorizing the heterogeneous spectrum of iatrogenic LPDs. Overlapping diagrams indicate histopathologic differential diagnostic challenges. (BL, Burkitt lymphoma; B-NHL, B-cell non-Hodgkin lymphoma; CHL, classic Hodgkin lymphoma; DLBCL, diffuse large B-cell lymphoma; EBV, Epstein-Barr virus; HGBCL, high-grade B-cell lymphoma; LBCL 11Q, large B-cell lymphoma with 11q aberration; LPD, lymphoproliferative disorder; LYG, lymphomatoid granulomatosis; MALT, mucosa-associated lymphoid tissue; MCU, mucocutaneous ulcer; PBL, plasmablastic lymphoma; T/NK, T-cell/natural killer cell. (Adapted from El-Mallawany NK, Kamdar KY. Evolving beyond morphology in pediatric PTLD. *Blood*. 2023;142(5):400-402.)

remains preserved, often evidenced by the presence of reactive germinal centers in the vicinity. In some fulminant IM-PTLD cases, the EBV+ immunoblasts may be very abundant, including foci of necrosis, and have small monoclonal or oligoclonal populations, making the differential diagnosis with Poly-PTLD or even EBV+ diffuse large B-cell lymphoma (DLBCL)-PTLD very challenging. The IM diagnosis is favored as long as the alterations are deemed acceptable within the context of immunocompetent individuals. Manifestations

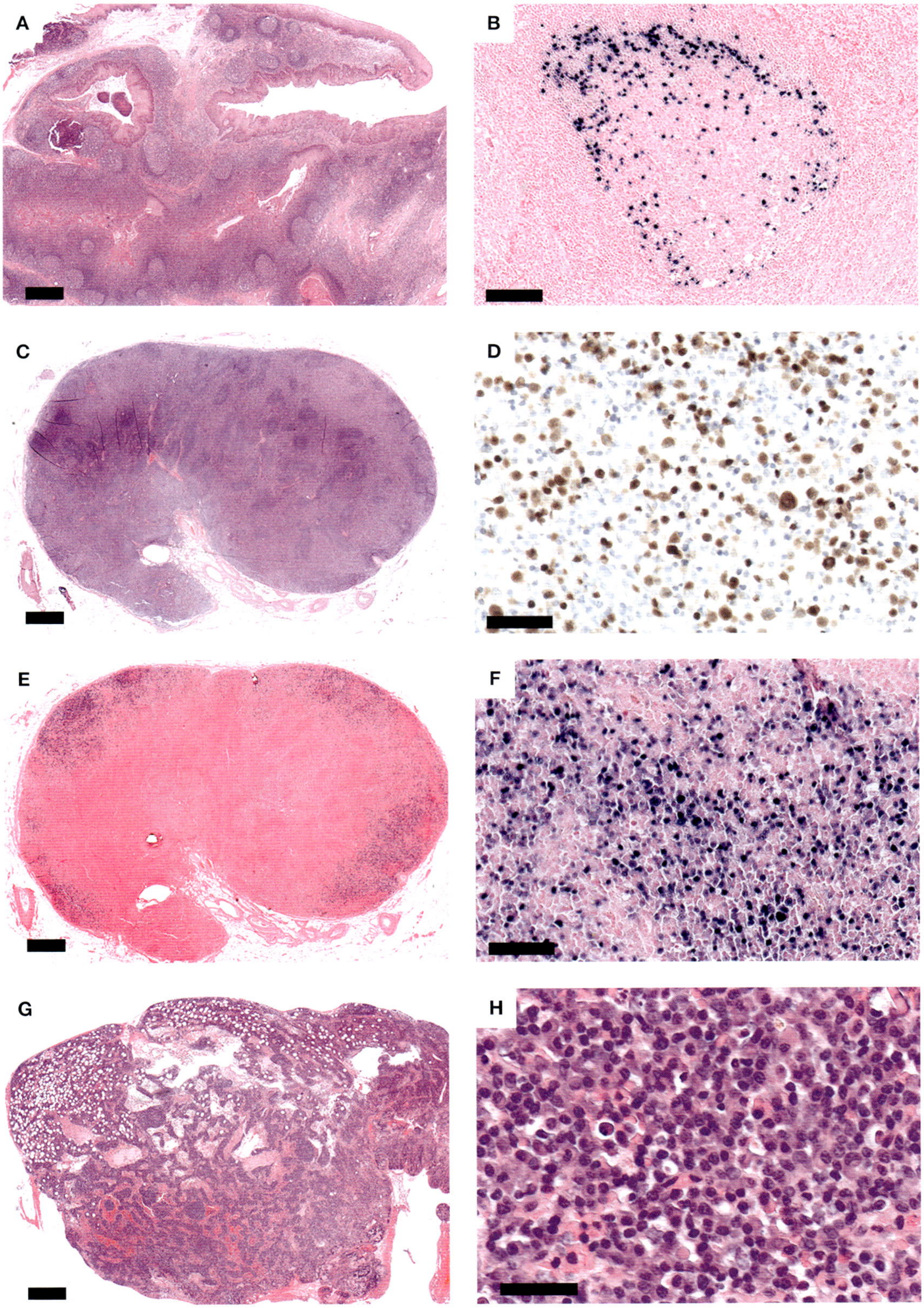

FIGURE 113.2 Histologic spectrum of nondestructive posttransplant lymphoproliferative disorders (PTLDs). **A** and **B:** Follicular hyperplasia PTLD in a tonsil in an 18-year-old man, 5 years after liver transplantation. **A:** Intact tonsillar architecture, with reactive follicles. **B:** Some of the follicles contain EBER+ germinal center B cells. **C-F:** Fulminant infectious mononucleosis PTLD in cervical lymph node of a 10-year-old renal allograft recipient. **C:** The overall nodal architecture is preserved, but there is paracortical expansion by a mixture of variably sized B cells, expressing PAX5 **(D)** and EBER **(E and F)**. **G-H:** Plasmacytic hyperplasia PTLD. **G.** The normal lymph node architecture is preserved. **H.** Numerous plasma cells are present.

of acute IM causing ulcerative tonsillar lesions should be distinguished from EBV+ MCU, based on clinical information (age and degree of illness in particular) and serological or monospot tests.

Plasmacytic hyperplasia

Histologically, there is an increase in the number of interfollicular, mature-appearing plasma cells in the affected tissue (see Figure 113.2G-H). These plasma cells may form aggregates or sheets but should express EBER and polytypic light chains and typically lack clonal immunoglobulin rearrangements on polymerase chain reaction (PCR).

Polymorphic PTLD

Poly-PTLD is a challenging variant in which there is obliteration of underlying tissue architecture by a heterogeneous infiltrate of lymphoid cells, plasma cells, and immunoblasts of varying sizes and cytologies, some closely resembling HRS cells (Figure 113.3). Differential diagnosis with CHL-PTLD is imperative, and differential diagnostic criteria are discussed herein. The EBV-infected B cells are interspersed with a notable presence of reactive histiocytes and T cells, but with a significant reduction in the functional natural killer (NK) and EBV-specific $CD8^+$ T-cell subsets responsible for controlling EBV infection.[13] The distinction between ND-PTLD and Poly-PTLD is based on whether the structural integrity of the affected tissue is maintained or not, although distinction between a fulminant IM-like PTLD and Poly-PTLD is not always possible on a biopsy specimen only.

In larger biopsy samples of a Poly-PTLD case, one might notice focal areas with a significant number of cytologically atypical EBV+ cells, even forming small sheets. Although stringent criteria are lacking, such lesions should not be considered as Mono-PTLD, even when necrosis and angioinvasion are present.

Poly-PTLDs have a chance to regress on withdrawal of IS. This is in contrast to Mono-PTLDs, which are lymphoid neoplasms driven by genetic changes and considered conceptually as different lesions. In challenging cases, the clinical presentation and anatomical site become crucial factors and effective communication with a hemato-oncologist is imperative. Emphasis should be placed on the time post transplant, as Mono-PTLD rarely occurs within a year of SOT. Molecular testing can be applied but should be used with extreme caution. While a polyclonal infiltrate supports the diagnosis of Poly-PTLD over

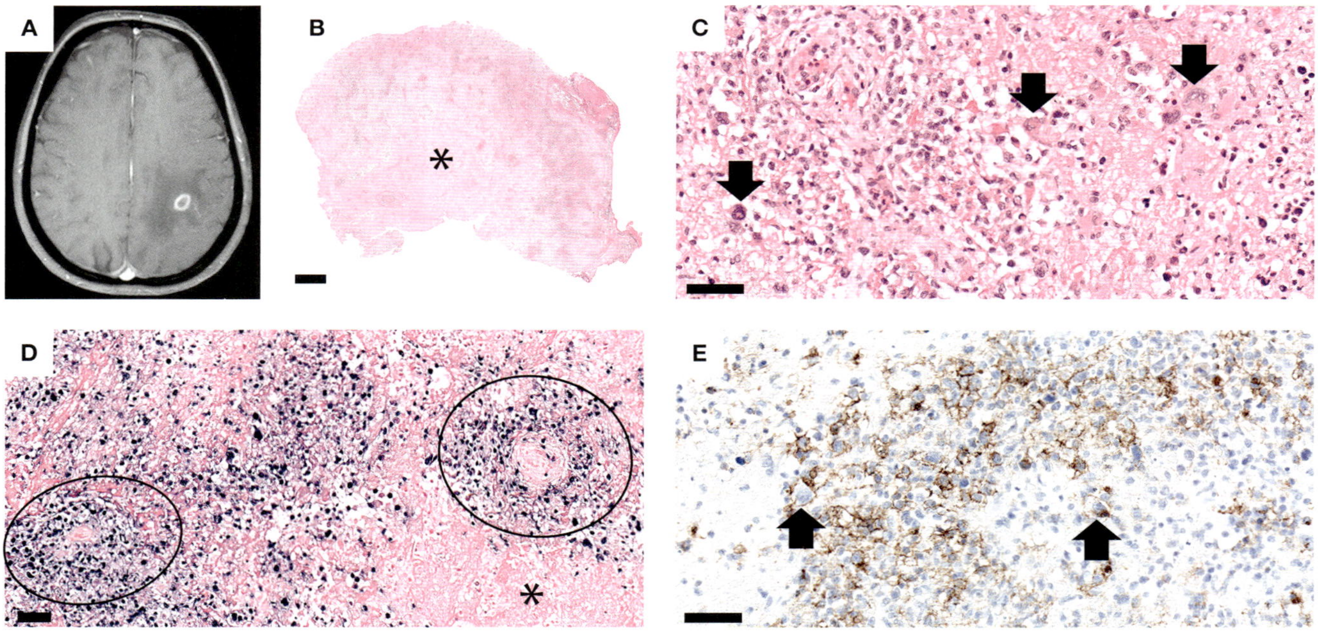

FIGURE 113.3 Polymorphic posttransplant lymphoproliferative disorder. A 64-year-old man develops a right-sided paralysis 10 months after cardiac transplant. The lesion regressed after reduction of immunosuppression and radiotherapy. **A:** Magnetic resonance imaging shows a subcortical ring-like contrast-enhancing tumor in the left frontoparietal lobe with perilesional edema. **B:** Brain biopsy shows areas of geographic type necrosis (*). **C:** The brain parenchyma is infiltrated with a polymorphic infiltrate including cells, resembling Hodgkin and Reed-Sternberg (HRS) cells (arrows). **D:** EBER in situ hybridization indicates a spectrum of variably sized cells, including small to medium-sized and HRS-like cells, with an angiotropic predilection (circled) necrosis (*). **E:** CD20 is often only partially expressed in the HRS-like cells (arrows).

Mono-PTLD, both conditions may exhibit a monoclonal population.

Extranodal disease with involvement of the lung, CNS, and skin is frequent in Poly-PTLD but also in lymphomatoid granulomatosis (LYG). While both conditions exhibit a polymorphic infiltrate and frequent necrosis, the proportion of EBV+ cells is notably lower in LYG, particularly within low-grade lesions. Since the organ damage in LYG may be linked not solely to the EBV-infected B cells but also to the host's immune response to EBV, look for the characteristic angiotropic T-cell infiltrate and vasculitis in LYG.

EBV+ mucocutaneous ulcer PTLD

When presented with a solitary, sharply demarcated mucosal or skin ulceration containing a polymorphic EBV+ infiltrate, the diagnosis of EBV+ MCU should be considered, particularly in the absence of other clinical symptoms and lymphadenopathy. A deep biopsy is essential in order to be able to evaluate the base of the lesion; EBV+ MCU is sharply defined by a rim of abundant reactive T cells. The absence of an elevation in EBV DNA in peripheral blood serves as a valuable criterion for distinguishing EBV+ MCU from poly- and monomorphic EBV+ DLBCL.[14]

Monomorphic PTLD

Mono-PTLD represents the most frequently observed subtype of PTLD, in which the tissue displays a malignant clonal proliferation of B, T, or NK cells, which meets diagnostic criteria for, and is indistinguishable from, lymphoid neoplasms originating in immunocompetent individuals. Further classification of Mono-PTLDs is required, based on their closest resembling lymphoma type in immunocompetent patients.

DLBCL is the most prevalent subtype, among the Mono-PTLD category, constituting 50% to 75% of cases. They include diverse cellular arrangements. At one end of the spectrum there may be uniform sheet-like proliferations of atypical B cells, similar to DLBCL not otherwise specified (NOS), or Burkitt-lymphoma in immunocompetent hosts. At the other end there are cases with sparse infiltration of large atypical cells, along with a variety of background inflammatory cells such as T cells and histiocytes, often resembling T-cell/histiocyte-rich large B-cell lymphoma in the immunocompetent host. Among the latter cases, the atypical cells can sometimes display a morphology reminiscent of HRS cells, creating differential diagnostic difficulties with Poly-PTLD or CHL-PTLD.

EBV+ DLBCL-PTLD will show morphological and immunophenotypic similarities to EBV+ DLBCL NOS and many exhibit angiodestruction and widespread coagulative geographic necrosis (Figure 113.4). As discussed earlier, cases with a background rich in immune cells can cause differential diagnostic issues with Poly-PTLD. EBV-negative DLBCL-PTLD will resemble DLBCL NOS in the immunocompetent host both morphologically and immunophenotypically[15-17] (Figure 113.5).

Identifying Burkitt lymphoma (BL)-PTLD holds significance due to the likelihood of necessitating immediate and aggressive therapeutic interventions in these patients.[18] Cases of what is currently termed large B-cell lymphoma with 11q aberration (previously referred to as Burkitt-like lymphoma) have been distinctly identified within the posttransplant context in the adult but not the pediatric population.[19,20]

While traditionally excluding cases resembling small B-cell lymphomas, the 2017 WHO revision incorporated EBV+ mucosa-associated lymphoid tissue (MALT) lymphomas as a PTLD subtype.[4] A recent study suggests adding EBV-negative marginal zone lymphomas, typically MALT type and frequently gastrointestinal, as a form of Mono-PTLD,[21] but this requires further confirmation.

Other lymphomas with plasmacytoid features, encountered in the posttransplant population, include plasmablastic lymphoma (PBL), plasmacytoma (Figure 113.6), and myeloma. It becomes crucial to differentiate more aggressive multiple myeloma-like cases from plasmacytoma-like cases, which might respond well even without aggressive treatment.

T- and NK cell PTLDs are infrequently observed, with only a small proportion of cases being associated with EBV.[22]

While infrequent in the posttransplant context (<5% of cases), certain PTLD cases show a CHL morphology and are in most cases EBV positive (Figure 113.7). The presence of HRS-like cells in many PTLDs of B-cell origin often complicates differentiation from EBV+ CHL. Nevertheless, identifying this particular CHL-PTLD type is important, as it requires prompt treatment with standard CHL therapy and demonstrates the most favorable prognosis among the destructive forms of PTLD.[12]

The descriptive terminology "Hodgkin-like" PTLD should not be used in the context of PTLD, and the diagnosis of CHL-PTLD should be made with caution, adhering to even stricter immunophenotypic criteria than in the immunocompetent host. Several helpful features can be used to distinguish Poly-PTLD from CHL-PTLD. First, in CHL the presence of typical HRS cells is a crucial diagnostic feature; HRS-like cells have

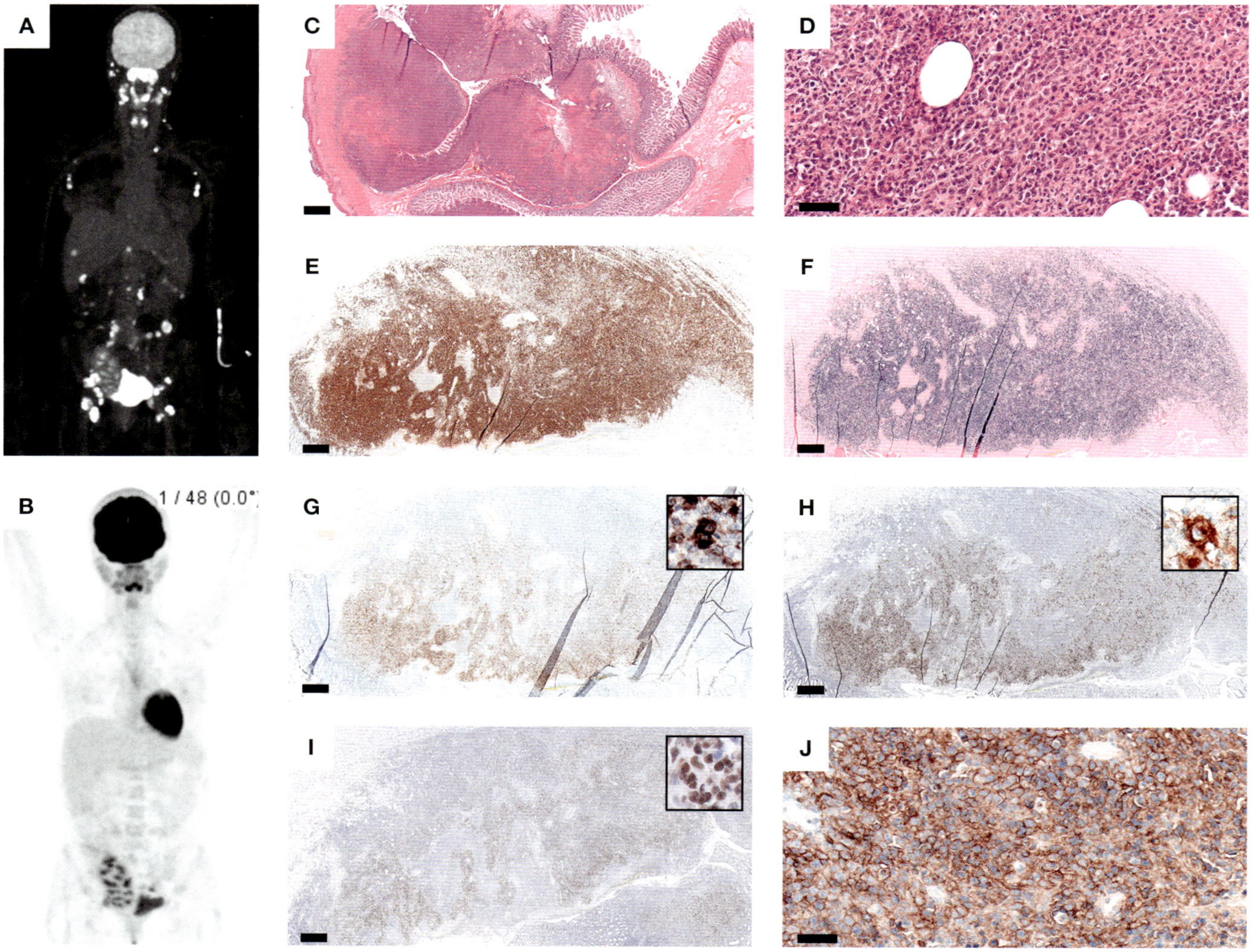

FIGURE 113.4 Monomorphic posttransplant lymphoproliferative disorder, EBV+ in a 42-year-old woman 12 years after kidney transplantation. **A:** Positron emission tomography (PET) scan at time of diagnosis showed bilateral tonsillar swelling, multiple infra- and subdiaphragmatic lymphadenopathies, as well as extranodal involvement. **B:** PET scan showed complete remission after reduction of immunosuppression and 8 cycles of anti-CD20 immunotherapy, with reduction of EBV titers in peripheral blood to an undetectable level. The patient is still in complete remission after 8 years. **C:** A diffuse transmural lymphoid infiltrate is present in the small bowel wall, including small foci of necrosis. **D:** The infiltrate consists of diffuse sheets of large atypical cells, some with Hodgkin/Reed-Sternberg (HRS)-like morphology, diffusely expressing CD20 **(E)**. **F:** EBER in situ hybridization is positive in >80% of the atypical B cells, while the expression of LMP1 **(G)** is only partial and largely corresponds to the CD30 **(H)** HRS-like cells (see insets). **I:** EBNA2, evidencing an EBV viral latency type III, is more diffusely expressed. **J:** Both neoplastic B cells, as well as tumor-associated macrophages in the background, diffusely express PD-L1, a manner to hijack the host immune response and a potential target for immune checkpoint inhibition.

a more variable presence in Poly-PTLD. Second, in CHL the EBV infection is confined to HRS cells, while in Poly-PTLD, EBV infection can affect various cell types, ranging from small lymphocytes to large B cells. Third, in CHL-PTLD, strict immunophenotypic criteria must be applied and HRS cells should be negative or only weakly/partially positive (but clearly less than 50% of HRS cells) for B-cell markers CD20, CD79A, and OCT2, while the majority of HRS cells will express CD15 and weak PAX5. The utilization of comprehensive B-cell antibody panels might be necessary in such scenarios.[23] Fourth, EBV+ CHL-type PTLD will express an EBV viral latency pattern II and thus the presence of EBNA2-expressing cells excludes the diagnosis of CHL. Lastly, correlation with the clinical manifestation is important as most CHL cases will present with mediastinal or cervical lymphadenopathy and will generally not be primarily in an extranodal location.

Immunophenotype

The immunophenotype of IM-like ND-PTLD and Poly-PTLD (see Figure 113.3) is subject to variabilities in the cytologic composition of the infiltrates, often

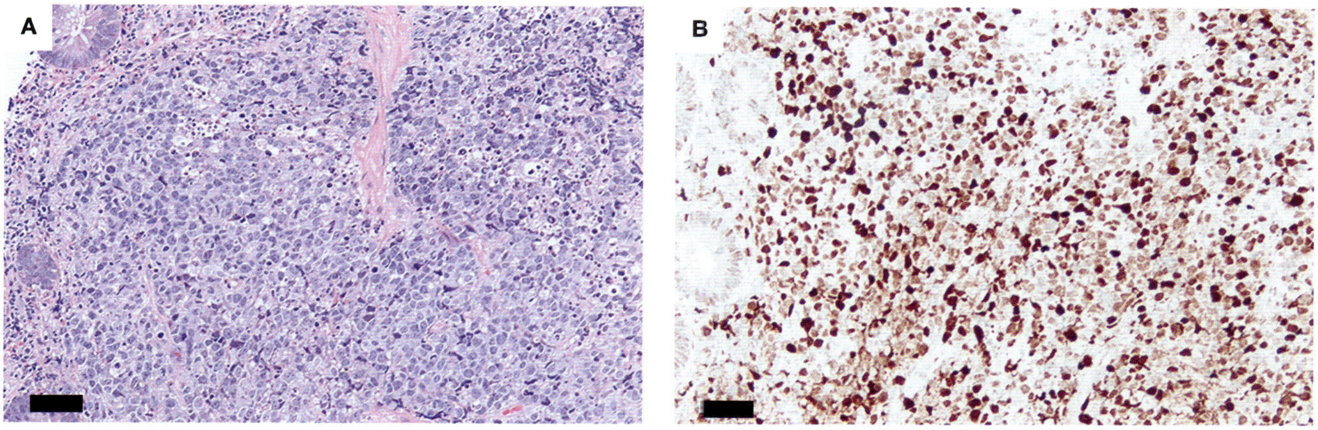

FIGURE 113.5 Monomorphic posttransplant lymphoproliferative disorder, diffuse large B-cell lymphoma (DLBCL) not otherwise specified. A 72-year-old man with a history of hepatitis C and hepatocellular carcinoma developed abdominal pain, nausea, and vomiting 3 years following an orthotopic liver transplant with evidence of ileal thickening. **A:** Biopsy of the ileal mass demonstrated large atypical lymphoid cells effacing tissue architecture. Immunophenotype was consistent with PT-DLBCL, germinal center type, and the neoplastic cells expressed increased p53 **(B)**. Molecular studies demonstrated a pathogenic *TP53* mutation.

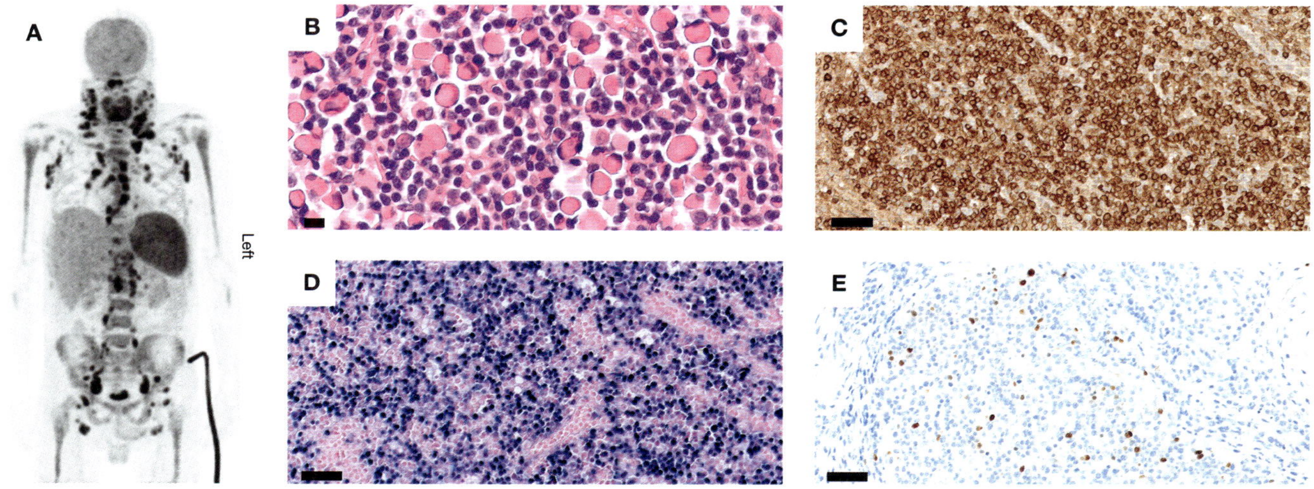

FIGURE 113.6 EBV+ plasmacytoma posttransplant lymphoproliferative disorder in a 58-year-old man 13 months after allogeneic stem cell transplantation for acute myeloid leukemia. **A:** Positron emission tomography scan showed generalized lymphadenopathies, including spleen and liver involvement. **B:** Lymph nodes were infiltrated by a diffuse plasmacytoid infiltrate containing multiple Russel bodies and expressing CD138 but no CD20. **C.** They were kappa light-chain restricted, and expressed EBER **(D)**. In addition to an EBV viral latency type III, many cells also expressed ZEBRA/BZLF1 **(E)**, corresponding to lytic replication.

leading to diagnostic challenge. Typically, there is at least partial positivity for CD45 on B cells and expression of the pan B-cell markers CD20, CD79a, PAX5, OCT2, and BOB1, in at least a subset of small and intermediate-sized B cells. Larger EBV-infected cells within the infiltrate frequently show partial downregulation of CD20. CD138 and MUM1 expression is seen on variable numbers of plasma cells and plasmacytoid immunoblastic cells. Aberrant T-cell marker expression has been observed, and therefore, multiple B-cell markers are required to indicate the cell of origin, particularly in cases lacking CD20 expression. CD30 is typically upregulated by EBV and HRS-like cells occasionally show CD15 positivity, complicating the differential diagnosis with CHL. Plasma cells in Poly-PTLD and ND-PTLD may be monotypic by kappa and lambda stains or flow cytometry but can be light chain negative. In some cases, oligoclonal populations or even monoclonal populations can be detected by PCR and do not preclude the diagnosis of Poly-PTLD or ND-PTLD. Ki-67 is variable and can be very high, even in ND-PTLD, and should not be used to classify PTLD.

Mono-PTLD should fulfill the immunophenotypic requirements set forth under the specific non-PTLD categories. The majority of EBV+ DLBCL-PTLDs (see Figure 113.4) are of non–germinal center B-cell origin,

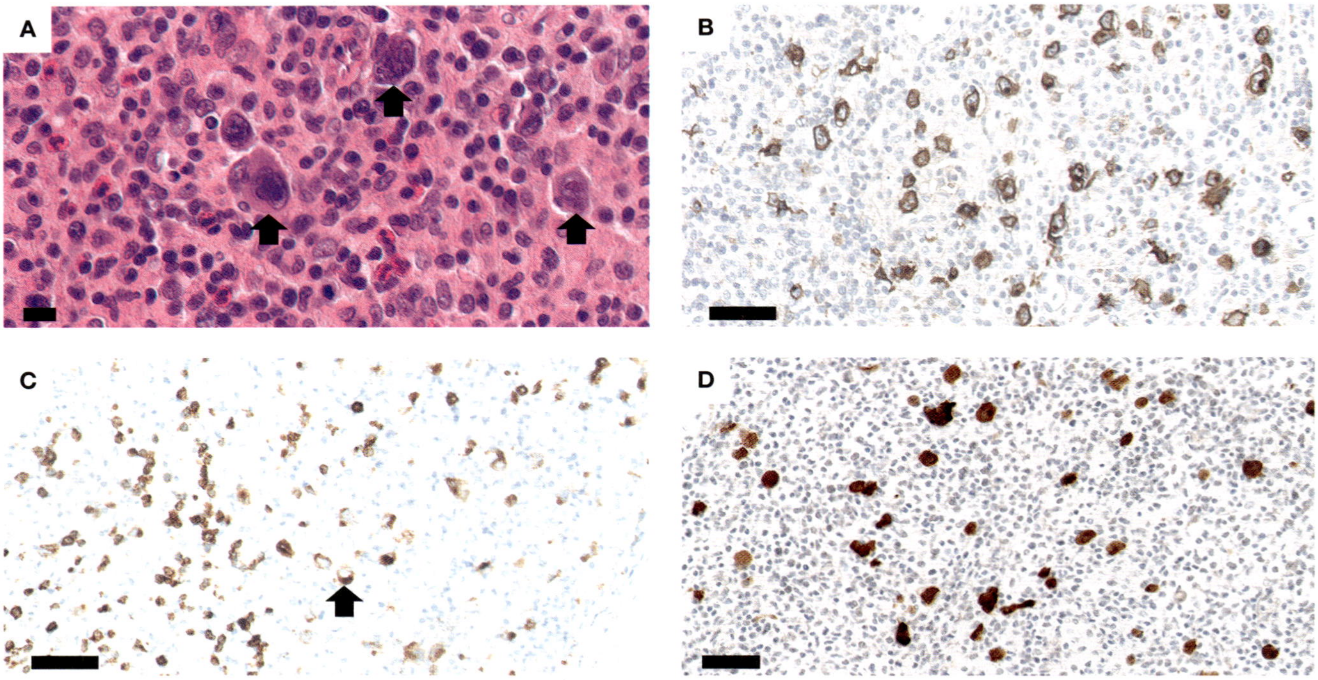

FIGURE 113.7 Classic Hodgkin posttransplant lymphoproliferative disorder, mixed cellularity subtype, developing in a mediastinal lymph node of a 35-year-old man, 3 years after a kidney transplantation. **A:** Arrows indicate the presence of Hodgkin/Reed-Sternberg cells in a mixed inflammatory background with eosinophils, plasma cells, and histiocytes. They express CD30 **(B)** and CD15 (see arrow) **(C)**, weak PAX5 and an EBV viral latency type II, illustrated by the presence of LMP1 **(D)** and the absence of EBNA2. Note that LMP1 expression is restricted to the HRS cells and it is not expressed by small or intermediate-sized lymphoid cells.

marked by MUM1 expression, absence of CD10, and variable BCL6 expression. Conversely, approximately 40% to 45% of EBV-negative DLBCL-PTLDs (see Figure 113.5) exhibit the germinal center B-cell phenotype. CD45 expression is variable, and some loss of pan B-cell antigen expression is common in EBV+ DLBCL-PTLD, as in EBV+ DLBCL NOS.

It is crucial to assess for EBV in every biopsy specimen of an SOT or SCT recipient, and EBER in situ hybridization is the gold standard. For the diagnosis of EBV+ DLBCL-PTLD, as per the definition, over 80% of viable malignant cells should demonstrate EBER expression. As this is an RNA-based assay the necrotic areas will typically not stain and should not be taken into account. Expression of EBV viral proteins LMP1 and EBNA2 is variable in PTLD and is suggestive of EBV latency II or III, the latter being more common among the most severely immunocompromised and pediatric PTLD cases. LMP1 expression is usually not detectable in all EBER+ neoplastic cells in posttransplant DLBCL but is often restricted to the larger $CD30^+$ HRS-like cells only (see Figure 113.4). EBNA2 on the other hand, if detectable, tends to be present in a wider variety of EBV-infected cells and defines a latency type III. The correlation between EBV latency pattern III and lytic replication (as evidenced by ZEBRA/BZLF1 expression) has been linked to notably reduced survival rates and early onset of aggressive PTLD, particularly after allogeneic SCT.[20,24] Integration of this aspect into the diagnostic reports should be taken into consideration.

Notwithstanding the immunosuppressive treatment administered to patients diagnosed with PTLD, these disorders often manifest within an immune cell–abundant, inflammatory tumor microenvironment. However, this environment is characterized by significantly reduced subsets of NK cells and $CD8^+$ T cells, responsible for controlling EBV infection.[25,26]

The PD-1/PD-L1 signaling pathway is dysregulated in EBV+ PTLDs, characterized by frequent PD-L1 expression in both tumor-associated macrophages and EBV+ neoplastic B cells, in the absence of PD-1 T-cells. PD-L1 expression is linked to the presence of EBV latency types II or III and PD-L1 copy number alterations (CNAs), likely indicating the presence of a proinflammatory tumor microenvironment.[27,28]

The BL-PTLDs have a similar immunophenotype as BL in immunocompetent hosts, including expression of germinal center B-cell markers CD10/BCL6, a 100% Ki-67 proliferative index, and MYC oncoprotein overexpression, related to a *MYC*-rearrangement, in the absence of BCL2 expression. The EBV+ PT-BL cases all show latency I/0, lacking expression of LMP1 and EBNA2.

PBL PTLD shares morphologic and immunophenotypic features of PBL in other states of immune dysregulation, like in the context of AIDS-related PBL, being EBER+ (with a latency I/0 pattern) and often characterized by a *MYC* rearrangement. Plasmacytoma-PTLD (see Figure 113.6) shows architectural effacement by uniform sheets of mature plasma cells that are monotypic and monoclonal. Differentiating EBV+ plasmacytoma cases from PBL can be very difficult if there is partial plasmablastic cytology. Starry sky pattern, coagulative tumor necrosis, high Ki-67 proliferation index, and absence of light chain expression favor PBL over plasmacytoma.[29] Clinical correlation is necessary to assess for features of multiple myeloma, regardless of the EBV status of the plasma cell infiltrate. Note that Poly-PTLD can contain sheets of monotypic plasma cells; however, they are mostly EBER negative, which complicates the differentiation from plasmacytoma or marginal zone lymphoma.

T-cell PTLDs of T/NK-cell origin share the immunohistochemical profiles with the corresponding lymphoma types in immunocompetent hosts and generally have a lower likelihood of being EBV positive than B-cell PTLDs.[22]

Genetics

When immune function is compromised due to iatrogenic IS after SOT or SCT, B cells that are latently infected with EBV can evade immune detection, allowing them to proliferate without restraint, facilitated by the growth impact of viral proteins they express. This uncontrolled growth can lead to different subtypes of PTLD. The underlying causes of EBV-negative PTLD are not yet fully understood, but potential mechanisms implicate viruses like human herpes virus 8 or cytomegalovirus in some cases. Other theories propose a "hit and run" infection scenario where incomplete integration of EBV into the host genome triggers disruptions in chromosomal structures at the site of integration, leading to the loss of EBV viral DNA. A more plausible explanation is that EBV-negative PTLDs are coincidentally arising in patients with a dysfunctional immune system but sharing in origin the same pathogenetic features as their respective EBV-negative counterparts in immunocompetent hosts.

Although the majority of nondestructive PTLD cases tend to be nonclonal, sporadic cases might display clonal populations with cytogenetic and mutational irregularities.[30] In the majority of polymorphic and monomorphic B-cell PTLDs, detectable clonal immunoglobulin rearrangements are observed. Poly-PTLDs might also show mutations, albeit not as frequently as observed in Mono-PTLDs.[31] Furthermore, due to a restricted T-cell repertoire, related to the IS drugs, approximately 50% of B-cell PTLDs exhibit oligoclonal TCR rearrangements, with monoclonal rearrangements being a rare occurrence. Most EBV+ DLBCL-PTLDs show somatic hypermutations (SHMs), although an aggressive subgroup, appearing very shortly after SCT, lacks SHM.[24]

Certain studies highlight notable differences in gene expression and mutational profiles between PTLD and lymphomas in immune-competent individuals, while others underscore the resemblances between EBV-negative PTLDs and EBV-negative DLBCL NOS.[17,31,32] CNA analysis and gene expression profiling revealed that EBV-negative PT-DLBCLs and DLBCL in immunocompetent individuals exhibit resemblances in terms of genomic and transcriptomic characteristics.[17] The separate genomic profiles between EBV+ and EBV-negative PT-DLBCLs particularly concern genes associated with inflammation and immune responses. The prevailing CNA observed in EBV+ PT-DLBCL is amplification of chromosome 9p24.1, linked to increased expression of PD-L1 and PD-L2 through the JAK2 pathway. The notable increase in the expression of these genes implies that EBV might play a role in promoting immune tolerance to viral infections of B cells by disrupting HLA regulation and impeding the infiltration of CD8 T lymphocytes. PD-L1, primarily expressed by antigen-presenting cells, initiates an inhibitory signaling cascade by binding to its receptor PD-1 on T cells, enabling evasion from T cell–mediated elimination. High PD-L1 expression serves as a mechanism to escape immune surveillance.[28] EBV+ PT-DLBCL cases exhibit elevated levels of PD-L1 expression in comparison with EBV-negative PT-DLBCL cases, and its expression is related to poor prognosis in the EBV+ group.[26] Consequently, targeting the PD-L1/PD-1 axis has emerged as a potential approach in EBV+ PTLD immunotherapy.[27,28]

EBV+ DLBCL-PTLD harbors fewer genomic aberrations and exhibits a lower frequency of driver mutations than EBV-negative DLBCL-PTLD or DLBCL in immunocompetent patients.[15,31] This observation reinforces the notion that the latent EBV genes and proteins possess an additional oncogenic potential, contributing to the lymphomagenesis. LMP1 is a constitutively active functional homologue for the human CD40 protein and essential to the transforming capability of EBV, while EBNA2 employs the Notch pathway for the immortalization of B cells.

Studies on the genomic landscape of PTLD are mainly focused on PT-DLBCL, and the observed genomic aberrations include gains of *MYC*, *BCL2*, and *BCL6* and loss of *TP53*. Next-generation sequencing studies identified worse outcomes for DLBCL-PTLD in association with somatic mutations in cell cycle and Notch molecular pathways. Adult EBV-negative DLBCL-PTLDs frequently contain *TP53* mutations,[15] and the mutational landscape of PT-DLBCL differs in the pediatric DLBCL-PTLDs, with a lack of mutations in *KMT2D* and *PIK3CD* and a lower frequency of *TP53* mutations. These findings suggest that early pediatric DLBCL-PTLD cases are marked by low genetic complexity and few CNAs and often achieve complete remission (CR) with reduction of immunosuppression (RIS) and rituximab alone.[20] Consequently, it is advisable to use caution in diagnosis of Mono-PTLD within the first year post transplantation.

The 11q gain/loss aberration is notably more common in adult PTLD than in immunocompetent patients, suggesting that IS may favor its formation. This was not observed in a pediatric cohort, neither were *IRF4* rearrangements.[19,20]

PTLDs of NK/T-cell origin are rare and different from B-cell PTLDs. The molecular and genomic changes identified in T/NK-PTLDs resemble those documented in T/NK-cell lymphomas found in immunocompetent individuals.[22]

Prognosis and Clinical Comment

There is no general consensus on prevention and treatment of PTLD.[3,5,33-37] However, the introduction of anti-CD20 immunotherapy (rituximab), treatment with lymphoma regimens specific to the histology, and improvements in supportive care have together led to improved outcomes in PTLD over time.[3,34,35]

Initial management of this heterogenous group of disorders, in patients who also have significant comorbidities, differs from standard approaches employed in immune-competent patients with lymphoma.[5,36,38] Approaches include RIS, single-agent anti-CD20 immunotherapy (rituximab monotherapy), chemotherapy, and/or immunochemotherapy regimens. Patients who are event free at 24 months, defined as no progression, relapse, retreatment, or death to any cause, do not have a similar outcome compared with normal age- and sex-matched population secondary to comorbidities, which is different from DLBCL in nonimmunocompromised patients.[12]

RIS is the initial step in the management of PTLD, regardless of histology, retaining the balance between partially restoring EBV-specific cellular immunity and preventing graft rejection.[5] RIS leads to regression in 20% to 80% of Poly- and EBV+ Mono-PTLDs, but EBV-negative DLBCL-PTLD is less responsive.[11] RIS is effective in 33% to 75% of plasmacytic PTLD.[5]

In contrast to DLBCL in nonimmunocompromised individuals, single-agent anti-CD20 monoclonal antibody therapy is the standard of treatment in patients with ND-PTLD, Poly-PTLD, or Mono-PTLD who fail or cannot undergo RIS. In retrospective analyses, the response rates were 44% to 79% with CR rates of 20% to 50%.[5] In a report with a median follow-up of 13 years in patients who achieved CR, the disease-specific survival was 94% at 5 years and 88% at 10 years.[39] In a prospective multicenter risk-stratified trial, the PTLD-1 trial, the CR rate in patients in the low-risk group was 25% (37/148) after 4 weekly doses of rituximab induction and these patients were treated with an additional 4 courses of rituximab every 21 days.[35] A CR predicted an improved overall survival (OS). All other patients, defined as the high-risk group not in CR, were treated with four cycles of R-CHOP (rituximab, cyclophosphamide, doxorubicin, vincristine, and prednisone). The CR rate was 70%. The median OS was 6.6 years. It remains unclear whether patients with Poly-PTLD experience superior prognosis compared with those with Mono-PTLD.[11,12]

The management of patients who relapse after immunochemotherapy is complicated. Autologous stem cell rescue in 21 patients resulted in a 3-year OS of 61% in a report from the Lymphoma Working Party of the European Bone Marrow Transplant Registry.[40] CD19 chimeric antigen receptor T-cell (CAR-T) treatment was reported in a retrospective analysis of 22 patients with DLBCL-PTLD with a CR rate of 55% and treatment-related mortality of 10%. Sixty-four percent of patients stopped IS prior to CAR-T, and three renal transplant patients had a loss of the allograft. The 2-year progression-free survival was 35%.[41] Because of the risk of allograft rejection, more data are needed. Adoptive immunotherapy strategies have been ongoing. Targeted cytotoxic lymphocytes against EBV exhibit promise for managing relapsed/refractory EBV+ PTLD; nevertheless, specialized clinical trials are imperative to ascertain the safe implementation of autologous CAR-T therapy in patients with PTLD.

Peripheral T-cell lymphoma NOS, BL, and CHL should be managed with standard recommended treatment regimens after RIS. In a cohort study of 192 patients with PT-CHL in the Scientific Registry of Transplant Recipients, 145 were treated with chemotherapy, which was associated with an improved disease-specific survival and OS.[42] After RIS, CNS-PTLD is managed with standard CNS-directed therapies.

Over the last two decades, the event-free survival rate for pediatric PTLD has consistently stood at 70% when treated with gentler approaches such as rituximab or low-dose chemoimmunotherapy-based methods.[43] Particularly in children who are EBV immune naïve, restoration of the immune response and EBV-directed therapeutic strategies proved to be curative, but accurately identifying patients necessitating intensive therapy has proven more challenging.[44]

Future research must be directed toward the development of a risk-stratification system, integrating traditional morphology with molecular data, to accurately identify a high-risk subset for whom intensive multiagent chemoimmunotherapy is warranted to improve chances of a cure. Simultaneously, it should effectively identify patients who can benefit from gentler rituximab-based or EBV-directed treatments, sparing them from the harsh side effects of intensive chemotherapy.[44]

References

1. Campo E, Jaffe ES, Cook JR, et al. The International consensus classification of mature lymphoid neoplasms: a report from the clinical advisory Committee. *Blood*. 2022;140(11):1229-1253.
2. Quintanilla-Martinez L, Swerdlow SH, Tousseyn T, Barrionuevo C, Nakamura S, Jaffe ES. New concepts in EBV-associated B, T, and NK cell lymphoproliferative disorders. *Virchows Arch*. 2023;482(1):227-244.
3. Allen UD, Preiksaitis JK; AST Infectious Diseases Community of Practice. Post-transplant lymphoproliferative disorders, Epstein-Barr virus infection, and disease in solid organ transplantation: guidelines from the American Society of transplantation infectious diseases community of practice. *Clin Transplant*. 2019;33(9):e13652.
4. WHO Classification of Tumours Editorial Board; Campo E, Harris NL, et al. WHO Classification of Tumours of Haematopoietic and Lymphoid Tissues (Medicine). World Health Organization; 2017. Revised.
5. Dierickx D, Habermann TM. Post-transplantation lymphoproliferative disorders in adults. *N Engl J Med*. 2018;378(6):549-562.
6. Maksten EF, Vase MØ, Kampmann J, et al. Post-transplant lymphoproliferative disorder following kidney transplantation: a population-based cohort study. *Transpl Int*. 2016;29(4):483-493.
7. de Fijter JW. Cancer and mTOR inhibitors in transplant recipients. *Transplantation*. 2017;101(1):45-55.
8. Francis A, Johnson DW, Teixeira-Pinto A, Craig JC, Wong G. Incidence and predictors of post-transplant lymphoproliferative disease after kidney transplantation during adulthood and childhood: a registry study. *Nephrol Dial Transplant*. 2018;33(5):881-889.
9. Crane GM, Powell H, Kostadinov R, et al. Primary CNS lymphoproliferative disease, mycophenolate and calcineurin inhibitor usage. *Oncotarget*. 2015;6(32):33849-33866.
10. Asleh R, Clavell AL, Pereira NL, et al. Incidence of malignancies in patients treated with sirolimus following heart transplantation. *J Am Coll Cardiol*. 2019;73(21):2676-2688.
11. Vergote VKJ, Deroose CM, Fieuws S, et al. Characteristics and outcome of post-transplant lymphoproliferative disorders after solid organ transplantation: a single center experience of 196 patients over 30 years. *Transpl Int*. 2022;35:10707.
12. King RL, Khurana A, Mwangi R, et al. Clinicopathologic characteristics, treatment, and outcomes of post-transplant lymphoproliferative disorders: a single-institution experience using 2017 WHO diagnostic criteria. *HemaSphere*. 2021;5(10):e640.
13. Natkunam Y, Goodlad JR, Chadburn A, et al. EBV-positive B-cell proliferations of varied malignant potential: 2015 SH/EAHP workshop report-Part 1. *Am J Clin Pathol*. 2017;147(2):129-152.
14. Kimura H, Kwong Y-L. EBV viral loads in diagnosis, monitoring, and response assessment. *Front Oncol*. 2019;9:62.
15. Courville EL, Yohe S, Chou D, et al. EBV-negative monomorphic B-cell post-transplant lymphoproliferative disorders are pathologically distinct from EBV-positive cases and frequently contain TP53 mutations. *Mod Pathol*. 2016;29(10):1200-1211.
16. Morscio J, Dierickx D, Ferreiro JF, et al. Gene expression profiling reveals clear differences between EBV-positive and EBV-negative posttransplant lymphoproliferative disorders. *Am J Transplant*. 2013;13(5):1305-1316.
17. Ferreiro JF, Morscio J, Dierickx D, et al. EBV-positive and EBV-negative posttransplant diffuse large B cell lymphomas have distinct genomic and transcriptomic features. *Am J Transplant*. 2016;16(2):414-425.
18. Bobillo S, Abrisqueta P, Sánchez-González B; Grupo Español de Linfomas/Trasplante Autólogo de Médula Ósea GEL/TAMO Cooperative Group, et al. Posttransplant monomorphic Burkitt's lymphoma: clinical characteristics and outcome of a multicenter series. *Ann Hematol*. 2018;97(12):2417-2424.
19. Ferreiro JF, Morscio J, Dierickx D, et al. Post-transplant molecularly defined Burkitt lymphomas are frequently MYC-negative and characterized by the 11q-gain/loss pattern. *Haematologica*. 2015;100(7):e275-e279.

20. Salmerón-Villalobos J, Castrejón-de-Anta N, Guerra-García P, et al. Decoding the molecular heterogeneity of pediatric monomorphic post-solid organ transplant lymphoproliferative disorders. *Blood.* 2023;142(5):434-445.
21. Galera P, Flavin R, Savage NM, et al. Epstein-barr virus-negative marginal zone lymphoma as an uncommon form of monomorphic posttransplant lymphoproliferative disorder. *Am J Surg Pathol.* 2020;44(10):1340-1352.
22. Margolskee E, Jobanputra V, Jain P, et al. Genetic landscape of T- and NK-cell post-transplant lymphoproliferative disorders. *Oncotarget.* 2016;7(25):37636-37648.
23. Tousseyn TA, King RL, Fend F, Feldman AL, Brousset P, Jaffe ES. Evolution in the definition and diagnosis of the Hodgkin lymphomas and related entities. *Virchows Arch.* 2023;482(1):207-226.
24. Morscio J, Finalet Ferreiro J, Vander Borght S, et al. Identification of distinct subgroups of EBV-positive post-transplant diffuse large B-cell lymphoma. *Mod Pathol.* 2017;30(3):370-381.
25. Overkamp M, Granai M, Bonzheim I, et al. Comparative analysis of post-transplant lymphoproliferative disorders after solid organ and hematopoietic stem cell transplantation reveals differences in the tumor microenvironment. *Virchows Arch.* 2021;478(6):1135-1148.
26. Marcelis L, Tousseyn T. The tumor microenvironment in post-transplant lymphoproliferative disorders. *Cancer Microenviron.* 2019;12(1):3-16.
27. Veloza L, Teixido C, Castrejon N, et al. Clinicopathological evaluation of the programmed cell death 1 (PD1)/programmed cell death-ligand 1 (PD-L1) axis in post-transplant lymphoproliferative disorders: association with Epstein-Barr virus, PD-L1 copy number alterations, and outcome. *Histopathology.* 2019;75(6):799-812.
28. Schiefer A-I, Salzer E, Füreder A, et al. PD-L1 and PD1 expression in post-transplantation lymphoproliferative disease (PTLD) of childhood and adolescence: an inter- and intra-individual descriptive study covering the whole spectrum of PTLD categories. *Cancer Med.* 2019;8(10):4656-4668.
29. Zhou T, Cheng J, Karrs J, et al. Clinicopathologic and molecular characterization of Epstein-Barr virus-positive plasmacytoma. *Am J Surg Pathol.* 2022;46(10):1364-1379.
30. Butzmann A, Sridhar K, Jangam D, et al. Mutations in JAK/STAT and NOTCH1 genes are enriched in post-transplant lymphoproliferative disorders. *Front Oncol.* 2021;11:790481.
31. Menter T, Juskevicius D, Alikian M, et al. Mutational landscape of B-cell post-transplant lymphoproliferative disorders. *Br J Haematol.* 2017;178(1):48-56.
32. Morscio J, Tousseyn T. Recent insights in the pathogenesis of post-transplantation lymphoproliferative disorders. *World J Transplant.* 2016;6(3):505-516.
33. Baker A, Frauca Remacha E, Torres Canizales J, et al. Current practices on diagnosis, prevention and treatment of post-transplant lymphoproliferative disorder in pediatric patients after solid organ transplantation: results of ERN TransplantChild Healthcare working group survey. *Children.* 2021;8(8):661.
34. Shah N, Eyre TA, Tucker D; Haemato-Oncology Task Force of the British Society for Haematology and the British Transplantation Society, et al. Front-line management of post-transplantation lymphoproliferative disorder in adult solid organ recipient patients—a British Society for Haematology Guideline. *Br J Haematol.* 2021;193(4):727-740.
35. Trappe RU, Dierickx D, Zimmermann H, et al. Response to rituximab induction is a predictive marker in B-cell post-transplant lymphoproliferative disorder and allows successful stratification into rituximab or R-CHOP consolidation in an International, prospective, multicenter phase II trial. *J Clin Oncol.* 2017;35(5):536-543.
36. Atallah-Yunes SA, Salman O, Robertson MJ. Post-transplant lymphoproliferative disorder: update on treatment and novel therapies. *Br J Haematol.* 2023;201(3):383-395.
37. Ohmoto A, Fuji S. Clinical features and treatment strategies for post-transplant and iatrogenic immunodeficiency-associated lymphoproliferative disorders. *Blood Rev.* 2021;49:100807.
38. Recently Updated Guidelines [Internet]. [cited 2023 September 15]. https://www.nccn.org/guidelines/recently-published-guidelines
39. González-Barca E, Capote FJ, Gómez-Codina J; GELTAMO Spanish Lymphoma Group and GOTEL Group of Oncology for Therapy and Study of Lymphomas, et al. Long-term follow-up of a prospective phase 2 clinical trial of extended treatment with rituximab in patients with B cell post-transplant lymphoproliferative disease and validation in real world patients. *Ann Hematol.* 2021;100(4):1023-1029.
40. Eyre TA, Caillard S, Finel H, et al. Autologous stem cell transplantation for post-transplant lymphoproliferative disorders after solid organ transplantation: a retrospective analysis from the Lymphoma Working Party of the EBMT. *Bone Marrow Transplant.* 2021;56(9):2118-2124.
41. McKenna M, Epperla N, Ghobadi A, et al. Real-world evidence of the safety and survival with CD19 CAR-T cell therapy for relapsed/refractory solid organ transplant-related PTLD. *Br J Haematol.* 2023;202(2):248-255.
42. Rosenberg AS, Klein AK, Ruthazer R, Evens AM. Hodgkin lymphoma post-transplant lymphoproliferative disorder: a comparative analysis of clinical characteristics, prognosis, and survival. *Am J Hematol.* 2016;91(6):560-565.
43. Rubinstein J, Toner K, Gross T, Wistinghausen B. Diagnosis and management of post-transplant lymphoproliferative disease following solid organ transplantation in children, adolescents, and young adults. *Best Pract Res Clin Haematol.* 2023;36(1):101446.
44. El-Mallawany NK, Kamdar KY. Evolving beyond morphology in pediatric PTLD. *Blood.* 2023;142(5):400-402.

Chapter 114

Other Iatrogenic Immunodeficiency-Associated Lymphoproliferative Disorders

Thomas A. Tousseyn, Genevieve M. Crane, Thomas M. Habermann, Elaine S. Jaffe, and Rebecca L. King

Definition

Following initial observation of the development of lymphoproliferative disorders (LPDs) in patients undergoing methotrexate (MTX) treatment of rheumatoid arthritis (RA), there has been a noticeable increase in reports documenting similar LPDs across various immunosuppressive (IS) and immunomodulatory (IM) drug regimens outside the posttransplant setting.[1-5] While the 2017 World Health Organization revision did not explicitly indicate histological subtyping within this category of diseases, we propose to categorize such other iatrogenic immunodeficiency-associated (OIIA)-LPDs in a manner similar to the post transplantation lymphoproliferative disorders (PTLD) scheme (see Table 113.1).[5] Similar to PTLD, the majority of cases are of B-cell lineage, encompassing a broad spectrum of conditions that range from benign to borderline Epstein-Barr virus–positive (EBV+) lesions, to overt malignant lymphomas that can be either EBV+ or EBV negative.[5] Indolent B-cell lymphomas have a higher incidence in patients with autoimmune disorders and should not be included in this category, except for EBV+ mucosa-associated lymphoid tissue. A subset of EBV+ mucocutaneous ulcers (MCUs) will belong to the OIIA-LPD category.[6]

More recently, similar LPDs were observed in patients after treatment of hematological and other malignancies. Such cancer therapy–related LPDs (CT-LPDs) are considered a form of secondary cancer or a complication of cancer therapy, including immunotherapy, multichemotherapy, and radiation therapy.[7] Since the pathology of CT-LPD closely resembles that of other LPDs developing in various immunodeficiency contexts and many are EBV related, implying these patients were in a immunocompromised state attributable to an iatrogenic etiology, CT-LPDs belong in the category of OIIA-LPDs.[7] However, for the diagnosis of CT-LPD, it is imperative to have a thorough understanding of the patient's clinical history and to rule out other causes of IS as outlined in the current classification.

With the ongoing emergence of new immunotherapeutic agents and a growing number of patients undergoing IM or IS treatments, it becomes increasingly important to raise awareness about this entity (Table 114.1). Hence, when a polymorphic EBV+ B-cell LPD is identified in a patient, it is advisable to conduct a comprehensive investigation of the patient's medical history to uncover any potential immune dysregulation, which should encompass a detailed assessment of drugs taken or past history of treated malignancies. On the other hand, it becomes crucial to avoid the overdiagnosis of malignancies in cases of polymorphic EBV+ B-cell LPDs that may, in fact, be benign and resolve upon withdrawal of the IS drug.

Synonyms

None.

Epidemiology

IS agents, typically used as disease-modifying agents in autoimmune conditions, predispose to the development of LPDs in patients with RA, dermatomyositis, Sjögren disease, systemic lupus erythematosus, inflammatory bowel disease (IBD), psoriasis, cutaneous atopic disorders, and other diseases. This is further complicated by the variable association of autoimmune disorders and non-Hodgkin lymphoma and Hodgkin lymphoma.[5] The standardized incidence ratio risk of LPD development in RA is two- to 20-fold compared with the control healthy population.[8,9]

MTX, thiopurines, calcineurin inhibitors, tumor necrosis factor (TNF) inhibitors, Janus kinase (JAK) inhibitors, cyclosporin, tacrolimus, fludarabine, mycophenolate mofetil (MMF), and other IS agents have been reported to be associated with LPD (see Table 114.1).[1,10-13] The incidence and prevalence of this

TABLE 114.1 List of reported drugs associated with OIIA-LPDs

Drug	Class	Type	Main mechanism of action	Indication
Methotrexate	IS	Antifolate	DNA synthesis inhibition	RA/psoriasis
Azathioprine/6-mercaptopurine	IS	Purine analogue	DNA synthesis inhibition	MS/RA/lupus/myasthenia/Crohn's
Mycophenolate mofetil	IS	Inosine-5′-MPDH inhibitor	DNA synthesis inhibition	Lupus/RA/Crohn's
Hydroxychloroquine	IS	TLR blocker	Inhibition of innate immune response	Lupus/RA
Leflunomide	IS	DHODH inhibitor	DNA synthesis inhibition	RA
Cyclosporin	IS	CNI	Inhibition of T-lymphocyte signaling	RA/lupus/psoriasis
Tacrolimus	IS	CNI	Inhibition of T-lymphocyte signaling	IBD/hepatitis
Aurothiopropanolsulfonate	IS	Gold-containing compound	Inhibition of reduction/oxidation enzymes	RA
Pirfenidone	IS	Small molecule	Anti-inflammatory	Idiopathic pulmonary fibrosis
Tofacitinib	IS	JAK1/3 inhibitor	Inhibition of cytokine signaling	RA/Sjögren
Mitoxantrone[a]	IS	Topoisomerase inhibitor	DNA synthesis inhibition	MS
Infliximab, adalimumab, etanercept[a]	IM	MoAb	Anti-TNF-α	RA/Crohn's/UC/psoriasis
Tocilizumab	IM	MoAb	Anti-IL6R	RA/giant cell arteritis
Canakinumab	IM	MoAb	Anti-IL 1β	CPS
Anakinra	IM	MoAb	Anti-IL 1R	RA/JIA
Ustekinumab	IM	MoAb	Anti-IL12 and anti-IL23	Psoriasis/Crohn's/UC
Vedolizumab	IM	MoAb	Anti-integrin α4/β7	Crohn's/UC
Natalizumab	IM	MoAb	Anti-α4β1 integrin: lymphocyte migration into CNS	MS/Crohn's
Efalizumab	IM	MoAb	Anti-CD11a	Psoriasis
Daclizumab	IM	MoAb	Anti-CD25	MS
Ipilimumab	CT	MoAb	Anti-CTLA4	Melanoma
Nivolumab	CT	MoAb	Anti-PD1	Melanoma
Alemtuzumab	CT/IM	MoAb	Anti-CD52	CLL/MS
Cyclophosphamide[a]	CT/IS	Alkylating agent	DNA synthesis inhibition	Lupus/RA/vasculitis
Imatinib	CT	Tyrosine kinase inhibitor	Inhibition of T-lymphocyte signaling	CML
Fludarabine	CT	Purine analogue	Inhibition of purine nucleotide synthesis	CLL
Temozolomide	CT	DNA methylation	Inhibition of DNA and cellular replication	Glioblastoma

CLL, chronic lymphocytic leukemia; CML, chronic myeloid leukemia; CNI, calcineurin inhibitor; CNS, central nervous system; CPS, cryopyrin-associated periodic syndromes; CT, cancer therapy; DHODH, dihydroorotate dehydrogenase; IBD, inflammatory bowel disease; IL, interleukin; IM, immunomodulatory; IS, immunosuppressive; JIA, juvenile idiopathic arthritis; MoAb, monoclonal antibody; MPDH, monophosphate dehydrogenase; MS, multiple sclerosis; RA, rheumatoid arthritis; TLR, Toll-like receptor; TNF, tumor necrosis factor; UC, ulcerative colitis.

[a]Agents only given in combination with other immunosuppressants.

disorder have not been well defined. Assessing the effect of a specific therapeutic agent is further complicated by the concurrent or sequential use of multiple drugs. MTX was the first reported and is the most common drug associated with the development of LPD. The risk of anti-TNFα inhibitors has been associated with the use of other immunomodulators, with an absolute risk that is low in patients treated for Crohn's disease.[5] Tofacitinib, an oral JAK inhibitor, has been reported to be associated with the development of lymphoma in patients with RA and Sjögren syndrome.[11]

Owing to the significant variations in therapeutic regimens tailored to individual patients, establishing correlations between specific drugs and LPDs within relatively small cohorts is challenging. No distinct associations between therapy types and underlying factors have been identified, except for reported correlation between hepatosplenic T-cell lymphoma (HSTCL) and the use of thiopurine and/or TNF antagonists for IBD.[5] Central nervous system involvement is mainly linked to azathioprine, MMF, MTX and natalizumab.[14] Gastrointestinal (GI) involvement is mainly observed in patients with IBD, followed by RA and treated lymphomas.[15,16]

Factors that can increase the risk of CT-LPDs include the type and intensity of cancer treatment, the use of IS drugs, the presence of certain viral infections (such as EBV or human herpesvirus-8), and the individual's overall health and immune function. The majority of patients diagnosed with CT-LPDs have a history of treatment of hematologic malignancies, and there is a relatively low occurrence in patients with solid tumors.[7]

General Clinical Features

Relevant history includes the rheumatologic, autoimmune, or other disorder and the type of IS treatment. The clinical features are overall similar to those of lymphoma in immunocompetent patients with the exception of more extranodal disease presentations. About 40% to 70% of patients with MTX-LPD have been reported to have extranodal disease.[4,8]

Morphology

At present, MTX is the predominant agent linked to the emergence of LPDs.[3] As a result, the prevalence of histological subtypes in MTX-LPD generally mirrors that found in other iatrogenic LPDs, including CT-LPDs.[10]

Most OIIA-LPDs are of B-cell origin, and the prevailing histological subtype is the diffuse large B-cell lymphoma (DLBCL) type, with or without EBV infection.[5] Additional prevalent subtypes include reactive follicular hyperplasia, polymorphic B-cell LPD (Poly-LPD), and classic Hodgkin lymphoma (CHL), and we advise to apply the same subclassification scheme as used for PTLDs (see Table 113.1).[6] Similar to PTLD, OIIA-LPDs can present synchronously (Figure 114.1) or metachronously with a different histologic subtype.

Nondestructive OIIA-LPDs (Figure 114.2) retain the architecture of the lymphoid tissue, and EBV-infected cells are typically detected in the interfollicular regions, as seen in acute mononucleosis, but they can also be found within hyperplastic lymphoid B follicles. Marked plasmacytic infiltration is a feature often observed, but if EBV negative, is most probably related to the underlying autoimmune disease.

In polymorphic OIIA-LPDs (see Figure 114.1A and B) the original tissue architecture is disrupted by the presence of EBV+ B cells and plasma cells exhibiting diverse sizes and maturation stages, including cells resembling Hodgkin and Reed-Sternberg cells. They share morphological and immunophenotypic features with CHL and mononucleosis-like lesions, and some clues to differentiate them are discussed in the PTLD chapter.

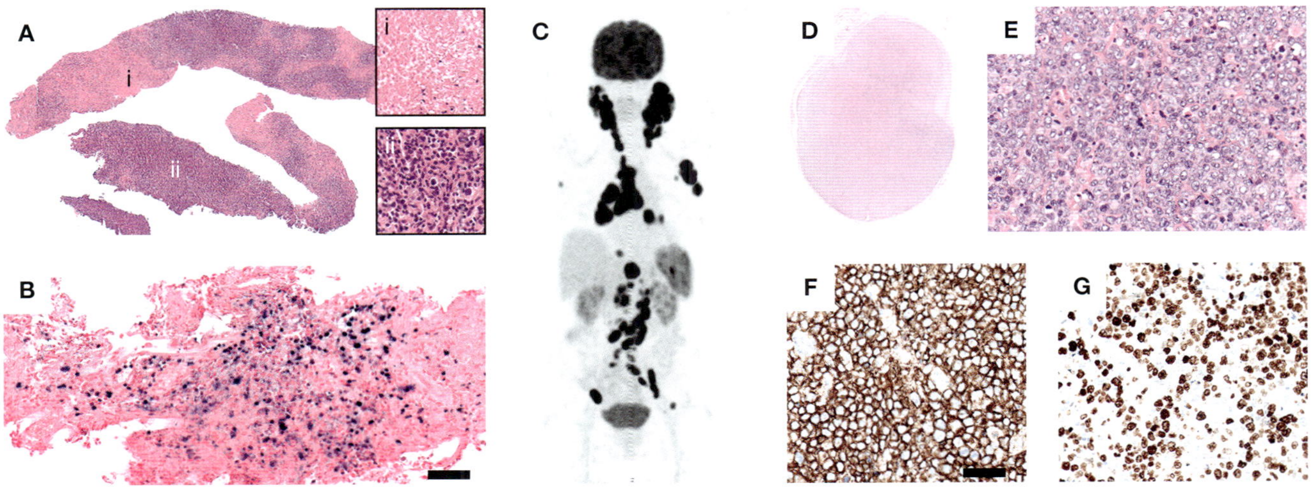

FIGURE 114.1 Synchronous appearance of clonally unrelated polymorphic and monomorphic OIIA-LPDs at distant sites in an 86-year-old woman treated with azathioprine for autoimmune hepatitis and Sjögren disease. **A:** A core needle biopsy taken in the parotid gland, clinically suspicious for mucosa-assisted lymphoid tissue lymphoma, showed tissue necrosis (i, inset) and infiltration by a polymorphic lymphoid infiltrate (ii, inset). **B:** EBER in situ hybridization illustrated a mixture of smaller, intermediate-sized cells and only some sparse larger atypical cells. **C:** Since the positron emission tomography scan showed widespread disease, an axillary lymph node excision was performed, showing a diffuse destruction **(D)** by a uniform high-grade proliferation of large cells **(E)**, expressing CD20 **(F)** and a high proliferation KI-67 index **(G)**. Immunoglobulin gene rearrangements by polymerase chain reaction showed that the lesions were clonally unrelated.

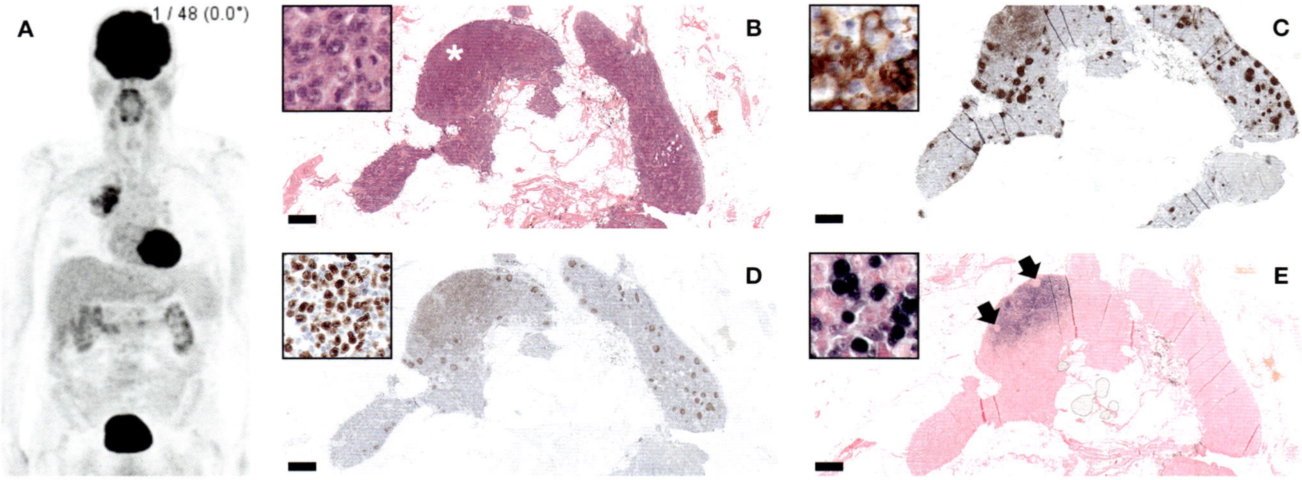

FIGURE 114.2 Nondestructive OIIA-LPD, infectious mononucleosis-type, in a 72-year-old male presenting with tonsillar swelling, during induction chemoradiotherapy and radiotherapy for a lung adenocarcinoma of the right upper lobe. **A:** One of the lymph nodes (position 4) provided at the time of pneumonectomy shows the incidental finding of focal (*) paracortical expansion by a mixture of small to medium sized B-immunoblasts, retaining the overall lymph node architecture, as evidenced by the H&E (**B**) and CD20 (**C**) stainings. **D:** Ki67 proliferation index can be worrisomely high, but corresponds to the proliferation of the EBER+ (**E**), B-blasts, leaving the B-cell follicles unaffected, as evidenced by the arrows.

EBV+ MCUs, particularly cutaneous and GI manifestations, are commonly linked to iatrogenic immunosuppression and in this clinical context should be designated as a type of OIIA-LPD.[6,13]

In monomorphic OIIA-LPDs, the affected tissue is disrupted due to the infiltration of large atypical cells, predominantly of B-cell origin, often accompanied by a variable number of inflammatory cells (see Figure 114.1D-G). DLBCL-like presentations constitute the most prevalent form among monomorphic OIIA-LPDs, including diverse cellular arrangements beyond just uniform sheets of large cells.

The precise frequency of small B-cell lymphomas in patients under IS/IM drug treatment is not known. However, since the majority of reported cases are EBV negative we advise to not designate them as OIIA-LPDs, particularly as low-grade B-cell lymphomas with plasma cell differentiation, eg, marginal zone lymphoma, may potentially be associated with the underlying autoimmune disorder. The exception is EBV+ marginal zone lymphomas, which are considered part of the OIIA-LPD spectrum since they have been linked to a variety of immunodeficiency scenarios.[17]

CHL is more often observed in OIIA-LPD than in the posttransplant context.[18] Similar to what was discussed for PTLD, the diagnosis of Poly-LPD should be favored over CHL in cases with expression of B-cell markers (CD20, OCT2, CD79A) in over 50% of atypical cells, exclusively extranodal manifestations, and/or EBV latency type III.

OIIA-LPDs of T-cell origin are rare, except for HSTCL that has been associated with the use of thiopurines and/or TNF antagonists in IBD (Figure 114.3).[19] No clear association with EBV has been described, and the criteria for diagnosis are similar to those employed in nonimmunocompromised patients.

Immunophenotype

The immunohistochemical findings resemble the previously delineated observations concerning PTLD (see earlier discussion).[6]

Even with an immunodeficiency background, only approximately 50% of the OIIA-DLBCLs have detectable EBV present, which is less than in PTLD (60%-80%). The distribution of viral latency profiles in EBV+ cases is within the same range for OIIA-LPD and PTLD, the majority of which carry a latency type II (59%) or III (29%).[3] Around two-thirds of OIIA-LPD cases classified as DLBCL belong to the non–germinal center B-cell type, defined by the Hans algorithm for cell of origin.

Genetics

The available research on OIIA-LPDs is considerably more limited than on PTLD, and mainly focused on MTX-LPD. The etiology of OIIA-LPDs is intricate and likely stems from a combination of multiple factors. Despite patients receiving IS medications being

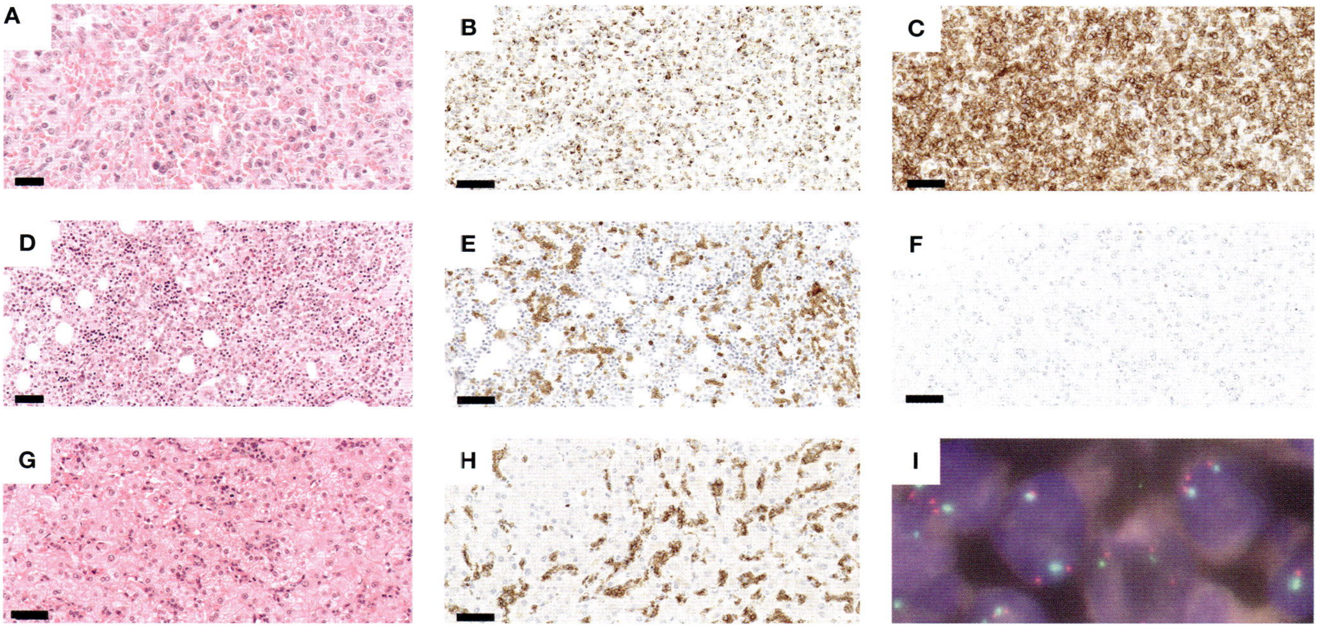

FIGURE 114.3 Hepatosplenic T-cell lymphoma in a 23-year-old patient under thiopurine treatment of inflammatory bowel disease. **A-C:** Diffuse splenic red pulp infiltration by atypical lymphoid cells, expressing cytotoxic marker TIA1 **(B)** and CD56 **(C)**. **D-F:** Intrasinusoidal bone marrow infiltration by atypical lymphoid cells, expressing CD2 **(E)** and lacking TCRbetaF1 **(F)**. **G-H:** Intrasinusoidal liver infiltration by atypical lymphocytes, expressing CD3. **I:** Fluorescence in situ hybridization confirms the presence of an isochromosome 7q.

in an immunocompromised state, it is important to note that the underlying autoimmune disease itself can contribute to the susceptibility of developing LPDs. It is conceivable to differentiate between pharmaceutical agents with IS and IM properties from an etiological standpoint.[1] IS drugs, such as methotrexate, inhibit immune cell proliferation, while IM drugs, like TNFα blockers (mainly monoclonal antibodies), alter the immune response by targeting cytokines. The relationship between these medications and LPDs is still under investigation, with indications that the underlying autoimmune disease activity may be more pivotal than the therapy's effects. Nevertheless, given that OIIA-LPDs can exhibit spontaneous regression upon cessation of the administered IS medication, it is evident that these therapeutic agents do indeed trigger the occurrence of LPDs within specific patient subsets.[9]

The scope of genetic alterations in patients with OIIA-LPD remains largely unexplored. Genomic features characteristic of MTX-DLBCL include gains in chromosomes 3q, 12q, and 20p, as well as loss in chromosome 13p.[20] Genes on 3q and 12q are related to the differentiation and maintenance of the tumor microenvironment (TME) in MTX-DLBCL, including the infiltration of M2-polarized macrophages and $CD8^+$ T cells into the TME. Similar to PTLD, there is a role for immune escape via the PD1/PD-L1 axis in MTX-DLBCL, particularly in EBV+ cases.

The long-term consequences of significant immune system disruptions, including a history of chemotherapy, remain inadequately understood. However, these disruptions could potentially render patients more susceptible to self-resolving B-cell LPDs associated with EBV, related to the suppression of the immune system by cancer therapies. The reasons behind the relatively low occurrence of CT-LPD in patients with solid tumors, compared with hematologic malignancies, remains unclear. Solid tumors might be less associated with tumor-induced host immunodeficiency and are seldom associated with EBV. Patients with solid tumors may receive fewer IS therapies and may have shorter lifespans and thus fewer chances for repeated IS treatments compared with those with hematologic malignancies.[7]

Prognosis and Clinical Comment

The risk and the prognosis is related to the type of IS/IM agent, primary disease, primary disease severity, accumulated inflammatory activity of the primary disease, degree of immune deficiency, histologic subtype (EBV+ MCU; superior), age (>70 years; unfavorable), and associated biology. The suitability of published clinical guidelines for managing PTLD in patients with OIIA-LPDs remains to be determined.[21,22] Regression of the LPD after withdrawal of immunosuppressive (WIS) drugs is the unique aspect of these disorders. LPD regression with MTX withdrawal has been observed in 20% to 86% of cases.[9] In patients who have responded to WIS, watchful waiting is the management strategy of choice. Over 50% of patients managed with WIS and watchful waiting do not require additional chemotherapy and have a superior overall survival. However, 33% of patients in one series relapsed. In a large Japanese study of MTX-LPD, LPD regression after MTX withdrawal comprised 86.2% of the 302 evaluable events.[9] The clinical patterns and management of MTX-LPD in this study included regression after discontinuing methotrexate, relapse after regression, and persistent disease in 225 patients including 66 EBV+ DLBCL; 50 DLBCL, not otherwise specified; 51 CHL; 17 Poly-LPD; 32 EBV+ MCU; and 9 nodular sclerosis-LPD.[9] EBV+ cases are more likely to respond to WIS than EBV-negative cases. The survival rates in all histologies ranged from 92% to 100% for those patients who responded to WIS, and 67% to 75% in the group with persistent disease managed with other strategies. In patients who have not responded to WIS, single-agent rituximab or immunochemotherapy agents are the treatment of choice. Patients developing HSTCL after thiopurine and TNF blockers have a very aggressive course. The management of patients who relapse or have persistent disease is that of the standard national and international practices for the histology of the disease and clinical prognostic factors.[23]

Treatment of CT-LPDs may involve a combination of strategies, including reducing or discontinuing IS medications, targeted therapies, chemotherapy, radiation therapy, and, in some cases, stem cell transplantation. The specific approach depends on the type and severity of the CT-LPD. Nevertheless, it is noteworthy that patients with CT-LPDs tend to experience a more unfavorable prognosis and higher mortality rates when compared with individuals with OIIA-LPDs for autoimmune disorders.[5,7]

References

1. Marcelis L, Berghen C, De Zutter A, et al. Other immunomodulatory agent-related lymphoproliferative diseases: a single-center series of 72 biopsy-confirmed cases. *Mod Pathol.* 2018;31(9):1457-1469. doi:10.1038/s41379-018-0054-2
2. Mercer LK, Regierer AC, Mariette X, et al. Spectrum of lymphomas across different drug treatment groups in rheumatoid arthritis: a European registries collaborative project. *Ann Rheum Dis.* 2017;76(12):2025-2030. doi:10.1136/annrheumdis-2017-211623
3. Momose S, Tamaru JI. Iatrogenic immunodeficiency-associated lymphoproliferative disorders of B-cell type that develop in patients receiving immunosuppressive drugs other than in the post-transplant setting. *J Clin Exp Hematop.* 2019;59(2):48-55. doi:10.3960/jslrt.19014
4. Ohmoto A, Fuji S. Clinical features and treatment strategies for post-transplant and iatrogenic immunodeficiency-associated lymphoproliferative disorders. *Blood Rev.* 2021;49:100807. doi:10.1016/j.blre.2021.100807
5. WHO Classification of Tumours Editorial Board; Campo E, Harris NL, et al. WHO Classification of Tumours of Haematopoietic and Lymphoid Tissues (Medicine). World Health Organization; 2017:585. Revised.
6. Campo E, Jaffe ES, Cook JR, et al. The international consensus classification of mature lymphoid neoplasms: a report from the clinical advisory committee. *Blood.* 2022;140(11):1229-1253. doi:10.1182/blood.2022015851
7. Pina-Oviedo S, Miranda RN, Medeiros LJ. Cancer therapy-associated lymphoproliferative disorders: an under-recognized type of immunodeficiency-associated lymphoproliferative disorder. *Am J Surg Pathol.* 2018;42(1):116-129. doi:10.1097/PAS.0000000000000954
8. Harigai M. Lymphoproliferative disorders in patients with rheumatoid arthritis in the era of widespread use of methotrexate: a review of the literature and current perspective. *Mod Rheumatol.* 2018;28(1):1-8. doi:10.1080/14397595.2017.1352477
9. Tokuhira M, Tamaru JI, Kizaki M. Clinical management for other iatrogenic immunodeficiency-associated lymphoproliferative disorders. *J Clin Exp Hematop.* 2019;59(2):72-92. doi:10.3960/jslrt.19007
10. Kurita D, Miyoshi H, Ichikawa A, et al. Methotrexate-associated lymphoproliferative disorders in patients with rheumatoid arthritis: clinicopathologic features and prognostic factors. *Am J Surg Pathol.* 2019;43(7):869-884. doi:10.1097/PAS.0000000000001271
11. Mariette X, Chen C, Biswas P, Kwok K, Boy MG. Lymphoma in the tofacitinib rheumatoid arthritis clinical development program. *Arthritis Care Res.* 2018;70(5):685-694. doi:10.1002/acr.23421
12. Natkunam Y, Goodlad JR, Chadburn A, et al. EBV-positive B-cell proliferations of varied malignant potential: 2015 SH/EAHP workshop report-part 1. *Am J Clin Pathol.* 2017;147(2):129-152. doi:10.1093/ajcp/aqw214
13. Pugh MR, Leopold GD, Morgan M, et al. Epstein-Barr virus-positive mucocutaneous ulcers complicate colitis

caused by immune checkpoint regulator therapy and associate with colon perforation. *Clin Gastroenterol Hepatol.* 2020;18(8):1785-1795.e3. doi:10.1016/j.cgh.2019.09.031

14. Tadipatri R, Ekhator C, Narayan R, et al. Iatrogenic immunodeficiency-associated lymphoproliferative disorders of the central nervous system: a treatment paradox. *Neurooncol Pract.* 2023;10(2):169-175. doi:10.1093/nop/npac098
15. Ishikawa E, Satou A, Nakamura M, Nakamura S, Fujishiro M. Epstein-Barr virus positive B-cell lymphoproliferative disorder of the gastrointestinal tract. *Cancers.* 2021;13(15):3815. doi:10.3390/cancers13153815
16. Zanelli M, Sanguedolce F, Palicelli A, et al. EBV-driven lymphoproliferative disorders and lymphomas of the gastrointestinal tract: a spectrum of entities with a common denominator (part 1). *Cancers.* 2021;13(18):4578. doi:10.3390/cancers13184578
17. Gong S, Crane GM, McCall CM, et al. Expanding the spectrum of EBV-positive marginal zone lymphomas: a lesion associated with diverse immunodeficiency settings. *Am J Surg Pathol.* 2018;42(10):1306-1316. doi:10.1097/PAS.0000000000001113
18. Miranda RN, Loo E, Medeiros LJ. Iatrogenic immunodeficiency-associated classical Hodgkin lymphoma: clinicopathologic features of 54 cases reported in the literature. *Am J Surg Pathol.* 2013;37(12):1895-1897. doi:10.1097/PAS.0000000000000095
19. Satou A, Tsuzuki T, Nakamura S. Other iatrogenic immunodeficiency-associated lymphoproliferative disorders with a T- or NK-cell phenotype. *J Clin Exp Hematop.* 2019;59(2):56-63. doi:10.3960/jslrt.19013
20. Carreras J, Yukie Kikuti Y, Miyaoka M, et al. Genomic profile and pathologic features of diffuse large B-cell lymphoma subtype of methotrexate-associated lymphoproliferative disorder in rheumatoid arthritis patients. *Am J Surg Pathol.* 2018;42(7):936-950. doi:10.1097/PAS.0000000000001071
21. Allen UD, Preiksaitis JK; AST Infectious Diseases Community of Practice. Post-transplant lymphoproliferative disorders, Epstein-Barr virus infection, and disease in solid organ transplantation: guidelines from the American society of transplantation infectious diseases community of practice. *Clin Transplant.* 2019;33(9):e13652. doi:10.1111/ctr.13652
22. Shah N, Eyre TA, Tucker D, et al. Front-line management of post-transplantation lymphoproliferative disorder in adult solid organ recipient patients—a British Society for Haematology Guideline. *Br J Haematol.* 2021;193(4):727-740. doi:10.1111/bjh.17421
23. Recently Updated Guidelines. Accessed September 15, 2023. https://www.nccn.org/guidelines/recently-published-guidelines

SECTION 14

Histiocytic and Dendritic Cell Neoplasms

Introduction to Histiocytic and Dendritic Cell Neoplasms

Laurence de Leval, Elaine S. Jaffe, and Stefano A. Pileri

Histiocytic and dendritic cell neoplasms comprise two groups of tumors: one group of neoplasms of hematopoietic origin, collectively named "histiocytoses,"[1] which are derived from myeloid cells and show characteristics of cells of the mononuclear phagocyte system, and another group of neoplasms that are derived from stromal cells of mesenchymal origin (Table 1 and Figure 1). Based on practice patterns and issues of differential diagnosis, the histiocytic and dendritic cell neoplasms are traditionally discussed alongside the mature lymphoid neoplasms, for several reasons: (1) many histiocytic and dendritic cell neoplasms present in the lymph nodes and should be differentiated from malignant lymphomas; (2) both myeloid-derived and mesenchymal cells of origin are usually regarded as "accessory" by taking part in the immune reaction; (3) the dendritic morphology (first described by Steinman and Cohn[2] and subsequently referred by Shortman and Liu[3] to a sparsely distributed, migratory group of elements specialized for the uptake, transport, processing, and presentation of antigens to T and B cells) is shown by tumors of different origin and is *per se* uncapable of clarifying the histogenesis of the process. Histiocytic and dendritic cell neoplasms are overall very rare accounting for less than 1% of lymph node tumors, but their true incidence is poorly characterized. In the International Consensus Classification, histiocytic and dendritic cell neoplasms include entities that were not listed in the former WHO4R classification, ie, Rosai-Dorfman-Destombes disease, which in the past was deemed a reactive or inflammatory condition; ALK-positive histiocytosis, which was first reported in 2008; and EBV-positive inflammatory follicular dendritic cell/fibroblastic reticular cell tumor formerly mentioned as inflammatory pseudotumor-like follicular/fibroblastic dendritic cell sarcoma.

TABLE 1 Histiocytic and dendritic cell neoplasms

Neoplasms of myeloid derivation
Histiocytic sarcoma
Langerhans cell histiocytosis
Langerhans cell sarcoma
Indeterminate dendritic cell histiocytosis[b]
Interdigitating dendritic cell sarcoma
ALK-positive histiocytosis[a]
Disseminated juvenile xanthogranuloma
Erdheim-Chester disease
Rosai-Dorfman-Destombes disease[a]
Neoplasms of mesenchymal derivation
Follicular dendritic cell sarcoma
Fibroblastic reticular cell sarcoma
EBV-positive inflammatory follicular dendritic cell/fibroblastic reticular cell tumor[a,b]

[a]Entities that were not listed in the WHO4R classification.
[b]Change in terminology.

Myeloid-Derived Histiocytic and Dendritic Cell Neoplasms

These tumors stemming from the myeloid axis collectively designated "histiocytoses" derive from macrophages, Langerhans cells, or myeloid dendritic cells, which are differentiated from embryonal progenitors or bone marrow–derived myeloid progenitors with divergent differentiation pathways and intermediate precursor cells circulating in the blood (ie, monocytes and precursor dendritic cells) (see Figure 1). Distinct neoplasms are classified according to their putative cell of origin. However, at the current time it is not possible to assign all dendritic cell neoplasms to one of the functional subtypes described later. Additionally, some neoplasms show variation in their phenotype and morphology leading to the existence of "mixed histiocytoses."[4] For example, Langerhans cell histiocytosis can coexist with Erdheim-Chester disease in the same patient in different lesions or at different points in time.

Tissue macrophages are effector cells displaying phagocytosis under some conditions of activation and play pivotal roles in tissue defense and homeostasis.

For a long time, the belief was that macrophages result from the differentiation of circulating monocytes entering tissues, but recent discoveries have changed our understanding of macrophage ontogeny.[5] It is now well accepted that most tissue-resident macrophages are long-lived cells with the ability to self-

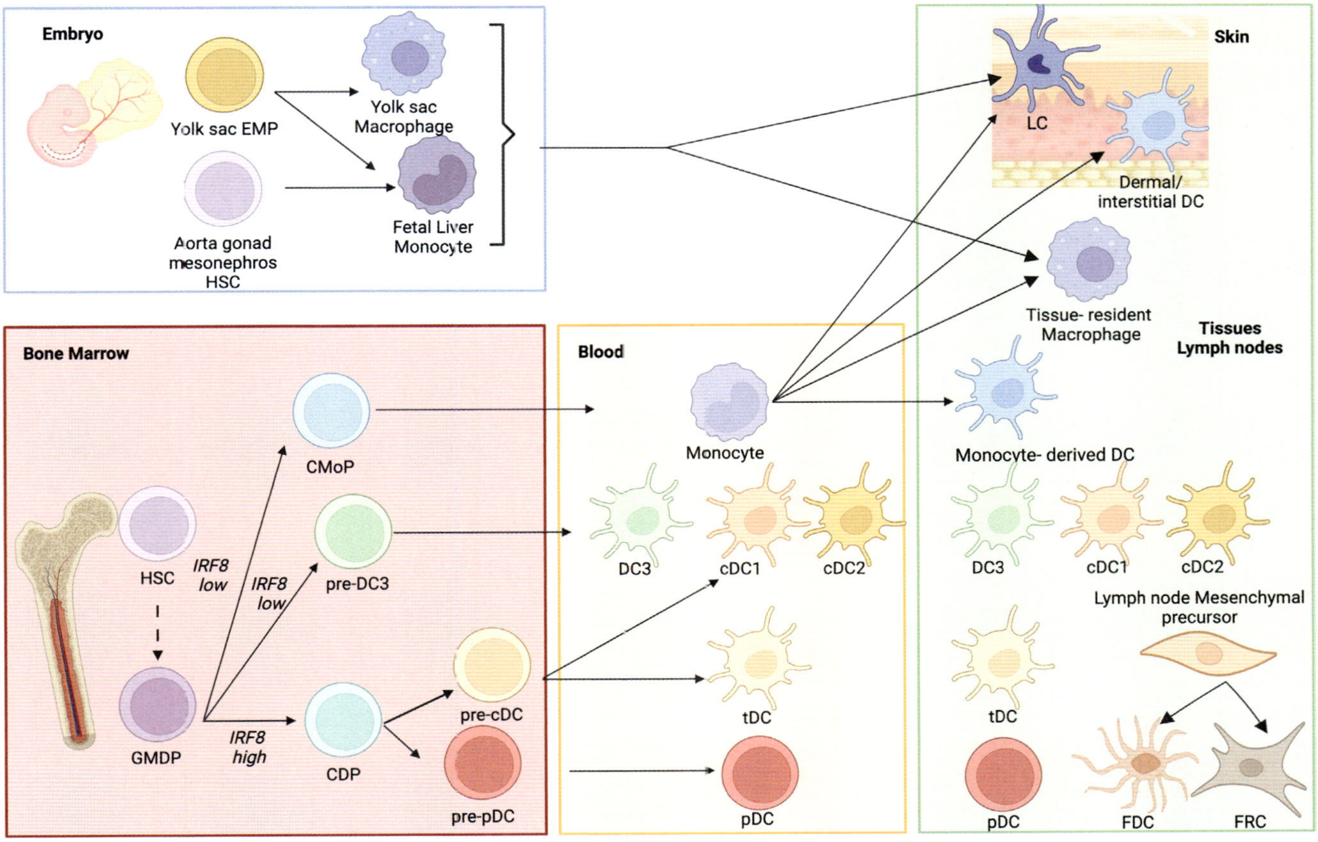

FIGURE 1 Representation of the human mononuclear phagocytic system and dendritic cells. cDC, classical DC; CDP, common dendritic cell progenitor; cMoP, common monocyte precursor; DC, dendritic cell; EMP, erythroid-myeloid progenitor; FDC, follicular dendritic cell; FRC, fibroblastic reticular cell; GMDP, granulocyte-monocyte and DC progenitor; HSC, hematopoietic stem cell; LC, Langerhans cell; pDC, plasmacytoid DC; tDC, transitional DC. (Created in BioRender. Sarkis R (2021) BioRender.com/g60t187.)

renew throughout the lifespan, derived from a transient hematopoietic wave of erythromyeloid progenitors emerging in the embryonal yolk sac. One pathway, c-Myb-independent, starts early in the embryonic life and gives rise to primitive macrophages in the yolk sac, which seed every tissue and will also give rise to microglia in the brain. In a subsequent pathway that requires c-Myb expression erythromyeloid progenitors colonize the fetal liver where they generate fetal monocytes, which migrate to every tissue outside the brain and gradually generate the major pool of adult tissue-resident macrophages. A third wave of hematopoietic stem cells–derived monocytes emerges from the fetal liver and contributes to the long-lived macrophage pool established at birth while the adult hematopoiesis is starting in the bone marrow. The precursor relationship between subsets of monocytes and macrophages remains an area of investigation. During the lifespan, circulating monocytes are required for macrophage network maintenance in the dermis, spleen, liver, and intestinal mucosa.

Neoplastic entities derived from macrophages include histiocytic sarcoma, ALK-positive histiocytosis, Rosai-Dorfman-Destombes disease, and Erdheim-Chester disease. Phenotypic markers of normal macrophages include CD4, CD68, CD163, and lysozyme; in addition, they variably express S100, factor XIII, and fascin. At variance with their normal counterparts, phagocytic activity is usually not a prominent feature of histiocytic neoplasms. Conversely, the hematophagocytic lymphohistiocytoses, which collectively designate a group of genetic or acquired nonneoplastic disorders characterized by macrophage proliferation and activation, typically are associated with conspicuous phagocytic activity.

Dendritic cells (DCs) represent a heterogeneous group of hematopoietic cells enriched in skin and mucosal surfaces and lymphoid organs. DCs are distinguished from macrophages by their morphology and their superior capacity to process and present antigen and stimulate antigen-specific T cells, effectively bridging innate and adaptive immune responses, and they can migrate from tissues to lymph nodes.

Human DC subsets are defined based on their developmental pathways (ontogeny) and phenotype (for review[6]). In recent years, high-throughput single-cell studies have revealed further heterogeneity.[7] Human DCs are classified into the following types: classical DC type 1 (cDC1), cDC type 2 (cDC2), DC3, plasmacytoid DC (pDC), and monocyte-derived DC (mo-DC). A population of transitional DC (AXL+ SIGLEC6+) combining phenotypic and gene expression characteristics of pDCs and cDC2, and functionally closer to cDC2, is also described. pDC and pre-cDC arise from a common dendritic cell progenitor stemming out of an IRF8-high granulocyte-monocyte-DC progenitor.

cDC1 ($CD1c^-$ $CD11c^+$ $CD141^{++}$) are found in the blood, tissues, and T-cell areas of lymph nodes. They secrete type III interferons, are specialized in the presentation of necrotic cell–associated material, can activate $CD4^+$ T cells along Th1 and Th2 differentiation, and also promote the differentiation of cytotoxic $CD8^+$ T cells. **cDC2** ($CD1c^+$ $CD11c^{++}CD141^+$) are found in the blood and lymphoid tissues with a preferential distribution at the border between B and T zones. They are most efficient in the presentation of soluble antigens *in vitro*, and while being able to induce cytotoxic $CD8^+$ T cells and most T helper cell subsets, they are the most potent inductors of follicular helper T cells (TFH cells). cDC2 secrete IL23 and IL12p70. **DC3** have a mixed cDC2/monocyte transcriptomic signature and cytokine secretion profile (IL23 and IL12p70 plus IL-1β), coexpress CD1c and CD163, and can differentiate to cDC2 in vitro. **Mo-DC** ($CD1c^+$ $CD14^+$ $CD11c^+$) have overlapping features with monocyte-derived macrophages, include a subset of cells present in the steady state in some tissues including the dermis (interstitial/dermal DCs), and otherwise are recruited to tissues during inflammation and preferentially induce the differentiation of Th17 or Th1 cells from $CD4^+$ cells, and induce the differentiation of effector cytotoxic $CD8^+$ T cells. **pDCs** are characterized by the expression of CD123 (IL-3R), CD303 (BDCA2), CD304 (BDCA4), and TCF4 and can produce large amounts of type I interferons in response to viral infections. In addition to their role in antiviral immune responses, they have a role in systemic autoimmunity and are expanded in conditions like systemic lupus erythematous. There is controversy regarding the origin of pDC, with emerging data suggesting that they may derive from a lymphoid progenitor and that these interferon-producing cells should rather be assigned to a subcategory of innate lymphocytes.[8]

cDCs represent the cell origin of interdigitating dendritic cell sarcoma, and juvenile xanthogranuloma is believed to derive from interstitial/dermal monocyte-derived DCs. Neoplasms derived from monocytes, ie, leukemias with monocytic or monoblastic differentiation, as well as neoplasms of immature plasmacytoid dendritic cells (blastic plasmacytoid dendritic cell neoplasms) are in the section of myeloid disorders. Sometimes there can be intermediate stages or a continuum and the distinction between histiocytosis versus tissue infiltrates of leukemias can be difficult.

Langerhans cells are myeloid cells with dendritic cell morphology and properties, resident in the epidermis and other stratified epithelia. They are tissue-resident sentinels that are able to capture antigen, migrate to lymph nodes, and develop immunostimulatory capacity. Their typical immunophenotype is $CD4^+$ $CD1a^+$ $CD207(langerin)^+$ $S100^+$. There has been a conceptual shift in the understanding of their cellular origin, like described previously for macrophages. Langerhans cells were initially thought to derive from bone marrow progenitors, but more recent data indicate that, like tissue-resident macrophages, Langerhans cells represent bone marrow–independent cells derived from yolk sac macrophages and fetal liver monocytes.[9] The pool of Langerhans cells is self-renewing in the absence of inflammation. In case of skin inflammation resulting in increased turnover of Langerhans cells and exit to the draining lymph nodes, increased proliferation may replenish the pool of Langerhans cells, but in cases of severe inflammation and epithelial denudation, there is a recruitment of blood monocytes that have the potential to migrate to the epidermis and differentiate into Langerhans-like cells, retaining the expression of lysozyme while developing low expression of langerin.[10] More controversial is the differentiation of cDC progenitors of DC2 type to Langerhans cells. The DC origin of a subset of Langerhans cell is supported by the fact that it is possible to differentiate $CD1c^+$ blood DC into Langerhans cells in response to cocktails of cytokines or growth factors and that there is physiologically a small population of langerin+ DCs in certain tissues.

Langerhans cells are normal counterpart of Langerhans cell histiocytosis and Langerhans cell sarcoma. The relationship of indeterminate dendritic cell tumor to Langerhans cells and other dendritic cells remains uncertain.

Our understanding of histiocytoses has markedly evolved in recent years with their genetic characterization and the discovery of oncogenic mutations in the mitogen-activated protein kinase (MAPK) or phosphatidylinositol-3-kinase (PI3K) pathways genes (*BRAF,*

CSF1R, ALK, RET, NTRK, RAS, RAF, MAP2K1, PI3K1, PI3K2) representing a common pathogenic pathway across different entities.[11] None of these mutations are specific for histiocytoses, since they can occur in many tumors of different histogenesis. However, in histiocytoses, they arise in the setting of relatively few other mutations. In addition, part of these mutations are also found in hematopoietic precursors. Of note, many of the observed mutations, among which are highly recurrent *BRAF*^{V600E} mutations, for example, are not specific to any individual entity. This new knowledge has modified the diagnostic approach to these disorders and generated major advances in their therapy.[12]

The majority of histiocytic/dendritic cell neoplasms arise *de novo*, but in rare circumstances they occur in association with or subsequently to a precursor or mature lymphoid neoplasms, most commonly follicular lymphoma, chronic lymphocytic leukemia, and T- or B-lymphoblastic leukemia/lymphoma, and carry the same antigen receptor gene rearrangement.[13-16] The molecular dissection of the synchronous or metachronous tumors suggests divergent differentiation or transdifferentiation from a common lymphoid progenitor clone.[14,17]

Mesenchymally Derived Dendritic Cell Neoplasms

Neoplasms of follicular dendritic cells (FDCs) and fibroblastic reticular cells (FRCs) originate from mesenchymal cells in lymphoid tissues, and not from the mononuclear phagocyte system. FDCs and FRCs share a common stromal or mesenchymal precursor located in the perivascular spaces of the lymphoid organs and tissues.

FDCs reside within primary and secondary B-cell follicles and play a crucial role in adaptive immunity.[18] FDCs express markers such as CD21, CD23, CD35, clusterin, CXCL13, and D2-40 (podoplanin). They contribute to the formation of germinal centers and store antigens on their cell surface in the form of immune complexes, which are presented to B cells. This interaction is pivotal in the activation and maturation of B cells and the development of robust humoral immune responses.

FRCs are specialized cells characterized by the expression of smooth muscle actin and desmin providing structural support to the lymphoid stroma, regulating the positioning and trafficking of lymphocytes and other immune cells and modulating immune responses.[19] Some neoplasms display a hybrid phenotype and are not clearly designated as derived from FDC or FRC, which includes the EBV+ inflammatory FDC/FRC tumor.

References

1. Emile JF, Abla O, Fraitag S, et al. Revised classification of histiocytoses and neoplasms of the macrophage-dendritic cell lineages. *Blood.* 2016;127(22):2672-2681. doi:10.1182/blood-2016-01-690636
2. Steinman RM, Cohn ZA. Identification of a novel cell type in peripheral lymphoid organs of mice. I. Morphology, quantitation, tissue distribution. *J Exp Med.* 1973;137(5):1142-1162. doi:10.1084/jem.137.5.1142
3. Shortman K, Liu YJ. Mouse and human dendritic cell subtypes. *Nat Rev Immunol.* 2002;2(3):151-161. doi:10.1038/nri746
4. Bonometti A, Ferrario G, Parafioriti A, et al. MAP2K1-driven mixed Langerhans cell histiocytosis, Rosai-Dorfman-Destombes disease and Erdheim-Chester disease, clonally related to acute myeloid leukemia. *J Cutan Pathol.* 2021;48(5):637-643. doi:10.1111/cup.13918
5. Hoeffel G, Ginhoux F. Fetal monocytes and the origins of tissue-resident macrophages. *Cell Immunol.* 2018;330:5-15. doi:10.1016/j.cellimm.2018.01.001
6. Segura E. Human dendritic cell subsets: an updated view of their ontogeny and functional specialization. *Eur J Immunol.* 2022;52(11):1759-1767. doi:10.1002/eji.202149632
7. Villar J, Segura E. Decoding the heterogeneity of human dendritic cell subsets. *Trends Immunol.* 2020;41(12):1062-1071. doi:10.1016/j.it.2020.10.002
8. Ziegler-Heitbrock L, Ohteki T, Ginhoux F, Shortman K, Spits H. Reclassifying plasmacytoid dendritic cells as innate lymphocytes. *Nat Rev Immunol.* 2023;23(1):1-2. doi:10.1038/s41577-022-00806-0
9. Collin M, Milne P. Langerhans cell origin and regulation. *Curr Opin Hematol.* 2016;23(1):28-35. doi:10.1097/MOH.0000000000000202
10. Allen CE, Merad M, McClain KL. Langerhans-cell histiocytosis. *N Engl J Med.* 2018;379(9):856-868. doi:10.1056/NEJMra1607548
11. Emile JF, Cohen-Aubart F, Collin M, et al. Histiocytosis. *Lancet.* 2021;398(10295):157-170. doi:10.1016/S0140-6736(21)00311-1
12. de Leval L, Alizadeh AA, Bergsagel PL, et al. Genomic profiling for clinical decision making in lymphoid neoplasms. *Blood.* 2022;140(21):2193-2227. doi:10.1182/blood.2022015854
13. Feldman AL, Arber DA, Pittaluga S, et al. Clonally related follicular lymphomas and histiocytic/dendritic cell sarcomas: evidence for transdifferentiation of the follicular lymphoma clone. *Blood.* 2008;111(12):5433-5439. doi:10.1182/blood-2007-11-124792

14. Egan C, Lack J, Skarshaug S, et al. The mutational landscape of histiocytic sarcoma associated with lymphoid malignancy. *Mod Pathol.* 2021;34(2):336-347. doi:10.1038/s41379-020-00673-x
15. Shao H, Xi L, Raffeld M, et al. Clonally related histiocytic/dendritic cell sarcoma and chronic lymphocytic leukemia/small lymphocytic lymphoma: a study of seven cases. *Mod Pathol.* 2011;24(11):1421-1432. doi:10.1038/modpathol.2011.102
16. Castro EC, Blazquez C, Boyd J, et al. Clinicopathologic features of histiocytic lesions following ALL, with a review of the literature. *Pediatr Dev Pathol.* 2010;13(3):225-237. doi:10.2350/09-03-0622-OA.1
17. Feldman AL. Clonal relationships between malignant lymphomas and histiocytic/dendritic cell tumors. *Surg Pathol Clin.* 2013;6(4):619-629. doi:10.1016/j.path.2013.08.003
18. Aguzzi A, Kranich J, Krautler NJ. Follicular dendritic cells: origin, phenotype, and function in health and disease. *Trends Immunol.* 2014;35(3):105-113. doi:10.1016/j.it.2013.11.001
19. Li L, Wu J, Abdi R, Jewell CM, Bromberg JS. Lymph node fibroblastic reticular cells steer immune responses. *Trends Immunol.* 2021;42(8):723-734. doi:10.1016/j.it.2021.06.006

Chapter 115
Histiocytic Sarcoma

Stefano A. Pileri, Caoimhe Egan, and Jason L. Hornick

Definition

Histiocytic sarcoma (HS) is a malignant neoplasm with the morphological and immunophenotypic characteristics of mature tissue histiocytes/macrophages. Neoplastic proliferations associated with acute monocytic leukemia are excluded from this diagnosis.

Synonyms

Primary or secondary malignant histiocytosis, histiocytic subtype (Revised Classification of the Histiocyte Society, 2016) (not recommended).[1] True histiocytic lymphoma (now obsolete).

Epidemiology

HS is an extremely rare condition with a reported incidence of 0.17 per 1,000,000 adults in one study.[2] There is a slight male predominance, although significant variability is present in reported male to female ratios across cohorts. It mostly occurs in adults in the fifth or sixth decades and is also occasionally observed in children.

General Clinical Features

HS has an extranodal, nodal, and systemic presentation in about 55%, 27%, and 18% of cases, respectively. Extranodal presentations may involve the gastrointestinal tract, skin, and soft tissues. Hepato/splenomegaly and pancytopenia are usually recorded in systemic cases. The tumor may present with a solitary mass, and there may be systemic symptoms including fever and loss of weight. HS can occur de novo (primary HS) or be associated in about 20% of cases with a prior or metachronous lymphoid malignancy (secondary HS) usually a B-cell lymphoma, particularly follicular lymphoma or chronic lymphocytic leukemia/small lymphocytic lymphoma. More rarely, it is associated with T- or B-lymphoblastic leukemia, T-cell lymphoma or myelodysplasia. A subset of cases present in patients with a history of mediastinal germ cell tumor, most frequently a malignant teratoma, with or without a yolk sac tumor component.

Morphology

HS shows a cohesive and diffuse growth pattern, although it can diffuse through sinuses in the lymph node, liver, and spleen. It consists of large, predominantly epithelioid cells characterized by a central or eccentric round-oval nucleus with finely dispersed chromatin and multiple small nucleoli and a wide rim of acidophilic cytoplasm (Figure 115.1A). The number of mitotic figures is highly variable (10-30/10 HPF). At times, HS shows marked pleomorphism with fusiform and giant cells and striking mitotic activity (Figure 115.1B). Hemophagocytosis is minimal or absent, conversely to what is seen in hemophagocytic lymphohistiocytosis. Foci with a xanthomatous appearance can occasionally be detected (Figure 115.2). A variable number of reactive cells may be seen, including small lymphocytes, plasma cells, benign histiocytes, and eosinophils. Occasionally, the neoplastic cells are obscured by a heavy inflammatory infiltrate; this feature is particularly described in HS involving the central nervous system. The differential diagnosis includes diffuse large B-cell lymphoma, anaplastic large cell lymphoma, follicular dendritic cell sarcoma, melanoma, and carcinoma. Immunohistochemistry plays a pivotal role in the correct interpretation.

On electron microscopy, neoplastic cells show abundant cytoplasm with numerous lysosomes. Birbeck granules and cell junctions are not detected.

Immunophenotype

Neoplastic cells express one or more histiocytic markers including CD68 (as detected by both KP1 and PG-M1 antibodies), CD163, CD14, CD11c, lysozyme (in a granular fashion, corresponding to lysosomes on electron microscopy, at times the staining being accentuated in the Golgi area), CD4 (in about 50% of cases), and PU.1 (SPI1).[3] Other markers expressed include CD45RO, HLA-DR, CD45 (in most instances),

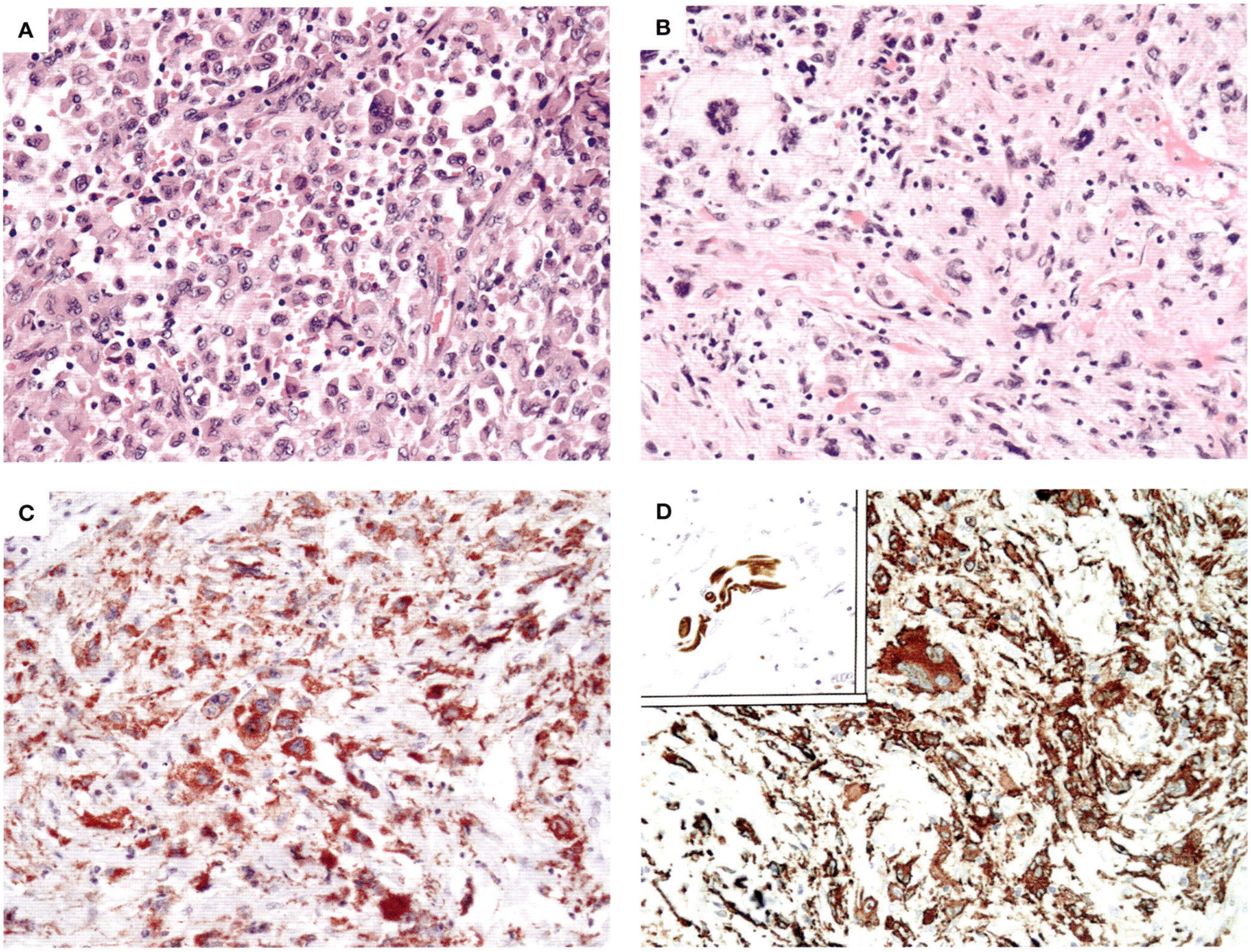

FIGURE 115.1 Histiocytic sarcoma. **A:** Intrasinusoidal diffusion in a lymph node, mimicking metastatic carcinoma; **B:** soft tissue localization: neoplastic cells vary in shape, from giant to fusiform; **C:** CD68/PGM1 staining; **D:** CD163 positivity (in the inset: negativity for S-100; the nerve represents the internal control).

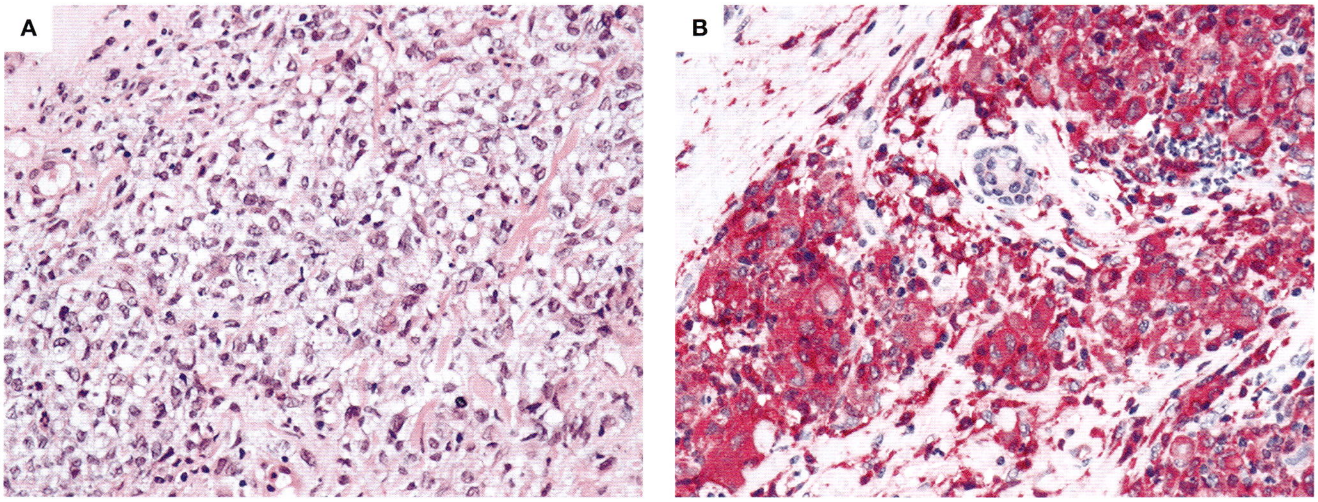

FIGURE 115.2 Histiocytic sarcoma. **A:** Skin involvement: neoplastic cells have a foamy appearance; **B:** in the same case, CD163 staining.

and S100 (weakly, if present) (Figure 115.1C and D). PD-L1 has been detected in some cases, a finding of potential therapeutic interest.[4] Other entities must be excluded, and HS is negative for B- and T-cell-specific markers (CD20, PAX5, CD19, CD3) and markers of Langerhans cells (CD1a, CD207/langerin), follicular dendritic cells (CD21, CD23, CD35), melanocytic cells (HMB.45, Melan A), and epithelial cells (cytokeratins). Myeloperoxidase, CD117, CD34, ALK protein, EBV, and CD30 (with rare exceptions) are also not expressed. The Ki-67 rate is variable (10%-50%).

Genetics

HS is characterized by frequent alterations in one or more genes of the MAPK pathway, including *KRAS, BRAF, MAP2K1, PTPN11, CBL, NRAS,* and *NF1*, as well as recurrent alterations in *CDKN2A, TP53,* and in genes of the PI3K-AKT-MTOR pathway, in particular *PTEN*.[5,6] Fusions involving *BRAF* and a *TPM3::NTRK1* fusion have also been described.

Clonal relatedness between secondary HS and a concurrent or previous B- or T-cell malignancy has been shown through the demonstration of identical immunoglobulin (IG) or T-cell receptor (TCR) genes rearrangements, common cytogenetic findings, and/or shared mutations in both tumors.[7] Evidence of a B-cell origin has also been shown in HS associated with B-cell lymphoma by the identification of somatic hypermutation or a mutational signature of somatic hypermutation in the HS. Cases of HS associated with follicular lymphoma have been shown to harbor the IGH::*BCL2* translocation and mutations in *CREBBP* or *KMT2D* that are shared with the lymphoma, suggesting origin of both tumors from a common precursor cell.[8] Evidence of divergent evolution between the HS and the associated malignancy may be apparent with differences in their respective molecular profiles, and the acquisition of a MAPK pathway mutation is associated with transdifferentiation to a histiocytic phenotype at least in some instances. HS harboring molecular alterations associated with B-cell lymphoma, or arising in patients with a history of B-cell lymphoma, is enriched for alterations in MAPK pathway genes and in *CDKN2A*.[8]

Occasional cases of apparently sporadic HS without a history of antecedent B-cell lymphoma have also been shown to carry clonal IG rearrangements and mutations in genes that are frequently mutated in B-cell malignancy and to have evidence of a mutational signature of aberrant somatic hypermutation suggesting that some primary HS may develop from a progenitor with B-lineage potential or arise in the setting of an occult B-cell neoplasm.

The rare cases arising in association with a mediastinal germ cell tumor may show an identical isochromosome 12p to the germ cell tumor or have other shared molecular alterations indicating a common clonal origin, such as shared *TP53* mutations.[9]

Prognosis and Clinical Comment

HS is an aggressive neoplasm, the optimal treatment of which still represents an unmet clinical need. More than half of patients experience rapid progression and die, reflecting the high stage at presentation (III/IV). About 30% achieve complete remission with CHOP/CHOP-like therapies, but usually relapse and die. Only 20% of individuals with HS are alive on long-term follow-up: they usually presented with a single mass and small tumor burden. In the era of targeted therapy, some case reports have documented a clinical or radiological response to treatments targeting the MAP kinase pathway including BRAF and MEK inhibitors such as trametinib, dabrafenib, and vemurafenib in patients with *MAP2K1, PTPN11,* and *BRAF*-mutated HS.[10] Immune checkpoint inhibitors have also been used with variable success.

References

1. Emile JF, Abla O, Fraitag S, et al. Revised classification of histiocytoses and neoplasms of the macrophage-dendritic cell lineages. *Blood*. 2016;127(22):2672-2681.
2. Kommalapati A, Tella SH, Durkin M, Go RS, Goyal G. Histiocytic sarcoma: a population-based analysis of incidence, demographic disparities, and long-term outcomes. *Blood*. 2018;131(2):265-268.
3. Pileri SA, Grogan TM, Harris NL, et al. Tumours of histiocytes and accessory dendritic cells: an immunohistochemical approach to classification from the International Lymphoma Study Group based on 61 cases. *Histopathology*. 2002;41(1):1-29.
4. Facchetti F, Pileri SA, Lorenzi L, et al. Histiocytic and dendritic cell neoplasms: what have we learnt by studying 67 cases. *Virchows Arch*. 2017;471(4):467-489.
5. Massoth LR, Hung YP, Ferry JA, et al. Histiocytic and dendritic cell sarcomas of hematopoietic origin share targetable genomic alterations distinct from follicular dendritic cell sarcoma. *Oncologist*. 2021;26(7):e1263-e1272.
6. Shanmugam V, Griffin GK, Jacobsen ED, Fletcher CDM, Sholl LM, Hornick JL. Identification of diverse activating mutations of the RAS-MAPK pathway in histiocytic sarcoma. *Mod Pathol*. 2019;32(6):830-843.

7. Feldman AL, Arber DA, Pittaluga S, et al. Clonally related follicular lymphomas and histiocytic/dendritic cell sarcomas: evidence for transdifferentiation of the follicular lymphoma clone. *Blood*. 2008;111(12):5433-5439.
8. Egan C, Lack J, Skarshaug S, et al. The mutational landscape of histiocytic sarcoma associated with lymphoid malignancy. *Mod Pathol*. 2021;34(2):336-347.
9. Taylor J, Donoghue MT, Ho C, et al. Germ cell tumors and associated hematologic malignancies evolve from a common shared precursor. *J Clin Invest*. 2020;130(12):6668-6676.
10. Tzankov A, Kremer M, Leguit R, et al. Histiocytic cell neoplasms involving the bone marrow: summary of the workshop cases submitted to the 18th Meeting of the European Association for Haematopathology (EAHP) organized by the European Bone Marrow Working Group, Basel 2016. *Ann Hematol*. 2018;97(11):2117-2128.

Chapter 116

Langerhans Cell Histiocytosis

Stefano A. Pileri, Carl E. Allen, and Alberto Zamò

Definition

Langerhans cell histiocytosis (LCH) is a clonal neoplastic proliferation of myeloid dendritic cells that express a mature Langerhans cell phenotype (eg, $CD207^{+}$) in lesions. The cell of origin is closer to a myeloid dendritic cell than to an epidermal Langerhans cell.[1]

Synonyms

Langerhans cell granulomatosis; histiocytosis X; eosinophilic granuloma; Hand–Schüller–Christian disease; Letterer-Siwe disease (not recommended).

Epidemiology

The annual incidence in children is about five cases per 1 million, whereas in adults it is one to two cases per 1 million people. The M:F ratio is 1 to 2:1. The disease is more common among individuals of European descent and Hispanics. LCH can also be associated with Erdheim-Chester disease or other histiocytic disorders, either concomitantly or asynchronously, with shared molecular alterations.[2-5]

General Clinical Features

LCH can be unifocal or multifocal within a single system or can be multisystemic. Unifocal LCH preferentially affects older children and adults, while multifocal LCH occurs preferentially in young children, and multisystem LCH is seen preferentially in infants. Single-system LCH predominantly involves the bone (skull, femur, vertebrae, pelvis, ribs, and mandible) and less commonly lymph nodes, skin, and lungs. In multisystemic LCH, the skin, bone, liver, spleen, and bone marrow are preferentially involved. Diabetes insipidus occurs in case of hypothalamic pituitary involvement. In multisystem LCH, cutaneous lesions may precede visceral compromise. The gonads and kidney appear to be spared even in disseminated cases.[2]

Morphology

On microscopic grounds (Figure 116.1A and B), LCH cells are oval and measure 10 to 15 µm. Their nuclei are characteristically grooved, folded, indented, or lobed, with fine chromatin, inconspicuous nucleoli, and thin nuclear membranes. Nuclear atypia is minimal, but mitotic activity is variable. The cytoplasm is abundant, slightly eosinophilic, and devoid of dendritic processes. The characteristic inflammatory milieu includes variable numbers of eosinophils, histiocytes, multinucleated giant cells, neutrophils, small lymphocytes, and plasma cells. Occasionally, eosinophilic microabscesses with central necrosis are found. In late lesions, LCH cells are decreased in number, with increased foamy macrophages and fibrosis.[6]

Involved lymph nodes have a sinus pattern with secondary infiltration of the paracortex. Spleen shows nodular red pulp involvement. Liver involvement has strong preference for intrahepatic biliary involvement with progressive sclerosing cholangitis. Bone marrow biopsy is preferred to aspiration for documentation of bone marrow involvement. Notably, LCH cells in bone marrow, liver, and brain may not express CD1a or CD207, but may be identified by immunohistochemistry for $BRAF^{V600E}$ with the VE-1 stain.[7,8] Large clusters or sheets of LCH cells accompanied by eosinophils can be found within other neoplastic lesions. They can represent a local reactive phenomenon or else the result of a transdifferentiation process (see below for follicular lymphoma and B- or T-lymphoblastic leukemia).[9,10]

The ultrastructural hallmark of LCH is the cytoplasmic Birbeck granule, which is 200 to 400 nm long and 33 nm wide, with a tennis-racket shape and a zipper-like appearance.[6]

Immunophenotype

LCH cells express the phenotype of mature LCs (Figure 116.1C and D), staining positive for CD1a, CD207/langerin, S100 protein, CD68, and HLA-DR. CD45 and lysozyme expression is low. B- and T-cell lineage markers (except for CD4), CD30, and follicular

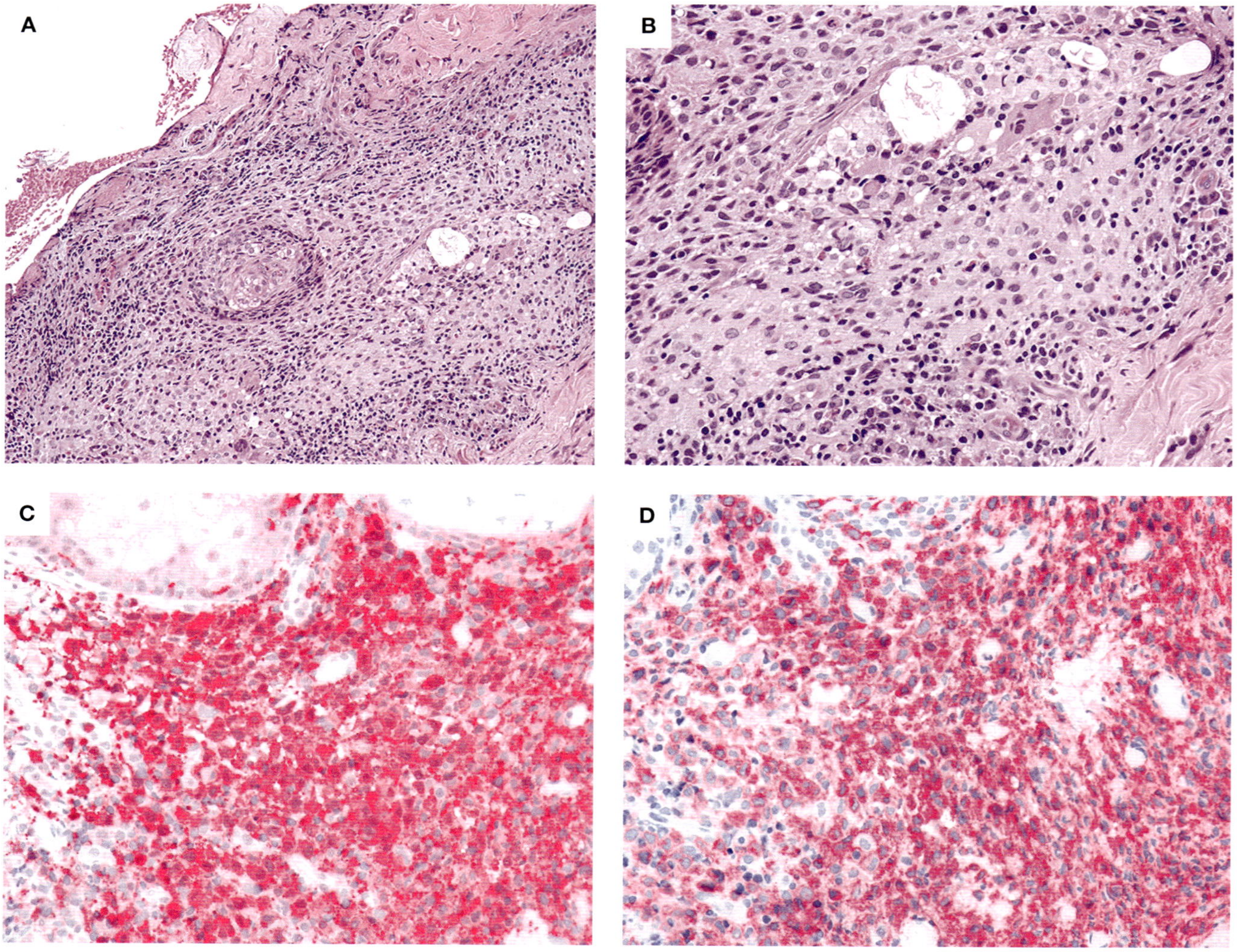

FIGURE 116.1 Cutaneous involvement by LCH. **A:** low magnification (H&E), **B:** cytological details (H&E), **C:** positivity for S100 protein, and **D:** Langerin.

dendritic cell markers are absent.[2,6] The *BRAF* V600E mutation can be identified by a specific antibody.[8] The Ki-67 proliferation index is typically comparable to background immune cells. PD-L1 is expressed in a percentage of cases; it can represent the target for immune checkpoint inhibitors.[11] OCT2 is positive in about 40% of cases, more commonly with weak staining intensity.[12]

Genetics

A misguided myeloid differentiation model has been proposed, in which the occurrence of activating MAPK pathway mutations either in a pluripotent hematopoietic, or in a tissue-restricted/local precursor drive high-risk multisystemic, multifocal low-risk, or unifocal LCH, respectively. These mutations, especially $BRAF^{V600E}$, may confer an advantage for tissue site accumulation via disrupted cell migration and apoptosis.[1,2]

LCH has been shown to be clonal by X-linked androgen receptor gene assay (HUMARA), except in some adult pulmonary lesions. Familial clustering has shown a high concordance rate for identical twins but not dizygotic twins, and no vertical inheritance. Rare familial cases are reported.[3] MAPK pathway gene mutations are identified in >85% of cases, and phospo-extracellular signal-regulated kinases is observed in almost all cases, representing the rationale for the therapeutic usage of specific inhibitors. Mutations affect *BRAF* (Figure 116.2) or alternatively *MAP2K1* or much more rarely *ARAF*, *ERBB3*, *NRAS*, and *KRAS*.[1-5,7,8] About 30% of the cases show clonal IGH, IGK, and/or TCR gene rearrangements.[13] Cases associated with follicular lymphoma or B- or T-lymphoblastic leukemia are considered examples of transdifferentiation and behave more aggressively.[9]

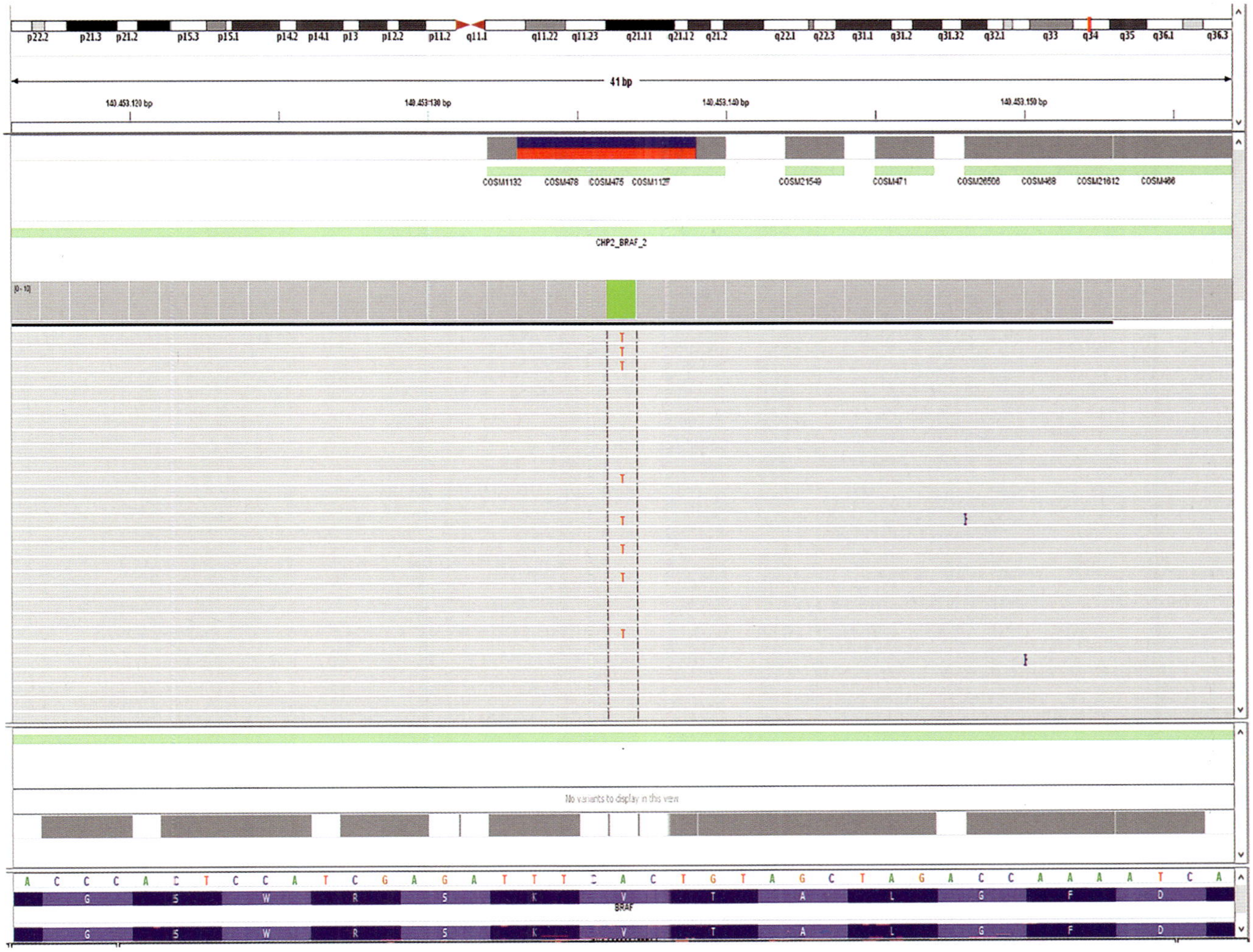

FIGURE 116.2 Detection of *BRAF*^{V600E} mutation by NGS.

Prognosis and Clinical Comments

The clinical course is related to staging at presentation, with a ≥99% survival rate for unifocal disease and >80% survival in cases with critical organ involvement (brain, liver, lung or bone marrow). Progression from initially focal to multisystem LCH can occur, most commonly in infants with hypothalamic pituitary involvement. Multisystem LCH can be complicated by macrophage activation syndrome. *BRAF* mutation is correlated with increased relapse risk and potentially worse clinical parameters, including resistance to first-line therapy and neurodegenerative CNS LCH.[14,15] Neurodegenerative CNS LCH is associated with the presence of *BRAF*^{V600E}+ myeloid cells, clonally related to systemic LCH lesion, in the brain.[16] In previously diagnosed LCH patients with *BRAF* mutation, additional systemic lesions demonstrating *BRAF*–positive, CD1a/CD207-negative histiocytes may still represent active disease.[17]

Langerhans Cell Sarcoma

Langerhans cell sarcoma (LCS) is an extremely rare high-grade neoplasm, characterized by overt cytologic atypia (Figure 116.3A). It has been mainly reported in adults with a female predominance. It more often occurs at extranodal sites (skin and soft tissue), although also lymph nodes, lung, spleen, liver, and bone may be involved. It is more commonly a multifocal disease.[6]

LCS shows the same phenotypic, ultrastructural and molecular characteristics as LCH (Figure 116.3B). However, LCS consists of frankly atypical large cells with prominent nucleoli, with only a few being still recognizable as LCH cells. The number of mitotic figures (often atypical) is high as is the Ki-67 index.[6] Unlike LCH, LCS is associated with recurrent loss of *CDK2NA* and *TP53* mutations.[18] It can also arise as a transdifferentiation phenomenon related to a lymphoid tumor. Diffusion through sinuses can be observed in

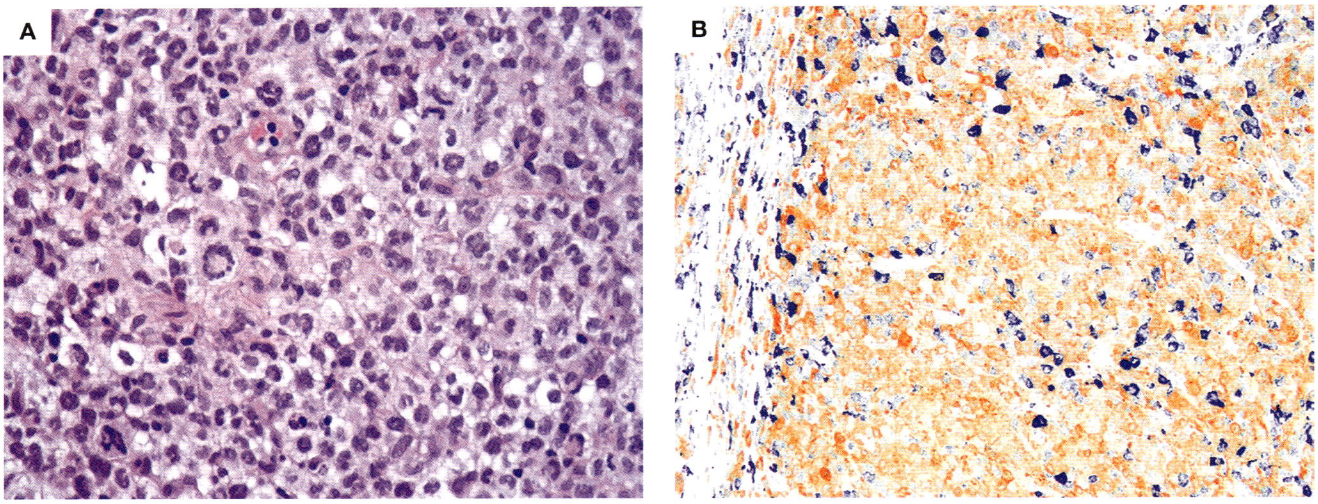

FIGURE 116.3 Langerhans cell sarcoma. **A:** The population is characterized by overt cytological atypia (H/E); **B:** double staining showing positivity for CD68 and Langerin (CD68, brown; langerin, blue).

the lymph nodes, liver, and spleen. LCS is a highly aggressive tumor. Half of the patients die of progressive disease. Forty percent of them respond to high-dose chemotherapies but quite soon relapse and die. Only a few are alive on the long-term follow-up.[6]

References

1. Allen CE, Li L, Peters TL, et al. Cell-specific gene expression in Langerhans cell histiocytosis lesions reveals a distinct profile compared with epidermal Langerhans cells. *J Immunol*. 2010;184(8):4557-4567.
2. Allen CE, Merad M, McClain KL. Langerhans-cell histiocytosis. *N Engl J Med*. 2018;379(9):856-868.
3. Emile JF, Abla O, Fraitag S, et al. Revised classification of histiocytoses and neoplasms of the macrophage-dendritic cell lineages. *Blood*. 2016;127(22):2672-2681.
4. McClain KL, Bigenwald C, Collin M, et al. Histiocytic disorders. *Nat Rev Dis Primers*. 2021;7(1):73-131.
5. Friedman JS, Durham BH, Reiner AS, et al. Mixed histiocytic neoplasms: a multicentre series revealing diverse somatic mutations and responses to targeted therapy. *Br J Haematol*. 2024;205(1):127-137.
6. Pileri SA, Grogan TM, Harris NL, et al. Tumours of histiocytes and accessory dendritic cells: an immunohistochemical approach to classification from the International Lymphoma Study Group based on 61 cases. *Histopathology*. 2002;41(1):1-29.
7. Berres ML, Lim KP, Peters T, et al. BRAF-V600E expression in precursor versus differentiated dendritic cells defines clinically distinct LCH risk groups. *J Exp Med*. 2014;211(4):669-683.
8. Ballester LY, Cantu MD, Lim KPH, et al. The use of BRAF V600E mutation-specific immunohistochemistry in pediatric Langerhans cell histiocytosis. *Hematol Oncol*. 2018;36(1):307-315.
9. Feldman AL, Berthold F, Arceci RJ, et al. Clonal relationship between precursor T-lymphoblastic leukaemia/lymphoma and Langerhans-cell histiocytosis. *Lancet Oncol*. 2005;6(6):435-437.
10. West DS, Dogan A, Quint PS, et al. Clonally related follicular lymphomas and Langerhans cell neoplasms: expanding the spectrum of transdifferentiation. *Am J Surg Pathol*. 2013;37(7):978-986.
11. Tandon S, Weitzman S, Joyce B, et al. Expression and clinical correlation of PD-1/PD-L1 and VE1(BRAFp.V600E) in pediatric Langerhans cell histiocytosis. *Mediterr J Hematol Infect Dis*. 2023;15(1):e2023035.
12. Ungureanu IA, Cohen-Aubart F, Héritier S, et al. OCT2 expression in histiocytoses. *Virchows Arch*. 2023;483(1):81-86.
13. Chen W, Wang J, Wang E, et al. Detection of clonal lymphoid receptor gene rearrangements in Langerhans cell histiocytosis. *Am J Surg Pathol*. 2010;34(7):1049-1057.
14. Héritier S, Emile JF, Barkaoui MA, et al. BRAF mutation correlates with high-risk langerhans cell histiocytosis and increased resistance to first-line therapy. *J Clin Oncol*. 2016;34(25):3023-3030.
15. Nann D, Schneckenburger P, Steinhilber J, et al. Pediatric langerhans cell histiocytosis: the impact of mutational profile on clinical progression and late sequelae. *Ann Hematol*. 2019;98(7):1617-1626.
16. McClain KL, Picarsic J, Chakraborty R, et al. CNS Langerhans cell histiocytosis: common hematopoietic origin for LCH-associated neurodegeneration and mass lesions. *Cancer*. 2018;124(12):2607-2620.
17. Lee LH, Gasilina A, Roychoudhury J, et al. Real-time genomic profiling of histiocytoses identifies early-kinase domain BRAF alterations while improving treatment outcomes. *JCI Insight*. 2017;2(3):e89473.
18. Massoth LR, Hung YP, Ferry JA, et al. Histiocytic and dendritic cell sarcomas of hematopoietic origin share targetable genomic alterations distinct from follicular dendritic cell sarcoma. *Oncologist*. 2021;26(7):e1263-e1272.

Chapter 117
Indeterminate Dendritic Cell Histiocytosis

Neval Ozkaya and Elaine S. Jaffe

Definition

Indeterminate dendritic cell histiocytosis (IDCH) is a rare histiocytic neoplasm histologically and immunophenotypically resembling Langerhans cell histiocytosis (LCH), positive for CD1a and S100 protein, but lacking Birbeck granules and/or Langerin/CD207 expression.[1] It was initially reported as a skin-limited disorder but can also occur in extracutaneous sites.[1-3]

Synonyms

Indeterminate cell histiocytosis, indeterminate dendritic cell tumor (both acceptable).

Epidemiology

The disease is more common in adults than in children (ratio approximately 5:1) and in males than in females (ratio approximately 2:1). A subset of cases occurs in infants. No definite ethnic or racial predisposition has been reported.[3]

General Clinical Features

The median age at diagnosis is 70 years. Cutaneous involvement is most common (approximately 70% of the cases) and can be in the form of single, multifocal, or generalized papules and/or nodules. Lymph node involvement has been reported in approximately one-third of the patients, with a small subset having both lymph node and cutaneous involvement. A few patients have been reported with involvement of other extranodal sites: colon, lung, spleen, bone, thyroid, and parotid. Approximately half of the cases arise in the setting of other hematolymphoid neoplasms (so-called secondary IDCH) with underlying myeloid diseases being more common than those of lymphoid origin. Patients with secondary IDCH tend to be older than patients with primary IDCH.[3,4]

Morphology

The histiocytes have single indented or folded nuclei and abundant eosinophilic cytoplasm resembling LCH (Figure 117.1A). However, unlike LCH, admixed eosinophils are rare to absent. In the skin biopsies, the neoplastic cells demonstrate infiltration within the superficial and deep dermis, mostly without epidermotropism. Occasionally, focal epidermal ulceration or epidermotropism can be seen. IDCH should be distinguished from cases of histiocytic sarcoma, which can occasionally exhibit a dendritic cell or Langerhans cell phenotype with expression of S100, CD1a,[5] and rarely Langerin.[6,7]

Immunophenotype

The neoplastic cells are consistently positive for CD1a and CD4, while negative for Langerin/CD207 (Figure 117.1B and C).[3] S100 protein is at least focally positive in most cases (Figure 117.1D), but its negativity does not exclude IDCH.[3,4] Expression of CD68 and/or CD163 can be seen in subset of the cases, but strong and uniform expression should raise concern for another histiocytic neoplasm. Some cases may show partial expression for Langerin/CD207 in lesional cells. This feature is seen most often in cases closely resembling LCH histologically and at the genomic level. As there are no established criteria for the percent of cells with langerin positivity in LCH, such cases might be considered LCH in the appropriate setting.[3]

Genetics

MAPK pathway alterations including point mutations or fusions are common in both primary and secondary IDCH cases. Mutually exclusive *KRAS* and *BRAF* V600E mutations are the most common. Although *KRAS* mutations are slightly more enriched in secondary IDCH in comparison with *BRAF* alterations, neither is exclusive for primary or secondary IDCH. More than half of the cases harbor additional

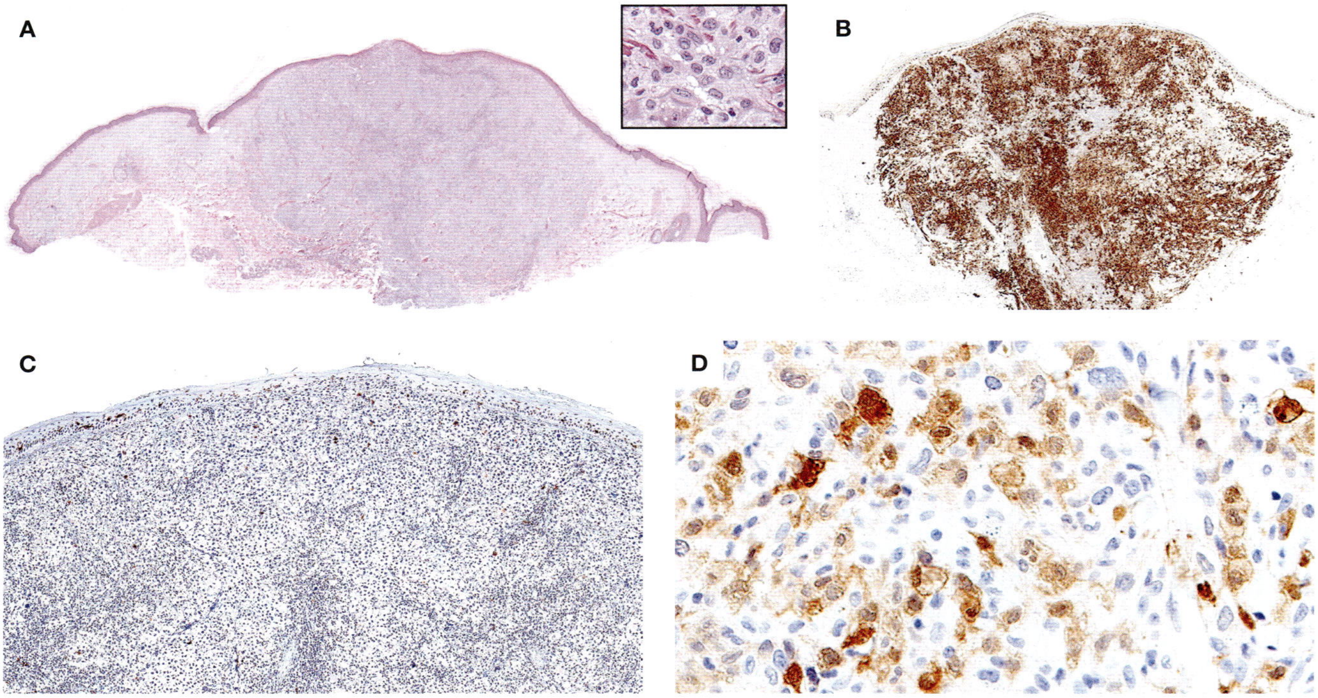

FIGURE 117.1 **A:** Skin involvement is very common in indeterminate dendritic cell histiocytosis. The infiltrate forms a nodular lesion in the superficial dermis. No epidermotropism is seen. The inset shows the typical cytological features. The cells have bland chromatin and grooved nuclei resembling Langerhans cells. **B:** The lesional cells are strongly positive for CD1a. **C:** Langerin is entirely negative in the lesional cells, but a few normal Langerhans cells are seen in the epidermis. **D:** There is partial positivity for S100.

myeloid neoplasm-associated mutations such as *TET2* and *DNMT3A* even in the absence of an overt myeloid malignancy.[3] Less frequently, an isolated *ETV3::NCOA2* fusion has been detected in IDCH; positive cases are associated with distinct clinicopathologic features including isolated skin involvement with absence of epidermotropism, complete absence of Langerin/CD207 expression, and absence of additional myeloid neoplasm-associated mutations. The *ETV3::NCOA2* fusion has been reported only in primary IDCH cases, both in the adult and pediatric age groups.[3,8]

Prognosis and Clinical Comment

Primary IDCH is an extremely indolent disease. In contrast, secondary IDCH cases generally have a poorer prognosis, which is generally linked to the subtype of accompanying hematologic neoplasm. The described treatment strategies in the literature are highly heterogeneous and hard to standardize. Some patients with primary IDCH were cured with surgical excision, while patients with secondary IDCH required systemic chemotherapy with dismal outcomes.[2-4]

References

1. Wood GS, Hu CH, Beckstead JH, Turner RR, Winkelmann RK. The indeterminate cell proliferative disorder: report of a case manifesting as an unusual cutaneous histiocytosis. *J Dermatol Surg Oncol.* 1985;11(11):1111-1119.
2. Rezk SA, Spagnolo DV, Brynes RK, Weiss LM. Indeterminate cell tumor: a rare dendritic neoplasm. *Am J Surg Pathol.* 2008;32(12):1868-1876.
3. Ozkaya N, Melloul Benizri S, Venkataraman G, et al. Indeterminate DC histiocytosis is distinct from LCH and often associated with other hematopoietic neoplasms. *Blood Adv.* 2024. doi: 10.1182/bloodadvances.2024013545
4. Zanella S, Berti E, Bonometti A; for Associazione Italiana Ricerca Istiocitosi ONLUS. Indeterminate cell histiocytosis: a systematic review of the literature with a comprehensive revision of clinical, histopathological, and molecular features. *J Eur Acad Dermatol Venereol.* Published online 2023.
5. Shao H, Xi L, Raffeld M, et al. Clonally related histiocytic/dendritic cell sarcoma and chronic lymphocytic leukemia/small lymphocytic lymphoma: a study of seven cases. *Mod Pathol.* 2011;24(11):1421-1432.

6. West DS, Dogan A, Quint PS, et al. Clonally related follicular lymphomas and Langerhans cell neoplasms: expanding the spectrum of transdifferentiation. *Am J Surg Pathol.* 2013;37(7):978-986.
7. Feldman AL, Minniti C, Santi M, Downing JR, Raffeld M, Jaffe ES. Histiocytic sarcoma after acute lymphoblastic leukaemia: a common clonal origin. *Lancet Oncol.* 2004;5(4):248-250.
8. Brown RA, Kwong BY, McCalmont TH, et al. ETV3-NCOA2 in indeterminate cell histiocytosis: clonal translocation supports sui generis. *Blood.* 2015;126(20):2344-2345.

Chapter 118
Interdigitating Dendritic Cell Sarcoma

Andrew L. Feldman and Wayne Tam

Definition

Interdigitating dendritic cell sarcoma (IDCS) is a neoplasm of spindled to ovoid cells with a phenotype similar to normal interdigitating dendritic cells.

Synonyms

Interdigitating dendritic cell tumor (not recommended).

Epidemiology

IDCS is very rare and occurs mostly in adults (median age, 53-58 years).[1,2] The male:female ratio is 1.5 to 1.7:1. Occasional cases are associated with B- or T-cell lymphomas, possibly representing transdifferentiation.[1,3,4] The causes of IDCS are otherwise unknown.

General Clinical Features

Patients typically present with an asymptomatic mass, often involving a solitary lymph node.[1] Systemic B symptoms are occasionally present. Extranodal sites of presentation include skin, soft tissue, spleen, liver, and testis. About 30% of patients present with disseminated disease, usually generalized lymphadenopathy and hepatosplenomegaly.

Morphology

In lymph nodes, IDCS typically involves the paracortex and may spare residual follicles.[1,5] The neoplastic cells are most commonly spindled and arranged in a fascicular and storiform pattern, sometimes resembling follicular dendritic cell sarcoma (Figure 118.1A). Other

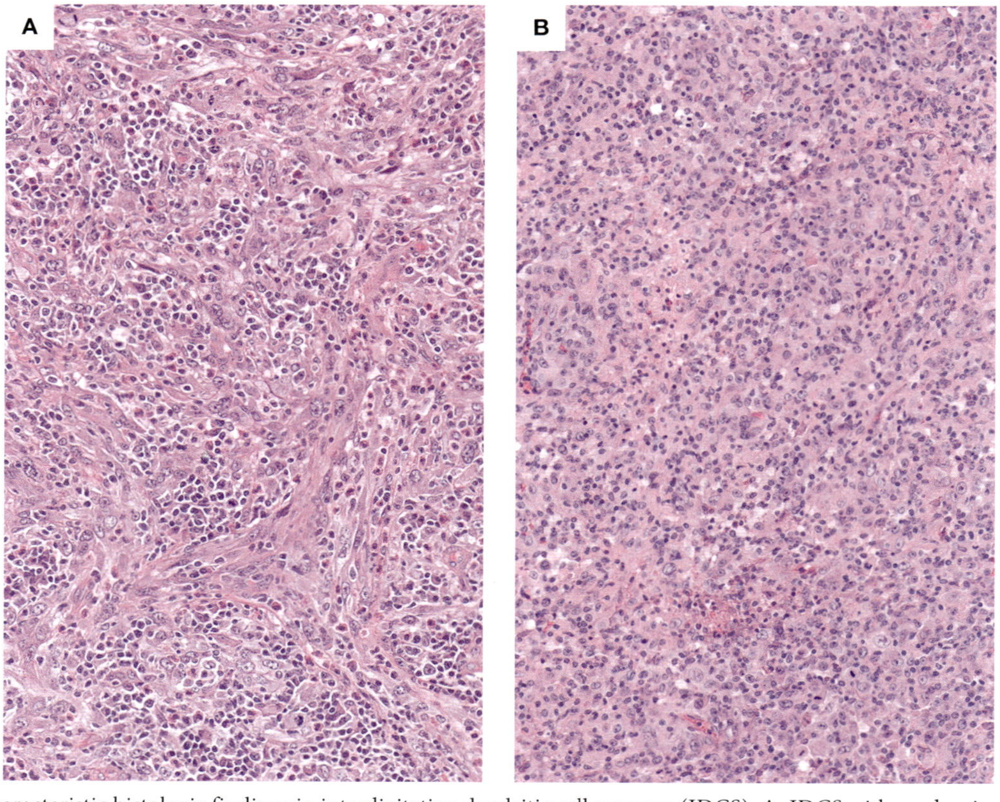

FIGURE 118.1 Characteristic histologic findings in interdigitating dendritic cell sarcoma (IDCS). **A:** IDCS with predominantly spindled neoplastic cells. **B:** IDCS with predominantly round to ovoid cells.

cases have predominantly ovoid cells, and occasionally sheets of round cells are present (Figure 118.1B). The cells show varying degrees of atypia and typically have abundant eosinophilic cytoplasm and oval nuclei with fine chromatin and distinct nucleoli. Multinucleated cells may be seen. Necrosis is generally absent. There are typically admixed small lymphocytes or, less frequently, plasma cells.

Immunophenotype

The tumor cells consistently express S100 (Figure 118.2A) and vimentin (Figure 118.2B) and often express fascin.[1,5] There is variable positivity for CD68 (Figure 118.2C), CD163 (Figure 118.2D), and CD45 (Figure 118.2E). Recent data suggest that cases expressing lysozyme and/or ZBTB46 may phenotypically resemble type 1 classical

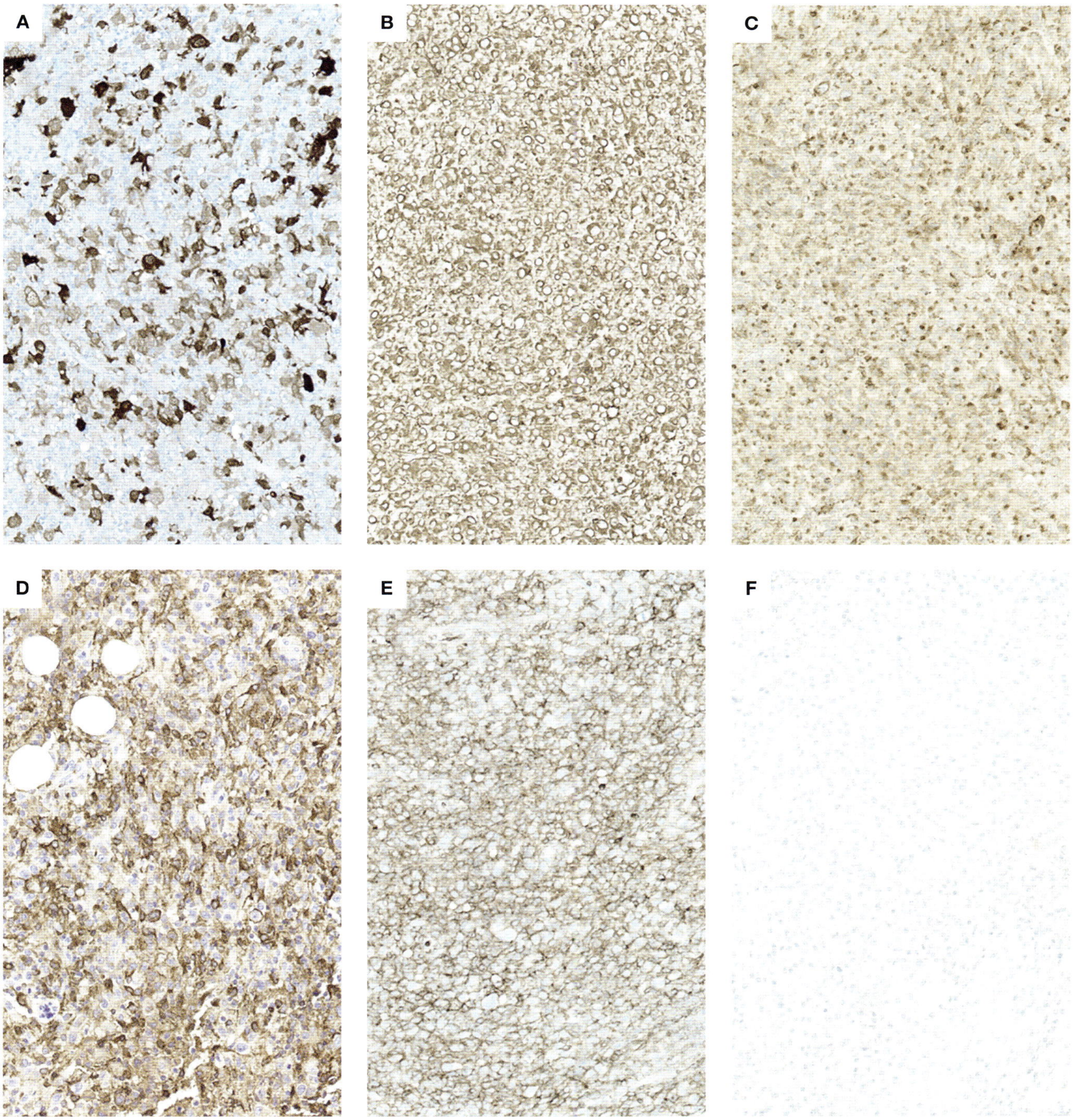

FIGURE 118.2 Characteristic phenotype of interdigitating dendritic cell sarcoma. Tumor shown in Figure 118.1B. The neoplastic cells are positive for S100 (**partial; A**), vimentin (**B**), CD68 (**C**), CD163 (partial; **D**), and CD45 (**E**). They are negative for CD1a (**F**).

dendritic cells (cDCs), while those expressing CD14 and/or OCT2 may resemble type 2 cDCs.[4] The tumor cells lack surface markers of B and T cells, Langerhans cells (CD1a [Figure 118.2F], langerin), and follicular dendritic cells (CD21, CD23, CD35), as well as CD30, CD34, MPO, EMA, and keratins. The proliferative rate by Ki-67 is typically 10% to 20%. The background small lymphocytes are characteristically T cells.

Genetics

Occasional cases may show monoclonal immunoglobulin gene rearrangements and/or *BCL2* rearrangements, particularly when associated with low-grade B-cell lymphoma (Figure 118.3).[3,4] More than half of IDCSs have mutations in MAPK pathway genes (eg, *NRAS*, *KRAS*, *MAP2K1*, *BRAF*), similar to other histiocytic and dendritic cell neoplasms.[4,6] Alterations of *TP53*, *TET2*, and *FBXW7* also have been reported.

Prognosis and Clinical Comment

Most cases are clinically aggressive, with a median overall survival (OS) of 35 months.[1,2] Optimal treatment is not well established, and 69% of patients relapse within 2 years. The mutational landscape suggests the possibility of targeted therapy with MAPK pathway inhibitors, but experience in IDCS is limited.[6,7] Clinical stage is an important prognostic factor, and patients presenting with disseminated disease have a median OS of only 10 months. Histological features have not been associated with outcome.

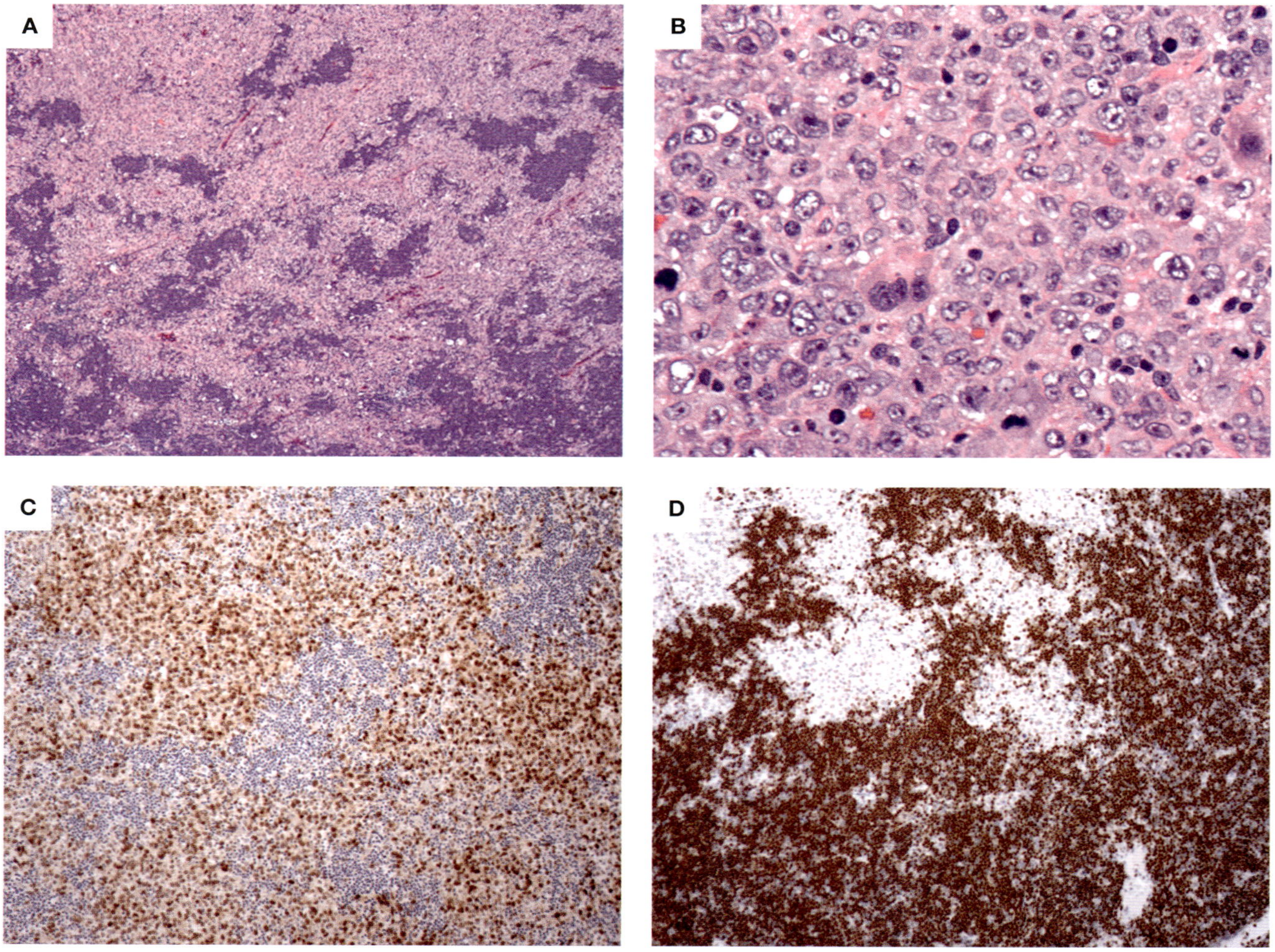

FIGURE 118.3 Interdigitating dendritic cell sarcoma (IDCS) clonally related to underlying chronic lymphocytic leukemia (CLL). **A:** Low-power image of lymph node, showing sheets and interconnecting cords of IDCS cells, with scattered islands of CLL cells. **B:** High-power image of IDCS cells, showing pleomorphic nuclei, sometimes with indentation or multilobation, and abundant cytoplasm. **C:** S100 is strongly positive in the IDCS cells. **D:** PAX5 highlights the CLL cells and is weakly positive in a subset of the IDCS cells. Both components showed identical IGH gene rearrangements and trisomy 12 (not shown).

References

1. Muhammed A, Ahmed ARH, Maysa H, Mohamed AES, Abd-El-Lateef AA, Elnakib E. New insights inside the interdigitating dendritic cell sarcoma-pooled analysis and review of literature. *Ann Hematol.* 2019;98(12):2641-2651.
2. Perkins SM, Shinohara ET. Interdigitating and follicular dendritic cell sarcomas: a SEER analysis. *Am J Clin Oncol.* 2013;36(4):395-398.
3. Feldman AL, Arber DA, Pittaluga S, et al. Clonally related follicular lymphomas and histiocytic/dendritic cell sarcomas: evidence for transdifferentiation of the follicular lymphoma clone. *Blood.* 2008;111(12):5433-5439.
4. Ravindran A, Dasari S, Ruan GJ, et al. Malignant histiocytosis comprises a phenotypic spectrum that parallels the lineage differentiation of monocytes, macrophages, dendritic cells, and Langerhans cells. *Mod Pathol.* 2023;36(10):100268.
5. Pileri SA, Grogan TM, Harris NL, et al. Tumours of histiocytes and accessory dendritic cells: an immunohistochemical approach to classification from the International Lymphoma Study Group based on 61 cases. *Histopathology.* 2002;41(1):1-29.
6. Massoth LR, Hung YP, Ferry JA, et al. Histiocytic and dendritic cell sarcomas of hematopoietic origin share targetable genomic alterations distinct from follicular dendritic cell sarcoma. *Oncologist.* 2021;26(7):e1263-e1272.
7. Di Liso E, Pennelli N, Lodovichetti G, et al. Braf mutation in interdigitating dendritic cell sarcoma: a case report and review of the literature. *Cancer Biol Ther.* 2015;16(8):1128-1135.

Chapter 119
ALK-Positive Histiocytosis

Elaine S. Jaffe and Benjamin H. Durham

Definition

ALK-positive histiocytosis is a non-Langerhans cell histiocytic neoplasm with overexpression of the ALK receptor tyrosine kinase based on the fusion involving *ALK* and a 5′ partner gene that is most commonly *KIF5B*.[1]

Synonyms

Xanthogranuloma (not recommended).

Epidemiology

The disease is most common in infants and children and is more common in females than in males (ratio approximately 2:1).[1-3] A subset of cases occurs in young adults, generally under 50 years of age.[4] No definite ethnic or racial predisposition has been reported to date.

General Clinical Features

Most cases in the pediatric age group present with multisystem disease, hepatosplenomegaly, and involvement of bone marrow.[2] Clinical manifestations include anemia, thrombocytopenia, and systemic symptoms.[5] Skin involvement has been reported but is not common. Neurological involvement is common, approximately 50%.[2,6] Patients with involvement of the central nervous system present with diverse symptomatology including seizures, ataxia, headache, and paresis. Infrequent presentations include localized disease involving bone, soft tissue, and skin (Figure 119.1). Adults may also present with multisystem disease but are more likely to present with isolated lesions involving breast, gastrointestinal tract, and soft tissue.[9,10] Involvement of lung and lymph nodes has been reported.

Morphology

The histological features resemble xanthogranuloma. The histiocytes have plump foamy cytoplasm.[2] However, the morphology is variable with some cases having cells with a more spindle-shaped appearance or epithelioid morphology (see Figure 119.1).[10,11] The nuclear features are generally bland with oval-to-indented nuclei, finely stippled chromatin, and small nucleoli. Touton-type giant cells may be present, and emperipolesis is occasionally seen.[3] However, other inflammatory cells including eosinophils are largely absent from the tissue microenvironment. A mildly fibrotic background is noted. The bone marrow is usually not diffusely involved. In the liver the cells tend to infiltrate the hepatic sinusoids.[1]

Immunophenotype

The cells display markers consistent with the histiocytic lineage with expression of CD4, CD68, CD163, and factor XIIIa.[3] Immunohistochemistry for ALK should identify cytoplasmic staining in the lesional cells. ALK immunostaining is recommended to be performed in all cases of *BRAF*^{V600E}-wild-type histiocytosis. S100 is positive in about 50% of cases, but CD1a and langerin are negative. Overexpression of OCT-2, p-ERK, and Cyclin D1 is often seen.[2]

Genetics

ALK rearrangements can be confirmed by RNA sequencing or fluorescence in situ hybridization (FISH) using an *ALK* break-apart probe (see Figure 119.1F). *KIF5B* (Kinesin Family Member 5B) serves as a microtubule-dependent motor involved in the normal distribution of mitochondria and lysosomes and is the most common 5′ fusion partner for *ALK* with several variable fusion breakpoints within *KIF5B* (most commonly involves exons 1-24), but *EML4::ALK*, *TPM3::ALK*, *SQSTM1::ALK*, *CLTC::ALK*, *TFG::ALK*, and *DCTN1::ALK* fusions have also been described (Figure 119.2). All the described ALK fusion proteins have an intact kinase domain (most commonly encoded by exons 20-27) fused with different 5′ partner genes where the N-terminal protein encoded by the 5′ partner gene has a coiled-coil or other heterodimerization domains. This can lead to ligand-independent

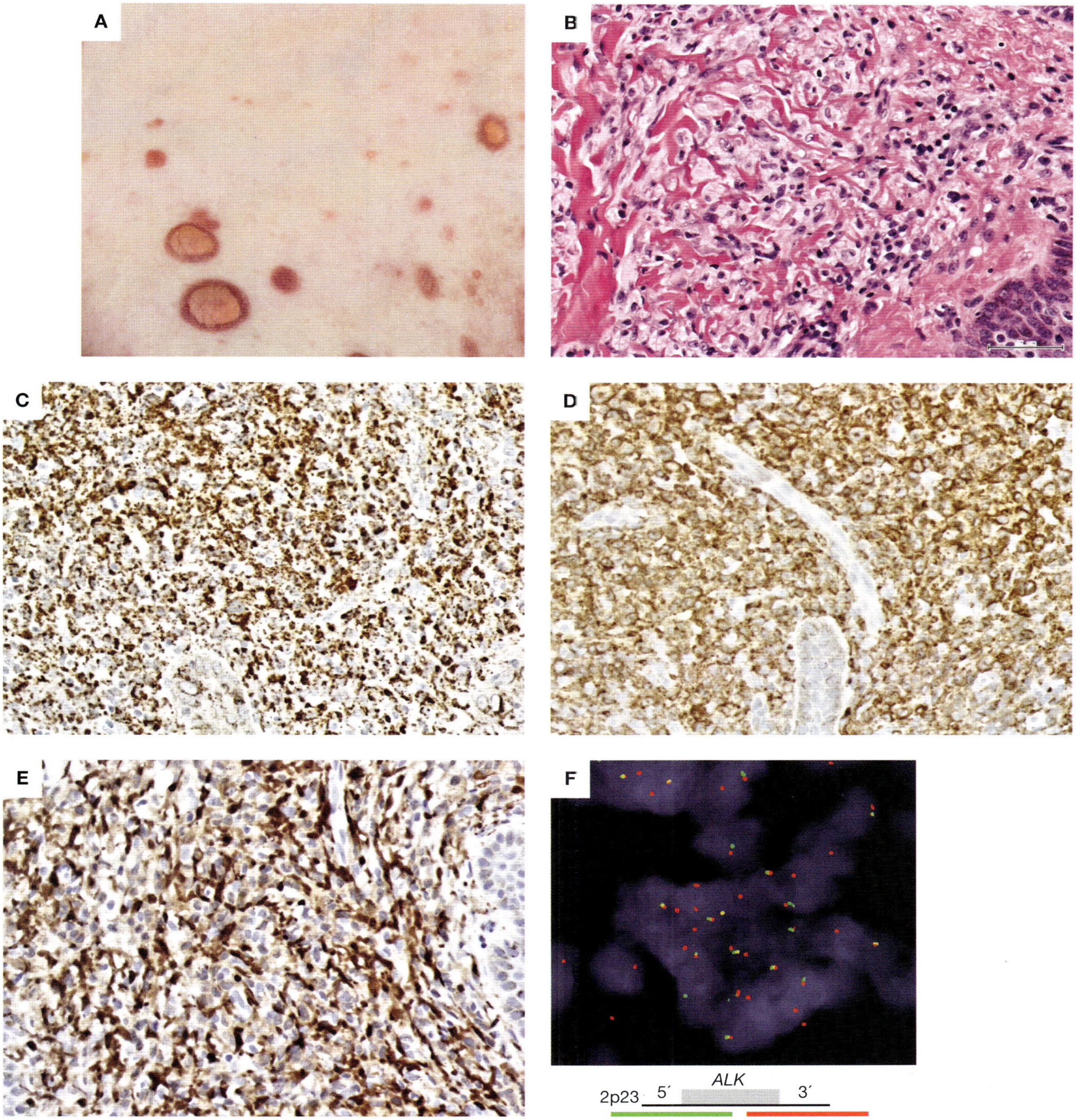

FIGURE 119.1 Example of clinical and histological features of ALK-positive histiocytosis. **A:** Diffuse xanthomatous skin lesions in a patient with multisystem involvement by *KIF5B::ALK*-rearranged histiocytosis. **B:** Xanthogranulomatous morphology with a monomorphic histiocytic infiltrate dissecting through the dermal collagen bundles (hematoxylin and eosin; original magnification ×400). **C:** CD68 immunohistochemical staining showing diffuse, granular cytoplasmic staining in the lesional histiocytes (original magnification ×400). **D:** CD163 immunohistochemical staining demonstrating strong, diffuse expression by the monomorphic histiocytic infiltrate (original magnification ×400). **E:** ALK immunohistochemical staining with strong cytoplasmic and membranous overexpression by the neoplastic histiocytes (original magnification ×400). **F:** *ALK* FISH break-apart probe (schematic beneath image) reveals an isolated red signal confirming the translocation of *ALK*.[2,7,8]

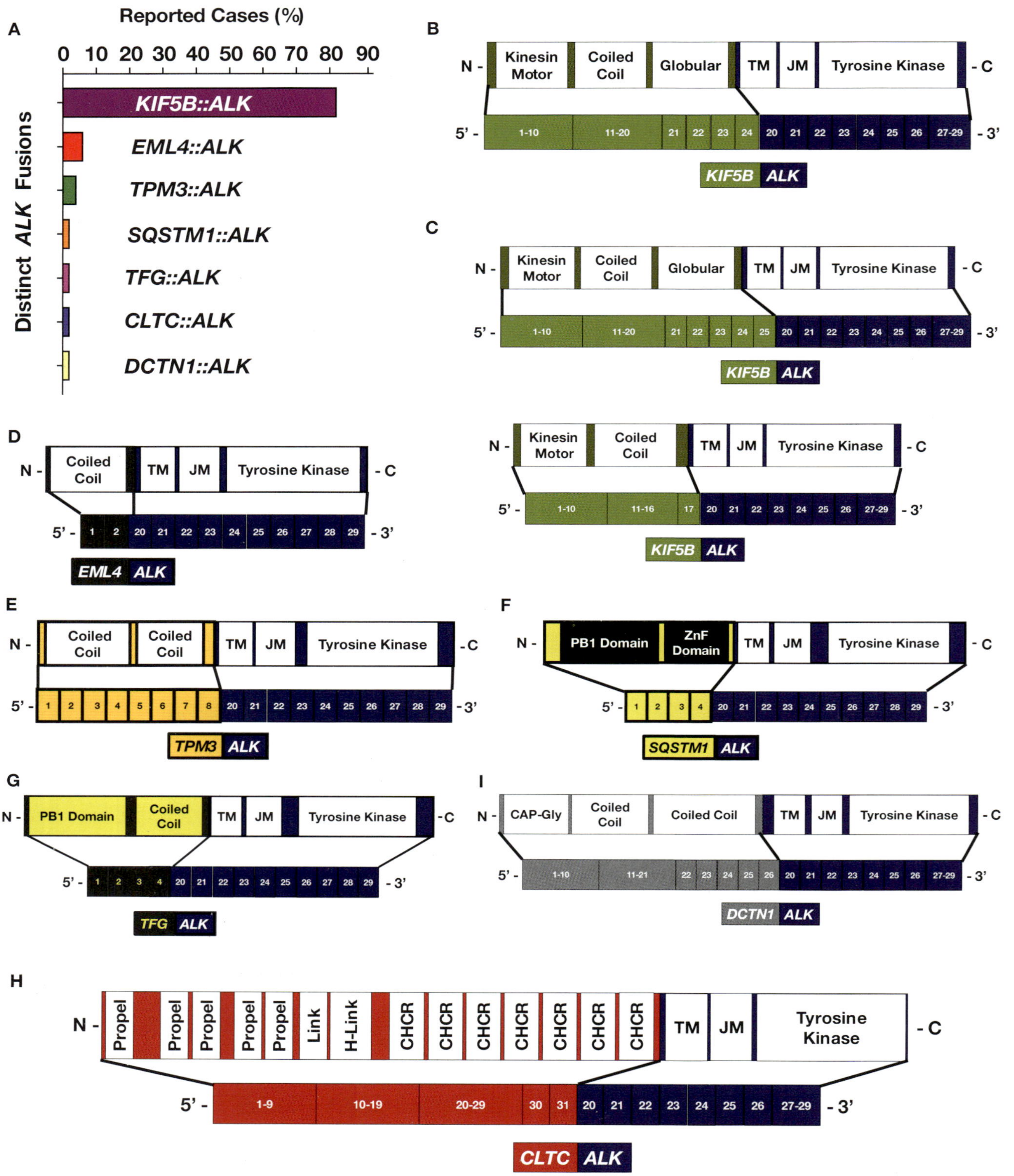

FIGURE 119.2 Summary of the *ALK* fusions uncovered in ALK-positive histiocytosis. **A:** Histogram showing the current frequencies of distinct *ALK* fusions in ALK-positive histiocytosis. **B:** Illustrations of the recurrent *KIF5B::ALK* fusions with the most common *KIF5B* (exons 1-24) and *ALK* (exons 20-27) fusion, as well as **C:** fusions with variant breakpoints involving *KIF5B* across the ALK-positive histiocytosis. Diagrams of the less common fusions: **D:** *EML4::ALK* fusions, **E:** *TPM3::ALK* fusions, **F:** *SQSTM1::ALK* fusion, **G:** *TFG::ALK* fusion, **H:** *CLTC::ALK* fusion, and **I:** *DCTN1::ALK* fusion.[1-3,7,8]

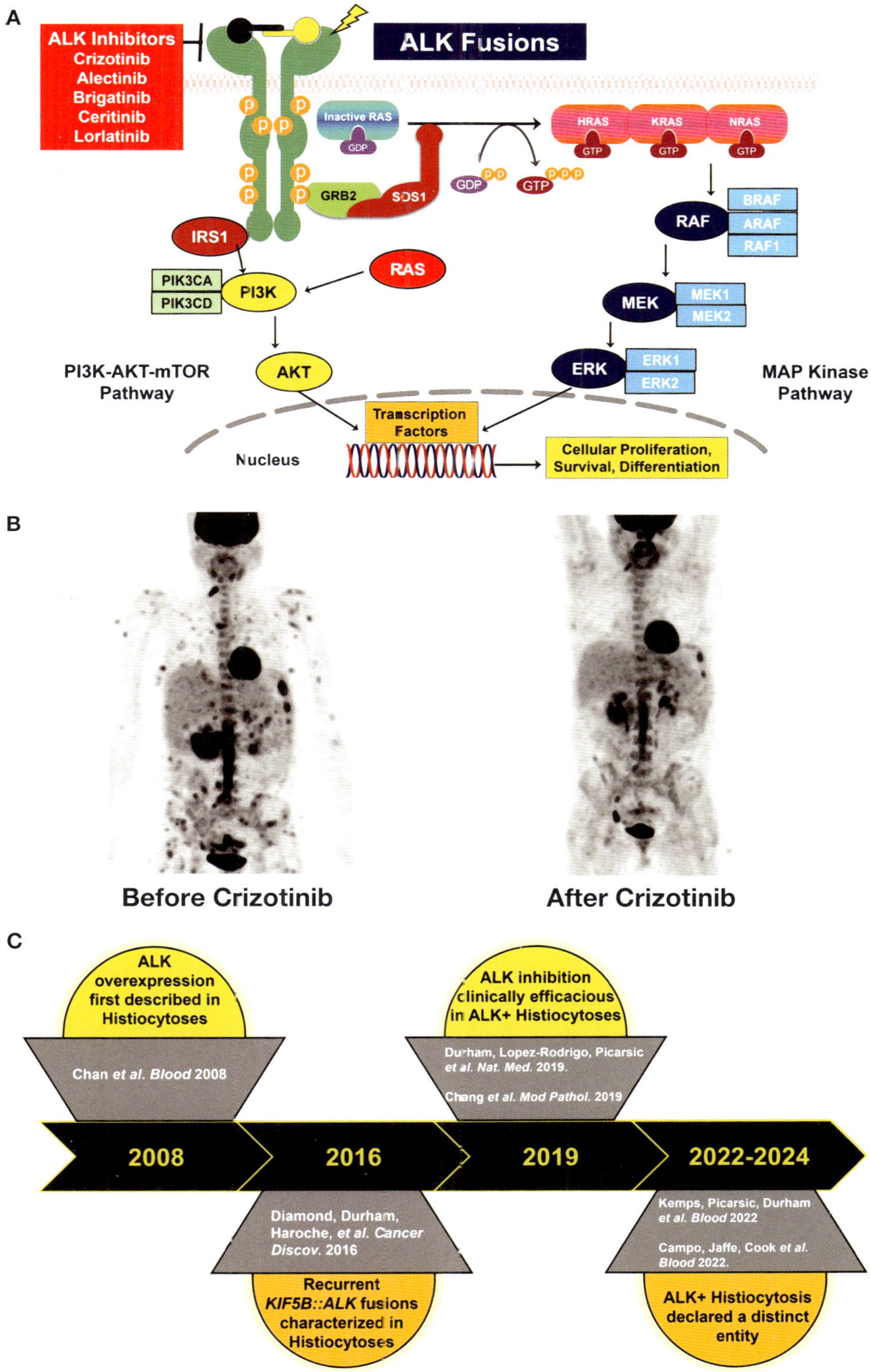

FIGURE 119.3 Schematic overviews of aberrant ALK signaling in ALK-positive histiocytosis, the benefit of ALK inhibition in *ALK*-rearranged histiocytic neoplasms, and a summary of the emergence of ALK-positive histiocytosis as a distinct hematological neoplasm. **A:** Schematic diagram of aberrant ALK signaling through the downstream MAPK and PI3K-AKT-mTOR signaling pathways in ALK-positive histiocytosis, as well as available clinical ALK inhibitors that have been utilized in *ALK*-rearranged neoplasia. **B:** Maximum-intensity projection images from [^{18}F]fluorodeoxyglucose positron emission tomography scans before and 12 to 13 months following treatment with crizotinib in a patient with multisystem, *KIF5B::ALK*-rearranged histiocytosis. **C:** Historical timeline documenting key milestones in the emergence of ALK-positive histiocytosis as a distinct and recognized subtype of histiocytic neoplasms over the past 14 years.[1-3,7,8]

constitutive activation of the intact, intracellular ALK kinase domain leading to inappropriate overexpression of ALK and constitutive activation of the MAPK and PI3K-AKT-mTOR signaling pathways within the neoplastic histiocytes.

Prognosis and Clinical Comment

In patients with single-system disease and localized lesions, surgical resection may be curative. Systemic chemotherapy has been employed in patients with systemic disease with or without corticosteroids. Specific ALK inhibitors have demonstrated promising clinical efficacy in patients with persistent and multisystem disease (Figure 119.3).[2,3,7,8] In young children, however, some patients appear to improve over time without aggressive therapy.[1]

References

1. Chan JK, Lamant L, Algar E, et al. ALK+ histiocytosis: a novel type of systemic histiocytic proliferative disorder of early infancy. *Blood.* 2008;112(7):2965-2968. doi:10.1182/blood-2008-03-147017
2. Kemps PG, Picarsic J, Durham BH, et al. ALK-positive histiocytosis: a new clinicopathologic spectrum highlighting neurologic involvement and responses to ALK inhibition. *Blood.* 2022;139(2):256-280. doi:10.1182/blood.2021013338
3. Chang KTE, Tay AZE, Kuick CH, et al. ALK-positive histiocytosis: an expanded clinicopathologic spectrum and frequent presence of KIF5B-ALK fusion. *Mod Pathol.* 2019;32(5):598-608. doi:10.1038/s41379-018-0168-6
4. Liu W, Liu HJ, Wang WY, et al. Multisystem ALK-positive histiocytosis: a multi-case study and literature review. *Orphanet J Rare Dis.* 2023;18(1):53. doi:10.1186/s13023-023-02649-x
5. Kemps PG, Hebeda KM, Pals ST, et al. Spectrum of histiocytic neoplasms associated with diverse haematological malignancies bearing the same oncogenic mutation. *J Pathol Clin Res.* 2021;7(1):10-26. doi:10.1002/cjp2.177
6. Bhatia A, Hatzoglou V, Ulaner G, et al. Neurologic and oncologic features of Erdheim-Chester disease: a 30-patient series. *Neuro Oncol.* 2020;22(7):979-992. doi:10.1093/neuonc/noaa008
7. Diamond EL, Durham BH, Haroche J, et al. Diverse and targetable kinase alterations drive histiocytic neoplasms. *Cancer Discov.* 2016;6(2):154-165. doi:10.1158/2159-8290.cd-15-0913
8. Durham BH, Lopez Rodrigo E, Picarsic J, et al. Activating mutations in CSF1R and additional receptor tyrosine kinases in histiocytic neoplasms. *Nat Med.* 2019;25(12):1839-1842. doi:10.1038/s41591-019-0653-6
9. Gupta GK, Xi L, Pack SD, et al. ALK-positive histiocytosis with KIF5B-ALK fusion in an adult female. *Haematologica.* 2019;104(11):e534-e536. doi:10.3324/haematol.2019.230094
10. Kashima J, Yoshida M, Jimbo K, et al. ALK-positive histiocytosis of the breast: a clinicopathologic study highlighting spindle cell histology. *Am J Surg Pathol.* 2021;45(3):347-355. doi:10.1097/PAS.0000000000001567
11. Osako T, Kurisaki-Arakawa A, Dobashi A, et al. Distinct clinicopathologic features and possible pathogenesis of localized ALK-positive histiocytosis of the breast. *Am J Surg Pathol.* 2022;46(3):344-352. doi:10.1097/pas.0000000000001794

Chapter 120
Juvenile Xanthogranuloma

John R. Goodlad and Sylvie Fraitag

Definition

Juvenile xanthogranuloma encompasses a spectrum of disease characterized by accumulations of histiocytes and Touton-type giant cells that display phenotypic features of both macrophage and dendritic cell differentiation. Evidence of clonal proliferation has been documented in a proportion cases. The putative cell of origin is a dermal/interstitial dendritic cell.

Synonyms

Adult xanthogranuloma (AXG), juvenile xanthogranuloma (JXG), benign cephalic histiocytosis (BCH), generalized eruptive histiocytosis (GEH), progressive nodular histiocytosis (PNH), xanthoma disseminatum (XD) (all not recommended).

Epidemiology

JXG is an uncommon disease with an estimated incidence of 0.5 in a million children.[1] Solitary dermal JXG is by far the most common presentation (80% of cases). Much less frequently, patients present with multiple lesions limited to skin (15%), or with widespread systemic disease (5%). The majority of patients are children under 10 years of age, with >50% occurring in the first year of life.[1,2]

General Clinical Features

The JXG family of histiocytoses display a broad range of clinical manifestations, and disease distribution has historically been reflected in the applied nomenclature.[3,4] The prototypic skin lesion is a red to yellow papule or nodule ranging from a few to 10 mm in diameter. JXG refers to the presence of one, several, or numerous skin-limited lesions that usually resolve spontaneously in the first few years of life (Figure 120.1A), while AXG has been used to label solitary lesions in adults. Less common manifestations include self-healing eruptions of papules limited to the head and neck area in children younger than 3 years (BCH) or the presence of numerous flesh-colored red macules and papules that develop in crops on the face, trunk, and arms of young adults (GEH). In the latter, lesions may persist for months to years but ultimately spontaneously resolve. PNH is a rare disorder of middle to old age. Patients present with hundreds of lesions, usually on the trunk, in the form of small yellow papules 2 to 10 mm diameter or large deep fibrous nodules up to 50 mm diameter. There may be conjunctival, oral, or laryngeal involvement. Lesions persist in most cases with only rare spontaneous resolution. A disseminated form of the disease (XD), mostly affecting young adult males, is occasionally encountered. It is characterized by numerous brown papules and nodules concentrated around flexor areas and the eyes, with mucosal lesions in 50%. There is also frequent central nervous system (CNS) and ocular involvement, with diabetes insipidus in 40%. Most patients are young adult males, and the disease runs a chronic, persistent course.[4] Finally, exceedingly rare cases of disseminated JXG have been described in children <2 years of age, including neonates. These patients present with multiple skin lesions and visceral involvement, often associated with liver failure and potentially fatal outcome.[5]

An association between JXG and neurofibromatosis type 1 has been described, as has a relationship with juvenile chronic myelomonocytic leukemia, although the latter remains subject to debate.

Morphology

Histological appearances are consistent regardless of clinical presentation and are in part dictated by the age of the lesion sampled. Lesions comprise a variable composition of histiocytes of differing size and morphology (see Figure 120.1B, C and D). Small mononuclear nonxanthomatized histiocytes are prominent in early lesions. These become increasingly lipidized, with foamy histiocytes predominating in more mature lesions. Scattered Touton-type giant cells are usually present in cutaneous

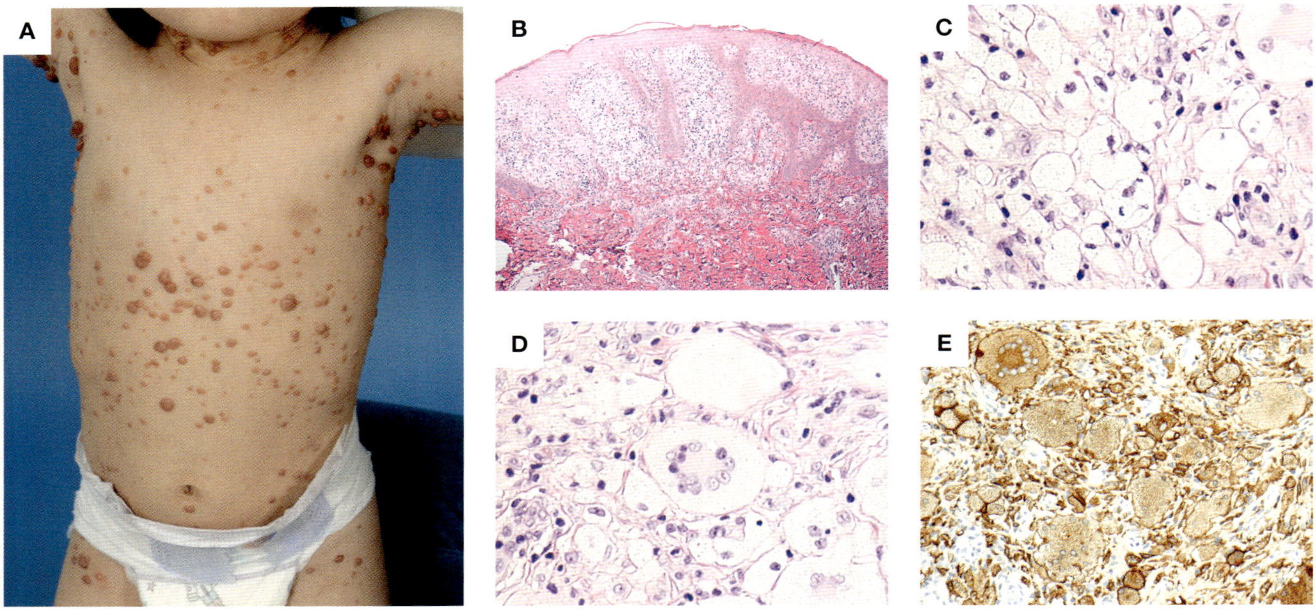

FIGURE 120.1 Juvenile xanthogranuloma. **A:** Juvenile xanthogranuloma in a 2-year old presenting with multiple skin lesions. **B:** Low-power view showing accumulation of histiocytes in the upper reticular and papillary dermis. **C:** Xanthomatous histiocytes form the bulk of the lesion. **D:** Touton-type giant cells can also be seen. **E:** Immunohistochemistry shows positive staining for CD163.

lesions but are less commonly seen at noncutaneous sites. Emperipolesis may be seen, particularly in large, S-100-positive cells. There is almost always an associated mixed inflammatory infiltrate comprising small lymphocytes, eosinophils, neutrophils, and/or plasma cells. As lesions regress, fibroblasts and fibrosis become more prominent.[4,5]

Immunophenotype

The phenotype is not specific. The histiocytes are positive for CD14, CD68, CD163 (see Figure 120.1E), and Fascin. FXIIIA is frequently but not always expressed, while S-100 is positive in <20% of cases. The cells are negative for CD1a, CD207, and ALK.[4,5]

Genetics

Activating mutations affecting the MAPK pathway genes *ARAF, NRAS,* and *MAPK1* have been documented in a proportion of JXG, as have mutations of *CSFR1* and *PIK3CD*, as well as *NTRK1* rearrangements.[6-8] *BRAF* mutations are not generally found in skin-limited JXG, but, along with *RNF11::BRAF*, fusions have been documented in CNS JXG, although, in adults, it is argued that such cases may be better classified as Erdheim-Chester disease.[3,7]

Prognosis and Clinical Comment

Surgery, usually undertaken as a diagnostic procedure, is curative for solitary JXG, while multiple lesions limited to skin typically undergo spontaneous resolution and require no treatment. Outcome in these situations is excellent. There is no standardized treatment for systemic/disseminated JXG, and various therapeutic approaches have been attempted. These include Langerhans cell histiocytosis–like chemotherapy with corticosteroids and vinca alkaloids, radiotherapy, and hematopoietic stem cell transplantation. Surgery is sometimes also indicated for individual lesions if function is compromised. Outcome is variable. While >50% of patients with systemic JXG are treated to good effect, a proportion (35%) have persistent disease and a minority (6%) die as a consequence of disease.[9] Going forward, targeted therapy may improve outcome and prognosis when suitable mutations are identified.

References

1. Janssen D, Harms D. Juvenile xanthogranuloma in childhood and adolescence: a clinicopathologic study of 129 patients from the kiel pediatric tumor registry. *Am J Surg Pathol.* 2005;29(1):21-28. doi:10.1097/01.pas.0000147395.01229.06

2. Fraitag S, Emile JF. Cutaneous histiocytoses in children. *Histopathology*. 2022;80(1):196-215. doi:10.1111/his.14569
3. Emile JF, Abla O, Fraitag S; Histiocyte Society, et al. Revised classification of histiocytoses and neoplasms of the macrophage-dendritic cell lineages. *Blood*. 2016;127(22):2672-2681. doi:10.1182/blood-2016-01-690636
4. Goodlad JR. Histiocytic and dendritic cell neoplasms. In: Brenn T, Goodlad J, Mentzel T, eds. Nonmelanocytic Tumors of the Skin. 5th ed. American Registry of Pathology; 2021:469-522.
5. Dehner LP. Juvenile xanthogranulomas in the first two decades of life: a clinicopathologic study of 174 cases with cutaneous and extracutaneous manifestations. *Am J Surg Pathol*. 2003;27(5):579-593. doi:10.1097/00000478-200305000-00003
6. Chakraborty R, Abdel-Wahab O, Durham BH. MAP-kinase-driven hematopoietic neoplasms: a decade of progress in the molecular age. *Cold Spring Harb Perspect Med*. 2021;11(5):a034892. doi:10.1101/cshperspect.a034892
7. Durham BH. Molecular characterization of the histiocytoses: neoplasia of dendritic cells and macrophages. *Semin Cell Dev Biol*. 2019;86:62-76. doi:10.1016/j.semcdb.2018.03.002
8. Durham BH, Lopez Rodrigo E, Picarsic J, et al. Activating mutations in CSF1R and additional receptor tyrosine kinases in histiocytic neoplasms. *Nat Med*. 2019;25(12):1839-1842. doi:10.1038/s41591-019-0653-6
9. Zou T, Wei A, Ma H, et al. Systemic juvenile xanthogranuloma: a systematic review. *Pediatr Blood Cancer*. 2023;70(5):e30232. doi:10.1002/pbc.30232

Chapter 121
Erdheim-Chester Disease

Neval Ozkaya and Ahmet Dogan

Definition

Erdheim-Chester disease (ECD) is a rare histiocytic neoplasm characterized by multiorgan accumulation of mature histiocytes in a background of inflammation and fibrosis.

Synonyms

Lipogranulomatosis; lipoid granulomatosis; lipid (cholesterol) granulomatosis; polyostotic sclerosing histiocytosis (all not recommended).

Epidemiology

ECD is a disease of middle-aged adults with a mean age of ~50 to 55 years, but it has also been rarely reported in children.[1-5] Childhood onset of ECD is mostly reported in association with Langerhans cell histiocytosis (LCH), known as mixed histiocytosis.[4,5] The disease is more common in males than in females (ratio approximately 3:1).[1-4] ECD is a clonal neoplastic disorder with no definite ethnic or racial predisposition.

General Clinical Features

ECD can affect virtually any organ system and therefore has diverse organ system manifestations. However, the lymph nodes, spleen, and liver are generally spared.[1-4] Patients can be asymptomatic but often present with bone pain (50%), exophthalmos (25%-30%), xanthelasma (20%-30%), and diabetes insipidus (25%-50%). Central nervous system (CNS) disease presents with either tumor mass or neurodegenerative-type symptoms.[1-4] Lung involvement is mostly asymptomatic or may cause cough and/or progressive dyspnea and is seen radiologically in ~50% of cases.[3] Renal dysfunction is usually secondary to obstructive uropathy rather than parenchymal involvement.[4] Rare cases present with cardiac tamponade or a painful abdominal mass.[2-4]

Approximately 10% to 15% of ECD cases are associated with different myeloid neoplasms. Patients with underlying myeloid neoplasms tend to be relatively older. It is important to rule out concomitant myeloid neoplasms among patients with ECD due to their high rates of co-occurrence as well as to avoid discordant treatment response with targeted therapies.[4,6] A bone marrow biopsy should be considered, especially in the context of otherwise unexplained cytopenias and/or monocytosis.[3,4,6] ECD can be associated with other histiocytic neoplasms including LCH, Rosai-Dorfman-Destombes disease (RDD), and indeterminate dendritic cell histiocytosis, as well as autoimmune disorders.[2-4,6-8]

On imaging symmetrical osteosclerosis of metadiaphysis of the lower-extremity bones is a defining feature of ECD. Although it is best visualized by bone scintigraphy (Figure 121.1A), (18F)-fluorodeoxyglucose (FDG) positron emission tomography (PET) is preferred as a diagnostic test by virtue of its ability to assess other organ involvement. It can also be seen on computed tomography (CT) or magnetic resonance imaging (MRI) while often missed on plain radiography.[3] Bilateral infiltration of perinephric fat (so-called hairy kidney appearance) on CT is frequent and can cause hydronephrosis. Imaging may also show a coated aorta, corresponding to a hypodense, plaque-like soft tissue thickening circumferentially involving the aorta and its branches (often the whole thoracoabdominal aorta) (Figure 121.1B).[3] Myocardial involvement in about one-third of the patients causes mass-like infiltration of the right atrium by MRI. Sclerosis of facial sinuses on CT scan can also be seen in ECD. CT of the chest may show pleural and septal thickening, as well as serous effusions.[3] Brain parenchymal lesions mainly affecting posterior cranial fossa and meningeal lesions mimicking meningioma on MRI are typical[3] (Figure 121.1C).

Morphology

Classic histopathologic findings include foamy histiocytes with small nuclei and Touton-type giant cells; however, ECD has a spectrum of histopathological

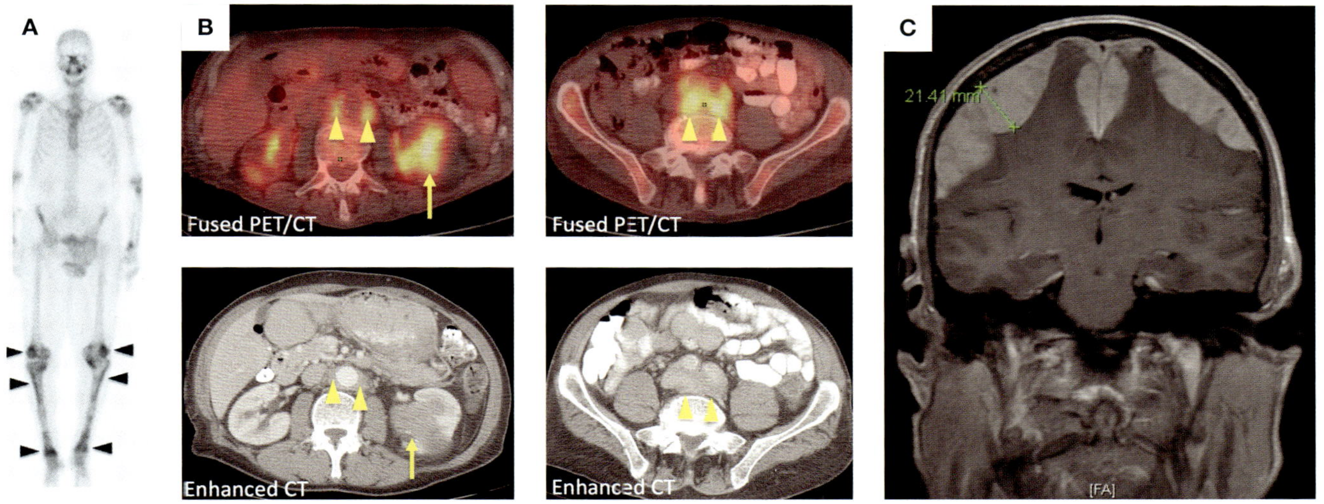

FIGURE 121.1 Imaging in Erdheim-Chester disease. **A:** Bone scintigraphy showing increased symmetric radionuclide uptake in distal femur, proximal tibia, and distal tibia. **B:** FDG-PET/CT and enhanced CT showing left perirenal (arrow) and para-aortic lesions (arrow heads) characteristic of ECD. **C:** Brain MRI showing multiple supratentorial mass-like dural involvement. (Images Courtesy of Dr Mariko Yabe, Memorial Sloan Kettering Cancer Center, NY.)

features (Figures 121.2, 121.3, 121.4A-B, and 121.5A). The lesional histiocytes can have foamy, lipid-laden, or eosinophilic cytoplasm associated with variable proportions of Touton-type giant cells, small lymphocytes, plasma cells, and rarely neutrophils.[2-4] The lesional histiocytes can be sparse and may have a distorted shape due to marked fibrosis. Therefore, absence of the classical description of foamy histiocytes and Touton-type giant cells does not preclude a diagnosis of ECD.[2-4] Variable degree of fibrosis is usually present and sometimes predominant, leading to interpretation of the lesion as a reactive fibroinflammatory process. Morphologically, it may be indistinguishable from xanthogranuloma.[2-4]

Immunophenotype

The neoplastic cells are consistently positive for CD163, CD68, and CD4, while negative for CD1a and Langerin/CD207 (Figure 121.4C-4E).[1-4] S100 protein is mostly negative (Figure 121.4F) but has been reported as focally positive in approximately one-third of the cases, which may cause diagnostic difficulty for the distinction from RDD.[4] In ECD, VE1 monoclonal antibody for the detection of *BRAF* V600E mutation is not sensitive or specific. Although a cytoplasmic staining with VE1 monoclonal antibody may imply presence of a *BRAF* V600E mutation (Figure 121.5B), it is recommended that the mutations are confirmed by molecular analysis.[1-4]

Genetics

Gain-of-function somatic alterations activating the mitogen-activated protein kinase (MAPK) cell signaling pathway have been identified in nearly all cases.[1-4] Demonstration of a corroborating genomic alteration may aid in diagnosis and treatment. *BRAF* V600E mutation is the most common and is present in 50% to 60% of cases.[2,4,9] Patients without *BRAF* V600E mutation frequently have other activating kinase mutations

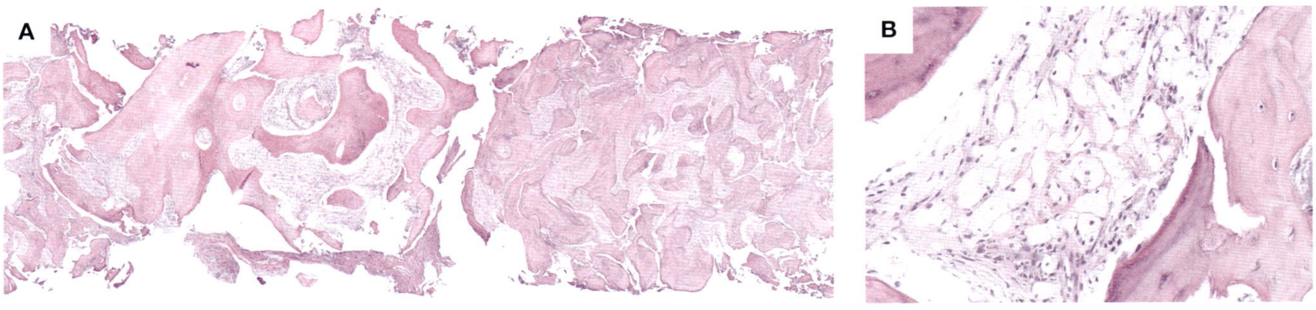

FIGURE 121.2 Histopathology of bone involvement in Erdheim-Chester disease. **A:** This tibial core biopsy shows extensive sclerosis of the bone, with marrow fibrosis and only small area with a cellular component. **B:** On high power, cellular area contains numerous histiocytic cells with foamy cytoplasm in a background of fine fibrosis and small number of inflammatory cells.

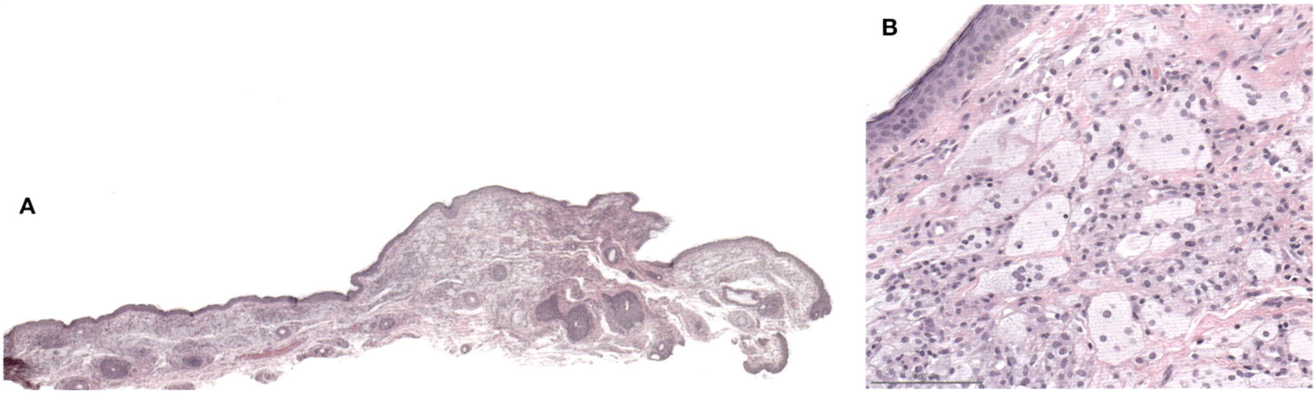

FIGURE 121.3 Histopathology of skin involvement in Erdheim-Chester disease. **A:** Skin shave biopsy shows a subtle lymphohistiocytic infiltrate in the superficial dermis. **B:** On high power the infiltrate is composed of numerous histiocytic cells with foamy cytoplasm and Touton-type giant cells in a background of fine fibrosis and small number of inflammatory cells.

or fusions involving *MAP2K1*, *NRAS*, *KRAS*, *ARAF*, or *BRAF*.[2,4,9] It should be noted that the allele frequency of mutations may be <5% in some cases, and thus, they are not detectable by less sensitive molecular methods.[10] An underlying clonal hematopoiesis has been described in 42% of patients in a reported series, which is significantly higher than that in the age-related general population.[11] A model with sequential acquisition of driver mutations leading to development of myeloid neoplasms and ECD from underlying clonal hematopoiesis has been proposed. However, most ECD cases present in the absence of detectable clonal hematopoiesis.

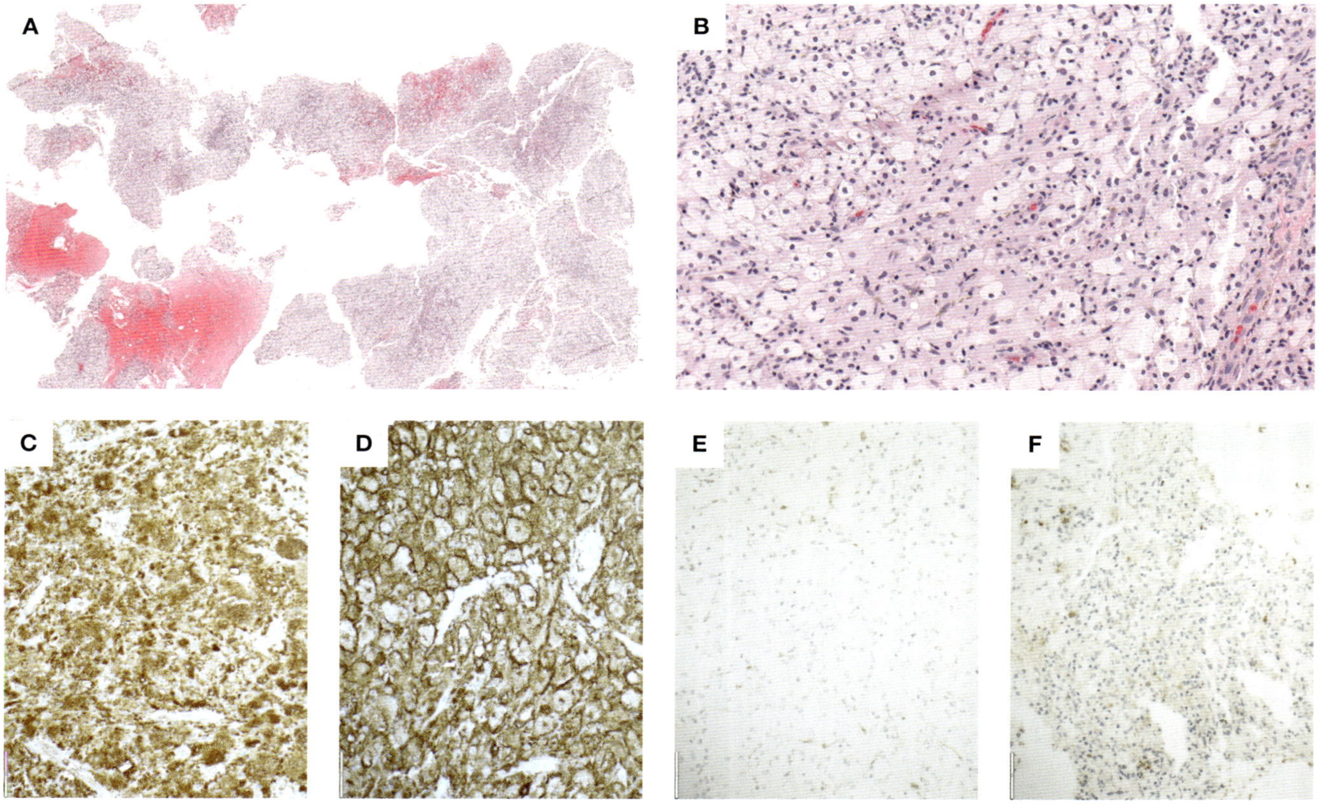

FIGURE 121.4 Histopathology and immunophenotypic features of Erdheim-Chester disease involving retroperitoneum. **A:** Low-power view shows multiple fragments of adipose tissue with a lymphohistiocytic infiltrate. **B:** On high power, the infiltrate is composed of numerous histiocytic cells with foamy or pale pink cytoplasm in a background of fine fibrosis, small vessels, and small number of inflammatory cells (H&E). **C-F:** Immunohistochemistry shows that the histiocytic cells express CD68 **(C)**, CD163 **(D)**, but not CD1A **(E)** or S100 protein **(F)**.

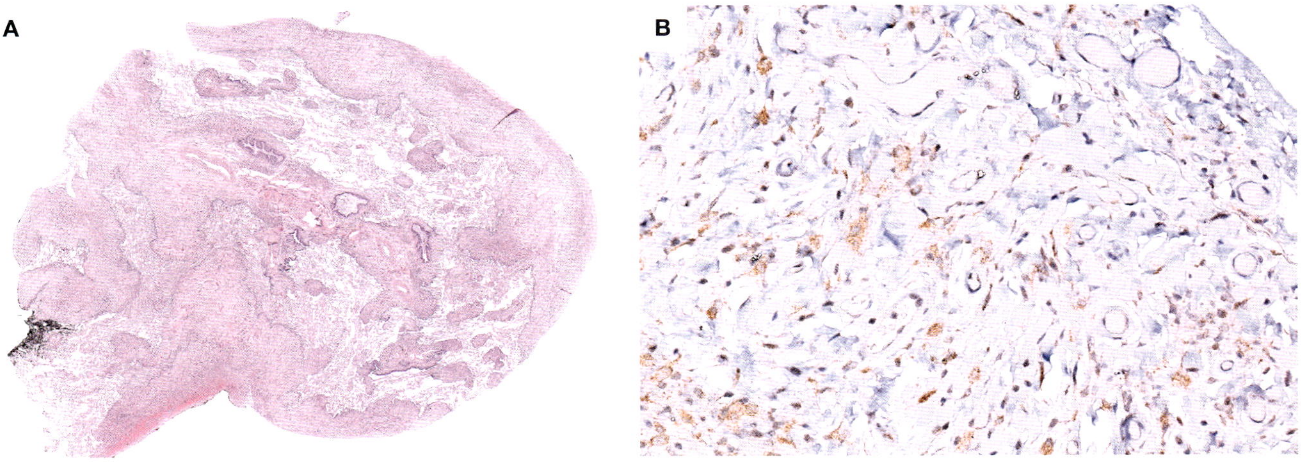

FIGURE 121.5 Histopathology of lung involvement in Erdheim-Chester disease. **A:** Low-power view shows characteristic involvement of pleura, interlobular septa, perivascular interstitium, and peribronchiolar areas, with areas of relatively normal alveolar parenchyma. **B:** BRAF V600E antibody (VE1) highlights subpleural neoplastic histiocytes in a fibroinflammatory background.

Prognosis and Clinical Comment

Prognosis depends on site and extent of the involvement.[3] CNS involvement is an independent poor prognostic factor. Baseline assessment with full-body FDG-PET, including the distal extremities, is recommended in all cases to aid in diagnosis and define the extent of disease; if FDG-PET cannot be performed, contrast-enhanced CT of the chest, abdomen, and pelvis; imaging of the lower extremities (CT, MRI, or 99Tc bone scan); and MRI of the brain with gadolinium can be performed.[3] Most patients require systemic therapy. Traditionally, interferon alfa-2a or pegylated interferon alfa has been used.[1] However, in recent years, MAPK pathway alterations have been recognized and targeted therapies with kinase inhibitors are frequently used. Recent studies reported a 43%-100% response rate and almost no disease progression with the use of BRAF and/or MEK inhibitors.[12-14]

References

1. Cohen-Aubart F, Emile JF, Carrat F, et al. Phenotypes and survival in Erdheim-Chester disease: results from a 165-patient cohort. *Am J Hematol.* 2018;93(5):E114-E117. doi:10.1002/ajh.25055
2. Estrada-Veras JI, O'Brien KJ, Boyd LC, et al. The clinical spectrum of Erdheim-Chester disease: an observational cohort study. *Blood Adv.* 2017;1(6):357-366. doi:10.1182/bloodadvances.2016001784
3. Goyal G, Heaney ML, Collin M, et al. Erdheim-Chester disease: consensus recommendations for evaluation, diagnosis, and treatment in the molecular era. *Blood.* 2020;135(22):1929-1945. doi:10.1182/blood.2019003507
4. Ozkaya N, Rosenblum MK, Durham BH, et al. The histopathology of Erdheim-Chester disease: a comprehensive review of a molecularly characterized cohort. *Mod Pathol.* 2018;31(4):581-597. doi:10.1038/modpathol.2017.160
5. Pegoraro F, Mazzariol M, Trambusti I, et al. Childhood-onset Erdheim-Chester disease in the molecular era: clinical phenotypes and long-term outcomes of 21 patients. *Blood.* 2023;142(13):1167-1171. doi:10.1182/blood.2023020569
6. Papo M, Diamond EL, Cohen-Aubart F, et al. High prevalence of myeloid neoplasms in adults with non-Langerhans cell histiocytosis. *Blood.* 2017;130(8):1007-1013. doi:10.1182/blood-2017-01-761718
7. Hervier B, Haroche J, Arnaud L, et al. Association of both Langerhans cell histiocytosis and Erdheim-Chester disease linked to the BRAFV600E mutation. *Blood.* 2014;124(7):1119-1126. doi:10.1182/blood-2013-12-543793
8. Roeser A, Cohen-Aubart F, Breillat P, et al. Autoimmunity associated with Erdheim-Chester disease improves with BRAF/MEK inhibitors. *Haematologica.* 2019;104(11):e502-e505. doi:10.3324/haematol.2018.214007
9. Diamond EL, Durham BH, Haroche J, et al. Diverse and targetable kinase alterations drive histiocytic neoplasms. *Cancer Discov.* 2016;6(2):154-165. doi:10.1158/2159-8290.CD-15-0913
10. Melloul S, Helias-Rodzewicz Z, Cohen-Aubart F, et al. Highly sensitive methods are required to detect mutations in histiocytoses. *Haematologica.* 2019;104(3):e97-e99. doi:10.3324/haematol.2018.201194
11. Cohen Aubart F, Roos-Weil D, Armand M, et al. High frequency of clonal hematopoiesis in Erdheim-Chester disease. *Blood.* 2021;137(4):485-492. doi:10.1182/blood.2020005101

12. Diamond EL, Subbiah V, Lockhart AC, et al. Vemurafenib for BRAF V600-mutant Erdheim-Chester disease and Langerhans cell histiocytosis: analysis of data from the histology-independent, phase 2, open-label VE-BASKET study. *JAMA Oncol.* 2018;4(3):384-388. doi:10.1001/jamaoncol.2017.5029
13. Cohen Aubart F, Emile JF, Carrat F, et al. Targeted therapies in 54 patients with Erdheim-Chester disease, including follow-up after interruption (the LOVE study). *Blood.* 2017;130(11):1377-1380. doi:10.1182/blood-2017-03-771873
14. Diamond EL, Durham BH, Ulaner GA, et al. Efficacy of MEK inhibition in patients with histiocytic neoplasms. *Nature.* 2019;567(7749):521-524. doi:10.1038/s41586-019-1012-y

Chapter 122

Rosai-Dorfman-Destombes Disease

Neval Ozkaya and Ahmet Dogan

Definition

Rosai-Dorfman-Destombes disease (RDD) is a histiocytic disorder characterized by proliferation of mature histiocytes with distinctive cytologic features and S100 protein expression in an inflammatory background.[1,2] Historically, it has been considered as a reactive histiocytic disorder, but a subset of the cases is neoplastic based on recently identified somatic mutations in the mitogen-activated protein kinase (MAPK) pathway.[3,4]

Synonyms

Rosai-Dorfman disease (acceptable); sinus histiocytosis with massive lymphadenopathy (not recommended).

Epidemiology

RDD is mostly a disease of young adults with a mean age of ~20 to 30 years with a wide age range.[1,5] The disease is more common in males than in females.[5] RDD affects all races but is reportedly more common in African Americans.[5] Rare patients have familial RDD in whom germline mutations in *SLC29A3* have been reported.[6] Some inherited conditions including heterozygous germline mutations in the *FAS* or *TNFRSF* genes, both responsible for autoimmune lymphoproliferative syndrome, may be associated with RDD-like changes, which are usually self-limited.[7]

General Clinical Features

Patients often present with painless, slow-growing lymph node enlargement with or without constitutional symptoms.[1,5] However, the clinical phenotype of RDD is heterogenous and any organ system can be affected.[1,8] Extranodal presentation and multisystem involvement can be seen in ~40% and 20% of RDD, respectively.[1] Central nervous system disease is rare (<5% of cases) and presents with intracranial (75%) or spinal lesions (25%).[9] It usually occurs in older patients and without lymphadenopathy.[5] Cutaneous involvement is mostly slow growing and painless in the form of nonpruritic nodules, plaques, or papules with coloration varying from yellow to red to brown and seen in ~10% of cases.[5,10] Involvement of the nasal cavity and paranasal sinuses occurs in ~10% of RDD cases.[1] Rare cases present with bone pain; however, bone fracture is rare.[1] Renal dysfunction can be seen secondary to either parenchymal involvement or obstructive uropathy.[1,5] Rare RDD cases can be associated with lymphomas of various types, other histiocytic neoplasms including Erdheim-Chester disease, and indeterminate dendritic cell histiocytosis as well as autoimmune disorders.[1,5,11,12]

Morphology

Classic histopathologic findings in lymph nodes include expanded sinuses filled by large histiocytes with pale eosinophilic cytoplasm containing central hypochromic nuclei and distinct, round nucleoli, which are associated with variable proportions of small lymphocytes and plasma cells[1] (Figure 122.1). The lesional histiocytes usually show emperipolesis manifested by the presence of intact lymphocytes and plasma cells within their cytoplasm.[1] Cytologic atypia and multinucleation are uncommon.[1] In lymph nodes, lymphoma-associated RDD lesions usually show focal involvement.[11] At extranodal sites, the morphology could be quite variable and in some cases lesional histiocytes can be sparse and emperipolesis can be rare or absent[9,13] (Figure 122.2). Therefore, absence of classical histopathologic findings as described previously does not preclude a diagnosis of RDD.

Immunophenotype

The lesional histiocytes strongly express S100 protein (both in the nucleus and cytoplasm) as well as CD68 and CD163 (with variable intensity), while they are negative for CD1a and Langerin/CD207[1,5,8,11,13,14] (Figure 122.3). Recent studies have shown that the OCT2 expression in the lesional histiocytes is also a consistent feature of RDD[14] (see Figure 122.3H). Background plasma cells are polytypic for immunoglobulin light chain

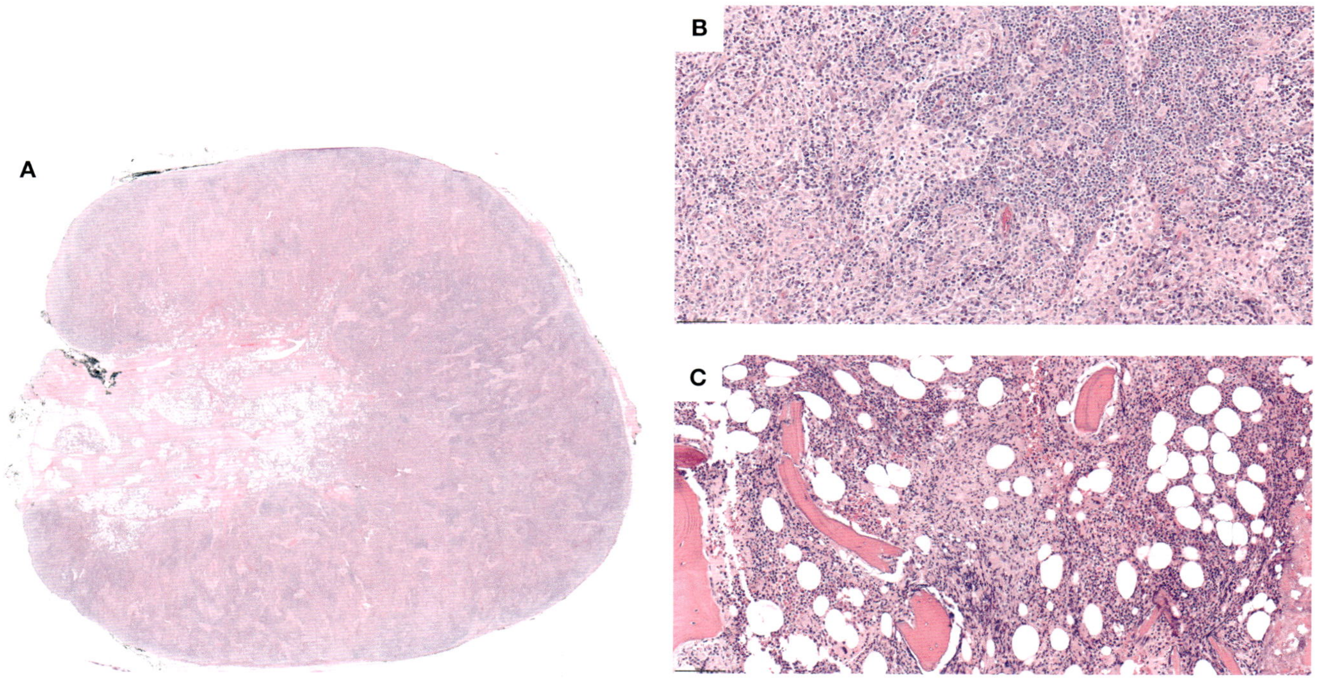

FIGURE 122.1 Histological features of Rosai-Dorfman-Destombes disease (RDD) in a lymph node. **A:** Low power of an excisional lymph node biopsy shows florid lymphohistiocytic infiltrate of the medulla and marked expansion of lymph node sinuses with similar cells (hematoxylin and eosin [H&E]). **B:** High-power view of the lymph node shows the details of the cytology. There are numerous large histiocytic cells with pale granular cytoplasm and oval nuclei with small prominent central nucleoli within the sinuses. These are intermixed with numerous small lymphocytes and plasma cells. Some of the histiocytic cells show marked emperipolesis of lymphocytes and plasma cells (H&E). **C:** Bone marrow biopsy from the same case showing focal involvement by RDD. There is a poorly defined aggregate of histiocytic cells with abundant pale cytoplasm in a background of otherwise normal hematopoiesis (H&E).

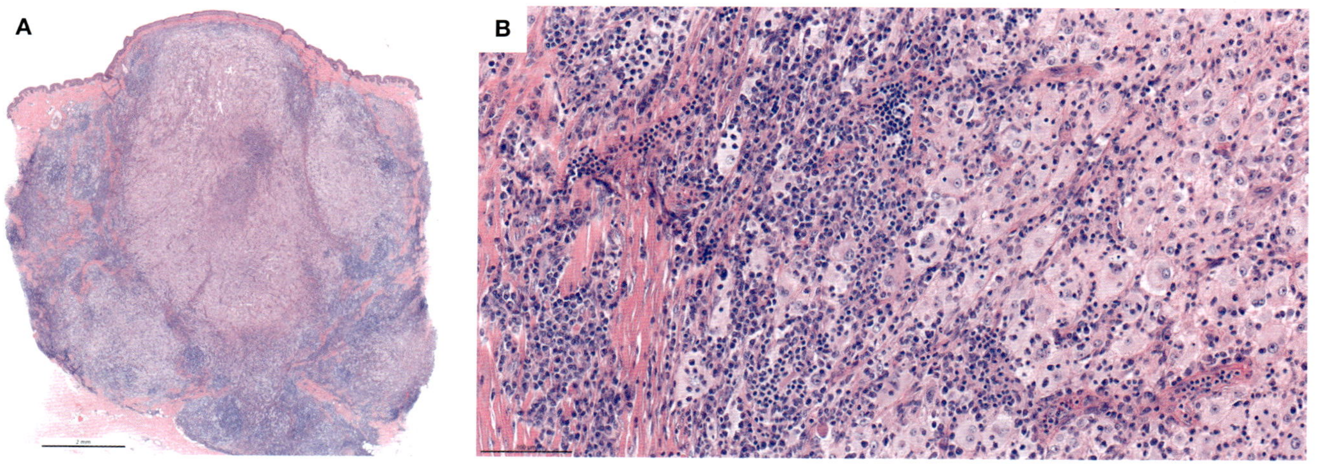

FIGURE 122.2 Cutaneous involvement by Rosai-Dorfman-Destombes disease. **A:** Low-power view shows a large lymphohistiocytic nodule occupying the full thickness of the dermis. The central part of the nodule is enriched by paler histiocytic cells, whereas the periphery predominantly contains darker staining lymphocytes and plasma cells (hematoxylin and eosin [H&E]). **B:** High-power view shows typical cytological features of RDD. There are numerous large histiocytic cells with pale granular cytoplasm and oval nuclei with small prominent central nucleoli. These are intermixed with numerous small lymphocytes and plasma cells (H&E).

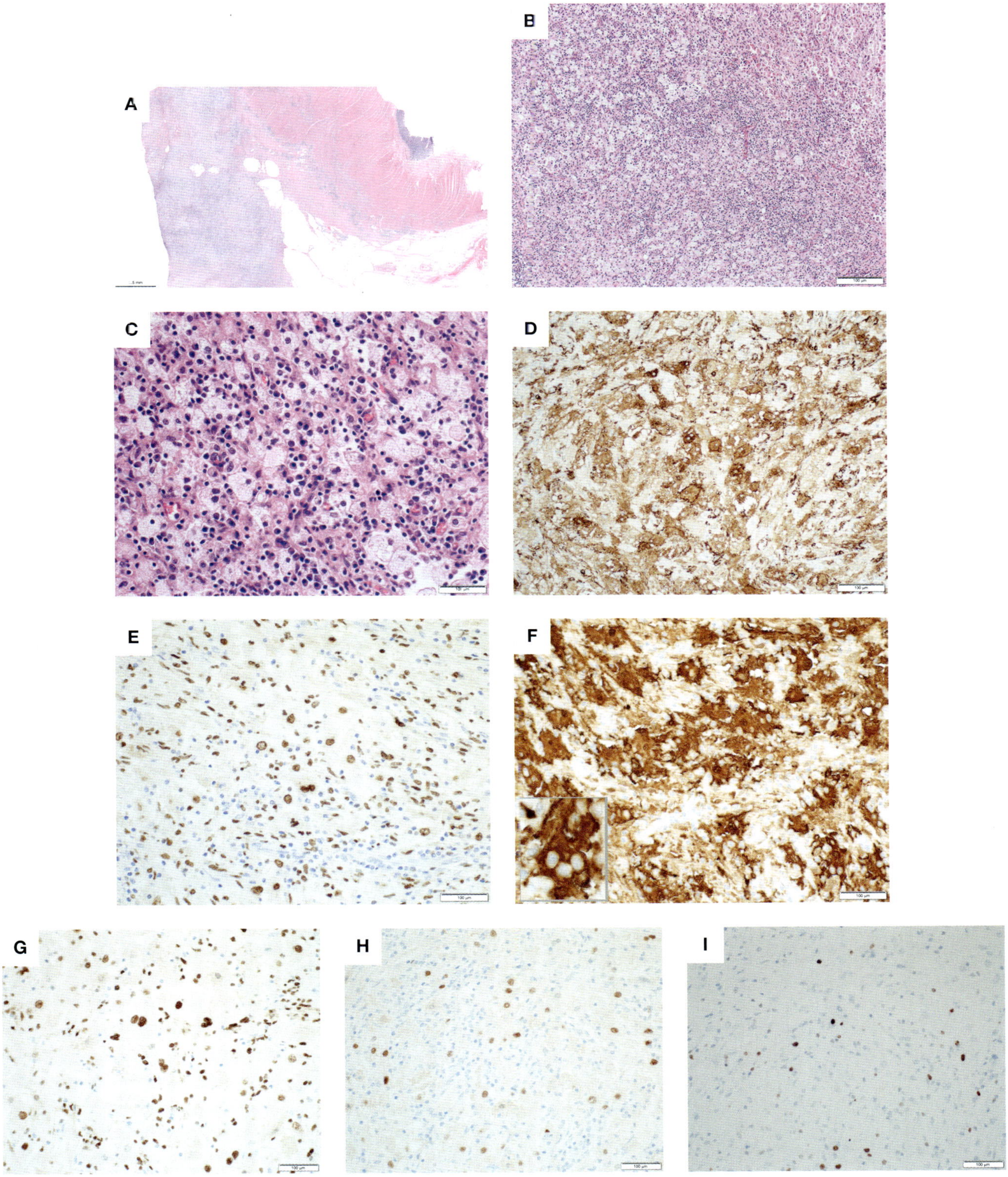

FIGURE 122.3 Immunophenotypic features of Rosai-Dorfman-Destombes disease (RDD) presenting with intestinal involvement. **A:** Low-power view shows an extensive lymphohistiocytic proliferation infiltrating the serosa and mesenteric fat (hematoxylin and eosin [H&E]). **B:** Intermediate-power view shows typical cytological features of RDD. There are numerous large histiocytic cells with pale granular cytoplasm and oval nuclei with small prominent central nucleoli. These are intermixed with numerous small lymphocytes and plasma cells (H&E). **C:** High-power view highlights emperipolesis (H&E). **D-I:** The histiocytic cells of RDD show characteristic phenotype expressing CD163 **(D)**, PU.1 **(E)**, S100 **(F:** F inset), OCT2 **(G)**, and Cyclin D1 **(H)** and show a low proliferation fraction with Ki67 **(I)**.

expression. In some cases IgG4-positive plasma cells can be numerous, which can make the diagnosis of RDD challenging.[15]

Genetics

Gain-of-function somatic alterations in genes including *KRAS, NRAS, MAP2K1,* and *ARAF,* activating the MAPK signaling pathway, have been identified in subset of cases (~50% of cases).[3,4] *BRAF* p.V600E mutations are rare. Mutations effecting the MAPK signaling pathway often lead to overexpression of Cyclin D1, which can be demonstrated by immunohistochemistry (see Figure 122.3I). Demonstration of a corroborating genomic alteration may aid in diagnosis and treatment.

Prognosis and Clinical Comment

Prognosis depends on site and extent of the involvement.[5] Therefore, baseline assessment should include evaluation of disease extent, as well as evaluation of conditions known to be associated with RDD as discussed earlier.[5] For patients with asymptomatic and limited disease, observation may be adequate.[5] A case series reported spontaneous remission in ~40% of cases.[16] However, a subset of patients has persistent disease, requiring therapy.[16] No uniform treatment approach has been delineated for RDD, and options may include complete excision, corticosteroids, or chemotherapy.[5] Recently, a few refractory cases showed substantial regression under the use of MEK inhibitors, which may be a helpful approach for this group of patients with RDD.[17]

References

1. Foucar E, Rosai J, Dorfman R. Sinus histiocytosis with massive lymphadenopathy (Rosai-Dorfman disease): review of the entity. *Semin Diagn Pathol.* 1990;7(1):19-73.
2. Destombes P. Adenitis with lipid excess, in children or young adults, seen in the Antilles and in Mali. (4 cases). *Bull Soc Pathol Exot Filiales.* 1965;58(6):1169-1175. Adenites avec surcharge lipidique, de l'enfant ou de l'adulte jeune, observees aux Antilles et au Mali. (Quatre observations).
3. Diamond EL, Durham BH, Haroche J, et al. Diverse and targetable kinase alterations drive histiocytic neoplasms. *Cancer Discov.* 2016;6(2):154-165. doi:10.1158/2159-8290.CD-15-0913
4. Garces S, Medeiros LJ, Patel KP, et al. Mutually exclusive recurrent KRAS and MAP2K1 mutations in Rosai-Dorfman disease. *Mod Pathol.* 2017;30(10):1367-1377. doi:10.1038/modpathol.2017.55
5. Abla O, Jacobsen E, Picarsic J, et al. Consensus recommendations for the diagnosis and clinical management of Rosai-Dorfman-Destombes disease. *Blood.* 2018;131(26):2877-2890. doi:10.1182/blood-2018-03-839753
6. Morgan NV, Morris MR, Cangul H, et al. Mutations in SLC29A3, encoding an equilibrative nucleoside transporter ENT3, cause a familial histiocytosis syndrome (Faisalabad histiocytosis) and familial Rosai-Dorfman disease. *PLoS Genet.* 2010;6(2):e1000833. doi:10.1371/journal.pgen.1000833
7. Maric I, Pittaluga S, Dale JK, et al. Histologic features of sinus histiocytosis with massive lymphadenopathy in patients with autoimmune lymphoproliferative syndrome. *Am J Surg Pathol.* 2005;29(7):903-911. doi:10.1097/01.pas.0000157997.61177.08
8. Goyal G, Ravindran A, Young JR, et al. Clinicopathological features, treatment approaches, and outcomes in Rosai-Dorfman disease. *Haematologica.* 2020;105(2):348-357. doi:10.3324/haematol.2019.219626
9. Sandoval-Sus JD, Sandoval-Leon AC, Chapman JR, et al. Rosai-Dorfman disease of the central nervous system: report of 6 cases and review of the literature. *Medicine (Baltim).* 2014;93(3):165-175. doi:10.1097/MD.0000000000000030
10. Al-Khateeb TH. Cutaneous Rosai-Dorfman disease of the face: a comprehensive literature review and case report. *J Oral Maxillofac Surg.* 2016;74(3):528-540. doi:10.1016/j.joms.2015.09.017
11. Garces S, Yin CC, Patel KP, et al. Focal Rosai-Dorfman disease coexisting with lymphoma in the same anatomic site: a localized histiocytic proliferation associated with MAPK/ERK pathway activation. *Mod Pathol.* 2019;32(1):16-26. doi:10.1038/s41379-018-0152-1
12. Razanamahery J, Diamond EL, Cohen-Aubart F, et al. Erdheim-Chester disease with concomitant Rosai-Dorfman like lesions: a distinct entity mainly driven by MAP2K1. *Haematologica.* 2020;105(1):e5-e8. doi:10.3324/haematol.2019.216937
13. Frater JL, Maddox JS, Obadiah JM, Hurley MY. Cutaneous Rosai-Dorfman disease: comprehensive review of cases reported in the medical literature since 1990 and presentation of an illustrative case. *J Cutan Med Surg.* 2006;10(6):281-290. doi:10.2310/7750.2006.00067
14. Ravindran A, Goyal G, Go RS, Rech KL; Mayo Clinic Histiocytosis Working Group. Rosai-dorfman disease displays a unique monocyte-macrophage phenotype characterized by expression of OCT2. *Am J Surg Pathol.* 2021;45(1):35-44. doi:10.1097/PAS.0000000000001617

15. Menon MP, Evbuomwan MO, Rosai J, Jaffe ES, Pittaluga S. A subset of Rosai-Dorfman disease cases show increased IgG4-positive plasma cells: another red herring or a true association with IgG4-related disease? *Histopathology.* 2014;64(3):455-459. doi:10.1111/his.12274
16. Pulsoni A, Anghel G, Falcucci P, et al. Treatment of sinus histiocytosis with massive lymphadenopathy (Rosai-Dorfman disease): report of a case and literature review. *Am J Hematol.* 2002;69(1):67-71. doi:10.1002/ajh.10008
17. Diamond EL, Durham BH, Ulaner GA, et al. Efficacy of MEK inhibition in patients with histiocytic neoplasms. *Nature.* 2019;567(7749):521-524. doi:10.1038/s41586-019-1012-y

Chapter 123
Follicular Dendritic Cell Sarcoma

Laurence de Leval, Caoimhe Egan, Elaine S. Jaffe, and Alberto Zamò

Definition

Follicular dendritic cell (FDC) sarcoma is a mesenchymally derived neoplastic proliferation of spindle to ovoid stromal cells showing morphologic and immunophenotypic features of FDCs.

Synonyms

Follicular dendritic cell tumor (acceptable), dendritic reticulum cell tumor (not recommended).

Epidemiology

FDC sarcoma is a rare neoplasm, which can occur at any age but predominantly affects adults at a median age of 50, with no sex predilection.[1] The etiology is unknown, but a subset of cases occurs in association with hyaline-vascular Castleman disease.

General Clinical Features

Patients present with slow-growing painless masses developing in lymph nodes, or more commonly occurring in extranodal sites (lung, tonsil, soft tissues, mediastinum, and others) (Figure 123.1A).[1,2] Likely most of the cases that have been reported in the liver, spleen, or gastrointestinal tract are EBV-positive and should be classified as Epstein-Barr virus (EBV)-positive inflammatory FDC tumors (see Chapter 125: EBV-positive inflammatory follicular dendritic cell/fibroblastic reticular cell tumor). Most patients have localized disease at presentation. Rarely, the disease may affect both nodal and extranodal sites. Systemic symptoms are uncommon. In a small subset of patients, the disease manifests with or may be complicated by paraneoplastic autoimmune manifestations, including paraneoplastic pemphigus, paraneoplastic autoimmune multiorgan syndrome, or myasthenia gravis.[3,4]

Morphology

Macroscopically, FDC sarcoma presents as a solid, well-limited or encapsulated tan-grey mass, ranging in size from 1 to >20 cm. Those presenting in extranodal sites tend to be larger than those involving lymph nodes.[5,6] Larger tumors may show necrosis or hemorrhage.[5] The tumor is composed of spindle to ovoid cells that form fascicles, whorls, or present a storiform pattern and form diffuse sheets of vague nodules (Figure 123.1B).[7,8] The neoplastic cells are usually cytologically relatively bland. They show indistinct cell borders, moderately abundant eosinophilic cytoplasm, and oval to elongated nuclei with usually finely dispersed chromatin, distinct small nucleoli and nuclear membrane (Figure 123.1C). There can be nuclear inclusions. Binucleated cells reminiscent of normal FDCs, or less commonly multinucleated neoplastic cells are often seen (Figure 123.1D). Some cases may show significant atypia. The mitotic rate, which is usually less than 5 per 10 high-power fields, can reach more than 30 in pleomorphic cases. The tumor is typically heavily infiltrated by small lymphocytes ± plasma cells sometimes aggregated around blood vessels. Focal or more extensive coagulative-type necrosis can occur.

Other cytomorphologic variants include epithelioid neoplastic cells (Figure 123.2A) comprising hyaline or clear cytoplasm, oncocytic cells, myxoid stroma, and cystic spaces, and admixed osteoclastic-type giant cells. Angiomatoid, biphasic, or inflammatory pseudotumor-like patterns have been described in rare cases.[7] In a subset of cases (<10%) that arise in association with hyaline-vascular Castleman disease, lymphoid tissue with features of Castleman disease may be seen around the tumor or in the background, and there can be associated dysplastic FDCs forming a continuum between the hyaline-vascular Castleman disease, dysplastic FDCs, and FDC sarcoma.[7]

Immunophenotype

FDC sarcoma expresses one or several markers characteristic of normal FDCs, such as CD21, CD23, CD35, CXCL13, podoplanin (recognized by D2-40 antibody), clusterin, and SSTR2 (see Figure 123.2).[7-9] The neoplastic cells are also usually positive for vimentin, fascin, EGFR, and HLA-DR. They may be positive for epithelial membrane antigen, CD30,

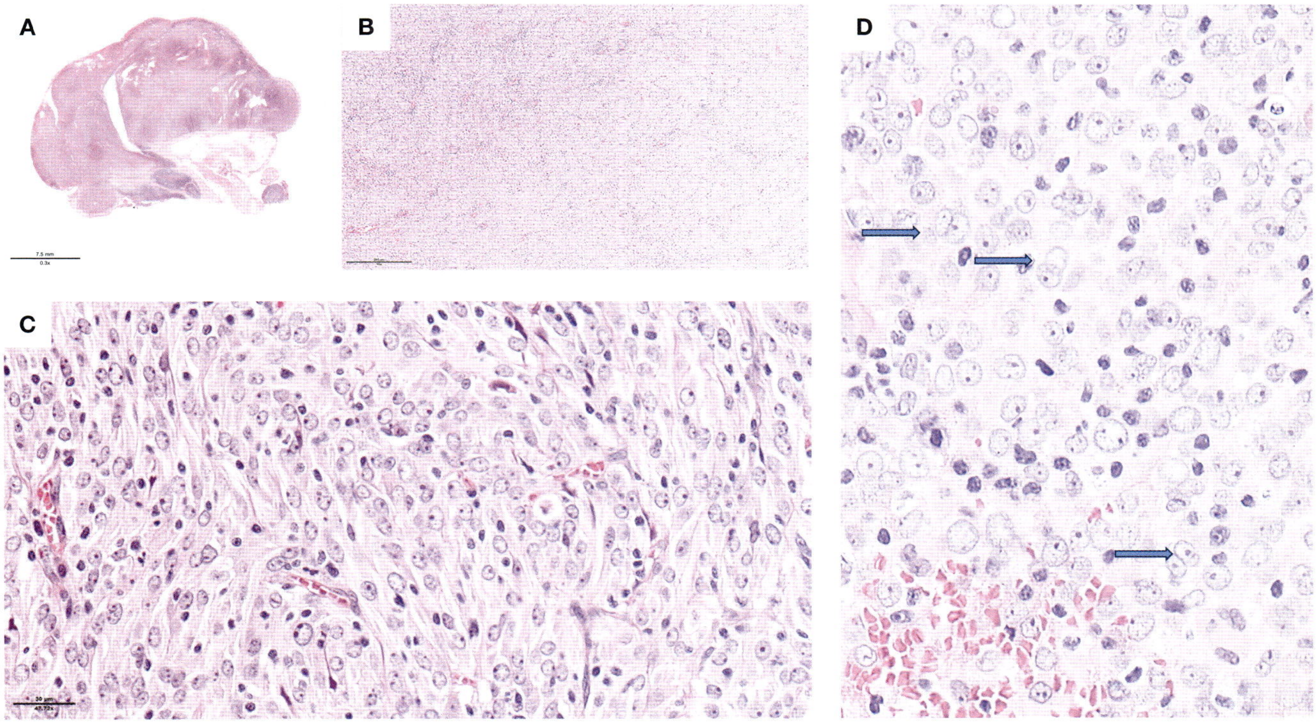

FIGURE 123.1 Morphology of follicular dendritic cell sarcoma. **A:** Low-power view of a case presenting as a tonsillar mass, replacing most of the lymphoid tissue. **B:** At medium power, the tumor is composed of pale eosinophilic cells arranged in fascicles and whorls. **C:** At high magnification, the neoplastic cells are spindled with oval bland nuclei, and there is a mild infiltrate of small lymphoid cells. **D:** Cytological features of another case showing more epithelioid morphology and comprising many binucleated cells (**A-D:** H&E stain).

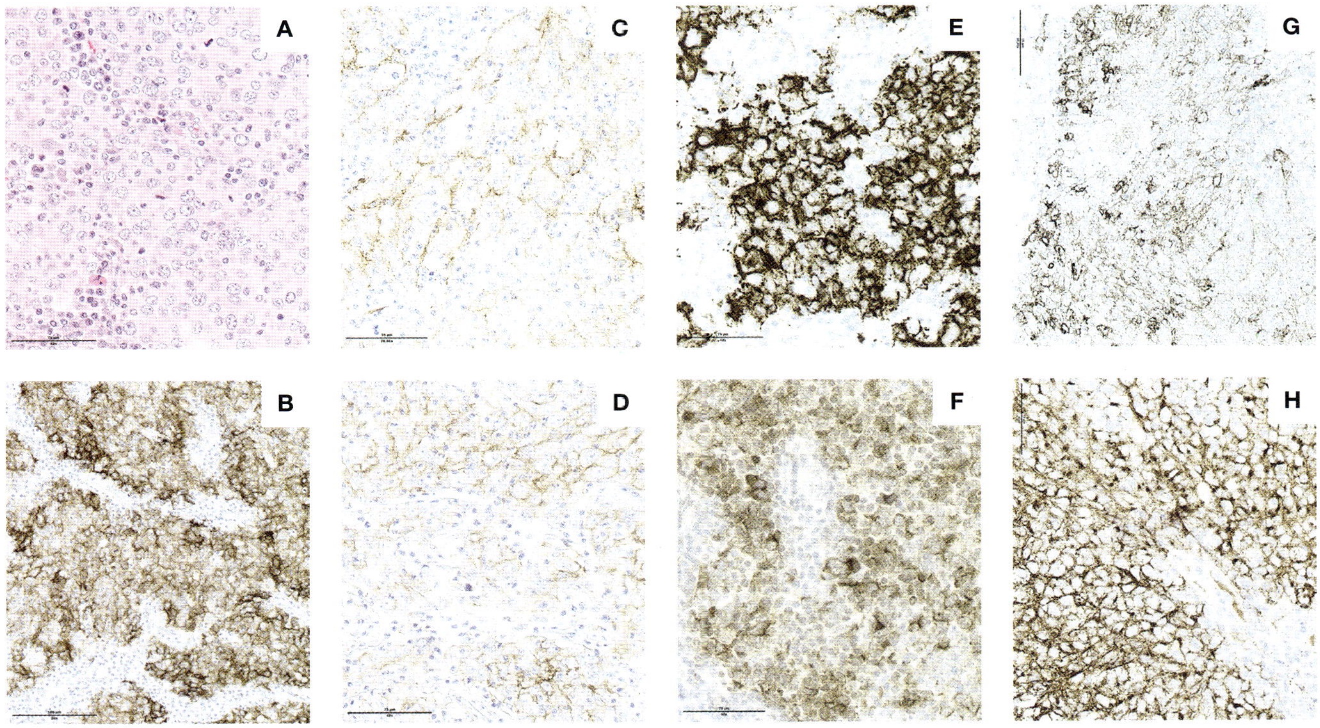

FIGURE 123.2 Immunophenotypic characteristics of follicular dendritic cell sarcoma. **A-F:** In this tumor composed of epithelioid cells with moderate cellular pleomorphism and showing numerous mitoses (**A:** H&E stain), the neoplastic cells are positive for CD21 (**B**), podoplanin (D2-40) (**C**), CD35 (**D**), CD23 (**E**), and CXCL13 (**F**). **G** and **H:** In another case, the neoplastic cells are partially positive for PD-L1 (**G**) and strongly positive for clusterin (**H**).

S100 protein, and CD68, but are usually negative for CD45, B- and T-cell markers, cytokeratin, CD1a, lysozyme, and myeloperoxidase.[7,8] Expression of PD-L1 and PD-L2 is reported in 50% to 100% of the cases, which may be a consequence of copy gain of chromosome 9p24 in some but not all instances (Figure 123.2G).[7,10-12] FDC-secreted protein and serglycin have been unveiled as specific markers of normal and neoplastic FDCs by whole transcriptome profiling, but they are generally not routinely used.[13] The admixed lymphoid component can be predominantly T or B cells, or an admixture of both. Up to 45% of cases contain immature T cells, which may sometimes be numerous; these indolent T-lymphoblastic proliferations comprising polyclonal terminal deoxynucleotidyl transferase-positive T cells may be associated with or predict paraneoplastic autoimmune complications (Figure 123.3).[4,14] FDC sarcoma is EBV-negative; EBV-positive neoplasms of FDCs or fibroblastic reticular cells are diagnosed as EBV-positive inflammatory FDC tumors (see Chapter 125: Epstein-Barr virus-positive inflammatory follicular dendritic cell/fibroblastic reticular cell tumor).

Genetics

Cytogenetic analyses, array-based studies, and whole genome sequencing performed in a few cases have documented variable ploidy levels, numerous copy number variations with more gains than losses in one study,[11] and structural variants in others.[11,12,15] *MYC* amplification or rearrangement is reported in one-third of the cases and associates with MYC overexpression.[16] Overall, the tumor mutational burden of FDC sarcoma is low.[12] FDC sarcoma shows recurrent alterations in genes of the NF-kappa B pathway (*BIRC3, NFKBIA, TRAF3, SOCS3, TNFAIP3, CYLD*) in up to 60% of the cases, and in cell-cycle regulators in up to 50% of the cases (*CDKN2A*, *RB1*, and *TP53*).[16,17] In addition to *RB1* and *TP53*, mutations in other genes related to homologous recombination DNA damage-repair, including *BRCA2* have been identified in a recent study, suggesting that as many as 70% of the cases overall might potentially benefit from poly-ADP ribose polymerase inhibition.[12] FDC sarcoma lacks mutations in genes of the MAPK pathway recurrently found in histiocytic and dendritic cell neoplasms.[16,17]

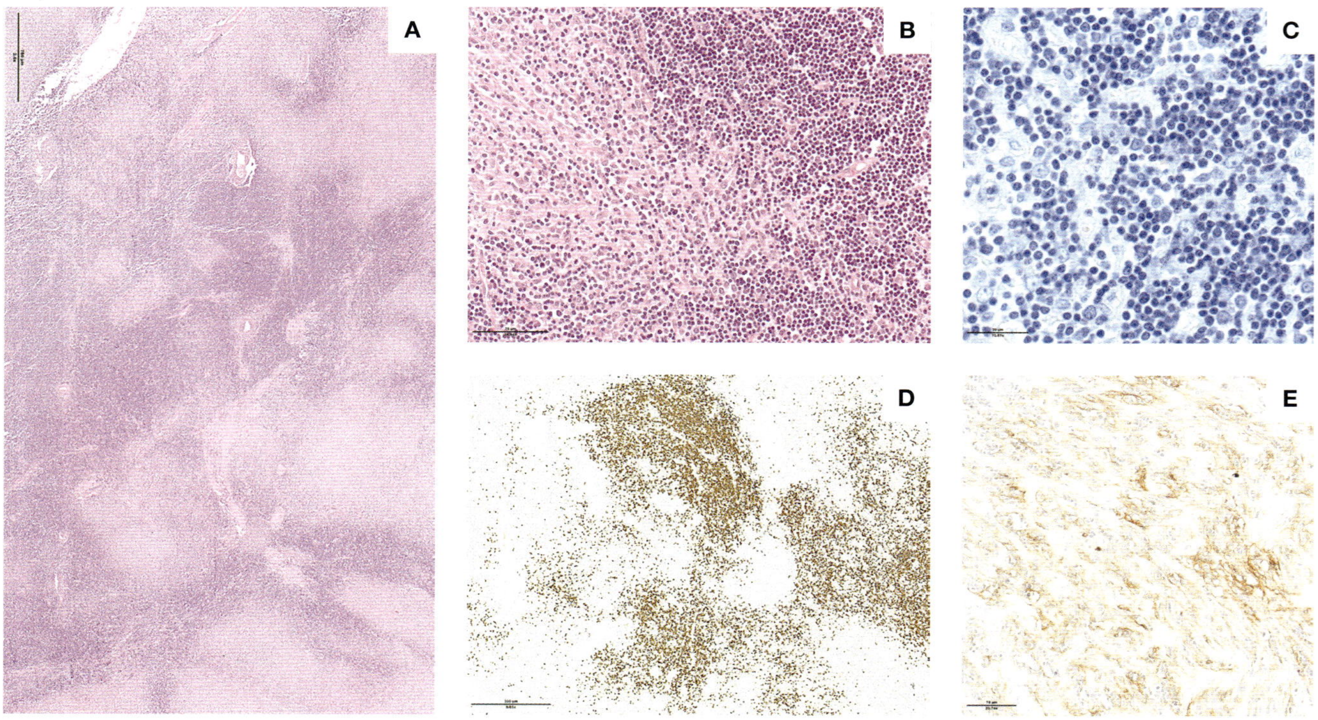

FIGURE 123.3 Follicular dendritic cell sarcoma with associated indolent T-lymphoblastic proliferation. This tumor was developed in the posterior mediastinum in a 35-year-old woman, who presented with myasthenia gravis. **A:** Low-power view of the tumor showing aggregates and larger nodules of pale neoplastic cells, alternating with dense lymphoid aggregates (H&E stain). **B:** A closer view shows spindled eosinophilic cells and aggregates of small lymphocytes (H&E stain). **C:** The neoplastic cells have pale oval bland nuclei with small nucleoli and the lymphoid component consists of monotonous small lymphocytes with round nuclei and fine dense chromatin (Giemsa stain). **D:** Terminal deoxynucleotidyl transferase (TdT) highlights the large lymphoid aggregates. **E:** The spindled cells show heterogeneous positivity for CD21.

Prognosis and Clinical Comment

FDC sarcoma is usually treated by surgical excision, with or without adjuvant radiation therapy or chemotherapy. FDC sarcoma is regarded as an intermediate grade malignancy with a rate of 25% to 30% local and distant recurrence.[1] Disease-related mortality, which varies in the reported series, is probably around 20%.[6,12] Young age at diagnosis (40 years or less), large tumor size (6 cm or more), lack of lymphocytic infiltrate, coagulative necrosis, high mitotic rate (5 or more per 10 high-power fields), and significant atypia have been associated with a worse prognosis.[1,6]

References

1. Saygin C, Uzunaslan D, Ozguroglu M, Senocak M, Tuzuner N. Dendritic cell sarcoma: a pooled analysis including 462 cases with presentation of our case series. *Crit Rev Oncol Hematol.* 2013;88(2):253-271. doi:10.1016/j.critrevonc.2013.05.006
2. Kaur R, Mehta J, Borges A. Extranodal follicular dendritic cell sarcoma-A review: "What the Mind Does Not Know the Eye Does Not See". *Adv Anat Pathol.* January 2021;28(1):21-29. doi:10.1097/PAP.0000000000000281
3. Hartert M, Strobel P, Dahm M, Nix W, Marx A, Vahl CF. A follicular dendritic cell sarcoma of the mediastinum with immature T cells and association with myasthenia gravis. *Am J Surg Pathol.* 2010;34(5):742-745. doi:10.1097/PAS.0b013e3181d7a2ee
4. Walters M, Pittelkow MR, Hasserjian RP, et al. Follicular dendritic cell sarcoma with indolent T-lymphoblastic proliferation is associated with paraneoplastic autoimmune multiorgan syndrome. *Am J Surg Pathol.* 2018;42(12):1647-1652. doi:10.1097/PAS.0000000000001158
5. Perez-Ordonez B, Erlandson RA, Rosai J. Follicular dendritic cell tumor: report of 13 additional cases of a distinctive entity. *Am J Surg Pathol.* 1996;20(8):944-955. doi:10.1097/00000478-199608000-00003
6. Li L, Shi YH, Guo ZJ, et al. Clinicopathological features and prognosis assessment of extranodal follicular dendritic cell sarcoma. *World J Gastroenterol.* 2010;16(20):2504-2519. doi:10.3748/wjg.v16.i20.2504
7. Facchetti F, Pileri SA, Lorenzi L, et al. Histiocytic and dendritic cell neoplasms: what have we learnt by studying 67 cases. *Virchows Arch.* 2017;471(4):467-489. doi:10.1007/s00428-017-2176-1
8. Facchetti F, Simbeni M, Lorenzi L. Follicular dendritic cell sarcoma. *Pathologica.* 2021;113(5):316-329. doi:10.32074/1591-951X-331
9. Tao LL, Huang YH, Chen YL, Yu GY, Yin WH. SSTR2a is a useful diagnostic marker for follicular dendritic cells and their related tumors. *Am J Surg Pathol.* 2019;43(3):374-381. doi:10.1097/PAS.0000000000001205
10. Xu J, Sun HH, Fletcher CD, et al. Expression of programmed cell death 1 ligands (PD-L1 and PD-L2) in histiocytic and dendritic cell disorders. *Am J Surg Pathol.* 2016;40(4):443-453. doi:10.1097/PAS.0000000000000590
11. Griffin GK, Sholl LM, Lindeman NI, Fletcher CD, Hornick JL. Targeted genomic sequencing of follicular dendritic cell sarcoma reveals recurrent alterations in NF-κB regulatory genes. *Mod Pathol.* 2016;29(1):67-74. doi:10.1038/modpathol.2015.130
12. Lorenzi L, Haferlach T, Mori L, et al. Massive parallel sequencing unveils homologous recombination deficiency in follicular dendritic cell sarcoma. *Haematologica.* 2024;109(6):1815-1824. doi:10.3324/haematol.2023.283669
13. Lorenzi L, Doring C, Rausch T, et al. Identification of novel follicular dendritic cell sarcoma markers, FDCSP and SRGN, by whole transcriptome sequencing. *Oncotarget.* 2017;8(10):16463-16472. doi:10.18632/oncotarget.14864
14. Ohgami RS, Zhao S, Ohgami JK, et al. TdT+ T-lymphoblastic populations are increased in Castleman disease, in Castleman disease in association with follicular dendritic cell tumors, and in angioimmunoblastic T-cell lymphoma. *Am J Surg Pathol.* 2012;36(11):1619-1628. doi:10.1097/PAS.0b013e318264e223
15. Udayakumar AM, Al-Bahri M, Burney IA, Al-Haddabi I. Follicular dendritic cell sarcoma: cytogenetics and pathological findings. *Sultan Qaboos Univ Med J.* 2015;15(3):e411-e414. doi:10.18295/squmj.2015.15.03.017
16. Frigola G, Buhler M, Marginet M, et al. MYC and TP53 alterations but not MAPK pathway mutations are common oncogenic mechanisms in follicular dendritic cell sarcomas. *Arch Pathol Lab Med.* 2023;147(8):896-906. doi:10.5858/arpa.2021-0517-OA
17. Massoth LR, Hung YP, Ferry JA, et al. Histiocytic and dendritic cell sarcomas of hematopoietic origin share targetable genomic alterations distinct from follicular dendritic cell sarcoma. *Oncologist.* 2021;26(7):e1263-e1272. doi:10.1002/onco.13801

Chapter 124
Fibroblastic Reticular Cell Sarcoma

Laurence de Leval, Caoimhe Egan, Elaine S. Jaffe, and Alberto Zamò

Definition

Fibroblastic reticular cell (FRC) sarcoma is a neoplasm of stromal derivation considered to originate from stromal FRCs, which are immunologically oriented specialized myofibroblasts found in the T-zones of lymph nodes.[1]

Synonyms

Fibroblastic reticular cell tumor (acceptable); reticulum cell sarcoma, cytokeratin-positive interstitial reticulum cell tumor, fibroblastic dendritic cell tumor (not recommended).

Epidemiology

FRC sarcoma is a very rare tumor.[2] In a recent review of 20 cases reported in the literature 60% of cases occurred in females and the mean age at diagnosis is 60 years.[3]

General Clinical Features

FRC sarcoma develops most commonly in lymph nodes, or less frequently in soft tissues, spleen, or various extranodal sites. It usually presents with slowly progressive painless swelling.

Morphology

FRC sarcoma is morphologically similar to follicular dendritic cell sarcoma or interdigitating dendritic cell sarcoma (see Chapter 123: Follicular dendritic cell sarcoma and Chapter 118: Interdigitating dendritic cell sarcoma).[4] It is composed of spindle to ovoid cells, arranged in whorls, sheets, or fascicles, or in a storiform pattern and accompanied by a lymphoplasmacytic infiltrate (Figure 124.1A and C). Epithelioid morphology has been occasionally described (Figure 124.1E).[5] There is usually moderate pleomorphism and atypia. Interspersed delicate collagen fibers are often seen (Figure 124.1F). Some tumors may show increased mitotic activity, marked pleomorphism, or necrosis.

Immunophenotype

FRC sarcoma expresses cytokeratin, vimentin, smooth muscle actin, and desmin in the majority of cases, and variably expresses epithelial membrane antigen or caldesmon (Figure 124.1B and D).[2] Histiocytic markers (CD68, CD14, CD163) have been described positive in a subset of reported cases, but further documentation is needed. Markers of follicular dendritic cells (CD21, CD23, CD35, CXCL13), Langerhans cells (CD1a, CD247/langerin), and/or interdigitating dendritic cells (S100) are negative.[4] Rare tumors with features of both follicular dendritic cells and fibroblastic reticular cells have been described.[6,7] Ki 67 proliferative index varies widely. EBV is negative.

Genetics

Cytogenetic or molecular genetic features have not been studied systematically. One case with a complex karyotype was reported.[7] Two cases of FRC sarcoma occurred in patients harboring germline mutations in *MLH1* or *JAK3*.[3]

Prognosis and Clinical Comment

Most patients present with localized disease, and more than half of them experience local recurrence or develop metastases.[2] The stage is the most important prognostic factor and patients with localized disease have a better survival than those with distant disease who have a median overall survival of 13 months.[2]

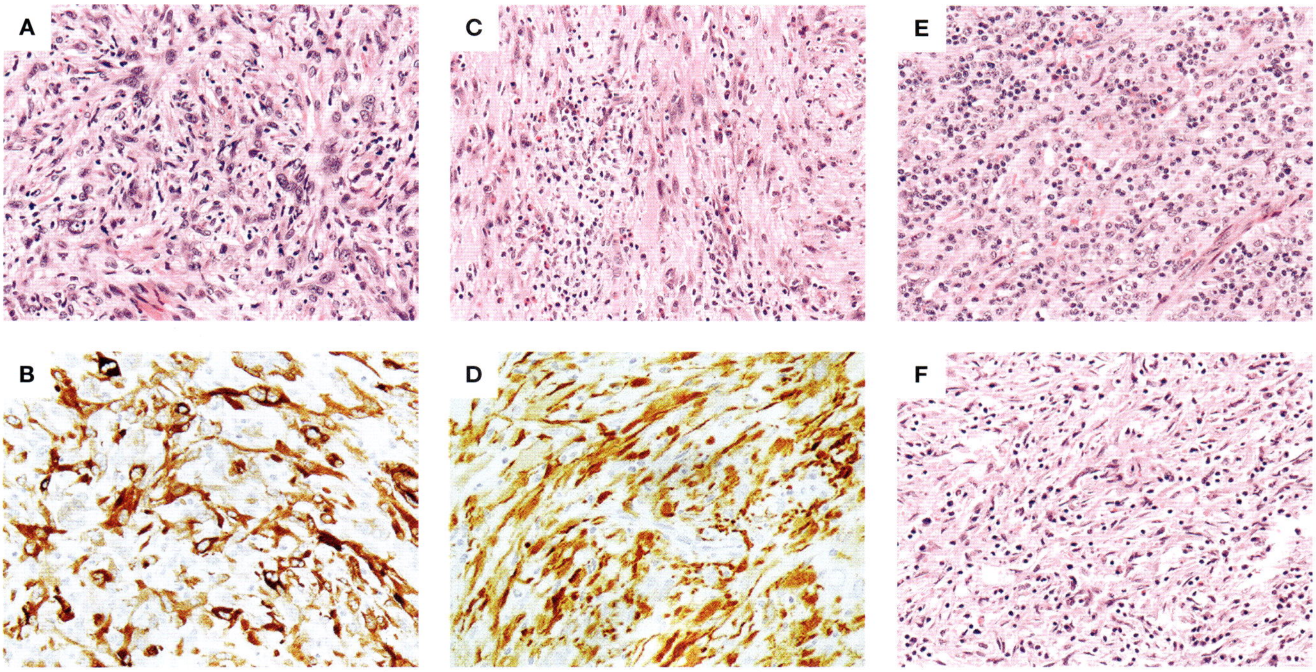

FIGURE 124.1 Morphology and immunophenotypic features of fibroblastic reticular cell sarcoma. **A** and **B:** This mediastinal tumor is composed of atypical pleomorphic spindle cells organized in whorls (**A:** H&E) and express smooth muscle actin (**B**). **C** and **D:** This tumor developed in the thigh is composed of elongated spindle cells organized in intersecting fascicles (**C:** H&E) and is positive for cytokeratin (**D**). **E:** This tumor shows epithelioid cytomorphology (H&E). **F:** This tumor is composed of short curved cells in an abundant stroma (H&E). (Images courtesy of Dr. Jason Hornick, the Brigham and Womens Hospital, Boston, MA.)

References

1. Fletcher AL, Acton SE, Knoblich K. Lymph node fibroblastic reticular cells in health and disease. *Nat Rev Immunol.* 2015;15(6):350-361. doi:10.1038/nri3846
2. Saygin C, Uzunaslan D, Ozguroglu M, Senocak M, Tuzuner N. Dendritic cell sarcoma: a pooled analysis including 462 cases with presentation of our case series. *Crit Rev Oncol Hematol.* 2013;88(2):253-271. doi:10.1016/j.critrevonc.2013.05.006
3. Pescia C, Lopez G, Gianelli U, Croci GA. Fibroblastic/cytokeratin-positive interstitial reticular cell tumor of the spleen with indolent behavior: a case report with review of the literature. *Virchows Arch.* 2023;482(6):1069-1077. doi:10.1007/s00428-022-03463-9
4. Andriko JW, Kaldjian EP, Tsokos M, Abbondanzo SL, Jaffe ES. Reticulum cell neoplasms of lymph nodes: a clinicopathologic study of 11 cases with recognition of a new subtype derived from fibroblastic reticular cells. *Am J Surg Pathol.* 1998;22(9):1048-1058. doi:10.1097/00000478-199809000-00002
5. Kaji S, Hiruta N, Sasai D, Nagashima M, Ohe R, Yamakawa M. Cytokeratin-positive interstitial reticulum cell (CIRC) tumor in the lymph node: a case report of the transformation from the epithelioid cell type to the spindle cell type. *Diagn Pathol.* 2020;15(1):121. doi:10.1186/s13000-020-01032-9
6. Goto N, Tsurumi H, Takami T, et al. Cytokeratin-positive fibroblastic reticular cell tumor with follicular dendritic cell features: a case report and review of the literature. *Am J Surg Pathol.* 2015;39(4):573-580. doi:10.1097/PAS.0000000000000362
7. Jones D, Amin M, Ordonez NG, Glassman AB, Hayes KJ, Medeiros LJ. Reticulum cell sarcoma of lymph node with mixed dendritic and fibroblastic features. *Mod Pathol.* 2001;14(10):1059-1067. doi:10.1038/modpathol.3880436

Chapter 125

Epstein-Barr Virus–Positive Inflammatory Follicular Dendritic Cell/Fibroblastic Reticular Cell Tumor

Daniel A. Arber, Laurence de Leval, Elaine S. Jaffe, and Alberto Zamò

Definition

Epstein-Barr virus (EBV)-positive inflammatory follicular dendritic cell/fibroblastic reticular cell tumor is a mesenchymally derived neoplastic proliferation of EBV-positive spindle cells with associated inflammation and fibrosis that is distinct from follicular dendritic cell sarcoma and most often involves the liver and spleen in adults.

Synonyms

Inflammatory pseudotumor-like follicular/fibroblastic dendritic cell sarcoma, EBV-positive inflammatory follicular dendritic cell sarcoma, inflammatory pseudotumor (all not recommended).

Epidemiology

EBV-positive inflammatory follicular dendritic cell/fibroblastic reticular cell tumor is a rare tumor, but the frequency is not well studied. It occurs most commonly in adult females at a median age of 52 years, and most cases have been reported in Asia.[1]

General Clinical Features

Patients may be asymptomatic. Symptomatic patients report abdominal pain and may demonstrate fever and weight loss. The tumors most commonly occur in the liver and/or spleen, but similar,[2] small polypoid lesions have been reported in the gastrointestinal tract.[3] The tumors are described as low-density lesions on plain or enhanced computed tomography and low-signal intensity on T2-weighted images and isointense on T1-weighted images by magnetic resonance imaging.

Morphology

The gross appearance of the liver and spleen typically reveals a single firm yellow-tan lesion without capsular extension, although multiple nodules are occasionally seen (Figure 125.1). Microscopically, a relatively bland spindle cell proliferation, often with collagen formation, may be obscured by abundant inflammatory cells that include lymphocytes, plasma cells, histiocytes, and eosinophils, similar to the background cells of classic Hodgkin lymphoma (Figure 125.2). Thick-walled vessels and foci of necrosis may be seen. The spindle cells

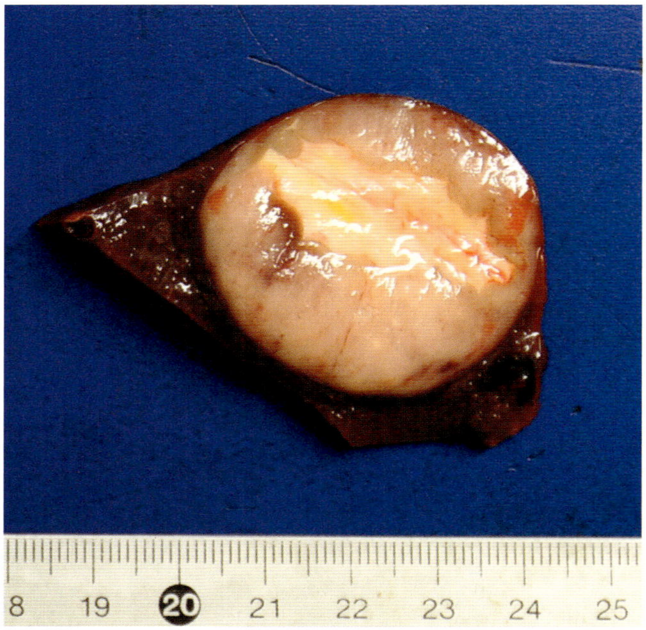

FIGURE 125.1 Gross appearance of a splenic EBV-positive inflammatory follicular dendritic cell/fibroblastic reticular cell tumor. The tumor typically forms a single, distinct, firm, tan nodule. (Image courtesy of Dr Bettina Bisig, Institute of Pathology, Lausanne University Hospital, Switzerland.)

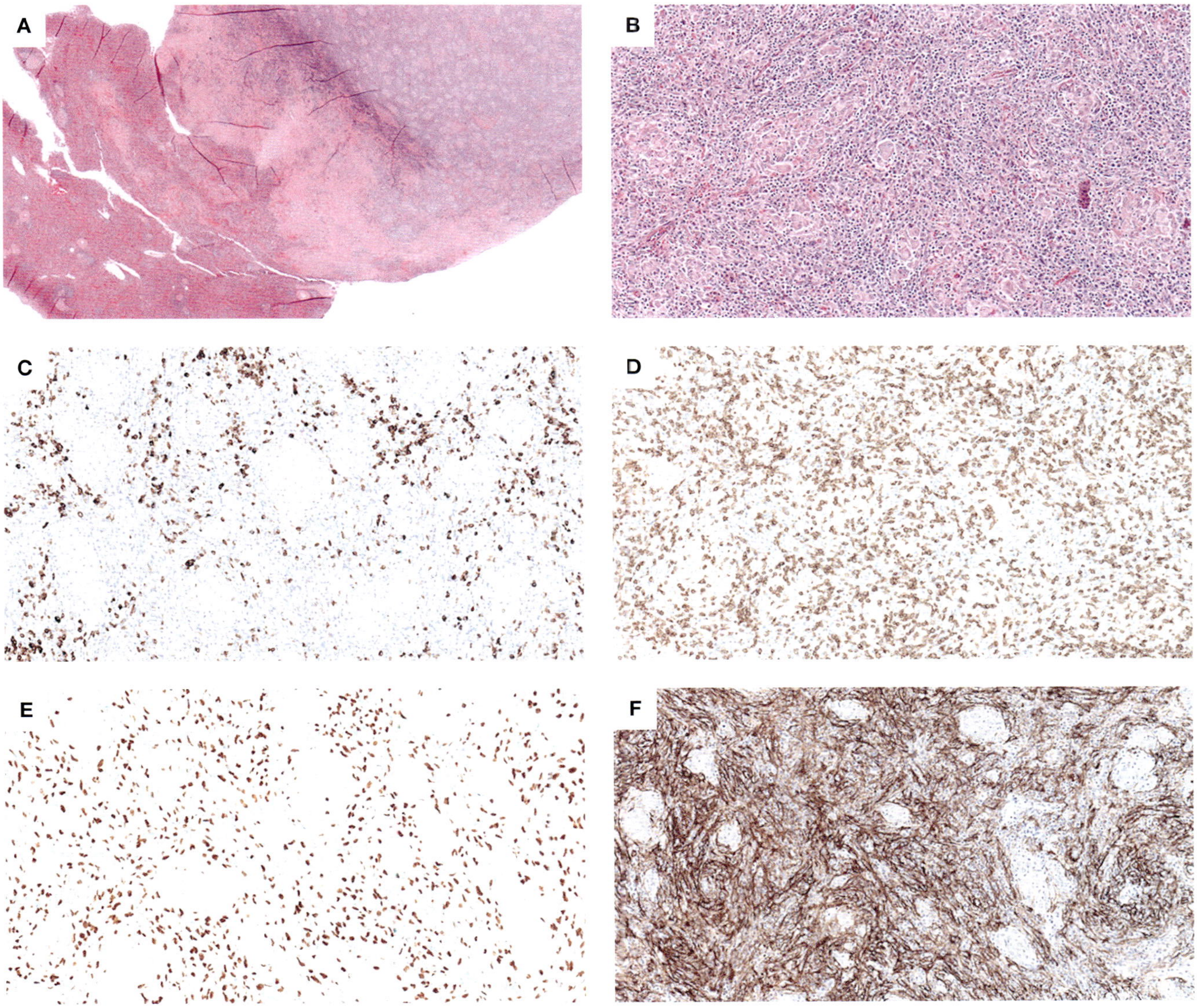

FIGURE 125.2 Hematoxylin and eosin–stained sections (**A** and **B**) showing adjacent normal spleen (**A**). Higher magnification of the tumor (**B**) demonstrates a mixed inflammatory infiltrate with thick collagenous bands. A mixture of CD79A-positive B cells (**C**) and CD3-positive T cells (**D**) are present. EBV-EBER in situ hybridization (**E**) is positive in the spindled cell nuclei. Smooth muscle actin (**F**) is also frequently positive.

have vesicular nucleoli and prominent nucleoli, and a subset of cells are often binucleated. Foci of dense fibrosis with thick-walled vessels but without inflammation and only sparse atypical spindled cells may occur. Recently, three histologic patterns have been described: *lymphoma-like*, with abundant, polytypic lymphoplasmacytoid cells; *classic type* with a mix of lymphocytes, vessels, and fibrosis; and *hemangioma-like* with abundant thick-walled vessels, fibrosis, and fewer lymphocytes.[1]

Immunophenotype

Follicular dendritic cells and fibroblastic reticular cells are mesenchymally derived stromal cells that exhibit plasticity, which results in immunophenotypic variation. Some cases express follicular dendritic cell markers, such as CD21, CD23, CD35, clusterin, and podoplanin (D2-40), but all may be negative. Some may express smooth muscle actin. All are positive for EBV (see Figure 125.2), and EBV positivity in the spindled cells is the most specific marker of this tumor. The spindled cells are consistently negative for CD8, CD34, and ALK1 but are reportedly PD-L1-positive. IgG4-positive plasma cells may be increased in the absence of features of IgG4-related disease.

Genetics

EBV-positive inflammatory follicular dendritic cell/fibroblastic reticular cell tumor is a clonal neoplasm,[4] but clonality studies are not performed diagnostically. Variable gene mutations have been reported in a small number of cases, with no clear recurring abnormalities yet identified.

Prognosis and Clinical Comment

EBV-positive inflammatory follicular dendritic cell/fibroblastic reticular cell tumor is treated with surgical excision. Although rare aggressive cases have been reported, splenectomy for splenic cases and polypectomy for gastrointestinal cases are usually curative. Hepatic cases may recur after incomplete resection, but recurrences tend to occur over years with an indolent behavior. For this reason, the designation "tumor" is preferred over the prior use of "sarcoma" for this entity.

References

1. Li Y, Yang X, Tao L, et al. Challenges in the diagnosis of Epstein-Barr virus-positive inflammatory follicular dendritic cell sarcoma: extremely wide morphologic spectrum and immunophenotype. *Am J Surg Pathol.* 2023;47(4):476-489.
2. Arber DA, Kamel OW, van de Rijn M, et al. Frequent presence of the Epstein-Barr virus in inflammatory pseudotumor. *Hum Pathol.* 1995;26(10):1093-1098.
3. Gong S, Auer I, Duggal R, Pittaluga S, Raffeld M, Jaffe ES. Epstein-Barr virus-associated inflammatory pseudotumor presenting as a colonic mass. *Hum Pathol.* 2015;46(12):1956-1961.
4. Selves J, Meggetto F, Brousset P, et al. Inflammatory pseudotumor of the liver. Evidence for follicular dendritic reticulum cell proliferation associated with clonal Epstein-Barr virus. *Am J Surg Pathol.* 1996;20(6):747-753.

Index

Note: Page numbers followed by *f* indicate figures and *t* indicate tables.

A

Acute basophilic leukemia, 241
  genetics, 242
  immunophenotype, 242
  morphology, 241–242, 242*f*
Acute leukemias of ambiguous lineage (ALALs), 16, 275, 276*f*, 276*t*
  diagnostic criteria, 275–280, 277*f*–278*f*
  epidemiology, 275
  genetics, 280–281
  prognosis and clinical outcome, 281
Acute lymphoblastic leukemia, germline predisposition, 178*t*
Acute myeloid leukemia (AML), 15–16, 56
  acute basophilic leukemia, 241
    genetics, 242
    immunophenotype, 242
    morphology, 241–242, 242*f*
  and acute myeloid leukemia/myelodysplastic syndrome with myelodysplasia-related gene mutations, 231
    clinical features, 231–232
    epidemiology, 231
    genetics, 232
    immunophenotype, 232
    morphology, 232
    prognosis and clinical comment, 232–233, 233*f*
  acute panmyelosis with myelofibrosis (APMF), 242
    genetics, 243
    immunophenotype, 243
    morphology, 242–243, 243*f*
  hierarchy of, 17*f*
  in-frame basic leucine zipper (bZIP) *CEBPA* mutations, 224
    clinical features, 224
    epidemiology, 224
    genetics, 225, 226*f*
    immunophenotype, 225
    morphology, 224, 225*f*
    prognosis and clinical comment, 225–227
  inv(16)(p13.1q22) or t(16;16)(p13.1;q22)/*CBFB::MYH11*, 198
    clinical features, 198
    epidemiology, 198
    genetics, 198–199, 200*f*
    immunophenotype, 198, 199*f*
    morphology, 198
    prognosis and clinical comment, 199–200
  inv(3)(q21.3q26.2) or t(3;3)(q21.3;q26.2)/*GATA2; MECOM(EVI1)*, 211
    clinical features, 211
    epidemiology, 211
    genetics, 212–213
    immunophenotype, 212
    morphology, 211–212, 212*f*–213*f*
    prognosis and clinical comment, 213
  KMT2A rearrangements
    clinical features, 204
    epidemiology, 204
    genetics, 204–206, 205*f*
    immunophenotype, 204
    morphology, 204
    prognosis and clinical comment, 206
  MECOM rearrangements, 213–214
  with mutated *NPM1*, 221
    clinical features, 221
    epidemiology, 221
    genetics, 222
    immunophenotype, 222
    morphology, 221, 221*f*
    prognosis and clinical comment, 222–223, 222*f*
  and myelodysplastic syndrome/acute myeloid leukemia, not otherwise specified, 237–238
    clinical features, 238
    cytologic and cytochemical features, 238*t*
    epidemiology, 238
    genetics, 238–239
    immunophenotype, 238
    morphology, 238
    prognosis and clinical comment, 239, 240*f*
  and myelodysplastic syndrome/acute myeloid leukemia with mutated *TP53*, 228
    clinical features, 228–229
    epidemiology, 228
    genetics, 229
    immunophenotype, 229
    morphology, 229, 229*f*
    prognosis and clinical comment, 230
  and myelodysplastic syndrome/acute myeloid leukemia with myelodysplasia-related cytogenetic abnormalities, 234, 234*t*
    clinical features, 234–235
    epidemiology, 234
    genetics, 235–236
    immunophenotype, 235
    morphology, 235
    prognosis and clinical comment, 236
  pure erythroid leukemia, 239
    clinical features, 239
    genetics, 241
    immunophenotype, 239
    morphology, 239, 241*f*
  rare recurring translocations, 215, 216*t*
    clinical features, 215
    epidemiology, 215
    genetics, 216–217
    immunophenotype, 215–216
    morphology, 215
    prognosis and clinical comment, 217
  t(9;22)(q34.1;q11.2)/*BCR::ABL1*, 218
    clinical features, 218, 219*t*
    epidemiology, 218
    genetics, 218–219
    immunophenotype, 218
    morphology, 218
    prognosis and clinical comments, 219
  t(6;9)(p22.3;q34.1)/*DEK::NUP214*, 208
    clinical features, 208
    epidemiology, 208
    genetics, 209–210
    immunophenotype, 209
    morphology, 208–209, 209*f*
    prognosis and clinical comment, 210
  t(9;11)(p21.3;q23.3)/*KMT2A::MLLT3*, 202
    clinical features, 202
    epidemiology, 202, 203*t*
    immunophenotype, 204
    morphology, 202, 203*f*
  t(8;21)(q22;q22)/*RUNX1::RUNX1T1*, 194
    clinical features, 194
    epidemiology, 194
    genetics, 195, 196*f*
    immunophenotype, 194–195
    morphology, 194, 195*f*
    prognosis and clinical comment, 196
Acute panmyelosis with myelofibrosis (APMF), 242
  genetics, 243
  immunophenotype, 243
  morphology, 242–243, 243*f*
Acute promyelocytic leukemia (APL)
  RARA translocations, 191–192, 192*f*, 192*t*
  t(15;17)(q24.1;q21.2)/*PML::RARA*, 190
    clinical features, 190
    epidemiology, 190
    genetics, 191
    immunophenotype, 191
    morphology, 190–191, 191*f*
    prognosis and clinical comment, 192–193, 193*f*
Acute undifferentiated leukemias (AULs), 275–276, 282
  epidemiology, 282
  genetics, 283
  immunophenotype, 282, 282*f*
  morphology, 282
  prognosis and clinical comment, 283
Adult T-cell leukemia/lymphoma (ATLL)
  clinical features, 604–605, 605*f*
  epidemiology, 604, 604*t*
  genetics, 608–611
  immunophenotype, 608
  morphology, 606–608, 606*f*–610*f*
  prognosis and clinical comments, 611
Age-adjusted bone marrow cellularity (adults), 6, 6*t*
Aggressive natural killer-cell leukemia (ANKL)
  clinical features, 635
  differential diagnosis, 620*t*, 670*t*
  epidemiology, 635
  genetics, 636–638
  immunophenotype, 636
  morphology, 635–636, 636*f*–637*f*
  prognosis and clinical comment, 638
Aggressive systemic mastocytosis, 94
ALALs. *See* Acute leukemias of ambiguous lineage (ALALs)
ALK-positive histiocytosis
  clinical features, 798, 799*f*
  epidemiology, 798
  genetics, 798–802, 800*f*–801*f*
  immunophenotype, 798
  morphology, 798, 799*f*
  prognosis and clinical comment, 802

ALK-positive large B-cell lymphoma (ALK+ LBCL)
  clinical features, 532
  epidemiology, 532
  genetics, 532
  immunophenotype, 532, 533*f*, 533*t*
  morphology, 532
  prognosis and clinical comment, 532
Alpha heavy chain disease (aHCD), 380–381, 382*f*
AML. *See* Acute myeloid leukemia (AML)
Amyloidosis, 390
Anaplastic large cell lymphoma, ALK negative (ALK− ALCL)
  clinical features, 741
  epidemiology, 741
  genetics, 743–744, 745*f*–747*f*
  immunophenotype, 742–743, 743*f*–744*f*
  morphology, 741, 742*f*
  prognosis and clinical comment, 744
Anaplastic large cell lymphoma, ALK positive (ALK+ ALCL)
  clinical features, 733
  epidemiology, 733
  genetics, 735
  immunophenotype, 734–735, 738*f*–739*f*
  morphology, 733–734, 734*f*–737*f*
  prognosis and clinical comment, 739
Atypical chronic myeloid leukemia (aCML), 110
  clinical features, 110
  diagnostic criteria for, 110*t*
  epidemiology, 110
  genetics, 111
  immunophenotype, 111
  morphology, 110–111, 112*f*
  prognosis and clinical comment, 111–113
  recurrent gene mutations in, 113*t*

B

B-cell prolymphocytic leukemia (B-PLL), 348, 349*f*
BCL2-rearrangement-negative, CD23-positive follicle center lymphoma (*BCL2*-R-, CD23+ FCL)
  clinical features, 441
  epidemiology, 441
  genetics, 443–444, 444*f*
  immunophenotype, 441–443
  morphology, 441, 442*f*–443*f*
  prognosis and clinical comment, 444
BCR::ABL1-negative myeloproliferative neoplasms (MPN), 31
  bone marrow fibrosis, grading of, 32–33, 33*t*, 34*f*
  clinical features of, 31, 32*t*
  diagnosis of, 31
  driver mutations, assessment of, 31
  essential thrombocythemia (ET), 38–42
  immunophenotype, 37–38
  morphological features of, 31, 32*t*
  polycythemia vera, 33–37
  primary myelofibrosis (PMF), 42–49
Blastic plasmacytoid dendritic cell neoplasm (BPDCN), 16, 256
  clinical features, 256, 257*f*
  diagnostic criteria for, 258*t*
  epidemiology, 256
  genetics, 258–259
  immunophenotype, 257–258, 258*t*, 259*f*
  morphology, 256–257, 257*f*
  prognosis and clinical comment, 259
Bloom syndrome, 184
B-lymphoblastic leukemia/lymphoma (B-ALL/LBL), 262, 265*f*, 289, 290*t*
  age distribution, 292*f*
  BCR::ABL1-like, *ABL1*-class rearranged, 301
  BCR::ABL1-like, JAK-STAT activated, 301–302, 302*f*
  BCR::ABL1-like, not otherwise specified, 302–303
  with coexisting *ZEB2* H1038R mutation and *IGH::CEBPE*, 310
  with *DUX4*-rearrangement, 304
  ETV6::RUNX1-like, 309
  flow cytometry analysis of, 267*f*
  gene expression clustering of, 291*f*
  with *HLF*-rearrangement, 307–308
  hyperdiploid, 296
    clinical features, 296
    epidemiology, 296
    genetics, 296–297, 298*f*
    immunophenotype, 296
    morphology, 296
    prognosis and clinical comment, 297
  with IKZF1 N159Y, 308–309
  with intrachromosomal amplification of chromosome 21, 303–304
  KMT2A-rearranged-like, 310–311
  low hypodiploid, 297
  with *MEF2D*-rearrangement, 305
  with *MYC*-rearrangement, 305–306
  myeloperoxidase, expression of, 268*f*
  near haploid, 297–299
  with NOS, 309
  with *NUTM1*-rearrangement, 306–307
  with PAX5 alteration, 310
  with PAX5 P80R, 308
  provisional entities, 309, 309*t*
  with recurrent genetic abnormalities, 289
  t(9;22)(q34.1;q11.2)/*BCR::ABL1* with lymphoid only involvement, 289–290, 292*f*
  t(9;22)(q34.1;q11.2)/*BCR::ABL1* with multilineage involvement, 290
    clinical features, 291
    epidemiology, 290
    genetics, 291
    immunophenotype, 291
    morphology, 291
    prognosis and clinical comment, 291–293
  t(12;21)(p13.2;q22.1)/*ETV6::RUNX1*, 294
    clinical features, 294
    epidemiology, 294
    genetics, 296
    immunophenotype, 295–296
    morphology, 295
    prognosis and clinical comment, 296
  t(5;14)(q31.1;q32.1)/*IGH::IL3*, 299
  t(v;11q23.3)/*KMT2A*-rearranged, 293
    clinical features, 293
    epidemiology, 293
    genetics, 293, 295*f*
    immunophenotype, 293
    morphology, 293
    prognosis and clinical comment, 293–294
  t(1;19)(q23;p13.3)/*TCF3::PBX1*, 299–300
  UBTF::ATXN7L3/PAN3,CDX2, 307
  with *ZNF384*-rearranged-like, 311
  with *ZNF384*-rearrangement, 304–305
Bone marrow fibrosis, grading of, 32–33, 33*t*, 34*f*
BPDCN. *See* Blastic plasmacytoid dendritic cell neoplasm (BPDCN)
Breast implant–associated anaplastic large cell lymphoma (BIA-ALCL)
  clinical features, 749
  epidemiology, 749
  genetics, 749–751
  immunophenotype, 749
  morphology, 749, 750*f*
  prognosis and clinical comment, 751
Burkitt lymphoma (BL)
  clinical features, 546–547
  epidemiology, 546
  genetics, 549, 549*f*–550*f*
  immunophenotype, 548, 548*f*
  morphology, 547–548, 547*f*–548*f*
  prognosis and clinical comment, 549–550

C

CCUS. *See* Clonal cytopenia of undetermined significance (CCUS)
Chronic active Epstein-Barr virus (CAEBV) disease, systemic
  clinical features, 618
  differential diagnosis, 620*t*
  epidemiology, 618
  genetics, 618–619
  immunophenotype, 618, 620*t*
  morphology, 618, 619*f*
  prognosis and clinical outcome, 621
Chronic eosinophilic leukemia, not otherwise specified (CEL, NOS), 56
  clinical features, 57
  diagnostic criteria for, 56*t*
  epidemiology, 56–57
  genetics, 59
  immunophenotype, 57–59
  morphology, 57, 58*f*
  prognosis and clinical comment, 59
Chronic lymphocytic leukemia (CLL), 340
  clinical features, 340
  epidemiology, 340
  genetics, 344–345, 344*f*, 345*t*
  immunophenotype, 341, 343*f*
  morphology, 340–341, 341*f*–342*f*
  prognosis and clinical comment, 346
Chronic lymphoproliferative disorder of natural killer cells (CLPDNK)
  clinical features, 600
  epidemiology, 600
  genetics, 602, 602*t*
  immunophenotype, 600–602
  morphology, 600, 601*f*
  prognosis and clinical comment, 602
Chronic myeloid leukemia (CML)
  clinical features, 22–23
  diagnosis of, 22
  epidemiology, 22
  genetics, 27–28
  immunophenotype, 27
  morphology
    accelerated phase, 24–25, 26*f*
    blast phase, 25–26, 26*f*
    chronic phase, 23–24, 23*f*, 24*t*, 25*f*
    extramedullary tissues, 26–27
  prognosis and clinical comment, 28
Chronic myeloid neoplasm (CMN), 68
Chronic myelomonocytic leukemia (CMML)
  clinical features, 103
  diagnostic criteria for, 102, 102*t*–103*t*
  epidemiology, 102–103
  genetics
    cytogenetics, 106
    molecular findings, 106–107
  immunophenotype, 106
  morphology, 103, 104*f*
    bone marrow, 103–105, 105*f*
    extramedullary tissues, 106
    peripheral blood, 103
  prognosis and clinical comment, 107
Chronic neutrophilic leukemia (CNL), 52
  clinical features, 52
  diagnostic criteria for, 52, 53*t*
  epidemiology, 52
  genetics, 54
  immunophenotype, 54
  morphology, 52–54, 53*f*
  prognosis and clinical comment, 54
Classic Hodgkin lymphoma (CHL)
  clinical features, 573–574
  epidemiology, 573
  genetics, 581–582
  immunophenotype, 578–581, 580*f*
  morphology, 574–578, 575*f*–578*f*
  prognosis and clinical comments, 582–583, 583*f*

Clinical Advisory Committee (CAC), 2
Clonal cytopenia of undetermined significance (CCUS), 127
  clinical features, 127–128, 128*t*
  epidemiology, 127
  genetics, 128–129
  immunophenotype, 128
  morphology, 128
  prognosis and clinical comment, 129
Clonal cytopenias, 13–14
Clonal monocytosis of undetermined significance (CMUS), 107
  clinical features, 107–108
  diagnostic criteria for, 107*t*
  epidemiology, 107
  genetics, 108
  immunophenotype, 108
  morphology, 108
  prognosis and clinical comment, 108
CML. *See* Chronic myeloid leukemia (CML)
CMML. *See* Chronic myelomonocytic leukemia (CMML)
CMUS. *See* Clonal monocytosis of undetermined significance (CMUS)
CNL. *See* Chronic neutrophilic leukemia (CNL)
Constitutional mismatch repair deficiency (CMMRD), 176
Core needle biopsy (CNB), 335
Cutaneous B-lymphoblastic lymphoma, 264*f*
Cutaneous mastocytosis (CM), 84
  clinical features, 90
  diagnosis, 90
  diffuse, 91
  epidemiology, 90
  genetics, 90–91
  immunophenotype, 90
  prognosis and clinical comment, 91
Cytochemical stains, 7, 7*t*
Cytopenia, 103

D
Diamond-Blackfan anemia (DBA), 183–184
Diffuse cutaneous mastocytosis, 91
Diffuse large B-cell lymphoma (DLBCL)
  clinical features, 472–473, 472*t*
  epidemiology, 472
  genetics
    antigen receptor genes, 476
    cell of origin, 475–476
    copy number alterations, 477
    functional subtypes, 476
    genomic subtypes, 477–479, 478*t*
    high-grade signatures, 476
    molecular subtypes, 475–476
    structural rearrangements, 476–477
    tumor microenvironment, 479
  immunophenotype, 474–475, 474*f*–475*f*
  morphology, 473–474, 473*f*
  prognosis and clinical comment, 479
Diffuse large B-cell lymphoma (DLBCL) associated with chronic inflammation (CI-DLBCL)
  clinical features, 519
  epidemiology, 518–519
  genetics, 520
  immunophenotype, 520
  morphology, 519, 519*f*
  prognosis and clinical comment, 520
Down syndrome, 184
  myeloid proliferations, 250–253
  transient abnormal myelopoiesis (TAM), 250–252
Duodenal-type follicular lymphoma (DTFL), 435–436
  clinical features, 436
  epidemiology, 436
  genetics, 437
  immunophenotype, 436
  morphology, 436, 437*f*
Dyserythropoiesis 146
Dyskeratosis congenita. *See* Telomere biology disorders (TBDs)
Dysmegakaryopoiesis, 208
Dysplasia, 208

E
EBV-positive polymorphic B-cell lymphoproliferative disorder, not otherwise specified (EBV+ polymorphic B-LPD NOS)
  clinical features, 527
  epidemiology, 527
  genetics, 530
  immunophenotype, 528, 530*f*
  morphology, 527–528, 528*f*, 529*t*
  prognosis and clinical comment, 530
Enteropathy-associated T-cell lymphoma (EATL)
  clinical features, 647
  differential diagnosis, 651*t*, 652*t*
  epidemiology, 646
  genetics, 648–650
  immunophenotype, 647, 649*f*–650*f*
  morphology, 647, 647*f*–649*f*
  prognosis and clinical comment, 650
Eosinophilia, 11, 68
Epstein-Barr virus (EBV)-associated T-cell and natural killer-cell lymphoproliferative disorders (LPD)
  chronic active Epstein-Barr virus (CAEBV) disease, systemic, 617–621
  hydroa vacciniforme lymphoproliferative disorder (HV-LPD), 613–616
  severe mosquito bite allergy (SMBA), 616–617
  systemic Epstein-Barr virus-positive T-cell lymphoma of childhood (SEBVTCL), 621–623
Epstein-Barr virus (EBV)-positive diffuse large B-cell lymphoma (DLBCL), not otherwise specified (NOS)
  clinical features, 514
  epidemiology, 514
  genetics, 515
  immunophenotype, 514–515, 515*f*
  morphology, 514, 515*f*, 516*f*
  prognosis and clinical comment, 516
Epstein-Barr virus (EBV)–positive inflammatory follicular dendritic cell/fibroblastic reticular cell tumor
  clinical features, 822
  epidemiology, 822
  genetics, 824
  immunophenotype, 823–824
  morphology, 822–823, 822*f*–823*f*
  prognosis and clinical comment, 824
Epstein-Barr virus (EBV)-positive mucocutaneous ulcer (EBV MCU)
  clinical features, 510
  epidemiology 510
  genetics, 512–513
  immunophenotype, 511–512, 512*f*
  morphology, 510–511, 511*f*
  prognosis and clinical comment, 513
Erdheim-Chester disease (ECD)
  clinical features, 806
  epidemiology, 806
  genetics, 807–808
  immunophenotype, 807, 808*f*–809*f*
  morphology, 806–807, 807*f*–809*f*
  prognosis and clinical comment, 809
Erythropoiesis, 35
Essential thrombocythemia (ET), 38
  clinical features, 38–39
  diagnostic criteria for, 39, 39*t*
  epidemiology, 38
  genetics, 42
  immunophenotype, 42
  morphology, 39
    accelerated and blast phase, 41–42
    bone marrow, 39–41, 40*f*–41*f*
    extramedullary tissues, 42
    peripheral blood, 39
    post-essential thrombocythemia myelofibrosis, 41, 42*t*
  prognosis and clinical comment, 42
ET. *See* Essential thrombocythemia (ET)
European Association for Haematopathology, 2
Extramedullary hematopoiesis (EMH), 31
Extranodal marginal zone lymphoma of mucosa-associated lymphoid tissue (MALT lymphoma), 409
  clinical features, 410, 411*f*
  epidemiology, 409–410, 410*t*
  genetics, 412–413
  immunophenotype, 411
  morphology, 410–411, 412*f*–415*f*
  prognosis and clinical comment, 413–416
Extranodal natural killer/T-cell lymphoma, nasal type (ENKTCL)
  clinical features, 627, 628*f*
  differential diagnosis, 620*t*, 651*t*–652*t*
  epidemiology, 627
    genetics
    epigenetic studies, 630–632
    Epstein-Barr virus (EBV), 630
    gene expression profiling, 630
    T-cell receptor (TCR) gene rearrangement, 630
  immunophenotype, 628–630, 629*f*
  morphology, 627–628, 628*f*
  prognosis and clinical comment, 632
Extraosseous plasmacytoma (EOP), 397–398, 398*t*

F
Fanconi anemia (FA), 182
Fibrin-associated diffuse large B-cell lymphoma (FA-DLBCL)
  clinical features, 520
  epidemiology, 520
  genetics, 522
  morphology, 520
  phenotype, 520
  prognosis and clinical comment, 522
Fibroblastic reticular cell (FRC) sarcoma
  clinical features, 820
  epidemiology, 820
  genetics, 820
  immunophenotype, 820, 821*f*
  morphology, 820
  prognosis and clinical comment, 820
Follicular dendritic cell (FDC) sarcoma
  clinical features, 816
  epidemiology, 816
  genetics, 818
  immunophenotype, 816–818, 817*f*–818*f*
  morphology, 816, 817*f*
  prognosis and clinical comment, 819
Follicular helper T-cell lymphoma (TFHL)
  clinical features, 721
  epidemiology, 721
  genetics, 728–729, 729*t*
  histological characteristics, 720*t*
  immunophenotype, 726–727, 728*f*
  morphology, 721–726, 722*f*–726*f*
  prognosis and clinical comment, 729–730
Follicular lymphoma (FL)
  clinical features
    clinical evaluation and staging, 427–428
    sites of involvement, 427
  early lesions

Follicular lymphoma (FL) *(Continued)*
duodenal-type follicular lymphoma (DTFL), 435–437
in situ follicular neoplasia (ISFN), 435
epidemiology, 427
genetics
antigen receptor genes, 432–433
other alterations, 433–434
grade 3B, 434
immunophenotype, 432
morphology
cytological variant of, 429, 429*f*
cytology, 428–429
grading, 429–431, 430*f*–431*f*
pattern, 431
tumor microenvironment, 431–432
prognosis and clinical outcome, 434–435

G

Gamma heavy chain disease (gHCD), 377
clinical features, 377
epidemiology, 377
genetics, 379
immunophenotype, 378
morphology, 377, 378*f*–379*f*
prognosis and clinical comment, 379
Granulocytes, 5
Granulocytic dysplasia, 147
Granulopoiesis, 35

H

Hairy cell leukemia (HCL), 356
clinical features, 356
genetics, 357
immunophenotype, 356, 358*f*
morphology, 356, 357*f*
prognosis and clinical comment, 357–358
Hairy cell leukemia variant (HCLv), 361
clinical features, 362
epidemiology, 362
genetics, 365
immunophenotype, 365
morphology, 362–365, 364*f*
prognosis and clinical comment, 365
Heavy chain diseases, 377, 378*f*
alpha heavy chain disease (aHCD), 380–381
gamma heavy chain disease (gHCD), 377–379
Mu heavy chain disease (mHCD), 379–380
Hematologic malignancies with germline predisposition, 171, 175*t*–178*t*, 180*f*–181*f*
acute lymphoblastic leukemia, 178*t*
clinical features, 172, 172*t*
with constitutional disorder affecting multiple organ systems, 179
bone marrow failure syndromes, 182–184
ERCC6L2 mutation, 182
GATA2 mutations, 179–180
SAMD9L mutations, 180–182
SAMD9 mutations, 180–182
with constitutional platelet disorder, 176–178
ANKRD26 mutation, 179
ETV6 mutation, 179
RUNX1 mutation, 178–179
epidemiology, 172
genetics, 173–185
immunophenotype, 173
morphology, 172–173, 173*t*
without constitutional disorder
CEBPA mutation, 174
constitutional mismatch repair deficiency (CMMRD), 176
DDX41 mutation, 174–175
Li-Fraumeni syndrome, 176
MBD4 mutation, 176
TP53 mutation, 176
Hepatomegaly, overt primary myelofibrosis (overt PMF), 46
Hepatosplenic T-cell lymphoma (HSTCL)
clinical features, 667
differential diagnosis, 670*t*
epidemiology, 667
genetics, 669–670
immunophenotype, 669
morphology, 667–669, 668*f*
prognosis and clinical comment, 670
Hepatosplenomegaly, 211
HHV8- and EBV-negative primary effusion-based lymphoma intravascular large B-cell lymphoma (IVLBCL)
clinical features, 508
epidemiology, 508
genetics, 508
immunophenotype, 508
morphology, 508, 509*f*
prognosis and clinical comment, 508
HHV8-positive diffuse large B-cell lymphoma, NOS (HHV8+ DLBCL)
clinical features, 543
epidemiology, 543
genetics, 543
immunophenotype, 543
morphology, 543
prognosis and clinical comment, 543
HHV8-positive germinotropic lymphoproliferative disorder (HHV8-positive GLPD)
clinical features, 541
epidemiology, 541
genetics, 542
immunophenotype, 541, 542*f*
morphology, 541, 542*f*
prognosis and clinical comment, 542
HHV8-positive multicentric castleman disease (HHV8+ MCD)
clinical features, 539–540
epidemiology, 539
genetics, 541
immunophenotype, 541
morphology, 540–541, 540*f*
prognosis and clinical comment, 541
High-grade B-cell lymphoma, not otherwise specified (HGBCL, NOS)
clinical features, 561
epidemiology, 561
genetics, 562
immunophenotype, 562
morphology, 561–562
prognosis and clinical comment, 562–563
High-grade B-cell lymphoma (HGBCL) with MYC and BCL2 rearrangements
clinical features, 552
epidemiology, 552
genetics, 554–555
immunophenotype, 554
morphology, 552–554
prognosis and clinical comment, 555–556
High-grade B-cell lymphoma (HGBCL) with MYC and BCL6 rearrangements
clinical features, 558
epidemiology, 558
genetics, 559–560
immunophenotype, 558–559
morphology, 558, 559*f*
prognosis and clinical comment, 560
Histiocytic and dendritic cell neoplasms, 778*t*
mesenchymally derived dendritic cell neoplasms, 781
myeloid-derived histiocytic and dendritic cell neoplasms, 778–781
Histiocytic sarcoma (HS)
clinical features, 783
epidemiology, 783
genetics, 785
immunophenotype, 783–785
morphology, 783, 784*f*
prognosis and clinical comment, 785
Hydroa vacciniforme lymphoproliferative disorder (HV-LPD)
clinical features, 615
epidemiology, 613–615, 614*t*
genetics, 616
immunophenotype, 615–616, 616*f*
morphology, 615, 615*f*–616*f*
prognosis and clinical outcome, 616
Hyperleukocytosis, 293
Hypogammaglobulinemia, 380

I

Iatrogenic immunodeficiency-associated lymphoproliferative disorders
clinical features, 756
epidemiology, 755–756
genetics, 765–766
immunophenotype, 760*f*–764*f*, 762–765
morphology, 756–762
prognosis and clinical comment, 766–767
ICC. *See* International Consensus Classification (ICC)
Idiopathic hypereosinophilic syndrome (iHES)
diagnostic criteria for, 56, 57*t*
morphological features of, 58*f*
IgM monoclonal gammopathy of undetermined significance (IgM MGUS)
clinical features, 373
diagnostic criteria for, 373, 373*t*
epidemiology, 373
genetics, 374
immunophenotype, 373–374
morphology, 373
plasma cell subtype of, 373, 373*t*
prognosis and clinical comment, 374
Immunoglobulin heavy chain gene rearrangement, 331*f*
Immunohistochemistry (IHC), 8
Indeterminate dendritic cell histiocytosis (IDCH)
clinical features, 791
epidemiology, 791
genetics, 791–792
immunophenotype, 791
morphology, 791
prognosis and clinical comment, 792
Indolent clonal T-cell lymphoproliferative disorder of the gastrointestinal tract (GIT)
clinical features, 662
differential diagnosis, 651*t*, 652*t*
epidemiology, 662
genetics, 664
immunophenotype, 662–664, 663*f*
morphology, 662, 662*f*
prognosis and clinical comment, 664
Indolent natural killer-cell lymphoproliferative disorder of the gastrointestinal tract
clinical features, 665
differential diagnosis, 651*t*, 652*t*
epidemiology, 665
genetics, 665
immunophenotype, 664*f*, 665
morphology, 664*f*, 665
prognosis and clinical comment, 665
Indolent systemic mastocytosis (ISM), 92–94
In situ follicular neoplasia (ISFN)
clinical features, 435
epidemiology, 435
genetics, 435
immunophenotype, 435
morphology, 435, 436*f*
Interdigitating dendritic cell sarcoma (IDCS)
clinical features, 794

epidemiology, 794
genetics, 796, 796*f*
immunophenotype, 795–796
morphology, 794–795
prognosis and clinical comment, 796
International Consensus Classification (ICC), 2–18
Intestinal T-cell lymphoma, not otherwise specified (ITCL, NOS)
clinical features, 660
differential diagnosis, 651*t*, 652*t*
epidemiology, 660
genetics, 661
immunophenotype, 660, 661*f*
morphology, 660, 661
prognosis and clinical comment, 661
Intravascular large B-cell lymphoma (IVLBCL)
clinical features, 505, 506*f*
epidemiology, 505
genetics, 506
immunophenotype, 505, 506*f*
morphology, 505, 506*f*
prognosis and clinical comment, 506
Iron stain, 8

J

JMML. *See* Juvenile myelomonocytic leukemia (JMML)
Juvenile myelomonocytic leukemia (JMML), 15, 160
clinical features, 160
diagnostic criteria for, 163*t*
epidemiology, 160
genetics, 163
immunophenotype, 161–163
like neoplasms, 164, 164*t*
morphology, 160–161, 161*f*–162*f*
Noonan syndrome–associated myeloproliferative disorder (MPD), 164
prognosis and clinical comment, 163–164
Juvenile xanthogranuloma
clinical features, 803
epidemiology, 803
genetics, 804
immunophenotype, 804
morphology, 803–804
prognosis and clinical comment, 804

L

Langerhans cell histiocytosis (LCH)
clinical features, 787
epidemiology, 787
genetics, 788, 789*f*
immunophenotype, 787–788
morphology, 787
prognosis and clinical comments, 789
Langerhans cell sarcoma (LCS), 789–790
Large B-cell lymphoma with *IRF4* rearrangement (LBCL-*IRF4*)
clinical features, 458
epidemiology, 458
genetics, 458–459, 460*f*
immunophenotype, 458, 460*f*
morphology, 458, 459*f*
prognosis and clinical comment, 459
Large B-cell lymphoma with 11q aberration (LBCL-11q)
clinical features, 481
epidemiology, 481
genetics, 482, 482*f*
immunophenotype, 482
morphology, 481–482, 481*f*
prognosis and clinical comment, 482
Leukocytosis, 110
Leukoerythroblastosis, 160
Li-Fraumeni syndrome, 176
Light chain and heavy chain deposition disease (LHCDD), 406–407, 407*f*
Lineage switch, 279–280
Localized immunoglobulin light chain amyloidosis, 405
LPL. *See* Lymphoplasmacytic lymphoma (LPL)
Lymphadenopathy, 106
Lymphoblastic neoplasms, 262
clinical features, 263–264, 264*f*
epidemiology, 262–263
etiology, 263
genetics, 269–270
immunophenotype, 266–268, 267*f*–270*f*
morphology, 264–266, 265*f*–267*f*
prognosis and clinical comment, 270–271
Lymphoid neoplasms, 328–338
B-cell development and subsets, 329–332, 330*f*–331*f*, 333*f*
immune response, 329
immunophenotyping, in lymphoma diagnosis, 335–336
molecular cytogenetic studies, 336–337, 337*t*
multiparameter approach, 335
T-cell subsets and NK cells, 332–334, 334*t*
tissue sampling considerations, 335
Lymphomatoid granulomatosis (LYG)
clinical features, 523
epidemiology, 523
genetics, 526
immunophenotype, 524–526
morphology, 523–524, 525*f*
prognosis and clinical comment, 526
Lymphomatoid papulosis
clinical features, 684, 685*f*
epidemiology, 684
genetics, 687–688
immunophenotype, 687
morphology, 684–686, 685*t*, 686*f*–691*f*
prognosis and clinical comment, 688
Lymphoplasmacytic lymphoma (LPL), 367
clinical features, 367
epidemiology, 367
genetics, 370, 371*f*
immunophenotype, 369–370
morphology
bone marrow and peripheral blood, 367–369, 367*f*–368*f*
lymph nodes and extramedullary tissues, 369, 369*f*–370*f*
prognosis and clinical comment, 370–371

M

Maculopapular cutaneous mastocytosis (MPCM), 91, 92*f*
Mantle cell lymphoma (MCL)
clinical features, 462
epidemiology 462
genetics
antigen receptor genes, 467
CCND2/D3 translocations, 467–468
CCND1 translocations, 467–468
mutational profile, 468
normal cell counterpart, 467
secondary genetic events, 468
SOX11, 468
immunophenotype, 464–466, 466*f*
morphology, 462–464, 464*f*–465*f*
prognosis and clinical comment, 468–470
in situ mantle cell neoplasia, 466–467
Mast cell leukemia (MCL), 94–95
Mast cell sarcoma (MCS)
clinical features, 98
epidemiology, 98
genetics, 99
immunophenotype, 99
morphology, 98–99, 98*f*
prognosis and clinical comment, 99
Mastocytoma of skin, 91–92, 93*f*
Mastocytosis, 12
classification, 84
clinical features, 85
cutaneous mastocytosis (CM), 90–91
diagnostic criteria, 84, 84*t*
epidemiology, 84–85
genetics, 88–89
immunophenotype, 87–88
morphology
cytology, 86, 86*f*
histology, 86–87, 87*f*–88*f*
variant, 87, 89*f*
prognosis and clinical comment, 90
subtypes (variants), 84, 84*t*
urticaria pigmentosa, 91
Mediastinal gray zone lymphoma (MGZL)
clinical features, 569
epidemiology, 569
genetics, 571
immunophenotype, 570–571
morphology, 569–570
prognosis and clinical comment, 571–572
Megakaryocytes, 148
cytology of, 5
morphology, 6, 6*t*
Megakaryopoiesis, 35, 161
Mixed-phenotype acute leukemias (MPALs), 275
B-cell component of, 277
B/myeloid MPAL with *ZNF384* rearrangement, 284–285
B/myeloid, not otherwise specified, 285
diagnostic criteria for, 275, 277*t*
flow cytometry analysis of, 267*f*
myeloid component of, 278–279, 279*f*–281*f*
t(9;22)(q34.1;q11.2), *BCR::ABL1*, 283
T-cell component of, 277–278
t(v;11q23.3); *KMT2A* rearranged, 283–284
T/myeloid MPAL, not otherwise specified, 286–287, 286*f*
T/myeloid MPAL with *BCL11B* alteration, 285
Monoclonal B-cell lymphocytosis (MBL), 340–346, 344*f*
Monoclonal immunoglobulin deposition diseases, 403
light chain and heavy chain deposition disease (LHCDD), 406–407
localized immunoglobulin light chain amyloidosis, 405
systemic immunoglobulin light chain amyloidosis, 403–405
Monocytosis, 105
Monomorphic epitheliotropic intestinal T-cell lymphoma (MEITL)
clinical features, 655
differential diagnosis, 651*t*, 652*t*
epidemiology, 655
genetics, 657, 658*f*
immunophenotype, 655–657, 656*f*–657*f*
morphology, 655, 656*f*
prognosis and clinical comment, 658
MPNs. *See* Myeloproliferative neoplasms (MPNs)
MS. *See* Myeloid sarcoma (MS)
Mu heavy chain disease (mHCD), 379
clinical features, 380
epidemiology, 380
genetics, 380
immunophenotype, 380
morphology, 380, 381*f*
prognosis and clinical comment, 380
Multiple myeloma (MM), 385–396
clinical features, 386
clinical variants, 387–388
imaging, 387
laboratory features, 387
POEMS syndrome, 388, 388*t*

Multiple myeloma (MM) *(Continued)*
staging of, 387, 387*t*
TEMPI syndrome, 388
cytogenetic subclassification of, 395*t*
diagnostic criteria for, 386*t*
epidemiology, 386
fluorescence in situ hybridization, 395*f*
genetics, 394–396
immunophenotype, 390–393, 391*f*–394*f*, 392*t*
morphology, 389–390, 389*f*–390*f*
prognosis and clinical comment, 396
Mycosis fungoides (MF)
clinical features, 672
epidemiology, 672
genetics, 675
immunophenotype
folliculotropic mycosis fungoides (FMF), 674
granulomatous slack skin, 675
pagetoid reticulosis, 674–675
morphology, 672–673, 673*f*
prognosis and clinical comment, 675–677, 678*t*
Myelodysplastic/myeloproliferative neoplasm not otherwise specified (MDS/MPN, NOS), 118
clinical features, 118
diagnostic criteria for, 118, 119*t*
epidemiology, 118
genetics, 119–121
with i(17q), 118, 119*t*
immunophenotype, 119
morphology, 118–119, 120*f*
prognosis and clinical comment, 121
Myelodysplastic/myeloproliferative neoplasm with ring sideroblasts and thrombocytosis, not otherwise specified (MDS/MPN-RS-T, NOS), 116
Myelodysplastic/myeloproliferative neoplasm with *SF3B1* mutation and thrombocytosis (MDS/MPN-*SF3B1*-T)
clinical features, 114
diagnostic criteria for, 114*t*
epidemiology, 114
genetics, 115
morphology
bone marrow, 115, 115*f*
peripheral blood, 114–115
prognosis and clinical comment, 115–116
Myelodysplastic syndrome/acute myeloid leukemia (MDS/AML), 153
clinical features, 153–154
diagnostic criteria for, 153*t*
epidemiology, 153
genetics, 155–156, 156*t*
immunophenotype, 154–155
morphology, 154, 154*f*–155*f*
prognosis and clinical comment, 156–157
Myelodysplastic syndrome, not otherwise specified (MDS-NOS), 145
clinical features, 146
diagnostic criteria for, 145, 145*t*
epidemiology, 145–146
genetics, 148
immunophenotype, 148
morphology, 146–148, 146*t*, 147*f*
prognosis and clinical comment, 148–149
Myelodysplastic syndromes (MDSs), 13–14, 124–125, 126*t*
hierarchy of, 17*f*
Myelodysplastic syndrome with del(5q) (MDS-del5q), 136
clinical features, 136
diagnostic criteria for, 136*t*
epidemiology, 136
genetics, 138, 138*t*
immunophenotype, 137
morphology, 136–137, 137*f*
prognosis and clinical comment, 138–139
Myelodysplastic syndrome with excess blasts (MDS-EB), 150
clinical features, 150
diagnostic criteria for, 151*t*
epidemiology, 150
genetics, 152
immunophenotype, 1502
morphology, 150, 151*f*
prognosis and clinical comment, 152
Myelodysplastic syndrome with mutated *SF3B1* (MDS-SF3B1), 132
clinical features, 132
epidemiology, 132
genetics, 133–134
immunophenotype, 133
morphology, 132–133, 133*f*, 133*t*
prognosis and clinical comment, 134
Myelodysplastic syndrome with mutated *TP53* (MDS-TP53), 140
allelic status, 143*f*
clinical features, 140
diagnostic criteria for, 142*t*
epidemiology, 140
genetics, 142–143
immunophenotype, 141–142
morphology, 140–141, 141*f*
prognosis and clinical comment, 143
Myeloid leukemia associated with Down syndrome (ML-DS), 252
epidemiology, 252
genetics, 253
immunophenotype, 253
morphology, 252–253
prognosis and clinical comment, 253
Myeloid/lymphoid neoplasms with eosinophilia and tyrosine kinase gene fusions (M/LN-eo-TK), 68–80, 69*f*
BCR::JAK2, 76–77, 77*f*
ETV6::ABL1, 78–79
clinical features, 79
epidemiology, 79
genetics, 80
immunophenotype, 80
morphology, 80
prognosis and clinical comment, 80
ETV6::JAK2, 76–77, 77*f*
FGFR1, rearrangement of, 74
clinical features, 74, 75*f*
epidemiology, 74
genetics, 74–75
immunophenotype, 74–75
morphology, 74–75
prognosis and clinical comment, 76
FLT3, rearrangement of, 77, 79*f*
clinical features, 78
epidemiology, 78
genetics, 78
immunophenotype, 78
morphology, 78
prognosis and clinical comment, 78
PCM1::JAK2, 76–77, 77*f*
PDGFRA, rearrangement of, 70
clinical features, 70
epidemiology, 70
genetics, 70–73, 72*t*
immunophenotype, 70
morphology, 70, 71*f*
prognosis and clinical comment, 73
PDGFRB, rearrangement of, 73
clinical features, 73
epidemiology, 73
genetics, 74
immunophenotype, 73–74
morphology, 73–74
prognosis and clinical comment, 74
Myeloid neoplasms
clinical features, 5
cytotoxic therapy, 4, 4*t*
germline conditions, 4
peripheral blood counts, 3
splenomegaly, 4
diagnostic qualifiers to, 16–18
disease groups, 10–16
genetics, 8–10, 9*t*
immunophenotypic analysis, 8
International Consensus Classification (ICC), 2–3, 3*f*
morphology
biopsy and aspirate smear, blasts in, 6–7, 7*t*
bone marrow aspirate specimen, 5
bone marrow trephine biopsy specimen, 5–6, 6*t*
cytochemical stains, 7, 7*t*
iron stain, 8
peripheral blood specimen, 5
reticulin and trichrome stains, 7
pediatric, 15
Myeloid precursors, 5
Myeloid sarcoma (MS), 245
clinical features, 245
epidemiology, 245
genetics, 247, 247*t*
immunophenotype, 246–247
morphology, 245–246, 246*f*
prognosis and clinical comment, 247–248
Myeloproliferative neoplasms (MPNs), 3, 10–11
Myeloproliferative neoplasms unclassifiable (MPN-U)
clinical features, 61
diagnostic criteria of, 61, 62*t*
epidemiology, 61
genetics, 63–64
immunophenotype, 63
morphology, 62–63, 62*f*–63*f*
phenotypic categories, 61
prognosis and clinical comment, 64

N

Next-generation sequencing (NGS), 8–9
NK-cell acute lymphoblastic leukemia (NK-LL)
clinical features, 323
diagnosis of, 323
epidemiology, 323
genetics, 324
immunophenotype, 324
morphology, 323, 324*f*
prognosis and clinical comment, 324
Nodal marginal zone lymphoma (NMZL)
clinical features, 421
epidemiology, 421
genetics, 424–425
immunophenotype, 422–424, 423*f*–425*f*
morphology, 421, 422*f*
prognosis and clinical comment, 425–426
Nodular lymphocyte predominant B-cell lymphoma (NLPBL)
clinical features, 484
epidemiology, 484
genetics, 487–488
immunophenotype, 486–487, 487*f*
morphology, 484–486, 484*f*–486*f*
prognosis and clinical comment, 488
Non-Hodgkin lymphoma (NHL), 329, 329*f*
Non-IgM monoclonal gammopathy of undetermined significance (non-IgM MGUS), 384
clinical features, 384–385
diagnostic criteria for, 384*t*
epidemiology, 384
genetics, 385
immunophenotype, 385
morphology, 385
prognosis and clinical comment, 385

Noonan syndrome–associated myeloproliferative disorder (MPD), 164
Nucleated red blood cells (nRBCs), 5

O

Optical genomic mapping (OGM), 8
Other iatrogenic immunodeficiency-associated lymphoproliferative disorders
- clinical features, 771
- epidemiology, 769–771
- genetics, 772–773
- immunophenotype, 772
- morphology, 771–772
- prognosis and clinical comment, 773–774

Overt primary myelofibrosis (overt PMF), 45–49
- clinical features, 46
- diagnostic criteria for, 46*t*
- genetics, 48
- immunophenotype, 48
- morphology, 46
  - accelerated and blast phase, 48
  - bone marrow, 46–48, 47*f*
  - extramedullary tissues, 48
  - peripheral blood, 46, 47*f*
- prognosis and clinical comment, 48–49

P

Paroxysmal nocturnal hemoglobinuria (PNH), 129, 130*f*
PCMZLPD. *See* Primary cutaneous marginal zone lymphoproliferative disorder (PCMZLPD)
Pediatric myelodysplastic syndrome, 166–170, 168*t*
- clinical features, 167

Pediatric myeloid neoplasms, 15
Pediatric-type follicular lymphoma (PTFL)
- clinical features, 450
- epidemiology, 450
- genetics, 451–452
- immunophenotype, 450–451
- morphology, 450, 451*f*–452*f*
- prognosis and clinical comment, 452

Peripheral blood counts, 3
Peripheral lymphadenopathy, 356
Peripheral T-cell lymphoma, not otherwise specified (PTCL, NOS)
- clinical features, 712
- epidemiology, 712
- genetics, 714–718
- immunophenotype, 713–714, 716*f*
- morphology, 713, 713*f*–715*f*
- prognosis and clinical comments, 718

Plasmablastic lymphoma (PBL)
- clinical features, 535
- epidemiology, 535
- genetics, 536–537
- immunophenotype, 535, 536*f*
- morphology, 535
- prognosis and clinical comment, 537

Plasma cell leukemia (PCL), 387–388
Plasma cell neoplasms, 384
- multiple myeloma (MM), 385–396
- non-IgM monoclonal gammopathy of undetermined significance (non-IgM MGUS), 384–385
- plasmacytoma, 396–398

Plasmacytoid dendritic cells (PDC), 105, 105*f*
Plasmacytoma, 396
- extraosseous plasmacytoma (EOP), 397–398, 398*t*
- solitary plasmacytoma of bone (SBP), 396–397

PMF. *See* Primary myelofibrosis (PMF)
POEMS syndrome, 388, 388*t*
Polycythemia vera, 36*f*
- clinical features, 33–34
- diagnostic criteria for, 35*t*
- epidemiology, 33
- genetics, 38
- immunophenotype, 37
- morphology, 35
  - accelerated and blast phase, 37
  - bone marrow, 35
  - extramedullary tissues, 37
  - peripheral blood, 35
  - post-polycythemia vera myelofibrosis (post-PV MF), 35–36
- prognosis and clinical comment, 38

Polymerase chain reaction (PCR), 89
Post-polycythemia vera myelofibrosis (post-PV MF), 34–36, 37*f*
- diagnostic criteria for, 36*t*

Post-polycythemic myeloid metaplasia, 34, 37*f*
Postremission therapy, 248
Posttransplant lymphoproliferative disorders (PTLDs)
- iatrogenic immunodeficiency-associated lymphoproliferative disorders
  - clinical features, 756
  - epidemiology, 755–756
  - genetics, 765–766
  - immunophenotype, 760*f*–764*f*, 762–765
  - morphology, 756–762
  - prognosis and clinical comment, 766–767

Prefibrotic primary myelofibrosis (pre-PMF), 43–45, 45*f*
- clinical features, 43–44
- genetics, 44
- immunophenotype, 44
- morphology, 44
- prognosis and clinical comment, 44–45

Premalignant clonal cytopenias, 124–125
Primary cold agglutinin disease (pCAD), 375
- clinical features, 375
- epidemiology, 375
- genetics, 376
- immunophenotype, 375
- morphology, 375, 376*f*
- prognosis and clinical comment, 376

Primary cutaneous acral CD8-positive T-cell lymphoproliferative disorder
- epidemiology, 706
- genetics, 708
- immunophenotype, 707–708, 707*f*
- morphology, 706–707, 706*f*–707*f*
- prognosis and clinical comment, 708

Primary cutaneous anaplastic large cell lymphoma (pcALCL)
- clinical features, 689, 692*f*
- epidemiology, 689
- genetics, 692
- immunophenotype, 690–692, 692*f*
- morphology, 690, 692*f*
- prognosis and clinical comment, 693

Primary cutaneous CD8-positive aggressive epidermotropic cytotoxic T-cell lymphoma (CD8^{+} AECTL)
- clinical features, 709
- epidemiology, 709
- genetics, 710
- immunophenotype, 710, 711*f*
- morphology, 710
- prognosis and clinical comment, 710
- synonyms, 709

Primary cutaneous CD4-positive small/medium T-cell lymphoproliferative disorder (pcSMTLPD)
- clinical features, 695
- epidemiology, 695
- genetics, 696
- immunophenotype, 696
- morphology, 695, 696*f*
- prognosis and clinical comment, 696

Primary cutaneous CD30-positive T-cell lymphoproliferative disorders (pcCD30^{+} T-LPDs)
- lymphomatoid papulosis, 684–688
- primary cutaneous anaplastic large cell lymphoma (pcALCL), 688–693

Primary cutaneous diffuse large B-cell lymphoma, leg type (PCDLBCL-LT)
- clinical features, 502, 502*f*
- epidemiology, 502
- genetics, 503
- immunophenotype, 502–503, 503*f*
- morphology, 502, 503*f*
- prognosis and clinical comment, 504

Primary cutaneous follicle center lymphoma (PCFCL)
- clinical features, 446, 447*f*
- epidemiology, 446
- genetics, 447
- immunophenotype, 446–447, 448*f*
- morphology, 446, 447*f*
- prognosis and clinical comment, 448

Primary cutaneous gamma-delta T-cell lymphomas (PCGDTCL)
- clinical features, 702
- epidemiology, 702
- genetics, 704
- immunophenotype, 703–704
- morphology, 703, 703*f*
- prognosis and clinical comment, 704–705

Primary cutaneous marginal zone lymphoproliferative disorder (PCMZLPD)
- clinical features, 417
- epidemiology, 417
- genetics, 418
- immunophenotype, 418, 419*f*
- morphology, 417, 418*f*
- prognosis and clinical comment, 418–419

Primary diffuse large B-cell lymphoma of the central nervous system (PCNS-DLBCL)
- clinical features, 494
- epidemiology, 494
- genetics, 495–496, 496*t*
- immunophenotype, 495
- morphology, 494, 495*f*
- prognosis and clinical comment, 496

Primary diffuse large B-cell lymphoma of the testis (PT-DLBCL)
- clinical features, 499
- epidemiology, 499
- genetics, 500–501
- immunophenotype, 499–500
- morphology, 499
- prognosis and clinical comment, 501

Primary effusion lymphoma
- clinical features, 543
- epidemiology, 543
- genetics, 544
- immunophenotype, 544
- morphology, 543, 544*f*–545*f*
- prognosis and clinical comment, 544

Primary mediastinal large B-cell lymphoma (PMBL)
- clinical features, 564, 564*f*
- epidemiology, 564
- genetics, 565–566, 567*f*
- immunophenotype, 565
- morphology, 564, 565*f*
- prognosis and clinical comment, 566

Primary myelofibrosis (PMF), 42–43
- epidemiology, 43
- overt primary myelofibrosis, 45–49
- prefibrotic primary myelofibrosis, 43–45

Primary nodal Epstein-Barr virus (EBV)-positive T- or NK-cell lymphoma (EBV+ nTNKL)
clinical features, 641
differential diagnosis, 620t
epidemiology, 640, 640t
genetics, 642, 642f
immunophenotype, 641–642, 641f–642f
morphology, 641, 641f
prognosis and clinical comment, 642
Promonocytes, 105
Promyelocytes, 7
Pronormoblasts, 5, 7
Pronounced neutrophilia, 52
Pure erythroid leukemia, 239
clinical features, 239
genetics, 241
immunophenotype, 239
morphology, 239, 241f

R
Refractory celiac disease (RCD), 644–646, 645f–646f. *See also* Type II refractory celiac disease
Refractory cytopenia of childhood (RCC), 15, 166, 168t
clinical features, 167
diagnostic criteria for, 166, 166t
epidemiology, 166
genetics, 169
immunophenotype, 167
morphology, 167, 168f–169f
prognosis and clinical comment, 169–170
Reticulin stain, 7
Richter transformation, 342f
Rosai-Dorfman-Destombes disease (RDD)
clinical features, 811
epidemiology, 811
genetics, 814
immunophenotype, 811–814, 813f
morphology, 811, 812f
prognosis and clinical comment, 814

S
Severe congenital neutropenias (SCNs), 183
Severe mosquito bite allergy (SMBA)
clinical features, 617, 617f
epidemiology, 616
genetics, 617
immunophenotype, 617, 617f
morphology, 617
prognosis and clinical outcome, 617
Sézary syndrome
clinical features, 680, 681f
epidemiology, 680
genetics, 681
immunophenotype, 681, 682f
morphology, 680–681, 682f
prognosis and clinical comment, 683
Shwachman-Diamond syndrome (SDS), 183
Small lymphocytic lymphoma (SLL), 340
clinical features, 340
epidemiology, 340
genetics, 344–345, 344f, 345t
immunophenotype, 341, 343f
morphology, 340–341, 341f–342f
prognosis and clinical comment, 346
Smoldering systemic mastocytosis, 94
SMZL. *See* Splenic marginal zone lymphoma (SMZL)
Solitary plasmacytoma of bone (SBP), 396–397
Splenectomy, 351
Splenic diffuse red pulp small B-cell lymphoma (SDRPL), 360
clinical features, 360
epidemiology, 360
genetics, 361
immunophenotype, 361
morphology, 360–361, 361f–363f
prognosis and clinical comment, 361
Splenic marginal zone lymphoma (SMZL), 351
clinical features, 351
epidemiology, 351
genetics, 353–354
immunophenotype, 353
morphology, 351–352, 351f–353f
prognosis and clinical comment, 354
Splenomegaly, 4, 22
overt primary myelofibrosis (overt PMF), 46
polycythemia vera, 34, 37
Subcutaneous panniculitis-like T-cell lymphoma (SPTCL)
clinical features, 697–698
epidemiology, 697
genetics, 699
immunophenotype, 698–699, 700f, 700t–701t
morphology, 698, 699f
prognosis and clinical comment, 699–701
Systemic Epstein-Barr virus-positive T-cell lymphoma of childhood (SEBVTCL)
clinical features, 621–622
differential diagnosis, 620t
epidemiology, 621
genetics, 623
immunophenotype, 623
morphology, 622–623, 622f–624f
prognosis and clinical outcome, 623
Systemic immunoglobulin light chain amyloidosis
clinical features, 403
epidemiology, 403
genetics, 405
morphology, 403–405, 404f
prognosis and clinical comment, 405
Systemic mastocytosis (SM)
aggressive systemic mastocytosis, 94
B-findings, 85t
C-findings, 85t
diagnostic criteria, 84t–85t
indolent systemic mastocytosis (ISM), 92–94
mast cell leukemia (MCL), 94–95
myeloid neoplasm, 95–98, 96f
peripheral blood abnormalities, 85
smoldering systemic mastocytosis, 94

T
TAM. *See* Transient abnormal myelopoiesis (TAM)
T-cell clones of uncertain significance (TCUS), 598
T-cell/histiocyte-rich large B-cell lymphoma (THRLBCL)
clinical features, 490
epidemiology, 490
genetics, 492
immunophenotype, 490–491, 491f–492f
morphology, 490
prognosis and clinical comment, 493
T-cell large granular lymphocytic leukemia (T-LGLL)
clinical features, 594
differential diagnosis, 670t
epidemiology, 594
genetics, 597
immunophenotype, 595–596
morphology, 594–595
prognosis and clinical comment, 597–598
T-cell clones of uncertain significance (TCUS), 598
T-cell prolymphocytic leukemia (T-PLL)
clinical features, 588–589
epidemiology, 588
genetics, 589–593
immunophenotype, 589, 591f
morphology, 589, 590f
prognosis and clinical comment, 593
Telomere biology disorders (TBDs), 182–183
TEMPI syndrome, 388
Testicular follicular lymphoma
clinical features, 454
epidemiology, 454
genetics, 455–456
immunophenotype, 455, 455f–456f
morphology, 454, 455f–456f
prognosis and clinical comment, 456
Therapy-related myeloid neoplasms (t-MN), 4, 4t
Tissue-based monoclonal B-cell lymphocytosis (tMBL), 340
T-lymphoblastic leukemia/lymphoma (T-ALL/LBL), 262, 267f, 315, 316t
BHLH, other, 320–321
early T-cell precursor lymphoblastic leukemia/lymphoma, *BCL11B*-activated
clinical features, 315
epidemiology, 315
genetics, 315–316, 317f
immunophenotype, 315, 316f
morphology, 315
prognosis and clinical comment, 316
early T-cell precursor lymphoblastic leukemia/lymphoma, NOS, 317–318
flow cytometry analysis of, 267t
HOXA dysregulated, 319
LMO1/2-rearranged, 319–320
NKX2-rearranged, 320
NOS, 318
SPI1-rearranged, 320
TAL1/2-rearranged, 318
TLX1-rearranged, 318–319
TLX3-rearranged, 319
Transient abnormal myelopoiesis (TAM), 250
clinical features, 250
epidemiology, 250
genetics, 252
immunophenotype, 251
morphology, 251, 251f
prognosis and clinical comment, 252
Trichrome stain, 7
Type II refractory celiac disease
clinical features, 644
differential diagnosis, 651t–652t
epidemiology, 644
genetics, 645, 646f
immunophenotype, 644–645, 646f
morphology, 644, 645f
prognosis and clinical comment, 645–646
Tyrosine kinase gene fusions, 11

U
Urticaria pigmentosa, 91

V
Variant allele frequency (VAF), 9–10
VEXAS syndrome, 129–130

W
Whole genome sequencing, 8
World Health Organization (WHO), 2
acute myeloid leukemia (AML), 16
blastic plasmacytoid dendritic cell neoplasm (BPDCN), 256
chronic neutrophilic leukemia (CNL), 52
lymphoplasmacytic lymphoma (LPL), 368
mastocytosis, 12
myelodysplastic syndrome with mutated *SF3B1* (MDS-*SF3B1*), 132
myeloid/lymphoid neoplasms, 12
myeloproliferative neoplasms (MPNs), 10–11

X
Xeroderma pigmentosa, 184